THE ESSENTIAL GUIDE TO PRESCRIPTION DRUGS

1999 EDITION

James J. Rybacki, Pharm. D.
James W. Long, M.D.

HarperPerennial
A Division of HarperCollins *Publishers*

Designed by C. Linda Dingler

Library of Congress Catalog Card Number 87–657561
ISSN 0894–7058

ISBN 0–06–271609–3   99 00 RRD 10 9 8 7 6 5 4 3 2 1
ISBN 0–06–273635–3 (pbk.) 99 00 RRD 10 9 8 7 6 5 4 3 2 1

Contents

Author's Note
for the 1999 Edition

This year, just as last year, great strides have been made in medicines. Over the past ten years many diseases or conditions that used to be fatal have become problems that can be controlled or actually cured. Medicines can very clearly make the difference between life and death. Unfortunately, the treatments themselves and the way that WE use (or combine) them can also make the difference between life and death. Fact: more than 100,000 Americans died last year because of adverse reactions to medicines. This makes it the fourth leading cause of death in the United States. An article by Dr. Classen which appeared in the *Journal of the American Medical Association* (JAMA) placed an estimate of the financial toll at **136 billion dollars a year** in 1997. Considering the loss of income and impact on people's jobs, I expect this will climb to more than **150 billion dollars in 1999.** That's greater than the cost of diabetes care in the United States and, unlike diabetes, is often preventable.

Who is to blame for these appalling statistics? Is it the patient, the doctor, the pharmacist, or the nurse who is at fault? Could it be all of us? I believe we each contribute to the problem and can also be part of the solution. I've coined the term Bad Med Syndrome (BMS) to describe lost treatment benefits, decreased quality of life, preventable hospitalizations, and deaths caused by medicines themselves or by the improper use of medicines. It doesn't mean the "meds" are bad, just that they need to be handled with care.

Has the Cure Become the Disease?

No one intentionally causes Bad Med Syndrome (see Glossary), yet year after year, we Americans continue to have a serious problem resulting from medicines. BMS comes from many sources: adverse drug reactions, allergies, medication errors, dosing errors, drug-drug interactions, prescribing errors, dispensing errors, and numerous other factors. Sometimes these problems are called adverse drug events, as if they were rare occurrences. A more inclusive name like BMS is needed to identify such errors as part of a larger problem, and prevent them from going unnoticed and unreported. Did you know that many researchers have found that less than 1 percent of serious drug reactions are reported to the FDA?

This means that problems resulting from medicines have been hidden, largely by omission and perhaps by failure to recognize that new symptoms may actually have been caused by the medicines themselves. Our current system REQUIRES manufacturers of medicines to report adverse effects, but such reporting is VOLUNTARY for health care professionals. I think this is a mistake. I've tried to increase public awareness via journals, on TV, in my newsletter and on my website (www.medicine info.com), much to the consternation of some of my colleagues. However, because problems arising from use and misuse of medicines have continued year after year with an increasing human and financial price tag, I decided that it was time for us as a nation to face reality. By giving this problem a name, we are one step closer to finding a solution.

Too many families (including my own) have been hurt because someone didn't use their medicine correctly, combined it with a dangerous second medicine or wasn't told about possible problems that the medicine itself might cause. My own father had a serious reaction to one of his heart medicines, and was actually given a sixth medicine to treat the life-threatening symptoms caused by a drug expected to control abnormal heartbeats. In short, all of his doctors missed the reaction—I know enough to prevent that now, something I think about often.

Another reality we need to face is that even our health care system itself may be part of the problem. President Clinton noted in his 1998 State of the Union Address that some 120 million Americans receive their health care from some kind of managed care organization (MCO). Some MCOs are good, but many have serious flaws. For example, many do not pay for education about medicines or chronic illnesses such as diabetes, or only pay for education for diabetics who require insulin—leaving more than 90 percent of their diabetics uneducated. They also frequently increase workload (either directly or indirectly) on health care professionals. For example, a typical "acute care" visit to the doctor's office is expected to be accomplished in ten minutes.

When considering a health maintenance organization (HMO), ask exactly how their results or outcomes compare with other providers of the same care. Ask if theirs is a restricted formulary and whether prescriptions must be filled by a mail-order pharmacy, versus your local pharmacy. If mail order is to be used, ask how you will be able to ask questions of a pharmacist, and who will review all of your medicines on a regular basis.

It is one thing to merely cut costs; it is very different to be able to contain costs while maintaining the same results or outcomes! I find it remarkable that a Patients' Bill of Rights was actually proposed in Congress to protect people from the health care system that is supposed to serve them. A health care system without a total plan for checking results is like a factory that never looks at the product it makes. It is a prescription for disaster.

Is there hope? Yes, there is always hope. Last year I mentioned the National Committee on Quality Assurance (NCQA). The NCQA has developed the Health Plan Employer Data and Information Set (HEDIS) in order to help tell how effective physicians are and how they compare to one another. It is perfectly acceptable for you to ask your doctor if he or she has been assessed using this measure, and how they compare to their colleagues. Recently, the NCQA took another bold step and joined forces with the American Medical Association (AMA) and the Joint Commission on Accreditation of Health Care Organizations (JCAHCO) in order to develop a joint effort to improve our health care system and actually measure results.

Never let health care be something that is done *to* you. Be an active participant. Rybacki's #1 recommendation: "It's always better to prevent a disease or condition than to have to treat it." Make each problem an opportunity to get the most from your medicines and improve your health:

- Ask about nutrients such as calcium supplements for osteoporosis that can help prevent disease. Aspirin can help prevent first heart attacks, strokes, and perhaps even intestinal cancer—your doctor can help decide if it makes sense for you.
- Find out if your condition or disease puts you at risk for other infectious diseases. Learn about available vaccines to prevent illnesses you may be prone to because of any recently diagnosed condition or advancing age.
- Remember, as we age our kidneys undergo a "natural" decline. This is commonly missed. Since many medicines are removed from the body by the kidneys, make certain you ask your doctor to adjust doses of medicines for the natural decline in kidney function if you are over 60 years old.
- I know it is difficult to give up any habit that you enjoy, but try to decrease ongoing risk. For example, **there are virtually no data to show that smoking is good for you.** That double or triple cheeseburger can add a lot of cholesterol. Limit how much fat you eat, and you may add years to your life.
- Many hospitals and clinics now have complementary care programs, using medicines as well as holistic and nontraditional approaches to helping prevent or cure diseases. Make use of them.
- Work with your doctor as a partner in health care, your nurse practitioner to keep and maintain your health, your pharmacist to make

certain you have the right medicine in the right dose at the right time. **Never assume that things are correct. ALWAYS** use the knowledge in this book to help protect you and your loved ones.

- Have all of your medicines mapped into your life for you (see Table 15). Well-mapped medicines can be a key to avoiding drug interactions, under-doses or overdoses and preventing or curing Bad Med Syndrome.
- TAKE CARE OF YOURSELF. That ten-minute visit in your doctor's office isn't meant to tell you all about the drugs that might be prescribed. Your medicines can make the difference between life and death. Never take them for granted and always take them just as they were prescribed.

As noted in each previous edition, no claim is made that *all* known actions, uses, side effects, adverse effects, precautions, interactions, etc., for a drug are included in the information provided in the sections that constitute this book. Although diligent care has been taken to ensure the accuracy of the information provided during the preparation of this revision, the continued accuracy and currentness are ever subject to change relative to the dissemination of new information derived from drug research, development, and general usage.

James Joseph Rybacki, Pharm. D.

Points for Consideration by the Patient

Never take any medicine for granted. I ask you this as a longtime member of the medical community, as a parent, and as a fellow human being. I think our cavalier attitude toward medicines leads to serious problems far more often than we know. Did you know that research on medicine use over the past 15 years shows that more than half of the people who get a prescription fail to take it correctly? This is a prescription for disaster.

Study after study finds similar results. Dr. Lucian L. Leape of Harvard found 334 drug errors in six months at two major teaching hospitals in the United States. Fourteen of these errors were life-threatening. A U.S. and Canadian study placed the financial cost at more than **9 billion dollars** in each country in 1996. A more recent study by Dr. Classen published in the *Journal of the American Medical Association* (JAMA) placed the expense at 136 billion dollars a year in 1997. The human cost cannot be calculated. Of course we must **do** something, rather than simply recording an ever-increasing toll.

If you are being treated for a recurrent or chronic disorder, such as asthma or diabetes, **learn as much as you can** about the nature and medical management of your condition. Dr. James Long's book, *The Essential Guide to Chronic Illness,* is a superb resource. Ask your doctor and pharmacist for written information, visit your local libraries for pertinent publications, and call local chapters of national organizations. The more you know about your disorder and its treatment, the more you'll be able to use your prescribed medications safely and effectively. Never be afraid to ask your doctor or pharmacist questions—you help them when you help yourself. Any competent physician or pharmacist will welcome the chance to help you understand your medicines, regardless of how busy they may be.

If they won't give you this critical time, find another physician or pharmacist.

Work with your doctor and pharmacist to ensure that any medicine prescribed is the most appropriate for you. **Share the responsibility** for safe and effective drug treatment. Make sure every prescriber and pharmacist who helps provide your health care is aware of **all** of the medicines you are taking. Include prescription, nonprescription, and any herbal or nutritional support you take. Television, newspaper, and radio ads can be seductive, but the use of any medicine is a very individual decision. A widely advertised or used medicine may not be the best choice for you. Ask your doctor or pharmacist for **printed information sheets** that offer unbiased information about the drug's benefits and risks—and its appropriateness for you.

Drug therapy **MUST** always be individualized, and also based on current research and studies. **NEVER** take someone else's medicine because your symptoms sound just like theirs.

When Your Doctor Prescribes a Drug for You

- ALWAYS ask that the prescription include both the **name of the drug** and the **disorder** for which the drug is taken. For example: Fosamax for osteoporosis or Zantac for heartburn. This helps avoid "sound-alike" errors. For example: over the phone, a person calling in Xanax may be understood to say Zantac. Zantac is for heartburn and ulcers. Xanax is for anxiety. IF the disorder being treated were on the label, it offers a second chance to discover an error.
- Tell your doctor about any known drug allergies and of any prior drug-induced adverse effects. This will let him or her check to see if they have inadvertently prescribed a medicine from the same chemical family.
- Always honestly talk about **all other drugs** (prescription, nonprescription, herbal, or nutritional) that you are taking. Include alcohol and marijuana. Remember that some herbal extracts contain the same ingredients found in prescription medicines. Make certain you tell your doctor about these.
- Many medicines **require** special precautions. Examples include avoiding certain foods, alcohol, exposure to sun, certain medicines, or even hazardous activities.
- Be sure you understand how long to take a medicine. Talk with your prescriber about this and, if applicable, when and how to stop it. I see many cases where patients thought they understood what do to, and actually stopped the wrong medicine.
- Ask your doctor to give you a **written summary** about the drug prescribed. Few people can remember all of the information and instructions that have been talked about. A concept I have pioneered is the Medication Map. Many medicine errors are made because people

forget, make incorrect combinations of medicines, mistake one pill for the other, or take medicine with food when it should not be. The Medication Map organizes all the medicines you are taking, and tells you how much, when, and with what the medicines should be taken. Take the Medicine Map from the back of this book to your doctor or pharmacist and ask him to fill in the form with you. This helps you fit the medicines realistically into your life, or even to show that the first medicine selected might not really be best for you. The best medicine in the world does absolutely no good if you can't or won't be able to take it. Get the most from your health care dollars.

- ALWAYS ask your doctor if the medicine prescribed offers the best balance of price and outcomes for you. This simple question will help focus a busy practitioner on his or her available choices. Remember to ask whether the dosing has been adjusted for any compromise in kidney or liver function or other chronic condition that you may have. Diseases can also "interact" with medicines.

- Many HMOs or health care insurers may not pay for some medicines. This can impact your doctor's prescribing authority and the pharmacist's ability to fill your prescription. Write the payer to complain. The Patient's Bill of Rights may restore your access to the medicine which will give the best results!

- Tell your doctor if new symptoms develop after you start taking the drug(s) prescribed. This can protect you from early stages of Bad Med Syndrome. Some problems caused by medicines themselves are easily reversible if they are caught early. If you are found to have had a reaction to a medicine, ask your doctor to report the problem to the Food and Drug Administration (FDA). This reporting is critical to maintaining safe and effective medicines.

- Keep follow-up appointments with your doctor and for laboratory tests. Many drugs must be monitored closely.

- If you go to any other health care provider, tell him or her of all medications you are taking currently—prescription and nonprescription. This is also a common source of problems—people often think that all doctors have all of their medical history simply because they are doctors. Doctors are not clairvoyant. Tell them your complete history in order to get the best possible results. Remember any herbal medicines you might be taking.

- This is controversial, but I think it is smart to ask your doctor if there is a gag rule he or she is working under which restricts him or her to a limited formulary and lower-cost medicines. There may be a conflict of interest in the advice he or she is giving you.

When You Get Your Prescription Drug(s) from Your Pharmacist

- OPEN THE BAG. Unfortunately, many people don't use the considerable education and help that their pharmacist can provide. Many prescription bags are stapled shut, with the brief patient information sheet on the inside.

- You'll be glad if you open the bag! This gives you a chance (on a refill prescription) to see if the pills look the same as before. It is also a chance to look over the dose and make sure you know how often to take it. Make sure you understand this. A few minutes reading the information about the medicine **can actually save your life.**
- READ THE LABEL carefully! This can be also be a lifesaving two minutes.
- Check that both the **name of the drug** and the **disorder** are specified. If these are missing, ask your pharmacist to call your doctor for permission to add them.
- If this is a refill, check to see that the drug in the bottle is the same as the drug in your original supply. If it is not the same, ask your pharmacist to explain the difference. (Generic drug products from different manufacturers often vary in size, shape, color, etc.)
- There are more than 1,000 drug names that "look alike" in print or "sound alike" in speech. Examples: Acutrim–Accutane, cyclosporine–cycloserine, Prilosec–Prozac, Xanax–Zantac. Mistaking one drug for the other can lead to serious problems. "Sound-alikes" cause problems when a prescription is given by telephone. Listing the **disorder** on the prescription will help the pharmacist realize the mistake. Also, many of the most-often prescribed drugs are pictured in the Color Chart insert in this book.
- Ask the pharmacist to give you **printed information sheets** about the drug(s) prescribed for you. Say YES if you are asked if you want counseling on your medicine! Make use of your pharmacist's training. Also ask him or her to fill out the **Medication Map** from the back of this book for you.
- Read the label. I've seen people pay more attention to a peanut butter label then they do to their prescription label. I've listed this twice because I think it is so important. These labels are a great opportunity to learn how to get the most from your medicines. They also tell about dosage forms that should not be altered (opened, crushed, or chewed), and about effects food may have.
- Use the same pharmacy for all of your medicines. Most pharmacies have a computer system. This can help prevent serious allergic reactions and significant drug interactions. Tell your pharmacist of all drugs (remember to include herbal remedies, megavitamins, alcohol, and nonprescription agents) you are currently taking.

Your Responsibilities—to Yourself—as a Patient

- Know both the generic and brand name of all drugs prescribed for you.
- If you are taking more than one drug, be sure that the label of **each** container includes the **name of the drug** and the **condition it treats**.

- Remember that foods can react with medicines. Something as simple as grapefruit juice is now known to interact with some high blood pressure medicines. The best liquid to take with most medicines is water. Be aware.
- Take a moment to make sure you understand the directions for using a drug. Ask if you're not sure.
- Many nonprescription medicines were once only prescription. Talk with your pharmacist or physician **BEFORE** combining any two drugs.
- Follow medicine instructions carefully and completely. **DO NOT** stop an antibiotic seven days into a ten-day prescription because you feel better. This can lead to serious illness. If you have trouble remembering to take your medications on time, ask for a dosing calendar or a weekly medication box.
- If you take medicines prescribed by more than one doctor, check the **generic names** for duplicate drugs with different brand names. This could cause serious overdoses.
- Ask your doctor or pharmacist if they offer "brown bag sessions" for your medicines. Put all the medicines you currently take, and have the pharmacist review them for potency, appropriateness, and dating.
- If you are looking at a new insurance plan or HMO, ask if there is a formulary. Find out if a mail-order pharmacy must be used. Finally, ask who will regularly review your medicines and how you will be able to contact a pharmacist for questions if a mail-order pharmacy must be used.
- Be certain all drugs you take are "in date" (have not expired).
- Effective and timely control of pain is a basic right to which you are entitled. The Agency for Health Care Policy and Research has released *Clinical Practice Guidelines* which outline management of cancer pain, but also apply to management of pain in general. Demand that your pain is respected as much as a high fever. The American Pain Society wants pain to be the fifth vital sign.
- If you are facing a terminal illness, ask if the hospital you are considering has a palliative care program as well as a hospice program.

Suggestions for Containing the Costs of Drug Therapy

- Cooperate fully with your doctor to ensure an accurate diagnosis. This helps ensure that the any medicines needed will be as safe and effective as possible.
- Ask your doctor to prescribe the drug that is most appropriate for you, selecting the product which offers the best balance of price and outcomes. If you have several chronic diseases at the same time, what appears to be a more expensive antibiotic may have a better **outcome** for you than a less costly one.
- Ask your doctor if an acceptable generic product is available.

- Ask your doctor if there are any vitamins or minerals (such as folic acid to help prevent some heart attacks or calcium for osteoporosis) that you should be taking based on family history.
- Follow your doctor and pharmacist's advice about your prescriptions.
- Many HMOs and physician groups use a concept called dual-product substitution. This is a measure that I agree with. For example: some prescription products are merely different names for **the same** medicine (Vanceril or Beclovent; Normodyne or Trandate). It makes perfect sense that the lowest-priced brand be freely substituted for a particular prescription. Ask your doctor about this idea when he or she is writing a prescription for you.
- Ask how the HMO or physician group measures up against other groups in your area. Remember, many groups are benchmarked or measured by groups such as the NCQA.

Points for Consideration by the Pharmacist

Adherence, adherence, adherence. I could probably end this section on this critical note. Half the people who get a prescription fail to take it correctly.

You can make a real difference by making sure that people understand how much to take, when to take it, and what to take it with. Remember, the current estimate is that adverse drug events or Bad Med Syndrome costs 136 billion dollars a year. Be a part of the solution! Many pharmacists are being paid for their expertise in medicines (cognitive services). In Veterans Administration hospitals some are even prescribing medicines via guidelines. Many states have given pharmacists the opportunity to provide vaccinations, and large numbers of you are starting to offer them. In a setting where the pressure of time is less restrictive, you can make a great difference in helping prevent some common illnesses.

Accept the FDA initiative to define your role and responsibility as counselor to consumers regarding the proper use of medicinal drugs. The FDA's position is that the patient has a right to demand and receive essential drug information, and that the pharmacist should offer it. The FDA recommends that **printed information** be dispensed with medicines to reinforce what the pharmacist says. Combined use of talking about prescriptions and giving printed materials gets the best results. I've often told patients that "We're always there for you" on the *Pharmacist Minute* radio series. Be there for your patients and make a difference. I've also told patients to "Take care of yourself" on my audiotapes and on my website. Rest assured that I'll be telling them what to look for to be a part of their health care!

The outcomes or results from medicines will be the hallmark of the use of medicines for the future. Pharmacists need to understand outcomes research; the FDA will be applying them to patient-directed advertising, physicians will be facing questions about who gets better on what medicine, and you will have a role in retrospective and potentially concurrent drug use review. Disease management and pharmacoeconomic principles will be widely applied.

Some pharmacists have made great inroads in clinical service by helping manage medicines for asthmatics, providing vaccines (where state law allows), offering smoking cessation groups, and helping monitor anticoagulation, blood sugar, and cholesterol. Contact your state board of pharmacy for more information. It's okay to accept appointments and charge a fee for cognitive services. Many stores are getting high rates of reimbursement. No one wants to contract Bad Med Syndrome and you can be there to help prevent it. I've created a Medication Map in this book (Table 15) which is also a perfect way for you to help patients realistically fit medicines into their lives.

I advise consumers to take the fullest advantage of their pharmacist's training and experience. It's a good idea to have a copy of the *Agency for Health Care Policy and Research Clinical Practice Guidelines Number 9* on the management of cancer pain, as well as copies of the patient guide on cancer pain. The Agency for Health Care Policy and Research is advocating effective and timely control of pain as a basic human right. The American Pain Society advocates pain as the fifth vital sign. This is also a clear opportunity for you to help in offering effective therapeutic options and superb pharmaceutical care. Call 1-800-422-6237 for more information.

When You Fill a Prescription

- Clarify with the prescriber any prescription information that is illegible, uncertain, or a potential source for erroneous interpretation—by you or the patient.
- Be alert to "look-alike" and "sound-alike" drug names. This is a significant cause of dispensing errors. In accepting prescriptions by telephone, ask the caller to spell the name of the drug, as appropriate.
- Include both the **name of the drug** and the **disorder** on the label (for example: Fosamax for osteoporosis) if the patient does not object, and consult with the prescribing physician when necessary. This will help (1) reduce dispensing errors caused by "look-alike" and "sound-alike" drug names; and (2) prevent confusion during concurrent use of multiple drugs: mistaken identity of drug and purpose, mistakenly altered dosing schedules, etc.
- Encourage your patients to look at the prescription label, **with you.** Paper clip the patient drug information to the bag. Take the lead in opening the bottle, showing the patient the medicine, and making sure they understand how much and when to take the medicine. This

also gives you a final chance to earn your place as the most trusted professional.

- Check the stock bottle for accurate identification and appropriate dating. If a technician fills the prescription, be certain you open the dispensing container as well as the completed prescription and check the drug personally.

When You Counsel the Patient as You Dispense the Filled Prescription

- Ask the patient to tell you how they are to take or give the medicine. Hearing them tell you about their medicines is a great way to make sure they really understand. Clarify any points of confusion or misunderstanding.
- Make sure that the patient recognizes the **name of the drug** and the **disorder being treated**. Explain what the drug is supposed to do.
- Review the details of dosing instructions: how much to take, when to take it, and for how long. It doesn't do them any good if it stays in the bottle. See if your computer vendor has a module for medication maps. If not, use the map provided in this book (Table 15). This can be a valuable cognitive service.
- Talk about possible side effects or adverse effects that may occur. Tell the patient about what to do if any of these occur. Encourage them to call their doctor if new symptoms develop.
- Precautions are critical. This includes possible interactions with foods, beverages, drugs, or restricted activities.
- Provide **written information** about the drug(s) dispensed and the patient's **disorder** (if available).
- Clarify how best to store the medicine. Tell them about refrigeration, and avoiding the humidity of a medicine chest. If a non-childproof lid is dispensed, remind them to keep the drug out of reach whenever children are visiting.
- Remind the patient that nonprescription (over-the-counter) drugs can interact with prescription drugs. Encourage them to call your pharmacy or their physician before combining any medicines.
- Always take a good medication history. Be certain to ask about any herbal remedies or megavitamins the patient may take.
- Encourage the patient to ask questions at the time of dispensing and later—whenever the need arises.

Suggestions for Containing the Costs of Drug Therapy

- As judgment dictates, fill the prescription with the most reasonably priced drug available—within legally possible and appropriate guidelines. Consult with the prescribing physician regarding generic substitution when feasible.

- If the patient is taking other drugs (prescribed by other physicians), look for drug duplications. Offer "brown bag sessions" where patients can bring in all their medicines and get your help regarding possible problems.

Points for Consideration by the Physician

Outcomes, benchmarking, and managed care. Three simple phrases that have significantly changed the way physicians practice medicine today. If you also add closed formularies and critical paths, in some senses clinical decision making has become more focused. I believe that a renewed focus on outcomes simply creates an atmosphere of continuous improvement and is just good medicine. One of the best colleagues to have in attaining the best results from any medicine is a fully informed patient.

Michael Weintraub, M.D., recognized this in 1991, when in his introduction to the *Yearbook of Drug Therapy* he stated, "In looking for trends in the medical literature, it is apparent that the need for the physician to be an educator of patients and their families is becoming greater and greater." In addition, citing an increased need for patient education, he summarized with the following opinion: "Treatment principles correctly applied by patients educated about their condition and involved in its management seem to be the wave of the future." More than ever before, the volume and characteristics of the drugs in use today require deliberate individualization of treatment. The overall effectiveness of any drug therapy depends on how carefully the drug is selected, dispensed, and administered. Responsible communication between physician, pharmacist, nurse, and patient must be achieved to the greatest extent possible. This process begins with the physician. It is absolutely unacceptable that current estimates put the expense of adverse drug events at some 136 billion dollars a year ... more than is spent on diabetes in the United States.

When You Evaluate a Patient for Drug Therapy

- Review the patient's drug history for known drug allergies and prior drug-induced adverse reactions.

- Ask if the patient is currently under treatment by other health care providers.
- Ask about all drugs used currently—prescription and over-the-counter. Remember that many over-the-counter agents were once prescription medicines. Make certain that you do not gloss over this aspect of the medicines your patient can take without ever obtaining your guidance.
- Remember the prevalence of herbal remedy and nutriceutical use. Include these substances in your questions.
- Consider a patient's history and lifestyle, think about diseases or conditions for which the patient is at risk, and vitamins (such as folic acid for heart disease) or minerals (calcium to prevent osteoporosis) that may be used to prevent the process. Rybacki's first recommendation: "It is always better to prevent a disease or condition than to have to treat it."
- Make certain that you are absolutely current. Many daily fax services are available which can be individualized to your practice and can easily be read after your morning rounds.
- Establish the nature and severity of the disorder under consideration for drug treatment.
- Elicit significant coexisting disorders—possible absolute contraindications for certain drugs.
- Evaluate any suspected or obvious organ dysfunction—possible relative contraindications for certain drugs. When creatinine values are available, take the time to calculate creatinine clearance. Many drugs have break points for adjustment of dosage at various levels of renal impairment. Even though an older patient's creatinine is within the "normal limits," their clearance will not be. For example, a 72-year-old, 70-kg man with a 1.4 creatinine will have a creatinine clearance of about 48.6 ml/min. This is **below the level where doses or intervals of renally eliminated medicines must be adjusted.** Hepatic disease will also impact doses or intervals for many drugs, particularly those which are highly protein-bound or heavily metabolized.
- Assess the patient's potential for adherence or nonadherence to the drug therapy. Remember the expense that a given prescription presents. The most brilliant prescription choice is totally ineffective if financial considerations prevent adherence to the medicine you choose. Once-a-day dosing is much easier to remember and, combined with a dosing calendar, gets excellent results. See if the patient's pharmacist offers a medication mapping service. If not, map your patient's medicines yourself.

When Selecting Drugs for Therapy

- Try to match the drug's power to the patient's problem. Avoid over-prescribing—medicinal "overkill." For example: mild to moderate stress reactions (situational anxiety–tension states) respond well to antianxiety drugs; they do not require antipsychotic medication. An uncomplicated urinary tract infection with a broadly sensitive single organism does not require a broad spectrum anti-infective drug.

- Obtain a copy of the *Agency for Health Care Policy and Research Clinical Practice Guidelines Number 9*. The AHCPR is advocating effective and timely pain control as a basic human right. Increase your awareness of the World Health Organization Pain Ladder and the use of the agents that are primary analgesics and adjuvants. AHCPR publications are great tools to help your patients understand their medicine and their disease. Push to make pain the fifth vital sign in your hospital.

- Always check for drug–drug, drug–food, and drug–disease interactions. Remember to take a "new" drug history periodically.

- Many new oral anti-infectives are effective against pathogens which historically required intravenous therapy. Although this allows you to avoid hospitalization, it makes the patient's adherence more critical.

- Consider the desired onset of drug action (immediate versus delayed) and the consequences or benefits of that effect.

- Choose the drug with the most favorable benefit-to-risk ratio: the best clinical effects with the fewest possible adverse reactions.

- When you prescribe narrow-therapeutic-window drugs that require periodic blood level, be certain that blood sampling is done after the drug has reached its steady state (usually five half-lives). Understand which level is preferable to measure: "peak" level (as for theophylline), "trough" level (as for digoxin), and "peak and trough" for aminoglycosides (such as tobramycin). Many clinical pharmacists (the author included) will willingly calculate the best dose and interval for you, and make a consultative recommendation.

- Give due consideration to the patient's prior experience with other drugs similar to the one you are considering and prescribe accordingly. Prescribing a second drug from the same drug class from which a patient already had an allergic or adverse drug effect that required discontinuation of therapy or provided no therapeutic benefit is not prudent.

- Remember individual patient factors such as age, education, and cultural factors (including genetic effects on medication elimination).

- Think about the desired extent of effect (systemic or local).

- If drug treatment fails after a reasonable trial with good adherence, change to a drug of another chemical class, or consider combination therapy with two medicines with different mechanisms of action. For example: if viral load decreases for a time, then increases in an AIDS patient, you MUST change treatment.

- Select the drugs you prescribe critically, utilizing independent, objective reviews of available information. The "most frequently prescribed" drug is not necessarily the best drug within its class. Slick, glossy detail pieces should always be confirmed by primary literature.

- Even "drugs of choice" in objective reviews can be poor choices when you consider the characteristics of individual patients. A renally compromised patient may better tolerate an "alternate drug" with dual elimination (hepatic and renal) than a "drug of choice" that is limited to renal elimination.
- Remember the pharmacokinetic and pharmacodynamic changes that occur in those over 65 can lead to accumulation and excessive responses to "normal" doses and dosing intervals.
- Be objective and discerning as you review the claims made for a newly released drug within a sizable class of drugs already available. Only 20 percent of newly approved drugs each year are classified by FDA as truly innovative or more advantageous than similar drugs in current use. The remaining 80 percent are largely "me too" drugs with a limited history of use and a potential for "surprises" after a period of general use. It is best to select drugs with established records showing them to be the best in their class.

When You Issue Prescriptions in Writing or by Telephone

- When prescribing for outpatient use, consider the advantage of including both the **name of the drug** and the **therapeutic indication** (the patient's disorder) on the prescription label. For example: Sinemet CR for Parkinson's. Putting the disorder on the label will help (1) reduce dispensing errors caused by "look-alike" and "sound-alike" drug names, and (2) prevent confusion that often occurs during concurrent use of multiple drugs, especially among the elderly: mistaken identity of drug and purpose, mistakenly altered dosing schedules, etc.
- Respect your patients' wishes as to whether or not they *want* the name of the disorder written on the prescription label. If they prefer you not include it, recommend that they write it on the label themselves *after* the prescription is filled.
- Keep dosing schedules as simple as possible. Once-a-day dosing improves adherence.
- Alert the pharmacist to "look-alike" and "sound-alike" drug names. Print the drug name on written prescriptions. Spell the drug name when prescribing by telephone.

When Counseling Patients About Drug Therapy

- Briefly explain the nature of the patient's disorder and its treatment. Use language that is readily understood by the average person.
- Provide written information or references for educational material

about the disorder. If the disorder is chronic in nature (diabetes, hypertension), explain the need to continue drug therapy indefinitely, possibly for life.

- Briefly explain the name and nature of the drugs you are prescribing. Stress the importance of strict adherence with the medicine. It is wise to tell the patient—in advance—about potential adverse effects. The patient who has such effects is more likely to be understanding and forgiving if they do not come as a surprise to them.

- To supplement your discussion, **provide a printed document** that summarizes the essential information the patient needs to use the drug(s) safely and effectively. This is comforting and will save you an amazing number of telephone calls. Be sure the patient knows what to do if a dose is missed. Look at an add-on program to your office management program that prints out relevant information for your patients to take home. Such services can provide detailed descriptions of drugs, general guidelines for drug use, and personalized instructions.

- Explain the need for follow-up visits to monitor the effects of drug treatment and the course of the disorder.

- Explain that drugs may not work in practice exactly as expected. Tell the patient to be alert to the possibility that a new symptom or sign *may* be drug related. If one of your patients does experience a novel adverse drug reaction, it is critical that you (or your designate) call the FDA MedWatch at 1-800-332-1088.

- This fulfills your voluntary obligation to Phase Four reporting and makes medication use safer for everyone. I admit that I am the one advocating mandatory reporting for everyone, not just the people who make the medicines. Encourage the patient to call as needed regarding any aspect of drug treatment. Recognize the need to adjust drug selection and/or dosage regimens to accommodate individual variability.

- Give special attention to the older patient on drug therapy. The elderly (1) generally use multiple drugs concurrently, and (2) are more prone to experience adverse drug effects.

- If you refer any of your patients to a specialist, be certain to take a repeat medication history when they are returned to your care. Check for duplications in medicines by cross-referencing brand or generic names.

- Every six months, ask your patients to bring in all the prescription, nonprescription, and herbal medicines that they routinely take. This kind of "brown bag session" can help you best understand all of the potential or actual interactions of therapies your patient is or will be taking. Remember: An informed patient can be your greatest ally in optimal therapeutics and the outcomes that will be benchmarked!

Suggestions for Containing the Costs of Drug Therapy

- When you have selected the most appropriate drug, consider its cost. If the patient requests an available generic product, direct the pharmacist to dispense one with certified bioequivalence. Because of generic product variability, caution the patient to have the prescription refilled with the identical generic (same manufacturer) each time.
- Avoid polypharmacy whenever possible. Limit the number of drugs that the patient is taking concurrently to the fewest required. Do not let the cure become the disease. Medicate serious, significant disorders; discourage the use of drugs for minor, transient complaints.
- Consider carefully any requests from patients for a prescription drug they have learned about through direct-to-consumer advertising. Explain to your patients the profit motive of the producer and assure them that you will prescribe the drug that, in your judgment, is the most appropriate one for them.
- When circumstances permit, use home intravenous drug therapy in preference to hospitalization.
- The move toward managed care and other health care reform initiatives brings increased scrutiny to the outcomes of your therapeutic and clinical decisions. Become more familiar with the expense of various medicinal options, as well as the specific patient populations where the benefit-to-risk and cost-to-outcome ratios make the most sense. Pharmacoeconomic and disease management approaches will bring the best balance of cost and outcome.

1

HOW TO USE THIS BOOK

2

GUIDELINES FOR SAFE AND EFFECTIVE DRUG USE OR HOW TO PREVENT BAD MED SYNDROME

3

TRUE BREAKTHROUGHS IN MEDICINES

1

How to Use This Book

A visit to your doctor's office can be a disconcerting experience. Many physicians face severe time constraints. Most of us have had the sense of our doctor needing, but not wanting, to hurry out of the exam room to see the next patient—this can be especially true in emergency departments in hospitals. You may be left with a prescription for yourself or a loved one.

This is innocent enough, but the problem lies in the fact that you may have been told very little about the medicines prescribed. In any case, even in the best circumstances, it will never be possible or practical for your doctor or other prescriber to provide you with *all* the information that could be considered appropriate and useful, or whatever information is given may be provided in complicated medical terms that may be difficult for you to remember.

Unfortunately, medical technology and medical research have advanced much more rapidly than our social ability to realize that there is such a thing as a good death. Comfort and palliation will need to replace extraordinary means and measures, which may actually become cruel when used to "help" the dying patient. In reality, few patients die at home and many die in pain. We should be shocked that there is a program called Project Death in America ... yet it is a start to make some needed changes. My stepfather, dying from cancer, looked at me from his deathbed and said, "Make a difference in people's pain." I hope this book will help do that.

I've rewritten this book to help cure Bad Med Syndrome, and to bring you current and important information to protect yourself and your family. I can help you become a partner in your health care and will always try to supplement the direction and guidance your doctor will offer about your medicines.

Your resource is arranged into six sections. The first section offers in-

1

sight into modern drug therapy, and gives you helpful tips on preventing Bad Med Syndrome. "True Breakthroughs in Medicines" will help identify completely new medicines that have gained FDA approval, or are the first new agents in many years to treat an existing disease or condition.

Section Two gives you detailed Drug Profiles covering more than 2,000 brand-name prescription drugs and nearly 400 widely used generic medicines. Selection of each drug is based on three criteria: the extent of its use, the urgency of the conditions it treats, and the volume and complexity of information essential to its proper use. You'll find that the Profiles are arranged alphabetically by generic name. Read carefully to be sure you have the correct medicine.

Each Profile is presented in the same way and once you become familiar with the format, you'll be able to quickly find specific information on any drug. Unlike other imitators, each Essential Drug Profile contains at least 45 helpful categories of information, including:

Year Introduced

Remember, the longer the drug has been in general use, the more likely all of its actions are known and the less likely ongoing use will produce new problems. This will help identify those medicines that are more likely to be more fully understood both because they have been in existence for a longer time period and have also been widely used.

Drug Class

Drug classes are like families—in fact, some of the profiles giving information about medicines from the same class have been arranged into Medication Family Profiles. Many actions, reactions, and interactions with other drugs are often shared by drugs of the same class. For example, *if you are allergic to one cephalosporin, you most likely will be allergic to a second cephalosporin. By the same logic, if a medicine in a certain class has not helped you, it is likely that a second one from the same class will do you little good.*

Prescription Required

Just because a medicine does not require a prescription (over-the-counter) does not mean the medicine is not strong. Remember, over the last ten years there has been a great shift in medicines from prescription to nonprescription. Current examples include medicines for yeast infections, patches and gum to help you stop smoking, as well as ulcer medicines (histamine H2 blockers) that can also be used to prevent or treat heartburn. Virtually all of these medicines were previously available only by prescription. Always mention nonprescription medicine use when asked about the "medicines" you take.

Controlled Drug

The Controlled Substances Act of 1970 assigned medicines with a potential for abuse to a specific schedule in the United States. A Canadian schedule is also given when applicable. A description of the schedules of controlled drugs is found at the back of your guide.

Available for Purchase by Generic Name

In general, costs can be greatly reduced by buying a generic equivalent of a brand-name product. The key word is "equivalent." It is important to make sure that "bioavailability and bioequivalence"—the comparative composition, quality, and effectiveness of the generic versus the brand-name drug product—is the same if a substitution is made. Further discussions of bioavailability and bioequivalence will be found in the Glossary (Section Five).

Brand Names

I realize that generic or chemical names of medicines can be complicated, so brand names are given to help. Brand names are listed for the United States and for Canada (✤). A combination drug (one with more than one active ingredient) is identified by [CD] following the brand name. Be careful! In some cases a name used in both the United States and Canada will represent entirely different generic drugs (in a single drug product), or a significantly different mixture of generic medicines. If you travel between the two countries, make sure that the brand name drug contains the same generic medicine(s).

Benefits versus Risks

This summarizes the "pros" and "cons" for each drug. Capital letters emphasize the drug's principal benefits and risks, while lowercase letters are used for less critical benefits and risks. One look reveals the "comparative weights" of the two columns and gives a first impression about how a drug's benefits relate to its potential risks. This is meant to help you become more circumspect in your use of medicines, and is not to be the sole basis for deciding whether or not to use a drug. **Failure to individualize drug selection and dose is probably the greatest weakness in current drug therapy.**

Principal Uses

A drug may be available as a single drug product or in combination with other drugs. "As a Single Drug Product" tells the primary use(s) of the drug when used alone. The "As a Combination Drug Product [CD]" tells primary use(s) when combined with other drugs in the same "pill." The uses are a consensus in the medical community and current research. Where appropriate, the logic for combining certain drugs is explained.

How This Drug Works

This section tells what a drug does to work. If a specific method of action has not been established, I tell you about the current theory.

Available Dosage Forms and Strengths

This gives you available manufacturers' dosage forms (tablets, capsules, elixirs, etc.) and strengths, without company identification. Dosage forms limited to hospital use are often not included. The entry on *dosage forms and strengths* in the Glossary can help with those few abbreviations used to describe strengths of each dosage form.

Usual Adult Dosage Range

Dosing information represents a consensus by appropriate authorities and is the currently recommended standard. It is a guide showing how much of the drug can reasonably be expected to be both effective and safe. Under certain circumstances, your doctor may decide to modify the "standard" dose. Some dosage forms are not covered (for example, extemporaneously made suppositories) and may require different doses than those listed.

Conditions Requiring Dosing Adjustments

Medical conditions can actually change the effect a medicine has on your body. This is a fact that is **often missed** in selecting a dose or dosing interval and can lead to Bad Med Syndrome. For example, people over 60 often have a decline in kidney function. This can mean that drugs stay in their bodies longer than younger patients. **It is critical to ask your doctor if any prescribed medicine dose has been adjusted for this age-related decline in how well your kidneys work.**

Dosing Instructions

Food and medicines can fight. Food can actually change how much medicine gets into your body, and this section tells you about them. Sometimes, when medicine is urgently needed, you may have to crush the tablet or open the capsule and mix the contents with a food or beverage. Some medicines should **NEVER** be crushed or altered in order to give them. This information category identifies those forms of each drug that may and those that should not be changed. Your pharmacist can once again be a great resource.

Usual Duration of Use

Many factors determine how long a medicine must be taken and this is often an area of great controversy: factors such as the nature and severity of symptoms, drug form and strength, ability of the patient to respond, and use of other drugs, among others. The focus here is to help you give the medicine an appropriate amount of time to work. Where appropriate, limitations in how long a medicine should be taken are given.

This Drug Should Not Be Taken If

These are the *absolute* contraindications to the use of the drug (see *contraindication* in the Glossary). By consensus, these are circumstances where the medicine should NEVER be taken. Tell your doctor **immediately** if any information in this category applies to you.

Inform Your Physician Before Taking This Drug If

This category tells you the *relative* contraindications to a medicine. One way to think of this information is as a relative benefit-to-risk decision. Here again, it is important that you tell your physician or other prescriber if these factors apply to you.

Possible Side Effects

Here you can learn about natural, expected, and usually unavoidable medicine actions—the normal and anticipated consequences of taking it. This gives a realistic perspective balancing side effects with goals of treatment.

Possible Adverse Effects

These are unusual, unexpected, and infrequent drug effects, which are often called adverse drug reactions or effects. These range from mild to serious. In the past, I've attempted to give set percentages to help you. These were often derived from Phase Three studies or current research. In order to more accurately define how frequently these effects happen, I've developed this system:

- Possible: An effect that has been documented for other drugs in the same family, but not the profiled drug. Also assigned when the effect occurs in some limited patient populations and not in others.
- Case reports: This means that an effect has been documented to happen, but only has been seen in isolated cases.
- Rare: This means that an effect is seen in less than 2 percent of patients. Another way to look at this is that 98 percent of people will take the medicine and NOT have the effect.

- Infrequent: An effect that is seen in 2 to 10 percent of patients.
- Frequent: These effects happen in more than 10 percent of patients.

Tell your doctor if you suspect you may be having an adverse drug effect. Serious adverse reactions may start with mild, unthreatening symptoms. It's also possible to have an adverse reaction that has not yet been reported. Don't discount an adverse effect just because it's not listed. *A properly selected drug usually has a comparatively small chance of producing serious harm.* Knowing that a drug can cause a serious adverse reaction should not deter you from using it when it has been properly selected and its use will be carefully supervised.

Possible Effects on Sexual Function

This information is often NOT something people want to discuss, or something that patients are told about. Currently available information (often inadequate and vague) from all reliable sources is presented. Both physician and patient are well advised to discuss frankly any potential effect that drug therapy could have on sexual expression.

Adverse Effects That May Appear Similar to Natural Diseases or Disorders

Medicines can actually cause effects similar to widely diagnosed diseases or disorders. Quite often this inadvertent error is compounded by prescribing another drug to relieve the "symptoms" of the first. My father was prescribed a medicine for his "arthritis" when he was actually having an adverse effect from a medicine for his heart rhythm. For milder symptoms (e.g., nasal congestion or diarrhea from reserpine), the oversight may not be too serious. But in the case of the Parkinson-like effects of some drugs, the mistake can be devastating. This section tells you about this common flaw.

Natural Diseases or Disorders That May Be Activated by This Drug

Many drugs can "activate" latent disorders that may not be recognized as drug induced. If a new and seemingly unrelated disorder starts during treatment with any new medicine, ask your doctor if it may be drug related.

Possible Effects on Laboratory Tests

Most drugs have significant effects on body chemistry and organ systems. Some effects are intended and beneficial (therapeutic); others are unintended, unavoidable, and potentially harmful. Timely use of laboratory tests lets us check how well a drug is working and the course of the condition being treated.

Caution

This category gives you information on aspects of drug action and/or drug use that require special emphasis. Occasionally these warnings may relate to information provided in other categories. When included here, such entries warrant being repeated.

Precautions for Use by Infants and Children

Doses often MUST be changed for infants and children under 12 years of age, and some drugs and/or treatment situations call for special precautions. When administering *any* prescription or over-the-counter drug, it is best to ask your doctor or pharmacist about needed precautions.

Precautions for Use by Those Over 60 Years of Age

Our bodies change as we age, and people age at different rates and in different ways. Assessment of "age" must be based upon individual mental and physical condition, and never upon years alone. In general, changes that accompany aging may affect the actions of the body on the drug, as well as actions of the drug on the body. Appropriate precautions are outlined in this category.

Advisability of Use During Pregnancy: Pregnancy Category

Information about the safe use of a particular drug during pregnancy was one of the most forceful concerns that led to the formal petitioning of the Food and Drug Administration in 1975 to make sure that information was disclosed to the public. The FDA definitions of the five pregnancy categories are listed at the back of this book. The FDA does not make the initial category assignment; this is the responsibility of the manufacturer that markets the drug. The initial designation is then subject to review and modification by the FDA. The "Pregnancy Category" designations presented in each Profile were determined after thorough review of pertinent literature and consultation with appropriate authorities. They are offered at this time for initial guidance only. They are in no sense "official" and do not have the endorsement of either the manufacturer or the FDA.

Advisability of Use if Breast-Feeding

This section tells you about effects of the drug on milk production, if the drug goes into human milk, and the possible effects of the drug on the nursing infant. Prudent recommendations are given where appropriate. Also included are impacts of disease where appropriate.

Suggested Periodic Examinations While Taking This Drug

Getting the best results from your medicines often means that your doctor may ask you to get periodic examinations while taking the drug(s) he or she has prescribed. Which exams and when they are made depends on your past and present medical history, the nature of the condition being treated, the dose and duration of drug use, and your doctor's observations of your response. There may be many occasions when he or she will feel no examinations are necessary. Always tell your doctor about all developments you think may be drug related.

While Taking This Drug, Observe the Following: Marijuana Smoking

The widespread "social" use of marijuana by virtually all age groups and the approval of medicinal smoking of marijuana in two states has led to inquiries about interactions between the active chemicals in marijuana smoke and medicines in common use. Currently available literature on the health aspects of marijuana use contains very little practical information concerning the potential for drug interactions. The limited information presented in this category of selected Drug Profiles represents those *possible interactions* considered likely to occur in view of the known pharmacological effects of the principal components of marijuana and of the medicine reviewed in the Profile. In most instances, the interaction statements are not based on documented evidence since very little is available. However, the conclusions stated—derived by logical inductive reasoning—represent the concurrence of authorities with expertise in this field.

While Taking This Drug, Observe the Following: Other Drugs

This confusing and often controversial area of drug information is divided into five subcategories of possible interactions between drugs. Look carefully at the wording of each subcategory heading (see also *interaction* in the Glossary). Some of the drugs listed do not have a representative Profile. If you are using one of these drugs, ask your doctor or pharmacist for help about potential interactions. A brand name (or names) that follows the generic name of an interacting drug is given as an example only. It is not intended to mean that the particular brand(s) named have interactions that are different from other brands of the same generic drug. If you are taking the generic drug, *all* brand names under which it is marketed MUST be considered as possible interactants. Medicines in the same or similar families may also interact.

Driving, Hazardous Activities

Clearly, medicines can change coordination and alertness. In addition to driving motor vehicles, the information in this category applies to any activity of a dangerous nature, such as operating machinery, working on ladders, using power tools, and handling weapons. Your individual response and degree of reaction may vary from others. Talk with your doctor or pharmacist if you take a medicine which may impair your abilities.

Aviation Note

Military pilots enjoy the expert guidance and surveillance provided by the flight surgeon, but no tightly structured control system exists for their civilian counterparts. However, the need for practical information regarding the possible effects of medicinal drugs on flight performance is the same for pilots in all settings. This section can tell civilian pilots how a particular drug may affect his or her eligibility to fly and when it is advisable or necessary to consult a designated aviation medical examiner or an FAA medical officer.

Occurrence of Unrelated Illness

Some medicines such as "blood thinners" or anticoagulants require careful regulation of daily doses to maintain a constant drug effect within critical limits. In this section of your book, emphasis is given to those illnesses that might affect drug use.

Discontinuation

How and when to stop is often as important as ever starting a medicine in the first place. Unfortunately, this aspect of drug use is often overlooked when a medicine is first discussed. Often, it is mandatory that the patient be fully informed on *when* to discontinue, when *not* to discontinue, and precisely *how* to stop use of the drug. When one medicine is stopped, other drugs being taken at the same time may also need to be adjusted. The doctor who is primarily responsible for your overall management must be kept informed of *all* the drugs you are taking at a given time.

I believe that the remaining information categories in the Drug Profiles are self-explanatory, but I always welcome your letters and questions. I have also started a web site called **medicineinfo** and can be reached at www.medicineinfo.com. Section Three, "The Leading Edge," offers what are, in my opinion, medicines that show great promise and are just over the horizon from FDA approval. Some of these medicines may not actually be approved, but they give such significant hope that they're worth consideration. The information may actually let patients facing serious diseases ask to be included in scientific studies and get the medicine prior to actual approval. Section Four is a presentation of drug classes arranged alphabetically by their chemical or therapeutic (generic) class. Because of chemical composition and biological activities, some drugs appear in two or more classes. For example, the drug product with the brand name Diuril will be represented by its generic name, chlorothiazide, in three drug classes: the Thiazide Diuretics (a chemical classification), the Diuretics (a drug action classification), and the Antihypertensives (a disease-oriented classification).

Frequently in the Drug Profiles in Section Two you are advised to "see

(a particular) Drug Class." This alerts you to a possible drug contraindication, or to possible interactions with certain foods, alcohol, or other
drugs. In each case, you can find the more readily recognized brand
names for each drug listed generically within a drug class by looking at the
appropriate Drug Profile. Timely use of these references can help you to
avoid many possible hazards of medication.

Section Five is a glossary of drug-related terms used throughout the
book. The preferred use of each term is explained. Frequent references to
the Glossary are made in the Drug Profiles. Use of the Glossary will help
you understand how to recognize and interpret significant drug effects.

Section Six offers tables of drug information. The title and introductory material explain the content and purpose of each table. The information emphasizes pertinent aspects of drug behavior. The tables give
you another source of ready reference. The Medication Map in this section
is a way for you to use your doctor's or pharmacist's expertise to arrange
all of the medicines you take into a reasonable schedule. Take the time to
have them help you get the most from your medicines. A new table (Table
16) identifies medicines that have been removed from the market. This
may help protect you from medicines that may still be available in other
countries. The index of brand and generic names in the back of the book
is a single alphabetical listing that provides page references to the appropriate Drug Profile(s) for all drugs found in this book. It will be more useful if you first read the introductory explanation of the special features of
this combined index.

2

Guidelines for Safe and Effective Drug Use

DO NOT

- pressure your doctor to prescribe drugs that, in his or her judgment, you do not need. A pill is not always the answer.
- blindly accept care from any provider. Ask your HMO or medical group how their results or outcomes compare to other groups in the area and the country.
- assume that all doctors know all the drugs you take. Always ask your doctor or pharmacist BEFORE combining any other medicine with medicines already prescribed.
- pick up a stapled prescription bag. ALWAYS open a stapled bag, check the brief patient information that may be inside the bag and make sure you understand it. While you are in the pharmacy, read the prescription label and make sure it makes sense. Look at the pills, and (especially on refill drugs) check to see that they look the same as they did before. On new prescriptions, ask that the prescription be checked to make sure it is the correct medicine.
- take prescription drugs on your own or on the advice of friends and neighbors because your symptoms are "just like theirs." Drug therapy must be individualized, based on liver and/or kidney function, medicines you currently take, and many other factors.
- offer drugs prescribed for you to anyone else without a physician's guidance.
- change the dose or timing of any drug without the advice of your physician (except when the drug appears to be causing adverse effects).
- leave it to a guess that you've taken your medicine. ALWAYS get a dosing calendar or make one so that you can check off **each dose** as you take it.

- continue to take a drug that you feel is causing problems, until you are able to talk with your doctor.
- store your medicines in a bathroom medicine cabinet. This is often an area of high humidity which can (even though the bottle is closed) enter the medicine and degrade the active drug. Select a lockable kitchen cabinet out of reach of children.
- take *any* drug (prescription or nonprescription) while pregnant or nursing an infant until you talk to your doctor or pharmacist. Many herbal combinations may have active ingredients similar to those found in prescription medicines.
- take any more medicines than are absolutely necessary. (The greater the number of drugs taken at the same time, the greater the likelihood of adverse effects.)
- withhold from your doctor information about previous prescription or nonprescription drug use. He or she will want to know what has helped and what has caused problems.
- take any drug in the dark. Identify every dose of medicine carefully in adequate light to be certain you are taking the intended drug.
- keep drugs on a bedside table. Drugs for emergency use, such as nitroglycerin, are an exception. It is best to have only one such drug at the bedside for use during the night.

DO

- talk with your doctor about the results or outcomes expected from any medicine being considered. Understand that taking the medicine EXACTLY as it is prescribed is critical. Missing one pill in a three times a day regimen may cause you to lose the benefits of all of the medicine.
- talk with your HMO or medical group every year about how their results or outcomes compare to other providers of health care in the area and in the country. This is especially important for businesses since the preferred provider they choose impacts the health of many people.
- ask your HMO or medical group what their disease management programs are, and how any specific disease or condition that you may have is addressed within the scope of their disease management plan. Find out how the results or outcomes of the program compare with other programs in the area or the country.
- know the name (and correct spelling) of the drug(s) you are taking. It is best to know both the brand name and the generic name.
- open the prescription bag and the bottle WHILE YOU ARE STILL IN THE PHARMACY. This will give you a chance to best use the training and experience of your pharmacist and will also let you make sure you understand how to best take your medicine. If the prescription is a refill, make sure the pills are the same as the ones originally prescribed. If they are not, ask why.

- read the package labels of all nonprescription drugs so you know what is in them.
- take the medicine exactly as prescribed. If you think there will be a change in your ability to take the medicine, call your doctor before you make any change. For example, taking one dose of a medicine that should be taken three times a day often will NOT give one-third of the desired effect. I've been asked this kind of question often. Taking a medicine less frequently than prescribed will often give no beneficial effects, especially for those medicines where a relatively constant blood level determines how well the medicine will work.
- put a dosing calendar or a reminder note on the refrigerator or near your car keys. Get a watch with an alarm and set it for the times when you need to take your medicine.
- thoroughly shake all liquid suspensions of drugs to ensure uniform distribution of ingredients.
- use a standardized measuring device for giving liquid medicines by mouth. The household "teaspoon" varies greatly in size.
- follow your doctor's advice on dietary or other measures designed to help the prescribed drugs work their best. For example, decreasing or eliminating salt when taking high blood pressure medicines may help achieve desired drug effects with smaller doses.
- tell your anesthesiologist, surgeon, and dentist of *all* drugs you are taking, before any surgery.
- tell your doctor if you become pregnant while you are taking any drugs from any source.
- keep a written record of *all* drugs (prescription and nonprescription), vaccines, and herbal remedies you take during your entire pregnancy—name, dose, dates taken, and reasons for use.
- keep a written record of *all* drugs (and vaccines) to which you become allergic or have an adverse reaction to. This should be done for each member of the family, especially the elderly or infirm.
- keep a written record of *all* drugs (and vaccines) to which *your children* become allergic or experience an adverse reaction.
- fill out "Your Personal Drug Profile" (Table 14). Get the number of your Poison Control Center **today** and post it by your telephone. The worst time to try to find an emergency number is while there is a dire need for it. Fill in the Medication Map (Table 15), and ask your doctor if the times selected and combinations of medicines are appropriate.
- tell your doctor of all known or suspected allergies, especially allergies to drugs. Be sure that allergies are a part of your medical record. People with allergies are four times more prone to drug reactions.
- call your doctor immediately if you think you are having an overdose, side effect, or an adverse effect from a drug.
- ask if it is safe to drive a car, operate machinery, or engage in other hazardous activities while taking the drug(s) prescribed.
- ask if it is safe to drink alcoholic beverages while taking the drug(s) pre-

scribed. We often forget that alcohol is a drug with its own pharmacology and drug–drug interactions.

- find out if any particular foods, beverages, or other prescription or non-prescription medicines should be avoided while taking the drug(s) prescribed.
- keep all appointments for follow-up examinations or laboratory tests.
- ask for help to understand any point that confuses you. If you are concerned about remembering information or instructions for use, ask for written materials.
- throw away all outdated drugs.
- ask your doctor if a prescribed medicine offers the best balance of cost and outcomes for you.
- store all drugs for intermittent use out of the reach of children. This is critical for those of you with grandchildren who visit infrequently.

PREVENTING ADVERSE DRUG REACTIONS

It is always better to prevent a condition or disease than to have to treat it. This is especially true in the case of adverse drug reactions where the cure can become the disease. As our understanding of drug actions and reactions has expanded, we learned that many adverse effects are, to some extent, predictable and preventable. Several contributing factors are now well recognized, and these fall into 11 categories.

Previous Adverse Reaction to a Drug

People who have had an adverse drug reaction in the past are more likely to have adverse reactions to other drugs, even though the drugs are unrelated. This suggests that some people may have a genetic (inborn) predisposition to unusual or abnormal drug responses. *Always tell your doctor about any history of prior adverse drug experiences.*

Allergies

Some people are allergic by nature (have hay fever, asthma, eczema, hives) and are more likely to develop allergies to drugs. The allergic patient must be watched very closely when medicines are used. Known drug allergies must be written in the medical record. Patients must tell every health care provider that he or she is allergic by nature and is allergic to specific drugs. *Provide this information without waiting to be asked.* Your doctor will then be able to avoid prescribing those drugs that could provoke an allergic reaction, as well as related (cross-sensitivity) drugs.

Contraindications

Both patient and physician must strictly observe contraindications to any drug under consideration. *Absolute contraindications* include those conditions and situations that prohibit the use of the drug for any reason. *Relative contraindications* are those conditions that, in the judgment of the physician, do not preclude the use of the drug, but make it essential that special care be given to its use. Often, dosing adjustments, additional supportive measures, and close supervision are needed.

Precautions in Use

Patients should know any special precautions needed while taking a drug. This includes advisability of use during pregnancy or while nursing; precautions on sun exposure (or ultraviolet lamps); avoidance of extreme heat or cold, heavy physical exertion (such as with fluoroquinolone antibiotics), etc.

Dose

It is important to take any medicine exactly as prescribed. *This is most important with those drugs that have narrow margins of safety.* Even once-a-day medications should be taken at the same time of day or night to ensure the most constant blood levels. Call your doctor if nausea, vomiting, diarrhea, or other problems interfere with taking your medicine as prescribed.

Interactions

Some drugs can interact with foods (including vitamins and some herbal remedies), alcohol, and other drugs (prescription and nonprescription) to cause serious adverse effects. *The patient must be told about all likely interactants.* If, during the course of treatment, you feel you have discovered a new interaction, tell your doctor so that its full significance can be determined.

Warning Symptoms

Many drugs will cause symptoms that are early warnings of a developing adverse effect: for example, severe headaches or visual disturbances *before* a stroke in a woman taking oral contraceptives. *It is imperative that you know symptoms and signs that could be early warnings of adverse reactions.* The patient is then empowered to act in his or her own behalf by calling their doctor **before** taking another dose of their medicine. Adverse reactions should be reported to the FDA following their current guidelines.

Examinations to Monitor Drug Effects

Many drugs in common use can damage vital body tissues (such as bone marrow, liver, kidney, eye structures, etc.)—especially when these drugs are used for a long time or in high doses. Sometimes these adverse effects are not discovered until a newly approved drug has been in wide use for a long time. This damage may be reversible if found quickly. *Cooperate fully with your doctor when he or she asks for periodic exams to check for adverse drug effects.*

Advanced Age and Debility

When we age or as some disease processes progress, vital organs may not work as well, and can greatly influence the body's response to drugs. These patients often poorly tolerate drugs with inherent toxic potential and frequently need smaller doses at longer intervals. *The effects of drugs on the elderly and severely ill are often unpredictable.* Great care must be taken to prevent or minimize adverse effects.

Appropriate Drug Choice

The use of any medicine is always a benefit-to-risk decision. The medication used should offer the best balance of overall cost (including lab tests) and outcomes (including quality of life). Many adverse reactions can be prevented if both physician and patient exercise good judgment and restraint.

Polypharmacy

Unfortunately, the cure can become the disease. Patients who are cared for by several physicians may end up with several drugs prescribed separately by more than one physician for different disorders—often without appropriate communication between patient and prescriber. This frequent practice can lead to serious drug–drug interactions. *The patient should routinely talk to* **each** *health care provider about all the drugs—prescription and nonprescription—that he or she may be taking.* It is **mandatory** that each prescriber has this information before prescribing additional drugs.

DRUGS AND THE ELDERLY

Advancing age brings changes that can alter how you react to medicines. An impaired digestive system may interfere with drug absorption. Declines in liver and kidney ability to metabolize and remove drugs may lead to toxic drug levels. We slowly lose the ability to maintain "steady state" (or homeostasis), and face increased sensitivity of many tissues to the actions of drugs, even in "normal" drug doses. If aging causes a decline in understanding, memory, vision, or coordination, these patients may not always use drugs safely and effectively. Adverse reactions to drugs occur three times more frequently in the older population. An unwanted drug response can change an independent older person into a confused or helpless patient. For these reasons, drug treatment in the elderly must **always** be accompanied by the most careful consideration of the individual health and tolerances. Once-daily dosing may be the only viable option.

Guidelines for the Use of Drugs by the Elderly

- Be certain that drug treatment is necessary. Many health problems of the elderly can be managed **without** the use of drugs.
- Avoid (if possible) the use of many drugs at one time.
- Dosing schedules should be as simple as possible. Once a medicine is selected, ask your doctor if a once- or twice-a-day formulation is available and appropriate.
- Treatment with most drugs is often best started by using less-than-standard doses. Maintenance doses should also be individualized and are often smaller for those over 60 years of age.
- Avoid large tablets and capsules if other dosage forms are available. Liquid forms are easier for the elderly or debilitated to swallow.
- Have all drug containers labeled with the drug name and directions for use in large, easy-to-read letters.
- Ask the pharmacist to package drugs in easy-to-open containers. Avoid childproof caps and stoppers.
- Do not take any drug in the dark. Identify each dose of medicine carefully in adequate light to be certain you are taking the intended drug.
- To avoid taking the wrong drug or an extra dose, do not routinely leave medicines on a bedside table. Drugs for emergency use, such as nitroglycerin, are an exception. It is best to have only one such drug at the bedside for use during the night.
- Drug use by older people may require supervision; watch constantly to ensure safe and effective use.
- Remember the adage: "Start low, go slow, and (when appropriate) learn to say no."

Drugs Best Avoided by the Elderly Because of Increased Possibility of Adverse Reactions

antacids (high sodium)*	diethylstilbestrol	oxyphenbutazone
barbiturates*	estrogens	phenacetin
benzodiazepines (long-acting)	indomethacin	phenylbutazone
cyclophosphamide	monoamine oxidase (MAO) inhibitors*	tetracyclines*

Drugs That Should Be Used by the Elderly in Reduced Dosages Until Full Effect Has Been Determined

anticoagulants (oral)*	colchicinecortisone-like drugs*	nalidixic acid
antidepressants*		narcotic drugs
antidiabetic drugs*	digitalis preparations*	prazosin
antihistamines*	diuretics* (all types)	pseudoephedrine
antihypertensives*	ephedrine	quinidine
anti-inflammatory drugs*	epinephrine	sleep inducers (hypnotics)*
barbiturates*	haloperidol	terbutaline
beta-blockers*	isoetharine	thyroid preparations

Drugs That May Cause Confusion and Behavioral Disturbances in the Elderly

acyclovir
albuterol
amantadine
anticholinergics*
antidepressants*
antidiabetic drugs*
antihistamines*
anti-inflammatory drugs*
asparaginaseatropine*
  (and drugs containing
  belladonna)
barbiturates*
benzodiazepines*
beta-blockers*

bromocriptine
carbamazepine
cimetidine
digitalis preparations*
diuretics*
ergoloid mesylates
famotidine
haloperidol
levodopa
meprobamate
methocarbamol
methyldopa
narcotic drugs
nizatidine

pentazocine
phenytoin
primidone
quinidine
ranitidine
reserpine
sedatives
sleep inducers
  (hypnotics)*
thiothixene
tranquilizers (mild)*
trihexyphenidyl

Drugs That May Cause Orthostatic Hypotension in the Elderly

antidepressants*
antihypertensives*
diuretics* (all types)

neuroleptics*
phenothiazines*
sedatives

selegiline
tranquilizers (mild)*
vasodilators*

Drugs That May Cause Sluggishness, Unsteadiness, and Falling in the Elderly

barbiturates*
beta-blockers*
chlordiazepoxide
clorazepate

diazepam
diphenhydramine
flurazepam
halazepam

methyldopa
prazepam
sleep inducers
  (hypnotics)*

Drugs That May Cause Constipation and/or Retention of Urine in the Elderly

acebutolol
amantadine
amiodarone
androgens
anticholinergics*
antidepressants*
anti-parkinsonism drugs*
atropinelike drugs*

calcium
cholestyramine
epinephrine
ergoloid mesylates
famotidine
iron (some forms)
isoetharine
ketorolac

metoclopramide
narcotic drugs
phenothiazines*
ranitidine
sucralfate
terbutaline

Drugs That May Cause Loss of Bladder Control (Urinary Incontinence) in the Elderly

diuretics* (all types)
sedatives
sleep inducers
  (hypnotics)*

tacrine
thioridazine

tranquilizers (mild)*

*See Section Four: Drug Classes.

THERAPEUTIC DRUG MONITORING
Measuring Drug Levels in Blood

The ability to accurately measure how much medicine is in your blood has evolved since the early 1970s. People vary greatly in nature and degree of their responses to drugs, and blood levels can help find the best dose. For many drugs, the clinical response clearly shows that the drug is working as intended. However, for some drugs—especially those with narrow safety margins—toxic reactions may closely resemble the symptoms being treated. In many cases, the patient's expected response is not in keeping with his or her clinical condition. By measuring blood levels at appropriate times, the physician or clinical pharmacist can adjust dosing schedules more accurately, reduce the risk of toxicity, and achieve the best results or outcomes.

Some medications require both a peak and trough level to ensure best results, and timing of blood sampling is critical. Sampling should be avoided during the two hours after an oral dose because during this absorption period, blood levels do not represent tissue levels of the drug, and the tissue is where many medicines actually work. The peak, or highest, level of the drug can measure several things: how effectively bacteria are killed or toxic levels within the body, for instance. The trough, or lowest, level tells how effectively a medicine is cleared from the body between doses. This can also be important because if too much drug remains toxicity can result, and if too little, it may not work well.

The following drugs are those most suitable for therapeutic drug monitoring. If you are using any of these on a regular basis, ask your doctor about checking blood levels. These numbers are ranges where effects are *usually* seen, but people react differently. Therapeutic ranges listed are not absolute fixed levels where lack of effect or toxicity definitely occur. Some have a therapeutic response at a level lower than the low end of the range. Generally in this case, the level should be followed closely and left alone. A blood level higher than the high end of the range is not always toxic, but is a level higher than desirable, and dosing changes should be made. Fortunately most physicians "treat the patient, not the level."

Generic Name/Brand Name	*Blood Level Range*
acetaminophen/Tylenol, etc.	10–20 mcg/ml
amikacin/Amikin	12–25 mcg/ml (peak)
	5–10 mcg/ml (trough)
amitriptyline/Elavil, etc.	120–250 ng/ml
(combined with nortriptyline)	
amoxapine/Asendin	200–500 ng/ml
aspirin (other salicylates)	100–250 mcg/ml
carbamazepine/Tegretol	5–10 mcg/ml
chloramphenicol/Chloromycetin	10–25 mcg/ml
chlorpromazine/Thorazine	50–300 ng/ml

Generic Name/Brand Name	Blood Level Range
ciprofloxacin/Cipro	0.94–3.4 mcg/ml
clonazepam/Klonopin	10–50 ng/ml
cyclosporine/Sandimmune	100–150 ng/ml
desipramine/Norpramin, Pertofrane	150–300 ng/ml
digitoxin/Crystodigin	15–30 ng/ml
digoxin/Lanoxin	0.5–2.0 ng/ml
diltiazem/Cardizem	100–200 ng/ml
disopyramide/Norpace	2.0–4.5 mcg/ml
doxepin/Adapin, Sinequan	100–275 ng/ml
ethosuximide/Zarontin	40–100 mcg/ml
flecainide/Tambocor	0.2–1.0 mcg/ml
flucytosine/Ancobon	50–100 mcg/ml
gentamicin/Garamycin	4–10 mcg/ml (peak)
	less than 2 mcg/ml (trough)
gold salts/Auranofin, etc.	1–2.0 mcg/ml
imipramine/Janimine, Tofranil, etc.	150–300 ng/ml
kanamycin/Kantrex	25–35 mcg/ml
lidocaine/Xylocaine, etc.	2–5 mcg/ml
lithium/Lithobid, Lithotabs, etc.	0.3–1.3 MEq/L
mephobarbital/Mebaral	1–7 mcg/ml
methotrexate/Mexate	up to 0.1 mcmol/L
methsuximide/Celontin	up to 1 mcg/ml
metoprolol/Lopressor	20–200 ng/ml
mexiletine/Mexitil	0.75–2.0 mcg/ml
nifedipine/Procardia	25–100 ng/ml
nortriptyline/Aventyl, Pamelor	50–150 ng/ml
combined with amitriptyline	125–250 ng/ml
phenobarbital/Luminal, etc.	10–25 mcg/ml
phenytoin/Dilantin	10–20 mcg/ml
primidone/Mysoline	6–12 mcg/ml
procainamide/Pronestyl	4–10 mcg/ml
(NAPA metabolite)	4–10 mcg/ml
propranolol/Inderal	50–100 ng/ml
protriptyline/Vivactil	70–250 ng/ml
quinidine/Quinaglute, etc.	1–4 mcg/ml
(specific to quinidine test method)	
sulfadiazine/Microsulfon	100–120 mcg/ml
sulfamethoxazole/Gantanol	90–100 mcg/ml
theophylline/Aminophylline, etc.	10–20 mcg/ml
thioridazine/Mellaril	50–300 ng/ml
tobramycin/Nebcin	4–10 mcg/ml (peak)
	less than 2 mcg/ml (trough)
tocainide/Tonocard	5–12 mcg/ml
trimethadione/Tridione	10–30 mcg/ml
trimethoprim/Proloprim	1–3 mcg/ml
valproic acid/Depakene	50–100 mcg/ml
vancomycin/Vancocin	30–40 mcg/ml (peak)
	5–10 mcg/ml (trough)
verapamil/Calan	50–200 ng/ml

3

True Breakthroughs in Medicines

Advances are being made in medicines. This section tells you about some of the best medicines that have recently been FDA approved, identifies novel treatment approaches, and gives truly new uses of existing medicines. I want to distinguish here between the "me too" products (that may simply be an existing drug with minor chemical changes) and forward-looking advances. This section can help make certain you are getting the latest treatment.

ADHERENCE (COMPLIANCE) PROGRAMS

The best medicine in the world will not do you any good at all if it stays in the bottle. I have had many consults asking me why a given medicine failed to help a particular patient, only to find out that the medicine itself was being incorrectly taken. Programs that encourage and explain exactly how much and when to take medicines help people get the best results from any medicine.

The American Heart Association has some excellent brochures that can be helpful. (You can reach them at 1-800-553-6321.)

ALENDRONATE (FOSAMAX)

This bisphosphonate was featured in last year's "True Breakthroughs" section, and has since gained FDA approval for **prevention** of post-menopausal osteoporosis. It is always better to prevent a disease or condition than to have to treat it.

AMAP, JCAHCO AND NCQA ALLIANCE

It is one thing to say that results or outcomes must be improved in our health care system, and quite a task to actually measure what is being

21

done. A landmark collaboration between the Joint Commission on Accreditation of Health Care Organizations, the National Committee on Quality Assurance, and the American Medical Accreditation Program will seek to make sure that measurement programs work well and are useful in helping make health care decisions.

ANTI-LEUKOTRIENE DRUGS

Zafirlukast (Accolate) is a leukotriene receptor antagonist that blocks the action of leukotrienes. It belongs to a completely new type of chemical family and may be especially useful in mild to moderate asthma where patients are aspirin sensitive. Zileuton (Zyflo) is the latest anti-leukotriene to be approved, and prevents the formation of leukotrienes.

ASPIRIN

I include aspirin once again in this section, because the indications for using this very old medicine have been broadened. It appears to prevent first heart attacks, limit damage from heart attacks that happen, have a role in preventing strokes, and may also help prevent bowel cancer. Talk to your doctor to see if regular use of aspirin makes sense for you.

ATORVASTATIN CALCIUM (LIPITOR)

The newest HMG-CoA reductase inhibitor to be approved. This medicine is now the most potent drug in lowering LDL cholesterol. The added benefit that atorvastatin offers is that it also lowers triglyceride levels as well!

HMG-COA REDUCTASE INHIBITORS

Two medicines from this class have now been approved for PREVENTION of strokes. This means that in addition to preventing heart attacks, these medicines can also help prevent a widely suffered problem.

INFLIXIMAB (AVAKINE)

Tumor necrosis factor (TNF) is implicated in numerous conditions. Centocor received FDA approval for use of infliximab in treating Chron's disease. Since TNF is also involved in some aspects of arthritis and AIDS, it appears that this newly approved medicine will have broader applications than its original approval.

LYME DISEASE VACCINE

This is the first vaccine to be FDA approved to PREVENT Lyme disease. The Smith Kline Beecham product (LYMErix) is the first of two vaccines that are pending approval.

PROTEASE INHIBITORS

I include this class (see *Protease Inhibitors*) again this year because more than any other medicines in the history of the AIDS epidemic, the protease inhibitors have offered the prospect (as combination therapy with other HIV medicines) of making HIV infection a long-term, survivable disease.

REPAGLINIDE (PRANDIN)

Meglitinides are a new class of medicines to fight diabetes. This drug is the first to be FDA approved, and offers a new chemical entity.

SLIDENAFIL (VIAGRA)

This drug has sparked more interest than any other medicine since the FDA started approving medicines. Presently, it offers hope to many men who have faced injections or implants in the past. The full story on interactions with other medicines is still unfolding. I've included a broad group of possible interacting medicines for you in the new profile.

DRUG PROFILES

Drugs Reviewed
in This Section

Included are detailed Drug Profiles of **more than 2,000 brands** and 300 drugs of major importance. The criteria are that the medicine:

1. is used to treat or prevent a prevalent, relatively serious or significant disease or disorder;

2. is recognized by experts to be among the "best choices" in its class;

3. has a current benefit-to-risk ratio that compares favorably with those in its class;

4. requires special information and guidance for both the health care practitioner (physician, dentist, pharmacist, nurse) and the consumer (patient and family) for safe and effective use;

5. is suitable (safe and practical) for use in an outpatient setting (home, work site, school, etc.). It can be self-administered, or may require dosing by trained medical personnel (as with home intravenous therapy, or freestanding cancer, emergency, or pain centers).

ACARBOSE (a KAR boz)

Introduced: 1996   **Class:** Antidiabetes agent, oral; alpha glucosidase inhibitor   **Prescription:** USA: Yes   **Controlled Drug:** USA: No; Canada: No   **Available as Generic:** No
Brand Name: Precose

BENEFITS versus RISKS	
Possible Benefits	*Possible Risks*
EFFECTIVE LOWERING OF BLOOD SUGAR	Gas and abdominal pain (often decreases over time)
DECREASED RISK OF HIGH BLOOD PRESSURE, HEART DISEASE, OR OTHER LONG-TERM DAMAGE OF HIGH BLOOD SUGAR (WITH BETTER CONTROL)	Mild decreases in hematocrit (was only seen in clinical trials)
COMBINED TREATMENT WITH SULFONYLUREA IF NEEDED	

▷ **Principal Uses**

As a Single Drug Product: Uses currently included in FDA-approved labeling: (1) Used with diet in diabetics who don't require insulin, yet don't have good blood sugar control with diet alone; (2) can be combined with a sulfonylurea (see Drug Classes) if diet plus acarbose or diet and sulfonylurea do not control blood sugar as well as needed.

Other (unlabeled) generally accepted uses: None at present.

How This Drug Works: By blocking the enzymes intestinal alpha glucosidase and pancreatic alpha amylase, this medicine impairs sugar digestion, and actually keeps sugar low after meals.

Available Dosage Forms and Strengths

Tablets — 25 mg, 50 mg, 100 mg

▷ **Recommended Dosage Ranges:** (Actual dose and schedule must be determined individually for each patient.)

Infants and Children: Safety and effectiveness not established in those less than 18 years old.

18 to 65 Years of Age: To start—25 mg three times daily, taken at the start of each meal (after first bite). Dose increases are made at 4 to 8 week intervals to achieve blood sugar control while minimizing intestinal side effects (using 50 mg three times daily at the start of each meal). If response is not acceptable, patients weighing more than 132 pounds (60 kg) may be given doses up to 100 mg three times daily. Those weighing less than 60 kg should NOT be given be given more than 50 mg three times daily. If a dose increase doesn't give better sugar control, consider dose decrease.

Over 65 Years of Age: No specific recommendations unless kidney function is very limited.

Conditions Requiring Dosing Adjustments

Liver Function: Specific dosing changes do not appear to be needed.

Kidney Function: Increases in drug blood levels occur. Dose decreases may be needed.

Specific guidelines not available. Only about 2% is usually absorbed.

▷ **Dosing Instructions:**   Take this pill after starting breakfast, lunch, and dinner—after the first bite of a meal has been eaten. Gas (flatulence) or diarrhea are common side effects, but often decrease over time. Limiting sucrose can also help.

If dose changes are made at 4- to 8-week intervals, the best sugar response and the least potential gas (flatulence) or diarrhea are realized. Often blood sugar is checked one hour after a meal (one hour postprandial) and the dose adjusted to get the best balance of blood sugar and side effects.

Usual Duration of Use: Dosing must be individualized. Peak drug response happens in about an hour. Dosing changes are made at 4 to 8-week intervals if needed. Regular use required to give better blood glucose control. Since noninsulin-dependent diabetes is a chronic condition, use of acarbose will be ongoing. Periodic hemoglobin A1C (glycosylated hemoglobin) tests and physician follow-up are needed. Keeping the sugar close to normal can minimize diabetic problems.

Possible Advantages of This Drug

May be used in combination with sulfonylurea oral hypoglycemics (see Drug Classes) to get the best control of blood sugar. Uses a different (novel) mechanism than other oral hypoglycemic drugs.

▷ **This Drug Should Not Be Taken If**

- you have had an allergic reaction to it previously.
- you are in diabetic ketoacidosis.
- your history includes intestinal obstruction or you have a partial obstruction of the intestine.
- you have inflammatory bowel disease or colon ulceration.
- serum creatinine is over 2 mg/dl (talk to your doctor).
- you have cirrhosis of the liver.
- you have an intestinal condition that may worsen (such as a megacolon or bowel obstruction) if increased gas (flatus) forms.
- you have a long-standing (chronic) intestinal disease altering digestion or your ability to absorb materials from the intestine.
- you are pregnant or are breast-feeding your infant (no data exists on use in pregnancy or breast-feeding).

▷ **Inform Your Physician Before Taking This Drug If**

- you do not know what the symptoms of hypoglycemia are.
- you have a history of kidney or liver disease.
- you will have surgery with general anesthesia.
- you forgot to tell your doctor about all drugs you take.
- you are unsure of how much to take or how often to take acarbose.

▷ **Possible Side Effects** (natural, expected, and unavoidable drug actions)

Gas (flatulence) or diarrhea (results from bacterial action on sugars), and tends to decrease over time.

▷ **Possible Adverse Effects** (unusual, unexpected, and infrequent reactions)

If any of the following develop, consult your physician promptly for guidance.

Mild Adverse Effects
    Allergic reactions: skin rash, itching.
    Sleepiness, headache, dizziness—of questionable causation.
    Pain or swelling of the belly (abdomen)—frequent.
    Gas (flatulence) or diarrhea—frequent (often eases).
    Increased liver enzymes—case reports—probably dose related.
Serious Adverse Effects
    Low blood sugar if combined with sulfonylureas—possible.
    Anemia—rare and occurred in some studies and not in others.
    Ileus—case reports and in those with prior bowel blockage history.
▷ **Possible Effects on Sexual Function:**   None reported.

Possible Effects on Laboratory Tests
    Hemoglobin A1C: trending more toward normal (good effect).
    Blood sugar one hour after eating (postprandial): decreased.
    Serum lipids: variable effect.
    Liver enzymes: increased (in up to 15% of people).

CAUTION
    1. This medicine itself does not cause hypoglycemia. Low sugar may result
       if combined with insulin or sulfonylureas.
    2. Infections may cause loss of sugar control and require temporary insulin
       use.
    3. This medicine is part of the total management of diabetes. A properly pre-
       scribed diet and regular exercise are still required for best control of
       blood sugar.
    4. If your kidneys fail or worsen, tell your doctor. This drug should not be
       used if serum creatinine is greater than 2 mg/dl.

Precautions for Use
    By Infants and Children: Safety and effectiveness for those under 18 not estab-
       lished.
    By Those Over 60 Years of Age: Specific recommendations are not made at this
       time.
▷ **Advisability of Use During Pregnancy**
    Pregnancy Category: B. See Pregnancy Risk Categories at the back of this
       book.
    Animal studies: No significant increase in birth defects in rats or rabbits.
    Human studies: Adequate studies of pregnant women are not available.
    Insulin is often the drug of first choice for blood sugar control in pregnancy.
       Ask your doctor for help.

Advisability of Use If Breast-Feeding
    Presence of this drug in breast milk: Yes, in rats. No human data available.
    Avoid drug or refrain from nursing.

Habit-Forming Potential: None.

Effects of Overdose: Temporary gas (flatus), abdominal discomfort and diar-
       rhea.

Possible Effects of Long-Term Use: Beneficial effects on blood sugar.

Suggested Periodic Examinations While Taking This Drug (at physician's dis-
       cretion)
    Periodic blood sugar tests one hour after eating. Hemoglobin A1C levels. Liver

function tests (transaminases)—every 3 months during first year of treatment and then periodically. Serum iron or iron-binding capacity prudent if anemia develops.

▷ **While Taking This Drug, Observe the Following**

Foods: Closely follow the diet your doctor has prescribed. Blood sugar control can help avoid or delay diabetes problems!

Beverages: No restrictions. May be taken with milk.

▷ *Alcohol:* No interaction with acarbose. If you also take a sulfonylurea (see Drug Classes), alcohol can exaggerate lowering of blood sugar or cause a disulfiramlike (see glossary) reaction.

Tobacco Smoking: No interactions expected, but I advise everyone to stop smoking.

▷ *Other Drugs*

Acarbose may *increase* the effects of
- sulfonylureas (see Drug Classes), causing too low blood sugars (not an acarbose effect). This may be used for therapeutic benefit.
- warfarin (Coumadin)—INR testing more often is advisable.

Acarbose *taken concurrently* with
- clofibrate (Atromid-S) may result in hypoglycemia.
- digestive enzyme products that contain amylase or lipase may result in loss of blood sugar control.
- digoxin (Lanoxin) may cause lower (subtherapeutic) blood levels of digoxin and loss of benefits (one case report).
- disopyramide (Norpace) may result in hypoglycemia.
- high-dose aspirin or other salicylates and some NSAIDs (nonsteroidal anti-inflammatory drugs; see Drug Classes) may result in hypoglycemia.
- insulin (see Profile) increases risk of low blood sugar.
- sulfonamide antibiotics (see Drug Classes) may pose an increased risk for low blood sugar (hypoglycemia).

The following drugs may *decrease* the effects of acarbose:
- adrenocortical steroids (see Drug Classes).
- beta-blockers (see Drug Classes).
- calcium channel blockers (see Drug Classes).
- furosemide (Lasix) and bumetanide (Bumex).
- isoniazid (INH).
- monoamine oxidase (MAO) inhibitors (see Drug Classes)
- nicotinic acid.
- phenytoin (Dilantin).
- rifampin (Rifadin, others).
- theophylline (Theo-Dur, others).
- thiazide diuretics (see Drug Classes).
- thyroid hormones (see Drug Classes).

▷ *Driving, Hazardous Activities:* Use caution until degree of drowsiness you may experience is known.

Aviation Note: Diabetes *is a disqualification* for piloting. Consult a designated aviation medical examiner.

Exposure to Sun: No restrictions.

Heavy Exercise or Exertion: Caution advised because this drug lowers peak in blood sugar after meals. Talk over dosing changes with your doctor.

Occurrence of Unrelated Illness: Illness can change blood sugar control. Temporary use of insulin may be **required**.

Discontinuation: **Never** stop acarbose before calling your doctor.

ACEBUTOLOL (a se BYU toh lohl)

Introduced: 1973   **Class:** Antihypertensive, heart rhythm regulator, beta-adrenergic blocker   **Prescription:** USA: Yes   **Controlled Drug:** USA: No; Canada: No   **Available as Generic:** Yes

Brand Names: Sectral, ✤Monitan, ✤Rhotral

BENEFITS versus RISKS	
Possible Benefits	*Possible Risks*
EFFECTIVE ANTIHYPERTENSIVE (mild-moderate high pressure)	CONGESTIVE HEART FAILURE in advanced heart disease
MAY DECREASE DEATHS OCCURRING AFTER A HEART ATTACK	Masking of low blood sugar (hypoglycemia) in diabetics
LONG-TERM USE CAN DECREASE DEATH AND HEART PROBLEMS	Rare lupus erythematosus syndrome

▷ **Principal Uses**

As a Single Drug Product: Uses currently included in FDA-approved labeling: (1) Treats mild to moderate high blood pressure alone or in combination; (2) used to prevent premature ventricular heartbeats.

Other (unlabeled) generally accepted uses: (1) Stabilizes angina pectoris; (2) used after a heart attack to help prolong life; (3) may have a role in easing the symptoms of panic attacks.

How This Drug Works: It blocks sympathetic nervous system effects and slows the rate and force of the heart, reducing the extent of blood vessel contraction, expanding the walls and lowering blood pressure. Also slows nerve impulse speed through the heart, which helps ease some heart rhythm disorders.

Available Dosage Forms and Strengths

Capsules — 100 mg (in Canada), 200 mg, 400 mg

▷ **Recommended Dosage Ranges:** (Actual dose and schedule must be determined for each patient individually.)

Infants and Children: Not indicated.

18 to 65 Years of Age: High blood pressure: 200 mg a day works for some, but most require 400 to 800 mg a day, rarely 1,200. Heart selectivity decreases as doses increase.

Arrhythmias: 400 mg daily, as 200 mg taken morning and evening (12 hours apart). Increased as needed and tolerated. Total dose should not exceed 1200 mg every 24 hours (600 mg twice a day.)

Angina: 600 to 1600 mg are divided into two or three equal doses spaced 8 to 12 hours apart.

Over 65 Years of Age: Bioavailability (amount taken into your body) doubles. Lower ongoing doses are needed. 800 mg a day **maximum**.

Conditions Requiring Dosing Adjustments

Liver Function: Used with caution in compromised liver function.

Kidney Function: Dose must be decreased by up to 75% in severe kidney failure.

▷ **Dosing Instructions:** May be taken without regard to eating. Capsule may be opened when taken. NEVER stop this drug abruptly.

Usual Duration of Use: Use on a regular schedule for 5 to 10 days may be required to see peak benefits in lowering blood pressure or stopping premature heartbeats. Long-term use determined by sustained benefit and response to a combined program (weight decrease, salt restriction, smoking cessation, etc.).

Possible Advantages of This Drug

Slows the heart less than most other beta-blocker drugs, and low doses are less likely to cause asthma in asthmatics.

▷ **This Drug Should Not Be Taken If**
- you have had an allergic reaction to it previously.
- you are in heart failure (overt).
- you have a severely slow (bradycardia) heart rate or serious heart block (second or third degree).
- you are taking, or took in the past 14 days, any monoamine oxidase (MAO) type A inhibitor drug (see Drug Classes).

▷ **Inform Your Physician Before Taking This Drug If**
- you have had an adverse reaction to any beta-blocker (see Drug Classes).
- you have serious heart disease or episodes of heart failure (this drug may aggravate it).
- you have hay fever (allergic rhinitis), asthma, chronic bronchitis, or emphysema.
- you have an overactive thyroid function (hyperthyroidism).
- you have problems with circulation to your arms and legs (peripheral vascular disease or intermittent claudication).
- you have a history of low blood sugar (hypoglycemia).
- you have impaired liver or kidney function.
- you have diabetes or myasthenia gravis.
- you take digitalis, quinidine, or reserpine, or any calcium blocker (see Drug Classes).
- you will have surgery with general anesthesia.
- you do not know how much to take or how often to take acebutolol.
- you have not asked if the dose was adjusted for age-related kidney decline or kidney disease.

Possible Side Effects (natural, expected, and unavoidable drug actions)

Lethargy and fatigability, cold extremities—rare; slow heart rate, lightheadedness in upright position (see ***orthostatic hypotension*** in Glossary)—possible.

▷ **Possible Adverse Effects** (unusual, unexpected, and infrequent reactions)

If any of the following develop, consult your physician promptly for guidance.

Mild Adverse Effects

Allergic reactions: skin rash, itching.

Fatigue—frequent.

Headache, dizziness, insomnia, fatigue, or abnormal dreams—infrequent.

Indigestion, nausea, constipation, diarrhea—infrequent.

Decreased tearing with long-term use—case reports.

Increased frequency and painful or nighttime urination—infrequent.

Joint and muscle discomfort, fluid retention (edema)—infrequent.

Serious Adverse Effects

Allergic reactions may be more severe or less responsive.

Mental depression or low blood sugar—rare.

Liver toxicity—case reports.

Chest pain, shortness of breath, precipitation of congestive heart failure—rare.

Bronchial asthma attack (in people with asthma)—possible.

Positive ANA and lupus erythematosus—infrequent to frequent, up to 33%.

▷ **Possible Effects on Sexual Function:** Impotence, decreased libido, Peyronie's disease (see Glossary)—case reports.

Possible Effects on Laboratory Tests

Antinuclear antibodies (ANA) and LE cells: often positive after 3 to 6 months. Free fatty acids (FFA): decreased.

Glucose tolerance test (GTT): decreased; abnormal tests at 60 and 120 minutes.

Potassium: mild increases.

CAUTION

1. ***Do not stop this drug suddenly*** without the knowledge of and help from your physician. Carry a note that says that you take this drug.
2. Nasal decongestants may cause sudden and SEVERE increases in blood pressure. Call your physician or pharmacist before using nasal decongestants and ask if they should ever be used.
3. Report the any tendency to emotional depression.
4. This medicine may worsen preexisting kidney insufficiency.

Precautions for Use

By Infants and Children: Safety and effectiveness for those under 12 years not established. If this drug is used, watch for fainting as a sign of low blood sugar (hypoglycemia) if a meal is skipped.

By Those Over 60 Years of Age: All antihypertensive drugs should be used ***cautiously***. High blood pressure should be lowered slowly, avoiding the risks (such as stroke or heart attack) of excessively low blood pressure. Small doses and frequent blood pressure checks needed. Total daily dose should not exceed 800 mg. Watch for dizziness, falling, confusion, hallucinations, depression, or frequent urination.

▷ **Advisability of Use During Pregnancy**

Pregnancy Category: B. See Pregnancy Risk Categories at the back of this book.

Animal studies: No significant increase in birth defects in rats or rabbits.

Human studies: Adequate studies of pregnant women are not available.

Use this drug only if clearly needed. Ask your doctor for help.

Advisability of Use If Breast-Feeding

Presence of this drug in breast milk: Yes, and concentrated.

Avoid drug or refrain from nursing.

Habit-Forming Potential: None.

Effects of Overdose: Weakness, slow pulse, low blood pressure, fainting, cold and sweaty skin, congestive heart failure, possible coma, and convulsions.

Possible Effects of Long-Term Use: Decreased heart reserve and heart failure in some people with advanced heart disease.

Suggested Periodic Examinations While Taking This Drug (at physician's discretion)
Blood pressure checks, heart and liver function tests.

▷ **While Taking This Drug, Observe the Following**
Foods: No restrictions. Avoid excessive salt intake. Ginseng may increase blood pressure.
Beverages: No restrictions. May be taken with milk.
▷ *Alcohol:* Alcohol may exaggerate lowering of blood pressure and may increase its mild sedative effect.
Tobacco Smoking: Nicotine may reduce this drug's effectiveness and can worsen closing of bronchial tubes seen in regular smokers. I advise everyone to quit smoking.
▷ *Other Drugs*
Acebutolol may *increase* the effects of
- other antihypertensive drugs and excessively lower the blood pressure. Dose adjustments may be necessary.
- reserpine (Ser-Ap-Es, etc.) and cause sedation, depression, slow heart rate, and low blood pressure.
Acebutolol *taken concurrently* with
- amiodarone (Cordarone) may result in severe slowing of the heart leading to sinus arrest. Use with great caution.
- calcium channel blockers such as mibefradil (Posicor) or verapamil (Calan) may lead to increased risk of abnormal heart rate or rhythm.
- clonidine (Catapres) may cause rebound high blood pressure if clonidine is withdrawn while acebutolol is still being taken.
- digoxin (Lanoxin) may change heart conduction.
- diltiazem (Cardizem) may result in increased acebutolol effects.
- fluoxetine (Prozac), fluvoxamine (Luvox), paroxetine (Paxil), or venlafaxine (Effexor) may decrease the rate or removal of acebutolol from the body (not reported as yet). Caution is advised.
- insulin may cause low blood sugar (hypoglycemia).
- NSAIDs (nonsteroidal anti-inflammatory drugs; see Drug Classes) may result in decreased lowering of blood pressure.
- oral antidiabetic drugs (see Drug Classes) may result in slow recovery from low blood sugar.
- ritonavir (Norvir) and perhaps other protease inhibitors may increase the metabolism of this medicine and blunt therapeutic benefits of acebutolol.
- The following drugs may *decrease* the effects of acebutolol:
- indomethacin (Indocin) and some other "aspirin substitutes" (NSAIDs) can blunt acebutolol's antihypertensive effect.
▷ *Driving, Hazardous Activities:* Use caution—may cause drowsiness.
Aviation Note: The use of this drug *is a disqualification* for piloting. Consult a designated aviation medical examiner.
Exposure to Sun: No restrictions.

Exposure to Heat: Hot environments can exaggerate the effects of this drug.

Exposure to Cold: Elderly need to prevent hypothermia (see Glossary).

Heavy Exercise or Exertion: This drug can intensify increased blood pressure (hypertensive) response to isometric exercise. Talk to your doctor about how much and how to exercise.

Occurrence of Unrelated Illness: Fevers can lower blood pressure and require decreased doses. Nausea or vomiting may interrupt the dosing schedule. Ask your doctor for help.

Discontinuation: **DO NOT** stop the drug suddenly. Dose decreases over 2-3 weeks are recommended. Ask your doctor for help.

ACETAZOLAMIDE (a set a ZOHL a mide)

Introduced: 1953   **Class:** Anticonvulsant, antiglaucoma, diuretic, sulfon-amides   **Prescription:** USA: Yes   **Controlled Drug:** USA: No; Canada: No   **Available as Generic:** USA: Yes; Canada: No

Brand Names: ✦Acetazolam, Ak-Zol, ✦Apo-Acetazolamide, Dazamide, Diamox, Diamox Sustained release, Diamox Sequels, Storzolamide, Novo-zolamide

BENEFITS versus RISKS	
Possible Benefits	*Possible Risks*
REDUCTION OF INTERNAL EYE PRESSURE in some glaucoma cases	Rare bone marrow, liver, or kidney injury
CONTROL OF ABSENCE (PETIT MAL) SEIZURES	Acidosis with long-term use—possible
	Increased risk of kidney stones
TREATMENT OF PERIODIC PARALYSIS	Tingling in the arms and legs (paresthesia)
REDUCES FLUID IN CONGESTIVE HEART FAILURE OR DRUG-INDUCED EDEMA	Paralysis—rare
	Bone weakening (with long-term use)—possible
PREVENTION OR LESSENING OF SYMPTOMS OF ACUTE MOUNTAIN SICKNESS	

▷ **Principal Uses**

As a Single Drug Product: Uses currently included in FDA-approved labeling: (1) Treatment of some kinds of glaucoma—especially in combination drugs; (2) used with other drugs to manage petit mal epilepsy; (3) treats familial periodic paralysis and prevents altitude (acute mountain) sickness; (4) used as a test showing blood flow (cerebrovascular reserve) patients have in their brains; (5) used to correct metabolic problems (acid–base) in people with chronic obstructive pulmonary disease (COPD).

Other (unlabeled) generally accepted uses: (1) Taken by mouth to help prevent uric acid kidney stones from recurring; (2) given intravenously to increase removal of some drug overdoses; (3) helps patients on ventilators by correcting chemical imbalances.

How This Drug Works: By blocking carbonic anhydrase enzyme, it slows fluid formation (the aqueous humor) in the eye and increases urine amount. It causes fluid loss by increasing elimination of bicarbonate (a basic chemical), potassium, sodium, and water.

Author's note: This profile has been shortened to make room for more widely used medicines.

ACETIC ACIDS
(Nonsteroidal Anti-Inflammatory Drug Family)

Diclofenac (di KLOH fen ak)   **Etodolac** (e TOE doh lak)   **Indomethacin** (in doh METH a sin)   **Ketorolac** (KEY tor o lak)   **Nabumetone** (na BYU me tohn) **Sulindac** (sul IN dak)   **Tolmetin** (TOHL met in)

Introduced: 1976, 1986, 1963, 1991, 1984, 1976, 1976, respectively
Class: NSAID, mild analgesic   **Prescription:** USA: Yes   **Controlled Drug:** USA: No; Canada: No   **Available as Generic:** USA: Yes: indomethacin, sulindac, tolmetin; Canada: No

Brand Names: Indomethacin: ✦Apo-Indomethacin, Indameth, ✦Indocid, ✦Indocid-SR, ✦Indocid PDA, Indocin, Indocin-SR, ✦Novomethacin, ✦Nu-Indo, Zendole; Diclofenac: ✦Apo-Diclo, Arthrotec [CD], Cataflam, ✦Novo-Difenac, ✦Nu-Diclo, Voltaren, Voltaren SR, Voltaren Ophthalmic; Etodolac: Lodine, Lodine XL; Ketorolac: Toradol, Acular (ketorolac ophthalmic); Nabumetone: Relafen; Sulindac: ✦Apo-Sulin, Clinoril, ✦Novo-Sundac; Tolmetin: Tolectin, Tolectin DS, Tolectin 600

BENEFITS versus RISKS	
Possible Benefits	*Possible Risks*
EFFECTIVE RELIEF OF MILD TO MODERATE PAIN AND INFLAMMATION	Gastrointestinal pain, ulceration, bleeding
	Liver or kidney damage
Easy change from the IM or IV form to the oral form (ketorolac)	Fluid retention
	Bone marrow depression
Decreased stomach (GI) problems (etodolac)	Pneumonitis (sulindac)
	Aseptic meningitis (diclofenac)
	Possible severe skin reactions (diclofenac, etodolac, ketorolac, and sulindac)

▷ **Principal Uses**

As a Single Drug Product: Uses currently included in FDA-approved labeling: (1) All of the drugs in this class except ketorolac are approved to treat osteoarthritis; (2) all of the drugs in this class except ketorolac and etodolac are approved to relieve rheumatoid arthritis; (3) etodolac and ketorolac are used to treat mild to moderate pain; (4) diclofenac and sulindac are useful in ankylosing spondylitis; (5) sustained-release form of indomethacin as well as the immediate-release form of sulindac help symptoms of tendonitis, bursitis, and acute painful shoulder; (6) tolmetin eases symptoms of juvenile rheumatoid arthritis; (7) sulindac therapy is useful in acute gout; (8) ophthalmic form of diclofenac is useful after cataract surgery and refractive surgery of the cornea (decreasing pain and sensitivity to light; (9) ketorolac is approved (ophthalmic form) for use in decreasing pain and sensitivity to light (photophobia) after refractive surgery.

Other (unlabeled) generally accepted uses: (1) Diclofenac used intramuscularly is effective in acute migraine headache and kidney colic; (2) indomethacin helps reduce systemic reactions in kidney transplants, and addresses low-grade neonatal intraventricular hemorrhage; (3) ketorolac has been helpful in reducing swelling after cataract surgery and treating reflex sympathetic dystrophy by injection; (4) sulindac is effective in treating colon polyps (Gardner's syndrome) and easing diabetic neuropathic pain.

How These Drugs Work: These drugs reduce prostaglandins (and related compounds), chemicals that cause inflammation and pain.

Available Dosage Forms and Strengths

Indomethacin:

Capsules — 25 mg, 50 mg, 75 mg
Gelatin capsule (Canada) — 25 mg, 50 mg
Capsules, SR (prolonged action) — 75 mg
Oral suspension — 25 mg/5 ml
Suppositories — 50 mg, 100 mg

Diclofenac sodium:

Suppositories — 50 mg, 100 mg (Canada)
Tablets — 25 mg, 50 mg
Tablets, prolonged action — 50 mg, 75 mg, 100 mg (Canada)
Ophthalmic solution — 1 mg/1 ml

Etodolac:

Capsules — 200 mg, 300 mg
Tablets, extended-release form— 400 mg, 600 mg

Ketorolac:

Tablets — 10 mg
Ophthalmic solution — 3 ml, 5 ml and 10 ml (0.5%)
Injection — 15 mg, 30 mg

Nabumetone:

Tablets — 500 mg, 750 mg

Sulindac:

Tablets — 150 mg, 200 mg

Tolmetin:

Capsules — 400 mg, 492 mg
Gelatin capsules — 400 mg (Canada)
Tablets — 200 mg, 600 mg

▷ **Usual Adult Dosage Range:** Indomethacin: For arthritis and related conditions: 25 to 50 mg two to four times daily. If needed and tolerated, dose may be increased by 25 or 50 mg per day at intervals of 1 week. For acute gout: 100 mg initially; then 50 mg three times per day until pain is relieved. Maximum daily dose is 200 mg.

SR form: 75 mg daily for ankylosing spondylitis or rheumatoid arthritis.

Diclofenac potassium: Maximum daily dose is 200 mg.

Diclofenac sodium: 100 to 200 mg daily to start in two to five divided doses. Reduction to the minimum effective dose is advisable. Maximum daily dose is 225 mg.

Etodolac: For osteoarthritis: A starting dose of 800 to 1200 mg is given in divided doses. The lowest effective dose is advisable, and effective treatment has been accomplished with 200 to 400 mg daily.

Etodolac is available in an extended release form (Lodine XL), which allows once-a-day dosing for many patients. Dosing range is 400 to 1000 mg daily. Maximum dose is 1000 mg daily.

Ketorolac: 10 mg is used every 4 to 6 hours for short-term treatment of pain. Maximum daily dose is 40 mg orally. Ophthalmic dosing: one drop 4 times daily for allergic conjunctivitis.

Nabumetone: 1000 mg daily as a single dose is given. Dose is increased as needed and tolerated to 1500 mg daily. The lowest effective daily dose is advisable. Maximum daily dose is 2000 mg.

Sulindac: Therapy is started with 150 to 200 mg twice daily taken 12 hours apart. Maximum daily dose is 400 mg.

Tolmetin: 400 mg three times daily is started, with usual ongoing doses of 600 to 1600 mg as needed and tolerated. Total daily dose should not exceed 1600 mg for osteoarthritis or 2000 mg for rheumatoid arthritis.

Children 2 years of age or older may be given 20 mg per kg of body mass orally, divided into three or four doses daily. The dose may be increased as needed and tolerated to a maximum daily dose of 30 mg per kg of body mass.

Note: Actual dose and dosing schedule must be determined for each patient individually.

Conditions Requiring Dosing Adjustments

Liver Function: These drugs are extensively metabolized in the liver. They should be used with caution in patients with liver compromise.

Kidney Function: All nonsteroidal anti-inflammatory drugs may inhibit prostaglandins and alter kidney blood flow in patients with kidney (renal) compromise. Use with caution or not at all in patients with kidney compromise.

▷ **Dosing Instructions:**   Take with or following food to prevent stomach irritation. Take with a full glass of water and remain upright (do not lie down) for 30 minutes. Regular-release tablets may be crushed, but not extended-release forms. The regular capsules may be opened, but not the prolonged-action capsules. Food actually increases absorption of nabumetone. Ketorolac ophthalmic should NOT be used while soft contacts are worn.

Usual Duration of Use: Continual use on a regular schedule for 1 to 2 weeks is usually necessary to determine drug benefit in relieving arthritic discomfort. The usual length of treatment for bursitis or tendonitis for indomethacin or sulindac is 7 to 14 days. Ketorolac oral or IV is used for short-term pain treatment (5 days only), while ophthalmic dosing is open ended. Long-term use of the other agents in this class requires physician supervision and periodic evaluation.

These Drugs Should Not Be Taken If

- you have had an allergic reaction to them previously.
- you are subject to asthma or nasal polyps caused by aspirin.
- you are pregnant (all NSAIDs during the last 3 months of pregnancy) or you are breast-feeding.
- you have active peptic ulcer disease or any form of gastrointestinal ulceration or bleeding.

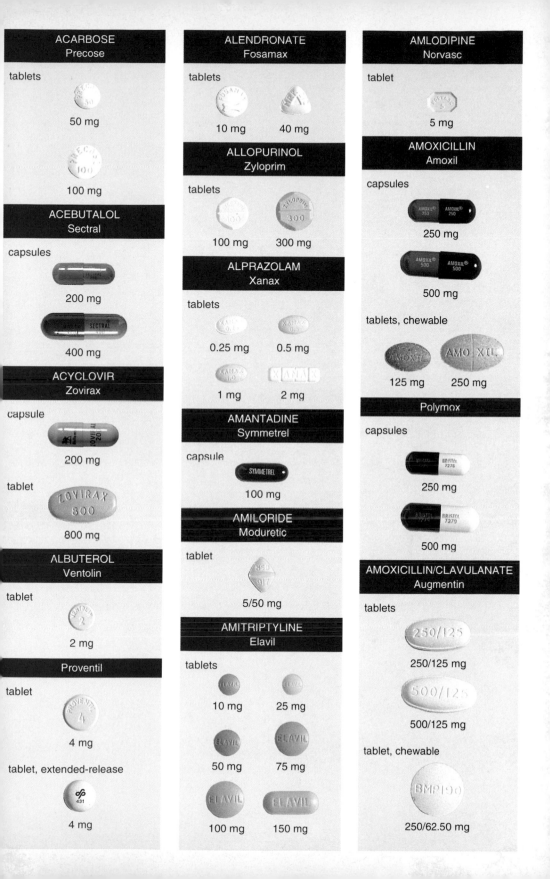

ACARBOSE
Precose

tablets

50 mg

100 mg

ACEBUTALOL
Sectral

capsules

200 mg

400 mg

ACYCLOVIR
Zovirax

capsule

200 mg

tablet

ZOVIRAX 800

800 mg

ALBUTEROL
Ventolin

tablet

2 mg

Proventil

tablet

4 mg

tablet, extended-release

4 mg

ALENDRONATE
Fosamax

tablets

10 mg   40 mg

ALLOPURINOL
Zyloprim

tablets

100 mg   300 mg

ALPRAZOLAM
Xanax

tablets

0.25 mg   0.5 mg

1 mg   2 mg

AMANTADINE
Symmetrel

capsule

SYMMETREL

100 mg

AMILORIDE
Moduretic

tablet

5/50 mg

AMITRIPTYLINE
Elavil

tablets

10 mg   25 mg

50 mg   75 mg

100 mg   150 mg

AMLODIPINE
Norvasc

tablet

5 mg

AMOXICILLIN
Amoxil

capsules

250 mg

500 mg

tablets, chewable

125 mg   250 mg

Polymox

capsules

250 mg

500 mg

AMOXICILLIN/CLAVULANATE
Augmentin

tablets

250/125 mg

500/125 mg

tablet, chewable

250/62.50 mg

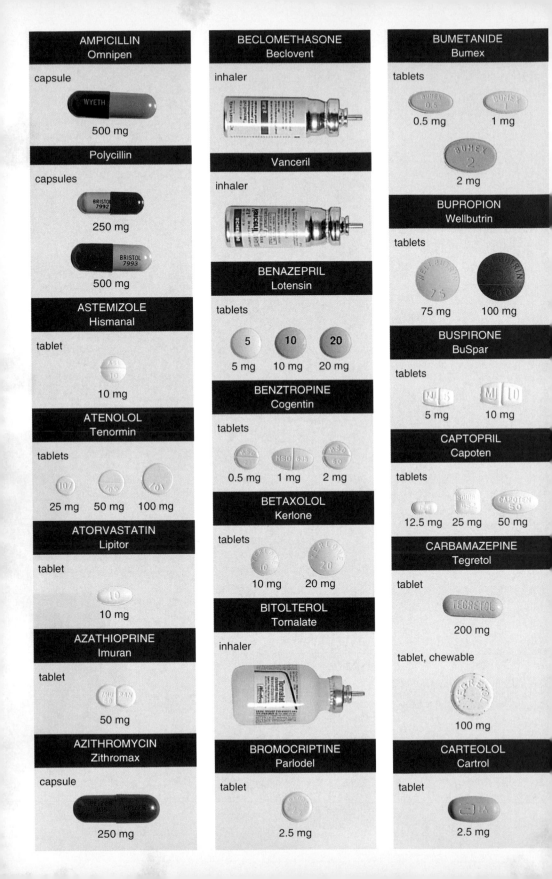

AMPICILLIN
Omnipen
capsule

500 mg

Polycillin
capsules

250 mg

500 mg

ASTEMIZOLE
Hismanal
tablet

10 mg

ATENOLOL
Tenormin
tablets

25 mg 50 mg 100 mg

ATORVASTATIN
Lipitor
tablet

10 mg

AZATHIOPRINE
Imuran
tablet

50 mg

AZITHROMYCIN
Zithromax
capsule

250 mg

BECLOMETHASONE
Beclovent
inhaler

Vanceril
inhaler

BENAZEPRIL
Lotensin
tablets

5 10 20

5 mg 10 mg 20 mg

BENZTROPINE
Cogentin
tablets

0.5 mg 1 mg 2 mg

BETAXOLOL
Kerlone
tablets

10 mg 20 mg

BITOLTEROL
Tornalate
inhaler

BROMOCRIPTINE
Parlodel
tablet

2.5 mg

BUMETANIDE
Bumex
tablets

0.5 mg 1 mg

2 mg

BUPROPION
Wellbutrin
tablets

75 mg 100 mg

BUSPIRONE
BuSpar
tablets

5 mg 10 mg

CAPTOPRIL
Capoten
tablets

12.5 mg 25 mg 50 mg

CARBAMAZEPINE
Tegretol
tablet

200 mg

tablet, chewable

100 mg

CARTEOLOL
Cartrol
tablet

2.5 mg

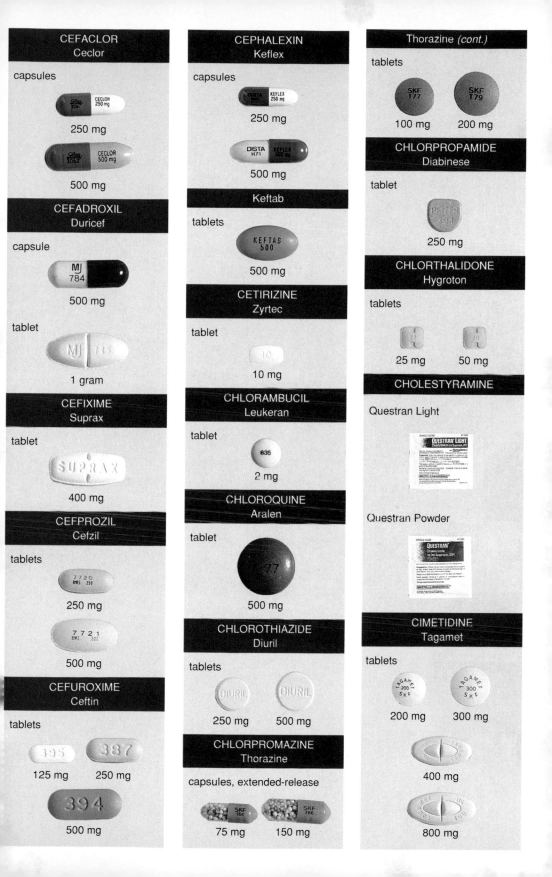

CEFACLOR
Ceclor

capsules

250 mg

500 mg

CEFADROXIL
Duricef

capsule

MJ 784

500 mg

tablet

MJ 785

1 gram

CEFIXIME
Suprax

tablet

SUPRAX

400 mg

CEFPROZIL
Cefzil

tablets

7720 BMS 250

250 mg

7721 BMS 500

500 mg

CEFUROXIME
Ceftin

tablets

395

125 mg

387

250 mg

394

500 mg

CEPHALEXIN
Keflex

capsules

DISTA H69 / KEFLEX 250 mg

250 mg

DISTA H71 / KEFLEX 500 mg

500 mg

Keftab

tablets

KEFTAB 500

500 mg

CETIRIZINE
Zyrtec

tablet

10

10 mg

CHLORAMBUCIL
Leukeran

tablet

635

2 mg

CHLOROQUINE
Aralen

tablet

177

500 mg

CHLOROTHIAZIDE
Diuril

tablets

DIURIL

250 mg

DIURIL

500 mg

CHLORPROMAZINE
Thorazine

capsules, extended-release

SKF T64

75 mg

SKF T66

150 mg

Thorazine *(cont.)*

tablets

SKF T77

100 mg

SKF T79

200 mg

CHLORPROPAMIDE
Diabinese

tablet

PFIZER 394

250 mg

CHLORTHALIDONE
Hygroton

tablets

25

25 mg

20

50 mg

CHOLESTYRAMINE

Questran Light

QUESTRAN LIGHT

Questran Powder

QUESTRAN POWDER

CIMETIDINE
Tagamet

tablets

TAGAMET 200 SKF

200 mg

TAGAMET 300 SKF

300 mg

400 mg

800 mg

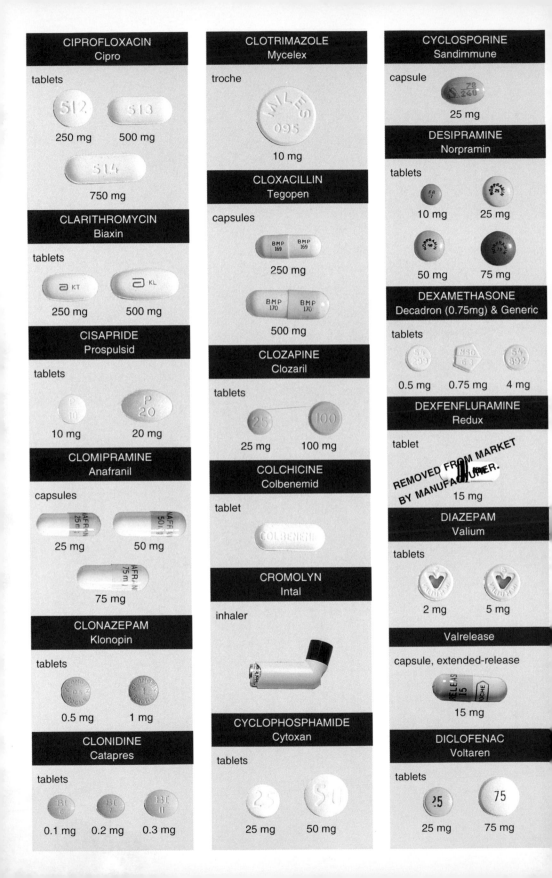

CIPROFLOXACIN
Cipro

tablets

512 — 250 mg
513 — 500 mg
514 — 750 mg

CLARITHROMYCIN
Biaxin

tablets

KT — 250 mg
KL — 500 mg

CISAPRIDE
Prospulsid

tablets

P 10 — 10 mg
P 20 — 20 mg

CLOMIPRAMINE
Anafranil

capsules

ANAFRANIL 25 — 25 mg
ANAFRANIL 50 — 50 mg
ANAFRANIL 75 — 75 mg

CLONAZEPAM
Klonopin

tablets

KLONOPIN 0.5 — 0.5 mg
KLONOPIN 1 — 1 mg

CLONIDINE
Catapres

tablets

BI 6 — 0.1 mg
BI 7 — 0.2 mg
BI 11 — 0.3 mg

CLOTRIMAZOLE
Mycelex

troche

MILES 095 — 10 mg

CLOXACILLIN
Tegopen

capsules

BMP 169 — 250 mg
BMP 170 — 500 mg

CLOZAPINE
Clozaril

tablets

25 — 25 mg
100 — 100 mg

COLCHICINE
Colbenemid

tablet

COLBENEMID

CROMOLYN
Intal

inhaler

CYCLOPHOSPHAMIDE
Cytoxan

tablets

25 — 25 mg
50 — 50 mg

CYCLOSPORINE
Sandimmune

capsule

78 240 — 25 mg

DESIPRAMINE
Norpramin

tablets

68 7 — 10 mg
NORPRAMIN — 25 mg
NORPRAMIN — 50 mg
NORPRAMIN — 75 mg

DEXAMETHASONE
Decadron (0.75mg) & Generic

tablets

54 299 — 0.5 mg
MSD 63 — 0.75 mg
54 892 — 4 mg

DEXFENFLURAMINE
Redux

tablet

REMOVED FROM MARKET BY MANUFACTURER.

15 mg

DIAZEPAM
Valium

tablets

2 — 2 mg
5 — 5 mg

Valrelease

capsule, extended-release

RELEASE 15 / ROCHE — 15 mg

DICLOFENAC
Voltaren

tablets

25 — 25 mg
75 — 75 mg

DIDANOSINE
Videx

tablet

VIDEX BL

25 mg

DIFLUNISAL
Dolobid

tablets

DOLOBID   DOLOBID

250 mg   500 mg

DIGOXIN
Lanoxicaps

capsules

0.1 mg   0.2 mg

Lanoxin

tablets

0.125 mg   0.25 mg   0.5 mg

DILTIAZEM
Cardizem

tablets

17   17

30 mg   60 mg

90 mg

120 mg

Cardizem CD

capsules

cardizem 180 mg

180 mg

Cardizem CD
capsules *(cont.)*

240 mg

300 mg

Cardizem SR

capsules

cardizem 60   cardizem 90

60 mg   90 mg

120 mg

DIPHENHYDRAMINE
Benadryl

capsules

PD 471

25 mg   50 mg

DISOPYRAMIDE
Norpace

capsules

SEARLE 2754   NORPACE 100 MG.   SEARLE 2762   NORPACE 150 MG.

100 mg   150 mg

Norpace CR

capsules, extended-release

SEARLE 2732   RPACE CR 100 mg

100 mg

150 mg

DISULFIRAM
Antabuse

tablets

ANTABUSE 250   500 ANTABUSE

250 mg   500 mg

DONEPEZIL
Aricept

tablet

5

5 mg

DOXAZOSIN
Cardura

tablets

1 mg   2 mg

4 mg   8 mg

DOXEPIN
Sinequan

capsules

10 mg   25 mg

50 mg

DOXYCYCLINE
Zenith generic

tablet

3626

100 mg

ENALAPRIL
Vasotec

tablet

2.5 mg

ERGOTAMINE
Ergostat

tablet

2 mg

ERYTHROMYCIN
Ery-Tab

tablet, delayed-release

EH

333 mg

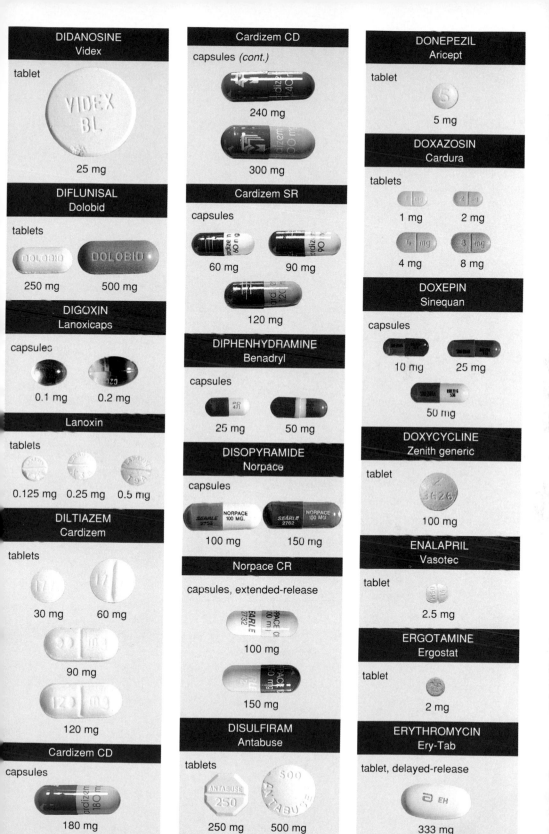

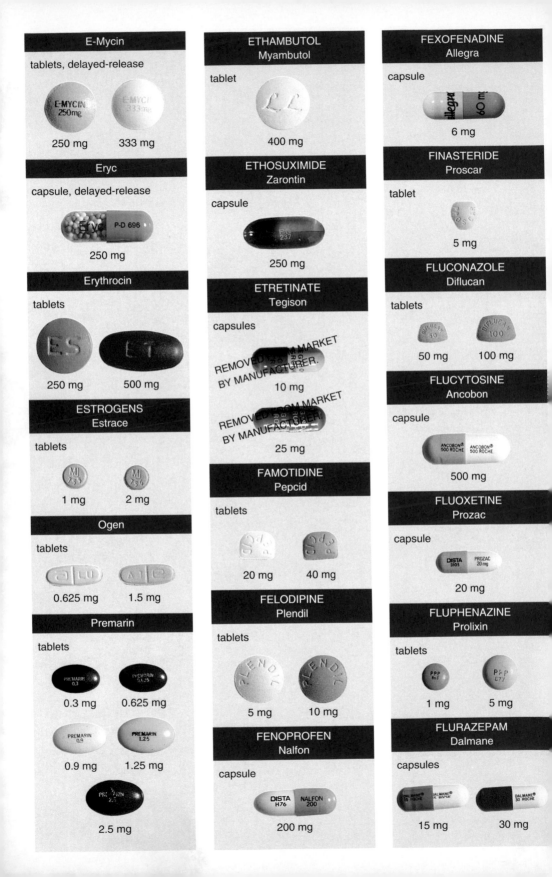

E-Mycin

tablets, delayed-release

250 mg 333 mg

Eryc

capsule, delayed-release

P-D 696

250 mg

Erythrocin

tablets

250 mg 500 mg

ESTROGENS
Estrace

tablets

1 mg 2 mg

Ogen

tablets

0.625 mg 1.5 mg

Premarin

tablets

0.3 mg 0.625 mg

0.9 mg 1.25 mg

2.5 mg

ETHAMBUTOL
Myambutol

tablet

400 mg

ETHOSUXIMIDE
Zarontin

capsule

250 mg

ETRETINATE
Tegison

capsules

REMOVED FROM MARKET BY MANUFACTURER.

10 mg

REMOVED FROM MARKET BY MANUFACTURER.

25 mg

FAMOTIDINE
Pepcid

tablets

20 mg 40 mg

FELODIPINE
Plendil

tablets

5 mg 10 mg

FENOPROFEN
Nalfon

capsule

DISTA H76 NALFON 200

200 mg

FEXOFENADINE
Allegra

capsule

6 mg

FINASTERIDE
Proscar

tablet

5 mg

FLUCONAZOLE
Diflucan

tablets

50 mg 100 mg

FLUCYTOSINE
Ancobon

capsule

ANCOBON 500 ROCHE ANCOBON 500 ROCHE

500 mg

FLUOXETINE
Prozac

capsule

DISTA 3105 PROZAC 20 mg

20 mg

FLUPHENAZINE
Prolixin

tablets

1 mg 5 mg

FLURAZEPAM
Dalmane

capsules

15 mg 30 mg

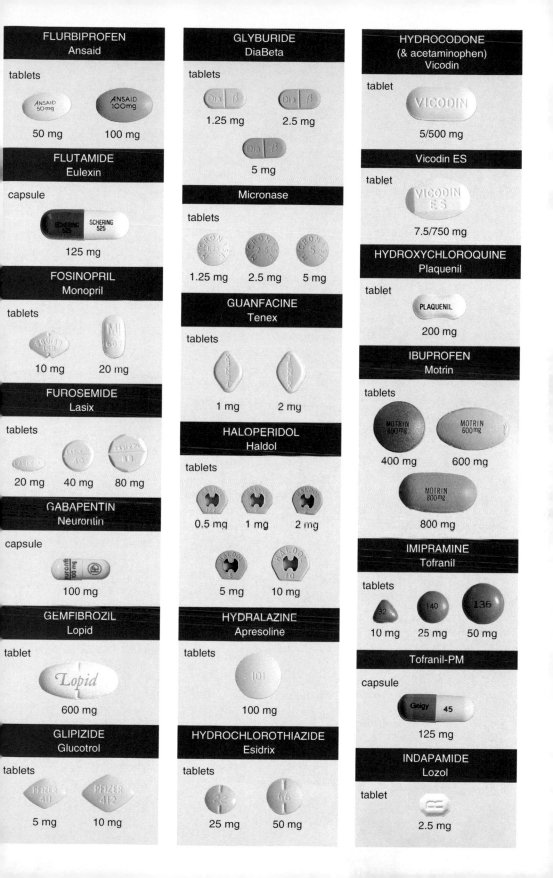

FLURBIPROFEN
Ansaid

tablets

ANSAID 50 mg — 50 mg
ANSAID 100mg — 100 mg

FLUTAMIDE
Eulexin

capsule

SCHERING 525 — 125 mg

FOSINOPRIL
Monopril

tablets

SQUIBB 158 — 10 mg
MI 609 — 20 mg

FUROSEMIDE
Lasix

tablets

LASIX 20 — 20 mg
LASIX 40 — 40 mg
LASIX 80 — 80 mg

GABAPENTIN
Neurontin

capsule

Neurontin 100 mg — 100 mg

GEMFIBROZIL
Lopid

tablet

Lopid — 600 mg

GLIPIZIDE
Glucotrol

tablets

PFIZER 401 — 5 mg
PFIZER 412 — 10 mg

GLYBURIDE
DiaBeta

tablets

Dia β — 1.25 mg
Dia β — 2.5 mg
Dia β — 5 mg

Micronase

tablets

MICRONASE 1.25 — 1.25 mg
MICRONASE 2.5 — 2.5 mg
MICRONASE 5 — 5 mg

GUANFACINE
Tenex

tablets

TENEX — 1 mg
TENEX — 2 mg

HALOPERIDOL
Haldol

tablets

HALDOL — 0.5 mg
HALDOL — 1 mg
HALDOL — 2 mg
HALDOL 5 — 5 mg
HALDOL 10 — 10 mg

HYDRALAZINE
Apresoline

tablets

101 — 100 mg

HYDROCHLOROTHIAZIDE
Esidrix

tablets

22 — 25 mg
46 — 50 mg

HYDROCODONE
(& acetaminophen)
Vicodin

tablet

VICODIN — 5/500 mg

Vicodin ES

tablet

VICODIN ES — 7.5/750 mg

HYDROXYCHLOROQUINE
Plaquenil

tablet

PLAQUENIL — 200 mg

IBUPROFEN
Motrin

tablets

MOTRIN 400mg — 400 mg
MOTRIN 600mg — 600 mg
MOTRIN 800mg — 800 mg

IMIPRAMINE
Tofranil

tablets

32 — 10 mg
140 — 25 mg
136 — 50 mg

Tofranil-PM

capsule

Geigy 45 — 125 mg

INDAPAMIDE
Lozol

tablet

2.5 mg

INDINAVIR
Crixivan

capsule

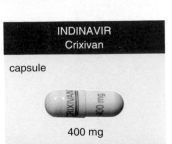

400 mg

INDOMETHACIN
Indocin

capsules

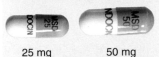

25 mg   50 mg

Indocin SR

capsule

75 mg

IODOQUINOL
Yodoxin

tablet

210 mg

ISONIAZID
INH

tablet

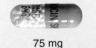

100 mg

ISOSORBIDE DINITRATE
Isordil

tablets

   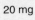

5 mg   10 mg   20 mg

30 mg   40 mg

Isordil *(cont.)*

tablet, extended-release

40 mg

tablet, sublingual

5 mg

ISOSORBIDE MONONITRATE
Ismo

tablet

20 mg

ISOTRETINOIN
Accutane

capsules

20 mg   40 mg

ISRADIPINE
DynaCirc

capsules

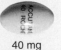

2.5 mg   5 mg

KETOCONAZOLE
Nizoral

tablet

200 mg

KETOPROFEN
Orudis

capsules

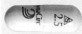

50 mg   75 mg

KETOROLAC
Toradol oral

tablet

10 mg

LABETALOL
Normodyne

tablets

100 mg   200 mg   300 mg

LATANOPROST
Xalatan

solution

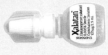

2.5 ml

LEVODOPA/CARBIDOPA
Sinemet

tablets

10/100 mg   25/100 mg

25/250 mg

Sinemet CR

tablet, sustained-release

50/200 mg

LEVOTHYROXINE
Synthroid

tablets

0.025 mg   0.05 mg   0.075 mg

0.1 mg   0.112 mg   0.125 mg

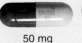

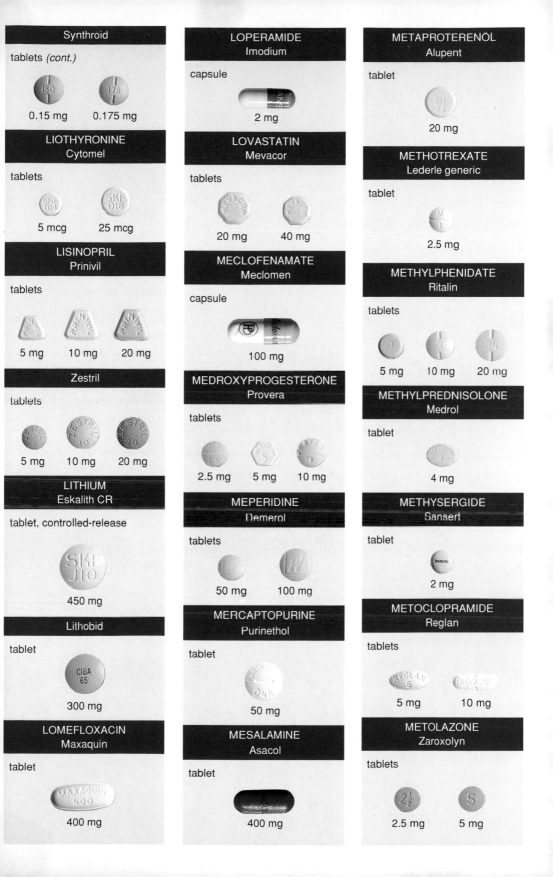

Synthroid
tablets *(cont.)*

0.15 mg   0.175 mg

LIOTHYRONINE
Cytomel
tablets

5 mcg   25 mcg

LISINOPRIL
Prinivil
tablets

5 mg   10 mg   20 mg

Zestril
tablets

5 mg   10 mg   20 mg

LITHIUM
Eskalith CR
tablet, controlled-release

450 mg

Lithobid
tablet

300 mg

LOMEFLOXACIN
Maxaquin
tablet

400 mg

LOPERAMIDE
Imodium
capsule

2 mg

LOVASTATIN
Mevacor
tablets

20 mg   40 mg

MECLOFENAMATE
Meclomen
capsule

100 mg

MEDROXYPROGESTERONE
Provera
tablets

2.5 mg   5 mg   10 mg

MEPERIDINE
Demerol
tablets

50 mg   100 mg

MERCAPTOPURINE
Purinethol
tablet

50 mg

MESALAMINE
Asacol
tablet

400 mg

METAPROTERENOL
Alupent
tablet

20 mg

METHOTREXATE
Lederle generic
tablet

2.5 mg

METHYLPHENIDATE
Ritalin
tablets

5 mg   10 mg   20 mg

METHYLPREDNISOLONE
Medrol
tablet

4 mg

METHYSERGIDE
Sansert
tablet

2 mg

METOCLOPRAMIDE
Reglan
tablets

5 mg   10 mg

METOLAZONE
Zaroxolyn
tablets

2.5 mg   5 mg

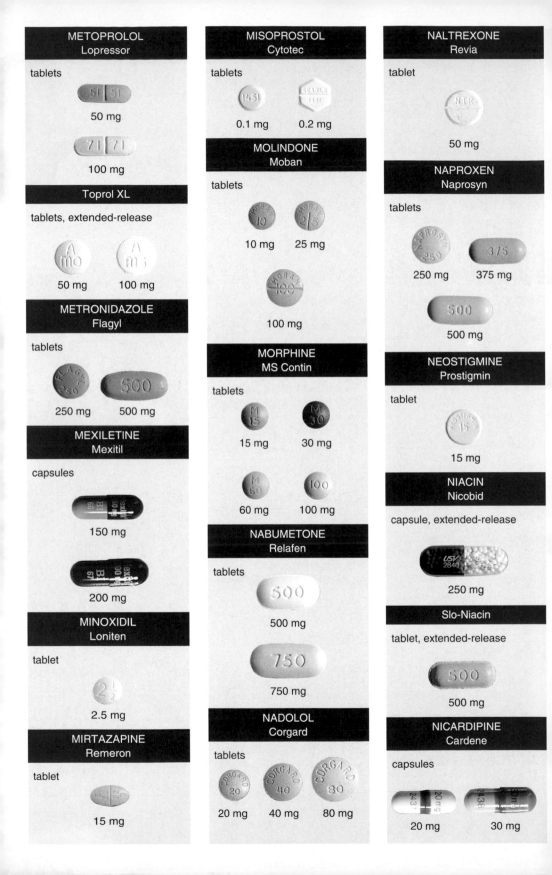

METOPROLOL
Lopressor

tablets

50 mg

100 mg

Toprol XL

tablets, extended-release

50 mg   100 mg

METRONIDAZOLE
Flagyl

tablets

250 mg   500 mg

MEXILETINE
Mexitil

capsules

150 mg

200 mg

MINOXIDIL
Loniten

tablet

2.5 mg

MIRTAZAPINE
Remeron

tablet

15 mg

MISOPROSTOL
Cytotec

tablets

0.1 mg   0.2 mg

MOLINDONE
Moban

tablets

10 mg   25 mg

100 mg

MORPHINE
MS Contin

tablets

15 mg   30 mg

60 mg   100 mg

NABUMETONE
Relafen

tablets

500 mg

750 mg

NADOLOL
Corgard

tablets

20 mg   40 mg   80 mg

NALTREXONE
Revia

tablet

50 mg

NAPROXEN
Naprosyn

tablets

250 mg   375 mg

500 mg

NEOSTIGMINE
Prostigmin

tablet

15 mg

NIACIN
Nicobid

capsule, extended-release

250 mg

Slo-Niacin

tablet, extended-release

500 mg

NICARDIPINE
Cardene

capsules

20 mg   30 mg

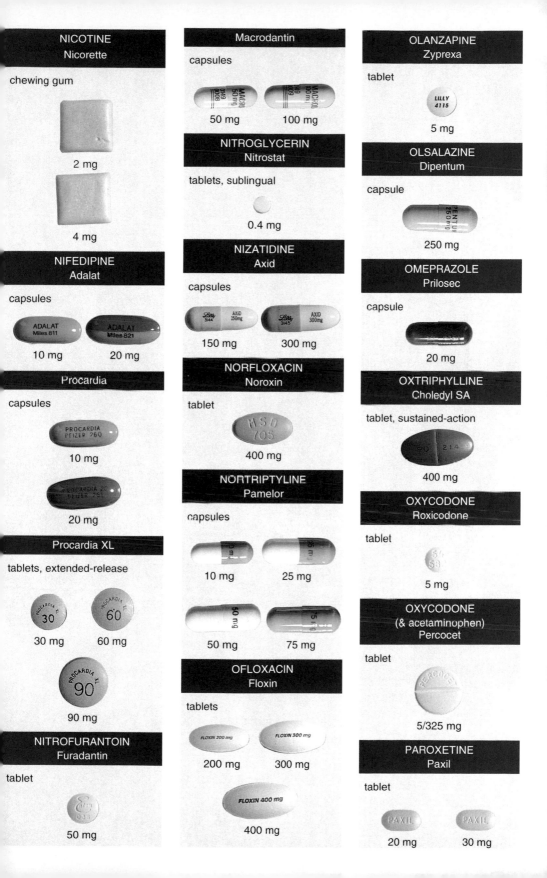

NICOTINE
Nicorette

chewing gum

2 mg

4 mg

NIFEDIPINE
Adalat

capsules

ADALAT Miles 811 — 10 mg

ADALAT Miles 821 — 20 mg

Procardia

capsules

PROCARDIA PFIZER 260 — 10 mg

PROCARDIA 20 PFIZER 751 — 20 mg

Procardia XL

tablets, extended-release

PROCARDIA XL 30 — 30 mg

PROCARDIA XL 60 — 60 mg

PROCARDIA XL 90 — 90 mg

NITROFURANTOIN
Furadantin

tablet

50 mg

Macrodantin

capsules

50 mg

100 mg

NITROGLYCERIN
Nitrostat

tablets, sublingual

0.4 mg

NIZATIDINE
Axid

capsules

Lilly 3144 — AXID 150mg — 150 mg

Lilly 3145 — AXID 300mg — 300 mg

NORFLOXACIN
Noroxin

tablet

MSD 705 — 400 mg

NORTRIPTYLINE
Pamelor

capsules

10 mg

25 mg

50 mg

75 mg

OFLOXACIN
Floxin

tablets

FLOXIN 200 mg — 200 mg

FLOXIN 300 mg — 300 mg

FLOXIN 400 mg — 400 mg

OLANZAPINE
Zyprexa

tablet

LILLY 4115 — 5 mg

OLSALAZINE
Dipentum

capsule

PENTUM 250 mg — 250 mg

OMEPRAZOLE
Prilosec

capsule

20 mg

OXTRIPHYLLINE
Choledyl SA

tablet, sustained-action

2 1 4 — 400 mg

OXYCODONE
Roxicodone

tablet

54 58 — 5 mg

OXYCODONE
(& acetaminophen)
Percocet

tablet

PERCOCET — 5/325 mg

PAROXETINE
Paxil

tablet

PAXIL — 20 mg

PAXIL — 30 mg

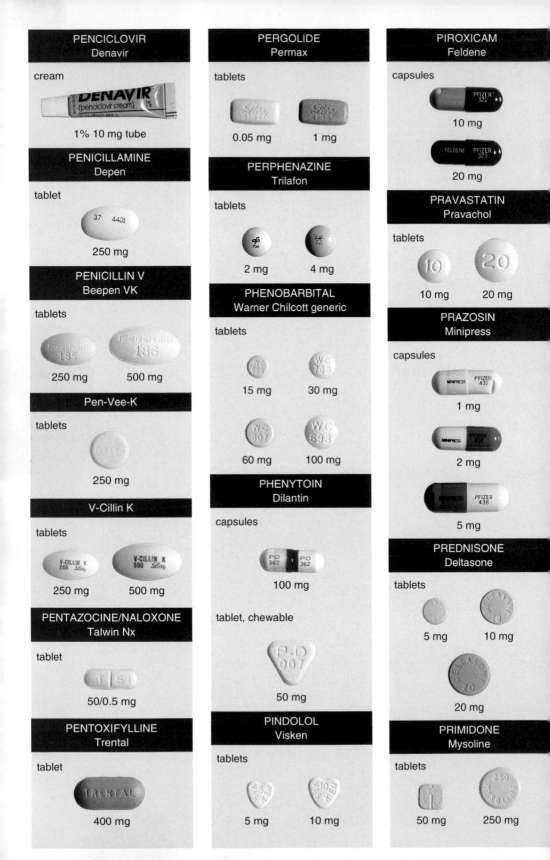

PENCICLOVIR
Denavir

cream

1% 10 mg tube

PENICILLAMINE
Depen

tablet

250 mg

PENICILLIN V
Beepen VK

tablets

250 mg   500 mg

Pen-Vee-K

tablets

250 mg

V-Cillin K

tablets

250 mg   500 mg

PENTAZOCINE/NALOXONE
Talwin Nx

tablet

50/0.5 mg

PENTOXIFYLLINE
Trental

tablet

400 mg

PERGOLIDE
Permax

tablets

0.05 mg   1 mg

PERPHENAZINE
Trilafon

tablets

2 mg   4 mg

PHENOBARBITAL
Warner Chilcott generic

tablets

15 mg   30 mg

60 mg   100 mg

PHENYTOIN
Dilantin

capsules

100 mg

tablet, chewable

50 mg

PINDOLOL
Visken

tablets

5 mg   10 mg

PIROXICAM
Feldene

capsules

10 mg

20 mg

PRAVASTATIN
Pravachol

tablets

10 mg   20 mg

PRAZOSIN
Minipress

capsules

1 mg

2 mg

5 mg

PREDNISONE
Deltasone

tablets

5 mg   10 mg

20 mg

PRIMIDONE
Mysoline

tablets

50 mg   250 mg

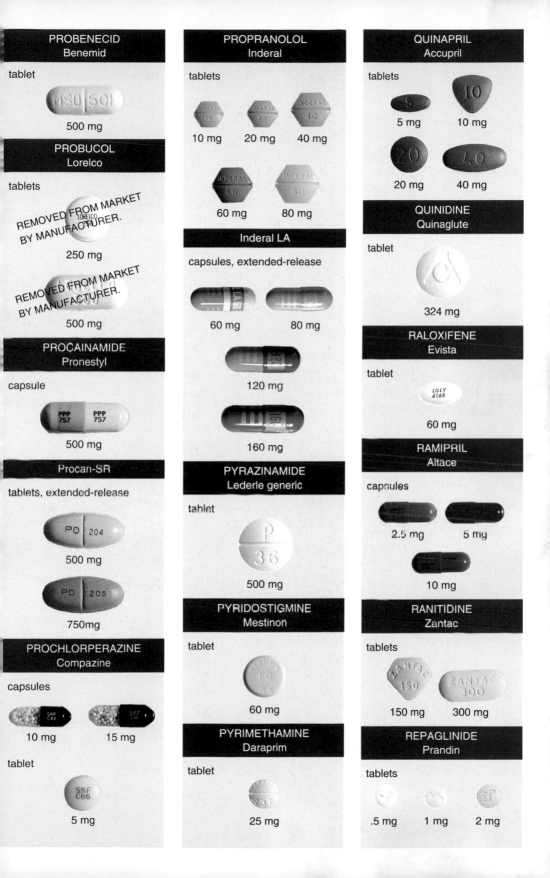

PROBENECID
Benemid

tablet

500 mg

PROBUCOL
Lorelco

tablets

REMOVED FROM MARKET BY MANUFACTURER.

250 mg

REMOVED FROM MARKET BY MANUFACTURER.

500 mg

PROCAINAMIDE
Pronestyl

capsule

PPP 757   PPP 757

500 mg

Procan-SR

tablets, extended-release

PD 204

500 mg

PD 205

750mg

PROCHLORPERAZINE
Compazine

capsules

SKF C44

10 mg

SKF C46

15 mg

tablet

SKF C66

5 mg

PROPRANOLOL
Inderal

tablets

INDERAL 10   INDERAL 20   INDERAL 40

10 mg   20 mg   40 mg

INDERAL 60   INDERAL 80

60 mg   80 mg

Inderal LA

capsules, extended-release

LA 60

60 mg   80 mg

120

120 mg

160

160 mg

PYRAZINAMIDE
Lederle generic

tablet

P 36

500 mg

PYRIDOSTIGMINE
Mestinon

tablet

MESTINON 60

60 mg

PYRIMETHAMINE
Daraprim

tablet

DARAPRIM A3A

25 mg

QUINAPRIL
Accupril

tablets

5

5 mg

10

10 mg

20

20 mg

40

40 mg

QUINIDINE
Quinaglute

tablet

324 mg

RALOXIFENE
Evista

tablet

LILLY 4165

60 mg

RAMIPRIL
Altace

capsules

2.5 mg   5 mg

10 mg

RANITIDINE
Zantac

tablets

ZANTAC 150

150 mg

ZANTAC 300

300 mg

REPAGLINIDE
Prandin

tablets

.5 mg   1 mg   2 mg

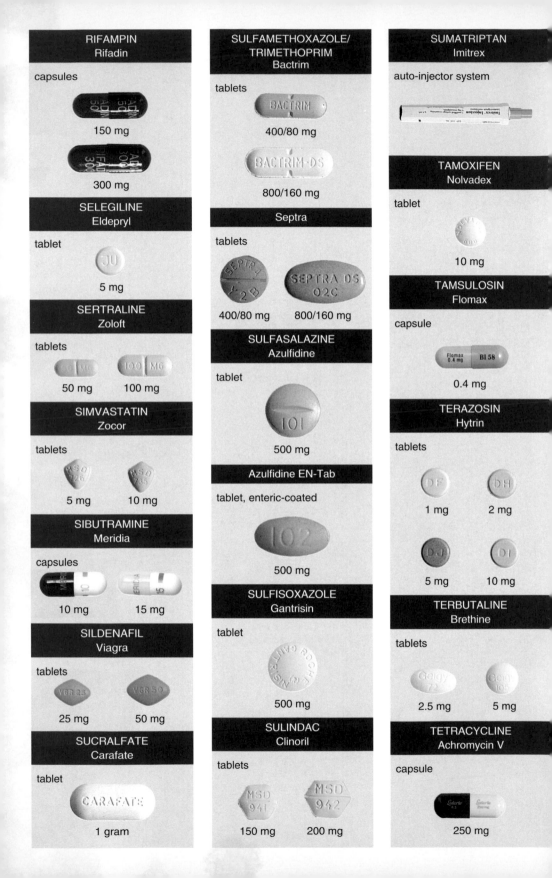

RIFAMPIN
Rifadin

capsules

150 mg

300 mg

SELEGILINE
Eldepryl

tablet

JU

5 mg

SERTRALINE
Zoloft

tablets

50 mg   100 mg

SIMVASTATIN
Zocor

tablets

5 mg   10 mg

SIBUTRAMINE
Meridia

capsules

10 mg   15 mg

SILDENAFIL
Viagra

tablets

25 mg   50 mg

SUCRALFATE
Carafate

tablet

CARAFATE

1 gram

SULFAMETHOXAZOLE/ TRIMETHOPRIM
Bactrim

tablets

400/80 mg

800/160 mg

Septra

tablets

400/80 mg   800/160 mg

SULFASALAZINE
Azulfidine

tablet

500 mg

Azulfidine EN-Tab

tablet, enteric-coated

500 mg

SULFISOXAZOLE
Gantrisin

tablet

500 mg

SULINDAC
Clinoril

tablets

150 mg   200 mg

SUMATRIPTAN
Imitrex

auto-injector system

TAMOXIFEN
Nolvadex

tablet

10 mg

TAMSULOSIN
Flomax

capsule

0.4 mg

TERAZOSIN
Hytrin

tablets

1 mg   2 mg

5 mg   10 mg

TERBUTALINE
Brethine

tablets

2.5 mg   5 mg

TETRACYCLINE
Achromycin V

capsule

250 mg

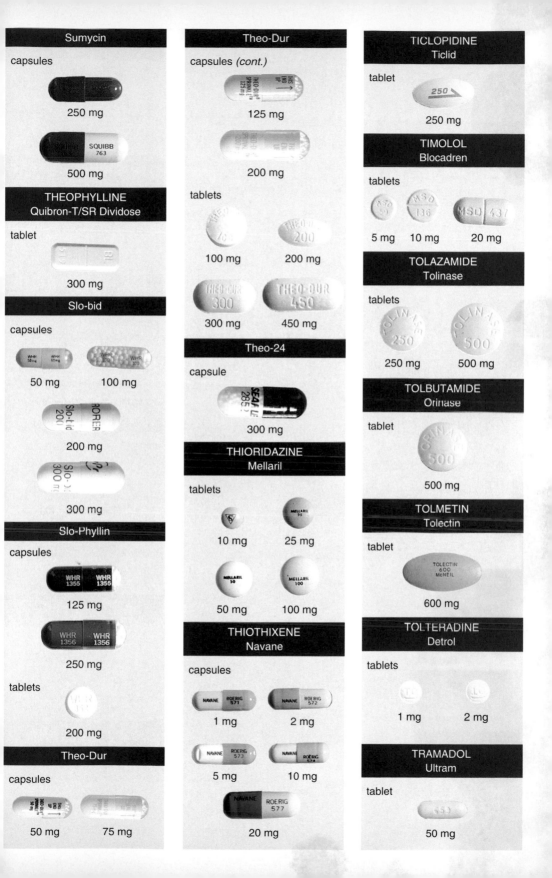

Sumycin

capsules

250 mg

500 mg

THEOPHYLLINE
Quibron-T/SR Dividose

tablet

300 mg

Slo-bid

capsules

50 mg   100 mg

200 mg

300 mg

Slo-Phyllin

capsules

125 mg

250 mg

tablets

200 mg

Theo-Dur

capsules

50 mg   75 mg

Theo-Dur

capsules (cont.)

125 mg

200 mg

tablets

100 mg   200 mg

300 mg   450 mg

Theo-24

capsule

300 mg

THIORIDAZINE
Mellaril

tablets

10 mg   25 mg

50 mg   100 mg

THIOTHIXENE
Navane

capsules

1 mg   2 mg

5 mg   10 mg

20 mg

TICLOPIDINE
Ticlid

tablet

250 mg

TIMOLOL
Blocadren

tablets

5 mg   10 mg   20 mg

TOLAZAMIDE
Tolinase

tablets

250 mg   500 mg

TOLBUTAMIDE
Orinase

tablet

500 mg

TOLMETIN
Tolectin

tablet

600 mg

TOLTERADINE
Detrol

tablets

1 mg   2 mg

TRAMADOL
Ultram

tablet

50 mg

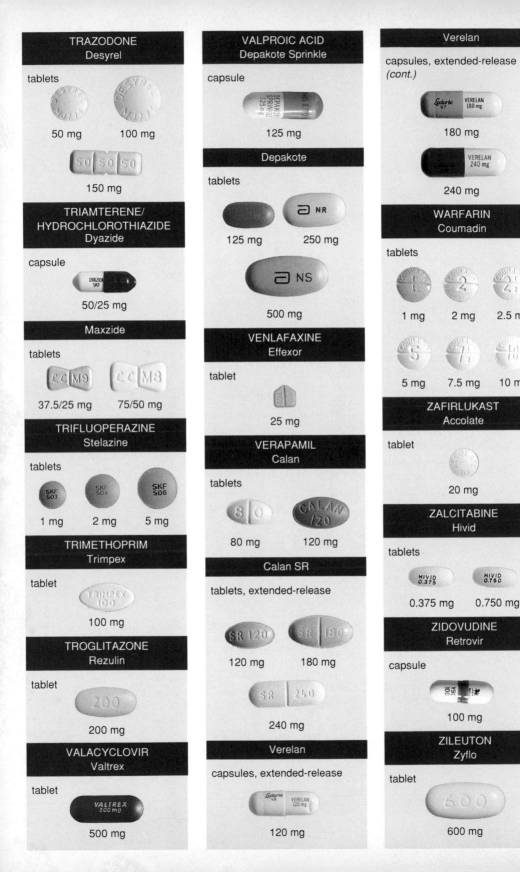

TRAZODONE
Desyrel

tablets

50 mg   100 mg

150 mg

TRIAMTERENE/ HYDROCHLOROTHIAZIDE
Dyazide

capsule

50/25 mg

Maxzide

tablets

37.5/25 mg   75/50 mg

TRIFLUOPERAZINE
Stelazine

tablets

1 mg   2 mg   5 mg

TRIMETHOPRIM
Trimpex

tablet

100 mg

TROGLITAZONE
Rezulin

tablet

200 mg

VALACYCLOVIR
Valtrex

tablet

500 mg

VALPROIC ACID
Depakote Sprinkle

capsule

125 mg

Depakote

tablets

125 mg   250 mg

500 mg

VENLAFAXINE
Effexor

tablet

25 mg

VERAPAMIL
Calan

tablets

80 mg   120 mg

Calan SR

tablets, extended-release

120 mg   180 mg

240 mg

Verelan

capsules, extended-release

120 mg

Verelan

capsules, extended-release
(cont.)

180 mg

240 mg

WARFARIN
Coumadin

tablets

1 mg   2 mg   2.5 mg

5 mg   7.5 mg   10 mg

ZAFIRLUKAST
Accolate

tablet

20 mg

ZALCITABINE
Hivid

tablets

0.375 mg   0.750 mg

ZIDOVUDINE
Retrovir

capsule

100 mg

ZILEUTON
Zyflo

tablet

600 mg

- you have active liver disease.
- you have a bleeding disorder or a blood cell disorder.
- you have severe impairment of kidney function.
- you have a history (indomethacin suppositories) of rectal bleeding or proctitis.
- you have porphyria (diclofenac, indomethacin).

▷ **Inform Your Physician Before Taking This Drug If**
- you are allergic to aspirin or to other aspirin substitutes.
- you have a history of peptic ulcer disease, Crohn's disease, ulcerative colitis, or any type of bleeding disorder.
- you have a history of epilepsy, Parkinson's disease, or mental illness (psychosis).
- you have impaired liver or kidney function.
- you have high blood pressure or a history of heart failure.
- you are taking acetaminophen, aspirin, or other aspirin substitutes or anticoagulants.

Possible Side Effects (natural, expected, and unavoidable drug actions)
Drowsiness, ringing in ears, fluid retention.

▷ **Possible Adverse Effects** (unusual, unexpected, and infrequent reactions)
If any of the following develop, consult your physician promptly for guidance.

Mild Adverse Effects
Allergic reactions: skin rash, hives, itching, localized swellings of face and/or extremities.
Headache—infrequent to frequent (indomethacin); dizziness, feelings of detachment—infrequent.
Mouth sores, indigestion, nausea, vomiting, diarrhea—infrequent.
Ringing in the ears—possible.
Temporary loss of hair (indomethacin)—case reports.

Serious Adverse Effects
Allergic reactions: worsening of asthma, difficult breathing, mouth irritation.
Blurred vision, confusion, depression—rare.
Active peptic ulcer, with or without bleeding—possible.
Liver damage with jaundice (see Glossary)—case reports.
Kidney damage with painful urination, bloody urine, reduced urine formation—rare.
Bone marrow depression (see Glossary): fatigue, fever, sore throat, bleeding, or bruising—case reports.
Severe skin rash (Stevens-Johnson syndrome—diclofenac, ketorolac, etodolac, sulindac)—case reports.
Fluid retention, increased blood pressure, or edema—possible with all.
Congestive heart failure (indomethacin)—case reports.
Peripheral neuritis (see Glossary): numbness, pain in extremities (indomethacin)—rare.
Lung fibrosis (nabumetone)—case reports.
Pancreatitis (sulindac)—rare; (indomethacin)—case reports.
Pneumonitis (sulindac)—rare.
Aseptic meningitis (diclofenac)—rare.
Seizures (indomethacin only)—case reports.

▷ **Possible Effects on Sexual Function:** Enlargement and tenderness of both male and female breasts (indomethacin, sulindac)—rare.
Nonmenstrual vaginal bleeding (indomethacin)—rare.
Impotence (indomethacin, diclofenac, nabumetone)—rare.
Decreased libido (indomethacin)—rare.
Uterine bleeding (etodolac, sulindac)—rare.

Possible Delayed Adverse Effects: Mild anemia due to "silent" blood loss from the stomach.

Adverse Effects That May Mimic Natural Diseases or Disorders
Liver reactions may suggest viral hepatitis. Pancreatitis has occurred with sulindac.

Natural Diseases or Disorders That May Be Activated by These Drugs
Peptic ulcer disease, ulcerative colitis.

Possible Effects on Laboratory Tests
Complete blood cell counts: decreased red cells, hemoglobin, white cells, and platelets—rare.
INR (prothrombin time): increased.
Blood lithium level: increased.
Liver function tests: increased liver enzymes (ALT/GPT, AST/GOT and alkaline phosphatase), increased bilirubin.
Blood sugar (glucose): increased (indomethacin only)—rare.
Kidney function tests: increased blood creatinine and urea nitrogen (BUN) levels (kidney damage).
Fecal occult blood test: positive.
Urine protein (tolmetin only) may be falsely positive.

CAUTION
1. Dose should be limited to the smallest amount that produces reasonable improvement.
2. These drugs may mask early signs of infection. Tell your doctor if you think you are developing an infection of any kind.

Precautions for Use
By Infants and Children: Indomethacin: This drug frequently impairs kidney function in infants. Fatal liver reactions are possible in children between 6 and 12 years of age; avoid the use of this drug in this age group. Note: This medicine is used in infants (patent ductus arteriosus intravenously).
Diclofenac, etodolac, ketorolac, nabumetone, sulindac: Safety and efficacy for those under 12 years of age not established.
Tolmetin: Safety and efficacy for those under 2 years of age not established.
By Those Over 60 Years of Age: Small doses are advisable until tolerance is determined. Watch for any signs of liver or kidney toxicity, fluid retention, dizziness, confusion, impaired memory, depression, peptic ulcer, or diarrhea, often with rectal bleeding.

▷ **Advisability of Use During Pregnancy**
Pregnancy Category: Indomethacin, diclofenac, tolmetin: B. Indomethacin, etodolac, ketorolac, nabumetone, and sulindac: D. (Indomethacin is category D if used after 34 weeks or for more than 48 hours); see Pregnancy Risk Categories at the back of this book.

Animal studies: Indomethacin: significant toxicity and birth defects reported in mice and rats.

Diclofenac: Mouse, rat, and rabbit studies reveal toxic effects on the embryo but no birth defects.

Ketorolac: Rat and rabbit studies did not reveal teratogenicity, however, oral dosing after the 17th day of pregnancy caused increased pup mortality.

Nabumetone, tolmetin: Rat and rabbit studies revealed no defects.

Human studies: Indomethacin: adequate studies of pregnant women are not available. However, birth defects have been attributed to the use of this drug during pregnancy.

The manufacturer recommends that indomethacin not be taken during pregnancy.

Diclofenac, nabumetone, sulindac, tolmetin: Adequate studies of pregnant women are not available. Avoid this drug completely during the last 3 months of pregnancy. Use it during the first 6 months only if clearly needed. Ask your doctor for guidance.

Ketorolac: Adequate studies of pregnant women are not available. Ask your doctor for guidance.

Etodolac: Adequate studies of pregnant women not available. The manufacturer advises that this drug be avoided during pregnancy.

Advisability of Use If Breast-Feeding

Presence of these drugs in breast milk: Yes (all).

Avoid drugs or refrain from nursing (may have bad effects on infant's nervous system).

Habit-Forming Potential: None.

Effects of Overdose: Drowsiness, agitation, confusion, nausea, vomiting, diarrhea, disorientation, seizures, coma.

Possible Effects of Long-Term Use: Indomethacin and tolmetin: eye changes—deposits in the cornea, alterations in the retina.

Suggested Periodic Examinations While Taking These Drugs (at physician's discretion)

Complete blood cell counts, liver and kidney function tests, complete eye examinations if vision is altered in any way.

While Taking These Drugs, Observe the Following

Foods: No restrictions. These medicines are taken with food to decrease stomach irritation.

Nutritional Support: Indomethacin: Take 50 mg of vitamin C (ascorbic acid) daily.

Beverages: No restrictions. May be taken with milk.

▷ *Alcohol:* Use with caution. Alcohol can irritate the stomach lining, and when this is added to irritation from these drugs, can increase the risk of stomach ulceration and/or bleeding.

Tobacco Smoking: No interactions expected. I advise everyone to quit smoking.

▷ *Other Drugs*

Medicines in this class may *increase* the effects of

- aminoglycoside antibiotics (amikacin, others—see Drug Classes) by increasing blood levels.
- anticoagulants such as warfarin (Coumadin), and increase the risk of bleeding; monitor INR (prothrombin time), adjust dose accordingly.

- cyclosporine (Sandimmune) and cause toxicity.
- digoxin (Lanoxin)—indomethacin only.
- lithium, and cause lithium toxicity (except sulindac, which may decrease lithium levels).
- methotrexate (Mexate, others) and cause toxic levels.
- phenytoin (Dilantin) because of increased drug levels.
- thrombolytics such as streptokinase or TPA.
- zidovudine (AZT) and lead to toxicity of either medicine (indomethacin).

Medications in this class may **decrease** the effects of
- ACE inhibitors (see Drug Classes).
- beta-blocker drugs (see Drug Classes), and reduce their antihypertensive effectiveness.
- bumetanide (Bumex).
- captopril (Capoten).
- ethacrynic acid (Edecrin).
- furosemide (Lasix) and other loop diuretics.
- thiazide diuretics (see Drug Classes).

Medications in this class **taken concurrently** with the following drugs may increase the risk of bleeding or serious side effects; avoid these combinations:
- aspirin or other NSAIDs.
- dicumarol.
- diflunisal (Dolobid).
- dipyridamole (Persantine).
- probenecid (Pro-Biosan, others).
- sulfinpyrazone (Anturane).
- valproic acid (Depakene).
- warfarin (Coumadin).

▷ *Driving, Hazardous Activities:* These drugs may cause drowsiness, dizziness, or impaired vision. Restrict activities as necessary.

Aviation Note: The use of these drugs **may be a disqualification** for piloting. Consult a designated aviation medical examiner.

Exposure to Sun: Caution. Several medicines in this class have caused increased sensitivity (photosensitivity—see Glossary).

ACYCLOVIR (ay SI kloh ver)

Other Name: Acycloguanosine
Introduced: 1979   **Class:** Antiviral   **Prescription:** USA: Yes   **Controlled Drug:** USA: No; Canada: No   **Available as Generic:** Yes (capsule, suspension, and tablets)
Brand Name: Zovirax

BENEFITS versus RISKS

Possible Benefits	*Possible Risks*
FASTER RECOVERY FROM INITIAL EPISODE OF GENITAL HERPES	Nausea, vomiting, diarrhea
PREVENTION OF RECURRENCE OF GENITAL HERPES	Joint and muscle pain
TREATMENT OF CHICKEN POX	Seizures or coma with IV use (rare)
TREATMENT OF SUDDEN (ACUTE) SHINGLES (HERPES ZOSTER)	

Author's Note: This medication was again rejected by the FDA for a change to nonprescription "over-the-counter" (OTC) status. This was based on fear of development of viral resistance—NOT safety issues.

▷ **Principal Uses**

As a Single Drug Product: Uses currently included in FDA-approved labeling: (1) Treats or helps prevent genital herpes; (2) used to treat varicella (chicken pox) in children over a year old who have a chronic lung disease or skin condition, who take aspirin regularly, who are receiving short courses of corticosteroids via the lungs, or are over 13 years old and are otherwise healthy **(must be started within 24 hours of symptoms)**; (3) treats shingles (herpes zoster); (4) treats skin and mucous membrane infections (mucocutaneous) caused by herpes simplex in patients with immune problems; (5) used to treat brain infections caused by herpes simplex; (6) used to prevent herpes simplex virus infections in bone marrow transplant patients.

Other (unlabeled) generally accepted uses: (1) Acyclovir helps treat herpes simplex infections of the eye and rectum, and pneumonia caused by the chicken pox (varicella) virus; (2) some data support its use in nonmalignant skin growths in the throat (laryngeal papillomatosis); (3) it is a trial (in combination) AIDS treatment; (4) can prevent recurrent erythema multiforme that may occur with herpes simplex infections.

How This Drug Works: By blocking genetic material formation of the herpes simplex virus, this drug stops viral multiplication and spread, reducing severity and duration of the herpes infection.

Available Dosage Forms and Strengths

Capsules — 200 mg, 400 mg, 800 mg
Intravenous — 500 mg, 1 g
Oral suspension — 200 mg/5 ml
Tablets — 200 mg, 400 mg and 800 mg
Ointment — 5%, 50 mg/g (Canada)

▷ **Recommended Dosage Ranges** (Actual dose and schedule must be determined for each patient individually.)

Infants and Children: Safety and efficacy of oral use in children younger than 6 weeks of age has NOT been established. Topical acyclovir use data in children less than 10 is lacking; however, the drug would be expected to follow the same patterns of side effects and risk-to-benefit decisions as the oral formulation.

18 to 65 Years of Age: For first episode of genital herpes: 200 mg every 4 hours for a total of five capsules daily for 7 to 10 days (or until what your doctor describes as "clinical resolution" happens). Some clinicians use 400 mg three times a day for 7 to 10 days. For intermittent recurrence: 200 mg every 4 hours for a total of five capsules daily for 5 consecutive days (total dose of 25 capsules) or 400 mg three times a day for 5 days. Start treatment at the earliest sign of recurrence. For prevention of frequent recurrence: 400 mg taken twice daily for up to 12 months, and then evaluation of ongoing need for this medicine. For the ointment form: Cover all infected areas every 3 hours for a total of six times daily for 7 consecutive days. Start treatment at the **earliest sign** of infection.

In attempting to decrease the pain of herpes zoster: 800 mg five times daily (every 4 hours) for 7–10 days. Ointment use 6 times a day for 10 days helps the crusts form sooner! Treatment of chicken pox (for those 2 or older): 20 mg per kg of body mass (do not exceed 800 mg) orally, four times a day for 5 days. If over 40 kg: 800 mg four times daily for 5 days. **Start treatment at the first** symptom or sign.

Over 65 Years of Age: The dose **must** be adjusted if the kidneys are impaired.

Conditions Requiring Dosing Adjustments

Liver Function: Specific adjustment in liver dysfunction is not defined.

Kidney Function: The dose **MUST** be adjusted in people with compromised kidney function. For example: creatinine clearance of 25–50 ml/min gets usual dose every 12 hours; 10–25 ml/min gets usual dose once daily.

Obesity: Dosing (intravenous form) should be made on ideal body weight and given as 10 mg per kg of body mass. Maximum dose is 500 mg per square meter every 8 hours.

▷ **Dosing Instructions:**   May be taken without regard to food. Capsule may be opened. The maker of this medicine recommends drinking 1 liter of water for each gram (1000 mg) of this medicine that is taken. Take the full course of the exact dose prescribed. Use a finger cot or rubber glove to apply the ointment.

Usual Duration of Use: Use on a regular schedule for 10 days is usually needed to see this drug's effect in reducing the severity and duration of the initial infection. Continual use for 6 months may be needed to prevent frequent recurrence of herpes eruptions.

▷ **This Drug Should Not Be Taken If**
- you have had an allergic reaction to it previously.

▷ **Inform Your Physician Before Taking This Drug If**
- your liver, kidney or nerve function is impaired.
- you take other medicines that may cause kidney damage.
- you think you are dehydrated and cannot or will not drink water.
- you are unsure of how much to take or how often to take acyclovir.

Possible Side Effects (natural, expected, and unavoidable drug actions)
With use of capsules—none. With IV—irritation of the vein up to 9%. With use of ointment—mild pain or stinging at site of application.

▷ **Possible Adverse Effects** (unusual, unexpected, and infrequent reactions)
If any of the following develop, consult your physician promptly for guidance.

Mild Adverse Effects
Allergic reaction: skin rash.
Headache, dizziness, nervousness, confusion, insomnia, depression, fatigue—rare.

Nausea, vomiting, diarrhea—infrequent with IV form.

Joint pains, muscle cramps—rare.

Acne, hair loss—rare.

Serious Adverse Effects

Superficial thrombophlebitis—infrequent with IV form.

Seizures or coma with IV use—rare.

Kidney problems—rare—especially if adequate water is taken.

Low platelets or red or white blood cells—case reports rare.

Colitis—case reports.

▷ **Possible Effects on Sexual Function:** No recent data.

Possible Effects on Laboratory Tests

Complete blood cell counts: decreased red or white cells, or hemoglobin—rare.

Blood urea nitrogen (BUN)/creatinine: increased—rare (5–10% fast IV).

Liver function tests: increased—rare.

CAUTION

1. This drug does **not** eliminate all herpes virus and is **not a cure**. Recurrence is possible. Resume treatment at the earliest sign of infection.
2. Avoid intercourse if herpes blisters and swelling are present.
3. Do not exceed the prescribed dose.
4. If severity/frequency of infections don't improve, call your doctor.
5. The manufacturer recommends drinking 1 liter (1000 ml) of fluid for each gram (1000 mg) of oral or intravenous form taken.
6. Other medicines that can form damaging crystals in the urine may lead to added kidney problem risk if combined with acyclovir.

Precautions for Use

By Infants and Children: Specific dosing required. Fluid intake must be adequate.

By Those Over 60 Years of Age: Avoid dehydration. Drink 2 to 3 quarts of liquids daily.

▷ **Advisability of Use During Pregnancy**

Pregnancy Category: C. See Pregnancy Risk Categories at the back of this book. A pregnancy registry exists at 1-800-722-9292 ext. 58465.

Animal studies: No birth defects found in mouse, rat, or rabbit studies.

Human studies: The pregnancy registry has followed more than 400 cases to date. No pattern of birth defects. The sample patient number is still too small to detect small (less than twofold) increases in risk. Talk with your doctor about use.

Advisability of Use If Breast-Feeding

Presence of this drug in breast milk: Yes.

Ask your physician for guidance (it's often OK to breast-feed).

Habit-Forming Potential: None.

Effects of Overdose: Possible impairment of kidney function.

Possible Effects of Long-Term Use: Development of acyclovir-resistant strains of herpes virus. Treatment will fail if this occurs.

Suggested Periodic Examinations While Taking This Drug (at physician's discretion)

Kidney function tests.

▷ **While Taking This Drug, Observe the Following**
  Foods: No restrictions.
  Beverages: No restrictions. May be taken with milk. **Drink 2 to 3 quarts of liquids** (if not contraindicated for you) **daily.**
▷ *Alcohol:* Use caution; dizziness or fatigue may be accentuated.
  Tobacco Smoking: No interactions expected. I advise everyone to quit smoking.
▷ *Other Drugs*
  The following drugs may *increase* the effects of acyclovir:
  • cyclosporine (Sandimmune): Use may result in increased risk of kidney toxicity.
  • probenecid (Benemid): May delay acyclovir elimination.
  Acyclovir *taken concurrently* with
  • meperidine (Demerol) may result in neurologic problems.
  • varicella vaccine (Varivax) will blunt the vaccine effectiveness.
  • zidovudine (AZT) may result in severe fatigue and lethargy.
▷ *Driving, Hazardous Activities:* Use caution if dizziness or fatigue occurs.
  Aviation Note: The use of this drug *may be a disqualification* for piloting. Consult a designated aviation medical examiner.
  Exposure to Sun: No restrictions; however, some data indicates that sun exposure may trigger release of herpes simplex from its dormant state (from the optic nerve).

ALBUTEROL (al BYU ter ohl)

Other Name: Salbutamol

Introduced: 1968   **Class:** Antiasthmatic, bronchodilator   **Prescription:** USA: Yes   **Controlled Drug:** USA: No; Canada: No   **Available as Generic:** Yes

Brand Names: ✤Apo-Salvent, Combivent [CD], ✤Novo-Salmol, Proventil HFA, Proventil Inhaler, Proventil Repetabs, Proventil Tablets, ✤Salbutamol, ✤Ventodisk, Ventolin Inhaler, Ventolin Nebules, Ventolin Rotacaps, Ventolin Syrup, Ventolin Tablets, Volmax Controlled-Release Tablets, Volmax Extended-Release Tablets

BENEFITS versus RISKS	
Possible Benefits	*Possible Risks*
VERY EFFECTIVE RELIEF OF BRONCHOSPASM	Increased blood pressure or heart rate
	Fine hand tremor
	Angina in patients with coronary artery disease
	Irregular heart rhythm and fatalities (with excessive use)
	Paradoxical spasm of the bronchi

▷ **Principal Uses**
  As a Single Drug Product: Uses currently included in FDA-approved labeling: (1) Relieves acute bronchial asthma and reduces frequency and severity of chronic, recurrent asthmatic attacks; (2) helps prevent exercise-induced bronchospasm.

Other (unlabeled) generally accepted uses: (1) May have a role (nebulized) where blood potassium is too high; (2) limited use in patients with leukemia who also have long-standing (chronic) cough.

How This Drug Works: By increasing cyclic AMP, this drug relaxes constricted bronchial muscles to relieve asthmatic wheezing.

Available Dosage Forms and Strengths

Aerosol	— 90 mcg per press (actuation)
	— 100 mcg per press (Canada)
	— 120 mcg per press
Capsules for inhalation (technique is important)	— 200 mcg, 400 mcg (Canada)
Nasal inhaler (Canada)	— 100 mcg/dose
Solution for inhalation	— 0.83% and 0.5%
Syrup	— 2 mg/5 ml
	— 2.4 mg/5 ml
Rotacaps	— 200 mcg
Tablets	— 2 mg, 4 mg
Tablets, sustained release	— 4 mg, 4.8 mg, 8 mg and 9.6 mg
Tablets, timed release	— 4 mg, 8 mg
Ventodisk (Canada)	— 200 mcg and 400 mcg per disk

▷ **Recommended Dosage Ranges** (Actual dose and schedule must be determined for each patient individually.)

Inhaler—Adults and children 12 or older: Two inhalations repeated every 4 to 6 hours. For some patients, one inhalation every 4 hours may be enough. Taking a larger number of inhalations is **not** recommended. If the dose that previously worked does not provide relief, call your doctor **immediately**. The status of your asthma must be examined.

Author's note: Proventil repetabs and Volmax are FDA approved to treat bronchospasm in patients 6 years old or older.

Tablets (immediate release)—2 to 4 mg three to four times daily, every 4 to 6 hours; (sustained release)—1 or 2 tablets every 12 hours.

Do not exceed eight inhalations (720 mcg) every 24 hours, or 32 mg (tablet form). Some manufacturers limit this to 16 mg) every 24 hours.

Conditions Requiring Dosing Adjustments

Liver Function: Use with caution and in low doses in people with liver compromise.

Kidney Function: No specific changes in dosing are available.

Coronary Artery Disease: A maximum starting dose should be 1 mg in order to avoid chest pain (angina).

Thyroid Disease: People with low (hypoactive) thyroids may require increased doses.

▷ **Dosing Instructions:**   May be taken on empty stomach or with food or milk. Nonsustained-release tablets may be crushed. Sustained-release forms should NEVER be crushed. For inhaler, follow the written instructions carefully. Do not use excessively.

Usual Duration of Use: Do not use beyond the time necessary to stop episodes of asthma.

▷ **This Drug Should Not Be Taken If**
- you have had an allergic reaction to any dosage form of it.
- you have an irregular heart rhythm.
- you have an overactive thyroid (hyperthyroid).
- you are taking, or took in the past 2 weeks, any monoamine oxidase (MAO) type A inhibitor (see Drug Classes).

▷ **Inform Your Physician Before Taking This Drug If**
- you have a heart or circulatory disorder, especially high blood pressure, coronary heart disease, or aneurysms.
- you have diabetes.
- you are take any form of digitalis or any stimulant drug.
- you take other prescription or nonprescription medications that weren't discussed when albuterol was prescribed.
- you are going to have a baby (this medicine may make contractions difficult to have).
- you are unsure how much to take or how often to take albuterol.

Possible Side Effects (natural, expected, and unavoidable drug actions)
Aerosol: dryness or irritation of mouth/throat, altered taste.
Tablet: nervousness, palpitation, fast heart rate (tachycardia)—infrequent.

▷ **Possible Adverse Effects** (unusual, unexpected, and infrequent reactions)
If any of the following develop, consult your physician promptly for guidance.
Mild Adverse Effects
Itching—rare.
Headache, dizziness, restlessness, insomnia—infrequent.
Fine hand tremor—frequent.
Nausea—rare.
Leg cramps, flushing of skin—rare.
Difficulty urinating—rare.
Rapid heart rate—infrequent.
Decreased platelets—possible, but not clinically significant.
Serious Adverse Effects
Heart attack—case reports after intravenous use.
Abnormal heart beats—possible.
Chest pain—possible with higher doses in patients with coronary artery disease.
Hallucinations or convulsions (with excessive dosing)—possible.
Decreased blood potassium (hypokalemia)—possible and dose related.
High blood sugar (hyperglycemia)—possible and more likely with intravenous use.

▷ **Possible Effects on Sexual Function:**   None reported.

Natural Diseases or Disorders That May Be Activated by This Drug
Latent coronary artery disease, diabetes, or high blood pressure.

Possible Effects on Laboratory Tests
Blood aldosterone: increased.
Blood HDL cholesterol level: increased.
Blood glucose level: increased.

Blood potassium: decreased.
Blood platelets: decreased (with high doses).

CAUTION
1. This drug may be dangerous if patients increase their dose and/or frequency, as it may result in rapid or irregular heart rhythm and fatalities with overuse.
2. Use of this drug by inhalation with beclomethasone aerosol (Beclovent, Vanceril) may increase the risk of fluorocarbon propellant toxicity. Use albuterol aerosol 20 to 30 minutes *before* beclomethasone aerosol to reduce toxicity and enhance the penetration of beclomethasone.
3. Serious heart rhythm problems or cardiac arrest can result from excessive or prolonged inhalation.
4. Call your doctor if you begin to increase the number of times you use this drug on a daily basis. Tolerance to the effects of this drug has been reported.

Precautions for Use
By Infants and Children: Used to help prevent bronchospasm caused by exercise in children ages 4–11.
By Those Over 60 Years of Age: Avoid excessive and continual use. If asthma is not relieved promptly, other drugs will have to be tried. Watch for nervousness, palpitations, irregular heart rhythm, and muscle tremors. Doses of 2 mg by mouth 3 or 4 four times daily prudent.

▷ **Advisability of Use During Pregnancy**
Pregnancy Category: C. See Pregnancy Risk Categories at the back of this book.
Animal studies: Cleft palate reported in mice.
Human studies: Adequate studies of pregnant women are not available.
Avoid use during first 3 months if possible.

Advisability of Use If Breast-Feeding
Presence of this drug in breast milk: Unknown.
Avoid drug or refrain from nursing.

Habit-Forming Potential: A few cases of dependency and abuse have been described. These may be cases of use for the effect of the propellants or the drug itself.

Effects of Overdose: Nervousness, palpitation, rapid heart rate, life-threatening arrhythmias, sweating, headache, tremor, vomiting, chest pain.

Possible Effects of Long-Term Use: Loss of effectiveness.

Suggested Periodic Examinations While Taking This Drug (at physician's discretion)
Blood pressure measurements, evaluation of heart status.

▷ **While Taking This Drug, Observe the Following**
Foods: No restrictions.
Beverages: Avoid excessive caffeine as found in coffee, tea, cola, chocolate.
▷ *Alcohol:* No interactions expected.
Tobacco Smoking: Smoking may interact with theophylline. I advise everyone to quit.
▷ *Other Drugs*
Albuterol *taken concurrently* with
• amphetamines may worsen of cardiovascular side effects.
• bendroflumethiazide (Corzide, Naturetin) and other thiazide and loop di-

uretics (see Drug Classes) may result in additive lowering of blood potassium.
- beta-blockers such as propranolol (Inderal) result in loss of effect of both medications.
- dopamine (Intropin) may worsen adverse effects on the heart. Avoid this combination.
- ephedrine (Bronkaid, Tedrigen) may result in excessive heart effects.
- ipratropium (Atrovent) can result in better (longer time) opening of the bronchi (beneficial interaction).
- isoproterenol (Isuprel) may result in worsening of heart (cardiac) side effects.
- monoamine oxidase (MAO) type A inhibitor drugs can cause very high blood pressure and undesirable heart stimulation.
- phenylephrine (Dimetapp, Dristan, others) may worsen bad effects on the heart (adverse reaction), and the combination is not recommended.
- phenylpropanolamine (Acutrim, Alka-Seltzer Plus, Contac, others) may worsen bad effects on the heart (adverse reaction). Do not combine.
- pseudoephedrine (Sudafed, others) may worsen adverse heart effects. DO NOT COMBINE.
- theophylline (Theo-Dur, others) may result in rapid removal of theophylline and loss of therapeutic theophylline effect.
- tricyclic antidepressants (see Drug Classes) may cause a severe increase in blood pressure.

▷ *Driving, Hazardous Activities:* Use caution if excessive nervousness or dizziness occurs.

Aviation Note: The use of this drug *is a disqualification* for piloting. Consult a designated aviation medical examiner.

Exposure to Sun: No restrictions.

Heavy Exercise or Exertion: Use caution. Excessive exercise can cause (induce) asthma in some asthmatics.

ALENDRONATE (a LEN druh nate)

Introduced: 1996   **Class:** Aminobisphosphonate   **Prescription:** USA: Yes   **Controlled Drug:** USA: No   **Available as Generic:** No
Brand Name: Fosamax

BENEFITS versus RISKS	
Possible Benefits	*Possible Risks*
EFFECTIVE TREATMENT OF OSTEOPOROSIS	Esophageal irritation
INCREASE IN BONE MASS	Minor muscle pain
EXPECTED PREVENTION OF OSTEOPOROSIS	
DECREASED RISK OF BONE FRACTURES	
SYMPTOM RELIEF IN PAGET'S DISEASE	
PREVENTION OF POSTMENOPAUSAL OSTEOPOROSIS	

▷ **Principal Uses**

As a Single Drug Product: Uses currently included in FDA-approved labeling: (1) Treatment of postmenopausal osteoporosis; (2) treatment of Paget's disease; (3) prevention of postmenopausal osteoporosis.

Other (unlabeled) generally accepted uses: Expected to work in the prevention and treatment of male osteoporosis.

How This Drug Works: This medicine works at the brush border of the osteoclast cell. This prevents this cell from resorbing (gobbling up) bone while the osteoblast (bone-building cell) continues to work. This results in bone building and decreased fracture risk.

Available Dosage Forms and Strengths

Tablets — 5 mg, 10 mg, and 40 mg

▷ **Recommended Dosage Ranges:** (Actual dose and schedule must be determined for each patient individually.)

Infants and Children: Efficacy and safety are not established.

18 to 65 Years of Age: In female postmenopausal osteoporosis: 10 mg taken once daily.

Osteoporosis prevention: 5 mg once daily.

I strongly recommend an appropriate amount of dietary calcium and/or calcium supplementation to ensure adequate calcium *every day*. Discuss the need for vitamin D with your doctor. Calcium and vitamin D are critical in osteoporosis prevention and treatment.

Paget's disease: 40 mg once daily for 6 months.

Over 65 Years of Age: Same as in those 18 to 65 years old.

Conditions Requiring Dosing Adjustments

Liver Function: No changes needed.

Kidney Function: Lower doses for patients with kidney compromise. Patients with creatinine clearances (see Glossary) less than 35 ml/min **should not** be given this medicine.

▷ **Dosing Instructions:**   TAKE THIS MEDICINE WITH 6 TO 8 OUNCES OF TAP WATER TO GET THE BEST RESULTS. DO NOT take this drug with food or other drugs; the therapeutic benefit will be decreased. Take it at least half an hour before the first food or liquids (other than plain tap water) of the day. Avoiding food or drink for more than 30 minutes lets more medicine get into your body to go to work. **DO NOT** lie down for 30 minutes (wait preferably an hour) after taking this drug (this decreases risk of irritation or ulceration of the esophagus).

Usual Duration of Use: In Paget's disease, this medicine is used once daily for 6 months, with recheck after that. In treating osteoporosis after menopause, many doctors get a bone mineral density test (DEXA is presently the most widely used) to help decide to start therapy, and then get a second test 2 years later to check results or outcome of therapy. Further study is needed to find the best dosing strategies in long-term (greater than 4 years) use of alendronate. Prevention of osteoporosis after menopause involves similar tests and appropriate follow-up.

Possible Advantages of This Drug

This drug increases bone mass more than other (anti-resorptive) drugs, which then decreases the risk of fractures.

This medicine also helps form normal bone (microarchitecture).

Better side-effect profile than earlier bisphosphonates.

▷ **This Drug Should Not Be Taken If**
- you are allergic to the drug or its components.
- you have a low blood calcium (hypocalcemia). Talk to your doctor.
- you have a significant kidney disease (medicine should NOT be taken if creatinine clearance is less than 35 ml/min—no data).
- you are unable to sit or stand for 30 minutes after taking this medicine (increased risk of esophageal problems).
- you are pregnant or are nursing your infant.
- you have esophageal disease (abnormal esophagus) or difficulty emptying the esophagus.

▷ **Inform Your Physician Before Taking This Drug If**
- you have ulcers or inflammation of the duodenum.
- you have difficulty swallowing.
- you have a vitamin D deficiency.
- you have a diet poor in calcium (low calcium diet).

Possible Side Effects (natural, expected, and unavoidable drug actions)
Irritation of the esophagus and potential ulceration—rare. This effect is worsened if patients lie down soon after taking drug.

▷ **Possible Adverse Effects** (unusual, unexpected, and infrequent reactions)
If any of the following develop, consult your physician promptly for guidance.
Mild Adverse Effects
Allergic reactions: rare skin rash or redness.
Headache—infrequent.
Gas (flatulence), diarrhea, or constipation—infrequent.
Pain in the muscles or skeleton (musculoskeletal)—infrequent.
Mild calcium decrease—2% decrease in some patients taking 10 mg daily.
Mild decrease in phosphorous—up to 6%.
Mild muscle pain—infrequent with the 10-mg dose.
Fever (drug fever) with intravenous use—rare.
Serious Adverse Effects
Allergic reactions: none reported.
Esophageal ulceration—rare. (Increased risk if you lie down after taking this drug. Best NOT to lie down for at least half an hour after taking this medicine.) One case report of a patient with a history of peptic ulcer disease who had stomach surgery and who was also taking aspirin developed an ulcer (anastomotic) and had mild hemorrhaging.

▷ **Possible Effects on Sexual Function:**   None reported.

Possible Effects on Laboratory Tests
Serum calcium or phosphorous: lowered—infrequent.
Liver function tests: increased—rare (with intravenous form)(asymptomatic and transient).

CAUTION
1. A "dear doctor" letter was sent out by the FDA warning of increased occurrence of esophageal ulceration. This may have been caused by patients taking the medicine with less water than directed. DO NOT LIE DOWN for 30 minutes after taking this drug. Patients should eat BEFORE they lie down.
2. Patients who take more than 10 mg of alendronate a day should avoid as-

pirin and aspirin-containing compounds because upper gastrointestinal adverse effects may be increased in this situation if the medicines are combined.

3. Other causes of osteoporosis besides estrogen or aging (secondary osteoporosis) must be ruled out.
4. Depression may be a risk factor for osteoporosis. Talk with your doctor about an osteoporosis test if depression is a problem for you.

Precautions for Use
By Infants and Children: Safety and efficacy in this age group have not been established.

By Those Over 65 Years of Age: The amount that goes into the body (bioavailability) and the places alendronate goes (disposition) are similar to those less than 65. No specific dosing changes needed. Increased sensitivity to this drug is possible.

Advisability of Use During Pregnancy
Pregnancy Category: C. See Pregnancy Risk Categories at the back of this book. Studies in rats have shown toxicity to the mother as well as neonatal death following dosing of alendronate during pregnancy. Adequate studies of pregnant women are not available. Avoid this medicine during pregnancy.

Advisability of Use If Breast-Feeding
Presence of this drug in breast milk: Yes in rats; unknown in humans. Avoid drug or refrain from nursing.

Habit-Forming Potential: None.

Effects of Overdose: Nausea, vomiting, hypocalcemia, and hypophosphatemia. Heartburn, ulceration of the upper gastrointestinal tract.

Possible Effects of Long-Term Use: Increased bone density and decreased fracture risk (beneficial).

Suggested Periodic Examinations While Taking This Drug (at physician's discretion)
Tests of bone mineral density, check of lab tests of bone lossor formation. Blood calcium.
Measurement of height.

▷ **While Taking This Drug, Observe the Following**
Foods: DO NOT TAKE THIS DRUG WITH FOOD. Adequate elemental calcium is needed. Calcium supplements should be taken at least half an hour **after** taking alendronate.

Beverages: Any liquid other than water will decrease the amount of alendronate that gets into your body to help you. It is critical that this medicine only be taken with 6 to 8 ounces of water.

▷ *Alcohol:* Alcohol (especially in high doses) may act as a bone-forming cell (osteoblast) poison and excessive use is a risk factor for osteoporosis. Alcohol may also irritate the stomach lining.

Tobacco Smoking: Tobacco may be a risk factor for osteoporosis. I advise everyone to stop smoking.

▷ *Other Drugs*
Alendronate *taken concurrently* with
• antacids may decrease the total absorption of alendronate and decrease its therapeutic benefit.

- aspirin or aspirin-containing products or salicylates may pose an increased risk of upper gastrointestinal adverse effects if more than 10 mg of alendronate is taken daily. Although other NSAIDs (nonsteroidal anti-inflammatory drugs; see Drug Classes) were not presented as potential problems with alendronate doses greater than 10 mg, caution is advised.
- estrogens (various) taken by a few women in clinical trials did not have problems. Combination not presently recommended due to lack of specific data. Trials are ongoing to see benefits.
- foscarnet (Foscavir) may result in an additive decrease in calcium.
- medicines in general should NOT be taken at the same time as alendronate. Separate any dose of alendronate and any other medicine by at least half an hour.
- ranitidine (Zantac) (intravenous form and perhaps oral form) may double how much alendronate gets into your body. The clinical importance of this is not yet known.

The following drugs may *decrease* the effects of alendronate:

- Because a small amount of alendronate gets into the body under the best conditions, take alendronate with a full 6 to 8 ounces of water and take any other drugs at least half an hour after alendronate.

▷ *Driving, Hazardous Activities:* No specific limitations.

Aviation Note: The use of this drug *is probably not a disqualification* for piloting. Consult a designated aviation medical examiner.

Exposure to Sun: No restrictions.

Heavy Exercise or Exertion: If your bone density is low, heavy aerobic exercise may not be a good idea. Discuss this with your doctor. In general, weight-bearing exercise stimulates receptors (mechanoreceptors) to release factors that result in increased bone strength.

Discontinuation: Talk with your doctor **before** stopping this medicine.

ALLOPURINOL (al oh PURE i nohl)

Introduced: 1963   **Class:** Anti-gout   **Prescription:** USA: Yes   **Controlled Drug:** USA: No; Canada: No   **Available as Generic:** USA: Yes; Canada: No

Brand Names: ✲Alloprin, ✲Apo-Allopurinol, Lopurin, ✲Novopurol, ✲Purinol, Zurinol, Zyloprim

BENEFITS versus RISKS	
Possible Benefits	*Possible Risks*
EFFECTIVE CONTROL OF GOUT	Increased frequency of acute gout
CONTROL OF HIGH BLOOD URIC	initially
ACID due to polycythemia,	Peripheral neuritis
leukemia, cancer, and	Allergic reactions in skin, lung, blood
chemotherapy	vessels, and liver
	Bone marrow depression
	Kidney toxicity

▷ **Principal Uses**

As a Single Drug Product: Uses currently included in FDA-approved labeling: (1) Long-term gout therapy to *prevent* acute gout (does not relieve sudden gout attacks); (2) helps prevent high blood levels of uric acid in people who have recurrent uric acid or calcium oxalate kidney stones, people getting chemotherapy or radiation for cancer, or who take thiazide diuretics (see Drug Classes).

Other (unlabeled) generally accepted uses: (1) May decrease pain and occurrence of mouth sores in people receiving 5-fluorouracil chemotherapy; (2) may help prostate swelling (nonbacterial prostatitis) not caused by bacteria; (3) early data show benefits in blood circulation damage (ischemic tissue damage).

How This Drug Works: By blocking the enzyme xanthine oxidase, it decreases uric acid formation.

Available Dosage Forms and Strengths

Tablets — 100 mg, 300 mg (and 200 mg in Canada)

▷ **Usual Adult Dosage Range:**   Starts as 100 mg every 24 hours. Increase by 100 mg every 24 hours (1 week apart) until uric acid blood level is 6 mg/dl or less. Usual dose is 200 to 300 mg every 24 hours for mild gout, and 400 to 600 mg every 24 hours for moderate to severe gout. Daily doses of 300 mg or less may be taken as a single dose. Doses exceeding 300 mg daily should be divided into two or three equal portions. For high uric acid levels associated with cancer, 600 to 800 mg every 24 hours, divided into three equal portions (with high water intake). Kidney stone (calcium oxalate) recurrence prevention: 200–300 mg per day.

Note: Actual dosage and schedule must be determined for each patient individually.

Conditions Requiring Dosing Adjustments

Liver Function: Dose adjustment in liver compromise is not documented.

Kidney Function: Dosing **must** be adjusted in kidney compromise.

Malnutrition: Malnourished patients or those on low protein diets will not remove this drug normally and are at risk for toxicity. Doses **must** be decreased.

▷ **Dosing Instructions:**   Best taken with food or milk to reduce stomach irritation. Tablet may be crushed. **Drink 2 to 3 quarts of liquids daily.**

Usual Duration of Use: Blood uric acid levels often decrease in 48 to 72 hours and may reach normal range in 1 to 3 weeks. Regular use for several months may be needed to prevent acute gout attacks. Ongoing use for years often needed for adequate control.

▷ **This Drug Should Not Be Taken If**

• you have had an allergic reaction to it previously.
• you are having an acute gout attack.

▷ **Inform Your Physician Before Taking This Drug If**

• you have a family history of hemochromatosis.
• you have a history of liver or kidney disease.
• you have had a blood cell or bone marrow disorder.
• you have a seizure or convulsive disorder (epilepsy).
• you take other prescription or nonprescription medications not discussed when allopurinol was prescribed.

- you are unsure how much to take or how often to take allopurinol.
- you are on a low protein diet.
- you are pregnant.

Possible Side Effects (natural, expected, and unavoidable drug actions)

Frequency and severity of episodes of acute gout may still happen during the first several weeks of therapy. Ask your doctor about using other drugs during this period.

▷ **Possible Adverse Effects** (unusual, unexpected, and infrequent reactions)

If any of the following develop, consult your physician promptly for guidance.

Mild Adverse Effects

Allergic reactions: skin rash, hives, itching—frequent; drug fever.

Confusion, headache, dizziness, drowsiness—rare.

Nausea, vomiting, diarrhea, stomach cramps—rare.

Taste disturbance—possible.

Loss of scalp hair—rare.

Serious Adverse Effects

Allergic reactions: severe skin reactions—infrequent.

High fever, chills, joint pains, swollen glands, kidney damage—rare.

Hepatitis with or without jaundice (see Glossary): yellow eyes and skin, dark-colored urine, light-colored stools (may be part of allergy)—rare.

Kidney damage—possible (case reports).

Bone marrow depression (see Glossary)—rare.

Blood vessel inflammation/damage—rare (risk increased in kidney failure and thiazide diuretic use at the same time).

Peripheral neuritis—rare.

Bronchospasm (part of hypersensitivity)—rare.

Eye damage (macular), cataract formation—rare.

▷ **Possible Effects on Sexual Function:** Less than 1% and questionable cause: male infertility, male breast enlargement, impotence.

Adverse Effects That May Mimic Natural Diseases or Disorders

Toxic liver reaction may suggest viral hepatitis.

Severe skin reactions may resemble the Stevens-Johnson syndrome (erythema multiforme).

Possible Effects on Laboratory Tests

Complete blood cell counts: decreased red cells, hemoglobin, and platelets; increased eosinophils.

Liver function tests: increased ALT/GPT, AST/GOT, and alkaline phosphatase.

CAUTION

1. Call your doctor immediately if you develop a rash. This can be the first sign of an allergic reaction. Prompt action may avoid a more serious reaction.
2. In the first few weeks of therapy, frequency of gout attacks may increase. These subside with ongoing therapy.
3. Drug should not be started in acute gout. It does not help.
4. Vitamin C in doses of 2 g or more daily can increase the risk of kidney stone formation during the use of allopurinol.
5. Patients with kidney function decline are more likely to have allergic reactions to this drug.

6. Frequency of rash may be increased in patients also taking a penicillin.
7. Allergic-type kidney damage can result if thiazide diuretics (see Drug Classes) are taken with allopurinol. Avoid this combination.
8. Patients on low protein diets will not eliminate allopurinol normally. Doses must be decreased.

Precautions for Use

By Infants and Children: Not used in children except for increased uric acid caused by malignant growths. Watch closely for allergic skin reactions and blood cell disorders. The toxicity of azathioprine (Imuran) or mercaptopurine (Purinethol) may be increased in children receiving chemotherapy.

By Those Over 60 Years of Age: Smaller starting and ongoing doses of this drug must be used.

▷ **Advisability of Use During Pregnancy**

Pregnancy Category: C. See Pregnancy Risk Categories at the back of this book.
Animal studies: Results are conflicting and inconclusive.
Human studies: Adequate studies of pregnant women are not available.
Avoid use of drug during the first 3 months. Use during the last 6 months only if clearly needed.

Advisability of Use If Breast-Feeding

Presence of this drug in breast milk: Yes.
Avoid drug or refrain from nursing.

Habit-Forming Potential: None.

Effects of Overdose: Nausea, vomiting, or diarrhea. Hypersensitivity reactions, kidney and liver function decline.

Possible Effects of Long-Term Use: None identified.

Suggested Periodic Examinations While Taking This Drug (at physician's discretion)

Blood uric acid levels, complete blood cell counts, liver and kidney function tests. Eye examinations (possible cataract formation or macular damage).

▷ **While Taking This Drug, Observe the Following**

Foods: Talk to your doctor about a low-purine diet. A low PROTEIN diet may increase toxicity risk if dose isn't decreased.

Beverages: No restrictions. May be taken with milk.

▷ *Alcohol:* No interactions expected.

Tobacco Smoking: No interactions expected. I advise everyone to quit smoking.

▷ *Other Drugs*

Allopurinol may *increase* the effects of
  • azathioprine (Imuran) and mercaptopurine (Purinethol), making dose decreases necessary.
  • oral anticoagulants (see Drug Classes) such as warfarin (Coumadin). INR should be checked more often.
  • theophylline (aminophylline, Elixophyllin, Theo-Dur, etc.).

Allopurinol *taken concurrently* with
  • ampicillin (and perhaps other penicillins) may increase the incidence of skin rash.
  • antacids containing aluminum will decrease the therapeutic effect of allopurinol.

- captopril (Capoten) or other ACE inhibitors (see Drug Classes) can increase the likelihood of allergic reactions.
- cyclophosphamide (Cytoxan, Neosar) may result in cyclophosphamide toxicity.
- cyclosporine (Sandimmune) can cause cyclosporine toxicity.
- iron salts may lead excess liver iron. Avoid combining.
- mercaptopurine (Purinethol) increases toxicity risk.
- tamoxifen (Nolvadex) may result in increased allopurinol levels and increased risk of liver toxicity.
- thiazide diuretics (see Drug Classes) may decrease kidney function.
- theophylline (Theo-Dur, etc.) may cause toxic theophylline levels.
- vidarabine (Vira-A) may increase risk of neurotoxicity.

▷ *Driving, Hazardous Activities:* Drowsiness may occur in some people. Use caution.

Aviation Note: The use of this drug *may be a disqualification* for piloting. Consult a designated aviation medical examiner.

Exposure to Sun: No restrictions.

Discontinuation: If you have a seizure disorder, this medicine dose should be slowly decreased and then stopped.

ALPRAZOLAM (al PRAY zoh lam)

Introduced: 1973   **Class:** Antianxiety drug, benzodiazepines   **Prescription:** USA: Yes   **Controlled Drug:** USA: C-IV*; Canada: No   **Available as Generic:** Yes

Brand Names: Alprazolam Intensol, ✦Apo-Alpraz, Novo-Alprazol, Nu-Alpraz, Xanax

Warning: The brand names Xanax and Zantac are similar and can lead to **serious** medication errors. Xanax is alprazolam. Zantac is ranitidine, which treats peptic ulcers and heartburn. Make sure your prescription was filled correctly.

BENEFITS versus RISKS

Possible Benefits	*Possible Risks*
RELIEF OF ANXIETY AND NERVOUS TENSION	Habit-forming potential with prolonged use
EFFECTIVE TREATMENT OF PANIC DISORDER	Minor impairment of mental functions with therapeutic doses
Wide margin of safety with therapeutic doses	Tachycardia and palpitations
May have some antidepressant activity	

▷ **Principal Uses**

As a Single Drug Product: Uses currently included in FDA-approved labeling: (1) Used for short-term relief of mild to moderate anxiety and nervous tension;

*See Controlled Drug Schedules at the back of this book.

(2) helps relieve anxiety associated with neurosis; (3) decreases frequency and severity of panic disorder.

Other (unlabeled) generally accepted uses: (1) Can help control extreme PMS symptoms; (2) lessens a variety of types of cancer pain when given with various narcotics; (3) eases agoraphobia; (4) decreases symptoms in essential tremor; (5) decreases loudness of ear ringing in tinnitus; (6) can be helpful in alcohol withdrawal; (7) eases irritable bowel syndrome; (8) eases anxiety sometimes seen with depression.

How This Drug Works: Calms by enhancing the action of the nerve transmitter gamma-aminobutyric acid (GABA), which in turn blocks higher brain centers.

Available Dosage Forms and Strengths
      Tablets — 0.25 mg, 0.5 mg, 1 mg, 2 mg
Oral solution — 0.25 mg, 0.5 mg, 1 mg/5 ml
           — 0.25 mg/2.5 ml

▷ **Usual Adult Dosage Range:**   For anxiety and nervous tension: 0.25 mg to 0.5 mg three times daily. Maximum dose is 4 mg every 24 hours, taken in divided doses.

For panic disorder: Initially 0.5 mg three times daily; increase dose by 1 mg every 3 to 4 days as needed and tolerated. Some patients stopped having panic attacks with 6 mg a day. Maximum daily dose is 10 mg. **Note: Actual dose and schedule must be determined for each patient individually.**

Conditions Requiring Dosing Adjustments
Liver Function: A starting dose of 0.25 mg is prudent in patients with advanced liver disease. Slow increase in dose only if needed.
Kidney Function: The manufacturer does not define specific dose reductions.
Obesity: Takes a longer time to reach final concentrations in obese people. Doses should be calculated based on ideal rather than actual body weight.
▷ *Alcoholism:* Because of some of the physiological and liver changes in alcoholism, removal of drug from the body may be delayed. Lower doses/longer times (intervals) between doses are needed.

▷ **Dosing Instructions:**   May be taken on empty stomach or with food or milk. Tablet may be crushed. Do not stop this drug abruptly if taken for more than 4 weeks (stop slowly by decreasing 0.5 mg every 3 days or longer).

Usual Duration of Use: Several days to several weeks. Avoid prolonged/uninterrupted use. Continual use should not exceed 8 weeks without evaluation by your doctor.

Author's note: The National Institute of Mental Health has a new information page on anxiety. It can be found on the World Wide Web at www.nimh.nih.gov/anxiety

▷ **This Drug Should Not Be Taken If**
• you have had an allergic reaction to it previously.
• you are pregnant (first 3 months).
• you have acute narrow-angle glaucoma.
• you have myasthenia gravis.

▷ **Inform Your Physician Before Taking This Drug If**
• your history includes palpitations or tachycardia (may be worsened).
• you are allergic to benzodiazepines (see Drug Classes).

- you are pregnant (last 6 months) or planning pregnancy.
- you are breast-feeding your infant.
- you have a history of depression or serious mental illness (psychosis).
- you have a history of alcoholism or drug abuse.
- you have impaired liver or kidney function.
- you have open-angle glaucoma.
- you have a seizure disorder (epilepsy).
- you have severe chronic lung disease.
- you take other prescription or nonprescription medications that were not discussed when alprazolam was prescribed for you.
- you are unsure how much to take or how often to take alprazolam.

Possible Side Effects (natural, expected, and unavoidable drug actions)
Drowsiness, light-headedness—frequent.

▷ **Possible Adverse Effects** (unusual, unexpected, and infrequent reactions)
If any of the following develop, consult your physician promptly for guidance.
Mild Adverse Effects
Allergic reactions: skin rash, hives.
Headache, dizziness, fatigue, blurred vision, dry mouth—infrequent.
Drowsiness—frequent, up to 50%.
Nausea, vomiting, constipation—infrequent.
Increased salivation—infrequent.
Serious Adverse Effects
Confusion, hallucinations, depression, excitement, agitation (paradoxical reaction)—rare.
Tachycardia and palpitations—infrequent.
Increased liver enzymes—rare.
Low blood pressure (hypotension)—case report.

▷ **Possible Effects on Sexual Function:** Rare but documented: inhibited female orgasm (5 mg/day); impaired ejaculation (3.5 mg/day); decreased libido, impaired erection (4.5 mg/day); altered timing and pattern of menstruation (0.75–4 mg/day).

Possible Effects on Laboratory Tests
Liver function tests: increased ALT/GPT, AST/GOT—rare and insignificant.
Urine screening tests for drug abuse: may be **positive** (depends upon amount of drug taken and testing method).

CAUTION
1. **Do not** stop taking this drug abruptly if it has been taken continually for more than 4 weeks.
2. Some nonprescription drugs with antihistamines (allergy and cold medicines, sleep aids) can cause excessive sedation.

Precautions for Use
By Infants and Children: Safety and effectiveness for those under 18 not established.
By Those Over 60 Years of Age: Starting dose should be 0.25 mg two or three times daily. Watch for excessive drowsiness, dizziness, unsteadiness, and incoordination (possible low blood pressure).

▷ **Advisability of Use During Pregnancy**
Pregnancy Category: D. See Pregnancy Risk Categories at the back of this book.
Animal studies: Diazepam (a closely related benzodiazepine) can cause cleft palate in mice and skeletal defects in rats. No data on alprazolam.
Human studies: Some studies suggest an association between diazepam use and cleft lip and heart deformities. Adequate studies in pregnant women not available.
Avoid use during entire pregnancy if possible.

Advisability of Use If Breast-Feeding
Presence of this drug in breast milk: Yes.
Avoid drug or refrain from nursing.

Habit-Forming Potential: This drug can cause psychological and/or physical dependence (see Glossary), especially if used in large doses for an extended period of time.

Effects of Overdose: Marked drowsiness, weakness, feeling of drunkenness, staggering gait, tremor, stupor progressing to deep sleep or coma.

Possible Effects of Long-Term Use: Psychological and/or physical dependence.

Suggested Periodic Examinations While Taking This Drug (at physician's discretion)
None required for short-term use.

▷ **While Taking This Drug, Observe the Following**
Foods: No restrictions.
Beverages: Avoid excessive caffeine-containing beverages: coffee, tea, cola (counteracts effects). This drug may be taken with milk.
▷ *Alcohol:* Use with extreme caution. Alcohol may increase the sedative effects of alprazolam. Alprazolam may increase the intoxicating effects of alcohol. Avoid alcohol completely—throughout the day and the night—if you find it necessary to drive or engage in *any* hazardous activity.
Tobacco Smoking: Heavy smoking may reduce calming. I advise quitting smoking.
Marijuana Smoking: Occasional (once or twice weekly): Increased sedative effect.
Daily: Marked increase in sedative effect.
▷ *Other Drugs*
Alprazolam may *increase* the effects of
• digoxin (Lanoxin), and cause digoxin toxicity.
Alprazolam may *decrease* the effects of
• levodopa (Sinemet, etc.), and reduce its effect in treating Parkinson's disease.
The following drugs may *increase* the effects of alprazolam:
• azole antifungals, such as itraconazole (Sporanox) or ketoconazole (Nizoral).
• birth control pills (oral contraceptives—various kinds).
• cimetidine (Tagamet).
• disulfiram (Antabuse).
• fluoxetine (Prozac).
• fluvoxamine (Luvox).

- isoniazid (INH, Rifamate, etc.).
- macrolide antibiotics (such as erythromycin, clarithromycinor, azithromycin—see Drug Classes).
- omeprazole (Prilosec).
- paroxetine (Paxil).
- propoxyphene (Darvon, etc.)
- ritonavir (Norvir) and perhaps other protease inhibitors (see Drug Classes).
- sertraline (Zoloft).
- valproic acid (Depakene).

The following drugs may *decrease* the effects of alprazolam:
- carbamazepine (Tegretol).
- rifampin (Rimactane, etc.).
- theophylline (aminophylline, Theo-Dur, etc.).

Alprazolam *taken concurrently* with
- alcohol (ethanol) will worsen coordination and mental abilities.
- benzodiazepines (see Drug Classes) can cause increased central nervous system (CNS) depression.
- buspirone (Buspar) can result in additive CNS depression.
- central nervous system active agents (see *antihistamine* and *antipsychotic drug* classes) can cause increased central nervous system (CNS) depression.
- narcotics (morphine, meperidine, and others) will result in additive CNS depression.
- nefazidine (Serzone) may double the blood level.
- tricyclic and other kinds of antidepressants (see Drug Classes) results in additional CNS depression.

▷ *Driving, Hazardous Activities:* This drug can impair mental alertness, judgment, physical coordination, and reaction time. Avoid hazardous activities accordingly.

Aviation Note: The use of this drug *is a disqualification* for piloting. Consult a designated aviation medical examiner.

Exposure to Sun: Use caution; rare photosensitivity reports (see Glossary).

Discontinuation: If this drug has been taken for an extended period of time, do not stop it abruptly. Slowly reduce dose by 1 mg per week until a total daily dose of 4 mg is reached; by 0.5 mg per week until a total daily dose of 2 mg is reached; then by 0.25 mg per week thereafter. Ask your doctor for help.

AMANTADINE (a MAN ta deen)

Introduced: 1966   **Class:** Anti-parkinsonism, antiviral   **Prescription:** USA: Yes   **Controlled Drug:** USA: No; Canada: No   **Available as Generic:** USA: Yes; Canada: No

Brand Names: Symadine, Symmetrel

BENEFITS versus RISKS	
Possible Benefits	*Possible Risks*
Partial relief of rigidity, tremor, and impaired motion in all forms of parkinsonism	Skin rashes, mild to severe
	Confusion, hallucinations
	Congestive heart failure
Prevention and treatment of respiratory infections caused by influenza type A viruses*	Increased prostatism (see Glossary)
	Abnormally low white blood cell counts

▷ **Principal Uses**

As a Single Drug Product: Uses currently included in FDA-approved labeling: (1) Treats all forms of parkinsonism; (2) prevents or treats respiratory tract infections caused by influenza type A virus (rimantadine is the drug of first choice because of amantadine's more frequent CNS side effects); (3) eases drug-induced extrapyramidal symptoms.

Other (unlabeled) generally accepted uses: (1) Small role helping manage behavioral problems after some brain injuries; (2) some success reversing symptoms of mild dementia; (3) eases some resistant myoclonic or absence seizures; (4) may help bed-wetting (enuresis) in children; (5) eases fatigue in multiple sclerosis (MS). May help MS patients who have fatigue that keeps them from living normally.

How This Drug Works: It increases a nerve transmitter (dopamine) in some nerve centers and reduces muscular rigidity, tremor, and impaired movement associated with parkinsonism. By keeping the influenza from entering cells, it prevents the flu.

Available Dosage Forms and Strengths

Capsules (gelatin and softgel) — 100 mg

Syrup — 50 mg/5 ml

▷ **Usual Adult Dosage Range:**   Anti-parkinsonism: 100 mg once or twice daily. The total daily dose should not exceed 300 mg.

Antiviral: 200 mg once daily; or 100 mg every 12 hours.

Children 1 to 9 years old: Treatment of type A flu: 4.4 to 8.8 mg per kg of body mass per day, up to a maximum of 150 mg once daily. **Note: Actual dose and schedule must be determined for each patient individually.**

Conditions Requiring Dosing Adjustments

Liver Function: No dosing changes currently thought to be needed.

Kidney Function: Must be carefully adjusted to blood levels in people with kidney problems. Those with creatinine clearances of 30–50 ml/min should receive 100 mg daily. Those with 15–29 clearance should receive 100 mg every other day. Those with clearances less than 15 should receive 200 mg once a week.

Epilepsy: Doses of 200 mg/day should be avoided, as seizure risk may increase.

▷ **Dosing Instructions:**   May be taken with or following meals. Can open the capsule to take it.

Usual Duration of Use: Use on a regular schedule for up to 2 weeks usually needed to see best effect in relieving Parkinson's symptoms. Long-term use

---

*Does **NOT** prevent or treat viral infections other than those caused by influenza type A viruses.

(months to years) requires periodic check of response and dose changes. See your doctor on a regular basis.

Following exposure to influenza type A, protection requires continual daily doses for at least 10 days. During influenza epidemics, this drug may be given for 6 to 8 weeks.

▷ **This Drug Should Not Be Taken If**
- you have had an allergic reaction to it previously.

▷ **Inform Your Physician Before Taking This Drug If**
- you have any type of seizure disorder.
- you have a history of a serious emotional or mental disorder.
- you have a history of heart disease, especially previous heart failure.
- you have impaired liver or kidney function.
- you have a history of lowering of blood pressure when you stand (orthostatic hypotension).
- you have a history of peptic ulcer disease.
- you have eczema or recurring eczemalike skin rashes.
- you are taking any drugs for emotional or mental disorders.
- you take other prescription or nonprescription medicines not discussed when amantadine was prescribed for you.
- you have a history of low white blood cell counts.
- you are unsure how much to take or how often to take this medicine.

Possible Side Effects (natural, expected, and unavoidable drug actions)
Light-headedness, dizziness, weakness, feeling faint (see *orthostatic hypotension* in Glossary). Dry mouth, constipation. Reddish-blue pattern or patchy skin discoloration on your legs or feet (livedo reticularis). Transient and unimportant.

▷ **Possible Adverse Effects** (unusual, unexpected, and infrequent reactions)
If any of the following develop, consult your physician promptly for guidance.

Mild Adverse Effects
Allergic reaction: skin rash.
Headache, nervousness, irritability, inability to concentrate, insomnia, nightmares—rare to infrequent.
Unsteadiness, visual disturbances, slurred speech—infrequent.
Swelling (fluid retention) of arms, feet, or ankles—case report.
Difficulty breathing—possible.
Urine retention—rare.
Loss of appetite, nausea, vomiting—infrequent.

Serious Adverse Effects
Allergic reaction: severe eczemalike skin rashes.
Idiosyncratic reactions: confusion, depression, hallucinations, aggression—case reports to rare.
Increased seizure activity in (epileptics)—possible.
Congestive heart failure—rare.
Aggravation of prostatism (see Glossary)—possible.
Elevated liver function tests—rare.
Low white blood cell counts: fever, sore throat, infection—rare.
Catatonia or seizures (if abruptly stopped).
Myasthenia gravis—case reports.

▷ **Possible Effects on Sexual Function:**   None reported.

Adverse Effects That May Mimic Natural Diseases or Disorders
Mood changes, confusion, or hallucinations may suggest a psychotic disorder. Swelling of the legs and feet may suggest (but not necessarily indicate) heart, liver, or kidney disorder.

Natural Diseases or Disorders That May Be Activated by This Drug
Latent epilepsy, incipient congestive heart failure.

Possible Effects on Laboratory Tests
Liver function tests: increased (AST/GOT, alkaline phosphatase).
Kidney function tests: brief increase—blood urea nitrogen (BUN).

CAUTION
1. NARROW margin of safety. Do not exceed a total dose of 400 mg every 24 hours. Watch closely for adverse effects with doses over 200 mg every 24 hours.
2. Initial anti-parkinsonism benefit may last 3 to 6 months. If this happens, ask your doctor if a new drug or dose is needed.
3. May increase susceptibility to German measles. Avoid exposure to anyone with active German measles.
4. Watch for early signs of congestive heart failure: shortness of breath on exertion or during the night, mild cough, swelling of feet or ankles. Report these promptly to your doctor.

Precautions for Use
By Infants and Children: Safety and effectiveness for those under one not established.
By Those Over 60 Years of Age: Confusion, delirium, hallucinations, and disorderly conduct may develop. Prostatism may be aggravated.

▷ **Advisability of Use During Pregnancy**
Pregnancy Category: C. See Pregnancy Risk Categories at the back of this book.
Animal studies: Birth defects reported in rat studies; no defects reported in rabbit studies.
Human studies: Adequate studies of pregnant women are not available. Single case of heart lesions. Ask your doctor for help.

Advisability of Use If Breast-Feeding
Presence of this drug in breast milk: Yes.
Nursing infant may develop skin rash, vomiting, or urine retention. Avoid drug or refrain from nursing.

Habit-Forming Potential: This drug has a potential for abuse because of its ability to cause euphoria, hallucinations, and feelings of detachment.

Effects of Overdose: Hyperactivity, disorientation, confusion, visual hallucinations, aggressive behavior, severe toxic psychosis, seizures, heart rhythm disturbances, drop in blood pressure.

Possible Effects of Long-Term Use: Livedo reticularis (see "Possible Side Effects" above). Congestive heart failure in predisposed people.

Suggested Periodic Examinations While Taking This Drug (at physician's discretion)
White blood cell counts, liver and kidney function tests.
Evaluation of heart function.

▷ **While Taking This Drug, Observe the Following**

Foods: No restrictions.

Beverages: No restrictions. May be taken with milk.

▷ *Alcohol:* This combination may impair mental function and lower blood pressure excessively.

Tobacco Smoking: No interactions expected. I advise everyone to quit smoking.

Marijuana Smoking: Added drowsiness.

▷ *Other Drugs*

Amantadine may *increase* the effects of

- atropinelike drugs used to treat parkinsonism, especially benztropine (Cogentin), orphenadrine (Disipal), and trihexyphenidyl (Artane). Amantadine can increase results, but if doses are too large, these drugs (taken with amantadine) may cause confusion, delirium, hallucinations, and nightmares.
- levodopa (Dopar, Larodopa, Sinemet, etc.), and enhance results. Combination may cause acute mental disturbances.

The following drugs may *increase* the effects of amantadine:

- amphetamine and amphetamine-like stimulant drugs may cause excessive stimulation and adverse behavioral effects.
- hydrochlorothiazide with triamterene may increase the blood level of amantadine and cause toxicity.

Amantadine taken *concurrently* with

- cotrimoxazole may increase risk of CNS stimulation or arrhythmias.
- hydrochlorothiazide (Dyazide, Esidrix, others) may increase risk of amantadine toxicity.
- sulfamethoxazole may increase risk of CNS stimulation or arrhythmia.
- trimethoprim may increase risk of CNS stimulation or arrhythmias.

▷ *Driving, Hazardous Activities:* May cause drowsiness, dizziness, blurred vision, or confusion. If these drug effects occur, avoid hazardous activities.

Aviation Note: The use of this drug *may be a disqualification* for piloting. Consult a designated aviation medical examiner.

Exposure to Sun: No restrictions.

Exposure to Cold: Use caution. Excessive chilling may enhance the development of livedo reticularis (see "Possible Side Effects" above).

Discontinuation: When used to treat parkinsonism, this drug should not be stopped abruptly. Sudden discontinuation may cause an acute parkinsonian crisis. When used to treat influenza A infections, this drug should be continued for 48 hours after the disappearance of all symptoms.

AMILORIDE (a MIL oh ride)

Introduced: 1967   **Class:** Diuretic   **Prescription:** USA: Yes   **Controlled Drug:** USA: No; Canada: No   **Available as Generic:** Yes

Brand Names: ✤Apo-Amilzide, Midamor, ✤Moduret [CD], Moduretic [CD], ✤Novamilor[CD], ✤Nu-Amilzide [CD]

```
┌─────────────────────────────────────────────────────────────────┐
│                    BENEFITS versus RISKS                          │
│       Possible Benefits              Possible Risks               │
│   EFFECTIVE DIURETIC WITH       ABNORMALLY HIGH BLOOD             │
│     DECREASED POTASSIUM LOSS       POTASSIUM with excessive use   │
│                                 Rare heart arrhythmias            │
│                                 Rare kidney toxicity              │
│                                 Rare liver toxicity               │
└─────────────────────────────────────────────────────────────────┘
```

▷ **Principal Uses**

As a Single Drug Product: Uses currently included in FDA-approved labeling: (1) Eliminates excessive fluid (edema) seen in congestive heart failure; (2) treats high blood pressure, especially those prone to low potassium; (3) thiazide-caused low blood pressure.

As a Combination Drug Product [CD]: Combined with other thiazide diuretics to prevent excess potassium loss.

Other (unlabeled) generally accepted uses: (1) May be able to help dissolve kidney stones in patients unable to tolerate surgery; (2) can help correct increased urination that occurs in patients taking lithium.

How This Drug Works: This drug promotes loss of sodium and water from the body and potassium retention by altering kidney enzymes that control urine formation.

Available Dosage Forms and Strengths

Tablets — 5 mg

▷ **Usual Adult Dosage Range:** One 5-mg dose a day, preferably in the morning. May increase up to 15 mg daily as needed and tolerated. Should not exceed 20 mg every 24 hours. **Note: Actual dose and schedule must be determined for each patient individually.**

Conditions Requiring Dosing Adjustments

Liver Function: Extreme caution in patients with severe liver disease.

Kidney Function: Should NOT be used in patients who can't make urine or who have acute kidney failure or creatinine clearance less than 50 ml/min.

▷ **Dosing Instructions:** Best taken when you wake up, with food. Tablet may be crushed for administration.

Usual Duration of Use: Ongoing long-term use to treat high blood pressure. As needed to lose abnormal fluid. Intermittent or every other day use to minimize imbalance of sodium and potassium.

▷ **This Drug Should Not Be Taken If**
- you have had an allergic reaction to it before.
- your blood potassium level is above the normal range.
- you have diabetic nerve damage (diabetic nephropathy).
- your kidneys are not making urine.

▷ **Inform Your Physician Before Taking This Drug If**
- you are allergic any similar drug.
- you have diabetes or glaucoma.
- you have kidney disease or impaired kidney function.
- you take any other diuretic, blood pressure drug, any form of digitalis, or lithium.
- you don't know how much to take or how often to take it.

Possible Side Effects (natural, expected, and unavoidable drug actions)
Abnormally high blood potassium level—infrequent.
Abnormally low blood sodium level, dehydration, decreased blood magnesium, constipation—possible.
Dizziness on standing (orthostatic hypotension)—possible.

▷ **Possible Adverse Effects** (unusual, unexpected, and infrequent reactions)
If any of the following develop, consult your physician promptly for guidance.
Mild Adverse Effects
Allergic reactions: skin rash, itching—rare to infrequent.
Headache—infrequent.
Dizziness, weakness, fatigue, numbness, and tingling—case reports (related to electrolyte problems).
Dry mouth, nausea, vomiting, stomach pains, diarrhea—infrequent.
Decreased ability to taste salt—possible.
Loss of scalp hair—rare.
Serious Adverse Effects
Idiosyncratic reactions: joint and muscle pains.
Liver or kidney toxicity—rare.
Abnormally low sodium level—case reports.
Increased internal eye pressure (of concern in glaucoma)—rare.
Depression, visual disturbances, ringing in ears, tremors—infrequent.
Bone marrow depression—rare (questionable cause).
Palpitations and arrhythmias—rare.

▷ **Possible Effects on Sexual Function:**   Decreased libido or impotence (5 to 10 mg per day)—rare.

Adverse Effects That May Mimic Natural Diseases or Disorders
Nervousness, confusion, or depression may mimic spontaneous mental disorder.

Natural Diseases or Disorders That May Be Activated by This Drug
Preexisting peptic ulcer, latent glaucoma.

Possible Effects on Laboratory Tests
Blood cholesterol level: decreased.
Blood creatinine level: increased with long-term use.
Blood potassium level: possibly increased.
Blood uric acid level: decreased with long-term use.
Blood sodium level: possibly decreased.

CAUTION
1. Do **NOT** take potassium supplements or eat more high potassium foods.
2. More frequent potassium levels are needed if you take digitalis compounds.
3. Do not stop this drug abruptly unless your doctor says you must.

Precautions for Use
By Infants and Children: Oral dosing with 0.625 mg per kg of body mass daily has been used to promote water loss (diuresis) in young patients weighing from 6 to 20 kg.
By Those Over 60 Years of Age: Declines in kidney function may make it likely that you will retain potassium. Limit use of this drug to periods of 2 to 3

weeks if possible. The dose MUST be reduced. May cause too much water loss, possible increased tendency of the blood to clot and increased risk of clots (thrombosis, heart attack, stroke).

▷ **Advisability of Use During Pregnancy**

Pregnancy Category: B. See Pregnancy Risk Categories at the back of this book.
Animal studies: No birth defects reported.
Human studies: Adequate studies of pregnant women are not available.
Use only if clearly needed.

Advisability of Use If Breast-Feeding

Presence of this drug in breast milk: Unknown, but probably present. This drug may suppress milk production.
Avoid drug if possible. If use is necessary, watch nursing infant closely and stop drug or nursing if adverse effects develop.

Habit-Forming Potential: None.

Effects of Overdose: Thirst, drowsiness, fatigue, weakness, nausea, vomiting, confusion, numbness and tingling of face and extremities, irregular heart rhythm, shortness of breath.

Suggested Periodic Examinations While Taking This Drug (at physician's discretion)

Complete blood counts; blood levels of sodium, potassium, magnesium, and chloride; kidney function tests; and check of water balance (state of hydration).

▷ **While Taking This Drug, Observe the Following**

Foods: Avoid excessive salt restriction and high potassium foods. Taking this drug with food may help nausea and stomach upset. Caution: Ginseng may increase blood pressure.

Beverages: No restrictions. May be taken with milk.

▷ *Alcohol:* Use caution. Alcohol can exaggerate the blood-pressure-lowering effect of this drug and cause orthostatic hypotension (see Glossary).

Tobacco Smoking: No interactions expected. I advise everyone to quit smoking.

▷ *Other Drugs*

Amiloride may ***increase*** the effects of
• other blood-pressure-lowering drugs. Dose decreases may be needed.

Amiloride may ***decrease*** the effects of
• digoxin (Lanoxin, etc.), and reduce its effect in treating heart failure.

Amiloride ***taken concurrently*** with
• ACE inhibitors (see Drug Classes) such as benazepril, or angiotensin II antagonists such as valsartan (Diovan), etc., may result in abnormally high blood potassium.
• lithium (Lithobid) may cause lithium toxicity.
• metformin (Glucophage) may increase glucophage levels and increase lactic acidosis or excessively lowered blood sugar hypoglycemia) risk.
• NSAIDs (nonsteroidal anti-inflammatory drugs; see Drug Classes) may decrease therapeutic effect.
• potassium supplements may result in extremely elevated blood potassium levels.
• spironolactone (Aldactone, Aldactazide) or triamterene (Dyrenium, Dyazide) may cause dangerously high potassium levels. Avoid these combinations.

▷   *Driving, Hazardous Activities:* May cause drowsiness, dizziness, and orthostatic hypotension. If these drug effects occur, avoid hazardous activities.

Aviation Note: The use of this drug **may be a disqualification** for piloting. Consult a designated aviation medical examiner.

Exposure to Sun: No restrictions.

Exposure to Heat: Caution is advised. Excessive sweating can cause water, sodium, and potassium imbalance. Hot environments can cause lowering of blood pressure.

Occurrence of Unrelated Illness: Call your doctor if you contract an illness causing vomiting or diarrhea.

Discontinuation: With high doses or prolonged use, withdraw this drug gradually. Excessive potassium loss may occur with sudden withdrawal.

AMINOPHYLLINE (am in OFF i lin)

Other Name: Theophylline ethylenediamine

Introduced: 1910   **Class:** Antiasthmatic, bronchodilator, xanthines   **Prescription:** USA: Yes   **Controlled Drug:** USA: No; Canada: No   **Available as Generic:** Yes

Brand Names: Aminophyllin, Mudrane [CD], Mudrane GG [CD], ✦Palaron, Phyllocontin, Somophyllin, ✦Somophyllin-12, Truphylline

Author's Note: This drug is actually (79%) theophylline. See the theophylline profile for further details.

AMITRIPTYLINE (a mee TRIP ti leen)

Introduced: 1961   **Class:** Antidepressant   **Prescription:** USA: Yes
Controlled Drug: USA: No; Canada: No   **Available as Generic:** Yes

Brand Names: Amitril, ✦Apo-Amitriptyline, Elavil, ✦Elavil Plus [CD], Emitrip, Endep, Enovil, Etrafon [CD], ✦Etrafon-A [CD], ✦Etrafon-D [CD], Etrafon-Forte [CD], ✦Levate, ✦Novo-Triptyn, PMS-Levazine [CD], SK-Amitriptyline, ✦Triavil [CD]

BENEFITS versus RISKS	
Possible Benefits	*Possible Risks*
EFFECTIVE RELIEF OF ENDOGENOUS DEPRESSION	ADVERSE BEHAVIORAL EFFECTS: Confusion, disorientation, hallucinations
Additive (adjunctive) therapy in some pain syndromes	CONVERSION OF DEPRESSION TO MANIA in manic-depressive disorders
	Irregular heart rhythms—possible
	Blood cell abnormalities—rare

▷ **Principal Uses**

As a Single Drug Product: Uses currently included in FDA-approved labeling: (1) Eases symptoms of spontaneous (endogenous) depression—should only be used to treat a true, significant primary depression; (2) helps depression resistant (refractory) to a single medicine.

Other (unlabeled) generally accepted uses: (1) Additive (adjuvant) therapy in chronic pain/pain syndromes; (2) eases agitation; (3) helps diabetic nerve (neuropathy) pain; (4) is an alternative in intractable hiccups; (5) combined with other medicines to ease the pain of postherpetic neuralgia; (6) some benefit in easing pain of chronic vulvar burning (vulvodynia); (7) used in fish (ciguatera) poisoning.

As a Combination Drug Product [CD]: Combined with chlordiazepoxide to relieve anxiety and depression.

Also available in combination with perphenazine, a phenothiazine,to relieve severe agitation that may occur with depression.

How This Drug Works: Eases depression by restoring normal levels of two nerve impulse chemicals (norepinephrine and serotonin).

Available Dosage Forms and Strengths

Injection — 10 mg/ml
Oral suspension — 10 mg/5 ml
Tablets — 10 mg, 25 mg, 50 mg, 75 mg, 100 mg, 150 mg

▷ **Usual Adult Dosage Range:** Intramuscular injection is given as 80 to 120 mg per day divided into four doses. Switch to oral form made as soon as possible. Oral dosing starts with 25 mg two to four times daily. May be increased cautiously as needed/tolerated by 10 to 25 mg daily at intervals of 1 week. Usual ongoing dose is 50 to 100 mg daily. Total dose should not exceed 150 mg daily. Once the best dose is found, it may be taken at bedtime as one dose. Some clinicians start with 50 mg at bedtime. **Note: Actual dose and schedule must be determined for each patient individually.**

Conditions Requiring Dosing Adjustments

Liver Function: Specific guidelines not available; however, low doses and a check of blood levels is prudent.

Kidney Function: Lower doses and blood level checks are needed with kidney failure (18% of drug is removed this way).

▷ **Dosing Instructions:** May be taken without regard to meals. Tablet may be crushed to take it.

Usual Duration of Use: Some benefit in 1 to 2 weeks, but peak benefit may take 30 days or longer. Long-term use should not exceed 6 months without follow-up evaluation.

▷ **This Drug Should Not Be Taken If**
- you are allergic to any of the brand names listed above.
- you are taking or have taken within the past 14 days any monoamine oxidase (MAO) type A inhibitor drug (see Drug Classes).
- you have heart-induced chest pain (angina pectoris).
- you have a rapid heart rate that occurs spontaneously (paroxysmal tachycardia).
- you have heart (cardiovascular) disease or abnormal heart rhythms, or are recovering from a recent heart attack.
- you have narrow-angle glaucoma.
- you are pregnant.
- you have congestive heart failure.

▷ **Inform Your Physician Before Taking This Drug If**
- you have a history of: diabetes, epilepsy (or other seizure disorder), glaucoma, heart disease, prostate gland enlargement, or overactive thyroid function.
- you will have surgery with general anesthesia.
- you take other prescription or nonprescription medicines not discussed when this drug was prescribed.
- you are unsure how much to take or how often to take it.
- you have a history of schizophrenia—this drug may worsen any paranoia.
- you have a history of prostate or sexual problems.
- you have a liver or kidney disorder.
- you have a blood cell disorder.
- you have a history of intestinal block (ileus).

Possible Side Effects (natural, expected, and unavoidable drug actions)
Drowsiness, blurred vision, dry mouth, constipation, impaired urination.

▷ **Possible Adverse Effects** (unusual, unexpected, and infrequent reactions)
If any of the following develop, consult your physician promptly for guidance.

Mild Adverse Effects
Allergic reactions: skin rash, hives, swelling of face or tongue, drug fever (see Glossary).
Headache, dizziness, weakness, fainting, unsteady gait, tremors—infrequent.
Peculiar taste, irritation of tongue or mouth, nausea, indigestion—rare to infrequent.
Fluctuation of blood sugar levels—possible.
Increased dental cavities (caries)—increased risk.
Restlessness and nightmares—rare.
Change in the ability to perceive tones—case report.

Serious Adverse Effects
Allergic reactions: hepatitis (see Glossary).
Idiosyncratic reactions: neuroleptic malignant syndrome (see Glossary).
Confusion or hallucinations—may be more likely in older patients and with higher doses.
Bowel obstruction (ileus)—rare.
SIADH (see Glossary)—rare.
Excessively low blood pressure (hypotension)—possible.
Seizures—rare.
Severe eye or other movement problems—case reports.
Heart palpitation and irregular rhythm—rare and more likely with increasing doses or overdose.
Bone marrow depression (see Glossary): fatigue, weakness, fever, sore throat, abnormal bleeding or bruising—rare.
Peripheral neuritis (see Glossary): numbness, tingling, pain, loss of arm or leg strength—possible.
Parkinson-like disorders (see Glossary): often mild and infrequent—more likely in the elderly.
Liver toxicity—rare.
Worsening of paranoid psychosis in schizophrenic patients—possible.

▷ **Possible Effects on Sexual Function:**   Decreased libido—rare; increased libido (possible antidepressant effect), inhibited female orgasm, inhibited ejaculation—case reports; male and female breast enlargement, milk production, swelling of testicles, impotence—case reports. These effects usually disappear within 2 to 10 days after discontinuation of the drug.

Adverse Effects That May Mimic Natural Diseases or Disorders
Liver toxicity may suggest viral hepatitis.

Natural Diseases or Disorders That May Be Activated by This Drug
Latent diabetes, epilepsy, glaucoma, impaired urination due to prostate.

Possible Effects on Laboratory Tests
Complete blood counts: decreased white cells and platelets; increased eosinophils.
Liver function tests: increased ALT/GPT, AST/GOT, alkaline phosphatase, increased bilirubin.
Blood glucose levels: increased or decreased (fluctuations).

CAUTION
1. Make sure you make follow-up visits to your doctor.
2. Best to withhold this drug if electroconvulsive therapy (ECT, "shock" treatment) is to be used.

Precautions for Use
By Infants and Children: Safety and effectiveness for those under 12 years old not established.
By Those Over 60 Years of Age: During the first 2 weeks watch for confusion, agitation, forgetfulness, delusions, and hallucinations. Decreased dose or stopping the drug may be needed. Unsteadiness may predispose to falling and injury. May worsen impaired urination seen with prostate gland enlargement (prostatism).

▷ **Advisability of Use During Pregnancy**
Pregnancy Category: D. See Pregnancy Risk Categories at the back of this book.
Animal studies: Skull deformities reported in rabbits.
Human studies: No defects reported in 21 exposures, one case report of a leg deformity in a woman also taking prochlorperazine. Adequate studies of pregnant women are not available. Avoid use of drug during first 3 months. Use during last 6 months only if clearly needed.

Advisability of Use If Breast-Feeding
Presence of this drug in breast milk: Yes, in small amounts.
Watch nursing infant closely and stop drug or nursing if adverse effects start.

Habit-Forming Potential: If prolonged therapy has been given, stopping this medicine suddenly can lead to headache, nausea, and weakness (malaise). Rare reports of hypomania or mania have been made 2 to 7 days after stopping therapy with tricyclic antidepressants.

Effects of Overdose: Confusion, hallucinations, marked drowsiness, heart palpitations, dilated pupils, tremors, stupor, deep sleep, coma, convulsions.

Suggested Periodic Examinations While Taking This Drug (at physician's discretion)
Complete blood cell counts, liver function tests, serial blood pressure readings, and electrocardiograms.

▷ **While Taking This Drug, Observe the Following**
Foods: Excessive vitamin C can blunt therapeutic benefit of this drug. May also increase appetite and cause excessive weight gain.

Beverages: No restrictions. May be taken with milk.

▷   *Alcohol:* Avoid completely. Can markedly increase the intoxicating effects of alcohol and brain function depression.

Tobacco Smoking: May hasten the removal of this drug from your body. I advise you to quit smoking.

▷   *Other Drugs*

Amitriptyline may ***increase*** the effects of

- albuterol or other direct sympathomimetic drugs (amphetamines, epinephrine).
- antihistamines (such as diphenhydramine—Benadryl, others) can increase the risk of urinary retention, chronic glaucoma, and bowel obstruction (ileus). This is especially problematic in the elderly.
- atropinelike drugs (see ***anticholinergic drugs*** in Drug Classes).
- cimetidine (Tagamet).
- disulfiram (Antabuse) if alcohol is consumed.
- phenytoin (Dilantin).

Amitriptyline may ***decrease*** the effects of

- clonidine (Catapres).
- guanethidine (Ismelin).
- guanfacine (Hytrin).
- methyldopa; can result in reduced amitriptyline and/or methyldopa benefits.

Amitriptyline ***taken concurrently*** with

- amphetamines can result in abnormally increased responses to amitriptyline.
- anticoagulants such as warfarin (Coumadin) may cause an increased risk of bleeding.
- carbamazepine (Tegretol) may decrease the blood level of amitriptyline.
- epinephrine may cause an increased risk of rapid heart rate and high blood pressure.
- estrogens (see Drug Classes) may increase amitriptyline drug levels.
- ethanol (alcohol) may result in additive toxicity to the central nervous system.
- fluoxetine (Prozac) can result in very high levels of amitriptyline.
- fluvoxamine (Luvox) can result in very high levels of amitriptyline.
- grepafloxacin (Raxar) may result in heart toxicity—DO NOT COMBINE.
- meperidine (Demerol) may worsen chances of breathing (respiratory) depression.
- monoamine oxidase (MAO) type A inhibitor drugs (see Drug Classes) may cause high fever, delirium, and convulsions.
- potassium (various) may lead to ulceration from potassium as amitriptyline may slow the intestine.
- quinidine (Quinaglute, etc.) can result in increased antidepressant blood levels.
- ritonavir (Norvir) and perhaps other protease inhibitors (see Drug Classes) can lead to amitriptyline toxicity.
- thyroid preparations may impair heart rhythm and function. Ask your doctor for help with adjustment of thyroid dose.
- tramadol (Ultram) may increase risk of seizures. This combination is not advised.

- venlafaxine (Effexor) can result in very high levels of amitriptyline.
- verapamil (Calan, others) can result in very high levels of amitriptyline.

▷ *Driving, Hazardous Activities:* This drug may impair mental alertness, judgment, physical coordination, and reaction time. Avoid hazardous activities.

Aviation Note: The use of this drug *is a disqualification* for piloting. Consult a designated aviation medical examiner.

Exposure to Sun: This drug may cause photosensitivity (see Glossary).

Exposure to Heat: This drug can inhibit sweating and impair the body's adaptation to hot environments, increasing the risk of heatstroke. Avoid saunas.

Exposure to Cold: The elderly should avoid conditions conducive to hypothermia (see Glossary).

Discontinuation: It is best to stop this drug gradually. Abrupt withdrawal after long-term use can cause headache, malaise, and nausea.

AMLODIPINE (am LOH di peen)

Introduced: 1986   **Class:** Anti-anginal, antihypertensive, calcium channel blocker   **Prescription:** USA: Yes   **Controlled Drug:** USA: No; Canada: No   **Available as Generic:** No

Brand Names: Lotrel [CD], Norvasc

Controversies in Medicine: Medicines in this class have had many conflicting reports. The FDA has held hearings on the calcium channel blocker (CCB) class. A study called ALLHAT is comparing amlodipine, an ACE inhibitor, a diuretic, and an alpha blocker (see Drug Classes) and should clarify adverse effects, mortality, and other issues relating to CCBs. **Amlodipine got the first FDA approval to treat high blood pressure or angina in people with congestive heart failure**. CCBs are currently second-line agents for high blood pressure, according to the JNC VI (see Glossary).

BENEFITS versus RISKS	
Possible Benefits	*Possible Risks*
EFFECTIVE PREVENTION OF BOTH MAJOR TYPES OF ANGINA EFFECTIVE TREATMENT OF HYPERTENSION	DOSE-RELATED CHANGES IN HEART RHYTHM Peripheral edema (fluid retention in feet and ankles) Dose-related palpitations Other medicines in the same family have: Rare concern about depression, memory loss, or malignancy

▷ **Principal Uses**

As a Single Drug Product: Uses currently included in FDA-approved labeling: (1) Treats angina pectoris due to spontaneous coronary artery spasm (Prinzmetal's variant angina) and is not associated with exertion; (2) classical angina-of-effort (caused by 'hardening' or atherosclerosis of coronary arteries) in people who don't respond or can't tolerate nitrates or beta-blockers; (3) mild to moderate hypertension; (4) hypertension or angina in people who also have congestive heart failure.

Other (unlabeled) generally accepted uses: (1) May keep early atherosclerotic lesions from getting worse; (2) can help stop premature labor; (3) helps some symptoms in cases of lung (pulmonary) hypertension.

As a Combination Drug Product [CD]: In combination with benazepril offers the benefits of an ACE inhibitor and a calcium channel blocker.

How This Drug Works: This drug blocks normal passage of calcium through cell walls, inhibiting coronary artery and peripheral arteriole narrowing. As a result, this drug

- prevents spontaneous coronary artery spasm (Prinzmetal's angina).
- decreases heart rate and contraction force in exertion, making effort-induced angina less likely.
- opens contracted peripheral arterial walls, lowering blood pressure (also lessens heart work and helps prevent angina).

Available Dosage Forms and Strengths
Lotrel tablets — 2.5/10 mg, 5/10 mg and 5/20 mg
    Tablets — 2.5 mg, 5 mg, 10 mg

▷ **Recommended Dosage Ranges** (Actual dose and schedule must be determined for each patient individually.)

Infants and Children: Dosage not established.

12 to 60 Years of Age: High blood pressure: 2.5 to 10 mg daily, in a single dose. Chronic angina: 5 to 10 mg daily; 10 mg may improve exercise ability in stable angina patients.

Congestive heart failure: 5 mg once daily for 2 weeks with increase to 10 mg as needed and tolerated.

Over 65 Years of Age: Lower doses (2.5 mg for high blood pressure and 5 mg for angina) are prudent and effective.

Conditions Requiring Dosing Adjustments

Liver Function: Patients with damaged livers started on a daily 2.5-mg dose for high blood pressure, 5 mg for angina. Then dosing may be slowly increased as needed or tolerated.

Kidney Function: No adjustment in dosing is needed.

Low Protein or Starvation: This drug is moved around the body by a protein called albumin. If protein is low, (in liver failure or starvation), increased effect may be seen with "normal" doses. Start therapy with low doses. Increased only if needed or tolerated.

▷ **Dosing Instructions:**   May be taken with or following food to reduce stomach irritation. The tablet may be crushed.

Usual Duration of Use: Regular use for 2 to 4 weeks often needed to see benefit in reducing angina frequency or severity of angina and in reducing high blood pressure control. Best to use the lowest dose that works for long-term use (months to years). Periodic evaluation by your doctor is needed.

Possible Advantages of This Drug
Slow onset and prolonged effect, allowing effective once-a-day treatment for both angina and high blood pressure.

▷ **This Drug Should Not Be Taken If**
- you have had an allergic reaction to it previously.
- you have active liver disease.
- you have low blood pressure—systolic below 90 mm Hg.

- you have atrioventricular block or sick sinus syndrome (talk to your doctor).
- your left heart ventricle doesn't work well (dysfunctional).
- you have a seriously contracted or narrowed (stenosed) aorta.

▷ **Inform Your Physician Before Taking This Drug If**
- you have had a bad reaction to any calcium blocker.
- you take digitalis or a beta-blocker (see Drug Classes).
- you are taking any drugs that lower blood pressure.
- you have had congestive heart failure, heart attack, or stroke.
- you are subject to disturbances of heart rhythm.
- you have a history of drug-induced liver damage.
- you develop a rash while taking this medicine.
- you are unsure how much to take or how often to take it.
- you have circulation problems in your hands.
- you have muscular dystrophy.

Possible Side Effects (natural, expected, and unavoidable drug actions)
Swelling of feet and ankles, flushing (4.5% in women and 1.5% in men) and sensation of warmth.
Impaired sense of smell.

▷ **Possible Adverse Effects** (unusual, unexpected, and infrequent reactions)
If any of the following develop, consult your physician promptly for guidance.
Mild Adverse Effects
Allergic reactions: skin rash (call your doctor, as persistent rashes may become serious).
Headache (up to 12%), dizziness (dose related)—infrequent; fatigue, nausea, or constipation—infrequent.
Dose-related palpitations: low dose—rare; 10 mg—infrequent.
Overgrowth of the gums (gingival hyperplasia)—up to 10% with drugs in the same class.
Increased urge to urinate at night—rare.
Visual changes (eye pain, double vision)—rare.
Ringing in the ears (tinnitus)—rare.
Cough, muscle pain—infrequent.
Dose-related flushing (4.5% in women and 1.5% in men)—infrequent.
Elevated liver enzymes (may be a hypersensitivity—usually resolves)—rare.
Serious Adverse Effects
Allergic reactions: none reported.
Idiosyncratic reactions: Parkinson-like symptoms—case report.
Dose-dependent edema (up to 6.2 % in those over 65)—infrequent.
Exfoliative dermatitis or erythema multiforme—rare.
Agranulocytosis (only with other medicines in this class—case reports).
Rebound angina—if drug is abruptly stopped.
Difficulty breathing (dyspnea)—infrequent.

▷ **Possible Effects on Sexual Function:** Sexual dysfunction—both men and women—1–2%.
Swelling and tenderness of male breast tissue (gynecomastia)—case report.

Adverse Effects That May Mimic Natural Diseases or Disorders
An allergic rash and swelling of the legs may resemble erysipelas.

Possible Effects on Laboratory Tests
    Liver function tests: transient increases in liver enzymes.

CAUTION
1. Make sure all your health care providers know you take this drug. List this drug on a card in your purse or wallet.
2. Nitroglycerin or other nitrate drugs can be used as needed to ease acute angina pain. If your attacks become more frequent or intense, call your doctor promptly.

Precautions for Use
    By Infants and Children: Safety and effectiveness for use by those under 12 not established.
    By Those Over 60 Years of Age May be more likely to be weak, dizzy, faint, or fall. Be careful to prevent injury. Low starting doses are prudent.

▷ **Advisability of Use During Pregnancy**
    Pregnancy Category: C. See Pregnancy Risk Categories at the back of this book.
    Animal studies: No information available.
    Human studies: Adequate studies of pregnant women are not available.
    Avoid this drug during the first 3 months. Use during the last 6 months only if clearly needed. Ask your physician for guidance.

Advisability of Use If Breast-Feeding
    Presence of this drug in breast milk: Unknown.
    Avoid drug or refrain from nursing.

Habit-Forming Potential: None.

Effects of Overdose: Weakness, fainting, fast pulse, low blood pressure, slow heartbeat, metabolic acidosis, low potassium and calcium, sinus arrest, heart attack, seizures.

Possible Effects of Long-Term Use: Possible overgrowth of the gums.

Suggested Periodic Examinations While Taking This Drug (at physician's discretion)
    Heart function tests: electrocardiograms, blood pressure check while supine, sitting, and standing.

▷ **While Taking This Drug, Observe the Following**
    Foods: One medicine in this class is increased by grapefruit or grapefruit juice. Avoid eating grapefruit for an hour after taking this medicine. Avoid excessive salt intake. Caution: Ginseng may increase blood pressure.
    Beverages: One medicine in this class is increased by grapefruit juice. Do not take this medicine with grapefruit juice. Avoid grapefruit juice for an hour after you take this medicine. May be taken with milk.
▷   *Alcohol:* Use caution. Alcohol may exaggerate the drop in blood pressure.
    Tobacco Smoking: Nicotine may reduce the effectiveness of this drug. I advise everyone to quit smoking.
    Marijuana Smoking: Possible reduced effectiveness of this drug; mild to moderate increase in angina; possible changes in electrocardiogram, confusing interpretation.
▷   *Other Drugs*
        Amlodipine *taken concurrently* with
        • adenosine (Adenocard) may cause extended problems with slow heart rate.
        • azole antifungals (such as fluconazole [Diflucan] or itraconazole [Spora-

nox]; see Drug Classes), and imidazoles such as ketoconazole (Nizoral) may lead to toxic amlodipine blood levels.
- beta-blocker drugs or digitalis preparations (see Drug Classes) may cause heart rate and rhythm problems.
- cyclosporine (Sandimmune) causes increased cyclosporine blood levels and increased risk of toxicity.
- delavirdine (Rescriptor) may cause increased amlodipine levels and toxicity.
- NSAIDs or oral anticoagulants such as warfarin (Coumadin; see *nonsteroidal anti-inflammatory drugs* in Drug Classes) may lead to increased risk of bleeding in the gastrointestinal (GI) tract.
- rifampin (Rifater, others) may result in decreased therapeutic benefit of amlodipine.
- ritonavir (Norvir) and probably other protease inhibitors (see Drug Classes) may lead to amlodipine toxicity.

The following drug may *increase* the effects of amlodipine
- cimetidine (Tagamet).

▷ *Driving, Hazardous Activities:* This drug may cause dizziness. Restrict activities as necessary.
Aviation Note: Coronary artery disease *is a disqualification* for piloting. Consult a designated aviation medical examiner.
Exposure to Sun: No restrictions.
Exposure to Heat: Caution is advised. Hot environments can exaggerate the blood-pressure-lowering effects of this drug. Observe for light-headedness or weakness.
Heavy Exercise or Exertion: This drug may improve your ability to be more active without resulting angina pain. Use caution.
Discontinuation: Do not stop this drug abruptly—gradual is often prudent. Watch for development of rebound angina.

AMOXAPINE (a MOX a peen)

Introduced: 1970   **Class:** Antidepressant   **Prescription:** USA: Yes
Controlled Drug: USA: No; Canada: No   **Available as Generic:** Yes
Brand Name: Asendin

BENEFITS versus RISKS	
Possible Benefits	*Possible Risks*
EFFECTIVE RELIEF OF PRIMARY DEPRESSIONS: Endogenous, neurotic, reactive	ADVERSE BEHAVIORAL EFFECTS: Confusion, delusions, disorientation, hallucinations
	CONVERSION OF DEPRESSION TO MANIA in manic-depressive disorders
	Rare blood cell abnormalities
	Rare movement disorders
	Rare seizures
	Rare liver toxicity

Author's Note: Since use of this medicine has declined in favor of newer medicines, the information in this profile has been shortened.

AMOXICILLIN (a mox i SIL in)

AMOXICILLIN/CLAVULANATE (a mox i SIL in/KLAV yu lan ayt)

AMPICILLIN (am pi SIL in)

See the penicillin family profile for further information on these medicines.

ANGIOTENSIN CONVERTING ENZYME (ACE) INHIBITOR FAMILY

Captopril (KAP toh pril)   **Enalapril** (e NAL a pril)   **Quinapril** (KWIN a pril) **Benazepril** (ben AY ze pril)   **Ramipril** (RAH mi pril)   **Fosinopril** (Foh SIN oh pril)   **Lisinopril** (li SIN oh pril)

Introduced: 1979, 1981, 1984, 1985, 1985, 1986, 1988   **Class:** Antihypertensive, ACE inhibitor   **Prescription:** USA: Yes   **Controlled Drug:** USA: No; Canada: No   **Available as Generic:** Yes (captopril and enalapril)

Brand Names: Captopril: ✦Apo-Capto, Capoten, Capozide [CD], ✦Novo-Captopril, ✦Nu-Capto, ✦Syn-Captopril; Enalapril: ✦Vaseretic (also in U.S.) [CD], Vasotec; Quinapril: Accupril; Benazepril: Lotensin, Lotensin HCT [CD], Lotrel [CD]; Ramipril: Altace; Fosinopril: Monopril; Lisinopril: Prinivil, Prinzide [CD], Zestoretic [CD], Zestril

BENEFITS versus RISKS	
Possible Benefits	*Possible Risks*
EFFECTIVE CONTROL OF MILD TO SEVERE HIGH BLOOD PRESSURE	Impaired white blood cell production—rare (none for ramipril)
USEFUL ADJUNCTIVE TREATMENT FOR CONGESTIVE HEART FAILURE	Bone marrow depression—rare (none for ramipril)
MAY DECREASE RISK OF KIDNEY PROBLEMS IN DIABETICS TAKING INSULIN	Allergic swelling of face, tongue, throat, vocal cords
MAY REDUCE RISK OF DEATH AFTER A HEART ATTACK (Captopril or Lisinopril are FDA approved for this)	Kidney damage—rare (enalapril, lisinopril, quinapril and ramipril lower risk)
MAY BE DRUGS OF FIRST CHOICE FOR PATIENTS WITH HIGH BLOOD PRESSURE WHO EXERCISE	Liver damage—rare (none for ramipril)

▷ **Principal Uses**

As Single Drug Products: Uses currently included in FDA-approved labeling: (1) Treats all degrees of high blood pressure; (2) may help prevent death after heart attacks; (3) used in advanced heart failure; (4) used in diabetics who have kidney problems; (5) helps people live longer (improves survival) in cases of congestive heart failure.

Author's note: Enalapril was studied in the ABCD trial and was found to control blood pressure and also decrease risk of heart attack in diabetics. More research is needed.

Other (unlabeled) generally accepted uses: (1) Helps relieve symptoms of cystinuria (captopril); (2) may ease rheumatoid arthritis symptoms (captopril or enalapril); (3) can help Raynaud's phenomenon symptoms (captopril); (4) lisinopril may help prevent migraines; (5) enalapril and quinapril may be helpful in aortic regurgitation.

Author's note: One large study found that patients using captopril had similar low rates of nonfatal and fatal heart (cardiovascular) events as patients taking beta-blockers or diuretics. Another study showed that fosinopril cut the risk of heart attack or stroke by 51% in people who have high blood pressure and diabetes.

As Combination Drug Products [CD]: In combination with hydrochlorothiazide, captopril, enalapril, lisinopril, and benazepril offer the benefits of an ACE inhibitor and a diuretic. Benazepril has also been combined with amlodipine, a calcium channel blocker.

How These Drugs Work: By blocking an enzyme system (ACE), these drugs relax arterial walls and lower pressure. This decreases the heart's workload and improves its performance. Benefits after heart attack result from blunting response to catecholamines, free-radical scavenging, and increased prostacyclin or bradykinin. Use in combination with a diuretic helps ease fluid load.

Available Dosage Forms and Strengths

Captopril:
Tablets — 12.5 mg, 25 mg, 50 mg, 100 mg
Enalapril:
Injection — 1.25 mg/ml
Tablets — 2.5 mg, 5 mg, 10 mg, 20 mg
Vaseretic:
Tablets — 10 mg enalapril and 25 mg of hydrochlorothiazide
Quinapril:
Tablets — 5 mg, 10 mg, 20 mg, 40 mg
Benazepril:
— 5 mg, 10 mg, 20 mg, 40 mg (Lotensin)
Ramipril:
Capsules — 1.25 mg, 2.5 mg, 5 mg, 10 mg
Fosinopril:
Tablets — 10 mg, 20 mg, 40 mg
Lisinopril:
Tablets — 5 mg, 10 mg, 20 mg, 40 mg
Prinzide, Zestoretic
— 20 mg lisinopril with 12.5 or 25 mg of hydrochlorothiazide

▷ **Recommended Dosage Range** Actual dose and schedule must be determined for each patient individually.

Children 12 or under: Captopril: One study used a starting dose of 0.01 to 0.25 mg per kg of body mass every 12 hours in infants; 0.05 to 0.5 mg per kg of body mass three times daily has been used in older children. Maximum dose is 2 mg/kg per dose up to 3 times a day.

Enalapril: Malignant Hypertension: 0.625 mg–1.25 mg per dose—given every 6 hours. Maximum dose is 5 mg every 6 hours intravenously.

Quinapril, benazepril, ramipril, fosinopril, and lisinopril: Dosage not established in infants and children.

12 to 60 Years of Age: For high blood pressure:

Captopril: 25 mg two or three times daily for 1–2 weeks. Dose may be increased to 50 mg three times daily if needed. If blood pressure still not acceptable, a diuretic or change to a combination form may be needed. Maximum daily dose is 450 mg.

Enalapril (if not also taking a diuretic): 5 mg once daily starting dose. Usual ongoing dose is 10 to 40 mg daily in a single dose or divided into two equal doses. Total daily dose should not exceed 40 mg if kidney function is impaired.

Quinapril, benazepril, lisinopril (12 to 60 years of age): 10 mg once daily for those not taking a diuretic; 5 mg once daily if taking a diuretic. Usual ongoing dose is 20 to 40 mg daily, taken in a single dose. If once-a-day dosing (for quinapril and benazepril) does not give stable blood pressure control over the day, divide the dose equally into morning and evening doses. Total daily maximum is 80 mg.

Ramipril: Initially 2.5 mg once daily for 2 to 4 weeks. Usual ongoing dose is 2.5 to 20 mg daily in a single dose or two divided doses. If taking diuretics: Either stop diuretic for 3 days before starting this drug, or begin treatment with 1.25 mg of this drug.

Fosinopril (18 to 60 years of age): Initially 10 mg once daily. Usual maintenance dose is 20 to 40 mg daily taken in a single dose. Total daily dosage should not exceed 80 mg.

▷ *For congestive heart failure (CHF):* Captopril: Doses of 25 mg three times daily are suggested. Lower doses (6.25 to 12.5 mg) three times daily reduces risk of excessively low blood pressure.

Enalapril: 2.5 to 10 mg once or twice daily. Usually combined with other medications. Maximum is 40 mg daily.

Fosinopril: Starting doses of 5 mg (especially for dehydrated patients or who have kidney failure) to 10 mg have been recommended. Some studies have used once-daily dosing. Dosing must be individualized.

After a heart attack:

Captopril: A test dose of 6.25 mg is given to see if excessive lowering of the blood pressure occurs. If the test is tolerated, 12.5 mg is given three times a day. This dose is then increased toward a goal of 50 mg three times a day.

Lisinopril: When hemodynamically stable: 5 mg may be given within 24 hours after symptoms started. If this dose is tolerated, a repeat dose is given 24 hours later and then increased to 10 mg a day. Therapy continues for at least 6 weeks.

For diabetic kidney problems (nephropathy) and eye problems (retinopathy):

Captopril: Success has been achieved with 50 mg twice daily in two large studies. The manufacturer suggests a starting dose of 25 mg three times a day.

Over 60 Years of Age: Quinapril: Same as 12 to 60 years of age, if kidney function is normal. If kidney function is significantly impaired, reduce dose by 50%. The total daily dose should not exceed 40 mg.

Benazepril: Same as 12 to 60 years of age, if kidney function is normal. If kidney function is significantly impaired, reduce dose by 50%. Total daily maximum is 40 mg in those with impaired kidneys.

Ramipril: Small doses are advisable until tolerance has been determined. Sudden and excessive lowering of blood pressure can predispose to stroke or heart attack in those with impaired brain circulation or coronary artery heart disease.

Fosinopril: Same as 18 to 60 years of age, but these patients may be more sensitive to fosinopril. Smaller and more gradual dose increases are prudent as needed and tolerated.

Lisinopril: Exercise tolerance was improved by 2.5 to 20 mg daily. Any needed dose increases should be made at longer intervals between adjustments.

Conditions Requiring Dosing Adjustments

Liver Function: Captopril: Must be used with extreme caution, and started at a lower dose in liver failure.

Enalapril: In patients with liver compromise, the dose may need to be **increased** because less of the drug is activated.

Quinapril, benazepril, and lisinopril: The liver is minimally involved removing these drugs.

Ramipril: Close monitoring for adverse effects is prudent.

Fosinopril: Is a prodrug, and is changed into fosinoprilat (the active form) by the liver. Used with caution and in lower doses by patients with liver compromise.

Kidney Function: Captopril: Increased blood level and risk of adverse effects (low blood counts and protein in the urine) if used in kidney failure. **Must decrease dose according to decreases in creatinine clearance.** The lowest effective dose must be used.

Enalapril: Patients with mild to moderate kidney failure can be given 5 mg/day. In severe kidney failure, maximum dose is 2.5 mg/day.

Quinapril: Patients with mild kidney failure can take 10 mg daily. Those with moderate kidney failure should take 5 mg daily. In severe kidney failure, 2.5 mg per day may be taken. If needed and tolerated, dose increases should only be made every 2 weeks.

Benazepril: For people with creatinine clearances of less than 30 ml/min., or serum creatinine greater than 3 mg/dl (ask your doctor), the starting dose should be 5 mg once daily.

Ramipril: For patients with moderate kidney failure or creatinine values of greater than 2.5 mg/dl, 1.25 mg of ramipril can be taken daily.

Lisinopril: Patients with moderate kidney failure should be started on 5 mg daily. In severe kidney failure, the patient can take 2.5 mg of lisinopril daily. This drug is contraindicated in kidney blood flow problems (renal artery stenosis).

Fosinopril: This drug undergoes liver and bile (dual hepatobiliary) and kidney (renal) elimination. Patients with renal compromise (especially those with renal artery stenosis) should start on a decreased dose, with slow dose increases if needed.

Diabetes: Enalapril: Patients with diabetes with decreased creatinine clearance and protein in the urine (proteinuria) should be given decreased.

▷ **Dosing Instructions:**   Captopril: Take on empty stomach, 1 hour before meals. Enalapril, quinapril benazepril, ramipril, fosinopril, and lisinopril may be taken without regard to food. All ACE drugs should be taken at the same time each day, and all ACE tablets may be crushed if needed to make them easier to take.

Usual Duration of Use: Several weeks of use on a regular schedule is usually needed to see high blood pressure control, and for other uses. Use may be continued for life for high blood pressure and in kidney disease.

Possible Advantages of These Drugs

Quinapril, benazepril, ramipril, fosinopril, and lisinopril: Controls blood pressure effectively with one daily dose with relatively low incidence of adverse effects (ramipril at present has the most favorable data). No adverse influence on asthma, cholesterol blood levels, or diabetes. Sudden withdrawal does not result in a rapid increase in blood pressure.

Captopril has a special chemical (sulfhydryl group) at its active site. This may help it ease intolerance to nitrates.

Lisinopril and captopril DO NOT require activation by the liver to work. They may be drugs of choice in situations where an ACE inhibitor is desirable and liver compromise is also present.

Quinapril goes into tissues well and may have a future role in treating or preventing problems (dysfunction) of the lining (endothelium) of blood vessels.

▷ **These Drugs Should Not Be Taken If**
- you have had an allergic reaction to them.
- you develop swelling of the tongue, face, or throat while taking the drug—call your doctor immediately.
- you are pregnant (last 6 months).
- you currently have a blood cell or bone marrow disorder.
- you have an abnormally high level of blood potassium.

▷ **Inform Your Physician Before Taking These Drugs If**
- you develop swelling of the tongue, face, or throat while taking this drug—call your doctor immediately.
- you are planning a pregnancy or to breast-feed your child.
- you have kidney disease or impaired kidney function.
- you have scleroderma or systemic lupus erythematosus.
- you have any form of heart or liver disease.
- you have diabetes.
- you have an elevated potassium level.
- you have a blood cell disorder.
- you take other antihypertensives, diuretics, nitrates, allopurinol (Zyloprim), Indocin, or potassium supplements.
- you will have surgery with general anesthesia.
- you have renal artery stenosis (ask your doctor).
- you are taking medicines that suppress the immune system.
- you are unsure how much to take or how often to take it.

Possible Side Effects (natural, expected, and unavoidable drug actions)

Dizziness, light-headedness, fainting (excessive drop in blood pressure).

Scalded mouth sensation for some class members. Impaired sense of smell—case reports for enalapril.

Nausea or constipation, increased blood potassium—all rare.

Cough—rare to infrequent.

▷ **Possible Adverse Effects** (unusual, unexpected, and infrequent reactions)
   If any of the following develop, consult your physician promptly for guidance.

Mild Adverse Effects

Allergic reactions: skin rash, psoriasis—rare to infrequent.

Swelling of face, hands, or feet; fever—rare.

Lost or altered (metallic or salty) taste, mouth or tongue sores—case reports.

Headache—infrequent.

Nightmares, joint pain—rare.

Increased temperature (hyperthermia)—case reports (captopril).

Rapid heart rate on standing—case reports.

Vulvovaginal itching—case reports (enalapril).

Serious Adverse Effects

Allergic reactions: Swelling (angioedema) of face, tongue, and/or vocal cords—rare; can be life-threatening—case reports.

Bone marrow depression (neutropenia, anemia, or aplastic anemia): weakness, fever, sore throat, bleeding or bruising—rare (infrequent in those with kidney failure and collagen vascular disease; not reported for ramipril).

Hemolytic or aplastic anemia—case reports (not for ramipril).

Kidney damage: water retention (edema)—case reports for some.

Elevated blood potassium (hyperkalemia)—case reports.

Rare accumulation of fluid around the heart (pericarditis)—case reports (captopril).

Hallucinations—rare (captopril).

Stevens-Johnson syndrome, lupus erythematosus, or other serious skin conditions (some members of this class)—rare.

Pancreatitis—case reports with some members of this class.

Liver damage (with or without jaundice)—rare.

▷ **Possible Effects on Sexual Function:**   Decreased male libido (20% to 30%) with recommended dose—captopril (other ACE inhibitors—rare). Impotence. Swelling and tenderness of male breast tissue (gynecomastia)—rare.

Possible Effects on Laboratory Tests

Complete blood counts: decreased red cells, hemoglobin, white cells, and platelets; increased eosinophils.

Blood antinuclear antibodies (ANA): increased (captopril, lisinopril).

Blood cholesterol and triglycerides: decreased (benazepril; 7.6–13.1%). No effects for the other listed ACEs.

Blood sodium level: decreased.

Blood urea nitrogen level (BUN): increased.

Liver function tests: increased liver enzymes (alkaline phosphatase, AST/GOT, LDH), increased bilirubin—possible.

Urine ketone tests: false positive results with Keto-Diastix and Chemstrip-6 (captopril).

Blood sugar (glucose): decreased—case reports (captopril).

Venereal Disease Research Laboratory (VDRL): rare false positive results (captopril).

Digoxin blood level: may read falsely low with fosinopril.

CAUTION

1. If possible, may be best to stop all other antihypertensive drugs (especially diuretics) for 1 week before starting.
2. **Tell your doctor immediately if you become pregnant.** These drugs should not be taken after the first 3 months of pregnancy.
3. **Report promptly** any signs of infection (fever, sore throat), and any indications of water retention (weight gain, swollen feet or ankles).
4. Many salt substitutes contain potassium; ask your doctor before using.
5. Blood counts and urine analyses are needed **before** taking these medicines.
6. The FDA has started to evaluate blood levels of ACE inhibitors (trough to peak ratios—T/P; see Glossary) to check how best these medicines should be dosed. Talk to your doctor about this concept.
7. High blood pressure rarely has symptoms. If this medicine is controlling your blood pressure, STAY ON IT—even if you never felt sick from your prior high blood pressure.

Precautions for Use

By Infants and Children: Enalapril, lisinopril, quinapril, fosinopril, benazepril, and ramipril: Safety and effectiveness not established.

By Those Over 60 Years of Age: In general, small starting doses are advisable. Sudden and excessive lowering of blood pressure can cause stroke or heart attack.

▷ **Advisability of Use During Pregnancy**

Pregnancy Category: C during the first 3 months; **D during the last 6 months** (last two trimesters). See Pregnancy Risk Categories at the back of this book.

Animal studies: Birth defects found in some animals for some ACE inhibitors.

Human studies: The use of ACE inhibitor drugs during the last 6 months of pregnancy is known to possibly cause very serious injury and possible death to the fetus; skull and limb malformations, lung defects, and kidney failure have been reported in over 50 cases captopril worldwide.

Avoid these drugs completely during the last 6 months. During the first 3 months of pregnancy, use this drug only if clearly needed. Ask your doctor for guidance.

Advisability of Use If Breast-Feeding

Presence of this drug in breast milk: Yes (captopril, enalapril and ramipril), in small amounts. Benazepril in very small amounts. Lisinopril, quinapril, fosinopril—unknown.

Monitor nursing infant closely and discontinue drug or nursing if adverse effects develop.

Habit-Forming Potential: None.

Effects of Overdose: Excessive drop in blood pressure—light-headedness, dizziness, fainting.

Possible Effects of Long-Term Use: Gradual increase in blood potassium level.

Suggested Periodic Examinations While Taking These Drugs (at physician's discretion)

Complete blood cell count, urine analysis, and blood potassium level before drug is started. Once started: blood counts during the first 3 months, then periodically. Urine protein every month for the first 9 months, then periodically. Periodic blood potassium tests. ANA titer.

▷ **While Taking This Drug, Observe the Following**
Foods: Talk to your doctor about salt intake. Ginseng may increase blood pressure.
Nutritional Support: **Do not** take potassium supplements unless directed by your physician. Case reports of zinc deficiency have been made (captopril). Large amounts of garlic, soy, and calcium may lower blood pressure.
Beverages: No restrictions. May be taken with milk.
▷ *Alcohol:* Alcohol can further lower blood pressure. Use with caution.
Tobacco Smoking: No interactions expected. I advise everyone to quit smoking.
▷ *Other Drugs*
These medicines *taken concurrently* with
- allopurinol (Zyloprim) may increase risk of serious skin reactions.
- azathioprine (Imuran) may result in severe anemia.
- cyclosporine (Sandimmune) may result in kidney failure that takes a while to appear (delayed acute renal dysfunction).
- interferons (alpha and beta) may greatly increase risk of blood problems with some members of this class. DO NOT combine (lisinopril, quinapril, benazepril case reports).
- lithium (Lithobid, others) may result in toxic blood lithium levels and **toxicity**.
- loop diuretics (such as Lasix or Bumex; see Drug Classes) may cause excessively low blood pressure on standing (postural hypotension).
- oral hypoglycemic agents (glyburide—Glynase, others) may result in decreased insulin resistance and the need to decrease the dose of the oral hypoglycemic agent (enalapril only).
- phenothiazines (see Drug Classes) may result in postural hypotension.
- potassium preparations (K-Lyte, Slow-K, etc.) will increase blood potassium with risk of serious heart rhythm disturbances.
- potassium-sparing diuretics—amiloride (Moduretic), spironolactone (Aldactazide), triamterene (Dyazide)—may increase blood levels of potassium with risk of serious heart rhythm disturbances.
- rifampin (Rifadin) or rifabutin (Mycobutin) may cause decreased therapeutic benefit from enalapril.
- thiazide diuretics (hydrochlorothiazide, others) may result (especially in older people) in increased levels of enalaprilat (the active medicine) and increased reduction in blood pressure. May be used to therapeutic benefit.
- cotrimoxazole (trimethoprim component)(Bactrim, Trimpex, others) may increase blood potassium (risk of serious heart rhythm disturbances).
The following drugs may *decrease* the effects of these medicines:
- antacids—by decreasing captopril (and perhaps other ACEs)absorption. Separate doses by 2 hours.
- ibuprofen (Motrin), indomethacin (Indocin), or other NSAIDs (nonsteroidal anti-inflammatory drugs; see Drug Classes).
- naloxone (Narcan).
- salicylates (aspirin, etc.) or other NSAIDs.

▷ *Driving, Hazardous Activities:* Usually no restrictions. Be aware of possible drops in blood pressure with resultant dizziness or faintness.

Aviation Note: The use of these drugs *may be a disqualification* for piloting. Consult a designated aviation medical examiner.

Exposure to Sun: Caution is advised. Some drugs in this class can cause photosensitivity.

Exposure to Heat: Caution is advised. Excessive perspiring may drop blood pressure.

Occurrence of Unrelated Illness: Call your doctor to report any disorder causing vomiting or diarrhea. Fluid and chemical imbalances must be corrected as soon as possible.

Discontinuation: Lisinopril, quinapril, fosinopril, and benazepril may be stopped abruptly without causing a sudden increase in blood pressure. Ask your doctor before stopping any drug for any reason.

ANTI-ALZHEIMER'S DRUG FAMILY

Donepezil (DON ep a zill)   **Tacrine** (TA kreen)

Introduced: 1993, 1996   **Class:** Acetylcholinesterase inhibitor, anti-alzheimer's drug   **Prescription:** USA: Yes   **Controlled Drug:** USA: No; Canada: No   **Available as Generic:** USA: No

Brand Names: Donepezil: Aricept; Tacrine: Cognex

BENEFITS versus RISKS	
Possible Benefits	*Possible Risks*
IMPROVEMENT OF MEMORY IN MILD TO MODERATE ALZHEIMER'S DISEASE IMPROVEMENT OF SYMPTOMS IN MILD TO MODERATE ALZHEIMER'S DISEASE	LIVER TOXICITY (tacrine) Nausea Dizziness

▷ **Principal Uses**

As a Single Drug Product: Uses currently included in FDA-approved labeling: Treats mild to moderate Alzheimer's disease symptoms (both medicines).

Author's Note: Guidelines from the American Psychiatric Association (APA) recommend use of vitamin E alone or in combination with donepezil as first-line therapy for delaying symptoms of patients with mild to moderate Alzheimer's. An early study of an herbal medicine called ginkgo biloba has also shown benefits in an early study.

Other (unlabeled) generally accepted uses: (1) Significant increases in protective white blood cells (CD4 lymphocytes) occurred when tacrine was used to treat AIDS dementia; (2) some early data indicated a benefit in movement disorders (tardive dyskinesia) for tacrine.

How These Drugs Work: Alzheimer's disease is thought to be caused by a loss of nerve cells that make a nerve transmitter (acetylcholine). Donepezil and tacrine act to increase levels of a neurotransmitter (acetylcholine) in the brain.

Available Dosage Forms and Strengths

Donepezil:
  Tablets — 5 mg, 10 mg
Tacrine:
  Capsules — 10 mg, 20 mg, 30 mg, 40 mg

▷ **Recommended Dosage Ranges** (Actual dosage and schedule must be determined for each patient individually.)

Infants and Children: No data are available on use of these drugs in infants and children.

18 to 60 Years of Age: Donepezil: Start with 5 mg once daily at bedtime, and keep at this dose for 6 weeks. As needed and tolerated, increase to 10 mg. The 10-mg dose has had increased GI side effects.

Tacrine: Starts at 10 mg four times a day (between meals). This can be increased at 6-week intervals if needed. Maximum daily dose is 160 mg.

Over 60 Years of Age: Same as 18 to 60 years of age.

Conditions Requiring Dosing Adjustments

Liver Function: Donepezil: decreased dose and blood levels prudent in patients with liver compromise. Tacrine used with great caution or not at all in liver compromise.

Kidney Function: Dose decreases in kidney compromise are not presently indicated.

▷ **Dosing Instructions:** The donepezil tablet may be crushed and is not affected by food. The tacrine capsule may be opened and is best taken 1 hour before meals. Food decreases the amount of tacrine that gets into your body by 30–40%.

Usual Duration of Use: Regular use for 3 to 4 weeks may be needed to see improvement from either medicine. Dose increases are made at 4- to 6-week intervals. Long-term use (months to years) requires periodic evaluation of response and dose. If benefits do not occur within 6 weeks, talk with your doctor about stopping these drugs.

Possible Advantages of These Drugs

Improvement of memory and other symptoms of mild to moderate Alzheimer's with fewer side effects than other agents. Donepezil has a more favorable side effect profile than tacrine, and also avoids liver damage.

Currently a "Drug of Choice"

Donepezil (fewer possible side effects) preferred for therapy symptoms in mild to moderate Alzheimer's disease.

These Drugs Should Not Be Taken If

Donepezil:
* you have had an allergic reaction to it previously.

Tacrine:
* you have had an allergic reaction to it previously.
* you have bronchial asthma.
* you have had tacrine liver toxicity and blood bilirubin levels greater than 3 mg/dl.
* you have an overly active thyroid (hyperthyroidism).
* you have peptic ulcer disease.
* you have an intestinal or urinary tract obstruction.

▷ **Inform Your Physician Before Taking These Drugs If**
- you have a history of seizure disorder.
- you have had liver disease.
- you have a history of peptic ulcer disease.
- you have a slow heartbeat (bradycardia), an abnormal electrical conduction system in your heart (AV conduction defect), or excessively low blood pressure.
- you take an NSAID (nonsteroidal anti-inflammatory drug; see Drug Classes).
- you take muscle relaxants.
- you have glaucoma (angle closure).
- you have a seizure disorder.

Possible Side Effects (natural, expected, and unavoidable drug actions)
Symptoms of cholinergic excess (abdominal upset, agitation).

▷ **Possible Adverse Effects** (unusual, unexpected, and infrequent reactions)
If any of the following develop, consult your physician promptly for guidance.

Mild Adverse Effects
Allergic reactions: skin rash.
Increased sweating—rare.
Increased urination—infrequent.
Muscle aches—infrequent.
Lowered blood pressure—possible.
Nausea or vomiting, belching and diarrhea, decreased appetite—infrequent to frequent.
Dizziness, confusion, and insomnia—infrequent.

Serious Adverse Effects
Allergic reactions: anaphylactoid reactions.
Dose-related increase in liver function tests (starts 6 to 8 weeks after therapy begins)—frequent for tacrine only.
Hallucinations—case report for tacrine.
Inner ear problems—rare for tacrine.
Purpura—infrequent for tacrine.
Severe decrease in white blood cells—one tacrine case report.
Anemia—infrequent for donepezil.
Slow heart rate (bradycardia) or abnormal rhythm—possible to rare.
Seizures—case reports for tacrine.

▷ **Possible Effects on Sexual Function:** Very rare effect of causing lactation for tacrine.

Possible Delayed Adverse Effects: Liver toxicity (tacrine only), rash, low white blood cell count (tacrine only).

Adverse Effects That May Mimic Natural Diseases or Disorders
Liver toxicity of tacrine may mimic acute hepatitis.

Natural Diseases or Disorders That May Be Activated by These Drugs
May worsen bronchial asthma and precipitate seizures. May exacerbate peptic ulcer disease.

Possible Effects on Laboratory Tests
Tacrine: Liver function tests: increased SGOT, SGPT, and CPK. Complete blood count: decreased white blood cells.
Donepezil: decreased hct or platelets.

CAUTION
1. These drugs should **NOT** be stopped abruptly. Sudden decline in thinking ability may happen (acute deterioration of cognitive abilities).
2. Changes in color of stools (light or very black—tacrine) should be promptly reported to your doctor.
3. These drugs do **NOT** alter the course of Alzheimer's disease. Over time, benefits may be lost.
4. The dose of tacrine **must** be decreased by 40 mg per day if the liver function levels (transaminases) rise to three to five times the upper normal value.
5. Females achieve 50% higher tacrine blood levels than men. Dose-related side effects may occur sooner (with lower doses) in women than in men. Beneficial doses may be lower for women than men.

Precautions for Use
By Infants and Children: Safety and effectiveness for those under 18 years of age not established.
By Those Over 60 Years of Age: No specific changes are presently indicated.

▷ **Advisability of Use During Pregnancy**
Pregnancy Category: C. See Pregnancy Risk Categories at the back of this book.
Animal studies: Data not available.
Human studies: Adequate studies of pregnant women are not available.
Consult your doctor.

Advisability of Use If Breast-Feeding
Presence of these drugs in breast milk: Unknown.
Monitor nursing infant closely and discontinue drug or nursing if adverse effects develop.

Habit-Forming Potential: None.

Effects of Overdose: May precipitate a cholinergic crisis—severe nausea and vomiting, slow heartbeat, low blood pressure, extreme muscle weakness, collapse, and convulsions.

Suggested Periodic Examinations While Taking These Drugs (at physician's discretion)
Assessment of mental status: periodically—check benefits or loss of benefits as Alzheimer's progresses. For tacrine, liver function tests should be checked every 2 weeks for the first 16 weeks of therapy, then monthly for 2 months, and then every 3 months ongoing if the same dose is used. If dose is increased, liver tests are checked weekly for 7 weeks and then on the above schedule. Tacrine and donepezil patients need complete blood counts periodically or if symptoms of low blood count occur.

While Taking These Drugs, Observe the Following
Foods: Tacrine is best **NOT** taken with food. Donepezil is not affected by food.
Beverages: No restrictions.
▷ *Alcohol:* Occasional small amounts of alcohol are acceptable. Frequent use of alcohol may worsen memory impairment and adversely affect liver enzymes.
Tobacco Smoking: No interactions expected. I advise everyone to quit smoking.
Marijuana Smoking: Additive dizziness may occur.
▷ *Other Drugs*
These medicines may *increase* the effects of

- bethanechol (Duvoid, others).
- theophylline (Theo-Dur, others) by doubling the drug level (reported for tacrine).
- succinylcholine (Anectine, others).

These medicines may *decrease* the effects of
- anticholinergic medications (see Drug Classes).

The following drug may *increase* the effects of these medicines:
- cimetidine (Tagamet).

These medicines *taken concurrently* with
- carbamazepine (Tegretol), dexamethasone, phenobarbital, phenytoin (Dilantin), or rifampin (Rifater, others) may decrease therapeutic benefits of the anti-Alzheimer drugs.
- ibuprofen (Motrin, others) was associated with delirium inone case report on tacrine.
- ketoconazole, quinidine, and perhaps ritonavir (Norvir) or other protease inhibitors (see Drug Classes) may lead to increased risk of donepezil or tacrine toxicity.
- NSAIDs (nonsteroidal anti-inflammatory drugs; see Drug Classes) may cause additive stomach upset.

▷ *Driving, Hazardous Activities:* These drugs may cause confusion or dizziness. Restrict activities as necessary.

Aviation Note: The use of these drugs *may be a disqualification* for piloting. See a designated aviation medical examiner.

Exposure to Sun: No restrictions.

Exposure to Heat: Increased sweating may occur rarely with tacrine. The combination of increased sweating and hot environments may lead to more rapid dehydration.

Discontinuation: These drugs should **NOT** be abruptly stopped. Some adverse effects are dose related, and may abate if the dose is decreased. Slow withdrawal of the drug is indicated if it is not tolerated.

ANTI-LEUKOTRIENE FAMILY

Montelukast (mon TELL oo cast) **Zafirlukast** (zah FUR lew kast) **Zileuton** (ZEYE loo ton)

Introduced: 1998, 1996, 1997 (respectively) **Class:** Anti-leukotriene, anti-asthmatic **Prescription:** USA: Yes **Controlled Drug:** USA: No; Canada: No **Available as Generic:** No

Brand Names: Montelukast: Singulair; Zafirlukast: Accolate; Zileuton: Zyflo

BENEFITS versus RISKS	
Possible Benefits	*Possible Risks*
EFFECTIVE PREVENTION AND CHRONIC TREATMENT OF BRONCHIAL ASTHMA	Headache Nausea Liver enzyme increase
Zafirlukast may have a role in treating bronchospasm caused by exercise	

▷ **Principal Uses**

As a Single Drug Product: Uses currently included in FDA-approved labeling: Used to prevent recurrence of asthmatic episodes and to chronically treat asthmatic episodes.

Author's Note: These medicines are indicated as Step Two medicines (alternatives to low-dose inhaled steroids, cromolyn, or nedocromil in mild persistent asthma) in the National Institutes of Health's (NIH, NHLBI) "Guidelines for Diagnosis and Management of Asthma."

Other (unlabeled) generally accepted uses: (1) Zafirlukast may have a role in preventing spasm of the bronchi caused by exercise; (2) zileuton may have a role in preventing allergic rhinitis or aspirin-sensitive asthma; (3) zileuton may also help symptoms of ulcerative colitis.

How These Drugs Work: Zafirlukast works by blocking (leukotriene receptor antagonist) action of chemicals called leukotrienes (slow-reacting substances of anaphylaxis). Zileuton works by blocking creation of (leukotriene pathway inhibitor) leukotrienes themselves. By inhibiting action or formation of leukotrienes, all medicines help keep the airways open.

Available Dosage Forms and Strengths

Montelukast:
Chewable tablet — 5 mg
      Tablet — 10 mg
Zafirlukast:
      Tablet — 20 mg
Zileuton:
      Tablet — 600 mg

▷ **Recommended Dosage Ranges** (Actual dosage and schedule must be determined for each patient individually.)

Children 6 to 14: Montelukast only: One 5 mg chewable tablet in the evening.

Patients 15 or Older: Montelukast only: One 10 mg tablet in the evening.

Children 12 or Older: Zafirlukast and zileuton: same as adult dose.

12 to 60 Years of Age: Zafirlukast: 20 mg twice daily.
Zileuton: 600 mg four times a day.

Over 60 Years of Age: Montelukast: No difference in safety or efficacy, but increased sensitivity to the drug can't yet be ruled out.

Zafirlukast: Maximum blood level can be twice that of younger patients. Prudent to lower doses, but specific guidelines have not been developed. Package insert notes that using typical dose did not result in adverse effects in clinical trials.

Zileuton: Same as those for 12 to 60 years old. **Note: These medicines may be continued during an acute worsening (exacerbation) of asthma, but are not to be used to treat a sudden (acute) asthma attack.**

Conditions Requiring Dosing Adjustments

Liver Function: Montelukast has NOT been studied in liver compromise.

Zafirlukast stays in the body up to 60% longer in patients with alcoholic cirrhosis. Lower doses and blood levels appear prudent. Zileuton should not be given if active liver disease is present.

Kidney Function: Dosage changes not needed for the medicines in this class.

▷ **Dosing Instructions:** Montelukast should be taken in the evening.
Zafirlukast should be taken on an empty stomach, 1 hour before or 2 hours

after a meal. Zileuton may be given with or without food. These medicines are NOT to be used to stop a sudden (acute) asthma attack.

Usual Duration of Use: Both zafirlukast and zileuton start to work in half an hour. Montelukast peaks and also starts to work in 3 to 4 hours. It lasts for 24 hours. Zafirlukast significantly relaxes bronchi in 30 minutes, and lasts for 12 hours after a typical dose. Zileuton peaks in 2 to 4 hours, and with multiple doses may last up to 7 days. Ongoing use requires periodic follow-up with your doctor.

These Drugs Should Not Be Taken If
- you have had an allergic reaction to them.
- you have active liver disease or increased liver enzymes (transaminases) greater than three times the upper normal limit (zileuton).

▷ Inform Your Physician Before Taking This Drug If
- you have a liver disease (montelukast or zafirlukast).
- you are having a sudden (acute) asthma attack.
- you have impaired kidney function (zafirlukast or zileuton).
- you drink large amounts of alcohol (zileuton).

Possible Side Effects (natural, expected, and unavoidable drug actions)
Not defined at present.

▷ Possible Adverse Effects (unusual, unexpected, and infrequent reactions)
If any of the following develop, consult your physician promptly for guidance.

Mild Adverse Effects
Allergic reactions: skin rash, hives.
Headache, fatigue, weakness—infrequent.
Dizziness—rare for zafirlukast, infrequent for zileuton.
Nausea or abdominal pain—infrequent.
Muscle pain—rare for zafirlukast, infrequent for zileuton.

Serious Adverse Effects
Allergic reactions: not reported as yet.
Idiosyncratic reactions: none reported as yet.
Liver toxicity (increased enzyme tests)—rare for zafirlukast, infrequent for zileuton.
Decreases in steroid doses may be followed by onset of Churg-Strauss syndrome (Zafirlukast only).

▷ Possible Effects on Sexual Function: None reported.

Natural Diseases or Disorders That May Be Activated by This Drug
Since both medicines may increase liver enzymes, hidden (subclinical) liver problems may be activated.

Possible Effects on Laboratory Tests
Liver function tests (SGPT, SGOT, LDH): may be increased.

CAUTION
1. The chewable montelukast tablet has phenylalanine (0.842 mg per 5 mg tablet). People with PKU MUST be advised.
2. Talk with your doctor about continuing other asthma drugs once you start one of these medicines.
3. Since zafirlukast and zileuton can (1.5% and 2% of the time) affect the

liver, it is critical that you have lab tests of liver function as your doctor orders them.

4. There is one case report of drug fever for zafirlukast.

Precautions for Use

By Children: Make certain that these medicines are taken in the amount and for the number of times they are ordered.

By Those Over 65 Years of Age: Zafirlukast goes to higher peak blood levels and remains in the body longer in those over 65. It appears that smaller starting doses are indicated. Montelukast and zileuton are not changed by age.

▷ **Advisability of Use During Pregnancy**

Pregnancy Category: Montelukast and zafirlukast: B; zileuton: C. See Pregnancy Risk Categories at the back of this book.

Animal studies: Montelukast: no teratogenicity at 320 times the maximum human dose in rats. Zafirlukast: no teratogenicity up to 160 times maximum recommended human dose given to mice. Zileuton: Adverse effects were seen in rats given 18 times the typical human dose.

Human studies: Adequate studies of pregnant women are not available.

Ask your doctor for guidance.

Advisability of Use If Breast-Feeding

Presence of this drug in breast milk: Zafirlukast—Yes. Montelukast and Zileuton—Unknown.

Avoid drug or refrain from nursing.

Habit-Forming Potential: None.

Effects of Overdose: No overdose experience in humans for montelukast or zafirlukast. Zileuton overdose experience is limited. One patient received 6.6 to 9.0 g of zileuton, which caused vomiting, and recovered without ill effects.

Possible Effects of Long-Term Use: Possible increased liver enzymes.

Suggested Periodic Examinations While Taking This Drug (at physician's discretion)

Periodic liver function tests.

▷ **While Taking This Drug, Observe the Following**

Foods: Zafirlukast should be taken on an empty stomach; no restrictions for montelukast or zileuton.

Beverages: No restrictions.

▷ *Alcohol:* May worsen drowsiness.

Tobacco Smoking: I advise everyone to quit smoking.

Marijuana Smoking: May cause additive drowsiness.

▷ *Other Drugs*

These medicines *taken concurrently* with

- aspirin (various brands) may cause zafirlukast toxicity.
- beta-blocker drugs (see Drug Classes) may cause beta-blocker toxicity if combined with zileuton.
- erythromycin (E-Mycin, Erythrocin, etc.) may decrease zafirlukast's benefits.
- terfenadine (Seldane) may decrease zafirlukast blood levels and its therapeutic benefits. Zileuton may decrease terfenadine (and perhaps other sim-

ilarly structured minimally sedating antihistamine levels) and lead to toxicity. DO NOT combine.
- theophylline (Theo-Dur, others) may decrease zafirlukast blood levels and its therapeutic benefits. Zileuton may result in doubling of theophylline levels and require reduced theophylline doses.
- warfarin (Coumadin) may lead to increased risk of bleeding. More frequent INRs are needed.

▷ *Driving, Hazardous Activities:* These drugs may cause dizziness. Restrict activities as necessary.

Aviation Note: The use of this drug **may be a disqualification** for piloting. Consult a designated aviation medical examiner.

Exposure to Sun: No restrictions.

Discontinuation: Do not stop this medicine without first talking with your doctor.

ASPIRIN* (AS pir in)

Other Names: ASA, acetylsalicylic acid

Introduced: 1899   **Class:** Analgesics, mild; antiplatelet; antipyretic; NSAIDs; salicylates   **Prescription:** USA: No   **Controlled Drug:** USA: No; Canada: No   **Available as Generic:** Yes

Brand Names: Added Strength Analgesic Pain Reliever, Adult Strength Pain Reliever [CD], Alka-Seltzer Effervescent Pain Reliever & Antacid [CD], Alka-Seltzer Night Time [CD], Alka-Seltzer Plus [CD], Alka-Seltzer Plus Cold [CD], Anacin [CD], Anacin Maximum Strength [CD], ✦Anacin w/Codeine [CD], ✦Ancasal, APC [CD], APC with Codeine [CD], ✦APO-ASA, Arthritis Pain Formula [CD], Arthritis Strength Bufferin, A.S.A. Enseals, ✦Asasantine [CD], Ascriptin [CD], Ascriptin A/D [CD], Aspergum, ✦Aspirin*, Asprimox, ✦Astrin, Axotal [CD], Azdone [CD], Bayer Aspirin, Bayer Children's Chewable Aspirin, Bayer Enteric Aspirin, Bayer Plus, BC Powder, Buffaprin, Bufferin [CD], Bufferin Arthritis Strength [CD], Bufferin Extra Strength [CD], Bufferin w/Codeine [CD], Cama Arthritis Pain Reliever [CD], Cardioprin, Carisoprodol Compound [CD], Cope [CD], Coricidin [CD], ✦Coryphen, ✦Coryphen-Codeine [CD], ✦C2 Buffered [CD], Darvon Compound [CD], Direct Formulary Aspirin, ✦Dristan [CD], Easprin, Ecotrin, 8-Hour Bayer, Empirin, Empirin w/Codeine No. 2, 4 [CD], ✦Entrophen, Excedrin [CD], Excedrin Extra Strength Geltabs [CD], Excedrin Migraine** [CD], Fiorinal [CD], ✦Fiorinal-C 1/4, -C 1/2 [CD], Fiorinal w/Codeine [CD], Genprin, Genacote, Goody's Headache Powder [CD], Halprin, Hepto [CD], Lortab ASA [CD], Low Dose Adult Chewable Aspirin, Marnal [CD], Maximum Bayer Aspirin, Measurin, Midol Caplets [CD], Momentum [CD], Norgesic [CD], Norgesic Forte [CD], Norwich Aspirin, ✦Novasen, Orphenadrine [CD], PAP with Codeine [CD], Percodan [CD], Percodan-Demi [CD], ✦Phenaphen

---

*In the United States *aspirin* is an official generic designation. In Canada *Aspirin* is the Registered Trademark of the Bayer Company Division of Sterling Drug Limited.

Author's note: Excedrin Migraine is the first nonprescription medicine to be FDA approved to treat mild to moderate migraine headaches.

[CD], ♣Phenaphen No. 2, 3, 4 [CD], Propoxyphene Compound [CD], ♣Riphen-10, Robaxisal [CD], ♣Robaxisal-C [CD], Roxiprin [CD], SK-65 Compound [CD], Soma Compound [CD], St. Joseph Children's Aspirin, ♣Supasa, Synalgos [CD], Synalgos-DC [CD], Talwin Compound [CD], Talwin Compound-50 [CD], ♣Tecnal tablet [CD], ♣Triaphen-10, ♣217 [CD], ♣217 Strong [CD], ♣292 [CD], ♣692 [CD], Vanquish [CD], Verin, Wesprin, Zorprin

---

BENEFITS versus RISKS

Possible Benefits	*Possible Risks*
EFFECTIVE RELIEF OF MILD TO MODERATE PAIN AND INFLAMMATION	Stomach irritation, bleeding, and/or ulceration
REDUCTION OF FEVER	Decreased numbers of white blood cells and platelets
PREVENTION OF BLOOD CLOTS	Hemolytic anemia—rare
PREVENTION OF HEART ATTACK	Liver toxicity—rare
PREVENTION OF STROKE	Bronchospasm in asthmatics—
PREVENTION OF COLON CANCER	possible
MAY ACT TO LIMIT THE SIZE AND SEVERITY OF A HEART ATTACK ONCE IT HAS STARTED	
TREATMENT OF MIGRAINE HEADACHES (EXCEDRIN MIGRAINE ONLY)	

▷ **Principal Uses**

As a Single Drug Product: Uses currently included in FDA-approved labeling: (1) Relieves mild to moderate pain and eases symptoms in conditions causing inflammation or high fever. Treats musculoskeletal disorders, especially acute and chronic arthritis, as well as painful menstruation (dysmenorrhea). Used selectively to: (2) reduce risk of first heart attack; (3) reduce the risk of repeat heart attack; (4) prevent platelet embolism to the brain (in men);(5) reduce risk of clots (thromboembolism) after heart attack and in people with artificial heart valves and after hip surgery (see *blood platelets* in Glossary); (6) help prevent a second stroke in people who have had a stroke; (7) help prevent strokes in people with transient ischemic attack (TIA) history; (8)help prevent migraine headaches (Excedrin Migraine only). Other (unlabeled) generally accepted uses: (1) long-term use may decrease the risk of colon polyps or colon cancer in women (may apply to men as well); (2) may limit size and severity of a heart attack if aspirin is taken immediately after symptoms are recognized and is continued for at least 30 days after the heart attack; (3) can help reduce flushing caused by niacin; (4) used after carotid artery surgery (endarterectomy) to prevent TIA or stroke; (5) general data supporting NSAID use and decreased Alzheimer's risk.

As a Combination Drug Product [CD]: Frequently combined with other mild or strong analgesic drugs to enhance pain relief. Also combined with antihistamines and decongestants in many cold preparations to relieve headache and general discomfort.

How This Drug Works: Reduces prostaglandins, chemicals involved in the production of inflammation and pain. By modifying the temperature-regulating center in the brain, dilating blood vessels, and increasing sweating, aspirin reduces fever. By preventing the production of thromboxane in blood platelets, aspirin inhibits formation of blood clots.

Available Dosage Forms and Strengths

Capsules, enteric coated —	500 mg
Capsules, enteric-coated granules —	325 mg
Gum tablets —	227.5 mg
Suppositories —	60 mg, 120 mg, 125 mg, 130 mg, 195 mg, 200 mg, 300 mg, 325 mg, 600 mg, 650 mg, 1.2 g
Tablets —	65 mg, 81 mg, 165 mg, 325 mg, 496 mg, 500 mg
Tablets, chewable —	81 mg
Tablets, enteric coated —	81 mg, 165 mg, 325 mg, 500 mg, 650 mg, 975 mg
Tablets, prolonged action —	80 mg (Canada), 650 mg, 800 mg, 975 mg

▷ **Usual Adult Dosage Range:**   For pain or fever—325 to 650 mg every 4 hours as needed. For arthritis (and related conditions)—3600 to 5400 mg daily in divided doses. For the prevention of blood clots—80 to 162 mg daily or every other day. Low-dose, long-term daily aspirin may also decrease risk of colon cancer or heart attacks. **Note: For long-term use, actual dosage and schedule must be determined for each patient individually.** FDA advocates 81–325 mg daily for unstable angina or a previous heart attack to reduce risk of death or another heart attack.

Conditions Requiring Dosing Adjustments

Liver Function: This medication should be avoided in severe liver disease.
Kidney Function: Avoided or used with caution in patients with kidney problems. NOT to be used in severe (creatinine clearance less than 10 ml/min) kidney failure.
Glucose-6-Phosphate Dehydrogenase (G6PD) Deficiency: May cause destruction of red blood cells in patients with G6PD deficiency.

▷ **Dosing Instructions:**   Take with food, milk, or a full glass of water to reduce stomach upset. Regular tablets may be crushed and capsules opened for administration. Enteric-coated tablets, prolonged-action tablets, A.S.A. Enseals, Cama tablets, and Ecotrin tablets should not be crushed.

Usual Duration of Use: Short-term use is recommended—3 to 5 days for fever or cold symptoms. Daily use should not exceed 10 days without physician supervision. Use on a regular schedule for 1 week usually needed to see benefit in relieving chronic arthritis symptoms. Response must be evaluated and dose adjusted in long-term use. Ongoing use for prevention of heart attack, colon cancer, or stroke REQUIRES ongoing supervision by your doctor, even though aspirin is not a prescription drug.

▷ **This Drug Should Not Be Taken If**
- you have had an allergic reaction to any form of aspirin.
- you have any type of bleeding disorder (such as hemophilia).
- you have active peptic ulcer disease.

- you are in the last 3 months of pregnancy.
- it smells like vinegar. This indicates decomposition of aspirin.

▷ **Inform Your Physician Before Taking This Drug If**
- you are taking any anticoagulant drug.
- you are taking oral antidiabetic drugs.
- you have a history of peptic ulcer disease or gout.
- you have lupus erythematosus.
- you are pregnant or planning pregnancy.
- you have asthma, carditis, or nasal polyps.
- you plan to have surgery of any kind.
- you take prescription or nonprescription medications not discussed when aspirin was recommended for you.
- you are unsure how much to take or how often to take it.
- you have a history of liver or kidney problems.
- you have a deficiency of glucose-6-phosphate dehydrogenase (G6PD).
- you have a history of vasospastic (Prinzmetalís) angina (may be worsened by this drug).

Possible Side Effects (natural, expected, and unavoidable drug actions)
Mild drowsiness in sensitive patients. Interference with usual blood clotting.

▷ **Possible Adverse Effects** (unusual, unexpected, and infrequent reactions)
If any of the following develop, consult your physician promptly for guidance.

Mild Adverse Effects
Allergic reactions: skin rash, hives, nasal discharge (resembling hay fever), nasal polyps.
Stomach irritation, heartburn, nausea, vomiting, constipation—infrequent to frequent.
Lowering of the blood sugar—rare.

Serious Adverse Effects
Allergic reactions: acute anaphylactic reaction (see Glossary), allergic destruction of blood platelets (see Glossary) and bruising—rare.
Idiosyncratic reactions: hemolytic anemia (see Glossary)—rare.
Stevens-Johnson syndrome—possible.
Erosion of stomach lining, with silent bleeding—may be dose and frequency related.
Activation of peptic ulcer, with or without hemorrhage—frequent with long-term nonenteric coated use.
Bone marrow depression (see Glossary): fatigue, weakness, fever, sore throat, abnormal bleeding or bruising—possible.
Hepatitis with jaundice (see Glossary): yellow skin and eyes, dark-colored urine, light-colored stool—possible, especially with daily use of more than 2 grams (2000 mg).
Hearing toxicity (ototoxicity)—more common with higher doses and long-term use.
Kidney function decline—possible in kidney failure patients who depend on prostaglandins for their kidneys to work.
Bronchospasm when used in patients with nasal polyps, asthma—possible.
May worsen angina attacks and increase their frequency—possible.
Reye's syndrome if used during viral illness—DO NOT USE.

▷ **Possible Effects on Sexual Function:**   None reported.

Adverse Effects That May Mimic Natural Diseases or Disorders

Liver damage may suggest viral hepatitis or reveal (unmask) low level (subclinical) liver disease.

Possible Effects on Laboratory Tests

Complete blood counts: decreased red cells, hemoglobin, white cells, and platelets.

Bleeding time: prolonged.

INR (prothrombin time): increased by large doses; decreased by small doses.

Blood glucose level: decreased.

Blood uric acid level: increased by small doses; decreased by large doses.

Liver function tests: increased ALT/GPT, AST/GOT, alkaline phosphatase.

Thyroid function tests: increased T_3 uptake, free T_3 and free T_4; decreased TSH, T_3, T_4, and free thyroxine index (FTI).

Urine sugar tests: false positive with Clinitest or Benedict's solution.

Fecal occult blood test: positive with large doses of aspirin.

CAUTION

1. **Aspirin is a drug**. Although it is one of our most useful drugs, we have an unrealistic sense of its safety and its potential for adverse effects.
2. Do NOT take more than 3 tablets (975 mg) at one time; allow at least 4 hours between doses; and do not take more than 10 tablets (3250 mg) in 24 hours without physician supervision.
3. Remember that aspirin can
   • cause new illnesses.
   • complicate existing illnesses.
   • complicate pregnancy.
   • complicate surgery.
   • interact unfavorably with other drugs.
4. When your doctor asks, "Are you taking any drugs?" the answer is **yes** if you are taking aspirin. This also applies to *any* nonprescription drug you may be taking (see *over-the-counter drugs* in Glossary).

Precautions for Use

By Infants and Children: Reye's syndrome (brain and liver damage in children, often fatal) can follow flu or chicken pox in children and teenagers. Some reports suggest that the use of aspirin by children with flu or chicken pox can increase the risk of developing this complication. Consult your physician before giving aspirin to a child or teenager with chicken pox, flu, or similar infection.

Usual dosage schedule for children:

Up to 2 years of age—consult physician.

2 to 4 years of age—160 mg/4 hours, up to 5 doses/24 hours.

4 to 6 years of age—240 mg/4 hours, up to 5 doses/24 hours.

6 to 9 years of age—320 mg/4 hours, up to 5 doses/24 hours.

9 to 11 years of age—400 mg/4 hours, up to 5 doses/24 hours.

11 to 12 years of age—480 mg/4 hours, up to 5 doses/24 hours.

Do not exceed 5 days of continual use without consulting your physician.

Give all doses with food, milk, or a full glass of water.

By Those Over 60 Years of Age: Watch for signs of high blood level: irritability, ringing in the ears, deafness, confusion, nausea, or stomach upset. Aspirin can cause serious stomach bleeding. This can occur as "silent" bleeding of small amounts over a long time. Sudden hemorrhage can occur, even without a history of stomach ulcer. Watch for gray- to black-colored stools, an indication of stomach bleeding.

▷ **Advisability of Use During Pregnancy**
Pregnancy Category: C. See Pregnancy Risk Categories at the back of this book. Animal studies: Significant birth defects due to this drug have been reported. Human studies: Information from studies of pregnant women indicates no increased risk of birth defects in 32,164 pregnancies exposed to aspirin. However, studies show that the regular use of aspirin during pregnancy is often detrimental to the health of the mother and the welfare of the fetus. Anemia, hemorrhage before and after delivery, and an increased incidence of stillbirths and newborn deaths have been reported. There are data that support use of aspirin in low doses to prevent toxemia of pregnancy in some women with a history of this problem. Ask your doctor for help. Avoid aspirin altogether during the last 3 months unless your doctor prescribes it.

Advisability of Use If Breast-Feeding
Presence of this drug in breast milk: Yes.
Avoid drug or refrain from nursing.

Habit-Forming Potential: Extended high dose use may cause a psychological dependence (see Glossary).

Effects of Overdose: Stomach distress, nausea, vomiting, ringing in the ears, dizziness, impaired hearing, blood chemistry imbalance, stupor, fever, deep and rapid breathing, twitching, delirium, shock, hallucinations, convulsions.

Possible Effects of Long-Term Use
A form of psychological dependence (see Glossary).
Anemia due to chronic blood loss from erosion of stomach lining.
The development of a stomach ulcer.
The development of "aspirin allergy"—nasal discharge, nasal polyps, asthma.
Kidney damage.
Prolonged bleeding time, critical in the event of injury or surgery.

Suggested Periodic Examinations While Taking This Drug (at physician's discretion)
Complete blood cell counts.
Kidney function tests and urine analyses.
Liver function tests.

▷ **While Taking This Drug, Observe the Following**
Foods: May decrease the total amount of aspirin per dose which is absorbed.
Nutritional Support: Do not take large doses of vitamin C while taking aspirin regularly.
Beverages: No restrictions. May be taken with milk.
▷ *Alcohol:* Use of alcohol and aspirin at the same time may increase risk of stomach damage and may prolong bleeding time.
Tobacco Smoking: No interactions expected. I advise everyone to quit smoking.
▷ *Other Drugs*
Aspirin may ***increase*** the effects of
  • adrenocortical steroids (see Drug Classes) leading to additive stomach irritation and bleeding.

- insulin (various brands) and require dosage adjustment.
- oral anticoagulants (see Drug Classes), such as warfarin (Coumadin), and cause abnormal bleeding.
- oral antidiabetic drugs (see Drug Classes), and cause hypoglycemia. Dosage adjustments are often necessary.
- heparin, and cause abnormal bleeding.
- methotrexate, and increase its toxic effects.
- tiludronate (Skelid) by increasing blood levels by 50%.
- valproic acid (Depakene).

Aspirin may *decrease* the effects of

- beta-adrenergic-blocking drugs (beta-blockers; see Drug Classes).
- captopril (Capoten).
- enalapril (Vasotec) by decreasing enalapril's beneficial increase in heart (cardiac) output.
- furosemide (Lasix).
- other NSAIDs (nonsteroidal anti-inflammatory drugs; see Drug Classes).
- phenytoin (Dilantin) (high aspirin doses) by decreasing phenytoin blood levels.
- probenecid (Benemid), and reduce its effectiveness in the treatment of gout—with aspirin doses of less than 2 g every 24 hours.
- spironolactone (Aldactazide, Aldactone, others), and reduce its diuretic effect.
- sulfinpyrazone (Anturane), and reduce its effectiveness in the treatment of gout—with aspirin doses of less than 2 g every 24 hours.

Aspirin *taken concurrently* with

- alendronate (Fosamax) may result in increased risk of stomach upset/diarrhea.
- cortisonelike drugs (see Drug Classes) increases risk of stomach ulcers.
- diltiazem (Cardizem) may result in increased risk of bleeding.
- high blood pressure (antihypertensive) medicines may blunt their therapeutic benefit, especially those that are diuretics such as furosemide (Lasix), spironolactone, or thiazides (see Drug Classes).
- intrauterine devices (IUDs) may result in decreased IUD effectiveness.
- lithium (Lithobid) may increase lithium blood levels.
- methotrexate (Mexate) may cause toxicity.
- niacin (various) may BENEFICIALLY decrease flushing fromniacin!
- valproic acid (Depakote) may cause toxic blood levels.
- varicella vaccine (Varivax) may result in Reye's syndrome. **Avoid aspirin and other salicylates for 6 weeks following Varivax inoculation.**
- verapamil (Calan, others) may cause increased bleeding risk.
- zafirlukast (Accolate) may increase zafirlukast blood levels and increase adverse effects.

The following drugs may *increase* the effects of aspirin:

- acetazolamide (Diamox).
- cimetidine (Tagamet).
- para-aminobenzoic acid (Pabalate).

The following drugs may *decrease* the effects of aspirin:

- antacids, with regular continual use.
- cholestyramine (Questran, others), by decreasing the amount of aspirin that goes to work—separate doses by 30 minutes.

- cortisonelike drugs (see Drug Classes).
- urinary alkalinizers (sodium bicarbonate, sodium citrate).

▷ *Driving, Hazardous Activities:* No restrictions or precautions.

Aviation Note: It is advisable to watch for mild drowsiness and restrict activities accordingly.

Exposure to Sun: Use caution; may cause photosensitivity.

Discontinuation: Aspirin should be stopped at least 1 week before surgery of any kind.

ATENOLOL (a TEN oh lohl)

Introduced: 1973 **Class:** Anti-anginal, antihypertensive, beta-adrenergic blocker **Prescription:** USA: Yes **Controlled Drug:** USA: No; Canada: No **Available as Generic:** Yes

Brand Names: ✦Apo-Atenolol, ✦Novo-Atenolol, ✦Nu-Atenolol, Tenoretic [CD], Tenormin

BENEFITS versus RISKS	
Possible Benefits	*Possible Risks*
EFFECTIVE ANTI-ANGINAL DRUG in the management of effort-induced angina EFFECTIVE, WELL-TOLERATED ANTIHYPERTENSIVE in mild to moderate high blood pressure	CONGESTIVE HEART FAILURE in advanced heart disease Worsening of angina in coronary heart disease (abrupt withdrawal) Masking of low blood sugar (hypoglycemia) in drug-treated diabetes Provocation of bronchial asthma (with high doses)

▷ **Principal Uses**

As a Single Drug Product: Uses currently included in FDA-approved labeling: (1) Treats classical, effort-induced angina pectoris; (2) used for mild to moderately severe high blood pressure (may be used alone or in combination with other antihypertensive drugs, such as diuretics); (3) used following heart attacks to prolong life, **helps decrease risk of a second heart attack**, decrease the size of the heart attack, and reduce risk of abnormal heartbeats.

Other (unlabeled) generally accepted uses: (1) Can help people with stage fright; (2) may have a role in preventing migraine headaches; (3) can have an adjunctive role in alcohol withdrawal; (4) helps congestive heart failure when used with fosinopril (Monopril).

As a Combination Drug Product [CD]: Used in combination with a thiazide diuretic to combine the benefits of a beta-blocker with the excess-fluid-losing properties of a thiazide. This attacks high blood pressure using two different mechanisms.

How This Drug Works: It blocks some actions of sympathetic nervous system, reducing heart rate and contraction force, reducing oxygen needs as the heart works; and it reduces blood vessel contraction, resulting in opening and lowering of blood pressure.

Available Dosage Forms and Strengths
Tablets — 25 mg, 50 mg, 100 mg

▷ **Usual Adult Dosage Range:**   Hypertension: Initially 50 mg once daily. Dose may be increased gradually at intervals of 7 to 10 days as needed and tolerated up to 100 mg every 24 hours. The usual maintenance dose is 50 to 100 mg every 24 hours. The total dose should not exceed 100 mg every 24 hours.

Angina: Starting dose is 50 mg once daily. May be gradually increased at 7 to 10 day intervals as needed and tolerated up to 100 mg every 24 hours. Usual ongoing dose is 50 to 100 mg every 24 hours. Some patients require 200 mg daily.

After a heart attack (post MI): Within 12 hours after the attack, 5 mg of this drug is given intravenously. This is followed by a second 5-mg intravenous dose 10 minutes later. Twelve hours after the second intravenous dose, 50 mg is given orally, followed by a second 50-mg dose 12 hours later. Oral dosing is continued at 100 mg orally for the next 10 days. **Note: Actual dose and schedule must be determined for each patient individually.**

Conditions Requiring Dosing Adjustments
Liver Function: No decreases needed (liver has a small removal role).
Kidney Function: The dose must be decreased with 25 mg a day as a maximum dose in some people.

▷ **Dosing Instructions:**   Food decreases the amount of drug that gets into your body by up to 20%. Better taken on an empty stomach. Tablet may be crushed to take it. **DO NOT** stop this drug abruptly.

Usual Duration of Use: Regular use for 3 to 7 days usually needed to see this drug's benefits in lowering blood pressure. Peak benefits may take two weeks. Meeting blood pressure goals will decide long-term use. Medicines are often coupled to an overall program of weight reduction, salt restriction, smoking cessation, etc. May take 3 months for peak chest pain benefits. See your doctor regularly.

Possible Advantages of This Drug: Least likely of all beta-blocker drugs to cause central nervous system adverse effects: confusion, hallucinations, nervousness, nightmares.

▷ **This Drug Should Not Be Taken If**
  • you have had an allergic reaction to it previously.
  • you are in heart failure (overt).
  • you have an abnormally slow heart rate or a serious form of heart block.
  • you are taking, or have taken within the past 14 days, any monoamine oxidase (MAO) type A inhibitor drug (see Drug Classes).
  • you are in cardiogenic shock.

▷ **Inform Your Physician Before Taking This Drug If**
  • you've had adverse reactions to beta-blockers (see Drug Classes).
  • you have a history of serious heart disease, with or without episodes of heart failure.
  • you have a history of hay fever (allergic rhinitis), asthma, chronic bronchitis, chronic obstructive pulmonary disease (COPD), or emphysema.
  • you have been taking clonidine.
  • you have a history of overactive thyroid function (hyperthyroidism).

- you have low blood sugar (hypoglycemia)—drug may hide some symptoms of hypoglycemia.
- you have impaired liver or kidney function.
- you have diabetes or myasthenia gravis.
- you take digitalis, quinidine, reserpine, or any calcium blocker (see Drug Classes).
- you will have surgery with general anesthesia.
- you take prescription or nonprescription drugs not discussed when atenolol was prescribed.
- you are unsure how much to take or how often to take it.

Possible Side Effects (natural, expected, and unavoidable drug actions)

Lethargy, fatigability, cold extremities, slow heart rate, light-headedness in upright position (see *orthostatic hypotension* in Glossary)—all reported during treatment.

▷ **Possible Adverse Effects** (unusual, unexpected, and infrequent reactions)

If any of the following develop, consult your physician promptly for guidance.

Mild Adverse Effects

Allergic reactions: skin rash, itching.

Headache, abnormal dreams—infrequent.

Dizziness, tiredness or depression—frequent.

Indigestion, nausea, diarrhea—infrequent.

Joint and muscle discomfort, fluid retention (edema)—possible.

Serious Adverse Effects

Allergic reactions: may contribute to seriousness and refractory allergic reactions.

Chest pain, shortness of breath, can lead to congestive heart failure—rare.

May lead to an asthma attack in asthmatic people—possible.

Angina or rebound hypertension—if abruptly stopped.

Difficulty walking (intermittent claudication)—controversial.

Psychosis—case reports.

Systemic lupus erythematosus—case reports.

▷ **Possible Effects on Sexual Function:**   Decreased libido and impaired potency (50 to 100 mg per day). This drug is less likely to cause reduced erectile capacity than most drugs of its class. Impotence—rare.

Possible Effects on Laboratory Tests

Blood cholesterol, LDL and VLDL cholesterol levels: no effect with doses of 50 mg/day; increased with doses of 100 mg/day.

Blood triglyceride levels: no effect with doses of 50 mg/day; increased with doses of 100 mg/day.

Blood HDL cholesterol levels: no effect with doses of 50 mg/day; decreased with doses of 100 mg/day.

CAUTION

1. Control your high blood pressure for life! Even though it usually does not have any signs or symptoms, high blood pressure does damage. Control your pressure and take your medicine.
2. ***DO NOT stop this drug suddenly*** without the guidance of your doctor. Carry a note in your purse or wallet that says you take this drug.
3. Talk to your doctor or pharmacist BEFORE using nasal spray or pill de-

congestants. These may cause sudden increases in blood pressure when combined with beta-blocker drugs.

4. Report any tendency to emotional depression to your doctor.

Precautions for Use

By Infants and Children: Safety and effectiveness by those under 12 years of age not established. However, if this drug is used, watch for development of low blood sugar (hypoglycemia), especially if meals are skipped.

By Those Over 60 Years of Age: Proceed ***cautiously*** with all antihypertensive drugs. High blood pressure should be reduced slowly, avoiding excessively low blood pressure. Small doses and frequent blood pressure checks are needed. Sudden and excessive decrease in blood pressure can predispose to stroke or heart attack. Maximum daily dosage is 100 mg. Watch for dizziness, unsteadiness, tendency to fall, confusion, hallucinations, depression, or urinary frequency.

▷ **Advisability of Use During Pregnancy**

Pregnancy Category: D. See Pregnancy Risk Categories at the back of this book. Animal studies: Increased resorptions of embryo and fetus reported in rats, but no birth defects.

Human studies: Adequate studies of pregnant women are not available, but the drug has caused fetal harm.

This drug has been used during the last three months of pregnancy; however, fetal growth may be slowed and the child may be born with low blood pressure and temperature. Ask your doctor for guidance.

Advisability of Use If Breast-Feeding

Presence of this drug in breast milk: Yes.

Avoid drug if possible. If drug is necessary, observe nursing infant for slow heart rate and indications of low blood sugar.

Habit-Forming Potential: None.

Effects of Overdose: Weakness, slow pulse, low blood pressure, fainting, cold and sweaty skin, congestive heart failure, possible coma, and convulsions.

Possible Effects of Long-Term Use: Reduced heart reserve or heart failure in some people with advanced heart disease.

Suggested Periodic Examinations While Taking This Drug (at physician's discretion)

Measurements of blood pressure, evaluation of heart function.

▷ **While Taking This Drug, Observe the Following**

Foods: Can decrease total atenolol absorption by 20%. Best to avoid excessive salt intake. Ginseng may increase blood pressure.

Beverages: No restrictions. May be taken with milk.

▷ *Alcohol:* Use caution. Alcohol may exaggerate this drug's ability to lower blood pressure and may increase its mild sedative effect.

Tobacco Smoking: Nicotine may reduce this drug's effectiveness. I advise everyone to quit smoking.

▷ *Other Drugs*

Atenolol may ***increase*** the effects of

• other antihypertensive drugs and cause excessive lowering of blood pressure. Dosage adjustments may be necessary.

- reserpine (Ser-Ap-Es, etc.) and cause sedation, depression, slowing of heart rate, and lowering of blood pressure.

Atenolol *taken concurrently* with

- amiodarone (Cordarone) may result in cardiac arrest.
- ampicillin or bacampicillin may result in lower blood levels of atenolol.
- calcium (various) may result in **large decreases** in atenolol blood levels.
- clonidine (Catapres) requires close monitoring for rebound high blood pressure if clonidine is stopped while atenolol is still being taken.
- digoxin (Lanoxin) may result in very slow heart rates.
- insulin requires close monitoring to avoid undetected hypoglycemia (see Glossary).
- oral antidiabetic drugs (see Drug Classes) may result in prolonged low blood sugar.
- phenothiazines (see Drug Classes) may increase the effects of both agents and result in phenothiazine toxicity or excessively low blood pressure.
- quinidine (Quinaglute) may cause additive lowering of the blood pressure.
- verapamil can result in undesirable slowing of the heart rate and excessively low blood pressure.

The following drugs may *decrease* the effects of atenolol:

- antacids, which can decrease atenolol absorption.
- fluvoxamine (Luvox).
- indomethacin (Indocin), and possibly other "aspirin substitutes," or NSAIDs, which may impair atenolol's blood-pressure-lowering (antihypertensive) effect.

▷ *Driving, Hazardous Activities:* Use caution until the full extent of drowsiness, lethargy, and blood pressure change has been determined.

Aviation Note: The use of this drug *is a disqualification* for piloting. Consult a designated aviation medical examiner.

Exposure to Sun: No restrictions.

Exposure to Heat: Caution is advised. Hot environments can lower blood pressure and exaggerate the effects of this drug.

Exposure to Cold: Caution is advised. Can enhance the circulatory deficiency that may occur with this drug. The elderly should be careful to prevent hypothermia (see Glossary).

Heavy Exercise or Exertion: Avoid exertion that causes light-headedness, excessive fatigue, or muscle cramping. This drug may worsen the blood pressure response to isometric exercise.

Occurrence of Unrelated Illness: Fever can lower blood pressure and require a decreased dose. Nausea or vomiting may interrupt the dosing schedule. Ask your physician for help.

Discontinuation: Avoid stopping this drug suddenly. If possible, gradual reduction of dose over a period of 2 to 3 weeks is recommended. During such reduction, physical activity is best kept to a Minimum. Ask your doctor for help.

ATORVASTATIN (a TOR va stat in)

Introduced: 1996   **Class:** Cholesterol-lowering agent, HMG-CoA reductase inhibitor   **Prescription:** USA: Yes   **Controlled Drug:** USA: No; Canada: No   **Available as Generic:** No
Brand Name: Lipitor

BENEFITS versus RISKS	
Possible Benefits	*Possible Risks*
REDUCTION OF TOTAL and LDL CHOLESTEROL	Drug-induced hepatitis (without jaundice)—rare
DECREASED TRIGLYCERIDES	Drug-induced myositis (muscle inflammation)—rare

▷ **Principal Uses**

As a Single Drug Product: Uses currently included in FDA-approved labeling: (1) Treats high blood cholesterol (in people with Types IIa and IIb hypercholesterolemia) due to increased fractions of low-density lipoprotein (LDL) cholesterol (used in conjunction with a cholesterol-lowering diet; should not be used until an adequate trial of nondrug methods has proved to be ineffective); (2) also helps familial hypercholesterolemia; (3) the only "statin" that also lowers triglycerides.

Other (unlabeled) generally accepted uses: None at present.

How This Drug Works: Blocks a liver enzyme that starts making cholesterol. Lowers low-density lipoproteins (LDL), the cholesterol fraction thought to increase risk of coronary heart disease. Since the amount of cholesterol is reduced in the liver, the VLDL fraction may also be decreased.

Available Dosage Forms and Strengths

Tablets — 10 mg, 20 mg, 40 mg

Recommended Dosage Ranges: (Actual dosage and schedule must be determined for each patient individually.)

Infants and Children: Data are not available.

18 to 65 Years of Age: Started with 10 mg once daily. Increased as needed and tolerated to a maximum of 80 mg daily. Lipid levels best rechecked within 2 to 4 weeks of starting or changing the dose.

Over 65 Years of Age: Some research shows that usual doses may result in higher levels than seen in younger patients. It appears prudent that the lowest dose (10 mg) be used and LDL-C levels be checked to guide any dose increases. Dose increases must be made after weighing the benefits and risks, mindful that any given dose may result in a higher than expected blood level.

Conditions Requiring Dosing Adjustments

Liver Function: Caution should be used in patients with liver compromise. In those with liver damage caused by alcohol, removal from the body has been prolonged. Ten-mg dose appears prudent. Like other HMG-CoA medicines, atorvastatin should not be given during active liver disease.

Kidney Function: The manufacturer does not recommend dosing changes.

Dosing Instructions: The tablet may be crushed. Better taken on an empty stomach.

Since cholesterol is made at the fastest rate between midnight and 5 A.M., many clinicians advise patients to take such medicines at bedtime.

Usual Duration of Use: Use on a regular schedule for 2 to 4 weeks usually determines the effectiveness of this drug in reducing blood levels of total and LDL-C cholesterol. Long-term use (months to years) requires periodic physician evaluation.

Possible Advantages of This Drug

Recent studies indicate that drugs of this class (HMG-CoA reductase inhibitors) are more effective and better tolerated than other drugs currently available for reducing total and LDL-C cholesterol. Head-to-head trials with other HMG-CoA medicines have not yet been done.

This Drug Should Not Be Taken If

- you have had an allergic reaction to it previously.
- you have active liver disease or increased liver function tests that are unexplained.
- you are pregnant or are breast-feeding your infant.

Inform Your Physician Before Taking This Drug If

- you have previously taken any other drugs in this class: lovastatin (Mevacor), simvastatin (Zocor).
- you have liver disease or impaired liver function.
- you have kidney disease.
- you are not using any method of birth control, or you are planning pregnancy.
- you regularly consume substantial amounts of alcohol.
- you develop unexplained muscle weakness, pain, or tenderness.
- you have any type of chronic muscular disorder.
- you plan to have major surgery in the near future.

Possible Side Effects (natural, expected, and unavoidable drug actions)

None with usual doses.

Possible Adverse Effects (unusual, unexpected, and infrequent reactions)

If any of the following develop, consult your physician promptly for guidance.

Mild Adverse Effects

Allergic reactions: skin rash—infrequent.

Headache—infrequent to frequent, rare drowsiness.

Flu-like syndrome—infrequent.

Diarrhea, constipation, or gas (flatulence)—infrequent.

Muscle pain (myalgia)—infrequent with 20-mg dose.

Serious Adverse Effects

Allergic reactions: not reported as yet.

Marked and persistent abnormal liver function tests (without jaundice): case reports—rare.

Acute myositis (muscle pain and tenderness)—rare to infrequent with 10- to 80-mg doses.

Rhabdomyolysis with sudden kidney failure—rarely reported with other HMG-CoA medicines.

One case report of euphoria, confusion, and short-term memory problems.

Possible Effects on Sexual Function: Decreased libido or impotence (2%).

Possible Delayed Adverse Effects: Rare muscle changes.

Natural Diseases or Disorders That May Be Activated by This Drug
    Latent liver disease.

Possible Effects on Laboratory Tests
    Blood total cholesterol, LDL cholesterol, and triglyceride levels: decreased.

CAUTION
    1. If pregnancy occurs while taking this drug, discontinue it immediately and consult your physician.
    2. Report promptly any development of muscle pain or tenderness, especially if accompanied by fever or malaise.
    3. Report promptly the development of altered or impaired vision so that appropriate evaluation can be made (visual changes have been reported with some other HMG-CoA medicines).
    4. If CPK levels become markedly elevated, this medicine should be stopped.

Precautions for Use
    By Infants and Children: Safety and effectiveness for those under 18 years of age not established.
    By Those Over 60 Years of Age: Blood levels for those over 65 may be higher than those reached by the same dose in younger people.

Advisability of Use During Pregnancy
    Pregnancy Category: X. See Pregnancy Risk Categories at the back of this book.
        Animal studies: Rat studies reveal decreased pup survival and maturity with high-dose studies.
        Human studies: Adequate studies of pregnant women are not available.
        This drug should be avoided during entire pregnancy.

Advisability of Use If Breast-Feeding
    Presence of this drug in breast milk: Yes, in rats; expected in humans.
    Avoid drug or refrain from nursing.

Habit-Forming Potential: None.

Effects of Overdose: Increased indigestion, stomach distress, nausea, diarrhea with other HMG-CoA medicines.

Possible Effects of Long-Term Use: Abnormal liver function tests.

Suggested Periodic Examinations While Taking This Drug (at physician's discretion)
    Blood cholesterol studies: total cholesterol, HDL, and LDL fractions.
    Liver function tests before treatment, every 6 weeks during the first 3 months of use, every 8 weeks for the rest of the first year, and at 6-month intervals thereafter have been recommended for other HMG-CoA inhibitors. Ask your physician for guidance.

▷ **While Taking This Drug, Observe the Following**
    Foods: Follow a standard low-cholesterol diet.
    Beverages: No restrictions. May be taken with milk.
    Alcohol: Excessive alcohol not recommended.
    Tobacco Smoking: No interactions expected. I advise everyone to quit smoking.
    Other Drugs
        Atorvastatin may *increase* the effects of
        • clofibrate (Atromid-S) and other fibric acid derivatives; has been associated with increased risk of muscle damage (rhabdomyolysis).

Atorvastatin *taken concurrently* with
- antacids decreases the amount of atorvastatin that gets into your body.
- azole antifungals (such as itraconazole or Sporanox) may increase the risk for muscle damage (myopathy).
- colestipol (Colestid) results in lowered atorvastatin blood levels, but better lowering of LDL-C.
- cyclosporine (Sandimmune) may increase the risk for myopathy.
- digoxin (Lanoxin, others) can decrease digoxin levels (and possibly therapeutic effects).
- erythromycin (and perhaps other macrolide antibiotics) may increase the risk for myopathy.
- mibefradil (Posicor) may lead to atorvastatin toxicity.
- niacin (various) may increase the risk for myopathy.
- oral contraceptives (norethindrone and ethinyl estradiol) may increases levels of the contraceptives. Increased monitoring for adverse effects is prudent.

Driving, Hazardous Activities: This drug may cause drowsiness. Restrict activities as necessary.

Aviation Note: The use of this drug *may be a disqualification* for piloting. Consult a designated aviation medical examiner.

Exposure to Sun: No restrictions.

Occurrence of Unrelated Illness:
Call your doctor if another physician (such as a specialist) diagnoses a sudden liver problem.

Discontinuation: Do not stop this drug without your doctor's knowledge and help. There may be a significant increase in blood cholesterol levels if this medicine is stopped.

AURANOFIN (aw RAY noh fin)

Introduced: 1976   **Class:** Antiarthritic   **Prescription:** USA: Yes
Controlled Drug: USA: No; Canada: No   **Available as Generic:**   Yes
Brand Name: Ridaura

BENEFITS versus RISKS	
Possible Benefits	*Possible Risks*
REDUCTION OF JOINT PAIN, TENDERNESS, AND SWELLING in active, severe RHEUMATOID ARTHRITIS	SIGNIFICANTLY REDUCED LEVELS OF RED AND WHITE BLOOD CELLS AND BLOOD PLATELETS
Effective when taken by mouth	LIVER DAMAGE WITH JAUNDICE
	Diarrhea
	Ulcerative colitis
	Skin rash
	Mouth sores
	Kidney toxicity (protein in the urine)
	Lung damage

▷ **Principal Uses**

As a Single Drug Product: Uses currently included in FDA-approved labeling: Used *only* for severe rheumatoid arthritis in adults who have had an inadequate response to aspirin, aspirin substitutes, or other antiarthritic drugs and treatment programs. Usually added to a well-established program of antiarthritic drugs.

Other (unlabeled) generally accepted uses: (1) May have a role in helping decrease the need for steroid use in people with asthma; (2) can ease the symptoms of nodular vasculitis.

How This Drug Works: Suppresses but does not cure arthritis. Works on T-cells and on other cells (macrophages), easing inflammation.

Available Dosage Forms and Strengths

Capsules — 3 mg

▷ **Usual Adult Dosage Range:** 6 mg daily, taken either as one dose every 24 hours or as two doses of 3 mg each every 12 hours. If 6 months of regular continual use does not produce an adequate response, the dose may be increased to 9 mg daily, taken as three doses of 3 mg each. If response remains inadequate after 3 months of 9 mg daily, this drug should be stopped. **Note: Actual dose and schedule must be determined for each patient individually.**

Conditions Requiring Dosing Adjustments

Liver Function: No dose decreases needed.

Kidney Function: Blood levels are recommended, and decreased doses may be needed.

▷ **Dosing Instructions:** Take with or following food to reduce stomach irritation. Take the capsule whole with milk or a full glass of water.

Usual Duration of Use: Regular use for 3 to 4 months is usually needed to see benefits in reducing joint pain, tenderness, and swelling associated with rheumatoid arthritis. Long-term use depends on benefits vs. adverse effects. See your doctor on a regular basis.

Author's Note: The information in this profile has been shortened to make room for medicines that are more widely used.

AZATHIOPRINE (ay za THI oh preen)

Introduced: 1965   **Class:** Antiarthritic, immunosuppressive   **Prescription:** USA: Yes   **Controlled Drug:** USA: No; Canada: No   **Available as Generic:** Yes

Brand Name: Imuran

BENEFITS versus RISKS	
Possible Benefits	*Possible Risks*
REDUCTION OF JOINT PAIN, TENDERNESS, AND SWELLING in active, severe RHEUMATOID ARTHRITIS	UNACCEPTABLE ADVERSE EFFECTS IN 15% OF USERS
	REDUCED LEVELS OF WHITE BLOOD CELLS
PREVENTION OF REJECTION IN ORGAN TRANSPLANTATION	REDUCED LEVELS OF RED BLOOD CELLS AND PLATELETS
	LIVER DAMAGE WITH JAUNDICE
	POSSIBLE INCREASED RISK OF MALIGNANCY

▷ **Principal Uses**
    As a Single Drug Product: Uses currently included in FDA-approved labeling: (1) Helps prevent transplanted organ rejection (mainly kidneys); (2) also used in active, severe rheumatoid arthritis (in adults) failing conventional treatment.
    Other (unlabeled) generally accepted uses: (1) Used to treat lupus erythematosus, ulcerative colitis, chronic active hepatitis, and other "autoimmune" disorders; (2) decreases rejection rates (combination therapy), preventing heart transplant failures; (3) very useful in actinic dermatitis.

How This Drug Works: It impairs metabolism of purines, DNA, and RNA. This blunts the immune reaction responsible for rheumatoid arthritis, lupus erythematosus, etc.

Available Dosage Forms and Strengths
    Injection — 100 mg per 20-ml vial
    Tablets — 50 mg

▷ **Usual Adult Dosage Range:** As immunosuppressant—3 to 5 mg per kg of body mass daily, 1 to 3 days before transplantation surgery; for ongoing postoperative use—1 to 2 mg per kg of body mass daily. In rheumatoid arthritis (RA)—1 mg per kg of body mass daily for 6 to 8 weeks; increased by 0.5 mg per kg of body mass every 4 weeks as needed.
    Maximal daily dose is 2.5 mg per kg of body mass. Total dose may be taken once daily or divided into equal doses taken 12 hours apart. Ongoing dose should be the lowest effective dose. **Note: Actual dose schedule must be determined for each patient individually.**

Conditions Requiring Dosing Adjustments
    Liver Function: The drug may need to be stopped if jaundice occurs. Liver function must be closely watched.
    Kidney Function: The dose must be decreased by up to 50% in kidney failure.

▷ **Dosing Instructions:** Take with or following food to reduce stomach upset. Tablet may be crushed.

Usual Duration of Use: Use on a regular schedule for 12 weeks is usually needed to determine this drug's effectiveness in helping rheumatoid arthritis. Successful use for more than a decade has been reported. See your physician regularly.

▷ **This Drug Should Not Be Taken If**
- you have had an allergic reaction to it previously.
- you are pregnant, and this drug is prescribed to treat rheumatoid arthritis.
- you have an active blood cell or bone marrow disorder.
- you are taking, or have recently taken, any form of chlorambucil (Leukeran), cyclophosphamide (Cytoxan), or melphalan (Alkeran).

▷ **Inform Your Physician Before Taking This Drug If**
- you have any kind of active infection.
- you have any form of cancer.
- you have gout or are taking allopurinol (Zyloprim).
- you have a history of blood cell or bone marrow disorders.
- you have impaired liver or kidney function.
- you are taking an ACE inhibitor (see Drug Classes). Use of azathioprine with these medicines has severely lowered white blood cell counts.

- you are taking any form of gold, penicillamine, or an antimalarial drug for arthritis.
- you plan pregnancy in the near future.
- you take other prescription or nonprescription medicines not discussed when azathioprine was prescribed.
- you are unsure how much to take or how often to take it.

Possible Side Effects (natural, expected, and unavoidable drug actions)
Development of infection.

▷ **Possible Adverse Effects** (unusual, unexpected, and infrequent reactions)
If any of the following develop, consult your physician promptly for guidance.

Mild Adverse Effects
Allergic reaction: skin rash—rare.
Loss of appetite, nausea, vomiting, diarrhea—infrequent.
Sores on lips and in mouth—possible.
Muscle aches—infrequent.

Serious Adverse Effects
Allergic reactions: drug fever (see Glossary), joint and muscle pain—rare.
Pancreatitis: severe stomach pain with nausea and vomiting—rare.
Bone marrow depression (see Glossary): fatigue, weakness, fever, sore throat, abnormal bleeding or bruising—dose dependent.
Liver damage: yellow eyes, dark urine (see **Hepatitis** and **Jaundice** in Glossary)—rare.
Drug-induced pneumonia: cough, shortness of breath—possible.
Development of cancer: skin cancer, reticulum-cell sarcoma, lymphoma, leukemia—possible.

▷ **Possible Effects on Sexual Function:**   Reversal of male infertility due to sperm antibodies; this drug suppresses autoantibodies and permits the normal accumulation of sperm. May also decrease sperm counts.

Possible Delayed Adverse Effects: Bone marrow depression may occur after stopping this drug.

Adverse Effects That May Mimic Natural Diseases or Disorders
Liver damage may suggest viral hepatitis.

Possible Effects on Laboratory Tests
Complete blood cell counts: decreased red cells, hemoglobin, white cells, and platelets.
Blood amylase and lipase levels: increased.
Blood uric acid levels: increased; decreased in gout patients.
Liver function tests: increased liver enzymes (ALT/GPT, AST/GOT, and alkaline phosphatase); increased bilirubin.
Sperm counts: decreased.

CAUTION
1. Promptly report infection—fever, chills, lip sores, etc.
2. Inform your physician promptly if you become pregnant.
3. Periodic blood counts are mandatory.
4. Talk to your doctor BEFORE you get any shots (vaccines).

Precautions for Use
By Infants and Children: Safety and effectiveness in those under 12 years of age not established.

By Those Over 60 Years of Age: The smallest effective dose should be used, as this reduces the risk of toxic reactions.

▷ **Advisability of Use During Pregnancy**
Pregnancy Category: D. See Pregnancy Risk Categories at the back of this book. Animal studies: Birth defects reported in rodent studies.
Human studies: This drug exhibits teratogenic effects and also poses a risk of suppression of the immune system of the newborn. Adequate studies of pregnant women are not available. **Avoid completely** during entire pregnancy if possible.

Advisability of Use If Breast-Feeding
Presence of this drug in breast milk: Yes.
Avoid drug or refrain from nursing.

Habit-Forming Potential: None.

Effects of Overdose: Immediate—nausea, vomiting, diarrhea. Delayed—lowered white blood cell and platelet counts, liver and kidney toxicity.

Possible Effects of Long-Term Use: Susceptibility to infection, bone marrow depression, development of malignancies.

Suggested Periodic Examinations While Taking This Drug (at physician's discretion)
Complete blood cell counts, liver function tests.

▷ **While Taking This Drug, Observe the Following**
Foods: No restrictions.
Beverages: No restrictions. May be taken with milk.
▷ *Alcohol:* No interactions expected.
Tobacco Smoking: No interactions expected. I advise everyone to quit smoking.
▷ *Other Drugs*
Azathioprine may *decrease* the effects of
• certain muscle relaxants (gallamine, pancuronium, tubocurarine), and make it necessary to increase their dosage.
• oral anticoagulants (warfarin, etc.), and requires increased doses.
The following drugs may *increase* the effects of azathioprine:
• allopurinol (Zyloprim); may increase its activity and toxicity and make it necessary to reduce its dosage.
Azathioprine *taken concurrently* with
• ACE inhibitors (see Drug Classes) such as captopril or enalapril may cause severe white blood cell count lowering or anemia.
• cotrimoxazole (Bactrim, others) can cause severe lowering of white blood cell counts.
• prednisolone will result in lower prednisolone blood levels and risk of decreased therapeutic benefit.
• warfarin (Coumadin) may result in decreased anticoagulant effectiveness.
▷ *Driving, Hazardous Activities:* No restrictions.
Aviation Note: The use of this drug *may be a disqualification* for piloting. Consult a designated aviation medical examiner.
Exposure to Sun: No restrictions.
Discontinuation: A gradual reduction in dosage is preferable. Consult your physician for a withdrawal schedule.

AZITHROMYCIN (a zith roh MY sin)

See the macrolide antibiotics profile for further information.

BACAMPICILLIN (bak am pi SIL in)

See the penicillin antibiotic family profile for further information.

BECLOMETHASONE (be kloh METH a sohn)

Introduced: 1976   **Class:** Antiasthmatic, cortisonelike drugs   **Prescription:** USA: Yes   **Controlled Drug:** USA: No; Canada: No   **Available as Generic:** No

Brand Names: ✦Beclodisk, ✦Becloforte, Beclovent, ✦Beclovent Rotacaps, ✦Beclovent Rotahaler, Beconase AQ Nasal Spray, Beconase Nasal Inhaler, ✦Propaderm, ✦Propaderm-C, Vancenase AQ Nasal Spray, Vancenase Nasal Inhaler, Vanceril

BENEFITS versus RISKS	
Possible Benefits	*Possible Risks*
EFFECTIVE RELIEF OF ALLERGIC RHINITIS	FUNGUS INFECTIONS OF THE MOUTH AND THROAT
EFFECTIVE CONTROL OF SEVERE, CHRONIC ASTHMA	Localized areas of "allergic" pneumonia
	Changes in lining of the nose (nasal mucosa)
	Increased cataract risk

▷ **Principal Uses**

As a Single Drug Product: Uses currently included in FDA-approved labeling: (1) Treats bronchial asthma in people who don't have sufficient response to bronchodilators and need cortisonelike drugs for asthma control; (2) prevents nasal polyp return after surgical removal; (3) treats seasonal and perennial rhinitis in children and adults (AQ nasal forms).

Other (unlabeled) generally accepted uses: (1) Helps lung disease (bronchopulmonary dysplasia), allowing smaller daily prednisone doses; (2) helps hoarseness seen in LE and juvenile rheumatoid arthritis.

How This Drug Works: It increases cyclic AMP, thus increasing epinephrine, which opens bronchial tubes and fights asthma. Also reduces local lung inflammation in the respiratory tract.

Available Dosage Forms and Strengths

Inhalant — 17 g (50 mcg)

Nasal inhaler — 16.8 g (42 or 82 mcg each)

Nasal spray — 0.042%, 42 mcg and 84 mcg per spray (52 mcg Canada)

Oral inhaler — 16.8 g (200 doses of 42 mcg each, 50 mcg in Canada)

Rotacaps (Canada) — 100- and 200-mcg capsules
Topical lotion (Canada) — 0.025%

▷ **Usual Dosage Ranges:**

Infants and Children: Data are not available for infants. Children 6–12 years old may receive: Nasal inhaler—one inhalation (42 mcg) in each nostril three times a day; oral inhalation—maximum is 10 inhalations (420 mcg).

18 to 65 Years of Age: Nasal inhaler—one to two inhalations (42-84 mcg) in each nostril twice daily. Oral inhaler (double strength)—two inhalations (of 84 mcg) twice daily. For severe asthma—6 to 8 inhalations daily. Maximum daily dose should not exceed 10 inhalations.

By Those Over 65 Years of Age: Doses similar to those used in younger patients have been effective and safe. In some cases, oral-steroid-dependent patients have been able to slowly taper, then stop, oral steroids while taking beclomethasone.

Note: Actual dose and schedule must be determined for each patient individually.

Conditions Requiring Dosing Adjustments

Liver Function: Use with caution in patients with liver compromise.
Kidney Function: No adjustments in dosing expected to be needed.

▷ **Dosing Instructions:**   May be used without regard to eating. Rinse the mouth and throat (gargle) with water thoroughly after each inhalation.

Usual Duration of Use: Regular use for 1 to 4 weeks is usually needed to see this drug's effectiveness in relieving severe, chronic allergic rhinitis and in controlling severe, chronic asthma. Long-term use must be physician supervised. See your doctor on a regular basis.

▷ **This Drug Should Not Be Taken If**
   • you have had an allergic reaction to any form of this drug.
   • you are having severe acute asthma or status asthmaticus that requires more intense treatment for prompt relief.
   • other antiasthmatic drugs that are not related to cortisone can control your asthma.
   • your asthma requires cortisonelike drugs infrequently for control.
   • you have a form of nonallergic bronchitis with asthmatic features.

▷ **Inform Your Physician Before Taking This Drug If**
   • you are now taking or have recently taken any cortisone-related drug (including ACTH by injection) for any reason (see Drug Classes).
   • you have a history of tuberculosis of the lungs.
   • you have chronic bronchitis or bronchiectasis.
   • you think you have an active infection of any kind, especially a respiratory infection.
   • you have recently been exposed to chickenpox or other viral illnesses.
   • you are prone to nosebleeds (epistaxis) (nasal forms).
   • you are unsure how much to take or how often to take it.

Possible Side Effects (natural, expected, and unavoidable drug actions)
   Fungus infections (thrush) of the mouth and throat.

▷ **Possible Adverse Effects** (unusual, unexpected, and infrequent reactions)
   If any of the following develop, consult your physician promptly for guidance.

Mild Adverse Effects
    Allergic reaction: skin rash—rare.
    Dryness of mouth, hoarseness, sore throat, cough—possible.
    Nosebleeds (epistaxis)—infrequent.
Serious Adverse Effects
    Allergic reaction: localized areas of "allergic" pneumonitis (lung inflammation).
    Bronchospasm, asthmatic wheezing—rare.
    Shrinking of the nasal tissues (nasal atrophy)—possible.
    Yeast infections (up to 41%)—frequent.
    Increased risk of cataracts with long-term (chronic) use.
    Osteoporosis (any corticosteroid can cause this)—possible.
▷ **Possible Effects on Sexual Function:**   None reported.
Natural Diseases or Disorders That May Be Activated by This Drug
    Cortisone-related drugs having systemic effects impair immunity and lead to reactivation of "healed" or dormant tuberculosis. People with a history of tuberculosis must be watched closely while using this drug.
Possible Effects on Laboratory Tests
    Blood cortisol levels: decreased.
CAUTION
    1. This drug should not be relied upon for immediate relief of acute asthma.
    2. If you required cortisonelike drugs **before** starting this inhaler, you may again require a cortisonelike drug if you are injured, have an infection or need surgery.
    3. If severe asthma returns while using this drug, call your doctor immediately. Cortisonelike drugs may be required.
    4. Carry a personal ID card saying that you have used (if true) cortisone-related drugs in the past year.
    5. Wait 5 to 10 minutes after using a bronchodilator inhaler like epinephrine, isoetharine, or isoproterenol (which should be used first) before this drug. This permits greater penetration of beclomethasone into the lung. The time between inhalations also reduces risk of adverse propellant effects.
    6. This drug does NOT replace systemic steroids, but may allow dosage decreases in some patients.
Precautions for Use
    By Infants and Children: Safety and effectiveness for use of the nasal inhaler or oral inhaler by those under 6 years of age have not been established. Maximum daily dose in children 6 to 12 years of age varies with the product being used.
    By Those Over 60 Years of Age: People with bronchiectasis should be watched closely for the development of lung infections.
▷ **Advisability of Use During Pregnancy**
    Pregnancy Category: C. See Pregnancy Risk Categories at the back of this book.
    Animal studies: Mouse, rat, and rabbit studies reveal significant birth defects due to this drug.
    Human studies: Adequate studies of pregnant women are not available.
    Avoid drug during the first 3 months. Use infrequently and only as clearly needed during the last 6 months.

Advisability of Use If Breast-Feeding
Presence of this drug in breast milk: Probably yes.
Avoid drug or refrain from nursing.

Habit-Forming Potential: With recommended dosage, a state of functional dependence (see Glossary) is not likely to develop. There have been a small number of cases reported where the aerosol was abused for the fluorocarbon propellants.

Effects of Overdose: Indications of cortisone excess (due to systemic absorption)—fluid retention, flushing of the face, stomach irritation, nervousness.

Suggested Periodic Examinations While Taking This Drug (at physician's discretion)
Inspection of nose, mouth, and throat for fungus infection. Inspection of the nose tissues for nasal atrophy. Assessment of adrenal function in people using cortisone-related drugs for an extended time prior to this drug. Lung X ray if a prior history of tuberculosis. Measures of bone mineral density and cataract check.

▷ **While Taking This Drug, Observe the Following**
Foods: No specific restrictions beyond those advised by your physician.
Beverages: No specific restrictions.
▷ *Alcohol:* No interactions expected.
Tobacco Smoking: No interactions expected. Smoking can reduce the benefits of this drug. I advise everyone to quit smoking.
▷ *Other Drugs*
The following drugs may *increase* the effects of beclomethasone:
• flunisolide (Nasalide).
• inhalant bronchodilators—epinephrine, isoetharine, isoproterenol.
• oral bronchodilators—aminophylline, ephedrine, terbutaline, theophylline, etc.
▷ *Driving, Hazardous Activities:* No restrictions.
Aviation Note: The use of this drug and the disorder for which this drug is prescribed *may be disqualifications* for piloting. Consult a designated aviation medical examiner.
Exposure to Sun: No restrictions.
Occurrence of Unrelated Illness: Acute infections, serious injuries, and surgery can create an urgent need for cortisone-related drugs. Call your doctor immediately in the event of new illness or injury.
Discontinuation: If this drug has made it possible to reduce or stop ongoing cortisonelike drugs, *do not* stop this drug abruptly. If you must stop this drug, call your doctor. You may need to resume cortisone medicines.
Special Storage Instructions: Store at room temperature. Avoid exposure to temperatures above 120 degrees F (49 degrees C). Do not store or use this inhaler near heat or open flame. Protect from light.

BENAZEPRIL (ben AY ze pril)

Class: Antihypertensive, ACE inhibitor
Please see the angiotensin converting enzyme inhibitor (ACE) combination profile for more information.

BENZTROPINE (BENZ troh peen)

Introduced: 1954   **Class:** Anti-parkinsonism, anticholinergic drugs   **Prescription:** USA: Yes   **Controlled Drug:** USA: No; Canada: No   **Available as Generic:** USA: Yes; Canada: Yes

Brand Names: ♣Apo-Benztropine, ♣Bensylate, Cogentin, ♣PMS Benztropine

BENEFITS versus RISKS	
Possible Benefits	*Possible Risks*
PARTIAL RELIEF OF SYMPTOMS OF PARKINSON'S DISEASE RELIEF OF DRUG-INDUCED EXTRAPYRAMIDAL REACTIONS	Atropinelike side effects: blurred vision, dry mouth, constipation, impaired urination Toxic psychosis—rare Tardive dyskinesia—rare

▷ **Principal Uses**

As a Single Drug Product: Uses currently included in FDA-approved labeling: (1) Used with other drugs to treat all types of parkinsonism—if relief is inadequate, more potent drugs (levodopa or bromocriptine) may supplement cogentin; (2) controls parkinsonian reactions from some antipsychotic drugs (such as phenothiazines); (3) eases parkinsonian symptoms after encephalitis.

Other (unlabeled) generally accepted uses: (1) helps sweaty palms (combined with psychotherapy); (2) can help drooling in developmentally disabled patients; (3) can relieve painful erections (priapism).

How This Drug Works: Restores a more normal balance of two brain chemicals (acetylcholine and dopamine), thereby decreasing parkinsonism symptoms.

Available Dosage Forms and Strengths

Injection — 1 mg/ml

Tablets — 0.5 mg, 1 mg, 2 mg

▷ **Usual Adult Dosage Range:** For Parkinson's disease: 0.5 to 2 mg daily, taken in a single dose at bedtime. For drug-induced parkinsonian reactions: 1 to 4 mg daily, either in a single dose or in two to three divided doses. The total daily dose should not exceed 6 mg. For Parkinson's symptoms after encephalitis: starting doses of 2 mg/day are used. May then be increased as needed or tolerated to 4 to 6 mg per day. **Note: Actual dosage and schedule must be determined for each patient individually.**

Conditions Requiring Dosing Adjustments

Liver Function: Use with caution in patients with impaired liver function.

Kidney Function: **Caution:** Decreased kidney function may lead to an increased blood level and an increased risk of adverse effects.

▷ **Dosing Instructions:** May be taken with or following food to reduce stomach irritation. Tablet may be crushed.

Usual Duration of Use: Regular use for 2 to 4 weeks usually needed to see peak benefit relieving symptoms of parkinsonism. Long-term use (months to years) requires physician supervision.

▷ **This Drug Should Not Be Taken If**

• you have had an allergic reaction to it.

• it is prescribed for a child under 3 years of age.

- you have tardive dyskinesia.
- you have narrow angle glaucoma.

▷ **Inform Your Physician Before Taking This Drug If**
- you have had an unfavorable reaction to atropine or atropinelike drugs.
- you have glaucoma or myasthenia gravis.
- you have heart disease or high blood pressure.
- you have a history of liver or kidney disease.
- you have difficulty emptying the urinary bladder, especially if due to an enlarged prostate gland.
- you are taking, or took in the past 2 weeks, any monoamine oxidase (MAO) type A inhibitor (see Drug Classes).
- you take prescription or nonprescription medicines not discussed when benztropine was prescribed for you.
- you are unsure how much to take or how often to take it.
- you will be exposed to extreme heat for extended periods, such as some iron smelters or tropical climates.
- you have a history of bowel obstructions.

Possible Side Effects (natural, expected, and unavoidable drug actions)
Nervousness, blurring of vision, dryness of mouth, constipation, impaired urination. (These often subside as drug use continues.)

▷ **Possible Adverse Effects** (unusual, unexpected, and infrequent reactions)
If any of the following develop, consult your physician promptly for guidance.
Mild Adverse Effects
Allergic reaction: skin rashes—rare.
Headache, dizziness, drowsiness, muscle cramps—possible.
Indigestion, nausea, vomiting—reported.
Fast heart rate (tachycardia)—infrequent.
Memory problems—possible.
Serious Adverse Effects
Idiosyncratic reactions: abnormal behavior, confusion, delusions, hallucinations, toxic psychosis—case reports.
Tardive dyskinesia—case reports.
Dystonia—rare.
Bowel obstruction—case reports.
Abnormal temperature (hyperthermia)—case reports.

▷ **Possible Effects on Sexual Function:**   Reversal of male impotence due to the use of fluphenazine (a phenothiazine antipsychotic drug).
Male infertility (0.5 to 6 mg per day).
May help treat priapism.

Natural Diseases or Disorders That May Be Activated by This Drug
Latent glaucoma, latent myasthenia gravis.

Possible Effects on Laboratory Tests
Prolactin: may be increased (especially if taken with haloperidol).

CAUTION
1. Many over-the-counter (OTC) drugs for allergies, colds, and coughs should NOT be combined with benztropine. Ask your doctor or pharmacist for help.

2. This drug may aggravate tardive dyskinesia (see Glossary). Ask your physician for guidance.

Precautions for Use

By Infants and Children: Safety and effectiveness for those under 3 years of age not established. Children are especially susceptible to the atropinelike effects.

By Those Over 60 Years of Age: Small starting doses are prudent. Increased risk of confusion, nightmares, hallucinations, increased internal eye pressure (glaucoma), and impaired urination associated with prostate gland enlargement (prostatism).

▷ **Advisability of Use During Pregnancy**

Pregnancy Category: C. See Pregnancy Risk Categories at the back of this book.
Animal studies: No data available.
Human studies: Adequate studies of pregnant women are not available.
Avoid use if possible, especially close to delivery. This drug can impair the infant's intestinal tract following birth.

Advisability of Use If Breast-Feeding

Presence of this drug in breast milk: Unknown.
Ask your doctor for help.

Habit-Forming Potential: Occasional reports of anti-parkinsonian drug abuse have been made. Sudden withdrawal of benztropine may lead to craving, restlessness, nervousness, and depression. Propranolol (20–80 mg three times daily) or diazepam (Valium) have been used to ease these symptoms.

Effects of Overdose: Weakness; drowsiness; stupor; impaired vision; rapid pulse; excitement; confusion; hallucinations; dry, hot skin; skin rash; dilated pupils.

Possible Effects of Long-Term Use: Increased internal eye pressure—possible glaucoma, especially in the elderly.

Suggested Periodic Examinations While Taking This Drug (at physician's discretion)

Measurement of internal eye pressure at regular intervals.

▷ **While Taking This Drug, Observe the Following**

Foods: No restrictions.
Beverages: No restrictions.
▷ *Alcohol:* Use caution. Alcohol may increase the sedative effects.
Tobacco Smoking: No interactions expected, but I advise everyone to quit smoking.
Marijuana Smoking: May increase heart rate to unacceptable levels. Avoid completely if this increased heart rate will be a problem for you.

▷ *Other Drugs*

Benztropine may *decrease* the effects of
- cisapride (Propulsid).
- haloperidol (Haldol).
- phenothiazines (Thorazine, others).

The following drugs may *increase* the effects of benztropine:
- antihistamines, which may add to the dryness of mouth and throat.
- monoamine oxidase (MAO) type A inhibitor drugs (see Drug Classes), which may intensify all effects of this drug.

- tricyclic antidepressants (Elavil, etc.), which may add to eye effects and further increase internal eye pressure (dangerous in glaucoma).

Benztropine *taken concurrently* with

- amantadine (Symmetrel) may cause increased confusion and possible hallucinations.
- clozapine (Clozaril) can cause increased risk of elevated temperatures, neurological adverse effects, and bowel obstruction (ileus).

▷ *Driving, Hazardous Activities:* Drowsiness and dizziness may occur in sensitive individuals. Avoid hazardous activities until full effects and tolerance have been determined.

Aviation Note: The use of this drug *is a disqualification* for piloting. Consult a designated aviation medical examiner.

Exposure to Sun: No restrictions.

Exposure to Heat: Use caution. This drug may reduce sweating, cause an increase in body temperature, and increase risk of heatstroke.

Heavy Exercise or Exertion: Use caution. Avoid in hot environments.

Discontinuation: Do not stop this drug abruptly. Ask your doctor how to reduce the dose gradually.

BETAXOLOL (be TAX oh lohl)

Introduced: 1983 **Class:** Antihypertensive, beta-adrenergic blocker **Prescription:** USA: Yes **Controlled Drug:** USA: No; Canada: No **Available as Generic:** No

Brand Names: Betoptic, Betoptic-Pilo [CD], Betoptic-S, Kerlone

BENEFITS versus RISKS	
Possible Benefits	*Possible Risks*
EFFECTIVE, WELL-TOLERATED ANTIHYPERTENSIVE in mild to moderate high blood pressure	CONGESTIVE HEART FAILURE in advanced heart disease
EFFECTIVE TREATMENT OF CHRONIC, OPEN-ANGLE GLAUCOMA	Worsening of angina in coronary heart disease (abrupt withdrawal)
	Masking of low blood sugar (hypoglycemia) in diabetes
PROLONGATION OF LIFE AFTER A HEART ATTACK	Provocation of bronchial asthma (with high doses)
Treatment of ocular hypertension	Rare anemia and low blood platelets

▷ **Principal Uses**

As a Single Drug Product: Uses currently included in FDA-approved labeling: Used to treat: (1) mild to moderate high blood pressure (alone or combined with other antihypertensive drugs, such as diuretics); (2) chronic open-angle glaucoma (eyedrops); (3) ocular hypertension; (4) Betoptic-Pilo: reduces elevated eye pressure in patients with primary open-angle glaucoma who have failed Betoptic-S therapy.

Other (unlabeled) generally accepted uses: (1) The oral form may help decrease death (mortality) from a heart attack; (2) helps decrease incidence and severity of chest pain (angina); (3) can ease aggressive behavior in selected psychiatric patients; (4) may help panic attacks; (5) can treat selected cases of stuttering.

How This Drug Works: By blocking some sympathetic nervous system actions, it reduces heart rate and contraction force, lowers blood ejection pressure, and reduces oxygen needed by the heart. Relaxes blood vessel walls, resulting in expansion and lower blood pressure. Reduces internal eye pressure.

Available Dosage Forms and Strengths
>   Eyedrops — 2.8 mg/ml
>   — 5.6 mg/ml
>   Tablets — 10 mg, 20 mg

▷ **Usual Adult Dosage Range:**   Hypertension: Initially 10 mg once daily. Dose may be increased at intervals of 7 to 14 days as needed and tolerated up to 20 mg every 24 hours. Usual ongoing dose is 10 to 15 mg daily. Some patients have tolerated 40 mg daily well, but had no benefit in reduced blood pressure. Total maximum is 20 mg daily.

For use in glaucoma: One or two drops of the 2.8 mg/ml solution or one drop of the 5.6 mg/ml.

Betoptic-Pilo: Reducing intraocular pressure in primary open-angle glaucoma failing Betoptic-S therapy: Follow label instructions. **Note: Actual dose and schedule must be determined for each patient individually.**

Conditions Requiring Dosing Adjustments
Liver Function: Use with caution; this drug is metabolized in the liver. Dose decreases not routinely needed.
Kidney Function: Starting dose is 5 mg. The dose is increased as needed and tolerated by 5 mg every 2 weeks for a maximum of 20 mg daily.

▷ **Dosing Instructions:**   May be taken without regard to eating. The tablet may be crushed. Do not stop this drug abruptly.

Usual Duration of Use: Regular use for 10 to 14 days usually needed to see this drug's effectiveness in lowering blood pressure. Long-term use is determined by success in lowering blood pressure and response to overall treatment program (weight reduction, salt restriction, smoking cessation, etc.). See your doctor regularly.

Possible Advantages of This Drug: Usually effective and well tolerated with a single dose daily, which is easier to remember to take.

▷ **This Drug Should Not Be Taken If**
- you have had an allergic reaction to it previously.
- you have heart (overt) failure.
- you have an abnormally slow heart rate or a serious heart block.
- you are taking, or took in the past 14 days, any monoamine oxidase (MAO) type A inhibitor (see Drug Classes).

▷ **Inform Your Physician Before Taking This Drug If**
- you have had an adverse reaction to any beta-blocker (see Drug Classes).
- you have serious heart disease or episodes of heart failure.
- you have a history of hay fever (allergic rhinitis), asthma, chronic bronchitis, or emphysema. Some drugs in this class are contraindicated in asthmatics.
- you have overactive thyroid function (hyperthyroidism).
- you have a history of low blood sugar (hypoglycemia).

- you have impaired liver or kidney function.
- you have narrowing of the vessels in your legs or arms (peripheral vascular disease). Discuss this with your doctor.
- you have diabetes or myasthenia gravis.
- you take digitalis, quinidine, or reserpine, or any calcium blocker drug (see Drug Classes).
- you will have surgery with general anesthesia.
- you take prescription or nonprescription medications not discussed when betaxolol was prescribed for you.
- you are unsure how much to take or how often to take it.

Possible Side Effects (natural, expected, and unavoidable drug actions)

Lethargy, fatigue (up to 10%), cold extremities—rare; slow heart rate, light-headedness in upright position (see **Orthostatic Hypotension** in Glossary).

▷ **Possible Adverse Effects** (unusual, unexpected, and infrequent reactions)

If any of the following develop, consult your physician promptly for guidance.

Mild Adverse Effects

Allergic reactions: skin rash, itching—rare.

Hair loss—rare.

Headache (up to 15%)—frequent.

Dizziness, fatigue—infrequent.

Insomnia or abnormal dreams—infrequent.

Indigestion, nausea, diarrhea—infrequent.

Joint and muscle discomfort—infrequent.

Fluid retention (edema)—rare.

Difficulty breathing—infrequent.

Serious Adverse Effects

Allergic reactions: May make allergic reactions more difficult to treat (refractory).

Mental depression or anxiety—rare.

Increased blood sugar (hyperglycemia) in non-insulin-dependent diabetics—possible.

Chest pain, shortness of breath, congestive heart failure—rare.

Induction of bronchial asthma (in asthmatic individuals)—possible.

Low blood platelets and anemia—rare.

Congestive heart failure—rare.

Angina (if pill form abruptly stopped).

Intermittent problems walking (intermittent claudication)—possible.

Heart attack (myocardial infarction)—rare.

Author's note: Adverse effects from eye drops happen rarely if at all versus pill form.

▷ **Possible Effects on Sexual Function:**   Decreased libido, impotence—rare.

Altered menstrual patterns (reported rarely with other medicines in this class)—possible.

Adverse Effects That May Mimic Natural Diseases or Disorders

Reduced blood flow to extremities may mimic Raynaud's disease (see Glossary).

Possible Effects on Laboratory Tests

Glaucoma-screening test (measurement of internal eye pressure): pressure is decreased (false low or normal value).

Antinuclear antibodies (ANA) test: positive in 5.3% of users.

Blood potassium: slightly increased.

Blood platelet counts and hemoglobin: decreased—rare.

Blood glucose: increased in non-insulin-dependent diabetics.

CAUTION

1. ***Do not stop this drug suddenly*** without calling your doctor. Always carry a note with you that says you are taking this drug.
2. Ask your physician or pharmacist before using nasal decongestants. These can cause sudden increases in blood pressure when combined with beta-blocker drugs.
3. Report any tendency to emotional depression.

Precautions for Use

By Infants and Children: Safety and effectiveness for those under 12 years of age not established.

By Those Over 60 Years of Age: **Caution**: High blood pressure should be slowly reduced, avoiding risks associated with excessively low blood pressure. Treatment should be started with 5 mg daily and blood pressure checked often. Sudden, rapid, and excessive reduction of blood pressure can cause stroke or heart attack. Total daily dosage should not exceed 10 to 15 mg. Watch for dizziness, unsteadiness, tendency to fall, confusion, hallucinations, depression, or urinary frequency. This age group is more prone to develop excessively slow heart rates and hypothermia.

▷ **Advisability of Use During Pregnancy**

Pregnancy Category: C. See Pregnancy Risk Categories at the back of this book.

Animal studies: Rat studies reveal increased resorptions of embryo and fetus, retarded growth and development of newborn, and mild skeletal defects.

Human studies: Adequate studies of pregnant women are not available.

Avoid use of drug during the first 3 months if possible. Avoid use during labor and delivery because of the possible effects on the newborn infant.

Advisability of Use If Breast-Feeding

Presence of this drug in breast milk: Yes.

Avoid drug if possible. If drug is necessary, observe nursing infant for slow heart rate and indications of low blood sugar.

Habit-Forming Potential: None.

Effects of Overdose: Weakness, slow pulse, low blood pressure, fainting, cold and sweaty skin, congestive heart failure, possible coma, and convulsions.

Possible Effects of Long-Term Use: Reduced heart reserve and eventual heart failure in susceptible individuals with advanced heart disease.

Suggested Periodic Examinations While Taking This Drug (at physician's discretion)

Measurements of blood pressure, evaluation of heart function.

▷ **While Taking This Drug, Observe the Following**

Foods: No restrictions. Avoid excessive salt intake. Ginseng may raise blood pressure.

Beverages: No restrictions. May be taken with milk.

▷   *Alcohol:* Use with caution. Alcohol may exaggerate lowering of blood pressure and may increase its mild sedative effect.

Tobacco Smoking: Nicotine may reduce this drug's effectiveness. High drug doses worsen bronchial constriction caused by regular smoking. I advise everyone to quit smoking.

▷ *Other Drugs*

Betaxolol may ***increase*** the effects of
- other antihypertensive drugs and cause excessive lowering of blood pressure. Dosage decreases may be necessary.
- reserpine (Ser-Ap-Es, etc.) and cause sedation, depression, slowing of heart rate, and lowering of blood pressure (light-headedness, fainting).
- verapamil and cause additive risk of congestive heart failure and slow heart rate (bradycardia).

Betaxolol ***taken concurrently*** with
- amiodarone (Cordarone) may result in extremely slow heart rate and arrest.
- calcium channel blockers (see Drug Classes) may cause severe lowering of blood pressure.
- clonidine (Catapres) requires close monitoring for rebound high blood pressure if clonidine is stopped while betaxolol is still being taken.
- fluoroquinolone antibiotics (see Drug Classes) may cause an increase in betaxolol blood levels and lead to toxicity.
- fluvoxamine (Luvox) may cause excessive slowing of the heart and very low blood pressure.
- insulin requires close supervision to avoid hypoglycemia (see Glossary).
- oral antidiabetic drugs (see Drug Classes) may prolong recovery from low blood sugars.
- phenothiazines (see Drug Classes) may result in additive blood-pressure-lowering effects.
- ritonavir (Norvir) and perhaps other protease inhibitors (see Drug Classes) may decrease betaxolol benefits.
- venlafaxine (Effexor) may cause excessive slowing of the heart and very low blood pressure.

The following drugs may ***decrease*** the effects of betaxolol:
- indomethacin (Indocin), and possibly other "aspirin substitutes" or NSAIDs, may impair betaxolol's antihypertensive effect.

▷ *Driving, Hazardous Activities:* Use caution until the full extent of drowsiness, lethargy, and blood pressure change has been determined.

Aviation Note: The use of this drug ***is a disqualification*** for piloting. Consult a designated aviation medical examiner.

Exposure to Sun: No restrictions.

Exposure to Heat: Caution is advised. Hot environments can lower blood pressure and exaggerate the effects of this drug.

Exposure to Cold: Caution is advised. Cold environments can enhance the circulatory deficiency in the extremities that may occur with this drug. The elderly should be careful to prevent hypothermia (see Glossary).

Heavy Exercise or Exertion: Talk with your doctor about an exercise program that is right for you mindful of this medicine and your physical condition.

Occurrence of Unrelated Illness: Fever can lower blood pressure and require dosing changes. Nausea or vomiting may interrupt dosing. Ask your doctor for help.

Discontinuation: DO NOT stop this drug suddenly. If possible, gradual dose reduction over 2 to 3 weeks is recommended. Ask your doctor to help you with this.

BITOLTEROL (bi TOHL ter ohl)

Introduced: 1985   **Class:** Antiasthmatic, bronchodilator   **Prescription:** Yes   **Controlled Drug:** No   **Available as Generic:** No   **Brand Name:** Tornalate

BENEFITS versus RISKS	
Possible Benefits	*Possible Risks*
EFFECTIVE PREVENTION AND RELIEF OF ASTHMA	Fine hand tremor
	Nervousness
	Throat irritation
	Irregular heart rhythm (with excessive use)

▷ **Principal Uses**

As a Single Drug Product: Uses currently included in FDA-approved labeling: (1) Relieves sudden (acute) asthma and frequency and severity of ongoing, recurrent asthmatic attacks; (2) helps asthmatics dependent on steroids.

Other (unlabeled) generally accepted uses: (1) May be more useful than other agents opening bronchi in chronic obstructive pulmonary disease (COPD); (2) helps prevent exercise-induced asthma in adults.

How This Drug Works: By increasing cyclic AMP, this drug relaxes bronchial muscles and relieves asthmatic wheezing.

Available Dosage Forms and Strengths

Aerosol inhaler — 15 ml (300 inhalations of 0.37 mg each)

Inhalation solution — 0.2 percent

▷ **Usual Adult Dosage Range:**   For acute bronchospasm—two inhalations at intervals of 1 to 3 minutes, followed by a third inhalation in 3 to 4 minutes if needed. Preventing bronchospasm—two inhalations every 8 hours. Maximum inhalation dose is two inhalations every 4 hours.

For children over 12: same as adult bronchospasm dose. **Note: Actual dose and schedule must be determined for each patient individually.**

Conditions Requiring Dosing Adjustments

Liver Function: Use with caution in severe liver compromise.

Kidney Function: Significant kidney removal; however, specific dosage guidelines are unavailable.

▷ **Dosing Instructions:**   May be used without regard to eating. Follow the written directions for use carefully. **Do not overuse.**

Usual Duration of Use: Do not use beyond time needed to stop acute asthma. Ask your doctor for help regarding prevention of asthma attacks.

▷ **This Drug Should Not Be Taken If**

• you have had an allergic reaction to it previously.

• you currently have an irregular heart rhythm.

• you are taking, or took a monoamine oxidase (MAO) type A inhibitor (see Drug Classes) in the past 2 weeks.

▷ **Inform Your Physician Before Taking This Drug If**

• you have any type of heart or circulatory disorder, especially high blood pressure or coronary heart disease.

- you have diabetes, epilepsy, or an overactive thyroid gland.
- you are taking any form of digitalis or any stimulant drug.
- you are unsure how much to take or how often to take it.
- you are pregnant and are nearing the time of delivery of your baby (may complicate labor and delivery).

Possible Side Effects (natural, expected, and unavoidable drug actions)
Dryness or irritation of mouth or throat.

▷ **Possible Adverse Effects** (unusual, unexpected, and infrequent reactions)
If any of the following develop, consult your physician promptly for guidance.
Mild Adverse Effects
Headache, dizziness, nervousness, insomnia—infrequent.
Fine tremor of hands—frequent.
Nausea, indigestion—infrequent.
Coughing—infrequent.
Fast heart rate (tachycardia)—rare.
Serious Adverse Effects
Excessive use can cause irregular heart rate or rhythm or increased blood pressure.
Paradoxical bronchospasm—rare.

▷ **Possible Effects on Sexual Function:**   None reported.

Natural Diseases or Disorders That May Be Activated by This Drug
Latent coronary artery disease, diabetes, or high blood pressure.

Possible Effects on Laboratory Tests
None reported.

CAUTION
1. Combination use of this drug by inhalation with beclomethasone aerosol (Beclovent, Vanceril) may increase the risk of toxicity due to fluorocarbon propellants. Use bitolterol aerosol 20 to 30 minutes *before* beclomethasone aerosol. This reduces toxicity risk and enhances penetration of beclomethasone.
2. Excessive or prolonged inhalation use can reduce benefits and cause serious heart rhythm disturbances.

Precautions for Use
By Infants and Children: Safety and effectiveness for children under 12 years of age not established.
By Those Over 60 Years of Age: Avoid excessive and continual use. If acute asthma is not relieved promptly, other drugs will be needed. Watch for nervousness, palpitations, irregular heart rhythm, and muscle tremors.

▷ **Advisability of Use During Pregnancy**
Pregnancy Category: C. See Pregnancy Risk Categories at the back of this book.
Animal studies: Cleft palate reported in mice.
Human studies: Adequate studies of pregnant women are not available.
Avoid use during first 3 months if possible.

Advisability of Use If Breast-Feeding
Presence of this drug in breast milk: Unknown.
Avoid drug or refrain from nursing.

Habit-Forming Potential: None.

Effects of Overdose: Nervousness, palpitation, rapid heart rate, sweating, headache, tremor, vomiting, abnormal heart rhythms, chest pain.

Possible Effects of Long-Term Use: Loss of effectiveness.

Suggested Periodic Examinations While Taking This Drug (at physician's discretion)

Blood pressure measurements, evaluation of heart status.

▷ **While Taking This Drug, Observe the Following**

Foods: No restrictions.

Beverages: Avoid excessive caffeine—coffee, tea, cola, chocolate.

▷ *Alcohol:* No interactions expected.

Tobacco Smoking: No interactions expected, but the smoke itself can irritate airways. I advise everyone to quit smoking.

▷ *Other Drugs*

Bitolterol *taken concurrently* with

• monoamine oxidase (MAO) type A inhibitors (see Drug Classes) may cause large increases in blood pressure and undesirable heart stimulation.

▷ *Driving, Hazardous Activities:* Use caution if excessive nervousness or dizziness occurs.

Aviation Note: The use of this drug *is a disqualification* for piloting. Consult a designated aviation medical examiner.

Exposure to Sun: No restrictions.

Heavy Exercise or Exertion: Use caution. Excessive exercise can induce an asthma attack.

BROMOCRIPTINE (broh moh KRIP teen)

Introduced: 1975   **Class:** Anti-parkinsonism, ergot derivative   **Prescription:** USA: Yes   **Controlled Drug:** USA: No; Canada: No   **Available as Generic:** No

Brand Names: Parlodel, Normatine

BENEFITS versus RISKS	
Possible Benefits	*Possible Risks*
PARTIAL RELIEF OF SYMPTOMS OF PARKINSON'S DISEASE	ABNORMAL INVOLUNTARY MOVEMENTS AND ALTERED
CORRECTION OF INFERTILITY AND ABSENT MENSTRUATION in women with high prolactin levels	BEHAVIOR in users taking high doses
	Raynaud's phenomenon (see Glossary) in users taking high doses
	Low blood pressure

▷ **Principal Uses**

As a Single Drug Product: Uses currently included in FDA-approved labeling: (1) Used to treat early-stage symptoms of Parkinson's disease (often used in conjunction with levodopa when levodopa benefits decrease, or the patient cannot tolerate levodopa and dose decrease or withdrawal is necessary); (2) treats disorders due to excessive prolactin from pituitary gland: absence of menstruation, infertility, and inappropriate production of milk; (3) adjunct to surgery in acromegaly; (4) eases breast engorgement and galactorrhea in stress-induced hyperprolactinemia; (5) can help functional infertility in females; (6) reduces size of pituitary tumors.

Other (unlabeled) generally accepted uses: (1) Can help stroke patients who have problems speaking; (2) may help cocaine withdrawal; (3) may return growth to normal in children experiencing abnormal skeletal growth; (4) sustained release form may help weight loss.

Author's Note: Bromocriptine is no longer FDA approved for the treatment of physiological lactation. This indication was withdrawn because the risks of the use of the drug outweigh the benefits for this indication.

How This Drug Works: This drug helps increase dopamine and relieve rigidity, tremor, and sluggish movement in Parkinson's disease. By keeping the body from making prolactin (anterior pituitary), this drug increases blood prolactin, blocking breast milk production; lowers high levels of prolactin, restoring levels that permit menstrual regularity and fertility.

Available Dosage Forms and Strengths
    Capsules — 5 mg
    Tablets — 0.8 mg, 2.5 mg
    Elixir — 4 mg/5 ml

▷ **Usual Adult Dosage Range:**   For Parkinson's disease—initially 1.25 mg twice daily. Benefit should be checked every 14 days. Dose may be increased as needed and tolerated by no more than 2.5 mg daily every 14 to 28 days. Usual range is 10 to 40 mg daily, not to exceed 100 mg daily. The lowest possible dose should be used. For absent menstruation and infertility—initially 2.5 mg one to three times daily with meals. Total dose can be increased by 2.5 mg every 3 to 7 days. Effective response may be seen at 2.5 to 15 mg per day. **Note: Actual dose and schedule must be determined for each patient individually.**

Conditions Requiring Dosing Adjustments
    Liver Function: The dose should be decreased or the dosing interval lengthened; however, specific guidelines are not available.
    Kidney Function: Use with caution in severe renal failure only.

▷ **Dosing Instructions:**   Take with food or milk to reduce stomach irritation. Capsule may be opened and tablet may be crushed.

Usual Duration of Use: Regular use for 3 to 4 months usually needed to determine benefit in controlling Parkinson's symptoms. Treatment for 4 to 12 weeks often restores fertility and normal menstruation; however, may take 6 to 12 months. Long-term use (up to 3 years or more) must be under a doctor's care.

▷ **This Drug Should Not Be Taken If**
  • you have had an allergic reaction to it.
  • you have had a serious adverse effect from any ergot preparation.
  • you have severe coronary artery disease or peripheral vascular disease.
  • you are pregnant.
  • you are nursing your infant (will disrupt milk formation).

▷ **Inform Your Physician Before Taking This Drug If**
  • you have constitutionally low blood pressure.
  • you are taking any antihypertensive drugs or phenothiazines (see Drug Classes).

- you have coronary artery disease, especially with a history of heart attack (myocardial infarction).
- you have a history of heart rhythm abnormalities.
- you have impaired liver function.
- you have a seizure disorder (epilepsy).
- you take prescription or nonprescription drugs not discussed when this medicine was prescribed.
- you have an ulcer.
- you have a history of mental illness.
- you take other medicines that can lower blood pressure.
- you are unsure how much to take or how often to take it.

Possible Side Effects (natural, expected, and unavoidable drug actions)

Fatigue, lethargy, light-headedness in upright position (see ***orthostatic hypotension*** in Glossary). Lowering of blood pressure (hypotension)—frequent. Swelling of feet and ankles (edema).

▷ **Possible Adverse Effects** (unusual, unexpected, and infrequent reactions)

If any of the following develop, consult your physician promptly for guidance.

Mild Adverse Effects

Allergic reaction: skin rash.

Headache, dizziness—frequent.

Fainting (syncope)—rare.

Nightmares—possible.

Nasal congestion, dry mouth—reported.

Loss of appetite, nausea—frequent.

Indications of "ergotism": numbness and tingling of fingers, cold hands and feet, muscle cramps of legs and feet—frequent.

Serious Adverse Effects

Abnormal involuntary movements—possible.

Hallucinations, psychosis—case reports.

Seizures—case reports.

Stroke—case reports.

Loss of urinary bladder control, inability to empty bladder—possible.

Retroperitoneal fibrosis—case reports.

May worsen existing ulcers.

Excessive lowering of blood pressure—possible.

Worsening of mania in manic patients—possible.

Abnormal heart rhythms—possible.

Vasospasms and potential for heart attack—very rare.

Lung changes (pulmonary fibrosis) with long-term use—rare.

▷ **Possible Effects on Sexual Function:**   Impotence—rare. However, this drug can correct impotence and reduced libido when the problem is due to high blood levels of prolactin (a pituitary hormone).

Adverse Effects That May Mimic Natural Diseases or Disorders

Effects on mental function and behavior may resemble psychotic disorders.

Natural Diseases or Disorders That May Be Activated by This Drug

Coronary artery disease with anginal syndrome, Raynaud's phenomenon.

Possible Effects on Laboratory Tests

Blood alkaline phosphatase level: increased.

White blood cell count and platelets: lowered (single case report).

CAUTION

1. During treatment of parkinsonism, avoid excessive and hurried activity as improvement occurs; this will reduce the risk of falls and injury.
2. The neurological and psychiatric disturbances due to this drug may last for 2 to 6 weeks after stopping it.
3. During treatment to reduce the blood level of prolactin and restore normal menstruation and fertility, it is mandatory that you use a barrier method of contraception to prevent pregnancy. Oral contraceptives should not be used while taking bromocriptine.
4. If pregnancy occurs, notify your physician **immediately**.

Precautions for Use

By Infants and Children: Safety and effectiveness for those under 15 years of age not established.

By Those Over 60 Years of Age: Your initial test dose should be 1.25 mg. Watch closely for light-headedness or faintness on attempting to stand after this first dose. You may be more susceptible to the development of impaired thinking, confusion, agitation, nightmares, hallucinations, nausea, or vomiting. Close monitoring and careful dosage adjustments are mandatory.

▷ **Advisability of Use During Pregnancy**

Pregnancy Category: B. See Pregnancy Risk Categories at the back of this book.

Animal studies: Rabbit studies reveal an increase in cleft lip.

Human studies: Serious birth defects have been reported in infants whose mothers took this drug during early pregnancy. Because the incidence of these defects does not exceed that reported for the general population, a cause-and-effect relationship is uncertain. Information from adequate studies of pregnant women is not available.

Ask your doctor for advice on stopping therapy.

Advisability of Use If Breast-Feeding

This drug prevents the production of milk and makes nursing impossible.

Habit-Forming Potential: Use to treat cocaine craving may result in a chemical dependence on bromocriptine.

Effects of Overdose: Weakness, low blood pressure, nausea, vomiting, diarrhea, confusion, agitation, hallucinations, loss of consciousness.

Possible Effects of Long-Term Use: Changes in lung tissue, thickening of the pleura and pleural effusion (fluid in the chest cage). These changes may reverse once the drug is stopped. Fibrosis (scar tissue formation) in the back abdominal wall and contractures of extremities have been reported.

Suggested Periodic Examinations While Taking This Drug (at physician's discretion)

Blood pressure measurements; CAT scan of the pituitary gland for enlargement due to tumor; pregnancy test; blood tests for anemia; evaluation of heart, lung, and liver functions.

▷ **While Taking This Drug, Observe the Following**

Foods: No restrictions.

Beverages: No restrictions. May be taken with milk.

▷   *Alcohol:* Caution—alcohol can exaggerate blood-pressure-lowering and sedative
effects of this drug. May worsen nausea and abdominal side effects.
Tobacco Smoking: May worsen symptoms of ergotism. I advise everyone to quit.

▷   *Other Drugs*
Bromocriptine ***taken concurrently*** with
  - antihypertensive drugs (and other drugs that can lower blood pressure) requires careful monitoring for excessive drops in pressure. Dosage adjustments may be necessary.
  - cyclosporine (Sandimmune) may lead to cyclosporine toxicity.
  - erythromycin or other macrolide antibiotics (see Drug Classes) may increase bromocriptine levels and toxicity risk.
  - phenylpropanolamine can result in bromocriptine toxicity.
The following drugs may ***decrease*** the effects of bromocriptine:
  - phenothiazines (see Drug Classes). It is probably best to avoid the concurrent use of these drugs until the results of further studies are available.

▷   *Driving, Hazardous Activities:* Be alert to the possible occurrence of orthostatic
hypotension, dizziness, drowsiness, or impaired coordination.
Aviation Note: Parkinsonism ***is a disqualification*** for piloting. The use of this
drug otherwise ***may be a disqualification*** for piloting. Consult a designated aviation medical examiner.
Exposure to Sun: No restrictions.
Discontinuation: Once this medicine is stopped, pituitary tumor regrowth and
symptoms of hyperprolactinemia may occur again.

BUMETANIDE (byu MET a nide)

Introduced: 1983   **Class:** Diuretic   **Prescription:** USA: Yes; Canada:
No   **Controlled Drug:** USA: No   **Available as Generic:** Yes
Brand Name: Bumex

BENEFITS versus RISKS	
Possible Benefits	*Possible Risks*
POTENT, EFFECTIVE DIURETIC BY MOUTH OR INJECTION	ABNORMALLY LOW BLOOD POTASSIUM with excessive use Decreased magnesium with chronic therapy Blood disorders—rare

▷ **Principal Uses**
As a Single Drug Product: Uses currently included in FDA-approved labeling: (1)
Removes fluid buildup in congestive heart failure, liver disease, or kidney
disease; (2) helps edema in patients who don't respond to or can't tolerate
furosemide.
Other (unlabeled) generally accepted uses: (1) Used as an adjunct to other
therapy in high blood pressure (hypertension); (2) can help older people decrease the number of times they must get up at night to urinate (nocturia);
(3) eases the amount of fluid that can build up in the lungs (pulmonary
edema).

How This Drug Works: Increases removal of salt and water from the body (through increased urine production). Reduces sodium and amount of fluid in the blood.

Available Dosage Forms and Strengths
Injection — 0.25 mg/ml (2-ml ampules)
Tablets — 0.5 mg, 1 mg, 2 mg

▷ **Usual Adult Dosage Range:**   0.5 to 2 mg daily, usually taken in the morning as a single dose. If needed, an additional second or third dose may be taken later in the day at 4- to 5-hour intervals. The total daily dose should not exceed 10 mg. Alternate-day dosage (every other day) may work for some people. **Note: Actual dose and schedule must be determined for each patient individually.**

Conditions Requiring Dosing Adjustments
Liver Function: Rapid body fluid removal can cause a coma in liver failure patients. Use of loop diuretics only done under close medical supervision (hospital or outpatient care center).
Kidney Function: **NOT** recommended for use in progressive renal failure.

▷ **Dosing Instructions:**   May be crushed when taken and given with or following food to reduce stomach irritation.

Usual Duration of Use: Two to three days of regular use often needed to see peak effect relieving fluid buildup (edema). Once peak benefit is realized, intermittent use reduces risk of sodium, potassium, magnesium, and water imbalance. Long-term use requires supervision by your doctor.

Possible Advantages of This Drug
Diuretic effect is usually complete in 4 hours; diuretic effect of furosemide usually lasts from 6 to 8 hours.

▷ **This Drug Should Not Be Taken If**
• you have had an allergic reaction to it.
• coma caused by liver failure is present.
• your kidneys are unable to produce urine.
• you have developed a marked increase in creatinine or blood urea nitrogen (BUN) while taking this drug.
• severe electrolyte or fluid imbalance.

▷ **Inform Your Physician Before Taking This Drug If**
• you are allergic to any form of "sulfa" drug.
• you are pregnant or planning pregnancy.
• you have a blood disorder.
• you have impaired liver or kidney function.
• you have diabetes, a diabetic tendency, or a history of gout.
• you have impaired hearing, or develop hearing loss during therapy.
• you are taking: cortisone, digitalis, oral antidiabetic drugs, insulin, probenecid (Benemid), indomethacin (Indocin), lithium, or drugs for high blood pressure.
• you will have surgery with general anesthesia.
• you are unsure how much to take or how often to take it.

Possible Side Effects (natural, expected, and unavoidable drug actions)
Light-headedness on arising from sitting or lying position (see ***orthostatic hypotension*** in Glossary).

Increase in level of blood sugar, affecting control of diabetes.

Increase in level of blood uric acid, affecting control of gout.

Decreased blood potassium and sodium with muscle weakness and cramping.

Decreased blood magnesium.

▷ **Possible Adverse Effects** (unusual, unexpected, and infrequent reactions)

If any of the following develop, consult your physician promptly for guidance.

Mild Adverse Effects

Allergic reactions: skin rashes, hives, itching.

Headache, dizziness, vertigo, fatigue, weakness, sweating, earache—rare.

Nausea, vomiting, stomach pain, diarrhea—infrequent.

Breast nipple tenderness, joint and muscle pains or cramps—rare.

Serious Adverse Effects

Serious skin rash (Stevens-Johnson syndrome)—case reports.

Liver coma (in preexisting liver disease)—possible.

Abnormally low magnesium, potassium, and sodium (electrolytes): possible with long-term or high-dose use—rare to frequent.

Low white blood cells and platelets (leukopenia and thrombocytopenia)—rare.

Kidney failure—rare.

Pseudoporphyuria—case report.

Pancreatitis—case reports.

Elevated blood glucose—infrequent.

Lung fibrosis—case reports.

Hearing toxicity (ototoxicity)—rare.

▷ **Possible Effects on Sexual Function:**   Difficulty maintaining an erection; premature ejaculation (0.5 to 2 mg daily)—rare.

Male breast enlargement and tenderness (gynecomastia)—case reports.

Natural Diseases or Disorders That May Be Activated by This Drug

Latent diabetes, gout.

Possible Effects on Laboratory Tests

White blood cell counts: increased—usual; decreased—rare.

Blood platelets: decreased.

Blood sugar (glucose): increased.

Blood lithium or uric acid levels: increased.

Blood potassium, magnesium, or chloride: decreased.

CAUTION

1. High doses can cause excessive excretion of water, sodium, and potassium, with loss of appetite, nausea, weakness, confusion, and profound drop in blood pressure (circulatory collapse).
2. May cause digitalis toxicity by depleting potassium. If you are taking a digitalis preparation (digitoxin, digoxin), ensure an adequate intake of high potassium foods.
3. People with cirrhosis of the liver must never increase their dose unless told to do so by their doctor. Excess dosing can cause liver coma.
4. People who take lithium may experience lithium toxicity.

Precautions for Use

By Infants and Children: Safety and effectiveness for those under 6 months of age not established. If 6 months or older, 0.015 mg per kg is used. If ongoing doses are needed, an intermittent schedule such as every other day or every 2–4 days is used.

By Those Over 60 Years of Age: Small starting doses are advisable. You may be more susceptible to the development of impaired thinking, orthostatic hypotension, potassium loss, and elevation of blood sugar. Overdose and prolonged use can cause excessive loss of body water, thickening of the blood, and an increased risk of blood clots, stroke, heart attack, or thrombophlebitis.

▷ **Advisability of Use During Pregnancy**

Pregnancy Category: C; D by one researcher. See Pregnancy Risk Categories at the back of this book.

Animal studies: Ten times the maximum therapeutic human dose caused bone defects in rabbits.

Human studies: Adequate studies of pregnant women are not available.

Only used in pregnancy if a very serious complication of pregnancy occurs for which this drug is significantly beneficial.

Advisability of Use If Breast-Feeding

Presence of this drug in breast milk: Unknown.

Avoid drug or refrain from nursing.

Habit-Forming Potential: None.

Effects of Overdose: Weakness, lethargy, dizziness, confusion, nausea, vomiting, muscle cramps, thirst, electrolyte disturbances, drowsiness progressing to deep sleep or coma, weak and rapid pulse.

Possible Effects of Long-Term Use: Impaired balance of water, salt, and potassium in blood and body tissues. Dehydration with possible increased blood viscosity and potential for abnormal clotting. Increased blood sugar in some patients.

Suggested Periodic Examinations While Taking This Drug (at physician's discretion)

Complete blood counts; blood levels of sodium, potassium, magnesium, chloride, sugar, uric acid; liver and kidney function tests.

▷ **While Taking This Drug, Observe the Following**

Foods: Salt restriction and a high potassium diet may be needed. Ask your doctor. See Section Six, Table 13, "High-Potassium Foods."

Beverages: No restrictions unless directed by your doctor. May be taken with milk.

▷ *Alcohol:* Alcohol can exaggerate the blood-pressure-lowering effect of this drug and cause orthostatic hypotension (see Glossary).

Tobacco Smoking: No interactions expected, but I advise everyone to quit smoking.

▷ *Other Drugs*

Bumetanide may *increase* the effects of

• antihypertensive drugs. Careful decreases in dose are needed to prevent excessive lowering of the blood pressure.

Bumetanide *taken concurrently* with

• ACE inhibitors (see Drug Classes) may result in severe lowering of blood pressure on standing (postural or orthostatic hypotension).

• aminoglycoside antibiotics (amikacin, gentamicin, kanamycin, neomycin, streptomycin, tobramycin, viomycin) increases the risk of hearing loss.

- cephalosporins (see Drug Classes) may increase risk of kidney toxicity.
- cortisone-related drugs may cause excessive potassium loss and also blunted therapeutic benefits.
- digitalis-related drugs (see Drug Classes) requires very careful monitoring to prevent serious disturbances of heart rhythm.
- lithium (Lithobid, others) may increase lithium toxicity risk.

The following drugs may *decrease* the effects of bumetanide:

- indomethacin (Indocin) or other NSAIDs (see Drug Classes), by reducing its diuretic effect.

▷ *Driving, Hazardous Activities:* **Caution**: Varying degrees of dizziness, weakness, or orthostatic hypotension (see Glossary) may occur.

Aviation Note: The use of this drug *may be a disqualification* for piloting. Consult a designated aviation medical examiner.

Exposure to Sun: No restrictions.

Occurrence of Unrelated Illness: Report vomiting or diarrhea promptly to your doctor.

Discontinuation: It may be advisable to stop this drug 5 to 7 days before major surgery. Ask your doctor for help.

BUPROPION (byu PROH pee on)

Other Name: Amfebutamone

Introduced: 1986   **Class:** Antidepressant   **Prescription:** USA: Yes
Controlled Drug: USA: No; Canada: No   **Available as Generic:** USA: No
Brand Names: Wellbutrin, Zyban

BENEFITS versus RISKS	
Possible Benefits	*Possible Risks*
ZYBAN IS APPROVED FOR USE IN SMOKING CESSATION	DRUG-INDUCED SEIZURES—rare
EFFECTIVE TREATMENT OF MAJOR DEPRESSIVE DISORDERS	Excessive mental stimulation: excitement, anxiety, confusion, hallucinations, insomnia
Offers a different class than tricyclic, MAO, or SSRI antidepressants	Conversion of depression to mania in manic-depressive disorders
May increase sexual desire in some people	

▷ **Principal Uses**

As a Single Drug Product: Uses currently included in FDA-approved labeling: (1) Helps smokers quit smoking (Zyban); (2) treatment of major depressive disorders.

Other (unlabeled) generally accepted uses: (1) May ease chronic fatigue syndrome symptoms; (2) can reduce cocaine craving when combined with psychotherapy; (3) drug of choice in people who have significant weight gain while taking tricyclic antidepressants; (4) can help some cases of low back pain that does not respond to other agents; (5) increased sexual desire in 77% of patients in one study.

How This Drug Works: Bupropion increases levels of two nerve transmitters (norepinephrine and dopamine). It is biochemically unique and works differently than other antidepressants (may be a benefit if other medicines have failed). How it works to help people quit smoking is unknown.

Available Dosage Forms and Strengths
Tablets, immediate release — 75 mg, 100 mg
Tablets, sustained release — 100 mg, 150 mg
Tablets, sustained release only — 150 mg

▷ **Recommended Dosage Ranges** (Actual dose and schedule must be determined for each patient individually.)

Infants and Children: Dosage not established for those under 18 years of age.

18 to 60 Years of Age: Depression: First 3 days: 100 mg in the morning and evening. On the fourth day, dose may be increased to 100 mg in the morning, at noon, and in the evening; total daily dose of 300 mg. This schedule of 100 mg, three times daily, 6 hours apart, is used for 3 to 4 weeks. If needed and beneficial, dose may be slowly increased to a maximum of 450 mg daily. Increases should not exceed 100 mg per day in a period of 3 days. No single dose should exceed 150 mg. If daily dose is 450 mg, take 150 mg in the morning, then 100 mg every 4 hours for three more doses.

The lowest effective dose should be used. Drug should be stopped if significant improvement is not seen after a trial of 450 mg daily. Doses higher than 450 mg daily may only increase risk of seizures.

Smoking cessation: 150 mg once a day for 3 days, then 150 mg twice daily for 7 to 12 weeks. If progress has not been made in 7 weeks, talk with your doctor.

Over 60 Years of Age: Same as 18 to 60 years of age.

Conditions Requiring Dosing Adjustments
Liver Function: Lower dosages and caution in monitoring should be used.
Kidney Function: The dose **must** be decreased in people with damaged kidneys or who develop kidney damage while taking this drug.

▷ **Dosing Instructions:**   May be taken with food to reduce stomach upset. Best to swallow the tablet whole, not chewing or crushing it; this drug has a bitter taste and a local numbing effect on the lining of the mouth. Sustained-release forms should never be crushed or altered.

Usual Duration of Use: Regular use for 3 to 4 weeks needed to realize benefits in depression. Long-term use (months to years) requires periodic evaluation of response and dose. For use in quitting smoking: use for 7 to 12 weeks. See your doctor regularly.

Possible Advantages of This Drug
Causes less atropinelike side effects: blurred vision, dry mouth, constipation, impaired urination.
Does not cause sedation or orthostatic hypotension (see Glossary).

▷ **This Drug Should Not Be Taken If**
• you have had an allergic reaction to it previously.
• you have a history of anorexia nervosa or bulimia (may be associated with increased seizure risk).
• you have a seizure disorder of any kind.
• you are taking, or took in the past 14 days, any monoamine oxidase (MAO) type A inhibitor (see Drug Classes).

▷ **Inform Your Physician Before Taking This Drug If**
- you have had any adverse effects from antidepressant drugs.
- you are pregnant or planning pregnancy.
- you are breast-feeding your infant.
- you have a history of mental illness, head injury, or brain tumor.
- you have a history of alcoholism or drug abuse.
- you have any kind of heart disease, especially a recent heart attack.
- you have impaired liver or kidney function.
- you take prescription or nonprescription drugs not discussed when bupropion was prescribed for you.
- you are unsure how much to take or how often to take it.

Possible Side Effects (natural, expected, and unavoidable drug actions)
Nervousness, anxiety, confusion, insomnia.
Weight loss of more than 5 pounds—frequent.

▷ **Possible Adverse Effects** (unusual, unexpected, and infrequent reactions)
If any of the following develop, consult your physician promptly for guidance.
Mild Adverse Effects
Allergic reactions: skin rash, itching—rare to infrequent.
Headache, dizziness, tremor, agitation (9.7% more than placebo), or blurred vision (4.3% more than placebo)—infrequent.
Indigestion, nausea and vomiting, constipation—infrequent.
Dry mouth—frequent.
Excessive sweating (diaphoresis)—frequent.
Ringing in the ears (tinnitus)—possible.
Serious Adverse Effects
Drug-induced seizures—rare, more common with high doses.
Change of depression to mania in manic-depressive disorders—possible.
Psychosis in patients with psychotic predisposition—possible.
Decreased (by 10–15%) white blood cell counts—possible.
Liver toxicity—case reports.

▷ **Possible Effects on Sexual Function:**   A study at the University of Alabama found 77% of patients experienced increased sexual desire. Impotence—infrequent; however, another study reported a decrease in sexual dysfunction when patients were switched from fluoxetine (Prozac) to bupropion; altered menstruation up to 3.6% more than placebo in clinical trials—infrequent.

Possible Delayed Adverse Effects: None reported.

Natural Diseases or Disorders That May Be Activated by This Drug
Latent epilepsy, latent psychosis, manic phase of bipolar affective disorder.

Possible Effects on Laboratory Tests
White blood cell count: decreased.

CAUTION
1. Take exactly the amount prescribed; rapid dose increases can cause seizures. Watch closely for excessive stimulation.
2. Ask your doctor or pharmacist BEFORE taking any other prescription or nonprescription drug.
3. Do not take any monoamine oxidase (MAO) type A inhibitor (see Drug

Classes) while taking this drug. If you have taken a MAO inhibitor, wait 2 weeks before starting bupropion.

Precautions for Use

By Infants and Children: Safety and effectiveness for those under 18 years of age not established.

By Those Over 60 Years of Age: Age-related liver or kidney function decline may require dose decreases.

▷ **Advisability of Use During Pregnancy**

Pregnancy Category: B. See Pregnancy Risk Categories at the back of this book.
Animal studies: Rat and rabbit studies reveal no significant birth defects.
Human studies: Adequate studies of pregnant women are not available.
Use this drug only if clearly needed. Ask your doctor for help.

Advisability of Use if Breast-Feeding

Presence of this drug in breast milk: Yes.
Avoid drug or refrain from nursing.

Habit-Forming Potential: Remote with use of recommended doses. Slight potential for abuse by those who abuse stimulant drugs.

Effects of Overdose: Headache, agitation, confusion, hallucinations, seizures, loss of consciousness.

Possible Effects of Long-Term Use: Not reported.

Suggested Periodic Examinations While Taking This Drug (at physician's discretion)

Liver and/or kidney function tests as appropriate.

▷ **While Taking This Drug, Observe the Following**

Foods: No restrictions.

Beverages: No restrictions. May be taken with milk.

▷ *Alcohol:* Avoid completely. Alcohol may predispose to the development of seizures.

Tobacco Smoking: No interactions expected. I advise everyone to quit smoking.

Marijuana Smoking: Avoid completely; it may lead to psychotic behavior.

▷ *Other Drugs*

The following drugs *taken concurrently* with bupropion may increase the risk of major seizures:

- antidepressants (tricyclic).
- clozapine (Clozaril).
- fluoxetine (Prozac).
- haloperidol (Haldol).
- lithium (Lithobid, others).
- loxapine (Loxitane).
- maprotiline (Ludiomil).
- molindone (Moban).
- phenothiazines (see Drug Classes).
- thioxanthenes (see *xanthines* Drug Classes).
- trazodone (Desyrel).

Bupropion *taken concurrently* with

- carbamazepine (Tegretol) may result in lowered carbamazepine levels.
- cimetidine (Tagamet) may lead to increased bupropion levels.
- levodopa results in increased nausea, restlessness, and tremor.

- monoamine oxidase (MAO) inhibitors (see Drug Classes) can lead to sudden toxicity. Do not combine.
- phenobarbital may result in decreased levels.
- phenytoin (Dilantin) may result in decreased phenytoin levels.
- ritonavir (Norvir) and probably other protease inhibitors may lead to increased blood levels of bupropion and toxicity—do not combine.

▷ *Driving, Hazardous Activities:* This drug may cause dizziness, drowsiness, or seizures. Restrict activities as necessary.

Aviation Note: The use of this drug *is a disqualification* for piloting. Consult a designated aviation medical examiner.

Exposure to Sun: No restrictions.

Discontinuation: Do not stop this drug abruptly. Ask your doctor for help.

BUSPIRONE (byu SPI rohn)

Introduced: 1979   **Class:** Antianxiety drug   **Prescription:** USA: Yes
Controlled Drug: USA: No; Canada: No   **Available as Generic:** Yes
Brand Name: Buspar

BENEFITS versus RISKS	
Possible Benefits	*Possible Risks*
EFFECTIVE RELIEF OF MILD TO MODERATE ANXIETY	Mild dizziness, faintness, or headache—uncommon
DECREASED RISK OF SEDATION OR DEPENDENCE THAN OTHER AGENTS	Tachycardia—rare
	Restlessness, depression, tremor, or rigidity (with high doses)—rare

▷ **Principal Uses**

As a Single Drug Product: Uses currently included in FDA-approved labeling: (1) Relieves mild to moderate anxiety and nervous tension—useful in the elderly, alcoholics, and addiction-prone people because of its lack of significant sedative effects or abuse potential; (2) helps control self-injurious behaviors or aggression in developmentally disabled adults.

Other (unlabeled) generally accepted uses: (1) May reduce alcohol craving in alcoholics; (2) can help aggression or hyperactivity in autistics; (3) may decrease symptoms in obsessive-compulsive disorder; (4) can help in sexual dysfunction in people with generalized anxiety disorder; (4) may help decrease smoking urge in smokers.

How This Drug Works: Changes brain chemicals (dopamine, norepinephrine, and serotonin), resulting in a calming effect. Also a partial agonist at serotonin reuptake sites (5HT1A).

Available Dosage Forms and Strengths

Tablets — 5 mg, 10 mg

▷ **Usual Adult Dosage Range:** Initially 7.5 mg twice daily; if needed, increase dose by 5 mg/day every 2 to 3 days, with individual doses every 6 to 8 hours. Maximum daily dose is 60 mg. **Note: Actual dose and schedule must be determined for each patient individually.**

Conditions Requiring Dosing Adjustments
> *Liver Function:* Use with caution in severe liver failure. Doses must be decreased.
> *Kidney Function:* Use with caution in severe kidney problems. Dose should be decreased to 25–50% of normal dose.

▷ **Dosing Instructions:**   The tablet may be crushed and taken without regard to food.

Usual Duration of Use: Regular use for up to 7 days may be needed to see full benefit in relieving anxiety and nervous tension.

Possible Advantages of This Drug
> Relieves anxiety or tension without severe sedation or impaired thinking. Does not cause withdrawal when it is stopped.
> Actually appears to improve driving-related skills in one study.

▷ **This Drug Should Not Be Taken If**
- you have had an allergic reaction to this medicine.
- you take, or took in the last 2 weeks, a monoamine oxidase (MAO) inhibitor (see Drug Classes). May increase blood pressure.

▷ **Inform Your Physician Before Taking This Drug If**
- you take other drugs that affect the brain or nervous system: tranquilizers, sedatives, hypnotics, analgesics, narcotics, antidepressants, antipsychotic drugs, anticonvulsants, or anti-parkinsonism drugs.
- you have impaired liver or kidney function.
- you take fluoxetine (Prozac) for depression.

Possible Side Effects (natural, expected, and unavoidable drug actions)
> Mild drowsiness (less than with benzodiazepines) (up to 16%)—frequent; lethargy is possible.

▷ **Possible Adverse Effects** (unusual, unexpected, and infrequent reactions)
> **If any of the following develop, consult your physician promptly for guidance.**
> *Mild Adverse Effects*
> Headache, faintness, excitement—infrequent.
> Dizziness—infrequent to frequent.
> Tingling and touch sensation changes (paresthesias)—rare.
> Insomnia and dream disturbances, depression—possible.
> Increased blood pressure—case reports.
> Nausea—infrequent.
> *Serious Adverse Effects*
> Tachycardia—infrequent.
> With high doses: dysphoria, restlessness, rigidity, tremors—possible.
> Movement disorders—case reports.

▷ **Possible Effects on Sexual Function:**   Increased or decreased libido, difficult or absent orgasm, inhibited ejaculation, impotence, breast milk production, altered timing or pattern of menstruation (10 to 40 mg daily)—all case reports.
> May increase prolactin; however no reports of male breast tenderness or enlargement have been reported.

Possible Effects on Laboratory Tests
> Growth hormone: conflicting increases or lack of effect on growth hormone levels. Blood prolactin levels: dose-related increase.

CAUTION
> This drug is reported to have very mild sedative effects and no abuse potential; however, it should be used with caution and only when clearly needed. Actual dysphoria has been reported with higher doses and may preclude its recreational use.

Precautions for Use
> *By Infants and Children:* Safety and effectiveness for those under 18 years of age not established.
> *By Those Over 60 Years of Age:* Expected to be tolerated much better than benzodiazepines and barbiturates. Watch for increased dizziness or weakness and avoid falls.

▷ **Advisability of Use During Pregnancy**
> *Pregnancy Category:* B. See Pregnancy Risk Categories at the back of this book.
> Animal studies: No birth defects found in rat and rabbit studies.
> Human studies: Adequate studies of pregnant women are not available.
> Discuss any use of this drug during pregnancy with your doctor.

Advisability of Use If Breast-Feeding
> Presence of this drug in breast milk: excreted in rat milk; probably also in humans.
> Avoid drug or refrain from nursing.

Habit-Forming Potential: Does not appear to cause addiction; however, more studies are needed. Higher doses result in a dysphoric reaction, which may keep it from becoming a drug involved in recreational use.

Effects of Overdose: Drowsiness, fatigue, nausea, dysphoria, tingling sensations (paresthesias), and a rare chance of seizures.

Possible Effects of Long-Term Use: None reported.

Suggested Periodic Examinations While Taking This Drug (at physician's discretion)
> Periodic check of heart rate.

▷ **While Taking This Drug, Observe the Following**
> *Foods:* No restrictions; taking with food may result in a clinically insignificant increase in absorption of this drug.
> *Beverages:* No restrictions.
▷ *Alcohol:* Milder problems than diazepam (Valium); however, avoid the combination.
> *Tobacco Smoking:* No interactions expected. I advise everyone to quit smoking.
> *Marijuana Smoking:* Additive increase in drowsiness.
▷ *Other Drugs:*
> Buspirone *taken concurrently* with
> - clozapine (Clozaril) may result in serious lowering of blood sugar and stomach bleeding.
> - fluoxetine (Prozac) may increase underlying anxiety or mental disorder such as obsessive-compulsive disorder. Do not combine.
> - fluvoxamine (Luvox) may result in serious slowing of the heart (bradycardia). Doses must be decreased.
> - monoamine oxidase (MAO) inhibitors (see Drug Classes) such as phenelzine (Parnate) may result in large blood pressure increases. Do not combine.

- narcotics such as oxycodone (Percodan) may result in additive sedation and potential decreases in breathing (respiratory depression).
- trazodone (Desyrel) may lead to liver toxicity. Liver tests should be obtained regularly if the two drugs are combined.
- venlafaxine (Effexor) may lead to decreased buspirone benefits or venlafaxine toxicity.

▷ *Driving, Hazardous Activities:* This drug may cause dizziness, faintness, or fatigue. Restrict activities as necessary.

Aviation Note: The use of this drug *may be a disqualification* for piloting. Consult a designated aviation medical examiner.

Exposure to Sun: No restrictions.

CALCITONIN (kal si TOH nin)

Other Names: Salcatonin, thyrocalcitonin

Introduced: 1977, nasal spray form 1995 **Class:** Anti-osteoporotic, hormones **Prescription:** USA: Yes **Controlled Drug:** USA: No; Canada: No **Available as Generic:** USA: No; Canada: No

Brand Names: Calcimar, Cibacalcin, Miacalcin Injection, Miacalcin Nasal Spray

BENEFITS versus RISKS	
Possible Benefits	*Possible Risks*
PARTIAL RELIEF OF SYMPTOMS OF PAGET'S DISEASE OF BONE	Nausea (with or without vomiting)
NASAL FORM CAN INCREASE BONE MASS	Allergic reactions
Effective adjunctive treatment of postmenopausal osteoporosis	
Effective adjunctive treatment of abnormally high blood calcium levels (associated with malignant disease)	

▷ **Principal Uses**

As a Single Drug Product: Uses currently included in FDA-approved labeling: (1) Treats Paget's disease of bone (excessive bone growth in skull, spine, and long bones); (2) treats postmenopausal osteoporosis, taken with calcium and vitamin D (also eases pain); (3) nasal form treats postmenopausal osteoporosis in women with low bone mass who had menopause 5 years previously; (4) add-on treatment of high blood calcium levels seen in bone cancer; (5) relieves symptoms of neurologic compression in Paget's disease.

Other (unlabeled) generally accepted uses: (1) Combination treatment of osteoporosis due to medicines, hormonal disorders, or immobilization, taken with calcium and vitamin D; (2) may help aneurysmal bone cysts when directly injected into the cyst; (3) may be of benefit in preventing migraine headaches and reduce or eliminate the need for prophylactic medicines; (4) useful adjunct in cancer pain; (5) very beneficial in treating pain that occurs when an arm or leg has been amputated (phantom limb); (6) several studies show this drug decreases risk of bone fractures in osteoporosis in the spine.

How This Drug Works: Slows abnormally accelerated "bone turnover" in Paget's disease. A more normal balance of bone is restored. In bone cancer, this drug slows bone destruction and decreases transfer of calcium from bone to bloodstream. In osteoporosis, this drug blocks resorption (inhibiting cells called osteoclasts), allowing bone-building cells to act. Intestinal effects (calcium absorption) and kidney benefits (decreased removal of calcium) may also play a role.

Available Dosage Forms and Strengths
Calcitonin-human
   Injection — 500 mcg (0.5 mg)
Calcitonin-salmon
   Injection — 200 IU per ml
Nasal spray — 200 IU per spray

▷ **Recommended Dosage Ranges** (Actual dosage and schedule must be determined for each patient individually.)

Skin Testing: Skin testing is accomplished by diluting 10 IU to 1 ml with 0.9% sodium chloride. 0.1 ml of this dilution is injected into the inner forearm (about 1 IU). A positive reaction occurs if more than mild skin reddening or a weal is seen within 15 minutes. The drug should NOT be used if this positive reaction is seen.

Infants and Children: Dosage not established.

12 to 60 Years of Age: Calcitonin-human: For Paget's disease—Initially 500 mcg (0.5 mg) daily, injected subcutaneously; after adequate response, dose may be decreased to 250 mcg (0.25 mg) daily, or 500 mcg (0.5 mg) two or three times per week. Severe cases may require 1 mg/day.

Calcitonin-salmon: For Paget's disease—50 to 100 IU daily or every other day, injected subcutaneously or intramuscularly; after adequate response, dose may be decreased to 50 IU daily, every other day, or three times per week.

For postmenopausal osteoporosis—100 IU daily, every other day, or three times per week, injected under the skin. If adverse effects are marked, reduce dose to 50 IU daily; then increase dose gradually over a period of 2 weeks.

Nasal spray: 200 IU (one spray) daily. Nostrils should be alternated daily to help avoid nasal irritation. Calcium and vitamin D replacement is strongly recommended—such replacement can help keep you from drawing on your "bone bank" (your bones) to maintain adequate calcium.

For high blood calcium levels—initially 4 IU per kg of body mass every 12 hours, injected subcutaneously or intramuscularly; as needed and tolerated, increase dose to 8 IU per kg of body mass every 12 hours; if necessary, the dose may be increased to a maximum of 8 IU per kg of body mass every 6 hours.

For adjunctive pain treatment: 100 to 200 IU daily, given intramuscularly or subcutaneously. Some clinicians use nasal spray form (200 IU daily) for adjunctive pain therapy.

Over 60 Years of Age: Same as 12 to 60 years of age.

Conditions Requiring Dosing Adjustments
Liver Function: No changes indicated.
Kidney Function: No changes needed.

▷ **Dosing Instructions:** **The nasal spray** form should be activated (as in package instructions), then the head placed upright, the spray tip placed firmly into the chosen nostril (remember to use a different nostril every day), and the pump depressed toward the bottle. Call your doctor if your nose becomes ulcerated. **Subcutaneous** (under the skin) injection is preferred for self-administration of the injectable form. Your doctor will teach you about proper injection technique. Daily dose may be given at bedtime on an empty stomach if you become nauseated.

Usual Duration of Use: Peak effect in treating Paget's disease is usually seen after 1–3 months of use on a regular schedule. If effective, the usual treatment is 6 months; and if response continues, the dose may be reduced during the next 6 months. Peak response may require treatment for up to 24 months. Long-term use (months to years) requires periodic physician evaluation. Bone mineral density testing is strongly recommended. Osteoporosis benefits should be checked by bone mineral density testing to measure ongoing success or need to change medicines.

Possible Advantages of This Drug
Calcitonin-human is less likely to induce allergic reactions than calcitonin-salmon, permitting treatment for longer periods of time.

▷ **This Drug Should Not Be Taken If**
- you have had an allergic reaction to it previously.
- you recently fractured a bone that has not healed completely.

▷ **Inform Your Physician Before Taking This Drug If**
- you are allergic by nature (history of eczema, hives, hay fever, asthma).
- you have known allergies to foreign proteins.
- you are unsure how much to take or how often to take it.
- you get sores in the nose after repeated intranasal use.
- you will be unable to have follow-up laboratory testing of blood calcium.

Possible Side Effects (natural, expected, and unavoidable drug actions)
Salty or metallic taste in mouth—possible.

▷ **Possible Adverse Effects** (unusual, unexpected, and infrequent reactions)
If any of the following develop, consult your physician promptly for guidance.
Mild Adverse Effects
Allergic reactions: skin rash, hives, itching—rare.
Headache, dizziness, weakness—rare.
Loss of appetite, nausea (frequent with injection), vomiting, stomach pain, diarrhea—infrequent.
Increased frequency of urination or urination at night (nocturia)—case reports.
Abnormal fluid accumulation (pedal edema)—rare.
Flushing of the face—may be frequent with human calcitonin injection.
Irritation of the nose (nasal spray use)—infrequent to frequent.
Serious Adverse Effects
Allergic reactions: flushing, redness, anaphylaxis—rare.
Sugar (glucose) intolerance—possible.
Excessive lowering of calcium and rigidity (tetany) of muscles due to lack of calcium—possible.
Severe ulceration of the nose (with nasal spray use)—rare.

▷ **Possible Effects on Sexual Function:**   None reported.

Possible Effects on Laboratory Tests

Blood alkaline phosphatase levels: decreased.
Blood calcium levels: decreased.
Urine hydroxyproline values: decreased.
Blood glucose: lack of diabetic control, glucose intolerance.
Bone mineral density: increased (beneficial effect).

CAUTION

1. It is best that your doctor perform a skin test before beginning treatment with calcitonin-salmon.
2. Eat a well-balanced diet with adequate calcium and vitamin D.
3. Tell your doctor if bone pain persists while taking this drug.
4. Try to decrease osteoporosis risk factors. Ask your doctor how much exercise is appropriate for you.

Precautions for Use

By Infants and Children: No specific information.

By Those Over 60 Years of Age: Watch fluid balance closely if this drug is given to lower blood calcium.

▷ **Advisability of Use During Pregnancy**

Pregnancy Category: C. See Pregnancy Risk Categories at the back of this book.

Animal studies: No drug-induced birth defects reported.

Human studies: Adequate studies of pregnant women are not available.

Ask your physician for help.

Advisability of Use if Breast-Feeding

Presence of this drug in breast milk: Yes.

Calcitonin taken in with breast milk is typically destroyed by infant stomach acids before it has any effect. Ask your doctor for guidance.

Habit-Forming Potential: None.

Effects of Overdose: Nausea, vomiting.

Possible Effects of Long-Term Use: Antibodies may cause resistance and loss of effect with pork or salmon calcitonin. This occurs in up to 70% of people after 2 to 18 months of treatment. Antibodies to human calcitonin are rare but have been reported.

Suggested Periodic Examinations While Taking This Drug (at physician's discretion)

Measurements of blood calcium, phosphate, and alkaline phosphatase levels.

Measurement of urine hydroxyproline content.

Measurement of bone mineral density (BMD) by DEXA scan.

▷ **While Taking This Drug, Observe the Following**

Foods: No restrictions.

Nutritional Support: Ensure adequate intake of calcium and vitamin D.

Beverages: No restrictions.

▷ *Alcohol:* No interactions expected, but alcohol (in higher doses) acts as a bone-forming cell (osteoblast) poison and is a risk factor for osteoporosis.

Tobacco Smoking: No interactions expected, but smoking is a risk factor for osteoporosis. I advise everyone to quit smoking.

▷ *Other Drugs*

Calcitonin *taken concurrently* with

• ketoprofen may inhibit the calcium and uric acid distribution in the urine by calcitonin of pig origin. Changes with other calcitonins are not defined.

- plicamycin will cause additive loss of calcium.

▷ *Driving, Hazardous Activities:* No restrictions.

Aviation Note: The use of this drug *may be a disqualification* for piloting. Consult a designated aviation medical examiner.

Exposure to Sun: No restrictions.

Heavy Exercise or Exertion: As defined by your doctor. Remember, weight-bearing exercise (if the doctor says it's okay) helps fight osteoporosis by stimulating receptors (mechanoreceptors) to release factors that structure healthy (normal architecture) bone.

Discontinuation: Your doctor should decide when to stop this drug.

Special Storage Instructions: Calcitonin-human: Store at a temperature below 77 degrees F (25 degrees C). Do not refrigerate. Protect from light.

Calcitonin-salmon: Store in refrigerator, between 36 and 46 degrees F (2 and 8 degrees C). Do not freeze.

Calcitonin-salmon nasal spray: Store unopened in the refrigerator. Once opened, bottle can be kept at room temperature for 2 weeks.

CAPTOPRIL (KAP toh pril)

Introduced: 1979   **Class:** Antihypertensive, ACE inhibitor
Please see the new angiotensin converting enzyme (ACE) inhibitor combination profile for more information.

CARBAMAZEPINE (kar ba MAZ e peen)

Introduced: 1962   **Class:** Anticonvulsant, antineuralgic, pain syndrome modifier   **Prescription:** USA: Yes   **Controlled Drug:** USA: No; Canada: No   **Available as Generic:** Yes

Brand Names: ✤Apo-Carbamazepine, Epitol, ✤Mazepine, ✤Novo-Carbamaz, ✤PMS Carbamazepine, Tegretol, Tegretol Chewable Tablet, Tegretol-XR

BENEFITS versus RISKS	
Possible Benefits	*Possible Risks*
RELIEF OF PAIN IN TRIGEMINAL NEURALGIA	BONE MARROW DEPRESSION (reduced formation of all blood cells)—RARE
EFFECTIVE CONTROL OF CERTAIN TYPES OF EPILEPTIC SEIZURES	Liver damage with jaundice—rare
Relief of pain in some rare forms of nerve pain (neuralgia)	

▷ **Principal Uses**

As a Single Drug Product: Uses currently included in FDA-approved labeling: (1) Pain relief in true trigeminal neuralgia (tic douloureux) or glossopharyngeal neuralgia; (2) for control of several types of epilepsy (grand mal, tonic-clonic, psychomotor/temporal lobe, complex partial and mixed seizure patterns). Precise diagnosis and careful management are mandatory.

Other (unlabeled) generally accepted uses: Beneficial in (1) bipolar affective disorders; (2) schizoaffective disorders; (3) resistant schizophrenia; (4) post-traumatic stress disorder; (5) tabes dorsalis; (6) diabetic neuropathy; (7) hemifacial spasm; (8) cocaine withdrawal; (9) aggression in some Alzheimer's patients; (10) helping hiccups and belching associated with flutter of the diaphragm; (11) treating nerve problems from thiamine deficiency; (12) possibly having a role in treating pain that occurs when an arm or leg is amputated (phantom limb pain); (13) eases a perceived repetitive ear noise called clicking tinnitus.

How This Drug Works: Reduces impulses at certain nerve terminals and relieves pain (of trigeminal neuralgia). Also reduces excitability of nerve fibers in the brain, decreasing likelihood, frequency and severity of seizures.

Available Dosage Forms and Strengths
>   Oral suspension — 100 mg/5 ml
>   Tablets — 200 mg (400 mg in Canada)
>   Tablets, chewable — 100 mg, 200 mg
> Tablets, extended release — 10 mg, 200 mg, 400 mg

▷ **Usual Dosage Ranges:**   *Adults:* Initially 200 mg every 12 hours (regular or extended-release tablets). Dose may be increased at weekly intervals by 200 mg daily as needed and tolerated. The dose is given twice daily for the extended-release tablets or three times daily for the regular tablets. Total daily dosage should not exceed 1200 mg.

Infants and Children: Children under age 6 are given 10 to 20 mg per kg of body mass. This dose is divided into three equal doses and is given three times daily. Increased as needed or tolerated based on clinical response and blood levels. Children 6–12 are given 100 mg twice daily or 50 mg of the suspension four times daily. The dose can then be increased by 100 mg a day after a week, as needed and tolerated. Maximum is 1000 mg or lower.

Note: Actual dosage and schedule must be determined for each patient individually. Dosing must be guided by blood levels.

Conditions Requiring Dosing Adjustments
Liver Function: Use with extreme caution, in lower doses and under close supervision. May have to be stopped in active liver disease.
Kidney Function: May be toxic to kidneys. Use with extreme caution and in smaller dose in patients with kidneys that already do not work well.
Heart Attack: Changes in blood distribution (perfusion) and protein binding may give much higher than expected blood levels. More frequent lab tests are needed to guide dosing and avoid toxicity.

▷ **Dosing Instructions:**   Take at same time each day, with or following food to reduce stomach irritation. Regular-release tablet may be crushed for administration. Extended-release tablet should not be altered.

Usual Duration of Use: Regular use for 3 months may be needed to see effect in easing of trigeminal neuralgia. Longer periods, with dose changes, may be required for control of epileptic seizures. Careful evaluation of tolerance and response should be made every 3 months during long-term treatment.

Currently a "Drug of Choice"
For patients with grand mal or partial seizures.

▷ **This Drug Should Not Be Taken If**
- you have had an allergic reaction to it previously.
- you have active liver disease.
- you currently have a blood cell or bone marrow disorder.
- you currently take, or have taken within the past 14 days, a monoamine oxidase (MAO) type A inhibitor (see Drug Classes).

▷ **Inform Your Physician Before Taking This Drug If**
- you have had an allergic reaction to any tricyclic antidepressant drug (see Drug Classes).
- you have taken this drug in the past.
- you have had any blood or bone marrow disorder, especially drug induced.
- you have a history of liver or kidney disease.
- you have depression or other mental disorder.
- you have had thrombophlebitis.
- you have high blood pressure, heart disease, or glaucoma.
- you take more than two alcoholic drinks a day.
- you take prescription or nonprescription drugs not discussed when carbamazepine was prescribed for you.
- you are unsure how much to take or how often to take it.
- you are pregnant or are breast-feeding your baby.

Possible Side Effects (natural, expected, and unavoidable drug actions)
Dry mouth and throat, constipation, impaired urination.

▷ **Possible Adverse Effects** (unusual, unexpected, and infrequent reactions)
If any of the following develop, consult your physician promptly for guidance.

Mild Adverse Effects
Allergic reactions: skin rash, hives, itching, drug fever—rare to infrequent.
Dizziness, drowsiness, unsteadiness—may be frequent when therapy is started, often eases.
Fatigue, blurred vision, confusion—infrequent.
Exaggerated hearing, ringing in ears—case reports.
Loss of appetite, nausea, vomiting, indigestion, diarrhea—may be frequent when starting therapy.
Decreased sense of taste—possible.
Aching of muscles and joints, leg cramps—case reports.

Serious Adverse Effects
Allergic reactions: severe dermatitis with peeling of skin, irritation of mouth and tongue, swelling of lymph glands—case reports.
Idiosyncratic reactions: lung inflammation (pneumonitis); cough, shortness of breath. Agranulocytosis may also be idiosyncratic—case reports.
Lowering of white blood cells (leukopenia): may be up to 10%—infrequent.
Low thyroid hormones—rare.
Bone marrow depression (see Glossary) (agranulocytosis, hemolytic or aplastic anemia) or thrombocytopenia: fatigue, weakness, fever, sore throat, abnormal bleeding or bruising—case reports.
Pseudolymphoma or systemic lupus erythematosus—case reports.
Abnormal heartbeats (bradyarrhythmias)—case reports.
Liver damage with jaundice (see Glossary): yellow eyes or skin, dark-colored urine, light-colored stools—case reports.

Kidney damage or porphyria—case reports.

Mental depression or agitation/psychosis or paradoxical increase in seizures—case reports.

Abnormally elevated urine output (SIADH)—case reports.

Neuroleptic malignant syndrome or aseptic meningitis—case reports.

Abnormal movement and muscle contractions—case reports.

Pancreatitis—case reports.

Retinopathy, visual hallucinations, peripheral neuritis (see Glossary)—case reports.

Vitamin D deficiency (especially if other risk factors are present). This may lead to osteoporosis.

▷ **Possible Effects on Sexual Function:**   Decreased libido and/or impotence—case reports. Possible male infertility. This drug is used to control hypersexuality (exaggerated sexual behavior) that can result from injury to the temporal lobe of the brain.

Adverse Effects That May Mimic Natural Diseases or Disorders

Liver reactions may suggest viral hepatitis. Lung reactions may suggest interstitial pneumonitis.

Natural Diseases or Disorders That May Be Activated by This Drug

Latent psychosis, systemic lupus erythematosus, osteoporosis.

Possible Effects on Laboratory Tests

Complete blood cell: decreased red cells, hemoglobin, white cells, and platelets; increased eosinophils, increased white cells.

Blood calcium level: decreased.

INR (prothrombin time): decreased.

Thyroid hormones: falsely decreased blood levels.

Blood urea nitrogen level (BUN): increased.

Liver function tests: increased liver enzymes (ALT/GPT, AST/GOT, and alkaline phosphatase), increased bilirubin.

Urine pregnancy tests: false negative or inconclusive results with Prepurex, Predictor, Gonavislide, Pregnosticon.

ANA: positive if SLE effect begins.

CAUTION

1. This drug should be used only after less toxic drugs have failed.
2. *Before* the first dose is taken, blood cell counts, liver function tests, and kidney function tests should be obtained.
3. Careful periodic testing for blood cell or bone marrow toxicity is *mandatory.*
4. *This drug should not be used* to prevent recurrence of trigeminal neuralgia when it is in remission.
5. *Do not stop this drug suddenly* if it is being used to control seizures.
6. If exposed to humidity, the tablet hardens, resulting in poor absorption and erratic control of seizures. Store in a cool, dry place; avoid bathrooms. Try a locking kitchen cabinet.

Precautions for Use

By Infants and Children: Careful testing of blood production and liver and kidney function must be performed regularly. This drug can reduce the effectiveness of other anticonvulsant drugs. Blood levels of all anticonvulsant drugs should be checked if this drug is added to the treatment program.

By *Those Over 60 Years of Age:* Can cause confusion and agitation. Watch for aggravation of glaucoma, coronary artery disease (angina), or prostatism (see Glossary).

▷ **Advisability of Use During Pregnancy**

Pregnancy Category: D. See Pregnancy Risk Categories at the back of this book.

Animal studies: Rat studies reveal significant birth defects.

Human studies: Adequate studies of pregnant women are not available.

Avoid completely during the first 3 months. Use during the last 6 months only if clearly needed.

Advisability of Use If Breast-Feeding

Presence of this drug in breast milk: Yes.

Avoid drug or refrain from nursing.

Habit-Forming Potential: None.

Effects of Overdose: Dizziness, drowsiness, disorientation, tremor, involuntary movements, nausea, vomiting, flushed skin, dilated pupils, stupor progressing to coma, cardiac arrest.

Possible Effects of Long-Term Use: Water retention (edema), impaired liver function, possible jaundice.

Suggested Periodic Examinations While Taking This Drug (at physician's discretion)

Complete blood counts weekly during the first 3 months, then monthly. Liver and kidney function tests. Eye examinations.

Bone mineral density tests (for osteoporosis).

▷ **While Taking This Drug, Observe the Following**

Foods: No restrictions. There may be a minor increase in absorption if taken with food.

Beverages: No restrictions. May be taken with milk.

▷ *Alcohol:* Avoid alcohol use, unless your doctor approves alcohol use.

Tobacco Smoking: No interactions expected. I advise everyone to quit smoking.

▷ *Other Drugs*

Carbamazepine may *increase* the effects of

- sedatives, tranquilizers, hypnotics, and narcotics, and enhance their sedative effects.

Carbamazepine may *decrease* the effects of

- adrenocortical steroids (see Drug Classes).
- antidepressants (see Drug Classes).
- birth control pills (oral contraceptives) and result in pregnancy.
- cyclosporine (Sandimmune).
- doxycycline (Doxy-II, Vibramycin, etc.).
- felodipine (Plendil).
- haloperidol (Haldol) or other phenothiazines.
- isradipine (DynaCirc).
- itraconazole (Sporanox).
- nelfinavir (Viracept).

- tetracyclines (see Drug Classes).
- valproic acid (Depakene, etc.).
- warfarin (Coumadin). Increased frequency of INR testing is indicated.

Carbamazepine *taken concurrently* with

- chlorpromazine (Thorazine) solution may form a rubbery orange precipitate that is passed in the stool. DO NOT combine.
- clozapine (Clozaril) may result in serious bone marrow suppression.
- felbamate (Felbatol) may result in decreased carbamazepine levels and seizures.
- lithium (Lithobid, others) may cause serious neurological problems: confusion, drowsiness, weakness, unsteadiness, tremors, and twitching.
- monoamine oxidase (MAO) type A inhibitor drugs (see Drug Classes) may cause severe toxic reactions.
- phenytoin (Dilantin, etc.) may cause unpredictable fluctuations of blood levels of both drugs and impair seizure control.
- terfenadine (Seldane), and perhaps other nonsedating antihistamines, may result in carbamazepine toxicity.
- theophylline (Theo-Dur, etc.) may reduce the effects of both drugs.
- thioridazine (Mellaril) solution may form a rubbery orange precipitate that is passed in the stool. DO NOT combine.

The following drugs may *increase* the effects of carbamazepine:

- cimetidine (Tagamet).
- danazol (Danocrine).
- diltiazem (Cardizem)—and perhaps other calcium channel blockers.
- flu shots (influenza vaccine).
- fluoxetine (Prozac); may lead to toxicity.
- fluvoxamine (Luvox); may result in toxicity.
- isoniazid (INH).
- macrolide antibiotics—erythromycins, clarithromycin, or troleandomycin (not azithromycin).
- nicotinamide (nicotinic acid amide).
- propoxyphene (Darvon, Darvocet, etc.).
- rifampin; may result in toxicity.
- ritonavir (Norvir) and perhaps other protease inhibitors (see Drug Classes).
- verapamil (Calan, Isoptin).

▷ *Driving, Hazardous Activities:* Can cause dizziness, drowsiness, or blurred vision. Adjust activities.

Aviation Note: The use of this drug *is a disqualification* for piloting. Consult a designated aviation medical examiner.

Exposure to Sun: This drug can cause photosensitivity (see Glossary). Use caution until sensitivity to sun is known.

Heavy Exercise or Exertion: Use caution if you have coronary artery disease. Can intensify angina and reduce tolerance for physical activity.

Occurrence of Unrelated Illness: You MUST tell all health care providers that you take this drug.

Discontinuation: If treating trigeminal neuralgia, every 3 months attempts to reduce the maintenance dose or to stop this drug are needed. If used to control epilepsy, this drug *must not be stopped abruptly.*

Special Storage Instructions: Store tablets in a cool, dry place. Protect from humid conditions **(do NOT store in a bathroom medicine cabinet).**

CARTEOLOL (KAR tee oh lohl)

Introduced: 1983   **Class:** Antihypertensive, beta-adrenergic blocker
Prescription: USA: Yes   **Controlled Drug:** USA: No; Canada: No   **Available as Generic:** No
Brand Names: Cartrol, Ocupress, Optipress

BENEFITS versus RISKS	
Possible Benefits	*Possible Risks*
EFFECTIVE, WELL-TOLERATED ANTIHYPERTENSIVE	Congestive heart failure
EFFECTIVE GLAUCOMA TREATMENT	Worsening of angina in coronary heart disease (abrupt withdrawal)
Prevention of angina	Masking of low blood sugar (hypoglycemia) in drug-treated diabetics
	Provocation of asthma in asthmatics

▷ **Principal Uses**

As a Single Drug Product: Uses currently included in FDA-approved labeling: (1) Treats mild to moderate high blood pressure, alone or in combination with other drugs, such as diuretics; (2) helps lower eye (intraocular) pressure in people with glaucoma.

Other (unlabeled) generally accepted uses: (1) Increases amount of exercise that can be performed before angina occurs; (2) can help decrease aggressive behavior; (3) decreases risk of abnormal heart rhythms; (3) other beta-blockers have shown benefits after heart attacks—however, studies using carteolol not yet performed; (4) may help lessen panic attacks.

How This Drug Works: Blocks certain actions of the sympathetic nervous system and:

- reduces the heart rate and contraction force, lowering ejection pressure of blood leaving the heart.
- reduces extent of blood vessel wall contraction, relaxing the walls and lowering blood pressure.
- reduces elevated eye pressure (intraocular) and relieves glaucoma symptoms.

Available Dosage Forms and Strengths
          Tablets — 2.5 mg, 5 mg
Ophthalmic solution — 5 ml, 10 ml (1%)

▷ **Usual Adult Dosage Range:**   High blood pressure (hypertension): Starts with 2.5 mg daily. Dose may be increased by 2.5 mg/day at intervals of 2 weeks, as needed and tolerated, up to 10 mg/day. Ongoing dose: 2.5 to 7.5 mg once daily is usually adequate. Maximum dose is 10 mg.

For glaucoma: One drop in the affected eye or eyes two times a day. **Note: Actual dose and schedule must be determined for each patient individually.**

Conditions Requiring Dosing Adjustments

Liver Function: Decreased doses needed in severe liver failure.

Kidney Function: Dosing interval **MUST** be decreased in kidney failure. In severe compromise, the drug is given every 48 to 72 hours.

▷ **Dosing Instructions:**   Tablet may be crushed and taken without regard to eating. Do not stop this drug abruptly.

Usual Duration of Use: Regular use for up to 3 weeks may be needed to see effectiveness in lowering blood pressure. Long-term use (months to years) is determined by lowering of blood pressure and response to an overall program (weight reduction, salt restriction, smoking cessation, etc). See your doctor on a regular basis.

Possible Advantages of This Drug
Adequate control of blood pressure with a single daily dose.
Causes less slowing of the heart rate than most other beta-blocker drugs.

▷ **This Drug Should Not Be Taken If**
• you have bronchial asthma.
• you have had an allergic reaction to it previously.
• you have congestive heart failure.
• you have an abnormally slow heart rate or a serious heart block.
• you have a dissecting aortic aneurysm (ask your doctor).

▷ **Inform Your Physician Before Taking This Drug If**
• you have had an adverse reaction to any beta-blocker (see Drug Classes).
• you have serious heart disease or episodes of heart failure.
• you have had hay fever (allergic rhinitis), asthma, chronic bronchitis, or emphysema.
• you have a history of overactive thyroid function (hyperthyroidism).
• you have a history of low blood sugar (hypoglycemia), diabetes, or myasthenia gravis.
• you have impaired liver or kidney function.
• you have a circulation problem (Raynaud's phenomenon, claudication pains in legs).
• you take any form of digitalis, quinidine, or reserpine, or any calcium blocker drug (see Drug Classes).
• you will have surgery with general anesthesia.

Possible Side Effects (natural, expected, and unavoidable drug actions)
Lethargy and fatigability, cold extremities, slow heart rate, light-headedness in upright position (see *orthostatic hypotension* in Glossary). Short-term itching or eye tearing with the ophthalmic drops—frequent.

▷ **Possible Adverse Effects** (unusual, unexpected, and infrequent reactions)
If any of the following develop, consult your physician promptly for guidance.
Mild Adverse Effects
Allergic reactions: skin rash—rare.
Headache, dizziness, nervousness, drowsiness—infrequent to frequent.
Indigestion, nausea, vomiting, constipation, diarrhea—infrequent.
Slight increase in blood potassium—possible.
Cough, wheezing, or sinusitis—rare.
Joint and muscle discomfort, numbness of fingers or toes—rare.
Episodic difficulty walking (intermittent claudication with peripheral vascular disease)—possible.
Tearing and irritation (with cye use)—infrequent to frequent.

Serious Adverse Effects
> Mental depression—possible, but less likely than some other beta-blockers.
>
> Chest pain, irregular heartbeat, shortness of breath; can cause congestive heart failure—possible.
>
> Induction of bronchial asthma (in asthmatic patients)—possible.
>
> Aggravation of myasthenia gravis—possible.
>
> May hide symptoms of low blood sugar.

▷ **Possible Effects on Sexual Function:**   Decreased libido, impotence—case reports.

Adverse Effects That May Mimic Natural Diseases or Disorders
> Decreased extremity blood flow may mimic Raynaud's phenomenon (see Glossary).

Natural Diseases or Disorders That May Be Activated by This Drug
> Raynaud's disease, intermittent claudication, myasthenia gravis.

Possible Effects on Laboratory Tests
> Blood creatine kinase level: increased.
>
> Blood potassium: slight increase.

CAUTION
> 1. ***Do not stop this drug suddenly*** without the knowledge of your doctor. Carry a note that says you are taking this drug.
> 2. Ask your physician or pharmacist before using nasal decongestants. These can cause sudden increases in blood pressure when combined with beta-blocker drugs.
> 3. Report any new tendency to emotional depression.

Precautions for Use
> *By Infants and Children:* Safety and effectiveness for those under 12 years of age not established.
>
> *By Those Over 60 Years of Age:* **Caution**: Unacceptably high blood pressure should be reduced without creating excessively low blood pressure. Small doses and frequent blood pressure checks are needed.
>
> Sudden or excessive lowering of blood pressure can lead to stroke or heart attack. Watch for dizziness, falling, confusion, depression, or urinary frequency.

▷ **Advisability of Use During Pregnancy**
> *Pregnancy Category:* C. See Pregnancy Risk Categories at the back of this book.
>
> Animal studies: No birth defects due to this drug found in rat or rabbit studies.
>
> Human studies: Adequate studies of pregnant women are not available.
>
> Use this drug only if clearly needed. Ask your physician for guidance.

Advisability of Use If Breast-Feeding
> Presence of this drug in breast milk: Unknown in humans; yes in animals. Avoid drug or refrain from nursing.

Habit-Forming Potential: None.

Effects of Overdose: Weakness, slow pulse, low blood pressure, fainting, cold and sweaty skin, congestive heart failure, possible coma, and convulsions.

Possible Effects of Long-Term Use: Reduced heart reserve and eventual heart failure in susceptible individuals with advanced heart disease.

Suggested Periodic Examinations While Taking This Drug (at physician's discretion)

Measurements of blood pressure, evaluation of heart function.

▷ **While Taking This Drug, Observe the Following**

Foods: No restrictions. Avoid excessive salt intake. Ginseng may increase blood pressure.

Beverages: No restrictions. May be taken with milk.

▷ *Alcohol:* Use caution. Alcohol may exaggerate blood pressure lowering and also increase the drug's mild sedative effect.

Tobacco Smoking: Nicotine may reduce benefits in treating high blood pressure. High doses may worsen bronchial constriction caused by regular smoking. I advise everyone to quit smoking.

▷ *Other Drugs*

Carteolol may ***increase*** the effects of

• other antihypertensive drugs, and cause excessive lowering of the blood pressure. Dosage adjustments may be necessary.

• reserpine (Ser-Ap-Es, etc.), and cause sedation, depression, slowing of the heart rate, and low blood pressure. This combination is best avoided.

• theophyllines (aminophylline, dyphylline, oxtriphylline, etc.).

• verapamil (Calan, Isoptin), and cause excessive depression of heart function; monitor this combination closely.

Carteolol ***taken concurrently*** with

• amiodarone (Cordarone) may cause severe slowing of the heart and sinus arrest. Do not combine these agents.

• clonidine (Catapres) requires close monitoring for rebound high blood pressure if clonidine is stopped while carteolol is still being taken. Severe rebound hypertension may occur.

• digoxin (Lanoxin) may lead to abnormal heart conduction. Caution is prudent.

• diltiazem (Cardizem) (like verapamil) may be very helpful in patients with normal heart function, but may result in AV conduction problems.

• epinephrine (Adrenalin, etc.) may cause sudden rise in blood pressure followed by slowing of the heart rate. Avoid this combination.

• ergot preparations (ergotamine, methysergide, etc.) may enhance serious ergot-induced constriction of peripheral circulation.

• fluoxetine (Prozac) may result in dangerous slowing of the heart or dangerously low blood pressure.

• fluvoxamine (Luvox) may result in dangerous slowing of the heart or dangerously low blood pressure.

• insulin requires close monitoring to avoid hypoglycemia (see Glossary).

• nifedipine (dihydroperidine) may result in excessive lowering of the blood pressure.

• oral antidiabetic drugs (see Drug Classes) may cause prolonged recovery from hypoglycemia should it occur.

• phenothiazines (see Drug Classes) can cause increased effects of both drugs.

• rifabutin (Mycobutin) may reduce carteolol's effectiveness.

• venlafaxine (Effexor) may lead to toxicity from either drug.

• zileuton (Zyflo) may result in increased toxicity risk from carteolol. Caution is advised.

The following drugs may *decrease* the effects of carteolol:
- indomethacin (Indocin), and possibly other "aspirin substitutes" or NSAIDs, may impair carteolol's antihypertensive effect.

▷ *Driving, Hazardous Activities:* Use caution until the full extent of fatigue, dizziness, and blood pressure change have been determined.

Aviation Note: The use of this drug *is a disqualification* for piloting. Consult a designated aviation medical examiner.

Exposure to Sun: No restrictions.

Exposure to Heat: Caution is advised. Hot environments can lower the blood pressure and exaggerate the effects of this drug.

Exposure to Cold: Caution is advised. The elderly should take precautions to prevent hypothermia (see Glossary).

Heavy Exercise or Exertion: Avoid exertion that produces light-headedness, excessive fatigue, or muscle cramping.

Occurrence of Unrelated Illness: Fever can lower blood pressure and require decreased doses. Illnesses that cause nausea or vomiting may interrupt the regular dosage schedule. Ask your physician for guidance.

Discontinuation: **DO NOT STOP this drug suddenly**. If possible, gradual reduction of dose over a period of 2 to 3 weeks is recommended. Ask your physician for help.

CARVEDILOL (KAR vi die lohl)

Introduced: 1997   **Class:** Antihypertensive, beta-adrenergic blocker
Prescription: USA: Yes   **Controlled Drug:** USA: No; Canada: No   **Available as Generic:** No
Brand Name: Coreg

BENEFITS versus RISKS	
Possible Benefits	*Possible Risks*
EFFECTIVE, WELL-TOLERATED ANTIHYPERTENSIVE	Worsening of heart failure (often responds to dose changes)
IMPROVES CONGESTIVE HEART FAILURE	Slow heart beat
DECREASES RISK OF HEART PROBLEMS AND DEATH (MORBIDITY AND MORTALITY)	Masking of low blood sugar (hypoglycemia) in drug-treated diabetics (possible)
WORKS ON TWO KINDS OF BETA RECEPTORS (B1 AND B2 AND ALPHA (ALPHA1) RECEPTORS AS WELL	Dizziness
	Provocation of asthma in asthmatics

▷ **Principal Uses**

As a Single Drug Product: Uses currently included in FDA-approved labeling: (1) Treats mild to moderate high blood pressure, alone or in combination with other drugs; (2) improves congestive heart failure.

Other (unlabeled) generally accepted uses: (1) Eases frequency and severity of angina; (2) may be of help in people with increased blood pressure in the liver blood circulation that stems from liver disease (portal hypertension);

(3) One study showed that this drug was beneficial when used after a heart attack.

DO NOT STOP this drug suddenly. If possible, gradual reduction of dose over a period of 2 to 3 weeks is recommended. Ask your physician for help.

Author's note: The information in this profile will be broadened as more information becomes available.

CEPHALOSPORIN ANTIBIOTIC FAMILY (SEF a low spoar ins)

Cefaclor (SEF a klor)   **Cefadroxil** (SEF a drox il)   **Cefixime** (SE fix eem)   **Cefprozil** (SEF proh zil)   **Ceftriaxone** (SEF try ax own)   **Cefuroxime** (SEF yur ox eem)   **Cephalexin** (SEF ah lex in)   **Loracarbef** (Lor ah KAR bef)

Introduced: 1979, 1977, 1986, 1991, 1984, 1974, 1969, 1992   **Class:** Antibiotics, cephalosporins   **Prescription:** USA: Yes   **Controlled Drugs:** USA: No; Canada: No   **Available as Generic:** Cefaclor: yes; cefadroxil: yes; cefixime: no; cefprozil: no; ceftriaxone: no; cefuroxime: yes; cephalexin: yes; loracarbef: no.

Brand Names: Cefaclor: Ceclor; Cefadroxil: Duricef, Ultracef; Cefixime: Suprax; Cefprozil: Cefzil; Ceftriaxone: Rocephin; Cefuroxime: Ceftin, Kefurox, Zinacef; Cephalexin: ✤Apo-Cephalex, Cefanex, ✤Ceporex, Keflet, Keflex, Keftab, Lorabid, ✤Novo-Lexin, ✤Nu-Cephalex; Loracarbef

BENEFITS versus RISKS	
Possible Benefits	*Possible Risks*
EFFECTIVE TREATMENT OF INFECTIONS due to susceptible microorganisms	ALLERGIC REACTIONS, mild to severe (may also be seen in those allergic to penicillin)
HOME INTRAVENOUS TREATMENT OF SERIOUS INFECTIONS (ceftriaxone)	Drug-induced colitis—rare Superinfections (see Glossary)
ONE INJECTION TREATMENT OF SOME CHILDHOOD EAR INFECTIONS	Low white blood cell or platelet counts (cefixime or ceftriaxone)—rare Anemia (ceftriaxone)—rare

▷ **Principal Uses**

As a Single Drug Product: Uses currently included in FDA-approved labeling: (1) To treat some infections of the skin and skin structures, the upper and lower respiratory tract (including middle ear infections—ceftriaxone has a one dose indication for bacterial otitis media—and "Strep" throat), some urinary tract and some postoperative wound infections; (2) treatment of advanced Lyme disease (stage 2 or 3) via home intravenous (home IV) services (ceftriaxone); (3) treatment of serious bone infections (osteomyelitis) via home IV; (4) treatment of gonorrhea (cefuroxime).

Other unlabeled, generally accepted uses: (1) May have an alternative role in helping prevent rheumatic fever if the bacteria are resistant to erythromycin (cefaclor); (2) may help treat resistant cervical infections (cefixime); part of combination treatment of Whipple's disease (cefixime); (3) treats sexual assault cases and chancroid (ceftriaxone); (4) used in *Shigella* infections; (5) used to change from an intravenous medicine to one taken by mouth in order to shorten hospital stays and preserve results (cefuroxime).

How These Drugs Work: These drugs destroy susceptible infecting bacteria by interfering with their ability to produce new protective cell walls as they multiply and grow.

Available Dosage Forms and Strengths
Cefaclor:

Capsules — 250 mg, 500 mg
Oral suspension — 125 mg, 187 mg, 250 mg, 375 mg/5 ml

Cefadroxil:

Capsules — 500 mg, 1000 mg
Gelatin capsules (Canada) — 500 mg
Oral suspension — 125 mg, 250 mg, 500 mg/5 ml
Tablets — 1000 mg (1 g)

Cefixime:

Oral suspension — 100 mg/5 ml
Tablets — 200 mg, 400 mg

Cefprozil:

Oral suspension — 125 mg, 250 mg/5 ml
Tablets — 250 mg, 500 mg

Ceftriaxone:

250 mg of Rocephin — Boxes of 1 or 10 vial(s)
500 mg of Rocephin — Boxes of 1 or 10 vial(s)
1 g of Rocephin — Boxes of 1 or 10 vial(s) or piggyback bottles of 10
2 g of Rocephin — Boxes of 10 vials, or piggyback bottles of 10
10 g of Rocephin — Box of one 1 g or 2 g ADD-Vantage packaging

Cefuroxime:

Tablets — 125 mg, 250 mg, 500 mg
Intravenous — 750 mg/10 ml
— 750 mg/50 ml
— 750 mg/100 ml
— 1.5 g/100 ml
— 1.5 g/50 ml
— 1.5 g/20 ml
— 7.5 g/127 ml
Oral suspension — 125 mg/5 ml

Cephalexin:

Capsules — 250 mg, 500 mg
Oral suspension — 125 mg, 250 mg/5 ml
Pediatric oral suspension — 100 mg/ml
Tablets — 250 mg, 500 mg, 1000 mg (1 g)

Loracarbef:

Capsules — 200 mg and 400 mg
Oral suspension — 100 mg, 200 mg/5 ml

▷ **Recommended Dosage Ranges:** Cefaclor: 250 to 500 mg every 8 hours. Maximum daily dose is 4 g (4000 mg).

Cefadroxil: Skin infections—500 mg every 12 hours, or 1 g daily. "Strep" throat—500 mg every 12 hours for 10 days. Urinary tract infections—500 mg to 1 g every 12 hours, or 1 to 2 g daily. Maximum daily dose 6 g (6,000 mg).

Cefixime: 400 mg daily, taken as a single dose or as 200 mg every 12 hours. For treatment of multidrug-resistant *Salmonella*: 20 mg per kg of body mass per day in equal doses every 12 hours, for at least 12 days. Uncomplicated gonorrhea: 400 to 800 mg as a single dose.

Cephalexin: 250 to 500 mg every 6 hours. Total daily dose should not exceed 4 g.

Loracarbef: 200–400 mg every 12 hours for 7–14 days depending on the infection being treated.

Infants and Children: Cefaclor: 20 to 40 mg per kg of body mass per day is given in divided doses every 8 hours. Maximum dose is 1 g (1000 mg) daily.

Cefadroxil: 30 mg per kg of body mass per day, given in divided doses every 12 hours.

Cefixime: For children over 6 months of age—8 mg per kg of body mass per day, all in one dose or divided into two doses.

Cefprozil: For otitis media (6 months to 12 years of age)—15 mg per kg of body mass every 12 hours, for 10 days.

Ceftriaxone: For neonates and children less than 12 for treatment of serious infections caused by susceptible organisms (other than CNS infections such as meningitis)—50 to 75 mg per kg of body mass per day, given in two equally divided doses 12 hours apart (not to exceed 2 g daily). Some clinicians use 50 mg per kg of body weight per day for neonates 1 week old or younger; neonates older than 1 week and weighing 2 kg or less also receive 50 mg per kg of body mass per day; and 50–75 mg per kg of body mass per day be given to neonates older than 1 week and weighing more than 2 kg.

For meningitis (caused by susceptible organisms) the dose for neonates and children 12 or younger is 100 mg per kg of body mass daily, divided into two equal doses given every 12 hours. The American Academy of Pediatrics suggests 80–100 mg per kg of body mass be given once daily or in two equally divided doses every 12 hours for children older than 1 month. Because the once-daily regimen is relatively new, I suggest that the 12-hour regimen be used. Serious CNS disease—children can be treated with 75–100 mg per kg of body mass IV daily for 21 days. Cardiac disease—children can be given 75–100 mg per kg of body mass per day IV. Treatment of serious arthritis, cardiac or neurologic complications of early or late (stage 2 or 3) Lyme disease: Arthritis—75–100 mg per kg of body mass per day IV. One recent article advocated a single dose of ceftriaxone for some childhood ear infections.

For otitis media: 75–100 mg per kg of body mass per day, in four divided doses.

Cefuroxime: For children over 2: oral—125 mg twice a day, 250 mg twice daily for treatment of otitis media. Intravenous: Those over 3 months should be given 50 to 100 mg per kg of body mass per day, divided every 6 to 8 hours. Maximum dose is 4 g.

Cephalexin: 25 to 50 mg per kg of body mass per day in two to four divided doses. Maximum dose is 4 g (4000 mg).

Loracarbef: For ear infection (otitis media)—30 mg per kg per day divided into equal doses and taken every 12 hours for 10 days (suspension only).

12 to 60 Years of Age: Cefprozil: Pharyngitis or tonsillitis—500 mg every 24 hours (once daily) for 10 days. Acute or chronic bronchitis—500 mg every 12 hours for 10 days. Bacterial pneumonia—250 mg three times a day for 14 days. Skin or skin structure infections—250 to 500 mg every 12 to 24 hours, for 10 days.

Ceftriaxone for most infections (caused by susceptible organisms) is: 1–2 g daily or in equally divided doses two times a day depending on the type and severity of the infection. Children over 12 are given the adult dose. Some clinicians use 4 G daily in CNS infections in adults. This is the maximum adult dosage recommended by the manufacturer. Uncomplicated gonor-rhea caused by penicillinase-producing strains of *Neisseria* gonorrhea (PPNG) or nonpenicillinase-producing strains may be treated by a single IM 250-mg dose of ceftriaxone. Disseminated gonococcal infection should be treated by 1 g of ceftriaxone IV or IM once a day for 7 days. Acute sexually transmitted epididymitis in adults may be treated with a single 250-mg IM dose of ceftriaxone followed by 7 days of oral tetracycline or erythromycin. For treatment of acute pelvic inflammatory disease (PID), a single 250-mg IM dose of ceftriaxone should be given and then followed by 100 mg of oral doxycycline two times a day for 10–14 days. Treatment of serious arthritis, cardiac or neurologic complications of early or late (stage 2 or 3) Lyme dis-ease: Arthritis—ceftriaxone at a dose of 2 g IV daily for adults. Serious CNS disease—ceftriaxone at a dose of 2 g IV daily for 21 days in adults. Cardiac disease—ceftriaxone 2 g IV per day for 21 days in adults. Surgical prophy-laxis—although ceftriaxone is FDA approved for surgical prophylaxis, we do not recommend its routine use. Other readily available agents are equally as effective, and much less expensive. Ceftriaxone use for surgical prophy-laxis also increases the potential for resistance to this drug, and could de-crease its usefulness in treating later infections.

Cefuroxime: Oral: 250 to 500 mg every 12 hrs. Total daily dosage should not exceed 4 g.

Intravenous: 750 mg to 1.5 g every 8 hours.

Over 60 Years of Age: Cefprozil: Same as 12 to 60 years of age. Decreased dose in kidney failure.

Ceftriaxone: Same as 12 to 60 years of age.

Loracarbef: Same as adult dose unless kidney function has declined.

Note: Actual dosage and schedule must be determined for each patient individually for ALL of these medicines.

Conditions Requiring Dosing Adjustments

Liver Function: Cefaclor, cefixime, cefprozil, cefuroxime, cephalexin or loracar-bef: No changes in dosing needed at present.

Cefadroxil: The liver is involved to a minimal degree, and no dosing changes are anticipated in liver compromise.

Ceftriaxone: Patients with both liver and kidney problems should have blood levels checked and a maximum dose of 2 g given.

Kidney Function: Cefaclor is 40–80% eliminated by the kidney. For creatinine clearances (CrCl) of 10–50 ml/min., 50–100% of the usual dose at the nor-mal interval is used. For creatinine clearances of less than 10 ml/min., 50% of the usual dose at the usual time is given.

Cefadroxil: With creatinine clearances of 10–50 ml/min., use the usual doses every 12 to 24 hours. For creatinine clearances less than 10 ml/min., usual doses are given every 24–48 hours.

Cefixime: Dose **must be decreased** in mild to moderate kidney problems. In severe failure, a single dose every 48 hours is often used.

Cefprozil: With severe kidney failure, **half** the dose can be given at the usual time.

Ceftriaxone: Patients with kidney compromise must be carefully followed for adverse effects.

Cefuroxime: 750 mg once daily for most kidney compromise. Dose must be repeated after dialysis, as this medicine is dialyzable.

Cephalexin: For creatinine clearances of 10–50 ml/min., usual dose every 6 hours. For creatinine clearances less than 10 ml/min., usual dose every 8–12 hours.

Loracarbef: Usual dose for creatinine clearances 50 ml/min. or greater. If the CrCl is 10-49 ml/min. half the usual dose is given at the usualtime.

Phenylketonuria (PKU): Cefprozil only: The suspension has 28 mg of phenylalanine in every 5 ml. This may preclude use of this drug in these patients.

▷ **Dosing Instructions:**   May be taken on an empty stomach or with food if stomach upset occurs. Loracarbef must be taken on an empty stomach.

Capsule (cefaclor, cefadroxil) may be opened and tablet forms crushed. Cefuroxime tablet can give a bitter taste that lingers. Shake suspension forms well before measuring (use a measured dose cup or calibrated dose measure). Intravenous forms should be brought to room temperature if they were refrigerated. Take the full course prescribed.

Usual Duration of Use: Regular use for 3 to 5 days is usually needed to see effectiveness of these drugs in controlling the infection. Response varies with the infection. Treatment time will vary from 1 (for some minor infections) to 6 (as in some bone infections) weeks. Some cases **require 10 consecutive days** of treatment to prevent rheumatic fever. Follow your doctor's instructions carefully. Many clinicians ask you to call them if symptoms worsen or fever persists for 24 to 48 hours after you start to take these medicines.

Possible Advantages of These Drugs

One time dosing (injection) of ceftriaxone guarantees that the medicine will be taken (adherence) by children with one kind of ear infection (acute otitis media).

These Drugs Should Not Be Taken If
- you are allergic to any cephalosporin (see Drug Classes).
- you have pseudomembranous colitis.

▷ **Inform Your Physician Before Taking These Drugs If**
- you have a history of allergy to any penicillin (see Drug Classes).
- you have a history of regional enteritis or ulcerative colitis.
- you have impaired kidney function.
- you have a history of blood clotting disorders.
- you have a history of low platelets or white blood cell count (cefprozil, cefixime, or ceftriaxone).

Possible Side Effects (natural, expected, and unavoidable drug actions)
Superinfections (see Glossary).

▷ **Possible Adverse Effects** (unusual, unexpected, and infrequent reactions)
If any of the following develop, consult your physician promptly for guidance.

Mild Adverse Effects
   Allergic reactions: skin rash, itching, hives.
   Nausea and vomiting or mild diarrhea—most common adverse effects.
   Sore mouth or tongue—possible.
   Mild and reversible decrease in white blood cells (neutrophils) (cefaclor).
   Confusion, nervousness, insomnia, dizziness—rare.
Serious Adverse Effects
   Allergic reactions: drug fever (see Glossary), anaphylactic reaction (see Glossary), Stevens-Johnson syndrome—rare.
   Idiosyncratic reactions: lowered white blood cell counts or platelets (cefixime, ceftriaxone, cefuroxime)—rare; rare and idiosyncratic (cephalexin).
   Extended time for blood to clot (reported with chronic use of other second- or third-generation cephalosporins in debilitated patients)—rare.
   Genital itching (may represent a fungus superinfection)—possible.
   Serum sickness (itching, joint pain, and irritated swellings)—rare.
   Increased blood urea nitrogen (BUN) or serum creatinine—rare.
   Gall bladder concretions (ceftriaxone)—rare.
   Severe diarrhea may be drug-induced colitis—rare.
   Increases in liver enzymes (cefadroxil and loracarbef) and jaundice (cholestatic—cefaclor)—rare.

▷ **Possible Effects on Sexual Function:**   None reported.

Adverse Effects That May Mimic Natural Diseases or Disorders
   Skin rash and fever may resemble measles.

Possible Effects on Laboratory Tests
   Blood platelet counts: decreased—rare (see above).
   INR: may be increased (cefixime, ceftriaxone)—rare.
   PTT: extended (cefprozil)—rare.
   Liver enzymes: increased (cefaclor, cefuroxime, cefprozil, ceftriaxone)—rare.
   BUN and creatinine: increased (cefaclor, cefprozil, cefuroxime, ceftriaxone)—rare.
   White blood cell counts: decreased (cefprozil, cefixime, cefuroxime, ceftriaxone, cephalexin)—rare.

CAUTION
   Some drugs in this class can cause a false positive test result for urine sugar when using Clinitest tablets, Benedict's solution, or Fehling's solution, but not with Tes-Tape.

Precautions for Use
   By Infants and Children: Not recommended for use in infants less than 1 month old (cefaclor), or 1 year old (cephalexin). The maximal dose in children should not exceed 1 g every 24 hours (cefaclor). Dosing of other medicines in this class is based on weight. Follow the dosing instructions exactly. Safety and effectiveness for those under 6 months not established (cefixime, cefprozil).
   By Those Over 60 Years of Age: Dosage must be carefully individualized and based upon evaluation of kidney function. Natural changes in the skin may predispose to severe and prolonged itching reactions in the genital and anal regions. Such reactions should be reported promptly. The natural decline in kidney function often requires a decrease in dose and achieves the same effect as a larger dose (all but ceftriaxone).

▷ **Advisability of Use During Pregnancy**
Pregnancy Category: B. See Pregnancy Risk Categories at the back of this book.
Animal studies: No birth defects reported.
Human studies: Information from adequate studies of pregnant women is not available.
Generally considered to be safe. Ask your physician for guidance.

Advisability of Use If Breast-Feeding
Presence of these drugs in breast milk: Yes, in small amounts (cefaclor, cefadroxil, ceftriaxone, cefuroxime, and cephalexin); unknown (cefixime, cefprozil and loracarbef).
Ask your doctor for advice.

Habit-Forming Potential: None.

Effects of Overdose: Nausea, vomiting, stomach cramps, and/or diarrhea.

Possible Effects of Long-Term Use: Superinfections (see Glossary).

Suggested Periodic Examinations While Taking These Drugs (at physician's discretion)
Complete blood cell counts.
Liver enzymes.
INR or PTT (for some of these medicines).
BUN and creatinine with long-term therapy.

▷ **While Taking These Drugs, Observe the Following**
Foods: Delays the absorption of these drugs and may result in decreased antibiotic effect (cefaclor). No restrictions (cefadroxil, cefprozil, cefixime, ceftriaxone, cefuroxime, or cephalexin).
Beverages: No restrictions. May be taken with milk.
▷ *Alcohol:* Ceftriaxone: May cause severe nausea and vomiting. Others: No interactions expected, but large amounts of alcohol may blunt the immune system.
Tobacco Smoking: No interactions expected. I advise everyone to quit smoking.
▷ *Other Drugs*
These medicines *taken concurrently* with
- any aminoglycoside antibiotic (see Drug Classes) may result in increased kidney (renal) toxicity.
- anticoagulants (blood thinners) such as heparin or warfarin (Coumadin) may have anticoagulant effects increased by some medicines in this class.
- birth control pills (oral contraceptives) may result in **decreased effectiveness** in preventing conception and pregnancy.
- cholestyramine may decrease cephalexin (and perhaps other drugs in this class) absorption and blunt the beneficial effects in fighting infection.
- loop diuretics such as ethacrynic acid may result in increased risk of kidney toxicity.
- nilvadipine (Escor) may increase cephalosporin blood levels.
- probenecid (Benemid) will slow the elimination of these drugs, resulting in higher blood levels and prolonged effect.
▷ *Driving, Hazardous Activities:* Usually no restrictions.
Aviation Note: The use of these drugs *may be a disqualification* for piloting. Consult a designated aviation medical examiner.
Exposure to Sun: No restrictions.

Special Storage Instructions: Oral suspensions should be kept at room temperature (cefixime or loracarbef). Oral suspensions should be refrigerated (cefaclor, cefadroxil, cefprozil, cephalexin, ceftriaxone IV form). Cefuroxime may be stored at room temperature or in the refrigerator.

Observe the Following Expiration Times: Do not take the oral suspension of this drug if it is older than 14 days (cefaclor, cefadroxil, cefprozil, cephalexin or loracarbef) or 10 days (cefuroxime).

CHLORAMBUCIL (klor AM byu sil)

Introduced: 1974   **Class:** Anticancer, immunosuppressant   **Prescription:** USA: Yes   **Controlled Drug:** USA: No; Canada: No   **Available as Generic:** USA: No; Canada: No

Brand Name: Leukeran

BENEFITS versus RISKS	
Possible Benefits	*Possible Risks*
EFFECTIVE PALLIATIVE TREATMENT FOR CHRONIC LYMPHOCYTIC LEUKEMIA	BONE MARROW DEPRESSION (see Glossary)
EFFECTIVE PALLIATIVE TREATMENT FOR HODGKIN'S DISEASE AND OTHER LYMPHOMAS	INCREASED SUSCEPTIBILITY TO INFECTIONS
	CENTRAL NERVOUS SYSTEM TOXICITY
Immunosuppression of nephrotic syndrome	Male and female sterility
Immunosuppression of rheumatoid arthritis	Drug-induced liver or lung damage
	Development of secondary cancers

▷ **Principal Uses**

As a Single Drug Product: Uses currently included in FDA-approved labeling: Treats (1) chronic lymphocytic leukemia; (2) Hodgkin's lymphoma and other malignant lymphomas.

Other (unlabeled) generally accepted uses: (1) Hairy cell leukemia; (2) multiple myeloma; (3) Letterer-Siwe disease; (4) nephrotic syndrome; (5) ovarian cancer; (6) may have a role in treating rheumatoid arthritis; (7) can have a short-term role in treating systemic lupus erythematosus.

How This Drug Works: This drug blocks genetic activity (impairs DNA and RNA), and inhibits production of essential proteins. This kills cancerous cells.

Available Dosage Forms and Strengths

Tablets — 2 mg

▷ **Usual Adult Dosage Range:** For leukemia and lymphoma: Initially (induction phase of 3–6 weeks) 0.1 to 0.2 mg per kg of body mass daily, or 3 to 6 mg per square meter of body surface daily (usually 4 to 10 mg daily) as a single dose or in divided doses. Intermittent doses (twice a week or monthly pulse therapy) for chronic lymphocytic leukemia have used an initial dose of 0.4 mg/kg (single dose) with the next doses increased by 0.1 mg/kg until the lymphocytes are controlled or toxicity is seen. Ongoing (maintenance) dose: often not used (increased leukemia risk).

For immunosuppression: 0.1 to 0.2 mg per kg of body mass daily, in a single dose, for 8 to 12 weeks.

Note: Actual dose and schedule must be determined for each patient individually.

Conditions Requiring Dosing Adjustments

Liver Function: Can cause liver damage. Use with extreme caution in liver compromise. Extensively metabolized.

Kidney Function: Can cause bladder inflammation; caution is advised in cases of compromised urine outflow.

▷ **Dosing Instructions:**   Tablet may be crushed; however, food may decrease absorption by up to 20%. Avoid this combination. See your doctor if vomiting prevents you from taking chlorambucil.

Usual Duration of Use: Regular use for 3 to 4 weeks is usually required to see benefits in controlling leukemia or lymphoma; several months are needed to assess immunosuppression.

▷ **This Drug Should Not Be Taken If**
- you have had an allergic reaction to it previously.
- you have a significant degree of bone marrow depression.
- you currently have an uncontrolled infection.

▷ **Inform Your Physician Before Taking This Drug If**
- you are allergic to melphalan (Alkeran).
- you are pregnant, planning pregnancy, or breast-feeding.
- you have had bone marrow depression or blood cell disorders.
- you have a history of gout or urate kidney stones.
- you have a seizure disorder of any kind.
- you have a history of porphyria.
- you have impaired liver or kidney function.
- you have had cancer chemotherapy or radiation therapy.
- you are taking drugs that can impair your immunity.
- you had or recently were exposed to chicken pox or herpes zoster.

Possible Side Effects (natural, expected, and unavoidable drug actions)

Decreased white blood cell and platelet counts.

Decreased immunity; susceptibility to infections.

Increased blood levels of uric acid, formation of kidney stones.

▷ **Possible Adverse Effects** (unusual, unexpected, and infrequent reactions)

If any of the following develop, consult your physician promptly for guidance.

Mild Adverse Effects

Allergic reactions: skin rash, itching, drug fever (see Glossary)—rare.

Mouth and lip sores, nausea, vomiting—infrequent.

Serious Adverse Effects

Allergic reactions: drug-induced hepatitis with jaundice—case reports.

Cataract formation with high-dose usage—case reports.

Central nervous system toxicity: agitation, confusion, hallucinations, seizures, tremors, paralysis—case reports.

Peripheral neuritis (see Glossary)—possible.

Lung damage: cough, shortness of breath—case reports.

Bone marrow damage, aplastic anemia (see Glossary)—possible (dose related and can be dose limiting).

Leukemia (may depend on dose and length of treatment)—possible.

Liver damage (hepatotoxicity and jaundice)—case reports.

Severe skin damage (toxic epidermal necrolysis)—case reports.

▷ **Possible Effects on Sexual Function:**   Can inhibit reproduction: stops sperm production (male sterility); altered menstrual patterns, blocks ovulation and menstruation (female sterility)—possible.

Possible Delayed Adverse Effects

Severe bone marrow depression (even after drug is stopped).

Secondary cancers (especially leukemia) have been reported.

Lung damage (pulmonary fibrosis).

Adverse Effects That May Mimic Natural Diseases or Disorders

Drug-induced seizures may suggest epilepsy.

Drug-induced jaundice may suggest viral hepatitis.

Natural Diseases or Disorders That May Be Activated by This Drug

Gout, urate kidney stones, porphyria, latent epilepsy.

Possible Effects on Laboratory Tests

Complete blood counts: decreased red cells, hemoglobin, white cells, and platelets.

Blood uric acid level: increased.

Liver function tests: increased liver enzymes (ALT/GPT, AST/GOT), increased bilirubin, increased icterus index.

Sperm counts: decreased or absent.

CAUTION

1. Long-term use of this drug in noncancerous conditions requires extreme caution. Risks include permanent sterility, lung damage, and the development of secondary cancers. It should only be used where less toxic medicines have failed.
2. Have dental work prior starting drug. Bone marrow depression could lead to gum infection, bleeding, and delayed healing.
3. If gout develops, allopurinol is the drug of choice for chlorambucil-caused gout symptoms.
4. Both killed or live virus vaccines will not work while you take this drug. Live virus vaccines may actually cause infection. It may take 3 months to a year for the immune system to recover after stopping this or similar drugs. People in close contact with chlorambucil patients should not get oral poliovirus vaccine. This eliminates risk of accidental exposure.
5. Immediately report: infection, unusual bruising or bleeding, excessive fatigue, tremors or muscle twitching, trouble walking, loss of appetite with nausea or vomiting.
6. It is advisable to avoid pregnancy while taking this drug. A nonhormonal method of contraception is recommended. Call your doctor promptly if you think pregnancy has occurred.

Precautions for Use

By Infants and Children: Dosage schedules and treatment monitoring should be supervised by a qualified pediatrician. Children with nephrotic syndrome can be more prone to drug-induced seizures.

By Those Over 60 Years of Age: Watch closely for central nervous system toxicity.

▷ **Advisability of Use During Pregnancy**
Pregnancy Category: D. See Pregnancy Risk Categories at the back of this book.
Animal studies: Rat studies reveal drug-associated defects of the nervous system, palate, skeleton, and urogenital system.
Human studies: Adequate studies of pregnant women are not available. There are two known cases of an infant born with an absent kidney and ureter following exposure to this drug during early pregnancy.
If possible, this drug should be avoided during pregnancy, especially the first 3 months.
A nonhormonal contraceptive is generally advisable during treatment with this and similar drugs.

Advisability of Use If Breast-Feeding
Presence of this drug in breast milk: Unknown.
Avoid drug or refrain from nursing.

Habit-Forming Potential: None.

Effects of Overdose: Fatigue, weakness, fever, sore throat, bruising, agitation, unstable gait, bone marrow depression, seizures.

Possible Effects of Long-Term Use: Permanent sterility; secondary cancers (leukemia); lung damage (pulmonary fibrosis).

Suggested Periodic Examinations While Taking This Drug (at physician's discretion) *Before* drug treatment and *periodically* during drug use: complete blood counts, uric acid levels, liver function tests, sperm counts.

▷ **While Taking This Drug, Observe the Following**
Foods: No restrictions.
Beverages: No restrictions. May be taken with milk. Drinking 2 to 3 quarts of liquids daily can reduce kidney stone risk. Ask your doctor.
▷ *Alcohol:* Use with caution. Avoid if platelet counts are low and there is a risk of stomach bleeding.
Tobacco Smoking: No interactions expected. I advise everyone to quit smoking.
Marijuana Smoking: Best avoided. Increases risk of central nervous toxicity. Some fungal infections (toxoplasmosis) may be contracted from marijuana itself if the immune system is weak.
Other Drugs
Chlorambucil *taken concurrently* with
• amphotericin B (Abelcet) may increase risk of bronchial spasm, low blood pressure, and kidney (nephrotoxicity) toxicity.
• antidepressant or antipsychotic (neuroleptic) drugs requires careful monitoring; these drugs lower the seizure threshold and increase the risk of chlorambucil-induced seizures.
• aspirin may increase the risk of bruising or bleeding; the platelet-reduction effects of chlorambucil and the antiplatelet action of aspirin are additive; avoid aspirin while taking chlorambucil.
• other immunosuppressant drugs can increase the risk of infection and the development of secondary cancers.
▷ *Driving, Hazardous Activities:* This drug may cause nervous agitation, confusion, hallucinations, or seizures. Restrict activities as necessary.

Aviation Note: The use of this drug *may be a disqualification* for piloting. Consult a designated aviation medical examiner.

Exposure to Sun: No restrictions.

Discontinuation: Many factors will determine when and how this drug should be stopped. Follow your doctor's advice to get the best results.

CHLORAMPHENICOL (klor am FEN i kohl)

Introduced: 1947   **Class:** Antibiotic   **Prescription:** USA: Yes   **Controlled Drug:** USA: No; Canada: No   **Available as Generic:** USA: Yes; Canada: No

Brand Names: Ak-Chlor, Chloracol, Chlorofair, Chloromycetin, Chloroptic, Chloroptic SOP, Econochlor, ✦Elase-Chloromycetin, I-Chlor, ✦Isopto Fenicol, ✦Minims, ✦Nova-Phenicol, ✦Novochlorocap, ✦Ocu-Chlor, Ophthochlor, ✦Ophtho-Chloram, Ophthocort, ✦PMS-Chloramphenicol, ✦Sopamycetin, Sopamycetin/HC

BENEFITS versus RISKS	
Possible Benefits	*Possible Risks*
VERY EFFECTIVE TREATMENT OF INFECTIONS due to susceptible microorganisms	BONE MARROW DEPRESSION APLASTIC ANEMIA (see Glossary) Peripheral neuritis (see Glossary) Liver damage, jaundice

Author's Note: Risks are largely as defined for systemic use, not ophthalmic.

▷ **Principal Uses**

As a Single Drug Product: Uses currently included in FDA-approved labeling: (1) Very effective in a broad spectrum of serious infections—however, because of serious toxicity (fatal aplastic anemia), it is now reserved for life-threatening infections (such as meningitis) caused by resistant organisms, and for infections in people who cannot tolerate other appropriate anti-infective drugs; (2) used in eye (intraocular) infections.

Available Dosage Forms and Strengths

Previously available capsules and oral suspensions are no longer made.

Cream — 1%

Eye/ear solutions — 0.5%

Eye ointment — 1%

Injection — 100 mg/ml

Ophthalmic/otic suspension — 2 mg/ml

▷ **Usual Adult Dosage Range:** Ophthalmic: Chloramphenicol plus hydrocortisone suspension or solution is given as two drops to the affected eye every 3 hours day and night for 48 hours. After this, the time between doses is usually lengthened and therapy continued until 48 hours after the eye appears normal. **Note: Actual dose and schedule must be determined for each patient individually.**

Author's Note: Because use of this medicine is largely limited to oph-

thalmic use, this profile has been shortened to make room for more widely used medicines.

CHLOROQUINE (KLOR oh kwin)

Introduced: 1964   **Class:** Amebecide, antimalarial   **Prescription:** USA: Yes   **Controlled Drug:** USA: No; Canada: No   **Available as Generic:** USA: Yes; Canada: No

Brand Names: Aralen, Kronofed-A-JR

Warning: The brand names Aralen and Arlidin are similar and can be mistaken for each other; this can lead to serious medication errors. These names represent very different drugs. Verify that you are taking the correct drug.

<table>
<tr><td colspan="2" align="center">BENEFITS versus RISKS</td></tr>
<tr><td align="center">Possible Benefits</td><td align="center">Possible Risks</td></tr>
<tr><td>EFFECTIVE PREVENTION AND TREATMENT OF CERTAIN FORMS OF MALARIA
EFFECTIVE COMBINATION TREATMENT OF SOME FORMS OF AMEBIC INFECTION
Possibly effective in palindromic rheumatism
Possibly effective in short-term treatment of systemic lupus erythematosus
Can be of help in refractory rheumatoid arthritis</td><td>INFREQUENT BUT SERIOUS DAMAGE OF CORNEAL AND RETINAL EYE TISSUES
RARE BUT SERIOUS BONE MARROW DEPRESSION; aplastic anemia, deficient white blood cells and platelets
Heart muscle damage—rare
Ear damage; hearing loss, ringing in ears—rare
Eye damage—rare</td></tr>
</table>

▷ **Principal Uses**

As a Single Drug Product: Uses currently included in FDA-approved labeling: (1) Treatment of acute attacks of certain types of malarial infection; (2) treatment for certain forms of amebic infection.

Other (unlabeled) generally accepted uses: (1) Reduces disease activity in refractory rheumatoid and juvenile arthritis; (2) suppresses disease activity in certain types of lupus erythematosus (patients are switched to hydroxychloroquine as soon as possible); (3) treatment of sarcoidosis, polymorphous light eruption, and porphyria; (4) may give dramatic results in palindromic rheumatism; (5) second-line agent for people traveling in areas where there is risk of malaria.

Author's Note: Because this medicine is not as widely used as other medicines, this profile has been shortened to make room for more widely used drugs.

CHLOROTHIAZIDE (klor oh THI a zide)

See the thiazide diuretics profile for further information.

CHLORPROMAZINE (klor PROH ma zeen)

Introduced: 1952   **Class:** Antipsychotic, strong tranquilizer, phenothiazines
Prescription: USA: Yes   **Controlled Drug:** USA: No; Canada: No   **Available as Generic:** Yes
Brand Names: ✤Chlorpromanyl, ✤Largactil, ✤Novochlorpromazine, Ormazine, Thora-Dex, Thorazine, Thorazine SR

BENEFITS versus RISKS

Possible Benefits	*Possible Risks*
EFFECTIVE CONTROL OF ACUTE MENTAL DISORDERS	Toxic effects on the brain with long-term use—rare but possible
Beneficial effects on thinking, mood, and behavior	Liver damage with jaundice—rare
Moderately effective control of nausea and vomiting	Rare blood disorders: hemolytic anemia, abnormally low white blood count
	Eye toxicity

▷ **Principal Uses**

As a Single Drug Product: Uses currently included in FDA-approved labeling: (1) Treats acute and chronic psychotic disorders such as agitated depression, schizophrenia, and mania; (2) can be used for presurgical anxiety; (3) helps reduce symptoms in porphyrias and tetanus; (4) is used to stop prolonged hiccups; (5) lessens or stops vomiting caused by toxic chemotherapy or a potent drug used to treat fungal infections (amphotericin B).

Other (unlabeled) generally accepted uses: (1) Can be of help in complicated drug withdrawal cases; (2) lessens the symptoms of Tourette's syndrome; (3) may be of help in combination therapy of tuberculosis; (4) can be used intravenously after some heart surgeries.

How This Drug Works: By inhibiting the action of dopamine, this drug acts to correct an imbalance of nerve impulses found in some mental disorders.

Available Dosage Forms and Strengths

Capsules, prolonged action — 30 mg, 75 mg, 150 mg, 200 mg, 300 mg
Concentrate — 30 mg/ml and 100 mg/ml
Oral drops — 40 mg/ml
Injection — 25 mg/ml
Suppositories — 25 mg, 100 mg
Syrup — 10 mg/5 ml
Tablets — 10 mg, 25 mg, 50 mg, 100 mg, 200 mg

▷ **Usual Adult Dosage Range:** Initially 10 to 25 mg three or four times daily. Dose may be increased by 20 to 50 mg at 3- to 4-day intervals as needed and tolerated. Usual dosage range is 300 to 800 mg daily. Extreme range is 25 to 2000 mg daily. Total daily dosage should not exceed 2000 mg. **Note: Actual dose and schedule must be determined for each patient individually.**

Conditions Requiring Dosing Adjustments

Liver Function: Use with caution and in decreased dose in patients with compromised livers. Can also be a cause of a specific kind of jaundice (cholestatic).
Kidney Function: Blood levels are recommended if used in severe kidney compromise.

▷ **Dosing Instructions:**   Tablets may be crushed and taken with or after meals to reduce stomach irritation. Prolonged-action capsules may be opened, but not crushed or chewed.

Usual Duration of Use: Use on a regular schedule for several weeks is usually needed to see this drug's effectiveness in controlling psychotic disorders. If benefits are not seen in 6 weeks, it should be stopped. Long-term use (months to years) requires periodic physician evaluation.

▷ **This Drug Should Not Be Taken If**
- you are allergic to any form of this drug.
- you have active liver disease.
- you have taken a large amount of alcohol or narcotics.
- you have cancer of the breast.
- you have a current blood cell or bone marrow disorder.

▷ **Inform Your Physician Before Taking This Drug If**
- you are allergic or very sensitive to any phenothiazine drug (see Drug Classes).
- you have impaired liver or kidney function.
- you have any type of seizure disorder.
- you have diabetes, glaucoma, or heart disease.
- you have a history of lupus erythematosus.
- you have had neuroleptic malignant syndrome.
- you work in extreme heat or are typically exposed to organophosphorous insecticides.
- you are taking any drug with sedative effects.
- you will have surgery with anesthesia (general or spinal).

Possible Side Effects (natural, expected, and unavoidable drug actions)

Drowsiness (usually during the first 2 weeks), orthostatic hypotension (see Glossary), blurred vision, dry mouth, nasal congestion, constipation, impaired urination.

Pink or purple coloration of urine, of no clinical significance.

▷ **Possible Adverse Effects** (unusual, unexpected, and infrequent reactions)

If any of the following develop, consult your physician promptly for guidance.

Mild Adverse Effects

Allergic reactions: skin rash, hives, low-grade fever—case reports.

Lowering of body temperature, especially in the elderly—possible.

Increased appetite and weight gain.

Weakness, agitation, insomnia, impaired day and night vision.

Chronic constipation, fecal impaction—possible.

Serious Adverse Effects

Allergic reactions: hepatitis with jaundice (see Glossary), usually between second and fourth week; high fever; asthma; anaphylactic reaction (see Glossary): case reports—rare.

Idiosyncratic reactions: neuroleptic malignant syndrome (see Glossary)—rare.

Depression, disorientation, seizures—possible.

Eye (ocular) toxicity—case reports.

Disturbances of heart rhythm—case reports.

Hemolytic or aplastic anemia (see Glossary)—case reports.

Low blood platelets or low white blood cells: fever, sore throat, infections—case reports.

Parkinson-like disorders (see Glossary): muscle spasms of face, jaw, neck, back, extremities—rare to frequent.

Prolonged drop in blood pressure with weakness, perspiration, and fainting or drop in blood pressure on standing (orthostatic hypotension)—infrequent.

▷ **Possible Effects on Sexual Function:**   Decreased libido and impotence (1200 mg/day); inhibited ejaculation (400 mg/day); priapism (see Glossary) (250 mg/day); male infertility (30 to 800 mg/day); enlargement of male breasts (gynecomastia)—case reports; enlargement of female breasts with milk production, cessation of menstruation (30 to 800 mg/day).

Adverse Effects That May Mimic Natural Diseases or Disorders

Nervous system reactions may suggest Parkinson's disease. Liver reactions may suggest viral hepatitis. Reactions resembling systemic lupus erythematosus can occur.

Natural Diseases or Disorders That May Be Activated by This Drug

Latent epilepsy, glaucoma, diabetes mellitus (25%), prostatism (see Glossary).

Possible Effects on Laboratory Tests

Complete blood counts: decreased red cells, hemoglobin, white cells, and platelets; increased eosinophils (often warns of jaundice).

Antinuclear antibodies (ANA): positive in 63% of long-term users.

Blood cholesterol level: increased (with liver damage).

Blood glucose level: increased with long-term use.

Glucose tolerance test (GTT): decreased; 40% abnormal with chronic use.

Partial thromboplastin time (PTT): increased.

Blood uric acid level: decreased.

Liver function tests: increased liver enzymes (ALT/GPT, AST/GOT, and alkaline phosphatase); increased bilirubin.

Urine pregnancy tests: false positive results with frog, rabbit, and immunological tests.

CAUTION

1. Many over-the-counter (OTC) medications (see Glossary) for allergies, colds, and coughs should not be combined with this drug. Ask your physician or pharmacist for help.

2. Antacids that contain aluminum and/or magnesium can lower absorption of this drug and reduce its effect.

3. Obtain prompt evaluation of any change or disturbance of vision.

4. This drug can cause false positive pregnancy test results.

Precautions for Use

By Infants and Children: This drug has been used in neonates. Younger children may require more frequent dosing. Do not use in children of any age with symptoms suggestive of Reye syndrome (see Glossary). Watch carefully for blood cell changes.

By Those Over 60 Years of Age: You may be more susceptible to the development of drowsiness, lethargy, constipation, lowering of body temperature (hypothermia), and orthostatic hypotension (see Glossary). Can worsen existing prostatism (see Glossary). Parkinson-like reactions and/or tardive dyskinesia (see discussion of these terms in Glossary) are more likely. Symptoms must be recognized early, since they may become irreversible.

▷ **Advisability of Use During Pregnancy**
Pregnancy Category: C. See Pregnancy Risk Categories at the back of this book.
Animal studies: No birth defects reported in rodent studies. However, rodent studies suggest possible permanent neurological damage to the fetus.
Human studies: No increase in birth defects reported in 284 exposures. Adequate studies of pregnant women are not available. Limit use to small and infrequent doses only when clearly needed. Avoid drug during the last month of pregnancy.

Advisability of Use If Breast-Feeding
Presence of this drug in breast milk: Yes, in small amounts.
Ask your doctor for advice.

Habit-Forming Potential: None.

Effects of Overdose: Marked drowsiness, weakness, tremor, agitation, unsteadiness, deep sleep, coma, convulsions.

Possible Effects of Long-Term Use: Tardive dyskinesia (see Glossary) in 10% to 20%; eye changes—cataracts and pigmentation of retina; gray to violet pigmentation of skin in exposed areas, more common in women; severe ulcerative colitis.

Suggested Periodic Examinations While Taking This Drug (at physician's discretion)
Complete blood counts, especially between 4 to 10 weeks of treatment.
Liver function tests, electrocardiograms.
Complete eye examinations—eye structures and vision.
Careful tongue inspection for fine, involuntary, wavelike movements that could be the beginning of tardive dyskinesia.

▷ **While Taking This Drug, Observe the Following**
Foods: No restrictions.
Nutritional Support: A riboflavin (vitamin B$_2$) supplement should be taken with long-term use. Vitamin C may blunt therapeutic benefits.
Beverages: Caffeine may lessen calming effect of drug. May be taken with milk.
▷ *Alcohol:* Avoid completely. Increases phenothiazine sedative action and accentuates their depressant effects on brain function and blood pressure. Phenothiazines can increase the intoxicating effects of alcohol.
Tobacco Smoking: Possible reduction of drowsiness from drug, but I advise everyone to quit smoking.
Marijuana Smoking: Moderate increase in drowsiness; worsened orthostatic hypotension; increased risk of precipitating latent psychoses.
▷ *Other Drugs*
Chlorpromazine may *increase* the effects of
• all atropinelike drugs, and cause nervous system toxicity.
• all sedatives or narcotics, especially meperidine (Demerol).
• zolpidem (Ambien).
Chlorpromazine may *decrease* the effects of
• guanethidine (Ismelin, Esimil), and reduce its effectiveness in lowering blood pressure.

- oral antidiabetic drugs (see Drug Classes).
- oral anticoagulants (warfarin or Coumadin).

Chlorpromazine *taken concurrently* with

- ACE inhibitors (see Drug Classes) causes excessive lowering of blood pressure.
- amphetamine will cause decreased effects of both drugs.
- beta-blockers (see Drug Classes) can intensify the effects of both drugs.
- birth control pills (oral contraceptives) may lead to increased chlorpromazine levels.
- lithium (Lithobid, others) may result in a decrease in lithium or chlorpromazine effectiveness.
- propranolol (Inderal) may cause increased effects of both drugs; watch drug effects closely—doses may have to be decreased.
- ritonavir (Norvir) and perhaps other protease inhibitors (see Drug Classes) may lead to chlorpromazine toxicity.
- tramadol (Ultram) may increase risk of seizures.
- sparfloxacin (Zagam) may lead to undesirable heart rhythms.
- valproic acid (Depakene) can result in elevated valproic acid blood levels and toxicity.

The following drugs may *decrease* the effects of chlorpromazine:

- antacids containing aluminum and/or magnesium.
- benztropine (Cogentin).
- trihexyphenidyl (Artane).

▷ *Driving, Hazardous Activities:* This drug can impair mental alertness, judgment, and physical coordination. Avoid hazardous activities.

Aviation Note: The use of this drug *is a disqualification* for piloting. Consult a designated aviation medical examiner.

Exposure to Sun: Use caution. Some phenothiazines cause photosensitivity (see Glossary).

Exposure to Heat: Use caution and avoid excessive heat. This drug can impair body temperature regulation and increase the risk of heatstroke.

Exposure to Cold: Use caution and dress warmly. Increased risk of hypothermia in the elderly.

Discontinuation: After long-term use, do not stop this drug suddenly. Gradually withdraw over 2 to 3 weeks. Do not stop this drug without your physician's knowledge and approval. Schizophrenia relapse rate after discontinuation is 50% to 60%.

CHLORPROPAMIDE (klor PROH pa mide)

Introduced: 1958   **Class:** Antidiabetic, sulfonylureas   **Prescription:** USA: Yes   **Controlled Drug:** USA: No; Canada: No   **Available as Generic:** Yes

Brand Names: ✤Apo-Chlorpropamide, ✤Chloronase, Diabinese, Glucamide

BENEFITS versus RISKS	
Possible Benefits	*Possible Risks*
Helps in regulating blood sugar in noninsulin-dependent diabetes (adjunctive to appropriate diet and weight control)	HYPOGLYCEMIA, severe and prolonged
	Allergic skin reactions (some severe)
	Water retention
Tight blood sugar control may avoid or delay blood vessel, heart, nerve, and vision damage possible with uncontrolled increased in blood sugar	Liver damage or blood cell and bone marrow disorders—rare

▷ **Principal Uses**

As a Single Drug Product: Uses currently included in FDA-approved labeling: Helps control mild to moderate type II diabetes mellitus (adult, maturity-onset) that does not require insulin, but is not adequately controlled by diet alone.

Other (unlabeled) generally accepted uses: (1) May be of help in easing abnormal urine output (SIADH); (2) can be used as a test to define some genetic characteristics of diabetes (CPAF test); (3) can be of benefit for some people who have an excessive reaction to sugar (reactive hypoglycemia).

How This Drug Works: This drug (1) stimulates the secretion of insulin if the pancreas is capable of responding to stimulation, and (2) enhances the utilization of insulin by appropriate tissues.

Available Dosage Forms and Strengths

Tablets — 100 mg, 250 mg

▷ **Usual Adult Dosage Range:** Initially 250 mg daily with breakfast. After 5 to 7 days, dose may be increased to 500 mg daily if needed and tolerated. Total daily dosage should not exceed 750 mg. **Note: Actual dosage and schedule must be determined for each patient individually.**

Conditions Requiring Dosing Adjustments

Liver Function: The dose **must** be decreased in patients with liver compromise.

Kidney Function: One researcher advocated a 50% decrease in dose in mild to moderate kidney failure and that this medicine should be avoided (and a different oral hypoglycemic used) in patients with moderate to severe kidney failure.

▷ **Dosing Instructions:** Tablet may be crushed when taken. Taking with food reduces stomach irritation.

Usual Duration of Use: Use on a regular schedule for 1 to 2 weeks is usually needed to see peak effect in controlling diabetes. Failure to respond to maximum doses in 1 month is a primary failure. Up to 15% of those who respond initially may develop secondary failure of the drug within a year. Periodic measurement of blood sugar is needed. See your physician on a regular basis.

Author's Note: Because this medicine is not as widely used as other medicines, this profile has been shortened to make room for more widely used drugs.

CHLORTHALIDONE (klor THAL i dohn)

See the thiazide diuretics profile for further information.

CHOLESTYRAMINE (koh LES tir a meen)

Introduced: 1959   **Class:** Anticholesterol   **Prescription:** USA: Yes
Controlled Drug: USA: No; Canada: No   **Available as Generic:** USA: No; Canada: No
Brand Names: Questran, Questran Light
> **Author's Note: Questran and Questran Light were proposed to the FDA to be changed from prescription to nonprescription status. Approval was not granted.**

BENEFITS versus RISKS

Possible Benefits	*Possible Risks*
EFFECTIVE REDUCTION OF TOTAL CHOLESTEROL AND LOW-DENSITY CHOLESTEROL IN TYPE IIa CHOLESTEROL DISORDERS	Constipation (may be severe)
	Reduced absorption of fat-soluble vitamins (A, D, E, K), folic acid, and niacin
Reduction of total cholesterol and reduction of LDL cholesterol	Reduced formation of prothrombin with possible bleeding
EFFECTIVE RELIEF OF ITCHING associated with biliary obstruction	
Effective binding of medicines in some drug overdoses	

▷ **Principal Uses**

As a Single Drug Product: Uses currently included in FDA-approved labeling: (1) Reduces high blood levels of total cholesterol and low-density (LDL) cholesterol in Type IIa cholesterol disorders; (2) relieves itching due to the deposit of bile acids in the skin associated with partial biliary obstruction; (3) reduces risk of heart disease in type II hyperlipoproteinemia; (4) reduces progression of disease in coronary arteries in people with type II hyperlipoproteinemia.

Other (unlabeled) generally accepted uses: (1) May be of help in biliary fistulas and skin irritations seen in colostomy; (2) can help lower thyroid hormone levels if too much thyroid hormone has been given in error; (3) may help treat cholesterol ester storage disease (CESD); (4) helps relapses of resistant diarrhea (pseudomembranous colitis); (5) eases diarrhea resulting from quinidine.

How This Drug Works: Binds bile acids and bile salts in the intestine, forming complexes which are then removed via feces. This process stimulates changeof cholesterol to bile acids to replace those removed, reducing cholesterol levels. By lowering bile acids, this drug reduces bile acids deposited in the skin and relieves itching.

Available Dosage Forms and Strengths
 Cans — 378 g
 Packets — 4 g, 9 g

▷ **Usual Adult Dosage Range:** Diarrhea (pseudomembranous colitis): 2–4 g two or three times daily.
 Hypercholesterolemia: 9 g of powder (equivalent to 4 g of cholestyramine) one to six times daily. Dose may be increased slowly as needed and tolerated. The total daily dose should not exceed 72 g of powder (32 g of cholestyramine).
 Itching: 4 grams (one packet) once or twice daily.
 Note: Actual dose and schedule must be determined for each patient individually.

Conditions Requiring Dosing Adjustments
 Liver Function: Removed in the feces—no liver involvement.
 Kidney Function: **Not** absorbed into the body.

▷ **Dosing Instructions:** Always take just before or with a meal; this drug is ineffective when taken without food. Mix the powder thoroughly in 4 to 6 ounces of water, fruit juice, milk, thin soup, or a soft food like applesauce; do not use carbonated beverages. **Do not take powder in its dry form.** Chewable bar should be chewed repeatedly before swallowing.

Usual Duration of Use: Regular use for up to 3 weeks may be needed to see benefits in lowering cholesterol. If an adequate response does not occur in 3 months, talk with your doctor about another medicine. Long-term use (months to years) requires ongoing follow-up by your doctor.

▷ **This Drug Should Not Be Taken If**
 • you have had an allergic reaction to it previously.
 • you have complete obstruction of the bile duct (biliary obstruction).
 • you have type III, IV, or V hyperlipoproteinemia (drug does not work in these conditions). Ask your doctor.

▷ **Inform Your Physician Before Taking This Drug If**
 • you are prone to constipation.
 • you have peptic ulcer disease.
 • you have a bleeding disorder of any kind.
 • you have impaired kidney function.
 • you have phenylketonuria (PKU), as Questran Light has aspartame.
 • you have a bleeding disorder.

Possible Side Effects (natural, expected, and unavoidable drug actions)
 Constipation; interference with normal fat digestion and absorption; reduced absorption of vitamins A, D, E, and K, folic acid or niacin. Possible tooth discoloration (do not swish this product in the mouth.)

▷ **Possible Adverse Effects** (unusual, unexpected, and infrequent reactions)
 If any of the following develop, consult your physician promptly for guidance.
 Mild Adverse Effects
 Allergic reactions: skin rash, hives, tongue irritation, anal itching—rare.
 Loss of appetite, heartburn, abdominal discomfort, excessive gas, nausea, vomiting, diarrhea—possible.
 Constipation—frequent.

Serious Adverse Effects

Allergic reaction: asthmalike wheezing.

Vitamin K lowering, increased bleeding tendency—case reports.

Impaired calcium absorption (osteoporosis risk higher)—possible.

Gallbladder colic—case reports.

Disruption of acid–base balance (acidosis, hyperchloremic)—case reports.

▷ **Possible Effects on Sexual Function:**   Increased libido (questionable).

Natural Diseases or Disorders That May Be Activated by This Drug

Peptic ulcer disease; steatorrhea (excessive fat in stools) with large doses.

Possible Effects on Laboratory Tests

Blood cholesterol and triglyceride levels: decreased (therapeutic effect).

Blood hemoglobin and iron levels: decreased (drug impairs absorption of iron).

INR (prothrombin time): increased (impaired vitamin K absorption).

Liver function tests: increased liver enzymes (ALT/GPT, AST/GOT) in a few cases; not thought to be liver damage.

Urine calcium: increased (drug impairs absorption of calcium from intestine).

CAUTION

1. The powder should never be taken in its dry form; always mix it thoroughly with a suitable liquid.
2. Use stool softeners and laxatives as needed if constipation develops. If you are prone to constipation, it may be prudent to start a stool softener before starting this drug.
3. This drug binds other drugs. Prudent to take *all other drugs* 1 to 2 hours before or 4 to 6 hours after taking cholestyramine.

Precautions for Use

By Infants and Children: Safety and effectiveness for those under 6 years of age not established. Watch carefully for development of acidosis and vitamin A or folic acid deficiency. (Ask your doctor for help.)

By Those Over 60 Years of Age: Increased risk of severe constipation. Impaired kidney function may increase acidosis risk.

▷ **Advisability of Use During Pregnancy**

Pregnancy Category: C. See Pregnancy Risk Categories at the back of this book.

Animal studies: No information available.

Human studies: Adequate studies of pregnant women are not available.

Use this drug only if clearly needed. Ensure adequate intake of vitamins and minerals. Ask your doctor for guidance.

Advisability of Use If Breast-Feeding

Presence of this drug in breast milk: No.

However, since it causes problems in absorbing fat-soluble vitamins, caution is advised.

Habit-Forming Potential: None.

Effects of Overdose: Progressive constipation.

Possible Effects of Long-Term Use

Deficiencies of vitamins A, D, E, and K and folic acid.

Calcium deficiency, osteoporosis.

Acidosis (excessive retention of chloride).

Suggested Periodic Examinations While Taking This Drug (at physician's discretion)

Measurements of blood levels of total cholesterol, low-density (LDL) cholesterol, and high-density (HDL) cholesterol. Complete blood cell count for possible anemia. Bone mineral density test to check for osteoporosis.

▷ **While Taking This Drug, Observe the Following**

Foods: Avoid foods that tend to constipate (cheeses, etc.).

Nutritional Support: Ask your doctor about the need for supplements of vitamins A, D, E, and K, folic acid, niacin, and calcium.

Beverages: Avoid carbonated beverages. Ensure adequate liquid intake (up to 2 quarts daily). This drug may be taken with milk.

▷ *Alcohol:* No interactions expected.

Tobacco Smoking: No interactions expected. I advise everyone to quit smoking.

▷ *Other Drugs*

Cholestyramine may *decrease* the effects of

- acetaminophen; take 2 hours before cholestyramine.
- digitoxin and digoxin; take 2 hours before cholestyramine.
- fluvastatin (Lescol).
- furosemide (Lasix).
- iron separate from cholestyramine doses by 4 hours.
- methotrexate (Mexate); take 3 hours before cholestyramine.
- metronidazole (Flagyl).
- NSAIDs (some acidic ones, such as piroxicam and sulindac; see Drug Classes).
- oral antidiabetic drugs (see Drug Classes).
- penicillin G (Pentids).
- phenobarbital; take 2 hours before cholestyramine.
- thiazide diuretics (see Drug Classes); take 2 hours before cholestyramine.
- thyroxin; take 5 hours before cholestyramine.
- warfarin; take 6 hours after cholestyramine.

Cholestyramine *taken concurrently* with

- amiodarone (Cordarone) can result in lowered amiodarone blood levels and decreased effectiveness.
- pravastatin (Pravachol) may work well in further lowering cholesterol if pravastatin dose is taken 1 hour before or 4 hours after cholestyramine is taken.

▷ *Driving, Hazardous Activities:* No restrictions.

Aviation Note: The use of this drug *is usually not a disqualification* for piloting. Consult a designated aviation medical examiner.

Exposure to Sun: No reports of problems at present.

Discontinuation: The dose of any potentially toxic drug taken concurrently must be reduced appropriately when this drug is discontinued.

CIMETIDINE (si MET i deen)

See the histamine (H₂) blocking drugs profile for further information.

CIPROFLOXACIN (sip roh FLOX a sin)

See the fluoroquinolone antibiotic family profile for more information.

CISAPRIDE (SIS a pryde)

Introduced: 1993   **Class:** Gastrointestinal drug   **Prescription:** USA:
Yes   **Controlled Drug:** USA: No; Canada: No   **Available as Generic:** USA:
No; Canada: No
Brand Names: ✤Prepulsid, Propulsid

BENEFITS versus RISKS	
Possible Benefits	*Possible Risks*
EFFECTIVE TREATMENT OF NOCTURNAL HEARTBURN	NEVER PRESCRIBED TO CONGESTIVE HEART FAILURE PATIENTS
FEW CENTRAL NERVOUS SIDE EFFECTS	HEART ARRHYTHMIAS (WHEN COMBINED WITH SEVERAL
May have a role in helping diabetic gastroparesis	OTHER MEDICINES AND MAY ALSO INCREASE RISK IN CERTAIN DISEASE STATES)
	Diarrhea, cramping
	Joint pain

▷ **Principal Uses**
As a Single Drug Product: Uses currently included in FDA-approved labeling: (1) Eases symptoms of reflux esophagitis; (2) decreases nocturnal heartburn caused by gastroesophageal reflux disease.
Other (unlabeled) generally accepted uses: (1) Improves delayed stomach emptying that may lead to anorexia nervosa; (2) can help children with chronic constipation; (3) hastens slowed stomach emptying (diabetic gastroparesis) seen in diabetes; (4) relieves slowed stomach emptying caused by morphine; (5) decreases pain and flatulence in irritable bowel syndrome; (6) helps gallbladder work better in patients with myotonic muscular dystrophy; (7) promotes defecation in spinal cord injury.

How This Drug Works: Increases the movement of the esophagus (by activating a specific muscarinic receptor) and increases contractions in the stomach and helps it to empty.

Available Dosage Forms and Strengths
Tablets — 10 mg, 20 mg
Oral suspension — 1 mg/ml

▷ **Recommended Dosage Ranges** (Actual dosage and schedule must be determined for each patient individually.)
Infants and Children: Safety and efficacy not established in children or infants.
12 to 60 Years of Age: For relief of nocturnal heartburn: 10 to 20 mg four times a day given 15 minutes before meals and at bedtime.
For reflux esophagitis: 10 mg four times a day combined with cimetidine (1 g a day).

For diabetic gastroparesis: 10 mg four times a day given 15 minutes before meals and at bedtime.

Over 60 Years of Age: Same as 12 to 60 years of age.

Conditions Requiring Dosing Adjustments

Liver Function: Prudent to give 50% usual dose to liver failure patients. Dose may then be increased (titrated upward) as needed/tolerated.

Kidney Function: Dose changes are not needed in kidney failure, but metabolites may accumulate.

▷ **Dosing Instructions:**   This medicine should be taken 15 minutes before meals and at bedtime for best effect.

Usual Duration of Use: Regular use for 8 to 12 weeks may be needed for peak benefit in chronic functional constipation. Up to 12 weeks may be needed for full therapeutic effect in reflux esophagitis. Long-term use (months to years) requires periodic physician evaluation of response and dose adjustment.

Possible Advantages of This Drug

Significant decrease in central nervous side effects compared to metoclopramide. Best reserved for treatment failures.

▷ **This Drug Should Not Be Taken If**
- you have had an allergic reaction to any dosage form.
- you have gastrointestinal obstruction, hemorrhage, or perforation.
- you are taking fluconazole, miconazole, itraconazole, ketoconazole, or macrolide antibiotics such as clarithromycin, erythromycin, or troleandomycin.
- you are taking protease inhibitors (see Drug Classes) or fluvoxamine (Luvox).
- you have advanced cancer, congestive heart failure, certain lung diseases (COPD), severe vomiting and dehydration (or other electrolyte disorders) or if you need sudden insulin or water pill (diuretic) therapy.

▷ **Inform Your Physician Before Taking This Drug If**
- you take a benzodiazepine drug (see Drug Classes).
- you have an abnormally fast heartbeat.
- you take prescription or nonprescription drugs not discussed when cisapride was prescribed.

Possible Side Effects (natural, expected, and unavoidable drug actions)

Sleepiness and fatigue—rare.

▷ **Possible Adverse Effects** (unusual, unexpected, and infrequent reactions)

If any of the following develop, consult your physician promptly for guidance.

Mild Adverse Effects

Allergic reactions: skin rash and itching—case reports.

Depression, somnolence or fatigueórare

Joint pain—rare.

Abnormal vision—rare.

Headache, dizziness, and sleep disturbances—infrequent.

Rhinitis, sinusitis, or coughing—rare.

Diarrhea, abdominal pain, joint pain—infrequent.

Urinary incontinence—rare.

Serious Adverse Effects

Allergic reactions: anaphylactic reaction (see Glossary)—case reports.

Rare increases in heart rate, palpitations, or abnormal heartbeat—case reports and intensified by drug interactions(see ìThis drug should not be taken ifî section above).

▷ **Possible Effects on Sexual Function:**   None reported.

Possible Delayed Adverse Effects: None defined.

Possible Effects on Laboratory Tests

Liver function tests: increased liver enzymes (SGOT, SGPT, and CPK).

CAUTION

1. May cause increased heart rate. Call your doctor.
2. Report promptly any increased tendency to depression.
3. **The FDA has recently strengthened warnings about some disease states or conditions that preclude use of this medicine.**

Precautions for Use

By Infants and Children: Safety and effectiveness for children not established.

By Those Over 60 Years of Age: Specific changes not required.

▷ **Advisability of Use During Pregnancy**

Pregnancy Category: C. See Pregnancy Risk Categories at the back of this book.

Animal studies: Has caused prolongation of breeding interval in female rats. Embryotoxic and fetotoxic in high-dose studies in rats.

Human studies: Adequate studies of pregnant women are not available. A benefit-to-risk decision in pregnancy. Ask your doctor for help.

Advisability of Use If Breast-Feeding

Presence of this drug in breast milk: Yes.

Monitor nursing infant closely and discontinue drug or nursing if adverse effects develop.

Habit-Forming Potential: None.

Effects of Overdose: Nausea, vomiting, flatulence, increased urination, and diarrhea.

Possible Effects of Long-Term Use: None defined.

Suggested Periodic Examinations While Taking This Drug (at physician's discretion)

Complete blood counts: Periodically.

▷ **While Taking This Drug, Observe the Following**

Foods: No restrictions, but food may actually increase the blood level obtained.

Beverages: No restrictions.

▷   *Alcohol:* Sedative effects of alcohol will be increased.

Tobacco Smoking: No interactions expected, but I advise everyone to quit smoking.

Marijuana Smoking: May cause additive drowsiness.

▷   *Other Drugs*

Cisapride *taken concurrently* with

- benzodiazepines (see Drug Classes) may result in increased blood levels and increased effects.
- cimetidine (Tagamet) or ranitidine (Zantac) results in increased cisapride

levels and potential cisapride toxicity. Cisapride dose may need to be decreased.

- diazepam (Valium) can lead to up to a 17% increase in the peak drug level.
- fluvoxamine (Luvox) may lead to heart (cardiac) toxicity. Do not combine.
- grepafloxacin (Raxar) and perhaps other fluoroquinolone antibiotics (see Drug Classes) may increase risk of heart toxicity.
- indinavir (Crixivan), nelfinavir (Viracept) saquinavir (Fortovase) or ritonavir (Norvir) may lead to major heart toxicity. DO NOT mix these medicines.
- ipratropium (Atrovent, Combivent) may blunt the benefits ofcisapride.
- itraconazole (Sporanox), ketoconazole (Nizoral), fluconazole (Diflucan), or miconazole (Monistat IV) can lead to cisapride toxicity and abnormal heart effects.
- macrolide antibiotics such as clarithromycin (Biaxin), erythromycin (E-Mycin, others), or troleandomycin can lead to cisapride toxicity. Do not combine.
- mibefradil (Posicor) may lead to major heart toxicity.
- nefazodone (Serzone) increases risk of heart (cardiac) toxicity. Do not combine.
- QT interval changing medicines (ask your doctor) may result in serious heart toxicity if combined with cisapride.
- warfarin (Coumadin) may lead to excessive lowering of prothrombin and increased risk of bleeding. More frequent INR testing is needed with warfarin dosing adjusted to lab results.

▷ *Driving, Hazardous Activities:* This drug may cause some drowsiness. Restrict activities as necessary.

Aviation Note: The use of this drug *may be a disqualification* for piloting. Consult a designated aviation medical examiner.

Exposure to Sun: No restrictions.

Discontinuation: If this medication is stopped and you have been taking an anticoagulant, INR (prothrombin time) testing will be needed.

CLARITHROMYCIN (klar ith roh MY sin)

See the macrolide antibiotic family profile for more information.

CLINDAMYCIN (klin da MY sin)

Introduced: 1973   **Class:** Antibiotic   **Prescription:** USA: Yes   **Controlled Drug:** USA: No; Canada: No   **Available as Generic:** USA: Yes; Canada: No

Brand Names: Cleocin, Cleocin Pediatric, Cleocin T, Cleocin Vaginal Cream, ✤Dalacin C, ✤Dalacin T

BENEFITS versus RISKS

Possible Benefits	*Possible Risks*
EFFECTIVE TREATMENT FOR SERIOUS INFECTIONS OF THE LOWER RESPIRATORY TRACT, ABDOMINAL CAVITY, GENITAL TRACT IN WOMEN, BLOODSTREAM (SEPTICEMIA), SKIN AND RELATED TISSUES caused by susceptible organisms	SEVERE DRUG-INDUCED COLITIS (fatalities reported—systemic use) Liver injury with jaundice—rare Reduction in white blood cell and platelet counts—rare
Combination treatment of *Pneumocystis carinii* pneumonia	
Effective for the local treatment of acne	

▷ **Principal Uses**

As a Single Drug Product: Uses currently included in FDA-approved labeling: (1) Treats serious and unusual infections of the lungs and bronchial tubes, organs and tissues within the abdominal cavity, the genital tract and pelvic organs in women, the skin and soft tissue structures, and generalized infections involving the bloodstream; (2) used in topical form to treat acne.

Other (unlabeled) generally accepted uses: (1) Treatment of resistant gum disease and malaria; (2) prevention of infection of the heart; (3) combination treatment of *Pneumocystis carinii* pneumonia (PCP), an infection associated with AIDS; (4) may have a role in combination therapy of toxoplasmosis infections of the brain in AIDS patients.

Author's note: This profile has been shortened to make room for more widely used medicines.

CLOMIPRAMINE (kloh MI pra meen)

Introduced: 1970   **Class:** Antidepressant   **Prescription:** USA: Yes
Controlled Drug: USA: No; Canada: No   **Available as Generic:** USA: Yes; Canada: No
Brand Name: Anafranil

BENEFITS versus RISKS

Possible Benefits	*Possible Risks*
EFFECTIVE TREATMENT OF SEVERE OBSESSIVE-COMPULSIVE NEUROSIS	DRUG-INDUCED SEIZURES—rare ADVERSE BEHAVIORAL EFFECTS
Effective relief of symptoms of some types of depression	Conversion of depression to mania in manic-depressive (bipolar) disorders
	Aggravation of schizophrenia
	Liver toxicity—rare
	Bone marrow depression and blood cell disorders—rare

▷ **Principal Uses**

As a Single Drug Product: Uses currently included in FDA-approved labeling: Relieves severe, disabling obsessive-compulsive disorder.

Other (unlabeled) generally accepted uses: (1) eases depression; (2) relieves symptoms of panic attacks; (3) helps some phobias; (4) may help repetitive symptoms in autistics; (5) could have a role in diabetic neuropathy; (6) can help premature ejaculation; (7) may relieve severity of hair pulling, nail biting, or arm burning in obsessive-compulsive patients; (8) can ease symptoms in severe premenstrual syndrome.

How This Drug Works: Increases brain nerve transmitters (mostly serotonin), reduces frequency and intensity of obsessive-compulsive behavior.

Available Dosage Forms and Strengths

Capsules — 10 mg (Canada only), 25 mg, 50 mg, 75 mg

▷ **Usual Adult Dosage Range:** Starts at 25 mg daily in the evening. If needed may be increased by 25 mg daily at 3 to 4 day intervals up to 100 mg daily (reached in 2 weeks). The 100 mg should be divided and taken after meals. Usual maintenance dose is 50 mg to 150 mg daily. Maximum daily dose is 250 mg. (Once identified, the daily dose may be given at bedtime as a single dose.) **Note: Actual dose and schedule must be determined for each patient individually.**

Conditions Requiring Dosing Adjustments

Liver Function: The dose should be decreased in patients with liver compromise.

Kidney Function: Changes in dose are not usually needed.

▷ **Dosing Instructions:** May be taken without regard to meals. If needed, the capsule may be opened and may be taken with or following food to reduce stomach upset.

Usual Duration of Use: Regular use for 3 to 4 weeks often needed to see benefits in controlling obsessive-compulsive behavior. Peak effect may take 3 or more months of use. Long-term use (months to years) requires periodic evaluation.

▷ **This Drug Should Not Be Taken If**

- you have had an allergic reaction to it previously.
- you are taking, or have taken within the past 14 days, any monoamine oxidase (MAO) type A inhibitor drug (see Drug Classes).
- you have active bone marrow depression or a current blood cell disorder.
- you have had a recent heart attack (myocardial infarction).
- you have narrow-angle glaucoma.

▷ **Inform Your Physician Before Taking This Drug If**

- you have had an adverse reaction to an antidepressant drug, especially one of the tricyclic class.
- you have a history of bone marrow or blood cell disorder.
- you have any type of seizure disorder.
- you have increased internal eye pressure.
- you have any type of heart disease, especially coronary artery disease or a heart rhythm disorder.
- you are subject to bronchial asthma.
- you have impaired liver or kidney function.

- you have any type of thyroid disorder or are taking thyroid medication.
- you have a history of suicide attempts.
- you have an adrenaline-producing tumor.
- you have prostatism (see Glossary).
- you have a history of alcoholism.
- you will have surgery with general anesthesia.

Possible Side Effects (natural, expected, and unavoidable drug actions)

Drowsiness, increased sweating, light-headedness, blurred vision, dry mouth, constipation, impaired urination.

▷ **Possible Adverse Effects** (unusual, unexpected, and infrequent reactions)

If any of the following develop, consult your physician promptly for guidance.

Mild Adverse Effects

Allergic reactions: skin rash, itching, drug fever (see Glossary)—case reports.

Headache, dizziness, nervousness, impaired memory, weakness, tremors, insomnia, muscle cramps, flushing—infrequent.

Sweating—infrequent.

Increased appetite, weight gain—infrequent.

Altered taste, indigestion, nausea, vomiting, diarrhea—infrequent.

Serious Adverse Effects

Allergic reactions: drug-induced hepatitis, with or without jaundice—case reports.

Idiosyncratic reactions: neuroleptic malignant syndrome (see Glossary)—case reports.

Adverse behavioral effects: confusion, delirium, delusions, hallucinations, paranoia—case reports.

Seizures; reduced control of epilepsy—case reports—rare.

Aggravated paranoid psychoses or schizophrenia—case reports.

Heart rhythm disturbances—case report.

Bone marrow depression (see Glossary): fatigue, weakness, fever, sore throat, infections, abnormal bleeding or bruising—case reports.

SIADH and severe lowering of blood sodium—case reports.

Liver toxicity—infrequent.

Serotonin syndrome—case reports.

▷ **Possible Effects on Sexual Function:** Altered libido, impaired (delayed) ejaculation, impotence, inhibited male orgasm, inhibited female orgasm, abnormal sperm formation, female breast enlargement with milk production, absence of menstruation—case reports.

Adverse Effects That May Mimic Natural Diseases or Disorders

Liver toxicity may suggest viral hepatitis.

Natural Diseases or Disorders That May Be Activated by This Drug

Latent epilepsy, glaucoma, prostatism, schizophrenia.

Possible Effects on Laboratory Tests

Complete blood cell counts: decreased red cells, hemoglobin, white cells, and platelets.

Liver function tests: increased liver enzymes (ALT/GPT, AST/GOT)—liver damage.

Thyroid function tests: decreased TT3 and FT3.

Blood sodium: severely lowered in cases of drug-induced SIADH.

CAUTION
1. Watch for toxicity: confusion, agitation, rapid heart rate, heart irregularity. Blood levels clarify the situation.
2. Use with caution in schizophrenia. Watch closely for deterioration of thinking or behavior.
3. Use with caution in epilepsy. Watch for any change in the frequency or severity of seizures.
4. Complete blood counts should be obtained in patients who develop sore throat or fever while taking this medicine.

Precautions for Use
By Infants and Children: Safety and effectiveness for those under 10 years of age not established. Dose and management should be supervised by a properly trained pediatrician. Total daily dosage should not exceed 200 mg or 3 mg per kg of body mass, whichever number is smaller.

By Those Over 60 Years of Age: Started with 10 mg at bedtime. Dose is increased as needed and tolerated to 75 mg daily in divided doses. During first 2 weeks, watch for behavioral reactions: restlessness, agitation, forgetfulness, disorientation, hallucinations. Unsteadiness or instability may predispose to falling. Prostate problems mayalso be aggravated.

▷ **Advisability of Use During Pregnancy**
Pregnancy Category: C. See Pregnancy Risk Categories at the back of this book.
Animal studies: No drug-induced birth defects reported in mouse or rat studies.
Human studies: Adequate studies of pregnant women are not available.
Use only if clearly needed. Avoid use during the last 3 months, if possible, to prevent withdrawal symptoms in the newborn infant: irritability, tremors, seizures.

Advisability of Use If Breast-Feeding
Presence of this drug in breast milk: Yes.
Avoid drug or refrain from nursing.

Habit-Forming Potential: Psychological or physical dependence is rare and unexpected. Withdrawal symptoms have been reported, and the drug should be tapered if it is to be stopped.

Effects of Overdose: Confusion, delirium, hallucinations, drowsiness, tremors, unsteadiness, heart irregularity, seizures, stupor, sweating, fever.

Possible Effects of Long-Term Use: Neuroleptic malignant syndrome (see Glossary): fever, fast or irregular heartbeat, fast breathing, sweating, weakness, muscle stiffness, seizures, loss of bladder control.

Suggested Periodic Examinations While Taking This Drug (at physician's discretion)
Monitoring of blood drug levels as appropriate.
Complete blood cell counts; liver and kidney function tests.
Serial blood pressure readings and electrocardiograms.
Measurement of internal eye pressure.

▷ **While Taking This Drug, Observe the Following**
Foods: No specific restrictions. May need to limit food intake to avoid excessive weight gain.
Beverages: No restrictions. May be taken with milk.

▷   *Alcohol:* Avoid completely. This drug can markedly increase the intoxicating effects of alcohol; the combination can depress brain function significantly.

Tobacco Smoking: May delay the elimination of this drug and require dosage adjustment. I advise everyone to quit smoking.

Marijuana Smoking: Increased drowsiness and mouth dryness; reduced effectiveness.

▷   *Other Drugs*

Clomipramine may *increase* the effects of

- all drugs with atropinelike effects (see *auticholinergic drugs* in Drug Classes).
- all sedating drugs. Watch for excessive sedation.

Clomipramine may *decrease* the effects of

- clonidine (Catapres).
- guanadrel (Hylorel).
- guanethidine (Ismelin, Esimil).

Clomipramine *taken concurrently* with

- anticonvulsants such as carbamazepine (Tegretol) (see Drug Classes) requires careful monitoring for changes in seizure patterns and the need to adjust anticonvulsant dosage.
- bepridil (Vascor) may lead to dangerous heart rhythms.
- grepafloxacin (Raxar) or sparfloxacin (Zagam) may lead to dangerous heart rhythms.
- monoamine oxidase (MAO) type A inhibitor drugs (see Drug Classes) may cause high fever, seizures and hypertension; avoid combining these drugs. Separate doses of either by 14 days.
- stimulant drugs (amphetamine, cocaine, epinephrine, phenylpropanolamine, etc.) may cause severe high blood pressure and/or high fever.
- thyroid preparations may increase risk of heart rhythm disorders.
- tramadol (Ultram) may increase seizure risk.
- warfarin (Coumadin) may cause an increased warfarin effect and bleeding. More frequent INR (prothrombin time) testing is needed.

The following drugs may *increase* the effects of clomipramine:

- ACE inhibitors (see Drug Classes).
- birth control pills (oral contraceptives).
- cimetidine (Tagamet).
- enalapril (Vasotec, Vaseretic).
- estrogens (various).
- fluoxetine (Prozac).
- fluvoxamine (Luvox).
- haloperidol (Haldol).
- methylphenidate (Ritalin).
- phenothiazines (see Drug Classes).
- quinidine (Quinaglute).
- ranitidine (Zantac).
- ritonavir (Norvir) and perhaps other protease inhibitors (see Drug Classes).
- sertraline (Zoloft).
- verapamil (Calan, others).

The following drugs may *decrease* the effects of clomipramine:

- barbiturates (see Drug Classes).
- carbamazepine (Tegretol).

- chloral hydrate (Noctec, Somnos, etc.).
- lithium (Lithobid, Lithotab, etc.).
- reserpine (Serpasil, Ser-Ap-Es, etc.).

▷ *Driving, Hazardous Activities:* This drug may cause seizures and impair alertness, judgment, physical coordination, and reaction time. Restrict activities as necessary.

Aviation Note: The use of this drug *is a disqualification* for piloting. Consult a designated aviation medical examiner.

Exposure to Sun: No restrictions.

Exposure to Heat: Use caution. This drug may impair the body's adaptation to hot environments, increasing the risk of heatstroke. Avoid saunas.

Exposure to Environmental Chemicals: This drug may mask the symptoms of poisoning due to handling certain insecticides (organophosphorous types). Read their labels carefully.

Discontinuation: It is best to slowly reduce the dose over 3 to 4 weeks. Abrupt withdrawal after prolonged use may cause nausea, vomiting, diarrhea, headache, dizziness, malaise, disturbed sleep, and irritability. Obsessive-compulsive behavior may worsen if drug is stopped. Other drug doses may need to be changed to adjust.

CLONAZEPAM (kloh NA ze pam)

Introduced: 1977   **Class:** Anticonvulsant, benzodiazepines   **Prescription:** USA: Yes   **Controlled Drug:** USA: C-IV*; Canada: No   **Available as Generic:** Yes

Brand Names: Klonopin, ✤Rivotril

Warning: Klonopin and the generic clonidine are similar and can be mistaken for each other—a serious error. Make sure you are taking the correct drug.

BENEFITS versus RISKS	
Possible Benefits	*Possible Risks*
EFFECTIVE CONTROL OF SOME TYPES OF PETIT MAL, AKINETIC, AND MYOCLONIC SEIZURES	Paradoxical reactions: excitement, agitation, hallucinations
Possibly effective in the management of panic disorders	Minor impairment of mental functions
Can help restless leg syndrome	Blood cell disorders: anemia, abnormally low white blood cell and platelet counts—rare
	Increased salivation (difficult with chronic lung disease)

▷ **Principal Uses**

As a Single Drug Product: Uses currently included in FDA-approved labeling: (1) Treats several types of epilepsy: petit mal variations, akinetic, myoclonic, and absence seizure patterns; (2) used in panic disorder.

Other (unlabeled) generally accepted uses: (1) Eases symptoms of Tourette's syndrome; (2) relieves trigeminal neuralgia; (3) helps resistant depression;

*See Controlled Drug Schedules at the back of this book.

(4) can ease drug-induced mania; (5) may be of help in restless leg syndrome (Ekbom syndrome); (6) may help essential tremor symptoms; (7) eases alprazolam withdrawal.

How This Drug Works: Increases the action of a nerve transmitter (gamma-aminobutyric acid or GABA), which blocks seizures.

Available Dosage Forms and Strengths

   Tablets — 0.125 mg, 0.25 mg, 0.5 mg, 1 mg, 2 mg

▷ **Usual Adult Dosage Range:**   Starts with 0.5 mg three times daily. Increased by 0.5 mg to 1.0 mg every 3 days, as needed and tolerated. Maximum daily dose 20 mg. **Note: Actual dose and schedule must be determined for each patient individually.**

Conditions Requiring Dosing Adjustments

   Liver Function: The dose **must** be decreased in liver compromise.

   Kidney Function: Watch for signs and symptoms of accumulation (see "Effects of Overdose" below).

▷ **Dosing Instructions:**   May be taken on empty stomach or with food or milk. The tablet may be crushed. Do not stop this drug abruptly if taken for seizure control, or if taken for more than 4 weeks to control panic attacks.

Usual Duration of Use: Regular use for 2 to 3 weeks may be needed to see benefit in reducing frequency or severity of seizures. Peak control requires dose adjustments over several months. Long-term use (months to years) requires evaluation by your doctor.

▷ **This Drug Should Not Be Taken If**
   • you have had an allergic reaction to it previously.
   • you have acute narrow-angle glaucoma.
   • you have active liver disease.

▷ **Inform Your Physician Before Taking This Drug If**
   • you are allergic to any benzodiazepine (see Drug Classes).
   • you have a history of alcoholism or drug abuse.
   • you are pregnant or planning a pregnancy.
   • you have palpitations, as this drug may worsen palpitations.
   • you have impaired liver or kidney function.
   • you have a history of serious depression or mental disorder.
   • you have any of the following: asthma, emphysema, chronic bronchitis, myasthenia gravis.
   • you have acute intermittent porphyria.

Possible Side Effects (natural, expected, and unavoidable drug actions)

   Drowsiness—frequent (may diminish with time); increased salivation.

▷ **Possible Adverse Effects** (unusual, unexpected, and infrequent reactions)

   If any of the following develop, consult your physician promptly for guidance.

   Mild Adverse Effects

   Allergic reactions: skin rash, hives, itching.

   Ataxia—frequent.

   Weight gain—frequent.

   Headache, dizziness, blurred vision, double vision, slurred speech, impaired memory, confusion, depression—possible.

   Muscle weakness, uncontrolled body movements—possible.

Palpitations or hair loss—rare.

Nausea, vomiting, constipation, diarrhea, impaired urination, incontinence—case reports in older patients.

Serious Adverse Effects

Idiosyncratic reactions: paradoxical responses of excitement, hyperactivity, agitation, anger, hostility—case reports.

Hallucinations, seizures—case reports.

Blood disorders: abnormally low platelet counts—case reports.

Porphyria—case reports.

Increased secretions and breathing problems, especially in those with chronic lung disease—case reports.

▷ **Possible Effects on Sexual Function:** Increased libido, enlargement of male breasts. May cause abnormally early (precocious) secondary sex characteristics in children—case reports.

Possible Effects on Laboratory Tests

Complete blood cell counts: decreased red cells, hemoglobin, white cells, and platelets.

Urine screening tests for drug abuse: may be *positive*. (Test results depend upon amount of drug taken and testing method used.) Liver function tests: increased.

CAUTION

1. Drug should not be stopped abruptly if controlling seizures.
2. Some over-the-counter products containing antihistamines (allergy and cold preparations, sleep aids) can cause excessive sedation if combined with clonazepam.
3. Adverse behavioral reactions are more common in people with brain damage, mental retardation, or psychiatric disorders.
4. Decreased drug response seen in about 30% of users 3 months after therapy starts. Dose increase often needed to restore seizure control.

Precautions for Use

By Infants and Children: This drug is used to treat infants and children of all ages. Careful dosage adjustment based on weight and age is mandatory. Abnormal behavioral responses are more common in children.

By Those Over 60 Years of Age: Smaller doses and longer intervals are suggested. Watch for lethargy, indifference, fatigue, unsteadiness, disturbing dreams, paradoxical excitement, agitation, anger, hostility, or rage.

▷ **Advisability of Use During Pregnancy**

Pregnancy Category: C. See Pregnancy Risk Categories at the back of this book.

Animal studies: This drug causes cleft palates, open eyelids, fused rib structures, and limb defects in rabbits.

Human studies: Adequate studies of pregnant women are not available.

Avoid drug during the first 3 months if possible. Frequent use in late pregnancy may cause the "floppy infant" syndrome in newborns: weakness, lethargy, unresponsiveness, low body temp, depressed breathing.

Advisability of Use If Breast-Feeding

Presence of this drug in breast milk: Yes.

Avoid drug or refrain from nursing.

Habit-Forming Potential: This drug can produce psychological and/or physical dependence (see Glossary) especially with large doses for extended periods.

Effects of Overdose: Marked drowsiness, weakness, confusion, slurred speech, staggering gait, tremor, stupor progressing to deep sleep or coma.

Possible Effects of Long-Term Use: Benefits versus risks must be considered carefully during the extended use of this drug in children. Possible adverse effects on physical or mental development may not be apparent for many years.

Suggested Periodic Examinations While Taking This Drug (at physician's discretion)

During long-term use: complete blood cell counts; liver function tests.

▷ **While Taking This Drug, Observe the Following**

Foods: No restrictions.

Beverages: No restrictions. May be taken with milk.

▷ *Alcohol:* Use with extreme caution. Alcohol may increase the depressant effects of this drug on the brain. It is advisable to avoid alcohol completely— throughout the day and night—if it is necessary to drive or to engage in any hazardous activity.

Tobacco Smoking: No interactions expected. I advise everyone to quit smoking.

Marijuana Smoking: Increased sedation and significant impairment of intellectual and physical performance.

▷ *Other Drugs*

Clonazepam *taken concurrently* with

- amiodarone (Cordarone) may decrease elimination of clonazepam and also worsen toxicity by causing low thyroid function.
- carbamazepine (Tegretol) may decrease blood levels and hence decrease benefits of both medications.
- desipramine, imipramine, and other tricyclic antidepressants (see Drug Classes) can decrease the tricyclic antidepressant blood level and lessen its therapeutic benefit.
- Monoamine oxidase (MAO) inhibitors (see Drug Classes) may result in very low blood pressure and worsening of sedation and respiratory depression.
- phenytoin (Dilantin) may result in decreased phenytoin levels.
- ritonavir (Norvir), and perhaps other protease inhibitors (see Drug Classes), may lead to clonazepam toxicity.
- valproic acid (Depakene, etc.) may cause continuous absence seizures.

The following drugs may *increase* the effects of clonazepam:

- antifungal medicines such as itraconazole (Sporonox) and ketoconazole (Nizoral).
- cimetidine (Tagamet).
- disulfiram (Antabuse).
- macrolide antibiotics such as azithromycin, clarithromycin, or erythromycin (see Drug Classes).
- omeprazole (Prilosec).
- oral contraceptives (birth control pills).

The following drugs may *decrease* the effects of clonazepam:

- rifampin (Rifater) or rifabutin (Mycobutin).
- theophylline (aminophylline, Theo-Dur, etc.).

▷   *Driving, Hazardous Activities:* This drug can impair mental alertness, judgment, physical coordination, and reaction time. Avoid hazardous activities accordingly.

Aviation Note: The use of this drug *is a disqualification* for piloting. Consult a designated aviation medical examiner.

Exposure to Sun: No restrictions.

Discontinuation: Do not stop clonazepam suddenly if it was controlling any type of seizure, or if it was taken for more than 4 weeks. Dosing should be slowly decreased (tapered) to prevent a withdrawal syndrome.

CLONIDINE (KLOH ni deen)

Introduced: 1969   **Class:** Antihypertensive   **Prescription:** USA: Yes
Controlled Drug: USA: No; Canada: No   **Available as Generic:** USA: Yes; Canada: No
Brand Names: ✦Apo-Clonidine, Catapres, Catapres-TTS, Combipres [CD], ✦Dixarit, ✦Nu-Clonidine

BENEFITS versus RISKS	
Possible Benefits	*Possible Risks*
EFFECTIVE ANTIHYPERTENSIVE in mild to moderate high blood pressure	ACUTE WITHDRAWAL SYNDROME (rebound hypertension) with abrupt discontinuation
Effective control of menopausal hot flashes (in selected cases)	Raynaud's phenomenon (cold fingers or toes)
Effective help in narcotic withdrawal	

▷ **Principal Uses**

   As a Single Drug Product: Uses currently included in FDA-approved labeling: Used in combination with other medicines to treat mild to moderate high blood pressure. May also be added later, replacing drugs causing marked orthostatic hypotension (see Glossary).

   Other (unlabeled) generally accepted uses: (1) Helps prevent migraine headache; (2) helps improve outcomes in some head injuries; (3) can aid menopausal hot flashes and severe menstrual cramps; (4) lessens symptoms of alcohol or narcotic drug withdrawal; (5) helps some Alzheimer's cases.

   As a Combination Drug Product [CD]: Available in combination with chlorthalidone. The different ways in which these drugs work complement each other, making the combination a more effective antihypertensive.

How This Drug Works: Decreases action of the brain (vasomotor center), limiting the sympathetic nervous system's constriction of blood vessels and blood pressure increases.

Available Dosage Forms and Strengths
   Patches — 2.5 mg, 5.0 mg, 7.5 mg
   Tablets — 0.1 mg, 0.2 mg, 0.3 mg

▷ **Recommended Dosage Range:**   Tablets—initially 0.1 mg twice daily. Increased by 0.1 to 0.2 mg daily as needed and tolerated. Usual range is 0.2 to 0.6 mg daily, taken in two doses. Maximum daily dose is 2.4 mg. Some clinicians set maximum of 1.2 mg daily. Patches are applied once a week. Hypertension in children has been treated with 5 to 10 mcg per kg of body mass per day, divided into two or three doses. **Note: Actual dose and schedule must be determined for each patient individually.**

Conditions Requiring Dosing Adjustments

Liver Function: This drug is changed into six active forms. The dose **must** be decreased in liver compromise.

Kidney Function: Some kidney patients may require higher ongoing doses to get the best blood pressure.

▷ **Dosing Instructions:** Tablets may be taken without regard to eating. The tablet may be crushed. Patches should not be altered.

Usual Duration of Use: Use on a regular schedule for 2 to 3 weeks is usually needed to see this drug's benefit in lowering high blood pressure. Long-term use (months to years) requires physician supervision and guidance.

▷ **This Drug Should Not Be Taken If**
- you have had an allergic reaction to it previously.
- you have a problem in your heart that impacts the timing of the heartbeat or transmission of electrical impulses through the heart.

▷ **Inform Your Physician Before Taking This Drug If**
- you have a circulatory disorder of the brain.
- you have angina or coronary artery disease.
- you have or have had serious emotional depression.
- you have a very slow heart rate.
- you have Buerger's disease or Raynaud's phenomenon.
- you are taking a tricyclic antidepressant (see Drug Classes).
- you are taking any sedative or hypnotic drugs or an antidepressant.
- you will have surgery with general anesthesia.

Possible Side Effects (natural, expected, and unavoidable drug actions)

Drowsiness, dry nose and mouth, constipation—common; decreased heart rate, mild orthostatic hypotension (see Glossary). Serious abnormal heartbeats possible if drug is stopped suddenly.

▷ **Possible Adverse Effects** (unusual, unexpected, and infrequent reactions)
If any of the following develop, consult your physician promptly for guidance.

Mild Adverse Effects

Allergic reactions: skin rash, hives, localized swellings, itching—rare to infrequent.

Drowsiness—infrequent to frequent.

Headache, dizziness, fatigue, anxiety, sleep disorders (nightmares or vivid dreaming), dry and burning eyes—possible.

Painful parotid (salivary) gland, nausea, vomiting—case reports.

Dry mouth—frequent.

Urination at night—rare.

Increased liver function tests—case reports.

Serious Adverse Effects
   Idiosyncratic reaction: Raynaud's phenomenon (see Glossary)—case reports.
   Aggravation of congestive heart failure, heart rhythm disorders—case reports.
   Depression, hallucinations, or psychosis—case reports.
▷ **Possible Effects on Sexual Function:**   Decreased libido in 10% (0.2 to 0.8
   mg/day); impotence in 8 to 24% (0.5 to 3.6 mg/day); impaired ejaculation—
   rare; enlargement of male breasts (gynecomastia) (0.2 to 0.8 mg/day)—rare.
   Precocious puberty in females.

Possible Effects on Laboratory Tests
   Blood cholesterol or triglyceride levels: no consistent or significant effects.
   Blood sodium level: increased.
   Liver function: Rare increases of enzymes (ALT/GPT, AST/GOT, alkaline phos-
   phatase).

CAUTION
   1. ***Do not stop this drug suddenly.*** Sudden withdrawal can cause a severe
      and possibly fatal reaction.
   2. Hot weather or fever can reduce blood pressure significantly. Dose ad-
      justments may be necessary.
   3. Report any tendency to depression.

Precautions for Use
   By Infants and Children: Initial doses of 5–10 mcg per kg of body mass per day,
      divided into two or three doses, have been used. A larger evening dose and
      smaller morning dose can help minimize sedation during school hours
      when used for ADHD.
   By Those Over 60 Years of Age: **Proceed cautiously** with this drug. High blood
      pressure should be reduced slowly without the risks associated with exces-
      sively low blood pressure. Low initial doses and frequent blood pressure
      checks are needed. Watch for development of light-headedness, dizziness,
      unsteadiness, fainting, and falling. Sedation and dry mouth occur in 50% of
      elderly users. Promptly report any changes in mood or behavior: depres-
      sion, delusions, hallucinations.

▷ **Advisability of Use During Pregnancy**
   Pregnancy Category: C. See Pregnancy Risk Categories at the back of this book.
      Animal studies: No birth defects reported. However, this drug is toxic to the
      embryo in low dosage.
      Human studies: Adequate studies of pregnant women are not available.
      The manufacturer recommends that women avoid this drug who are or who
      may become pregnant. Ask your physician for guidance.

Advisability of Use If Breast-Feeding
   Presence of this drug in breast milk: Yes.
   This drug may impair milk production. Monitor nursing infant Closely. Stop
      drug or nursing if adverse effects begin.

Habit-Forming Potential: A small number of reports regarding abuse of this
   drug have surfaced. It may cause extreme grogginess and lethargy when
   combined with diazepam (Valium).

Effects of Overdose: Marked drowsiness, weakness, dry mouth, slow pulse, low
   blood pressure, vomiting, stupor progressing to coma.

Possible Effects of Long-Term Use: Development of tolerance (see Glossary) with loss of drug effect; weight gain due to salt and water retention; temporary sexual impotence.

Suggested Periodic Examinations While Taking This Drug (at physician's discretion)

Blood pressure measurements, monitoring of body weight.

▷ **While Taking This Drug, Observe the Following**

Foods: Avoid excessive salt. Ask your doctor for help with salt restriction. Ginseng may raise blood pressure.

Beverages: No restrictions. May be taken with milk.

▷ *Alcohol:* Use with extreme caution. Combined effects can cause marked drowsiness and exaggerated reduction of blood pressure.

Tobacco Smoking: No expected interactions. I advise everyone to quit smoking.

▷ *Other Drugs*

Clonidine may *decrease* the effects of

- levodopa (Larodopa, Sinemet, etc.), causing an increase in parkinsonism symptoms.

Clonidine *taken concurrently* with

- beta-adrenergic-blocking drugs (Inderal, Lopressor, etc.) may increase rebound hypertension risk if clonidine is stopped first. It is best to stop the beta-blocker first, and then withdraw clonidine gradually.
- naloxone (Narcan, Talwin NX) may blunt the therapeutic effect of clonidine and result in a hypertensive response.
- niacin may decrease the facial flushing side effect of niacin.
- nonsteroidal anti-inflammatory drugs NSAIDs (see Drug Classes) may blunt blood-pressure-lowering benefits of clonidine.
- verapamil (Calan, others) may lead to problems in conduction of the heart.

The following drugs may *decrease* the effects of clonidine:

- tricyclic antidepressants (Elavil, Sinequan, etc.; see Drug Classes); may reduce its effectiveness in lowering blood pressure.

▷ *Driving, Hazardous Activities:* Use caution. Can cause drowsiness and impair alertness, judgment, and coordination.

Aviation Note: Hypertension (high blood pressure) *is a disqualification* for piloting. Consult a designated aviation medical examiner.

Exposure to Sun: No restrictions.

Exposure to Heat: Caution: Hot environments may reduce blood pressure, making orthostatic hypotension (see Glossary) more likely.

Exposure to Cold: Use caution. May cause painful blanching and numbness of the hands and feet on exposure to cold air or water (Raynaud's phenomenon).

Heavy Exercise or Exertion: Use caution. This drug may intensify the hypertensive response to isometric exercise. Ask your doctor for help.

Occurrence of Unrelated Illness: Fever may lower blood pressure. Repeated vomiting may prevent the regular use of this drug and cause an acute withdrawal reaction. Consult your physician.

*Discontinuation: **Do not stop this drug suddenly.*** A severe withdrawal reaction can occur within 12 to 48 hours after the last dose. It is best to gradually decrease the dose over 3 to 4 days, and check blood pressure often.

CLOTRIMAZOLE (kloh TRIM a zohl)

Introduced: 1976   **Class:** Antifungal   **Prescription:** USA: Yes, though some are nonprescription   **Controlled Drug:** USA: No; Canada: No   **Available as Generic:** USA: Yes; Canada: No

Brand Names: ✦Canesten, Clotrimaderm, Clotrimazole, Femcare, Gyne-Lotrimin (1% cream and insert are nonprescription), ✦Lotriderm, Lotrimin, Lotrimin AF (nonprescription), Lotrisone , Mycelex (1% vaginal cream is nonprescription), Mycelex-7, Mycelex-G, ✦Myclo, ✦Neo-Zol

Warning: The brand names Mycelex and Myoflex are similar. This can lead to serious errors. Make sure you are using the correct drug.

```
┌─────────────────────────────────────────────────────────────┐
│                   BENEFITS versus RISKS                      │
│     Possible Benefits              Possible Risks            │
│ EFFECTIVE TREATMENT AND       Skin and mucous membrane       │
│   PREVENTION OF CANDIDA          irritation due to sensitization (drug- │
│   (YEAST) INFECTIONS OF THE      induced allergy)            │
│   MOUTH AND THROAT (THRUSH)   Nausea, vomiting, stomach cramping, │
│ EFFECTIVE TREATMENT OF           diarrhea (when swallowed)   │
│   CANDIDA (YEAST) INFECTIONS                                 │
│   OF THE SKIN                                                │
│ EFFECTIVE TREATMENT OF                                       │
│   CANDIDA (YEAST) INFECTIONS                                 │
│   OF THE VULVA AND VAGINA                                    │
│ EFFECTIVE TREATMENT OF TINEA                                 │
│   (RINGWORM) INFECTIONS OF                                   │
│   THE SKIN                                                   │
└─────────────────────────────────────────────────────────────┘
```

▷ **Principal Uses**

As a Single Drug Product: Uses currently included in FDA-approved labeling: (1) Treats *Candida* (yeast) infections of skin, mouth, throat, vulva, and vagina; (2) treats tinea and related infections: ringworm of the body, groin (jock itch), or feet (athlete's foot), due to susceptible fungi.

Other (unlabeled) generally accepted uses: Prevention of *Candida* (yeast) infections of the mouth and throat in the management of AIDS.

How This Drug Works: It damages cell walls and blocks critical enzymes, inhibiting fungal growth (with low drug levels) and kills fungus (with high drug concentrations).

Available Dosage Forms and Strengths

Cream — 1% (10 mg/g)
Lotion — 1% (10 mg/g)
Topical solution — 1% (10 mg/ml)
Mouth lozenges — 10 mg
Vaginal cream — 1% (10 mg/g), 2%
Vaginal tablets — 100 mg, 200 mg, 500 mg

▷ **Recommended Dosage Ranges** (Actual dosage and schedule must be determined for each patient individually.)

Infants and Children: Use of lozenges not recommended for children under 5 years of age; for 5 years and older—dissolve one lozenge slowly and completely in mouth five times a day for 14 days, longer if necessary.

12 to 60 Years of Age: For *Candida* infections of mouth and throat—dissolve 1 lozenge slowly and completely in mouth five times a day for 14 days; extended treatment will be necessary for people with AIDS.

For *Candida* and tinea infections of skin—apply cream, lotion, or solution to infected areas twice a day, morning and evening.

For *Candida* infections of vulva and vagina—one applicatorful (5 g) of cream intravaginally at bedtime for 7 to 14 consecutive days; or one 100-mg tablet intravaginally at bedtime for 7 days; or two 100-mg tablets intravaginally at bedtime for 3 days; single-dose treatment: one 500-mg tablet intravaginally at bedtime, one time only.

Over 60 Years of Age: Same as 12 to 60 years of age.

Conditions Requiring Dosing Adjustments
Liver Function: This drug is removed via the bile—dose should be decreased if bile duct is blocked.
Kidney Function: Dosing changes are not needed.

▷ **Dosing Instructions:** Dissolve lozenge in mouth completely, swallowing saliva as it accumulates. Do not chew the lozenge or swallow it whole. Take full course prescribed. If symptoms persist after or worsen during a course of nonprescription forms, see your doctor. Many clinicians prefer multiple day regimens for more complicated or severe vulvovaginal yeast infections.

Usual Duration of Use: Regular use for 1 to 2 weeks usually needed to see benefit in controlling yeast or tinea infection. Some single-, 3-, or 7-day courses are appropriate for some creams or tablets. Long-term use (as in AIDS management) requires periodic physician evaluation. Treatment failure may indicate need for new combination HIV therapy.

Possible Advantages of This Drug
Reasonably effective with minimal toxicity.
More palatable than nystatin.

▷ **This Drug Should Not Be Taken If**
- you have had an allergic reaction to it previously.

▷ **Inform Your Physician Before Taking This Drug If**
- you are allergic to related antifungal drugs: fluconazole, itraconazole, ketoconazole, miconazole.
- you have liver problems and take oral clotrimazole troche.

Possible Side Effects (natural, expected, and unavoidable drug actions)
None.

▷ **Possible Adverse Effects** (unusual, unexpected, and infrequent reactions)
If any of the following develop, consult your physician promptly for guidance.
Mild Adverse Effects
Allergic reactions: skin rash, hives, itching, burning, swelling, blistering (not present prior to treatment)—possible.
Depression, disorientation, or drowsiness—may be frequent with oral therapy.
Nausea, vomiting, stomach cramping, diarrhea (when swallowed)—frequent.

Serious Adverse Effects

Allergic reactions: sensitization of tissues (where applied locally) that will react allergically with future drug application—possible.

Liver toxicity (with oral form)—infrequent.

Author's note: Side effects with topical forms are rare.

▷ **Possible Effects on Sexual Function:**   None.

Possible Delayed Adverse Effects: Local tissue sensitization to this drug.

Possible Effects on Laboratory Tests

Liver function tests: increased liver enzyme AST/GOT in 15% of oral form users.

CAUTION

1. Avoid contact of cream, lotion, and solution with the eyes.
2. Do not cover applied cream or lotion with an occlusive dressing.

Precautions for Use

By Infants and Children: Use of lozenges by those under 5 years of age is not recommended.

By Those Over 60 Years of Age: No specific problems reported.

▷ **Advisability of Use During Pregnancy**

Pregnancy Category: B. See Pregnancy Risk Categories at the back of this book.

Animal studies: No drug-induced birth defects were found in mouse, rat, or rabbit studies.

Human studies: Adequate studies of pregnant women are not available.

Use this drug only if clearly needed. Ask your physician for guidance.

Advisability of Use If Breast-Feeding

Presence of this drug in breast milk: Unknown.

Watch infant closely. Stop drug or nursing if adverse effects develop.

Habit-Forming Potential: None.

Effects of Overdose: Excessive use of lozenges may cause nausea, vomiting, or diarrhea.

Possible Effects of Long-Term Use: None reported.

Suggested Periodic Examinations While Taking This Drug (at physician's discretion)

Ongoing oral use: liver function tests.

▷ **While Taking This Drug, Observe the Following**

Foods: No restrictions.

Beverages: No restrictions.

▷ *Alcohol:* No interactions expected.

Tobacco Smoking: No interactions expected. I advise everyone to quit smoking.

▷ *Other Drugs:*

Clotrimazole (oral dosage forms) *taken concurrently* with

- amphotericin B lipid complex (Abelcet) may blunt benefits.
- betamethasone (Diprolene, others) may worsen infections.
- cyclosporine (Sandimmune) may result in cyclosporine toxicity.
- tacrolimus (Prograf) can result in kidney toxicity and increased potassium and glucose.
- trimexate (Neutrexin) may result in trimexate toxicity.

▷ *Driving, Hazardous Activities:* No restrictions.

Aviation Note: No restrictions.
Exposure to Sun: No restrictions.
Discontinuation: As directed by your doctor.

CLOXACILLIN (klox a SIL in)

See the new penicillin combination profile for more information.

CLOZAPINE (KLOH za peen)

Introduced: 1975   **Class:** Strong tranquilizer (antipsychotic)   **Prescription:** USA: Yes   **Controlled Drug:** USA: No   **Available as Generic:** USA: Yes

Brand Name: Clozaril

Note: In the United States, this drug is available only by special arrangement through the Clozaril Patient Management System, which was administered by Caremark Homecare Corporation, and is now administered by HMI. The toll-free number is 1-800-648-1975. Ask your doctor for help.

BENEFITS versus RISKS	
Possible Benefits	*Possible Risks*
EFFECTIVE CONTROL OF SEVERE SCHIZOPHRENIA that has failed to respond adequately to other appropriate drugs	SERIOUS BLOOD CELL DISORDERS: abnormally low white blood cell and platelet counts
Improvement in many refractory cases	DRUG-INDUCED SEIZURES (depending upon size of dose)
Useful in patients who have tardive dyskinesia	

▷ **Principal Uses**

As a Single Drug Product: Uses currently included in FDA-approved labeling: (1) Manages severe schizophrenia that fails to respond to adequate trials of other standard antipsychotic medicines. Because of potential for serious blood cell disorders and seizures, its use is reserved for severely ill schizophrenic patients.

Other (unlabeled) generally accepted uses: (1) Severe and refractory bipolar disorder; (2) severe tardive dyskinesia (dystonic subtype)—a syndrome that can happen after some medicines are used to treat psychosis; (3) psychosis occurring after labor with lactation.

How This Drug Works: By blocking the place (receptor) where dopamine works, this drug corrects an imbalance of nerve impulses causing schizophrenic thought disorders.

Available Dosage Forms and Strengths

Tablets — 25 mg, 100 mg

▷ **Usual Adult Dosage Range:** Initially 12.5 mg two times a day; the dose is gradually increased by 25 mg to 50 mg daily, as tolerated, to reach a dose of 300 mg to 450 mg daily (divided into three doses) by the end of 2 weeks. Later increases should be limited to 100 mg one or two times a week. Average dosage requirements are 600 mg daily. Daily maximum is 900 mg. **Note: Actual dose and schedule must be determined for each patient individually.**

Conditions Requiring Dosing Adjustments
Liver Function: Eliminated in the liver; however, no specific dosing guidelines are available.

Kidney Function: Patients with kidney failure should be watched closely for adverse effects.

▷ **Dosing Instructions:**   May be taken without regard to meals or with food if necessary to reduce stomach irritation. The tablet may be crushed.

Usual Duration of Use: Benefits may be seen after 2 to 4 weeks of regular use. Peak effect may require 3 to 12 months. If no significant benefit is seen in 6 to 8 weeks, the drug should be stopped. Long-term use requires periodic evaluation by your doctor.

Possible Advantages of This Drug
Rarely causes significant sexual dysfunction.

Low incidence of Parkinson-like reactions (see Glossary).

Only case reports of tardive dyskinesia (see Glossary).

Currently a "Drug of Choice"
For treatment of severe schizophrenia in patients who have not responded to other standard antipsychotic drugs.

▷ **This Drug Should Not Be Taken If**
- you have had an allergic reaction to it previously.
- you have had severe bone marrow depression (impaired white blood cell production) with previous use of this drug.
- you have a bone marrow or blood cell disorder.
- you take any other drug that can cause bone marrow depression (see Glossary).

▷ **Inform Your Physician Before Taking This Drug If**
- you have a history of any type of seizure disorder.
- you have a history of narrow-angle glaucoma.
- you have any type of heart or circulatory disorder, especially heart rhythm abnormalities or hypertension.
- your body is very depleted (cachectic).
- you have impaired liver or kidney function.
- you have prostatism (see Glossary).

Possible Side Effects (natural, expected, and unavoidable drug actions)
Drowsiness, sedation—frequent.

Weight gain—frequent.

Dizziness, light-headedness—infrequent to frequent.

Orthostatic hypotension (see Glossary)—possible.

Blurred vision, salivation, dry mouth, impaired urination, constipation—possible.

▷ **Possible Adverse Effects** (unusual, unexpected, and infrequent reactions)
If any of the following develop, consult your physician promptly for guidance.

Mild Adverse Effects
Allergic reactions: skin rash; drug fever (see Glossary), which usually occurs within the first 3 weeks of treatment and is self-limiting—rare.
Headache, tremor, fainting, sleep disorders, restlessness, confusion, depression—rare.
Increased salivation—frequent.
Rapid heartbeat, hypertension, chest pain—rare to infrequent.
Nausea, indigestion, vomiting, diarrhea—rare.
Serious Adverse Effects
Allergic reactions: asthmatic-type respiratory reaction—case reports.
Bone marrow depression: specific impairment of white blood cell production with potential for serious infection—rare.
Drug-induced seizures, dose related—rare.
Tardive dyskinesia—case reports.
Abnormally low blood pressure on standing (orthostatic hypotension)—possible.
Anticholinergic syndrome—rare.
Neuroleptic malignant syndrome—case reports.

▷ **Possible Effects on Sexual Function:** Decreased libido and impotence (infrequent and dose related—over 150 mg), abnormal ejaculation or priapism (see Glossary)—rare.

Adverse Effects That May Mimic Natural Diseases or Disorders
Drug-induced fever may suggest systemic infection. Because of the risk of bone marrow depression and secondary infection, any occurrence of fever must be carefully evaluated.
Drug-induced seizures may suggest the possibility of epilepsy.

Natural Diseases or Disorders That May Be Activated by This Drug
Latent glaucoma, prostatism.

Possible Effects on Laboratory Tests
White blood cell counts: decreased.

CAUTION
1. Baseline white blood cell counts must be checked before clozapine treatment is started; follow-up counts must be made every week during the entire course of treatment and for 4 weeks after discontinuation of clozapine.
2. Promptly report any signs of infection: fever, sore throat, flu-like symptoms, skin infections, painful urination, etc.
3. Report promptly light-headedness or dizziness on rising from a sitting or lying position; this could be orthostatic hypotension (see Glossary).
4. Call your doctor before taking any other medication. This includes all prescription and over-the-counter drugs.

Precautions for Use
By Infants and Children: An open label trial of 11 patients from 12 to 17 years old used 12.5 to 25 mg per day as a starting dose, and increased every 4 days by one or two times the starting dose. This dosing strategy was used to treat refractory childhood onset schizophrenia. Mean trial dose was 370 mg per day.

By Those Over 60 Years of Age: Starting doses of 6.25-12.5 mg are prudent. There is an increased risk of orthostatic hypotension, confusion, blood problems, and prostatism. Report related symptoms promptly.

▷ **Advisability of Use During Pregnancy**

Pregnancy Category: B. See Pregnancy Risk Categories at the back of this book.

Animal studies: No birth defects due to this drug reported.

Human studies: Adequate studies of pregnant women are not available.

Use this drug only if clearly needed.

Advisability of Use If Breast-Feeding

Presence of this drug in breast milk: Unknown.

Avoid drug or refrain from nursing.

Habit-Forming Potential: None, but a withdrawal syndrome has been reported after suddenly stopping long-term therapy.

Effects of Overdose: Marked drowsiness, delirium, hallucinations, rapid and irregular heartbeat, irregular breathing, fainting.

Possible Effects of Long-Term Use: Tardive dyskinesia—case report.

Suggested Periodic Examinations While Taking This Drug (at physician's discretion)

White blood and differential counts prior to starting therapy, every week during therapy, and for 4 weeks after stopping therapy.

Serial blood pressure measurements and electrocardiograms.

▷ **While Taking This Drug, Observe the Following**

Foods: No restrictions.

Beverages: No restrictions. May be taken with milk.

▷ *Alcohol:* Avoid completely. Alcohol increases sedation and accentuates its brain function and blood pressure depression. This drug can increase the intoxicating effects of alcohol.

Tobacco Smoking: May accelerate the elimination of this drug and require increased dosage. I advise everyone to quit smoking.

Marijuana Smoking: Moderate increase in drowsiness; worsening of orthostatic hypotension; increased risk of aggravating psychosis.

▷ *Other Drugs*

Clozapine may ***increase*** the effects of

- antihypertensive drugs; observe for excessive lowering of blood pressure.
- drugs with atropinelike actions (see ***anticholinergic drugs*** in Drug Classes).
- drugs with sedative actions; observe for excessive sedation.

Clozapine ***taken concurrently*** with

- cimetidine (Tagamet) can result in a toxic level of clozapine.
- erythromycin (E-Mycin, others) can result in increased clozapine concentrations and potential toxicity. This has been seen in a single case report, but caution is advised.
- fluoxetine (Prozac) can result in clozapine toxicity.
- fluvoxamine (Luvox) can result in clozapine toxicity.
- lithium (Lithobid, Lithotab, etc.) may increase the risk of confusional states, seizures, and neuroleptic malignant syndrome (see Glossary).
- monoamine oxidase (MAO) inhibitors (see Drug Classes) may cause abnormally low blood pressure and exaggerated central nervous system response.
- nefazodone (Serzone) may lead to clozapine toxicity.

- other bone marrow depressant drugs, such as carbamazepine (Tegretol), may increase the risk of impaired white blood cell production.
- paroxetine (Paxil) may lead to toxicity from either medicine.
- phenytoin (Dilantin) can cause a decreased clozapine level and result in breakthrough schizophrenia.
- risperidone (Risperdal).
- ritonavir (Norvir), and perhaps other protease inhibitors (see Drug Classes), may lead to increased risk of blood adverse effects or other adverse effects. DO NOT COMBINE.
- sertraline (Zoloft) can result in clozapine toxicity.
- tramadol (Ultram) may increase seizure risks.
- venlafaxine (Effexor) may lead to clozapine toxicity.

▷ *Driving, Hazardous Activities:* This drug may cause drowsiness, dizziness, blurred vision, confusion, and seizures. Restrict activities as necessary.

Aviation Note: The use of this drug *is a disqualification* for piloting. Consult a designated aviation medical examiner.

Exposure to Sun: No restrictions.

Exposure to Heat: Use caution. This drug can cause fever and can impair the body's adaptation to heat.

Occurrence of Unrelated Illness: Infections must be vigorously treated. White blood cell response to infection must be followed closely.

Discontinuation: If possible, this drug should be discontinued gradually over a period of 1 to 2 weeks. If abrupt withdrawal is necessary, observe carefully for recurrence of psychotic symptoms.

CODEINE (KOH deen)

Introduced: 1886   **Class:** Analgesic, opioid, narcotic   **Prescription:** USA: Yes   **Controlled Drug:** USA: C-II*; Canada: No   **Available as Generic:** Yes

Brand Names: A.B.C. Compound with Codeine [CD], AC & C [CD], Accopain, Actagen-C [CD], Actifed w/Codeine [CD], Afed-C [CD], Alamine-C [CD], Alamine Expectorant [CD], Ambenyl Expectorant [CD], Ambenyl Syrup [CD], Anacin 3 with Codeine #2–4, Anacin w/Codeine [CD], APC with Codeine [CD], Atasol-8, -15, -30 [CD], Ban-Tuiss C [CD], Benylin Syrup w/Codeine [CD], Bitex [CD], Bromanyl Cough Syrup [CD], Bromotuss, Bromphen DC [CD], Brontex [CD], Bufferin w/Codeine [CD], Butalbital Compound [CD], Chemdal Expectorant [CD], Chem-Tuss NE [CD], Chlor-Trimeton Expectorant [CD], Coactifed [CD], Codecon-C [CD], Codehist DH, Codehist Elixir, ✦Codeine Contin (timed release), ✦Coricidin with Codeine [CD], ✦Coryphen-Codeine [CD], ✦C2 Buffered, ✦C2 with Codeine, Deproist [CD], Dimetane Cough Syrup-DC [CD], Dimetane Expectorant-C [CD], Dimetapp-C [CD], Dimetapp w/Codeine [CD], Empirin w/Codeine No. 2, 4 [CD], ✦Empracet-30, -60 [CD], Empracet w/Codeine No. 3, 4 [CD], ✦Emtec-30 [CD], ✦Exdol-8, -15, -30 [CD], ✦Extra Strength Acetaminophen, ✦Fiorinal-C 1/4, -C 1/2 [CD], Fiorinal w/Codeine No. 1, 2, 3 [CD], Gecil [CD],

*See Controlled Drug Schedules at the back of this book.

Glydeine, Isoclor Expectorant [CD], ♣Lenoltec w/Codeine No. 1, 2, 3, 4 [CD], ♣Mersyndol, Naldecon-CX [CD], Normatane [CD], Novadyne DH [CD], ♣Novahistex C [CD], ♣Novo-Gesic, Nucochem [CD], Nucofed [CD], ♣Omni-Tuss [CD], Oridol-C [CD], Panadol with Codeine [CD], ♣Paveral, Pediacof [CD], Penntuss [CD], ♣Phenaphen No. 2, 3, 4 [CD], Phenaphen w/Codeine No. 2, 3, 4 [CD], Phenergan w/Codeine [CD], Poly-Histine [CD], Promethazine CS [CD], Pyra-Phed [CD], ♣Robaxacet-8, Robaxisal-C [CD], ♣Rounox w/Codeine [CD], SK-Apap [CD], Tamine Expectorant DC [CD], ♣Tecnal C [CD], Terpin Hydrate and Codeine [CD], Triafed with Codeine [CD], Triaminic Expectorant w/Codeine [CD], ♣Triatec-8, 30 [CD], ♣Tussaminic C Forte [CD], ♣Tussaminic C Ped [CD], ♣Tussi-Organidin [CD], ♣Tylenol w/Codeine [CD], Tylenol w/Codeine No. 1, 2, 3, 4 [CD], Tylenol w/Codeine Elixir [CD], ♣222 [CD], ♣282 [CD], ♣292 [CD], ♣318 A.C. & C. [CD], ♣VC Expectorant with Codeine, ♣Veganin [CD]

BENEFITS versus RISKS	
Possible Benefits	*Possible Risks*
EFFECTIVE RELIEF OF MODERATE TO SEVERE PAIN	Potential for habit formation (dependence)
VERY EFFECTIVE CONTROL OF COUGH	Mild allergic reactions—infrequent
	Nausea, constipation

▷ **Principal Uses**
   As a Single Drug Product: Uses currently included in FDA-approved labeling: (1) relieves moderate to severe pain; (2) controls cough. Its widest use is as an ingredient in analgesic preparations and cough remedies.
   Other (unlabeled) generally accepted uses: (1) limited role in controlling diarrhea; (2) treats migraine during pregnancy.
   As a Combination Drug Product [CD]: Codeine is combined with other analgesics (aspirin and acetaminophen) on the World Health Organization pain ladder to increase overall pain control. It is also added to cough mixtures containing antihistamines, decongestants, and expectorants.

How This Drug Works: By depressing some brain functions, this drug decreases pain perception, calms emotional responses to pain, and reduces cough reflex sensitivity.

Available Dosage Forms and Strengths
       Injection — 30 mg/ml, 60 mg/ml
          Tablets — 15 mg, 30 mg, 60 mg
    Tablets, soluble — 15 mg, 30 mg, 60 mg

▷ **Usual Adult Dosage Range:**   As analgesic—15 to 60 mg every 4 hours. Current pain theory says that the drug should be scheduled, not taken in response to pain. For cough—10 to 20 mg every 4 to 6 hours as needed. Maximum daily dose 200 mg for pain, 120 mg for cough. **Note: Actual dose and schedule must be determined for each patient individually.**

Conditions Requiring Dosing Adjustments
   Liver Function: The dose must be decreased in liver compromise.
   Kidney Function: Dose decreased by up to 50% in moderate to severe failure.

▷ **Dosing Instructions:**   Tablet may be crushed, then taken with or following food to reduce stomach irritation or nausea.

Usual Duration of Use: As required to control cough. Continual use should not exceed 5 to 7 days without reassessment of need.

▷ **This Drug Should Not Be Taken If**
- you have had an allergic reaction to any form of it.
- you are having an acute attack of asthma.
- your breathing is depressed (respiratory depression).

▷ **Inform Your Physician Before Taking This Drug If**
- you have a history of drug abuse or alcoholism.
- you have impaired liver or kidney function.
- you have gallbladder disease, a seizure disorder, or an underactive thyroid gland.
- you have chronic obstructive pulmonary disease (COPD) or other lung problems such as asthma.
- you have low blood calcium (increased sensitivity to this medicine).
- you have a history of porphyria.
- you tend to be constipated.
- you are taking any other drugs that have a sedative effect.
- you will have surgery with general anesthesia.

Possible Side Effects (natural, expected, and unavoidable drug actions)

Drowsiness, light-headedness, dry mouth, urinary retention—possible.

Constipation— frequent and dose related. Best to start a stool softener or related medicine before codeine is started if you are prone to constipation.

▷ **Possible Adverse Effects** (unusual, unexpected, and infrequent reactions)
If any of the following develop, consult your physician promptly for guidance.

Mild Adverse Effects

Allergic reactions: skin rash, hives, itching—case reports.

Dizziness, impaired concentration, sensation of drunkenness, confusion, depression, blurred or double vision—infrequent.

Nausea, vomiting—frequent and may be dose related.

Serious Adverse Effects

Allergic reactions: anaphylaxis, severe skin reactions—case reports.

Idiosyncratic reactions: delirium, hallucinations, excitement, increased pain sensitivity once the medicine wears off.

Seizures—rare.

Impaired breathing—dose related.

Porphyria—case reports.

Liver toxicity—case reports.

▷ **Possible Effects on Sexual Function:** Opiates have a variety of effects on sexual response. These may range from blunting of sexual response to increased response if anxiety has been a factor inhibiting response—case reports.

Adverse Effects That May Mimic Natural Diseases or Disorders

Paradoxical behavioral disturbances may suggest psychotic disorder.

Possible Effects on Laboratory Tests

Blood platelet counts: decreased.

Blood amylase and lipase levels: increased (natural side effect).

Urine screening tests for drug abuse: may be **positive**. (Test results depend upon amount of drug taken and testing method used.)

CAUTION

1. If you have asthma, chronic bronchitis, or emphysema, use of this drug may cause respiratory difficulty, thickening of secretions, and decrease of needed cough reflex.
2. Combining this drug with atropinelike drugs can increase the risk of urinary retention and reduced intestinal function.
3. Do not take this drug following acute head injury.

Precautions for Use

By Infants and Children: Do not use this drug in children under 2 years of age (possible life-threatening respiratory depression). Children 2 to 6 years old: 1 mg per kg of body mass per day, divided into four equal doses. Maximum dose is 30 mg per day. Children 6 to 12 years of age can receive 5 to 10 mg per dose every 4 to 6 hours, to a maximum of 60 mg every 24 hours.

By Those Over 60 Years of Age: Small starting doses and short-term use is indicated. Expect increased risk of drowsiness, dizziness, unsteadiness, falling, urinary retention, and constipation (often leading to fecal impaction).

▷ **Advisability of Use During Pregnancy**

Pregnancy Category: C; D if used in high doses or for prolonged periods near the time the baby is about to be born. See Pregnancy Risk Categories at the back of this book.

Animal studies: Skull defects reported in hamster studies.

Human studies: Adequate studies of pregnant women are not available. Some studies suggest an increase in significant birth defects when this drug is taken during the first 6 months of pregnancy. Codeine taken during the last few weeks before delivery can cause withdrawal symptoms in the newborn.

Use this drug only if clearly needed and in small, infrequent doses.

Advisability of Use If Breast-Feeding

Presence of this drug in breast milk: Yes, in small amounts.

Avoid drug or refrain from nursing.

Habit-Forming Potential: Psychological and/or physical dependence can develop with use of large doses for an extended period of time. However, true dependence is infrequent and unlikely with prudent use.

Effects of Overdose: Drowsiness, restlessness, agitation, nausea, vomiting, dry mouth, vertigo, weakness, lethargy, stupor, coma, seizures.

Possible Effects of Long-Term Use: Psychological and physical dependence, chronic constipation.

Suggested Periodic Examinations While Taking This Drug (at physician's discretion)

None.

▷ **While Taking This Drug, Observe the Following**

Foods: No restrictions.

Beverages: No restrictions. May be taken with milk.

▷   *Alcohol:* DO NOT COMBINE. Codeine intensifies alcohol, and alcohol intensifies codeine depressant effects on brain function, breathing, and circulation.

Tobacco Smoking: No interactions expected. Tobacco smoking may cause de-

creased pain tolerance and require an increased or more frequent dose of
codeine. I advise everyone to quit smoking.

Marijuana Smoking: Increased drowsiness and pain relief; mental and physical
performance will be impaired.

▷ *Other Drugs*

Codeine may *increase* the effects of
- atropinelike drugs, and increase the risk of constipation and urinary retention.
- monoamine oxidase (MAO) inhibitors and also increase central nervous symptoms and depression.
- other drugs with sedative effects.
- tramadol (Ultram).

Codeine *taken concurrently* with
- quinidine may decrease codeine pain control.
- rifabutin (Mycobutin) may decrease codeine's effectiveness.
- ritonavir (Norvir) may blunt codeine benefits.

▷ *Driving, Hazardous Activities:* This drug can impair mental alertness, judgment,
reaction time, and physical coordination. Avoid hazardous activities accordingly.

Aviation Note: The use of this drug *is a disqualification* for piloting. Consult a
designated aviation medical examiner.

Exposure to Sun: No restrictions.

Discontinuation: Best to limit use to short-term. If extended use occurs, gradualdecreases in dose are prudent to minimize possible withdrawal (usually
mild with codeine).

COLCHICINE (KOL chi seen)

Introduced: 1763   **Class:** Anti-gout   **Prescription:** USA: Yes   **Controlled Drug:** USA: No; Canada: No   **Available as Generic:** Yes
Brand Names: Colbenemid [CD], Col-Probenecid [CD], Cosalide , Proben-C
[CD]

BENEFITS versus RISKS	
Possible Benefits	*Possible Risks*
EFFECTIVE RELIEF OF ACUTE GOUT SYMPTOMS	Loss of hair
	Rare bone marrow depression (see
Prevention of recurrent gout attacks	Glossary)
Prevention of attacks of	Rare peripheral neuritis (see
Mediterranean fever	Glossary)
	Rare liver damage

▷ **Principal Uses**

As a Single Drug Product: Uses currently included in FDA-approved labeling: (1)
Reduces pain, swelling, and inflammation seen in acute gout attacks (many
clinicians prefer nonsteroidal anti-inflammatory drugs [(NSAIDs); see Drug
Classes] as drugs of first choice in acute gout); (2) also used in smaller
doses to prevent recurrent gout attacks.

Other (unlabeled) generally accepted uses: (1) Prevention and control of attacks of familial Mediterranean fever; (2) may have a role in easing symptoms of Behçet's disease; (3) limited use in cirrhosis of the liver; (4) damaged disk syndrome may be helped in some patients; (5) may have a role in recurrent pericarditis; (6) can be of help in pseudogout; (7) appears to be of benefit in some lung disease (idiopathic pulmonary fibrosis); (8) treats some cases of refractory immune thrombocytopenic purpura.

As a Combination Drug Product [CD]: Colchicine combined with probenecid enhances its ability to prevent recurrent attacks of gout. Colchicine is most effective in relieving acute gout; it has some effect in preventing recurrent and chronic discomfort. Probenecid increases removal of uric acid by the kidneys and reduces risk of acute gout. This dual action is more effective than either drug used alone in long-term management of gout.

How This Drug Works: Decreases joint tissue acid, lowering painful uric acid deposits and acute inflammation and pain. (Colchicine does not lower uric acid in the blood or increase urine removal.)

Available Dosage Forms and Strengths
    Injection — 1 mg/2 ml
    Tablets — 0.5 mg, 0.6 mg, O.65 mg (also 1 mg in Canada)

▷ **Usual Adult Dosage Range:**   For acute attack—0.5 to 1.2 mg, followed by 0.5 to 0.65 mg every 1 to 2 hours until pain eases or nausea, vomiting, or diarrhea occurs. Maximum total dose is 8 mg. For preventing recurrent attacks—0.5 to 0.65 mg, one to three times per day. Pericarditis: 1 mg daily to start, followed by 0.5 mg daily. **Note: Actual dose and schedule must be determined for each patient individually.**

Conditions Requiring Dosing Adjustments
    Liver Function: Caution must be used, and the dose decreased, if there is a bile obstruction. This drug should NOT be used in people with both liver and kidney compromise.
    Kidney Function: For severe kidney failure, 50% of the usual dose should be given. Ongoing preventive use NOT prudent in moderate (creatinine clearance less than 50 ml/min) kidney problems. Those with creatinine clearances less than 10 ml/min should NOT be given this medicine.

▷ **Dosing Instructions:**   The tablet may be crushed, then either taken on an empty stomach or with food to reduce nausea or stomach irritation. Start treatment at the first sign of an acute attack. Take the exact dose prescribed.

Usual Duration of Use: For acute attack—stop the drug when pain is relieved or when nausea, vomiting, or diarrhea occurs; do not start this drug for 3 days without asking your doctor. For prevention—use the smallest dose that works. Ask your doctor about dosing.

▷ **This Drug Should Not Be Taken If**
    • you have had an allergic reaction to it previously.
    • you have an active stomach or duodenal ulcer.
    • you have active ulcerative colitis.
    • you have a severe kidney or liver disorder.
    • you have a serious heart disorder.
    • you have a history of blood cell disorders.

▷ **Inform Your Physician Before Taking This Drug If**
- you have peptic ulcer disease or ulcerative colitis.
- you develop diarrhea and vomiting while taking this drug.
- you have any type of heart disease.
- you have impaired liver or kidney function.
- you plan to have surgery in the near future.

Possible Side Effects (natural, expected, and unavoidable drug actions)
Nausea, vomiting, abdominal cramping, diarrhea—frequent, especially with maximum doses.

▷ **Possible Adverse Effects** (unusual, unexpected, and infrequent reactions)
If any of the following develop, consult your physician promptly for guidance.
Mild Adverse Effects
Allergic reactions: skin rash, hives, fever—rare.
Hair loss—reported after overdoses.
Serious Adverse Effects
Allergic Reaction: Anaphylactic reaction (see Glossary)—case reports.
Bone marrow depression (see Glossary): fatigue, weakness, fever, sore throat, abnormal bleeding or bruising—case reports.
Peripheral neuritis (see Glossary): numbness, tingling, pain, weakness in hands and/or feet, or myopathy with nerve symptoms (facial palsy and weakness, especially with long-term use in patients with declines in kidney function)—case reports.
Rhabdomyolysis—case reports.
Porphyria—case reports.
Drooping of the eyes (ptosis)—case reports.
Inflammation of colon with bloody diarrhea—case reports.
Thrombophlebitis with intravenous use—case reports.

▷ **Possible Effects on Sexual Function:**   Reversible absence of sperm (azoospermia).

Possible Delayed Adverse Effects: Impaired production of sperm, possibly resulting in birth defects.
A rare combined muscle and nerve damage syndrome.

Natural Diseases or Disorders That May Be Activated by This Drug
Peptic ulcer disease, ulcerative colitis.

Possible Effects on Laboratory Tests
Complete blood cell counts: decreased red cells, hemoglobin, white cells, and platelets; increased white cells (follows initial decrease).
Prothrombin time: decreased (with concurrent use of warfarin).
Blood vitamin B_{12} level: decreased.
Liver function tests: increased liver enzymes (ALT/GPT, AST/GOT, and alkaline phosphatase), increased bilirubin.
Fecal occult blood test: positive.
Sperm counts: decreased (may be marked).

CAUTION
1. If this drug causes vomiting and/or diarrhea before relief of joint pain, stop it and call your doctor.

2. Try to limit each course of treatment for acute gout to 4 to 8 mg. Do not exceed 3 mg every 24 hours or a total of 10 mg per course.
3. Omit drug for 3 days between courses to avoid toxicity.
4. Carry this drug with you while traveling if you are subject to attacks of acute gout.
5. Surgical stress can cause a gout attack. Ask your doctor how much colchicine should be taken before and after surgery to prevent gout.
6. This medicine may inhibit healing of the cornea. Talk to your doctor about this if you will have eye surgery.

Precautions for Use

By Infants and Children: Use for preventing (prophylaxis) familial Mediterranean fever in children 6 to 13 years of age was given as 0.5 mg per day and increased by 0.5 mg per day, to symptom control or a maximum of 2 mg per day. For other uses in children, dosage has not been established. Ask your physician for guidance.

By Those Over 60 Years of Age: Because the dosage needed to relieve acute gout often causes vomiting and/or diarrhea, extreme caution is advised if you have heart or circulatory disorders, reduced liver or kidney function, or general debility.

▷ Advisability of Use During Pregnancy

Pregnancy Category: C by one manufacturer, and D by another. See Pregnancy Risk Categories at the back of this book.

Animal studies: This drug causes significant birth defects in hamsters and rabbits.

Human studies: Adequate studies of pregnant women are not available. However, it is reported that colchicine can cause harm to the fetus.

Avoid during entire pregnancy if possible. Ask your physician for guidance.

Advisability of Use If Breast-Feeding

Presence of this drug in breast milk: Yes.
Ask your doctor for help.

Habit-Forming Potential: None.

Effects of Overdose: Nausea, vomiting, abdominal cramping, diarrhea (may be bloody), burning sensation in throat and skin, weak and rapid pulse, progressive paralysis, inability to breathe.

Possible Effects of Long-Term Use: Hair loss, aplastic anemia (see Glossary), peripheral neuritis (see Glossary).

Suggested Periodic Examinations While Taking This Drug (at physician's discretion)

Complete blood cell counts, uric acid blood levels to monitor status of gout, sperm analysis for quantity and condition, liver function tests.

▷ While Taking This Drug, Observe the Following

Foods: Follow your doctor's advice about a low purine diet.

Beverages: Drink at least 3 quarts of liquids every 24 hours. This drug may be taken with milk. Some "herbal teas" (promoted as being beneficial for arthritis) contain phenylbutazone and other potentially toxic ingredients. Avoid herbal teas if you are not certain of their source, content, and medicinal effects.

▷ *Alcohol:* No interactions expected. Combination may increase the risk of gastrointestinal irritation or bleeding and raise uric acid blood levels.

Tobacco Smoking: No interactions expected. I advise everyone to quit smoking.

▷ *Other Drugs*

Colchicine *taken concurrently* with

- allopurinol (Zyloprim), probenecid (Benemid), or sulfinpyrazone (Anturane) can prevent attacks of acute gout that often occur when treatment with these drugs is first started.
- cyanocobalamin will decrease absorption of the vitamin B_{12}. Higher doses of oral cyanocobalamin may be required by patients on colchicine.
- cyclosporine (Sandimmune) may increase cyclosporine levels and result in toxicity.
- erythromycins (E.E.S., clarithromycin) can result in toxic colchicine blood levels.
- insulin may inhibit the response (biphasic) of the body to sugar.

▷ *Driving, Hazardous Activities:* Usually no restrictions when taken continually in small (preventive) doses. May cause nausea, vomiting, and/or diarrhea when taken in larger (treatment) doses.

Aviation Note: The use of this drug *may be a disqualification* for piloting. Consult a designated aviation medical examiner.

Exposure to Sun: No restrictions.

Exposure to Cold: This drug can lower body temperature. Use caution to prevent excessive lowering (hypothermia), especially in those over 60 years of age.

Occurrence of Unrelated Illness: Acute attacks of gout may result from injury or illness. Call your doctor for dosing adjustment if injury or new illness occurs.

COLESTIPOL (koh LES ti pohl)

Introduced: 1974   **Class:** Anticholesterol (cholesterol-reducing drugs)
Prescription: USA: Yes   **Controlled Drug:** USA: No; Canada: No
Available as Generic: USA: No; Canada: No
Brand Name: Colestid

BENEFITS versus RISKS	
Possible Benefits	*Possible Risks*
EFFECTIVE REDUCTION OF TOTAL CHOLESTEROL AND LOW-DENSITY CHOLESTEROL IN TYPE IIa CHOLESTEROL DISORDERS	Constipation (may be severe)
	Reduced absorption of fat, fat-soluble vitamins (A, D, E, and K), and folic acid
EFFECTIVE RELIEF OF ITCHING associated with biliary obstruction	Reduced formation of prothrombin with resultant bleeding
Treatment of some pseudomembranous colitis cases	

▷ **Principal Uses**

As a Single Drug Product: Uses currently included in FDA-approved labeling: (1) Used in combination with diet changes to decrease blood cholesterol and low-density (LDL) cholesterol in Type IIa cholesterol disorders; (2) eases itching due to deposit of bile acids in skin.

Other (unlabeled) generally accepted uses: (1) Data from one study showed that colestipol in combination with lovastatin actually caused regression of plaque buildup (atherosclerosis) inside blood vessels; (2) some data show that colestipol is useful in pseudomembranous colitis.

How This Drug Works: Binds bile acids and is removed in feces. Removal of bile acids stimulates conversion of cholesterol to bile acids, which then reduces cholesterol. By reducing levels of bile acids, this drug hastens removal of bile acids in the skin and relieves itching.

Available Dosage Forms and Strengths

Bottles — 250 g, 500 g

Packets — 5 g

Flavored Colestid Granules for oral suspension — 5 g per dose

▷ **Usual Adult Dosage Range:**   Starts with 5 g of powder mixed in an approved liquid (such as orange juice, apple juice, water, or grape juice) and taken three times daily. May be increased slowly as needed and tolerated to 30 g daily in two to four divided doses. **Note: Actual dose and schedule must be determined for each patient individually.**

Conditions Requiring Dosing Adjustments

Liver Function: No changes needed.

Kidney Function: No changes are needed.

▷ **Dosing Instructions:**   Always take just before or with a meal; drug does not work if taken without food. Mix the powder thoroughly in 4 to 6 ounces of water, fruit juice, tomato juice, milk, thin soup, or a soft food like applesauce. **Do not take it in its dry form.**

Usual Duration of Use: Regular use for up to a month may be needed to see peak benefits in lowering cholesterol. If no acceptable response in 3 months, the drug should be stopped. Long-term use (months to years) requires periodic follow-up with your doctor.

▷ **This Drug Should Not Be Taken If**
- you have had an allergic reaction to it previously.
- you have complete biliary obstruction.

▷ **Inform Your Physician Before Taking This Drug If**
- you are prone to constipation.
- you have low thyroid function (hypothyroidism).
- you have peptic ulcer disease.
- you have a bleeding disorder of any kind.
- you have impaired kidney function.

Possible Side Effects (natural, expected, and unavoidable drug actions)

Constipation; interference with normal fat digestion and absorption; reduced absorption of vitamins A, D, E, and K and folic acid. Binds to vitamin B_{12}—intrinsic factor complex.

▷ **Possible Adverse Effects** (unusual, unexpected, and infrequent reactions)

If any of the following develop, consult your physician promptly for guidance.

Mild Adverse Effects
 Allergic reactions: skin rash—rare; hives, tongue irritation, anal itching—case
  reports.
 Headache, dizziness, weakness, muscle and joint pains—possible.
 Constipation—most frequent.
 Loss of appetite, indigestion, heartburn, abdominal discomfort, excessive gas,
  nausea, vomiting, diarrhea—case reports.
Serious Adverse Effects
 Vitamin K deficiency and increased bleeding tendency—possible.
 Impaired absorption of calcium; predisposition to osteoporosis—possible.
 Hypothyroidism—possible.
 Disruption of normal acid–base balance of the body (metabolic acidosis)—
  possible with long-term use.

▷ **Possible Effects on Sexual Function:**   None reported.

Natural Diseases or Disorders That May Be Activated by This Drug
 Peptic ulcer disease; steatorrhea (excessive fat in stools) with large doses.

Possible Effects on Laboratory Tests
 Blood cholesterol and triglyceride levels: decreased (therapeutic effect).
 Blood thyroxine (T_4) level: decreased when colestipol and niacin are taken
  concurrently (in presence of normal thyroid function).

CAUTION
 1. Never take the dry powder; always mix thoroughly with a suitable liquid
   before swallowing.
 2. Watch carefully for constipation; use stool softeners and laxatives as
   needed.
 3. This drug may bind other drugs taken concurrently and impair their absorption. It is advisable to take **all other drugs** 1 to 2 hours before or 4
   to 6 hours after taking this drug.

Precautions for Use
 By Infants and Children: Safety and effectiveness for those under 12 years of age
  not established. Watch carefully for the possible development of acidosis
  and vitamin A or folic acid deficiency. (Ask your physician for guidance.)
 By Those Over 60 Years of Age: Increased risk of severe constipation. Impaired
  kidney function may predispose to the development of acidosis.

▷ **Advisability of Use During Pregnancy**
 Pregnancy Category: C. See Pregnancy Risk Categories at the back of this book.
 Animal studies: No information available.
 Human studies: Adequate studies of pregnant women are not available.
 Use this drug only if clearly needed. Ensure adequate intake of vitamins and
  minerals to satisfy needs of mother and fetus.

Advisability of Use If Breast-Feeding
 Presence of this drug in breast milk: None.
 Breast-feeding is permitted.

Habit-Forming Potential: None.

Effects of Overdose: Progressive constipation, skin changes (skin drying).

Possible Effects of Long-Term Use: Deficiencies of vitamins A, D, E, and K and
  folic acid. Calcium deficiency, osteoporosis. Acidosis due to excessive re-

tention of chloride. Binding of the B-12 intrinsic factor complex may lead to blood cell problems.

Suggested Periodic Examinations While Taking This Drug (at physician's discretion)

Measurements of blood levels of total cholesterol, low-density (LDL) cholesterol, and high-density (HDL) cholesterol. Hemoglobin and red blood cell studies for possible anemia. Thyroid function tests.

▷ **While Taking This Drug, Observe the Following**

Foods: Avoid foods that tend to constipate (cheeses, etc.).

Nutritional Support: Ask your doctor if you need supplements of vitamins A, D, E, and K, folic acid, and calcium.

Beverages: Ensure adequate liquid intake (up to 2 quarts daily). This drug may be taken with milk.

▷ *Alcohol:* No interactions expected.

Tobacco Smoking: No interactions expected. I advise everyone to quit smoking.

▷ *Other Drugs*

Colestipol may *decrease* the effects of

- acetaminophen (Tylenol); take 2 hours before colestipol.
- aspirin; take 2 hours before colestipol.
- digitoxin and digoxin (Lanoxin); take 2 hours before colestipol.
- folic acid; take 2 hours before colestipol.
- furosemide (Lasix); take 4 hours before colestipol.
- hydrocortisone; take 2 hours before colestipol.
- iron preparations; take 2 to 3 hours before colestipol.
- penicillin G; take 2 hours before colestipol.
- phenobarbital; take 2 hours before colestipol.
- pravastatin (Pravachol); take 2 hours before colestipol.
- tetracycline (Achromycin); take 2 hours before colestipol.
- thiazide diuretics (see Drug Classes); take 2 hours before colestipol.
- thyroxine (see *thyroid hormones* in Drug Classes); take 5 hours before colestipol.
- vitamin B_{12}.

▷ *Driving, Hazardous Activities:* No restrictions.

Aviation Note: The use of this drug *is usually not a disqualification* for piloting. Consult a designated aviation medical examiner.

Exposure to Sun: No restrictions.

Discontinuation: The dose of any toxic drug combined with colestipol must be reduced when this drug is stopped. Once colestipol is stopped, cholesterol levels usually return to pretreatment levels in 1 month.

CROMOLYN (KROH moh lin)

Other Names: Cromolyn sodium, sodium cromoglycate

Introduced: 1968   **Class:** Antiasthmatic drug, preventive   **Prescription:** USA: Yes   **Controlled Drug:** USA: No; Canada: No   **Available as Generic:** USA: No; Canada: No

Brand Names: Crolom, Gastrocrom, Intal, ✦Intal Spincaps, ✦Intal Syncroner, ✦Nalcrom, Nasalcrom, ✦Nove-cromolyn, Opticrom, , ✦Rynacrom

Author's note: Cromolyn sodium (4%) as Nasalcrom is available without a prescription.

BENEFITS versus RISKS

Possible Benefits	*Possible Risks*
LONG-TERM PREVENTION OF RECURRENT ASTHMA ATTACKS	Anaphylactic reaction (see Glossary)
Prevention of acute asthma due to allergens or exercise	Spasm of bronchial tubes, increased wheezing
Prevention and treatment of allergic rhinitis	Allergic pneumonitis (allergic reaction in lung tissue)
Prevention of bronchospasm	
RELIEF OF ALLERGIC CONJUNCTIVITIS	
Treatment of giant papillary conjunctivitis	

▷ **Principal Uses**

As a Single Drug Product: Uses currently included in FDA-approved labeling: (1) Prevents allergic reactions in the nose (allergic rhinitis, hay fever) and the bronchial tubes (bronchial asthma); (2) used to treat conjunctivitis (allergic); (3) helps prevent exercise- or environmentally-induced asthma; (4) treats mastocytosis and manages several allergy-related skin disorders.

Other (unlabeled) generally accepted uses: (1) Can be used to help stop cough from ACE inhibitors (see Drug Classes) ;(2) helps modify the reactions in food allergies; (3) may have a small part in therapy of Bell's palsy.

How This Drug Works: Blocks the release of histamine (and other chemicals) that worsen allergic reactions. Prevents sequence of events leading to swelling, itching, and constriction of bronchial tubes (asthma).

Available Dosage Forms and Strengths

Capsules, oral — 20 mg, 100 mg

Eyedrops — 2% and 4%

Inhalation aerosol — 0.8 mg per metered spray

Inhalation capsules (powder) — 20 mg

Inhalation solution — 20 mg per ampule

Nasal insufflation (powder) — 10 mg per cartridge

Nasal solution — 40 mg/ml

▷ **Usual Adult Dosage Range**

Eyedrops: one to two drops four to six times daily at regular intervals.

Inhalation aerosol: 1.6 mg (two inhalations) four times daily at regular intervals for prevention of asthma, or a single dose 10 to 15 minutes before exposure to prevent allergen-induced or exercise-induced asthma.

Inhalation powder: 20 mg (one capsule) four times daily at regular intervals for long-term prevention of asthma; 20 mg (one capsule) as a single dose 10 to 15 minutes before exposure to prevent acute allergen-induced or exercise-induced asthma. Total daily maximum dosage is 160 mg (eight capsules).

Inhalation solution: Same as inhalation powder.

Nasal insufflation: Initially 10 mg in each nostril every 4 to 6 hours as needed; reduce to every 8 to 12 hours for maintenance.

Nasal solution: 2.6 mg to 5.2 mg in each nostril three to six times daily as needed.

Oral powder: ALL of the contents of capsules for oral use are poured into 1/2 glass of hot water. This is stirred, and one half glass of cold water is added while mixing. Drink all the liquid and add more water to be sure you drink any leftover medicine. Mix cromolyn with water only, not with fruit juice, milk, or foods. **Note: Actual dose and schedule must be determined for each patient individually.**

Conditions Requiring Dosing Adjustments

Liver Function: If the bile duct is damaged by liver disease, the dose must be decreased.

Kidney Function: The dose should be decreased in kidney failure.

▷ **Dosing Instructions:**   Follow instructions provided with all of the dosage forms, especially inhalers. Do not swallow capsules intended for inhalation. (If the capsule is accidentally swallowed, drug will cause no beneficial or adverse effects.) Capsules for mouth (oral) use can be poured into 4 ounces (one half glass) of hot water as above.

Usual Duration of Use: Regular use for 6 weeks or more is often needed for benefits in preventing asthma attacks or allergic rhinitis. Long-term use (months to years) requires periodic evaluation.

Possible Advantages of This Drug

May be quite effective in the young asthmatic.

Usually well tolerated. Serious adverse effects are very rare.

▷ **This Drug Should Not Be Taken If**

• you have had an allergic reaction to any dosage form of it previously.

▷ **Inform Your Physician Before Taking This Drug If**

• you are allergic to milk, milk products, or lactose. (The inhalation powder contains lactose.)
• you have impaired liver or kidney function.
• you have soft contact lenses (these should not be worn while using the eyedrops).
• you have angina or a heart rhythm disorder. (The inhalation aerosol contains propellants that could be hazardous.)

Possible Side Effects (natural, expected, and unavoidable drug actions)

Unpleasant taste with use of inhalation aerosol.

Mild throat irritation, hoarseness, cough (minimized by a few swallows of water after each powder inhalation).

▷ **Possible Adverse Effects** (unusual, unexpected, and infrequent reactions)

If any of the following develop, consult your physician promptly for guidance.

Mild Adverse Effects

Allergic reactions: skin rash, hives, itching—possible.

Headache, dizziness, drowsiness—rare.

Nausea, vomiting, urinary urgency and pain (dysuria), joint pain—infrequent.

Muscle pain (myositis)—rare.

Stinging or burning of the eyes with ophthalmic use—possible.

Cough and bronchial irritation—rare.

Nosebleed or itching with nasal solution use—rare.

Serious Adverse Effects

Allergic reactions: rare anaphylactic reactions (see Glossary). Allergic pneumonitis (allergic reaction in lung tissue)—case reports.

Propellants in the metered dose inhaler may cause problems in patients with disease of the heart arteries or a history of abnormal heart rhythms—possible.

Inflammation of the arteries—case reports.

▷ **Possible Effects on Sexual Function:**   None reported.

Possible Effects on Laboratory Tests

None reported.

CAUTION

1. This drug only helps **prevent** bronchial asthma—used **before** the start of acute bronchial constriction (asthmatic wheezing).
2. ***Do not*** use during an acute asthma attack—may worsen and prolong asthmatic wheezing.
3. This drug does ***not*** block the benefits of drugs that relieve acute asthma attacks after they start. Cromolyn is used ***before and between*** acute attacks to help keep them from starting; bronchodilators are used ***during*** acute attacks.
4. If you are using a bronchodilator drug by inhalation, it is best to take it about 5 minutes before inhaling cromolyn.
5. If this drug has allowed you to decrease or eliminate steroids, and you are unable to tolerate it, ask your doctor about the need to start steroids once again.

Precautions for Use

By Infants and Children: Safety and effectiveness for those under 5 years of age not established for the metered dose inhaler. Inhalation capsules: For children 2 years and older—20 mg (contents of one capsule) inhaled four times a day. Young children may find a nebulized solution easier than the powder.

By Those Over 60 Years of Age: This drug does not work in the management of chronic bronchitis or emphysema.

▷ **Advisability of Use During Pregnancy**

Pregnancy Category: B. See Pregnancy Risk Categories at the back of this book.

Animal studies: Mouse, rat, and rabbit studies revealed no birth defects due to this drug.

Human studies: Adequate studies of pregnant women are not available.

Use this drug only if clearly needed.

Advisability of Use If Breast-Feeding

Presence of this drug in breast milk: Unknown.

Avoid drug or refrain from nursing.

Habit-Forming Potential: None.

Effects of Overdose: No significant effects reported.

Possible Effects of Long-Term Use: Allergic reaction of lung tissue (allergic pneumonitis)—very rare.

Suggested Periodic Examinations While Taking This Drug (at physician's discretion)

Sputum analysis and X ray if symptoms suggest allergic pneumonitis.

▷ **While Taking This Drug, Observe the Following**
Foods: Follow physician-prescribed diet. Avoid all foods to which you are allergic.
Beverages: Avoid all beverages to which you may be allergic.
▷ *Alcohol:* No interactions expected.
Tobacco Smoking: No interactions with the medicine, but smoking can irritate your airways. I advise everyone to quit smoking.
▷ *Other Drugs:* Cromolyn may allow reduced dosage of cortisonelike drugs in the management of chronic asthma. Ask your doctor about dosage adjustment.
▷ *Driving, Hazardous Activities:* This drug may cause dizziness. Restrict activities as necessary.
Aviation Note: The use of this drug ***may be a disqualification*** for piloting. Consult a designated aviation medical examiner.
Exposure to Sun: No restrictions.
Heavy Exercise or Exertion: This drug may prevent exercise-induced asthma if taken 10 to 15 minutes before exertion. It is most effective in young people.
Discontinuation: If cromolyn has made it possible to reduce or stop maintenance doses of cortisonelike drugs, and you find it necessary to discontinue cromolyn, watch closely for a sudden return of asthma. You may have to start a cortisonelike drug as well as other measures to control asthma.
Special Storage Instructions: Keep the powder cartridges in a dry, tightly closed container. Store in a cool place, but not in the refrigerator. Do not handle the cartridges or the inhaler when hands are wet.

CYCLOPHOSPHAMIDE (si kloh FOSS fa mide)

Introduced: 1959   **Class:** Anticancer, immunosuppressant   **Prescription:** USA: Yes   **Controlled Drug:** USA: No; Canada: No   **Available as Generic:** No

Brand Names: Cytoxan, Neosar, ✤Procytox

BENEFITS versus RISKS	
Possible Benefits	*Possible Risks*
CURE OR CONTROL OF CERTAIN TYPES OF CANCER	REDUCED WHITE BLOOD CELL COUNT
PREVENTION OF REJECTION IN ORGAN TRANSPLANTATION	SECONDARY INFECTION
	URINARY BLADDER BLEEDING
Possibly beneficial in rheumatoid arthritis or lupus erythematosus	HEART, LUNG, LIVER, OR KIDNEY DAMAGE
May help selected cases of childhood nephrotic syndrome	Loss of hair

▷ **Principal Uses**
As a Single Drug Product: Uses currently included in FDA-approved labeling: (1) Treats various cancers: malignant lymphomas, multiple myeloma, sarcomas, retinoblastomas, leukemias, as well as breast and ovarian cancers; (2) also used to prevent rejection in organ transplantation and in some autoimmune disorders; (3) treats some resistant forms of nephrotic syndrome. Other (unlabeled) generally accepted uses: (1) Used to prepare patients for au-

tologous bone marrow transplants; (2) part of several combination chemotherapy regimens; (3) helps overall survival in combination therapy of lung or fallopian tube cancers; (4) can be part of combination therapy for Ewing's sarcoma; (5) may be of help in patients with lupus erythematosus who have interstitial lung disease or nephritis; (6) secondary role in prostate cancer; (7) high-dose therapy of anemia (aplastic anemia); (8) helps in resistant rheumatoid arthritis.

How This Drug Works: Kills cancer cells during all phases of development. Suppresses primary growth and secondary spread (metastasis) of some types of cancer.

Available Dosage Forms and Strengths
Injection — vials of 100 mg, 200 mg, 500 mg, 1 g, and 2 g
Tablets — 25 mg, 50 mg

▷ **Usual Adult Dosage Range:**   Oral form: 60 to 120 mg per square meter of body surface area daily or 400 mg per square meter of body surface area on days 1 to 5, every 3 to 4 weeks. As therapy continues, the dose is adjusted according to how the tumor responds or unacceptable low white blood cell counts develop. Intravenous: 1000 to 1500 mg per square meter every 3 to 4 weeks, adjusted the same as the oral form. **Note: Actual dose and schedule must be determined for each patient individually.**

Conditions Requiring Dosing Adjustments
Liver Function: Dose changes are not required in liver compromise.
Kidney Function: In moderate to severe kidney problems, the dose is decreased by 25–50%.

▷ **Dosing Instructions:**   Tablets may be crushed, and are best taken on an empty stomach. If nausea or indigestion occurs, may be taken with or following food. Liquid intake should be no less than 3 quarts every 24 hours to reduce risk of bladder irritation.

Usual Duration of Use: Use on a regular schedule is required to achieve and maintain a significant cancer remission. Initial response often happens in one to three weeks. Duration depends on response of the cancer and patient tolerance of the drug.

▷ **This Drug Should Not Be Taken If**
• you have had an allergic reaction to it previously.
• you have an active infection of any kind.
• you have bloody urine for any reason.
• you have kidney (renal) failure with creatinine clearance less than 30 ml/min (talk with your doctor).
• you are pregnant.

▷ **Inform Your Physician Before Taking This Drug If**
• you have impaired liver or kidney function.
• you have a blood cell or bone marrow disorder.
• you have had previous chemotherapy or X-ray therapy for any type of cancer.
• you take, or have taken within the past year, any cortisonelike drug (adrenal corticosteroids).
• you have diabetes.
• you will have surgery with general anesthesia.

Possible Side Effects (natural, expected, and unavoidable drug actions)

Bone marrow depression (see Glossary)—low production of white blood cells and, to a lesser degree, red blood cells and blood platelets (see Glossary). Possible effects include fever, chills, sore throat, fatigue, weakness, abnormal bleeding or bruising.

Leukemia has been reported following cyclophosphamide therapy.

Impairment of natural resistance (immunity) to infection.

Weakening of the heart muscle (cardiomyopathy).

Excessive urination (SIADH).

Cystitis or hemorrhagic cystitis.

Up to ninefold increase in bladder cancer risk.

▷ **Possible Adverse Effects** (unusual, unexpected, and infrequent reactions)

If any of the following develop, consult your physician promptly for guidance.

Mild Adverse Effects

Allergic reaction: skin rash—rare.

Headache, dizziness, blurred vision—possible.

Loss of scalp hair (50% of users), darkening of skin and fingernails, transverse ridging of nails.

Nausea, vomiting (dose related)—frequent.

Ulceration of mouth, diarrhea (may be bloody)—possible.

Serious Adverse Effects

Idiosyncratic reaction: hemolytic anemia—case reports.

Liver damage with jaundice: yellow eyes and skin, dark-colored urine, light-colored stools—rare.

Kidney damage: impaired kidney function, reduced urine volume, bloody urine—case reports.

Severe inflammation of bladder: painful urination, bloody urine—infrequent to frequent.

Drug-induced damage of heart and lung (interstitial pneumonitis) tissue—case reports.

Pancreatitis—case reports.

▷ **Possible Effects on Sexual Function:** Suppression of ovarian function—irregular menstrual pattern or cessation of menstruation (18 to 57%, depending upon dose and duration of use).

Testicular suppression—reduced or no sperm production (100% of users).

Possible Delayed Adverse Effects

Development of other types of cancer (secondary malignancies). Development of severe cystitis with bleeding from the bladder wall. (May occur many months after the last dose.)

Possible Effects on Laboratory Tests

Complete blood cell counts: decreased red cells, hemoglobin, white cells, and platelets.

INR (prothrombin time): increased.

Liver function tests: increased liver enzymes (ALT/GPT, AST/GOT, and alkaline phosphatase), increased bilirubin.

CAUTION

1. This drug may interfere with the normal healing of wounds.
2. This drug can cause significant changes in genetic material in both men

and women (sperm and eggs or ova). Patients taking this drug **must** understand the potential for serious defects in children that are conceived during or following the course of medication.

3. This drug can suppress natural resistance (immunity) to infection, resulting in life-threatening illness.
4. Avoid live virus vaccines while taking this drug (talk with your doctor about this).

Precautions for Use

By Infants and Children: This drug should not be given if the child is dehydrated. Adequate fluid intake to ensure a copious urine volume for 4 hours following each dose is needed. Prevent exposure of child to anyone with active chicken pox or shingles. This drug may cause ovarian or testicular sterility.

By Those Over 60 Years of Age: Increased risk of serious bladder problems (chemical cystitis). Patients **MUST** drink large amounts of water in order to keep the bladder flushed. This may increase the risk of urinary retention in men with prostatism (see Glossary).

▷ **Advisability of Use During Pregnancy**

Pregnancy Category: D. See Pregnancy Risk Categories at the back of this book. Animal studies: Significant birth defects reported in mice, rat, and rabbit studies.

Human studies: Information from studies of pregnant women indicates that this drug can cause serious birth defects or fetal death.

Avoid completely during the first 3 months. Use of this drug during the last 6 months must be carefully individualized.

Advisability of Use If Breast-Feeding

Presence of this drug in breast milk: Yes.

Avoid drug or refrain from nursing.

Habit-Forming Potential: None.

Effects of Overdose: Nausea, vomiting, diarrhea, bloody urine, water retention, weight gain, severe bone marrow depression, severe infections.

Possible Effects of Long-Term Use: Development of fibrous tissue in lungs; secondary malignancies.

Suggested Periodic Examinations While Taking This Drug (at physician's discretion)

Complete blood cell counts, every 2 to 4 days during initial treatment; then every 3 to 4 weeks during maintenance treatment.

Liver and kidney function tests.

Thyroid function tests (if symptoms warrant).

▷ **While Taking This Drug, Observe the Following**

Foods: No restrictions.

Beverages: No restrictions. May be taken with milk.

▷ *Alcohol:* No interactions expected.

Tobacco Smoking: No interactions expected. I advise everyone to quit smoking.

▷ *Other Drugs*

Cyclophosphamide *taken concurrently* with

- allopurinol (Zyloprim) may increase the extent of bone marrow depression.
- amphotericin (Abelcet and others) may increase risk of kidney toxicity.
- chloramphenicol can decrease cyclophosphamide effectiveness.

- ciprofloxacin (Cipro) can result in lowered ciprofloxacin levels and the need for a larger than usual dose.
- digoxin may decrease digoxin absorption and impair digoxin's effectiveness.
- flu (influenza) vaccine, and perhaps other vaccines, may decrease the vaccine's ability to confer immunity.
- hydrochlorothiazide and other thiazide diuretics (see Drug Classes) may worsen the lowering of white blood cells (myelosuppression) caused by cyclophosphamide.
- indomethacin (Indocin) can cause fluid retention.
- live virus vaccines should be avoided.
- pentostatin may cause fatal heart damage.
- ritonavir (Norvir) may lead to cyclophosphamide toxicity.
- succinylcholine can result in succinylcholine toxicity.
- tamoxifen (Nolvadex) can increase blood clot risk.

▷ *Driving, Hazardous Activities:* Use caution if dizziness occurs.

Aviation Note: The use of this drug *may be a disqualification* for piloting. Consult a designated aviation medical examiner.

Exposure to Sun: No restrictions.

Occurrence of Unrelated Illness: Any signs of infection—fever, chills, sore throat, cough, or flu-like symptoms—must be promptly reported. This drug may have to be stopped until the infection is controlled. Consult your physician.

CYCLOSPORINE (SI kloh spor een)

Other Names: Ciclosporin, cyclosporin A

Introduced: 1983   **Class:** Immunosuppressant   **Prescription:** USA: Yes   **Controlled Drug:** USA: No; Canada: No   **Available as Generic:** USA: Yes, capsules; Canada: No

Brand Names: Neoral, , Sandimmune

BENEFITS versus RISKS	
Possible Benefits	*Possible Risks*
EFFECTIVE PREVENTION AND TREATMENT OF REJECTION IN ORGAN TRANSPLANTATION	MARKED KIDNEY TOXICITY DEVELOPMENT OF HYPERTENSION
Some use treating severe rheumatoid arthritis, psoriasis, and other inflammatory (autoimmune) conditions	HIGH BLOOD PRESSURE Liver toxicity Low white blood cell count Development of lymphoma Excessive hair growth

▷ **Principal Uses**

As a Single Drug Product: Uses included in FDA-approved labeling: (1) Helps prevent (in conjunction with cortisonelike drugs) organ rejection in kidney, liver, and heart transplantation; (2) helps treat rejection crisis; (3) the Neoral microemulsion form treats severe active rheumatoid arthritis; (4) treats refractory psoriasis.

Other (unlabeled) generally accepted uses: (1) Used in transplantation of the bone marrow; (2) used investigationally in a variety of diseases involving the immune system such as: Sjögren's, Crohn's, and Grave's diseases; psoriasis; myasthenia gravis; bullous pemphigoid; pulmonary fibrosis associated with rheumatoid arthritis; rheumatoid arthritis; Sweet's syndrome; insulin-dependent diabetes; lupus erythematosus; large granular lymphocytic leukemia; and some anemias; (3) treats severe, steroid-dependent asthma; (4) treats severe skin reactions (toxic epidermal necrolysis) to phenytoin (Dilantin).

How This Drug Works: By inhibiting some lymphocytes (white blood cells) and their growth factors, this drug suppresses the rejection of transplanted organs.

Available Dosage Forms and Strengths
  Capsules, soft gelatin — 25 mg, 100 mg
  Injection, intravenous — 50 mg/ml
  Oral solution (Note: The microemulsion, Neoral, is NOT the same as Sandimmune)   — 100 mg/ml

▷ **Usual Adult Dosage Range:**   Initially 5-6 mg per kg intravenously, taken 4 to 12 hours prior to transplantation surgery. 7-10 mg per hour is continued for an average of 26 hours. After 26 hours, blood levels are obtained, and dosing is adjusted to keep the cyclosporine levels between 350 to 450 ng/ml for a total of 7 days after the transplant. Lowest levels (trough) from day 7 after transplant onward can be expected to be 0.3 times the daily cyclosporine dose in milligrams.

   If a conversion is made from oral Sandimmune to Neoral, Neoral dose is usually started at the same daily dose as Sandimmune, given at the same time each day in two equally divided doses. Cyclosporine trough levels should be measured twice weekly in people who were taking more than 10 mg per kg of body mass per day of Sandimmune. **Note: Actual dose and schedule must be determined for each patient individually.**

Conditions Requiring Dosing Adjustments
  Liver Function: The dose must be adjusted (based on blood levels) in liver compromise. Much of the drug is eliminated in the bile.
  Kidney Function: This drug is capable of causing marked kidney toxicity. Caution is critical. Dosing usually does not change, but more frequent blood levels are indicated.
  Diabetes: People who are diabetic and subsequently have kidney or pancreatic transplants will need larger than usual doses.
  Hypercholesterolemia: If the blood cholesterol is 50% above normal, the dose must be decreased by 50% in order to avoid toxicity.
  Obesity: Dosing **must** be based on ideal body weight (a calculation that helps eliminate the weight that is fat).
  Cystic Fibrosis: It is very difficult to appropriately dose this medication in patients who have this disease. Some patients will require as much as two times the usual dose. The dose should be adjusted to drug levels.
  Multiple Organ Transplants: Patients with multiple transplants (such as pancreas and kidney) often need an increased dose of cyclosporine in order to achieve the desired effect. The dose should be determined based on blood levels.

▷ **Dosing Instructions:**   Preferably taken with or immediately following food to reduce stomach irritation. The capsule should be swallowed whole; do not open, crush, or chew. The oral solution should be mixed with milk, chocolate milk, or orange juice (at room temperature) in a glass or ceramic cup; do not use a wax-lined or plastic container. Stir well and drink immediately. It is advisable to take this drug at the same time each day to maintain steady blood levels.

Usual Duration of Use: Use on a regular schedule for several weeks is usually needed to prevent organ rejection or stop rejection already underway. Benefits in psoriasis or rheumatoid arthritis may take 4 to 8 weeks. Long-term use (months to years) requires follow-up by your doctor.

▷ **This Drug Should Not Be Taken If**
- you have had an allergic reaction to it previously.
- you are taking any immunosuppressant drug other than cortisonelike preparations.
- you have an active lymphoma of any type.
- you have an active, uncontrolled infection, especially chicken pox or shingles.

▷ **Inform Your Physician Before Taking This Drug If**
- you are pregnant or breast-feeding.
- you have a history of liver or kidney disease, or impaired liver or kidney function.
- you have a history of hypertension or gout.
- you have a chronic gastrointestinal disorder.
- you are taking a potassium supplement or drugs that can raise the blood level of potassium.
- you have a seizure disorder.
- you have a history of a blood cell disorder.
- you take other medicines toxic to the kidney.

Possible Side Effects (natural, expected, and unavoidable drug actions)
Predisposition to infections (such as pneumocystis).

▷ **Possible Adverse Effects** (unusual, unexpected, and infrequent reactions)
If any of the following develop, consult your physician promptly for guidance.
Mild Adverse Effects
Allergic reactions: skin rash, itching—case reports.
Excessive hair growth—frequent in transplant patients; acne—rare.
Headache, confusion—infrequent.
Tremors (dose dependent)—frequent.
Mouth sores—rare; gum overgrowth—frequent in some reports; nausea/vomiting, diarrhea—infrequent.
Changes in facial features (dysmorphosis)—possible with longer-term therapy.
Serious Adverse Effects
Allergic reactions: anaphylactic reaction (see Glossary) to intravenous solution—case reports.
Kidney injury (25% kidney transplant, 37% liver, and 38% heart)—frequent.
Hypertension, mild to severe (up to half)—frequent.
Seizures—rare to frequent (kidney—1.8%, bone marrow—5.5%, and up to 25% of liver transplant patients).

Cortical blindness—case reports.

Liver injury—infrequent.

Pancreatitis—rare.

Low white blood cell count (leukopenia)—infrequent.

Low blood platelets—rare.

High blood potassium levels, blood glucose, uric acid levels (and gout), increased blood cholesterol, or low blood magnesium—all possible.

Lymphoma, possibly drug induced—rare to infrequent.

Relapse of lupus erythematosus—case reports.

Increased risk of skin cancers (risk increased by sun or UV light exposure).

▷ **Possible Effects on Sexual Function:** Enlargement and tenderness of male breast (1 to 4%)—rare to infrequent.

Adverse Effects That May Mimic Natural Diseases or Disorders

Liver toxicity may suggest viral hepatitis.

Natural Diseases or Disorders That May Be Activated by This Drug

Latent infections, hypertension, gout.

Possible Effects on Laboratory Tests

Complete blood cell counts: decreased red cells, hemoglobin, and white cells.

Blood potassium level or uric acid level: increased.

Blood platelets, white cells, magnesium: decreased.

Liver function tests: increased liver enzymes (ALT/GPT, AST/GOT, and alkaline phosphatase), increased bilirubin.

Kidney function tests: blood creatinine and urea nitrogen levels (BUN) increased; urine casts present.

CAUTION
1. Report promptly any indications of infection of any kind.
2. Promptly report swollen glands, sores or lumps in the skin, abnormal bleeding or bruising.
3. Inform your physician promptly if you become pregnant.
4. Periodic laboratory tests are mandatory.
5. It is best to avoid immunizations and contact with people who have recently taken oral poliovirus vaccine.

Precautions for Use

By Infants and Children: This drug has been used successfully and safely in children of all ages. Dosing is made on the adult schedule in some cases, while others require increased dosing.

By Those Over 60 Years of Age: The dose must be adjusted to any decline in kidney function.

▷ **Advisability of Use During Pregnancy**

Pregnancy Category: C. See Pregnancy Risk Categories at the back of this book.

Animal studies: Rat and rabbit studies reveal that this drug is toxic to the embryo and fetus. No drug-induced birth defects were found.

Human studies: Adequate studies of pregnant women are not available.

Avoid this drug during entire pregnancy unless it is clearly needed.

Advisability of Use If Breast-Feeding

Presence of this drug in breast milk: Yes.

Avoid drug or refrain from nursing.

Habit-Forming Potential: None.

Effects of Overdose: Headache, pain, facial flushing, gum soreness and bleeding, high blood pressure, atrial fibrillation, respiratory distress, seizures, coma, hallucinations, neurotoxicity, electrolyte disturbances, liver toxicity.

Possible Effects of Long-Term Use: Irreversible kidney damage, severe hypertension, abnormal growth of gums.

Suggested Periodic Examinations While Taking This Drug (at physician's discretion)
    Cyclosporine blood levels. Complete blood counts. Liver and kidney function tests. Magnesium, potassium, and uric acid blood levels. Blood pressure checks.

▷ **While Taking This Drug, Observe the Following**
    Foods: Avoid excessive intake of high potassium foods (see Table 13, Section Six). Food may also increase the peak blood level of cyclosporine.
    Beverages: Grapefruit juice and other fruit juices increase blood levels. Milk may increase blood levels.
▷   *Alcohol:* Large amounts of alcohol may increase cyclosporine levels.
    Tobacco Smoking: This interaction has not been well studied. I advise everyone to quit smoking.
▷   *Other Drugs*
    Cyclosporine *taken concurrently* with
- ACE inhibitors (see Drug Classes) may increase the risk of kidney problems.
- aminoglycoside antibiotics (see Drug Classes) may increase kidney toxicity.
- amphotericin B (Abelcet, others) can cause serious kidney toxicity.
- aspirin substitutes (nonsteroidal anti-inflammatory drugs or NSAIDs) may increase kidney toxicity.
- azathioprine (Imuran) may increase immunosuppression.
- calcium channel blockers (see Drug Classes) may result in cyclosporine toxicity.
- ciprofloxacin (and other fluoroquinolones—see Drug Classes) may increase risk of kidney toxicity.
- cotrimoxazole (Bactrim, others) may result in decreased cyclosporine effectiveness as well as kidney toxicity.
- cyclophosphamide (Cytoxan) may increase immunosuppression.
- digoxin (Lanoxin) may result in serious digoxin toxicity.
- furosemide (Lasix) may result in increased risk of gout.
- ganciclovir (Cytovene) may result in increased kidney toxicity.
- histamine (H_2) blockers (see Drug Classes) and ketoconazole may result in decreased cyclosporine blood levels.
- imipenem/cilastatin (Primaxin) may result in neurotoxicity.
- lovastatin (Mevacor) and other HMG-CoA reductase inhibitors may increase risk of muscle toxicity (myopathy) or kidney failure.
- methylprednisolone (Medrol) may cause seizures.
- metronidazole (Flagyl) may result in increased cyclosporine levels and toxicity.
- nifedipine (Adalat) may worsen abnormal gum growth (gingival hyperplasia) and also cause nifedipine toxicity (low blood pressure and abnormal heartbeats).
- pravastatin (Pravachol) can cause myopathy.
- simvastatin (Zocor) may cause myopathy.

- sulfamethoxazole and/or trimethoprim (Septra) may increase kidney toxicity.
- tacrolimus (Prograf) can cause kidney toxicity.
- thiazide diuretics (see Drug Classes) may increase adverse effects on the blood (myelosuppression).
- vaccines may blunt the benefit of the vaccine.
- verapamil (Calan) may increase immunosuppression.

The following drugs may *increase* the effects of cyclosporine:
- acetazolamide.
- allopurinol (Zyloprim).
- amiodarone (Cordarone).
- ceftriaxone (Rocephin).
- clarithromycin (Biaxin).
- clotrimazole (Mycelex, Gyne-Lotrimin, others).
- colchicine (Colbenemid).
- danazol or other anabolic steroids.
- diltiazem (Cardizem).
- econazole (Spectazole).
- erythromycin (E.E.S., others).
- fluconazole (Diflucan).
- glipizide (Glucotrol) or glyburide (Diabeta).
- grepafloxacin (Raxar).
- itraconazole (Sporanox).
- ketoconazole (Nizoral).
- methotrexate (Rheumatrex).
- methyltestosterone.
- metoclopramide (Reglan).
- miconazole (Lotrimin, Micatin).
- oral contraceptives (birth control pills).
- ritonavir (Norvir).
- terconazole (Terazol).

The following drugs may *decrease* the effects of cyclosporine:
- carbamazepine (Tegretol).
- isoniazid (INH).
- nafcillin.
- octreotide (Sandostatin).
- phenobarbital.
- phenytoin (Dilantin).
- quinine.
- rifabutin (Mycobutin).
- rifampin (Rifadin).
- sulfadimidine, sulfadiazine, and/or trimethoprim.
- ticlopidine (Ticlid).
- warfarin (Coumadin).

▷ *Driving, Hazardous Activities:* This drug may cause confusion or seizures. Restrict activities as necessary.

Aviation Note: The use of this drug *may be a disqualification* for piloting. Consult a designated aviation medical examiner.

Exposure to Sun: Exposure to sunlight or other ultraviolet (UV) radiation may increase the risk of skin cancer.

Discontinuation: Do not stop this drug without your physician's guidance.

Special Storage Instructions: Keep the gelatin capsules in the blister packets until ready for use. Store below 77 degrees F (25 degrees C).

Keep the oral solution in a tightly closed container. Store below 86 degrees F (30 degrees C). Do not refrigerate.

Observe the Following Expiration Times: The oral solution must be used within 2 months after opening.

DESIPRAMINE (des IP ra meen)

Introduced: 1964   **Class:** Antidepressant   **Prescription:** USA: Yes
Controlled Drug: USA: No; Canada: No   **Available as Generic:** USA: Yes; Canada: Yes
Brand Names: Norpramin, Pertofrane

BENEFITS versus RISKS	
Possible Benefits	*Possible Risks*
EFFECTIVE RELIEF OF ENDOGENOUS DEPRESSION	ADVERSE BEHAVIORAL EFFECTS: confusion, disorientation, delusions, hallucinations
Possibly beneficial in other depressive disorders	CONVERSION OF DEPRESSION TO MANIA in manic-depressive (bipolar) disorders
	Aggravation of paranoia and schizophrenia
	Drug-induced heart rhythm disorders
	Abnormally low white blood cell and platelet counts

▷ **Principal Uses**

As a Single Drug Product: Uses currently included in FDA-approved labeling: Relieves severe depression (primary endogenous) and some secondary (exogenous) depression.

Other (unlabeled) generally accepted uses: (1) Chronic pain syndromes, including diabetic neuropathy; (2) treats attention deficit disorder (children over 6 and adolescents); (3) decreases symptoms of panic disorder; (4) treats resistant malaria; (5) may help reduce binge eating in bulimia.

How This Drug Works: Relieves depression by increasing brain levels of nerve impulse transmitters (serotonin and norepinephrine).

Available Dosage Forms and Strengths

Capsules — 25 mg, 50 mg

Tablets — 10 mg, 25 mg, 50 mg, 75 mg, 100 mg, 150 mg

▷ **Usual Adult Dosage Range:** Initially 25 mg two to four times daily. May be increased as needed and tolerated by 25 mg daily at intervals of 1 week. Usual ongoing dose is 100 mg to 200 mg daily. Maximum dose is 300 mg. (When determined, daily dose may be given at bedtime as a single dose.) **Note: Actual dose and schedule must be determined for each patient individually.**

Conditions Requiring Dosing Adjustments

Liver Function: The dose should be decreased in patients with compromised livers.

Kidney Function: Can cause urine retention—use with caution in kidney compromise with urine outflow problems.

▷ **Dosing Instructions:**   May be taken without regard to meals. The capsule may be opened and the tablet may be crushed.

Usual Duration of Use: Regular use for 3 to 4 weeks often needed to see start of effect in helping depression; peak response may require 3 months of use. Regular ongoing use is critical even if you feel better. Those people with delusions may require 7 weeks to benefit. Long-term use (months to years) requires periodic evaluation of response and dose adjustment.

▷ **This Drug Should Not Be Taken If**

• you have had an allergic reaction to it previously.
• you are taking, or have taken within the past 14 days, any monoamine oxidase (MAO) type A inhibitor drug (see Drug Classes).
• you have had a recent heart attack (myocardial infarction).
• you have narrow-angle glaucoma.

▷ **Inform Your Physician Before Taking This Drug If**

• you have had an adverse reaction to another antidepressant.
• you have any type of seizure disorder.
• you have increased internal eye pressure.
• you have any type of heart disease, especially a heart rhythm disorder.
• you have a thyroid disorder or take thyroid medication.
• you have thought about or attempted suicide.
• you have diabetes or sugar intolerance.
• you take levodopa (increased risk of heart rhythm problems with high desipramine doses).
• you have prostatism (see Glossary).
• you will have surgery with general anesthesia.

Possible Side Effects (natural, expected, and unavoidable drug actions)

Mild drowsiness, light-headedness (low blood pressure), blurred vision, dry mouth, constipation, impaired urination.

▷ **Possible Adverse Effects** (unusual, unexpected, and infrequent reactions)

If any of the following develop, consult your physician promptly for guidance.

Mild Adverse Effects

Allergic reactions: skin rash, hives, swelling of face or tongue, drug fever (see Glossary)—case reports.

Headache, dizziness, weakness, unsteadiness, tremors, fainting—infrequent.

Irritation of tongue or mouth, altered taste, difficulty talking—rare; indigestion, nausea—infrequent.

Fluctuations of blood sugar—possible.

Serious Adverse Effects

Allergic reactions: drug-induced hepatitis, with or without jaundice; anaphylactic reaction (see Glossary)—case reports.

Adverse behavioral effects: delusions, hallucinations—case reports.

Seizures; reduced control of epilepsy—case reports.

Aggravation of paranoid psychoses and schizophrenia—possible.

Heart rhythm disturbances, myocarditis—case reports.

Parkinson-like disorders, peripheral neuritis (see both terms in Glossary)—rare to infrequent.

Abnormally low white blood cell and platelet counts: fever, sore throat, infections, abnormal bleeding or bruising—case reports.

Neuroleptic malignant syndrome—case reports.

▷ **Possible Effects on Sexual Function:**   Decreased libido, increased libido (antidepressant effect), impotence, painful male orgasm, male breast enlargement (gynecomastia), female breast enlargement with milk production, swelling of testicles, decreased sperm viability—case reports.

Adverse Effects That May Mimic Natural Diseases or Disorders

Liver toxicity may suggest viral hepatitis.

Natural Diseases or Disorders That May Be Activated by This Drug

Latent diabetes, epilepsy, glaucoma, prostatism.

Possible Effects on Laboratory Tests

Complete blood cell counts: decreased red cells, hemoglobin, white cells, and platelets; increased eosinophils (allergic reaction).

Blood glucose levels: unexplained fluctuations.

Liver function tests: increased liver enzymes (ALT/GPT, AST/GOT, and alkaline phosphatase), increased bilirubin—all rare.

Thyroid function tests: decreased TSH and mean free thyroxin.

CAUTION

1. Should only be used when a true, primary, endogenous depression (not reactive) has been diagnosed.
2. Watch for toxicity: confusion, agitation, fast heart rate, heart irregularity. Blood levels will be needed.
3. It is advisable to withhold this drug if electroconvulsive therapy (ECT) is to be used to treat the depression.

Precautions for Use

By Infants and Children: Safety and effectiveness for those under 6 years of age not established. This drug is being used to treat children who have attention deficit disorder, with or without hyperactivity. Dose and management must be supervised by a properly trained pediatrician.

By Those Over 60 Years of Age: Start treatment with 25 mg one or two times daily to evaluate tolerance. During the first 2 weeks of treatment, watch for confusion, restlessness, agitation, forgetfulness, disorientation, delusions, or hallucinations. Also observe for unsteadiness and instability that may predispose to falling. This drug may aggravate prostatism.

▷ **Advisability of Use During Pregnancy**

Pregnancy Category: C. See Pregnancy Risk Categories at the back of this book.

Animal studies: Birth defects reported in rat and rabbit studies.

Human studies: Adequate studies of pregnant women are not available.

Use only if clearly needed. Avoid during the first 3 months if possible.

Advisability of Use If Breast-Feeding

Presence of this drug in breast milk: Yes, in small amounts.

Monitor nursing infant closely and discontinue drug or nursing if adverse effects develop.

Habit-Forming Potential: Psychological or physical dependence is rare and unexpected. Some patients may seek to abuse this medicine for its ability to create anticholinergic delirium.

Effects of Overdose: Confusion, hallucinations, drowsiness, tremors, heart irregularity, seizures, stupor, hypothermia (see Glossary).

Possible Effects of Long-Term Use: None reported.

Suggested Periodic Examinations While Taking This Drug (at physician's discretion)
> Complete blood cell counts, liver function tests.
> Serial blood pressure readings and electrocardiograms.

▷ **While Taking This Drug, Observe the Following**
> *Foods:* No specific restrictions. Limiting food intake may avoid excess weight gain.
> *Nutritional Support:* High doses of vitamin C may blunt the therapeutic effects of desipramine.
> *Beverages:* No restrictions. May be taken with milk.

▷   *Alcohol:* **Avoid completely.** This drug can markedly increase the intoxicating effects of alcohol; the combination can depress brain function.

> *Tobacco Smoking:* May accelerate the elimination of this drug and require increased doses. I advise everyone to quit smoking.
> *Marijuana Smoking:* Occasional (once or twice weekly): transient increase in drowsiness and mouth dryness as well as possible unacceptable increases in heart rate.
> Daily: persistent drowsiness and mouth dryness; possible reduced effectiveness of this drug.

▷   *Other Drugs*
> Desipramine may *increase* the effects of
> • all drugs with atropinelike effects (see **anticholinergic drugs** in Drug Classes).
> • all drugs with sedative effects; watch for excessive sedation.
> Desipramine may *decrease* the effects of
> • clonidine (Catapres).
> • guanethidine (Ismelin, Esimil).
> • guanfacine (Tenex).
> • levodopa, by decreasing absorption of the levodopa.
> Desipramine *taken concurrently* with
> • albuterol (Ventolin) may increase the effect of albuterol on the blood vessels.
> • anticonvulsants (carbamazepine–Tegretol or phenytoin–Dilantin are examples) requires careful monitoring for changes in seizure patterns (need to adjust anticonvulsant dose).
> • ethchlorvynol (Placidyl) may cause delirium; avoid concurrent use.
> • large doses (greater than 2 g/day) of vitamin C may lead to increased removal of desipramine and need to adjust dose.
> • monoamine oxidase (MAO) type A inhibitor drugs (see Drug Classes) may cause high fever, seizures, and high blood pressure; avoid combining. Wait 14 days between administration of either.
> • quinidine may cause desipramine toxicity.
> • stimulant drugs (amphetamine, cocaine, epinephrine, phenylpropanolamine, etc.) may cause severe high blood pressure and/or high fever.

- thyroid preparations may increase the risk of heart rhythm disorders.
- tramadol (Ultram) may increase seizure risk.
- warfarin may cause an increased risk of bleeding. Increased testing of INR is indicated.

The following drugs may *increase* the effects of desipramine:
- cimetidine (Tagamet).
- fluoxetine (Prozac).
- fluvoxamine (Luvox).
- methylphenidate (Ritalin).
- nefazodone (Serzone).
- phenothiazines (see Drug Classes).
- ritonavir (Norvir) and perhaps other protease inhibitors (see Drug Classes).

The following drugs may *decrease* the effects of desipramine:
- barbiturates (see Drug Classes).
- chloral hydrate (Noctec, Somnos, etc.).
- clonazepam (Klonopin).
- estrogen (see profile for brand names).
- lithium (Lithobid, Lithotab, etc.).
- oral contraceptives (birth control pills; see profile for brand names).
- reserpine (Serpasil, Ser-Ap-Es, etc.).

▷ *Driving, Hazardous Activities:* This drug may impair mental alertness, judgment, physical coordination, and reaction time. Restrict activities as necessary.

Aviation Note: The use of this drug *is a disqualification* for piloting. Consult a designated aviation medical examiner.

Exposure to Sun: Use caution. This drug may cause photosensitivity (see Glossary) and changes in iris and skin pigment color with sun exposure.

Exposure to Heat: Use caution. This drug can inhibit sweating and impair adaptation to hot environments, increasing the risk of heatstroke. Avoid saunas.

Exposure to Cold: The elderly should use caution and avoid conditions conducive to hypothermia (see Glossary).

Exposure to Environmental Chemicals: This drug may mask the symptoms of poisoning due to handling certain insecticides (organophosphorous types). Read labels carefully.

Discontinuation: Best to stop this drug gradually. Abrupt withdrawal after prolonged use may cause headache, malaise, and nausea. If this drug is stopped, doses of other drugs may be need adjustment.

DEXAMETHASONE (dex a METH a sohn)

Introduced: 1958   **Class:** Cortisonelike drugs   **Prescription:** USA: Yes
Controlled Drug: USA: No; Canada: No   **Available as Generic:** USA: Yes; Canada: Yes

Brand Names: Acroseb-Dex, ✤Ak-Dex, Ak-Trol [CD], Baldex, Dalalone, Dalalone DP, Dalalone LA, Decaderm, Decadron, Decadron Nasal Spray, Decadron-LA, Decadron Phosphate Ophthalmic, Decadron Phosphate Respihaler, Decadron Phosphate Turbinaire, Decadron w/Xylocaine [CD], Decaject, Decaject LA, Decaspray, Deenar [CD], ✤Deronil, Dex-4, Dexacen-4, Dexacen LA-8, Dexacidin[CD], Dexacort, Dexameth, Dexasone, Dexasone-LA, Dexo-

LA, Dexon, Dexone, Dexone-E, Dexone-LA, Hexadrol, Maxidex, Mymethasone, ✤Neodecadron Eye-Ear, Neodexair, Neomycin-Dex, Ocu-Trol [CD], ✤Oradexon, ✤PMS-Dexamethasone, ✤SK-Dexamethasone, ✤Sofracort, Solurex, Solurex-LA, ✤Spersadex, Tobradex, , Turbinaire

---

BENEFITS versus RISKS

Possible Benefits	*Possible Risks*
EFFECTIVE RELIEF OF SYMPTOMS IN A WIDE VARIETY OF INFLAMMATORY AND ALLERGIC DISORDERS EFFECTIVE IMMUNOSUPPRESSION in selected benign and malignant disorders	Long-term systemic use (exceeding 2 weeks) is associated with many possible adverse effects: ALTERED MOOD AND PERSONALITY, CATARACTS, GLAUCOMA, HYPERTENSION, ARRHYTHMIAS, PEPTIC ULCERS, PANCREATITIS, OSTEOPOROSIS, ASEPTIC BONE NECROSIS, INCREASED SUSCEPTIBILITY TO INFECTIONS

▷ **Principal Uses**

As a Single Drug Product: Uses currently included in FDA-approved labeling: (1) Used to manage serious skin disorders, asthma, allergic rhinitis, lymphoma, brain edema, shock, systemic lupus erythematosus, and all types of major rheumatic disorders including bursitis, systemic lupus erythematosus, tendonitis, and most forms of arthritis; (2) ulcerative disease of the colon; (3) topical cream is used to treat eczema, psoriasis, dermatitis, and lichen planus; (4) used in conjunction with antibiotics in meningitis; (5) helps ease swelling in otitis media.

Other (unlabeled) generally accepted uses: (1) Adrenal insufficiency; (2) acute airway obstruction; (3) mountain sickness; (4) vomiting caused by chemotherapy; (5) cardiopulmonary bypass; (6) refractory depression; (7) relief of brain cancer symptoms; (8) combination with other drugs in multiple myeloma; (9)cases of *Pneumocystis carinii* pneumonia; (10) can help suppress male hormones (androgens) in women with acne, hirsutism, or hair loss (androgenic alopecia) caused by androgens; (11) eases vomiting after cancer treatment (chemotherapy).

How This Drug Works: Inhibits defensive functions of certain white blood cells. It reduces the production of lymphocytes and some antibodies and acts as an immunosuppressant.

Available Dosage Forms and Strengths

Aerosol — 0.01% and 0.04%
Aerosol inhaler — 84 mcg per spray
Cream — 0.1%
Elixir — 0.5 mg/5 ml
Eye ointment — 0.05%
Eye solution — 0.1%
Gel — 0.1%
Injection — 4 mg/ml, 8 mg/ml, 10 mg/ml, 16 mg/ml, 20 mg/ml, 24 mg/ml
Oral solution — 0.5 mg/0.5 ml, 0.5 mg/5 ml

Solution — 0.1%
Spray, topical — 10 mg/25 g
Suspension — 0.1%
Tablets — 0.25 mg, 0.5 mg, 0.75 mg, 1 mg, 1.5 mg, 2 mg, 4 mg, 6 mg

▷ **Usual Adult Dosage Range:**   Turbinaire form: Two sprays in each nostril 2 or 3 times daily. Twelve sprays is the daily maximum. Oral: 0.75 to 9 mg daily divided into two to four doses.

Topical (0.1% cream): Apply thin film of medicine on the affected area three or four times a day.

Oral dose for children: 0.03 to 0.15 mg per kg of body mass per day, divided into equal doses given every 6 to 12 hours. Or 1–5 mg per square meter divided into equal doses and given every 6 to 12 hours. **Note: Actual dose and schedule must be determined for each patient individually.**

Conditions Requiring Dosing Adjustments

Liver Function: This drug is eliminated via the liver; however, no specific guidelines for dosing adjustments are available.

Kidney Function: Use with caution as it can cause alkalosis (a change toward a more basic condition in the body's chemistry).

Obesity: Dosing on a mg-per-kg-of-body-mass-per-day basis is recommended. It is best to measure free urinary cortisol as well.

▷ **Dosing Instructions:**   Tablet may be crushed and taken with or following food to prevent stomach irritation, preferably in the morning.

Usual Duration of Use: For acute disorders: 4 to 10 days. For chronic disorders: varies. Length of therapy should not exceed time needed for adequate symptomatic relief in acute self-limiting conditions, or time required to stabilize a chronic condition and permit gradual withdrawal. Because of its long duration of action, drug is not appropriate for alternate-day administration.

▷ **This Drug Should Not Be Taken If**
- you have had an allergic reaction to it previously.
- you have active peptic ulcer disease.
- you have an active herpes simplex infection of the eye.
- you have a systemic fungal infection (talk with your doctor).
- your sputum consistently grows *Candida albicans* (a yeast that may grow very quickly if steroids suppress your immune system).
- you have a psychoneurosis or psychosis.
- you have active tuberculosis.

▷ **Inform Your Physician Before Taking This Drug If**
- you have had unfavorable reactions to cortisonelike drugs.
- you have a history of peptic ulcer disease, thrombophlebitis, or tuberculosis.
- you have diabetes, glaucoma, high blood pressure, deficient thyroid function, or myasthenia gravis.
- you start to have restricted motion, increased pain, fever, or joint swelling; these may be early signs of a septic arthritis.
- you have osteoporosis.
- you plan to have surgery of any kind in the near future.

Possible Side Effects (natural, expected, and unavoidable drug actions)

Increased appetite, weight gain, retention of salt and water, excretion of potassium, increased susceptibility to infection (yeast infections can be frequent in cancer patients treated with a corticosteroid). Increased facial hair.

Increased white blood cell count (release from the bone marrow versus a sign of infection).

▷ **Possible Adverse Effects** (unusual, unexpected, and infrequent reactions)

If any of the following develop, consult your physician promptly for guidance.

Mild Adverse Effects

Allergic Reaction: Skin rash—case reports

Headache, dizziness, insomnia—possible.

Mild euphoria or depression—most common possible central nervous system (CNS) effects.

High blood pressure (more likely in older patients and those who already have high blood pressure; may be lessened by alternate-day therapy)—possible.

Acid indigestion, abdominal distention—possible.

Muscle cramping and weakness—case reports.

Easy bruising (ecchymosis) or acnelike lesions—case reports.

Vaginal itching—may be frequent with intravenous dosing.

Serious Adverse Effects

Allergic Reaction: Anaphylaxis—case reports.

Mental and emotional disturbances of serious magnitude—infrequent.

Reactivation of latent tuberculosis—possible. *Pneumocystis carinii* pneumonia—possible with immunosuppression and chronic use.

Development of peptic ulcer—rare, but risk increases with higher doses and preexisting ulcers.

Inflammation of the pancreas—rare.

Thrombophlebitis (inflammation of a vein with the formation of blood clot): pain or tenderness in thigh or leg, or swelling of the foot, ankle, or leg—possible with intravenous use.

Abnormal lipids (cholesterol, triglycerides, LDLs)—possible.

Abnormal heart rhythm—case reports.

Cushing's syndrome—possible with chronic use and high doses (supraphysiologic).

Suppression of the adrenal gland—possible with chronic use and more common with larger doses.

High blood sugar—risk increases with use in diabetics and with higher doses.

Excessively low blood potassium—case reports.

Abnormally slow heartbeat in infants—case reports.

Increased pressure in the eye or cataracts or glaucoma—rare to frequent.

Precipitation of porphyria—case reports.

Excessive thyroid function (questionable causality)—case reports.

Muscle changes (myopathy)—infrequent, but more likely with higher doses and some steroids.

Bone death (aseptic necrosis or avascular necrosis)—infrequent, but more likely with high initial doses.

Osteoporosis—more likely with long-term and higher-dose use.

▷ **Possible Effects on Sexual Function:**   Altered timing and pattern of menstruation—case reports.

Adverse Effects That May Mimic Natural Diseases or Disorders
Pattern of symptoms and signs resembling Cushing's syndrome.

Natural Diseases or Disorders That May Be Activated by This Drug
Latent diabetes, glaucoma, peptic ulcer disease, tuberculosis.

Possible Effects on Laboratory Tests
Blood amylase level: increased (possible pancreatitis).
Blood glucose level: increased.
Digoxin testing: may falsely increase digoxin results.
Glucose tolerance test (GTT): increased.
Blood potassium level: decreased.
Thyroid function tests: decreased.
Cholesterol: increased in some studies while decreased in others.

CAUTION
1. It is best to carry a card noting that you are taking this drug, if your course of treatment is to exceed 1 week.
2. Do not stop this drug abruptly if it is used for long-term treatment.
3. If vaccination against measles, rabies, smallpox, or yellow fever is required, stop this drug 72 hours before vaccination and do not resume it for at least 14 days after vaccination.
4. Children may be more sensitive to topical application since there is a larger skin surface area to body weight (ratio).

Precautions for Use
By Infants and Children: Avoid prolonged use if possible. During long-term use, watch for suppression of normal growth and the possibility of increased intracranial pressure. Following long-term use, the child may be at risk for adrenal gland deficiency during stress for as long as 18 months after cessation.
By Those Over 60 Years of Age: Avoid prolonged use of this drug. Continual use (even in small doses) can increase the severity of diabetes, enhance fluid retention, raise blood pressure, weaken resistance to infection, induce stomach ulcer, and accelerate the development of cataracts and osteoporosis.

▷ **Advisability of Use During Pregnancy**
Pregnancy Category: C. See Pregnancy Risk Categories at the back of this book.
Animal studies: Birth defects reported in mice, rats, and rabbits.
Human studies: Adequate studies of pregnant women are not available.
Avoid completely during the first 3 months. Limit use during the last 6 months as much as possible. If used, examine infant for possible deficiency of adrenal gland function.

Advisability of Use If Breast-Feeding
Presence of this drug in breast milk: Yes.
Avoid drug or refrain from nursing.

Habit-Forming Potential: Use to suppress symptoms over an extended period of time may produce a state of functional dependence (see Glossary). In treating asthma and rheumatoid arthritis, it is best to keep the dose as small as possible and to attempt drug withdrawal after periods of reasonable improvement. Such procedures may reduce the degree of "steroid rebound"—the return of symptoms as the drug is withdrawn.

Effects of Overdose: Fatigue, muscle weakness, stomach irritation, acid indigestion, excessive sweating, facial flushing, fluid retention, swelling of extremities, increased blood pressure.

Possible Effects of Long-Term Use: Increased blood sugar (possible diabetes), increased fat deposits on the trunk of the body ("buffalo hump"), rounding of the face ("moon face"), thinning and fragility of skin, loss of texture and strength of bones (osteoporosis, aseptic necrosis), cataracts, glaucoma, increased body hair (Hirsutism) retarded growth and development in children.

Suggested Periodic Examinations While Taking This Drug (at physician's discretion)

Measurements of blood pressure, blood sugar, and potassium levels.

Complete eye examinations at regular intervals. Chest X ray if history of tuberculosis.

Determination of the rate of development of the growing child to detect retardation of normal growth.

Bone mineral density testing to assess risk of osteoporosis.

▷ **While Taking This Drug, Observe the Following**

Foods: No interactions expected. Ask your physician about salt restriction or need for potassium-rich foods. During long-term use of this drug, it is advisable to eat a high protein diet.

Nutritional Support: During long-term use, take a vitamin D supplement and increase calcium. During wound repair, take a zinc supplement.

Beverages: No restrictions. Drink all forms of milk liberally.

▷ *Alcohol:* No interactions expected. Caution if you are prone to peptic ulcer disease.

Tobacco Smoking: Nicotine increases the blood levels of naturally produced cortisone and related hormones. Heavy smoking may add to the expected actions of this drug and requires close observation for excessive effects. I advise everyone to quit smoking.

Marijuana Smoking: May cause additional impairment of immunity, and also is a risk factor for toxoplasmosis.

▷ *Other Drugs*

Dexamethasone may *decrease* the effects of
- isoniazid (INH, Niconyl, etc.).
- salicylates (aspirin, sodium salicylate, etc.).
- vaccines (such as flu vaccine), by blunting the immune response to them.

Dexamethasone *taken concurrently* with
- birth control pills (oral contraceptives) may increase dexamethasone's therapeutic effects.
- carbamazepine (Tegretol) will reduce the effectiveness of dexamethasone.
- loop diuretics such as furosemide (Lasix) or bumetanide (Bumex) can result in additive potassium loss.
- oral anticoagulants may either increase or decrease their effectiveness; ask your doctor about prothrombin time testing and dose adjustment.
- oral antidiabetic drugs (see Drug Classes) will decrease their effectiveness.
- ritonavir (Norvir), saquinavir (Fortovase), and possibly other protease in-

hibitors (PI)(see Drug Classes), may decrease PI blood levels and increase dexamethasone blood levels.
- thiazide diuretics (see Drug Classes) will decrease their blood-pressure-lowering ability.

The following drugs may **decrease** the effects of dexamethasone:
- antacids—may reduce its absorption.
- barbiturates (Amytal, Butisol, phenobarbital, etc.).
- phenobarbital.
- phenytoin (Dilantin, etc.).
- primidone (Mysoline).
- rifabutin (Mycobutin).
- rifampin (Rifadin, Rimactane, etc.).

▷ *Driving, Hazardous Activities:* Usually no restrictions. Be alert to the rare occurrence of dizziness.

Aviation Note: The use of this drug **may be a disqualification** for piloting. Consult a designated aviation medical examiner.

Exposure to Sun: No restrictions.

Occurrence of Unrelated Illness: This drug may decrease natural resistance to infection. Call your doctor if you develop an infection of any kind. It may also reduce your body's ability to respond to the stress of acute illness, injury, or surgery. Keep your physician fully informed of any significant health changes.

Discontinuation: Do not stop this drug abruptly after chronic use. Ask your doctor for help about gradual withdrawal. For up to 2 years after stopping this drug, you may require it again if you have an injury, surgery or an illness.

DIAZEPAM (di AZ e pam)

Introduced: 1963   **Class:** Antianxiety drug (mild tranquilizer), benzodiazepines   **Prescription:** USA: Yes   **Controlled Drug:** USA: C-IV*; Canada: No   **Available as Generic:** Yes

Brand Names: ✤Apo-Diazepam, Diastat, ✤Diazemuls, Diazepam Intensol Oral Solution, ✤Meval, ✤Novodipam, ✤Rival, Valcaps, Valium, Valrelease, Vazepam, ✤Vivol, Zetran

BENEFITS versus RISKS	
Possible Benefits	*Possible Risks*
RELIEF OF ANXIETY AND NERVOUS TENSION	Habit-forming potential with prolonged use
Wide margin of safety with therapeutic doses	Minor impairment of mental functions
	Respiratory depression
	Jaundice—very rare

▷ **Principal Uses**

As a Single Drug Product: Uses included in FDA-approved labeling: (1) Provides short-term relief of mild to moderate anxiety; (2) relieves the symptoms of

*See Controlled Drug Schedules at the back of this book.

acute alcohol withdrawal (agitation, tremors, hallucinations, incipient delirium tremens); (3) eases skeletal muscle spasm; (4) provides short-term control of certain types of seizures (epilepsy, fever induced, and status epilepticus); (5) short-term relief of insomnia; (6) adjunctive use in endoscopic procedures; (7) decreases anxiety prior to electrical defibrillation of the heart (cardioversion); (8) eases severe muscle spasms.

Other (unlabeled) generally accepted uses: (1) Helps prevent LSD flashbacks; (2) short-term treatment of sleepwalking; (3) treatment of persistent hiccups; (4) adjunctive treatment of catatonia.

How This Drug Works: This drug calms higher brain centers by enhancing a nerve transmitter (gamma-aminobutyric acid, or GABA).

Available Dosage Forms and Strengths
Capsules, prolonged action (sustained release) — 15 mg
Concentrate — 5 mg/ml
Injection — 5 mg/ml
Oral solution — 5 mg/ml, 5 mg/5 ml
Tablets — 2 mg, 5 mg, 10 mg

▷ **Usual Adult Dosage Range:**   For anxiety: 2 to 10 mg, two to four times daily. Dose may be increased cautiously as needed and tolerated. After 1 week of continual use, the total daily dose may be taken at bedtime. Maximum daily dose is 60 mg. Sustained-release form can be given once daily if the total daily dose is 15 mg given as 5 mg three times daily. **Note: Actual dose and schedule must be determined for each patient individually.**

Conditions Requiring Dosing Adjustments
Liver Function: The dose **must** be decreased by 50% in patients with liver compromise.
Kidney Function: Caution—if 15 mg or more is given daily, diazepam metabolites may accumulate.
Obesity: Obese patients may take longer than nonobese patients to accumulate this medicine. The time that it takes to remove diazepam (elimination half-life) is prolonged in obese people. This means that obese people may take a much longer time to get the peak effect of diazepam and will also take a longer time to remove the drug from their bodies.

▷ **Dosing Instructions:**   The tablet may be crushed and taken on empty stomach or with food or milk. The prolonged-action capsule should not be opened. Do not stop this drug abruptly if taken for more than 4 weeks.

Usual Duration of Use: Regular use for 3 to 5 days is usually needed to see benefits in relieving moderate anxiety. Limit continual use to 1 to 3 weeks. Avoid uninterrupted and prolonged use.
Author's note: The National Institute of Mental Health has a new information page on anxiety. It can be found on the World Wide Web at www.nimh.nih.gov/anxiety

▷ **This Drug Should Not Be Taken If**
• you have had an allergic reaction to any dosage form of it previously.
• you have acute narrow-angle glaucoma.
• it is prescribed for a child under 6 months of age.

▷ **Inform Your Physician Before Taking This Drug If**
  • you are allergic to any benzodiazepine (see Drug Classes).
  • you have a history of alcoholism or drug abuse.
  • you are pregnant or planning pregnancy.
  • you have impaired liver or kidney function.
  • you have a history of serious depression or a mental disorder.
  • you have asthma, emphysema, epilepsy, or myasthenia gravis.

Possible Side Effects (natural, expected, and unavoidable drug actions)
  Drowsiness—frequent; lethargy, unsteadiness—rare; "hangover" effects on the
  day following bedtime use.

▷ **Possible Adverse Effects** (unusual, unexpected, and infrequent reactions)
  **If any of the following develop, consult your physician promptly for
  guidance.**
  Mild Adverse Effects
  Allergic reactions: rashes, hives—rare.
  Dizziness, fainting, blurred or double vision, slurred speech, sweating, nau-
  sea—possible.
  Ringing in the ears—case reports.
  Impaired motor skills (dose related to some extent)—frequency varies.
  Serious Adverse Effects
  Allergic reactions: liver damage with jaundice (see Glossary), kidney damage,
  abnormally low blood platelet count, anaphylaxis—case reports.
  Respiratory depression—dose related.
  Bone marrow depression: low white blood cells, fever, sore throat—case re-
  ports.
  Severe lowering of blood pressure, slow heart rate, and cardiac arrest has
  been reported after rapid intravenous dosing—case reports.
  Hip fracture—possible indirect effect of the medicine arising from unsteadi-
  ness.
  Amnesia—dose related.
  Obsessive-compulsive disorder following extended use and abrupt with-
  drawal—possible.
  Paradoxical responses of excitement, agitation, anger, rage—case reports.

▷ **Possible Effects on Sexual Function:**
  Altered timing and pattern of menstruation.
  Small doses (2 to 5 mg/day) may help the anxiety seen in many cases of im-
  potence in men and inhibited sexual responsiveness in women.
  Larger doses (10 mg/day or more) can decrease libido, impair potency in men,
  and inhibit orgasm in women.
  Swelling and tenderness of male breast tissue (gynecomastia). Abnormally
  prolonged erections (priapism)—case reports.

Adverse Effects That May Mimic Natural Diseases or Disorders
  Liver reaction with jaundice may suggest viral hepatitis.

Possible Effects on Laboratory Tests
  White blood cell counts: decreased.
  Blood thyroxine (T_4) level: decreased.
  Liver function tests: increased liver enzymes (ALT/GPT, AST/GOT, and alka-
  line phosphatase), increased bilirubin—all rare.

Urine sugar tests: no drug effect with Tes-Tape; low test results with Clinistix and Diastix.

Urine screening tests for drug abuse: may be **positive**. (Test results depend upon amount of drug taken and testing method used.)

CAUTION
1. This drug should not be stopped abruptly if it has been taken continually for more than 4 weeks.
2. Some nonprescription (over-the-counter or OTC) drug products that contain antihistamines (allergy and cold preparations, sleep aids) can cause excessive sedation if combined with diazepam.

Precautions for Use
By Infants and Children: This drug should not be used in hyperactive or psychotic children. Watch for excessive sedation and incoordination. Usual dose in children for muscle relaxation or sedation is 0.1 to 0.8 mg per kg of body mass per day, divided into equal doses and given every 8 hours or as often as every 6 hours. The drug has been used intravenously to help seizures in neonates.

By Those Over 60 Years of Age: Small doses are indicated. Observe for lethargy, indifference, fatigue, weakness, unsteadiness, disturbing dreams, nightmares, and paradoxical reactions of excitement, agitation, anger, hostility, and rage.

▷ Advisability of Use During Pregnancy
Pregnancy Category: D. See Pregnancy Risk Categories at the back of this book.
Animal studies: Cleft palate reported in mice; skeletal defects in rats.
Human studies: Available information is conflicting and inconclusive. Some findings of increased serious birth defects. Other studies have found no significant increase in birth defects.
Frequent use in late pregnancy can cause the "floppy infant" syndrome in the newborn: weakness, lethargy, unresponsiveness, depressed breathing, low body temperature.
Avoid use during entire pregnancy.

Advisability of Use If Breast-Feeding
Presence of this drug in breast milk: Yes.
Avoid drug or refrain from nursing.

Habit-Forming Potential: This drug can produce psychological and/or physical dependence (see Glossary), especially if used in large doses for an extended period of time.

Effects of Overdose: Marked drowsiness, weakness, feeling of drunkenness, staggering gait, tremor, stupor progressing to deep sleep or coma.

Possible Effects of Long-Term Use: Psychological and/or physical dependence, rare blood cell disorders.

Suggested Periodic Examinations While Taking This Drug (at physician's discretion)
Complete blood cell counts during long-term use.

▷ While Taking This Drug, Observe the Following
Foods: No restrictions.
Beverages: Avoid excessive intake of caffeine-containing beverages: coffee, tea, cola. May be taken with milk.

▷   *Alcohol:* **Avoid this combination**. Alcohol increases the absorption of this drug and adds to its depressant effects on the brain. It is advisable to avoid alcohol completely—throughout the day and night—if it is necessary to drive or to engage in any hazardous activity.

Tobacco Smoking: Heavy smoking may reduce the calming action of this drug. I advise everyone to quit smoking.

Marijuana Smoking: Increased sedation and impairment of intellectual and physical performance.

▷   *Other Drugs*

Diazepam may *increase* the effects of
- digoxin (Lanoxin), and cause digoxin toxicity.
- phenytoin (Dilantin), and cause phenytoin toxicity.

Diazepam may *decrease* the effects of
- levodopa (Sinemet, etc.), and reduce its effectiveness in treating Parkinson's disease.

Diazepam *taken concurrently* with
- fluoxetine (Prozac) may lead to diazepam toxicity.
- fluvoxamine (Luvox) can result in serious accumulation of diazepam and toxicity.
- macrolide antibiotics (see Drug Classes) may lead to toxicity.
- Monoamine oxidase (MAO) inhibitors (see Drug Classes) may exaggerate breathing depression.
- mirtazapine (Remeron) may worsen motor skills. Avoid operating dangerous machinery or tasks requiring coordination.
- narcotics or other centrally active medicines may cause additive respiratory depression or decreased levels of consciousness.

The following drugs may *increase* the effects of diazepam:
- birth control pills (oral contraceptives).
- cimetidine (Tagamet).
- cisapride (Propulcid).
- disulfiram (Antabuse).
- isoniazid (INH, Rifamate, etc.).
- itraconazole (Sporanox), ketoconazole (Nizoral).
- macrolide antibiotics such as erythromycin or clarithromycin.
- omeprazole (Prilosec).
- ritonavir (Norvir), and perhaps other protease inhibitors (see Drug Classes).
- sertraline (Zoloft).
- valproic acid (Depakene).

The following drugs may *decrease* the effects of diazepam:
- ranitidine (Zantac).
- rifampin (Rimactane, etc.).
- rifabutin (Mycobutin).
- theophylline (aminophylline, Theo-Dur, etc.).

▷   *Driving, Hazardous Activities:* This drug can impair mental alertness, judgment, physical coordination, and reaction time. Avoid hazardous activities accordingly.

Aviation Note: The use of this drug *is a disqualification* for piloting. Consult a designated aviation medical examiner.

Exposure to Sun: No restrictions.

Exposure to Heat: Because of reduced urine volume, this drug may accumulate in the body and produce effects of Overdose.

Discontinuation: Avoid stopping this drug suddenly if taken for over 4 weeks. Prudent to taper gradually to prevent a withdrawal syndrome (sweating, tremor, depression, hallucinations, seizures, and vomiting).

DICLOFENAC (di KLOH fen ak)

See the acetic acid (nonsteroidal anti-inflammatory drugs) profile for further information.

DIDANOSINE (di DAN oh seen)

Other Names: Dideoxyinosine, DDI

Introduced: 1991 **Class:** Antiviral **Prescription:** USA: Yes **Controlled Drug:** USA: No; Canada: No **Available as Generic:** USA: No; Canada: No

Brand Name: Videx

BENEFITS versus RISKS	
Possible Benefits	*Possible Risks*
DELAYED PROGRESSION OF DISEASE IN HIV-POSITIVE PATIENTS	DRUG-INDUCED PANCREATITIS DRUG-INDUCED PERIPHERAL NEURITIS
USE IN COMBINATION THERAPY OF AIDS	Drug-induced seizures Liver damage—rare
TWICE DAILY DOSING	

▷ **Principal Uses**

As a Single Drug Product: Uses currently included in FDA-approved labeling: (1) Treats human immunodeficiency virus (HIV) infections in adults and children (6 months of age or older); (2) treatment of advanced HIV infection in those failing zidovudine.

Author's Note: The *Panel on Clinical Practices for Treatment of HIV Infection Report* says that the preferred regimen is two nucleoside analogs and one potent protease inhibitor. Other (unlabeled) generally accepted uses: Used in combination with other antiretroviral medicines (such as protease inhibitors or hydroxyurea [Hydrea]) to treat HIV infection or AIDS.

How This Drug Works: By interfering with essential HIV enzyme systems, this drug prevents growth and reproduction of HIV particles in infected cells, limiting the severity and extent of HIV infection.

Available Dosage Forms and Strengths

Powder for oral solution — 2 g or 4 g per bottle

Powder for oral solution — packets of 100 mg, 167 mg, 250 mg, 375 mg

Tablets, chewable/dispersible — 25 mg, 50 mg, 100 mg, 150 mg

Author's Note: The company is actively investigating other formulations for this medicine.

▷ **Recommended Dosage Ranges** (Actual dose and schedule must be determined for each patient individually.)

Infants and Children: For those 6 months of age or older, dose is based on drug form and body surface area:

Pediatric oral solution (reconstituted and mixed with buffers)—125 mg (12.5 ml) every 12 hours for body surface area of $1.1–1.4$ m², 94 mg (9.5 ml) every 12 hours for body surface area of $0.8–1$ m², 62 mg (6 ml) every 12 hours for body surface area of $0.5–0.7$ m², 31 mg (3 ml) every 12 hours for body surface area of 0.4 m² or less. (Based on 200 mg/square meter per day.)

Chewable/dispersible tablets—100 mg every 12 hours for body surface area of $1.1–1.4$ m², 75 mg every 12 hours for body surface area of $0.8–1$ m², 50 mg every 12 hours for body surface area of $0.5–0.7$ m², 25 mg every 12 hours for body surface area of 0.4 m² or less. In children 1 year of age or older, each dose should be two tablets to ensure that adequate buffering is provided to prevent destruction (degradation) of the drug in stomach acid. In children younger than 1 year of age, one tablet will provide adequate buffering.

12 to 60 Years of Age: Adult oral solution (buffered)—250 mg every 12 hours for those weighing more than 60 kg, 167 mg every 12 hours for those weighing less than 60 kg.

Chewable/dispersible tablets—200 mg every 12 hours for body weight of 60 kg or more, 125 mg every 12 hours for body weight of less than 60 kg.

Over 60 Years of Age: Same as 12 to 60 group. Dose reduced in impaired liver or kidney function.

Conditions Requiring Dosing Adjustments

Liver Function: Increased risk of liver toxicity if used in people with compromised liver. Doses must be decreased in liver failure.

Kidney Function: Dose **must** be decreased in mild to moderate kidney failure. Also an increased risk of magnesium toxicity and drug-induced pancreatitis in patients with kidney problems.

▷ **Dosing Instructions:** Best taken on an empty stomach, 30 minutes before or 2 hours after eating.

Pediatric oral solution first reconstituted with water, then combined with equal amounts of antacid (such as Mylanta or Maalox). Shake this mixture thoroughly BEFORE you measure each dose.

Adult oral solution is made by stirring one packet into 120 ml (4 ounces) of water until the powder is dissolved; this may take up to 3 minutes. Do not mix powder with fruit juice or other acidic liquid. Swallow all of the 4-ounce solution immediately.

The chewable/dispersible buffered tablets should be thoroughly chewed, crushed, or dispersed in water before swallowing. To disperse the tablet(s), stir in at least 30 ml (1 ounce) of water until all the medicine is in the water. Swallow all of preparation immediately.

Author's Note: Current HIV therapy involves combination use of agents from different drug classes to attack the AIDS virus from different points and delay resistance. Many clinicians use viral load (see Glossary) to indicate success or failure of therapy.

Usual Duration of Use: Regular use for several months with repeat viral load and CD4 tests are needed to check benefits in slowing AIDS progression. Long-term use requires follow-up with your doctor.

Possible Advantages of This Drug

Does not cause serious bone marrow depression (production of blood cells). Less frequent liver toxicity. Twice daily dosing.

▷ **This Drug Should Not Be Taken If**

- you have had an allergic reaction to it previously.
- you have active liver disease.
- you have had pancreatitis recently.

▷ **Inform Your Physician Before Taking This Drug If**

- you have had allergic reactions to any drugs in the past.
- you are taking any other drugs currently.
- you have a history of pancreatitis or peripheral neuritis.
- you have a history of gout or high blood uric acid level.
- you have a history of alcoholism.
- you have a history of diarrhea.
- you have a history of phenylketonuria (PKU).
- you have a history of low blood platelets or blood disorder.
- you have a history of low blood potassium.
- you have a history of heart failure.
- you have a seizure disorder.
- you have impaired liver or kidney function.

Possible Side Effects (natural, expected, and unavoidable drug actions)

Mild decreases in red blood cell, white blood cell, and platelet counts in adults. Mild increases in blood uric acid levels. Increased magnesium levels in patients with kidney problems.

▷ **Possible Adverse Effects** (unusual, unexpected, and infrequent reactions)

If any of the following develop, consult your physician promptly for guidance.

Mild Adverse Effects

Allergic reactions: skin rash and itching—occasional in adults and common in pediatric patients.

Headache, dizziness, insomnia, nervousness, confusion—infrequent.

Visual disturbances—rare.

Nausea, vomiting—may be frequent in pediatrics; stomach pain and diarrhea (25% of adults and frequent in pediatric patients), dry mouth and altered taste, yeast infection of mouth—rare to infrequent.

Lowered blood pressure—rare to infrequent.

Loss of color in the retina (retinal depigmentation)—case reports.

Asthma, cough—infrequent.

Loss of hair, muscle and joint pains—rare to infrequent.

Serious Adverse Effects

Drug-induced pancreatitis, usually seen in the first 6 months—infrequent.

Drug-induced peripheral neuritis (see Glossary), usually occurring after 2 to 6 months of treatment. This effect also appears to be dose related—infrequent to frequent.

Electrolyte imbalance (low potassium, magnesium, or calcium)—variable.

Abnormal heart rhythm—infrequent.

High blood sugar—possible.

Excessive lowering of blood pressure and passing out (syncope)—case reports—infrequent.

Serious skin rash (Stevens-Johnson syndrome)—case reports.

Seizures (may be due to electrolyte problems)—rare.

Lowered white blood cell counts, lowered granulocyte (a specific white blood cell) counts, and lowered blood platelets (69%) in pediatric patients—infrequent to frequent.

Optic neuritis and blindness—case reports.

Liver damage—rare to infrequent.

Kidney damage—rare.

▷ **Possible Effects on Sexual Function:**   None reported.

Adverse Effects That May Mimic Natural Diseases or Disorders

Drug-induced liver reaction—rare at less than 0.2%—may suggest viral hepatitis.

Possible Effects on Laboratory Tests

Complete blood cell counts: decreased red cells and white cells—variable; decreased platelets—infrequent.

Blood amylase or uric acid level: increased—infrequent.

Blood electrolytes: low calcium, potassium, and magnesium.

Liver function tests: increased liver enzymes (ALT/GPT, AST/GOT, and alkaline phosphatase), increased bilirubin—infrequent in adults, higher in pediatric patients.

CAUTION

1. This drug **does not cure HIV infection.** Ongoing CD4 and viral load tests are prudent. The AIDS virus may still be passed to other people while you are taking this medicine.
2. Report stomach pain with nausea and vomiting to your doctor; this could indicate pancreatitis.
3. Report pain, numbness, tingling or burning in the hands or feet—could be peripheral neuritis. Drug may need to be stopped.
4. If your kidneys are damaged or your creatinine elevated, ask your doctor if accumulating magnesium will be a problem for you.

Precautions for Use

By Infants and Children: Safety and effectiveness for those under 6 months of age not established. Children are also at risk for developing pancreatitis and peripheral neuritis. It is recommended that detailed eye examinations be performed every 6 months and at any time that visual disturbance occurs.

By Those Over 60 Years of Age: Reduced kidney function may require dose reduction.

▷ **Advisability of Use During Pregnancy**

Pregnancy Category: B. See Pregnancy Risk Categories at the back of this book.

Animal studies: Rat and rabbit studies show no birth defects.

Human studies: Adequate studies of pregnant women not available.

Consult your physician for specific guidance.

Advisability of Use If Breast-Feeding

Presence of this drug in breast milk: Unknown.

Avoid drug or refrain from nursing.

Note: HIV has been found in human breast milk. Breast-feeding may result in transmission of HIV infection to the nursing infant.

Habit-Forming Potential: None.

Effects of Overdose: Nausea, vomiting, stomach pain, diarrhea, pain in hands and feet, irritability, confusion.

Possible Effects of Long-Term Use: Peripheral neuritis (see Glossary).

Suggested Periodic Examinations While Taking This Drug (at physician's discretion)

Complete blood cell counts before starting treatment and weekly thereafter until tolerance is established.

Electrolytes.

Blood amylase levels, fractionated for salivary gland and pancreatic origin.

Liver and kidney function tests.

Viral load or viral burden in order to assess success of treatment.

CD4 counts.

▷ **While Taking This Drug, Observe the Following**

Foods: Best taken on an empty stomach.

Beverages: No restrictions.

▷ *Alcohol:* No interactions expected.

Tobacco Smoking: No interactions expected. I advise everyone to quit smoking.

▷ *Other Drugs*

Didanosine may *increase* the effects of

• zidovudine (Retrovir), and enhance its antiviral effect against HIV.

Didanosine may *decrease* the effects of

• ciprofloxacin (Cipro), if taken at the same time; take ciprofloxacin at least 2 hours before taking didanosine.

• dapsone, and render it ineffective; avoid concurrent use.

• indinavir (Crixivan), and blunt therapeutic benefits; separate dosing by 2 hours.

• itraconazole (Sporanox). Separate dosing by at least 2 hours.

• ketoconazole (Nizoral), if taken at the same time; take ketoconazole at least 2 hours before taking didanosine.

• tetracyclines (see Drug Classes), if taken at the same time; take tetracyclines at least 2 hours before taking didanosine.

Didanosine *taken concurrently* with

• antacids will decrease didanosine absorption and lower its therapeutic benefit.

• delavirdine (Rescriptor) may lower both drug levels.

• histamine (H_2) blocking drugs (see Drug Classes)—cimetidine, etc.—may increase didanosine toxicity.

• pentamidine or sulfamethoxazole may increase the risk of drug-induced pancreatitis; watch for significant symptoms.

• triazolam (Halcion) may cause confusion.

• zalcitabine (Hivid) may cause increased neurotoxicity.

▷ *Driving, Hazardous Activities:* This drug may cause dizziness and impaired vision. Restrict activities as necessary.

Aviation Note: The use of this drug *is a disqualification* for piloting. Consult a designated aviation medical examiner.

Exposure to Sun: No restrictions.

Discontinuation: Do not stop this drug without your physician's knowledge and guidance.

DIFLUNISAL (di FLU ni sal)

See the acetic acids (nonsteroidal anti-inflammatory drugs) profile for further information.

DIGITOXIN (di ji TOX in)

See the digoxin profile for further information.

DIGOXIN (di JOX in)

Introduced: 1934   **Class:** Digitalis preparations   **Prescription:** USA: Yes   **Controlled Drug:** USA: No; Canada: No   **Available as Generic:** Yes
Brand Names: Lanoxicaps, Lanoxin, ✚Novodigoxin, SK-Digoxin

BENEFITS versus RISKS	
Possible Benefits	*Possible Risks*
EFFECTIVE HEART STIMULANT IN CONGESTIVE HEART FAILURE EFFECTIVE PREVENTION AND TREATMENT OF CERTAIN HEART RHYTHM DISORDERS	NARROW TREATMENT RANGE Frequent and sometimes serious disturbances of heart rhythm

▷ **Principal Uses**

As a Single Drug Product: Uses in current FDA-approved labeling: (1) Treats congestive heart failure; (2) restores and helps keep normal heart rate and rhythm in cases of atrial fibrillation (second-line agent behind verapamil, diltiazem, or a beta-blocker), atrial flutter, PAT, and atrial/supraventricular tachycardia.

Other (unlabeled) generally accepted uses: (1) postoperative arrhythmias; (2) helps to increase left ventricular function in patients with pacemakers; (3) may have a role in treating Wolff-Parkinson-White syndrome.

How This Drug Works: Increases force of heart muscle contraction. Delays electrical transmission through the heart helping restore normal rate and rhythm.

Available Dosage Forms and Strengths

Elixir, pediatric — 0.05 mg/ml
Capsules — 0.05 mg, 0.1 mg, 0.2 mg
Injection — 0.1 mg/ml, 0.25 mg/ml
Tablets — 0.0625 mg (Canada), 0.125 mg, 0.25 mg, 0.5 mg

Author's Note: Dosing and timing of doses is critical for this medicine. The difference between toxic blood levels and therapeutic blood levels is small. Be CERTAIN you understand how and when to take this medicine.

▷ **Usual Adult Dosage Range:**   Loading dose: 10 mcg per kilogram of lean body mass; 10–15 mcg per kg of body mass may be needed if digoxin is being used to control abnormal heart rhythms (such as atrial fibrillation). Loading dose can be given orally or intravenously. Once decided, is often given as 50% in the first dose with remainder divided into smaller doses and given at 6- to 8-hour intervals until the desired response is achieved. Usual ongoing dose after loading is 0.125 to 0.5 mg per day. In neonatal and pediatric patients, a similar loading and ongoing strategy is used, but the amount on a mg-per-kg-of-body-mass basis is very different. **Note: Actual dose and schedule must be determined for each patient individually.**

Conditions Requiring Dosing Adjustments
Liver Function: Use with caution; blood levels should be obtained more frequently.
Kidney Function: Dose **must** be adjusted in kidney compromise. Smaller doses and some cases of dosing every other day may be needed.

▷ **Dosing Instructions:**   Tablet may be crushed, and is best taken at the same time each day (to help keep blood levels about the same) on an empty stomach. Can be taken with or following food; milk and dairy products may delay absorption but do not reduce the amount of drug absorbed. The capsule should be swallowed whole.

Usual Duration of Use: Regular use for 7 to 10 days needed to see benefits in relieving heart failure or controlling heart rhythm disorders. Long-term use requires physician supervision.

▷ **This Drug Should Not Be Taken If**
• you have had an allergic reaction to any form of it.
• you are in ventricular fibrillation (a life-threatening heart rhythm).

▷ **Inform Your Physician Before Taking This Drug If**
• you have had an unfavorable reaction to digitalis.
• you have taken digitalis in the past 2 weeks.
• you take (or have recently taken) any diuretic drug.
• you have a history of severe lung disease.
• you have abnormal heart rhythms or certain aortic problems.
• you have had damage to the heart muscle (myocardium).
• you have a history of low blood potassium or magnesium.
• you have impaired liver or kidney function.
• you have a history of thyroid function disorder.

Possible Side Effects (natural, expected, and unavoidable drug actions)
Slow heart rate.
Enlargement or sensitivity of the male breast—rare.

▷ **Possible Adverse Effects** (unusual, unexpected, and infrequent reactions)
If any of the following develop, consult your physician promptly for guidance.
Mild Adverse Effects
Allergic reactions: skin rash, hives.
Headache, drowsiness, lethargy, confusion, changes in vision: "halo" effect, blurring, spots, double vision, yellow-green vision—infrequent.
Changes in vaginal tissue (vaginal cornification)—case reports.
Nightmares—case reports.

Loss of appetite, nausea, vomiting, diarrhea (early signs of adult toxicity)—frequent.

Serious Adverse Effects

Idiosyncratic reactions: hallucinations, facial neuralgias, peripheral neuralgias, blindness—case reports.

Low blood platelets—case reports and probably an immune reaction.

Psychosis and hallucinations—associated with toxic levels.

Seizures—rare.

Serious skin rash (Stevens-Johnson syndrome)—rare.

Disorientation, most common in the elderly.

Heart rhythm disturbances—possible and dose related.

▷ **Possible Effects on Sexual Function:**

Decreased libido and impotence in 35% of male users. Enlargement and tenderness of male breasts (gynecomastia)—case reports.

Both effects are attributed to digoxin's estrogenlike action.

Adverse Effects That May Mimic Natural Diseases or Disorders

Drug-induced mental changes may be mistaken for senile dementia or psychosis.

Possible Effects on Laboratory Tests

White blood cell counts: decreased.

Blood testosterone level: may be decreased with long-term use.

CAUTION

1. Take this medicine EXACTLY as prescribed.
2. If you take calcium supplements, ask your physician for help. Avoid large doses.
3. Prudent to carry a card that says you are taking this drug.
4. Avoid over-the-counter antacids and cold, cough, or allergy remedies without first asking your doctor or pharmacist.

Precautions for Use

By Infants and Children: Watch for indications of toxicity: slow heart rate (below 60 beats/min), irregular heart rhythms.

By Those Over 60 Years of Age: Reduced drug tolerance; smaller doses are prudent. Watch for toxicity: headache, dizziness, fatigue, weakness, lethargy, depression, confusion, nervousness, agitation, delusions, difficulty with reading. Call your doctor if these happen.

▷ **Advisability of Use During Pregnancy**

Pregnancy Category: C. See Pregnancy Risk Categories at the back of this book.

Animal studies: No birth defects reported.

Human studies: Adequate studies of pregnant women not available. However, no birth defects from the therapeutic use of this drug have been reported.

Use this drug only if clearly needed. Overdose can be harmful to the fetus.

Advisability of Use If Breast-Feeding

Presence of this drug in breast milk: Yes.

Monitor nursing infant closely and discontinue drug or nursing if adverse effects develop.

Habit-Forming Potential: None.

Effects of Overdose: Loss of appetite, excessive saliva, nausea, vomiting, diarrhea, serious disturbances of heart rate and rhythm, intestinal bleeding, drowsiness, headache, confusion, delirium, hallucinations, convulsions.

Possible Effects of Long-Term Use: None reported.

Suggested Periodic Examinations While Taking This Drug (at physician's discretion)

Measurements of blood levels of digoxin, calcium, magnesium, and potassium; electrocardiograms.

Time to sample blood for digoxin level: 6–8 hours after last dose, or just before next dose.

Recommended therapeutic range: 0.5–2.0 ng/ml.

▷ **While Taking This Drug, Observe the Following**

Foods: Talk to your doctor about high potassium foods. Peak level and rate digoxin enters your body will decrease if taken with food.

Beverages: Avoid excessive amounts of caffeine-containing beverages: coffee, tea, cola. May be taken with milk.

▷ *Alcohol:* No interactions expected.

Tobacco Smoking: Nicotine can cause heart muscle irritability and predispose to serious rhythm disturbances. I advise everyone to quit smoking.

Marijuana Smoking: Possible accentuation of heart failure; reduced digoxin effect; possible changes in electrocardiogram, confusing interpretation.

▷ *Other Drugs*

Digoxin *taken concurrently* with
- acarbose (Precose) may result in decreased digoxin blood levels and loss of digoxin's benefits.
- calcium (intravenously) may cause a fatal interaction.
- digoxin immune Fab (Digibind) will result in decreased blood levels. This is used to therapeutic advantage in digoxin toxicity.
- diuretics (except spironolactone or triamterene) can cause serious heart rhythm problems due to loss of potassium.
- metformin (Glucophage) may increase metformin levels and lead to excessively low blood sugar.
- propranolol or other beta-blocking medicines (see Drug Classes) may cause very slow heart rate.
- quinidine may result in decreased digoxin effectiveness and increased digoxin toxicity; careful dose adjustments are needed.
- succinylcholine may lead to abnormal heart rhythms.

The following drugs may *increase* the effects of digoxin:
- alprazolam (Xanax).
- amiloride (Midamor).
- amiodarone (Cordarone).
- amphotericin B (Abelcet, Fungizone).
- atorvastatin (Lipitor).
- benzodiazepines (Librium, Valium, etc.; see Drug Classes).
- captopril (Capoten, Capozide).
- cyclosporine (Sandimmune).
- diltiazem (Cardizem) and other calcium channel blockers (see Drug Classes).
- disopyramide (Norpace).
- erythromycin (E.E.S., Erythrocin, etc.). May also occur with clarithromycin and azithromycin.

- ethacrynic acid.
- flecainide (Tambocor).
- hydroxychloroquine.
- ibuprofen (Advil, Medipren, Motrin, Nuprin, etc.).
- indomethacin (Indocin) and other NSAIDs.
- itraconazole (Sporanox).
- methimazole (Tapazole).
- mibefradil (Posicor).
- nefazodone (Serzone).
- nifedipine (Adalat, Procardia).
- phenytoin (Dilantin).
- propafenone (Rythmol).
- propylthiouracil (Propacil).
- quinine.
- ritonavir (Norvir).
- tetracyclines (see Drug Classes).
- tolbutamide (Orinase).
- tramadol (Ultram).
- trazodone (Desyrel).
- verapamil (Calan, Verelan, others).

The following drugs may *decrease* the effects of digoxin:
- aluminum-containing antacids (Amphojel, Maalox, etc.).
- bleomycin (Blenoxane).
- carmustine (BiCNU).
- cholestyramine (Questran).
- colestipol (Colestid).
- cyclophosphamide (Cytoxan).
- cytarabine (Cytosar).
- doxorubicin (Adriamycin).
- fluvoxamine (Luvox).
- kaolin/pectin (Donnagel, others).
- methotrexate (Mexate).
- metoclopramide (Reglan).
- miglitol (Glyset).
- neomycin.
- penicillamine (Cuprimine, Depen).
- procarbazine (Matulane).
- rifampin or rifabutin.
- sucralfate (Carafate).
- sulfa antibiotics or sulfasalazine.
- thyroid hormones.
- vincristine (Oncovin).

▷ *Driving, Hazardous Activities:* Usually no restrictions. This drug may cause drowsiness, vision changes, and nausea. Restrict activities as necessary.

Aviation Note: Heart function disorders *are a disqualification* for piloting. Consult a designated aviation medical examiner.

Exposure to Sun: No restrictions.

Occurrence of Unrelated Illness: Vomiting or diarrhea can seriously alter this drug's effectiveness. Notify your physician promptly.

Discontinuation: This drug may be continued indefinitely. Do not stop it without consulting your physician.

DILTIAZEM (dil TI a zem)

Introduced: 1977   **Class:** Anti-anginal, antihypertensive, calcium channel blocker   **Prescription:** USA: Yes   **Controlled Drug:** USA: No; Canada: No   **Available as Generic:** Yes

Brand Names: ✤Apo-Diltiaz, Cardizem, Cardizem CD, Cardizem SR, Dilacor XR, Diltia XT, Diltiazem, ✤Novo-Diltiazem, ✤Nu-Diltiaz, ✤Syn-Diltiazem, Tiazac

Controversies in Medicine: Medicines in this class have had many conflicting reports. The FDA has held hearings on the calcium channel blocker (CCB) class. A study called ALLHAT is comparing amlodipine, an ACE inhibitor, a diuretic and an alpha blocker (see Drug Classes) and should clarify adverse effects, mortality and other issues relating to CCBs. CCBs are currently second line agents for high blood pressure according to the JNC VI.

BENEFITS versus RISKS	
Possible Benefits	*Possible Risks*
EFFECTIVE PREVENTION OF	Depression, confusion
BOTH MAJOR TYPES OF ANGINA	Low blood pressure
EFFECTIVE CONTROL OF MILD TO	Heart rhythm disturbance
MODERATE HYPERTENSION	Fluid retention
HELPS CONTROL ATRIAL	Liver damage—case reports
FIBRILLATION	Muscle damage—case reports

▷ **Principal Uses**

As a Single Drug Product: Uses currently included in FDA-approved labeling: Treats (1) angina pectoris (coronary artery spasm or spontaneous Prinzmetal's variant angina), which is associated with exertion; (2) classical angina-of-effort (due to atherosclerotic disease); (3) mild to moderate hypertension.

Other (unlabeled) generally accepted uses: (1) unstable angina; (2) congestive heart failure; (3) migraine prophylaxis; (4) prevention of abnormal protein excretion in the urine; (5) abnormal heart rhythms such as atrial fibrillation; (6) treats abnormal plaques inside blood vessels (atherosclerosis); (7) may help prevent abnormal growth of the left side of the heart (left ventricular hypertrophy) after a heart attack; (8) treats some esophageal disorders; (9) eases symptoms of an overactive thyroid gland (hyperthyroidism); (10) can ease symptoms of Raynaud's phenomenon; (11) can have a role in preserving function in kidney and heart transplant patients; (12) may protect against heart attacks or variant or unstable angina that can occur after (postoperatively) coronary artery bypass grafting.

How This Drug Works: This drug blocks normal passage of calcium through cell walls, inhibiting coronary artery and peripheral arteriole narrowing. As a result, this drug

- prevents spontaneous coronary artery spasm (Prinzmetal's angina).
- decreases heart rate and contraction force in exertion, making effort-induced angina less likely.
- opens contracted peripheral arterial walls, lowering blood pressure (also lessens heart work and helps prevent angina).{ebl}

Available Dosage Forms and Strengths

Tablets (immediate release) — 30 mg, 60 mg, 90 mg, 120 mg
Capsules (extended release) — 120 mg, 180 mg, 240 mg, 300 mg, 360 mg (Tiazac only)
Capsules (sustained release) — 60 mg, 90 mg, 120 mg

▷ **Usual Adult Dosage Range:**   Initially 30 mg, three or four times daily. Dose may be increased gradually at 1- to 2-day intervals as needed and tolerated. Sustained-release forms are dosed 120 or 180 mg daily. Daily maximum is 360 mg. **Note: Actual dose and schedule must be determined for each patient individually.**

Conditions Requiring Dosing Adjustments

Liver Function: Maximum daily dose in patients with liver compromise should be 90 mg. Rarely causes hepatoxicity, and a benefit-to-risk decision must be made.

Kidney Function: May be one of the best to use in kidney compromise (large liver and fecal removal). Caution must still be used. Drug can be a rare cause of kidney compromise.

▷ **Dosing Instructions:**   Immediate-release form may be crushed and is best taken before meals and at bedtime. Extended-release forms should NEVER be crushed or altered. Tiazac form may be taken with or without food.

Usual Duration of Use: Use for 2 to 4 weeks is required to see effectiveness in decreasing angina frequency and severity and in lowering blood pressure. Smallest effective dose should be used in long-term therapy (months to years).

Possible Advantages of This Drug

Often effective as single-drug therapy.
Does not reduce blood supply to kidneys.
Does not raise blood cholesterol levels.
Does not induce asthma in susceptible individuals.

▷ **This Drug Should Not Be Taken If**

- you have had an allergic reaction to it previously.
- you have "sick sinus" syndrome (and do not have an artificial pacemaker).
- you have second- or third-degree heart block.
- you have low blood pressure—systolic pressure below 90.
- you have heart failure (talk with your doctor).
- you have advanced stenosis of the aorta.

▷ **Inform Your Physician Before Taking This Drug If**

- you had an unfavorable response to any calcium blocker drug.
- you take digitalis or a beta-blocker (see Drug Classes).
- you have a history of congestive heart failure.
- you have atrial fibrillation (talk with your doctor).
- you have impaired liver or kidney function.
- you have a history of drug-induced liver damage.

Possible Side Effects (natural, expected, and unavoidable drug actions)
Fatigue—rare; light-headedness, heart rate and rhythm changes in some people—rare.

▷ **Possible Adverse Effects** (unusual, unexpected, and infrequent reactions)
If any of the following develop, consult your physician promptly for guidance.

Mild Adverse Effects
Allergic reactions: skin rash, hives, itching—rare.
Headache—may be self-limiting but frequent; drowsiness, dizziness—occasional and dose related; nervousness, sleep problems, depression, confusion, hallucinations—case reports.
Desire to be in constant motion (acathesia)—case reports.
Overgrowth of the gums (gingival hyperplasia)—may be frequent.
Impaired sense of smell—possible.
Increased urination—rare.
Flushing, palpitations, fainting, slow heart rate, low blood pressure—rare.
Nausea, indigestion, heartburn, vomiting, diarrhea, constipation—rare to infrequent.

Serious Adverse Effects
Serious skin rashes (Stevens Johnson Syndrome, others).
Serious disturbances of heart rate and/or rhythm, fluid retention (edema), congestive heart failure—rare.
Drug-induced myopathy or liver damage—rare.
Lowering of a specific kind of white blood cell (granulocytes)—case reports with other calcium channel blockers.
Lowering of blood platelets—case reports.

▷ **Possible Effects on Sexual Function:** Impotence is reported in less than 1% of users. Swelling or tenderness of the male breast tissue (gynecomastia)—case reports. One reported case of heavy vaginal bleeding.

Possible Effects on Laboratory Tests
Blood total cholesterol and triglyceride levels: no effects.
Blood HDL cholesterol level: increased.
Blood LDL and VLDL cholesterol levels: no effects.

CAUTION
1. Tell health care providers that you take this drug. Carry a card in your purse or wallet saying you take diltiazem.
2. Nitroglycerin and other nitrate drugs as needed may still be used to relieve acute angina pain. If your angina attacks become more frequent or intense, call your doctor promptly.

Precautions for Use
By Infants and Children: Safety and effectiveness for those under 12 years of age not established.
By Those Over 60 Years of Age: May be more likely to have weakness, dizziness, fainting, and falling. Take necessary precautions to prevent injury. Report promptly any changes in your pattern of thirst and urination.

▷ **Advisability of Use During Pregnancy**
Pregnancy Category: C. See Pregnancy Risk Categories at the back of this book.
Animal studies: Embryo and fetal deaths and skeletal birth defects reported in mice, rats, and rabbits.

Human studies: Adequate studies of pregnant women not available.
Avoid this drug during the first 3 months.
Use during the last 6 months only if clearly needed. Ask your physician for
    help.

Advisability of Use If Breast-Feeding
Presence of this drug in breast milk: Yes.
Avoid drug or refrain from nursing.

Habit-Forming Potential: None.

Effects of Overdose: Weakness, light-headedness, fainting, slow pulse, low.
    blood pressure, shortness of breath, congestive heart failure.

Possible Effects of Long-Term Use: None reported.

Suggested Periodic Examinations While Taking This Drug (at physician's dis-
    cretion)

Evaluations of heart function, including electrocardiograms; liver and kidney
    function tests, with long-term use.

▷ **While Taking This Drug, Observe the Following**
Foods: May increase absorption and cause a 30% increase in blood levels. Avoid
    excessive salt intake. Ginseng may increase blood pressure.
Beverages: No restrictions. May be taken with milk.
▷   *Alcohol:* Use with caution. Alcohol may exaggerate the drop in blood pressure.
Tobacco Smoking: Nicotine reduces benefits. I advise everyone to quit smoking.
Marijuana Smoking: Possible reduced effectiveness of this drug; mild to mod-
    erate increase in angina; possible changes in electrocardiogram, confusing
    interpretation.
▷   *Other Drugs*
Diltiazem *taken concurrently* with
- amiodarone (Cordarone) may lead to abnormal heart rhythm.
- aspirin can result in prolonged bleeding time or hemorrhage.
- beta-blocker drugs or digitalis preparations (see Drug Classes) may affect
    heart rate and rhythm. Careful physician monitoring is necessary if these
    drugs are combined.
- carbamazepine (Tegretol) may result in toxicity and seizures.
- cyclosporine (Sandimmune) may result in cyclosporine toxicity and kidney
    failure.
- digoxin (Lanoxin) can result in digoxin toxicity.
- lithium (Lithobid, others) can result in psychosis and neurotoxicity.
- oral antidiabetic drugs (see Drug Classes) such as glipizide (Glucotrol) may
    result in greater than expected lowering of blood sugar and hypoglycemia.
- phenytoin (Dilantin) decreases phenytoin metabolism and causes phenytoin
    toxicity.
- quinidine (Quinaglute, others) may lead to quinidine toxicity.
- rifabutin (Mycobutin) may decrease diltiazem blood levels.
- rifampin (Rifadin) may result in decreased diltiazem effectiveness.
- ritonavir (Norvir) and perhaps other protease inhibitors (see Drug Profiles)
    may lead to diltiazem toxicity.
- tacrolimus (Prograf) may result in tacrolimus accumulation and tacrolimus
    toxicity.
- theophylline (Theo-Dur, others) may lead to theophyllinetoxicity.

The following drugs may *increase* the effects of diltiazem:
- cimetidine (Tagamet).
- fluoxetine (Prozac).
- fluvoxamine (Luvox).
- ranitidine (Zantac).
- sertraline (Zoloft).

▷ *Driving, Hazardous Activities:* Usually no restrictions. This drug may cause drowsiness or dizziness. Limit activities as necessary.

Aviation Note: Coronary artery disease *is a disqualification* for piloting. Consult a designated aviation medical examiner.

Exposure to Sun: This drug may cause photosensitivity (see Glossary).

Exposure to Heat: Caution is advised. Hot environments can exaggerate the blood-pressure-lowering effects of this drug. Observe for light-headedness or weakness.

Heavy Exercise or Exertion: May improve ability to be more active without angina pain. Use caution and avoid excessive exercise that be excessive and yet might not result in warning pain.

Discontinuation: Do not stop this drug abruptly. Ask your doctor about gradual withdrawal.

DIPHENHYDRAMINE (di fen HI dra meen)

Introduced: 1946 **Class:** Hypnotic, antihistamines **Prescription:** USA: Varies **Controlled Drug:** USA: No*; Canada: No **Available as Generic:** Yes

This medicine is available without a prescription and is found in many products.

Brand Names: Acetaminophen-PM, AID to Sleep, Allerdryl, Allergy Capsules, Allergy Formula, Allermax, ✦Ambenyl Expectorant [CD], Ambenyl Syrup [CD], Anacin P.M. Aspirin-free, Banophen, Bayer Select, Beldin Syrup, Bena-D, Benahist, Benadryl, Benadryl 25, Benylin, ✦Benylin Decongestant [CD], ✦Benylin Pediatric Syrup, ✦Benylin Syrup w/Codeine [CD], ✦Caladryl [CD], Caldyphen Lotion, Children's Complete Allergy, Complete Allergy Medication, Compoz, Dermarest, Di-Delamine, Dihydrex, Diphendryl, Diphenhist, Dormarex 2, ✦Ergodryl [CD], Excedrin P.M. [CD], Extra Strength Tylenol PM, Gecil, Genahist, Gen-D-Phen, Hydramine, ✦Insomnal, Kolex, ✦Mandrax [CD], Maximum Strength Nytol, Medi-Phedryl, Midol-PM, Nervine Nightime Sleep, Nidryl Elixir, Nighttime Cold Medicine [CD], Nite-Time, Noradryl [CD], Noradryl 25, Nytol, Pain Relief PM [CD], Pathadryl, ✦PMS-Diphenhydramine, Sinutab Maximum Strength, SK-Diphenhydramine, Sleep, Sleep-Eze 3, ✦Sleep-Eze D, Sominex, Sominex 2, Theraflu Cold Medicine (Nighttime Strength) Twilite, Tylenol PM Extra Strength, Unisom Sleepgels, Valdrene, Valu-Dryl Allergy Medicine [CD], Wal-Ben, Wal-Dryl, Wehydryl

*Ambenyl Syrup is C-V. See Controlled Drug Schedules at the back of this book.

```
┌─────────────────────────────────────────────────────────────────────┐
│                       BENEFITS versus RISKS                         │
│     Possible Benefits                   Possible Risks              │
│  EFFECTIVE RELIEF OF ALLERGIC      Marked sedation                  │
│    RHINITIS AND ALLERGIC SKIN      Atropinelike effects             │
│    DISORDERS                       Accentuation of prostatism (see  │
│  EFFECTIVE, NONADDICTIVE             Glossary)                      │
│    SEDATIVE AND HYPNOTIC                                            │
│  Treatment of anaphylaxis                                          │
│  Prevention and relief of motion                                   │
│    sickness                                                        │
│  Partial relief of symptoms of                                     │
│    Parkinson's disease                                             │
└─────────────────────────────────────────────────────────────────────┘
```

▷ **Principal Uses**

As a Single Drug Product: Uses currently included in FDA-approved labeling: (1) Prevention or treatment of motion sickness (control of dizziness, nausea, and vomiting); (2) treatment of drug-induced parkinsonian reactions, especially in children or the elderly; (3) treatment of conditions caused by histamine release (such as allergic drug reactions); (4) used as a short-term sleep aid; (5) helps hives (urticaria) that have an unknown cause (idiopathic).

Other (unlabeled) generally accepted uses: (1) cough suppression; (2) eases the symptoms of the common cold; (3) can have a role in easing the discomfort of mucositis caused by radiation therapy.

As a Combination Drug Product [CD]: This drug may have a mild suppressant effect on coughing. It is combined with expectorants and codeine or dextromethorphan in some cough products.

How This Drug Works: Blocks the action of histamine. Its natural side effects are used to advantage: sedative action used to help people fall asleep; atropinelike action used in motion sickness and Parkinson-related disorders.

Available Dosage Forms and Strengths

Capsules — 25 mg (nonprescription), 50 mg (prescription)

Cream — 1%

Elixir — 12.5 mg/5 ml (14% alcohol)

Spray — 1%

Syrup — 12.5 mg, 13.3 mg/5 ml

Tablets — 25 mg (nonprescription), 50 mg (prescription)

▷ **Usual Adult Dosage Range:**   Antihistamine, to prevent motion sickness or in Parkinsonism: 25 to 50 mg every 6 to 8 hours. Maximum daily dose is 300 mg. Cough control (antitussive): 25 mg every 4 to 6 hours. Maximum daily dose is 150 mg. As a sleep aid (hypnotic), 50 mg at bedtime is often used. **Note: Actual dose and schedule must be determined for each patient individually.**

Conditions Requiring Dosing Adjustments

Liver Function: Caution—single doses are not expected to be a problem; however, the use of multiple doses in patients with liver compromise has not been studied.

Kidney Function: In mild kidney failure (creatinine clearance more than 50 ml/min) usual dose is given every 6 hours, every 6–12 hours in mild–moderate failure, and every 12–18 hours in severe kidney failure.

▷ **Dosing Instructions:** Tablet may be crushed and capsule may be opened, and is best taken with or following food.

Usual Duration of Use: Regular use for 2 to 3 days is needed to see effectiveness in easing allergic rhinitis and dermatosis symptoms. If it doesn't work after 5 days, this drug should be stopped. As a bedtime sedative (hypnotic), use only as needed. Avoid long-term use.

▷ **This Drug Should Not Be Taken If**
- you have had an allergic reaction to it previously.
- you are taking or took during the past 2 weeks, any monoamine oxidase (MAO) type A inhibitor (see Drug Classes).
- you have chicken pox.

▷ **Inform Your Physician Before Taking This Drug If**
- you have had an unfavorable response to any antihistamine.
- you have narrow-angle glaucoma.
- you have peptic ulcer disease, with any degree of pyloric obstruction.
- you have prostatism (see Glossary).
- you are subject to bronchial asthma or seizures (epilepsy).
- you have difficulty urinating.
- you have glucose-6-phosphate dehydrogenase (G6PD) deficiency.

Possible Side Effects (natural, expected, and unavoidable drug actions)
Drowsiness (diphenhydramine is the most sedating antihistamine); weakness; dryness of nose, mouth, and throat; constipation. Thickening of bronchial secretions.

▷ **Possible Adverse Effects** (unusual, unexpected, and infrequent reactions)
If any of the following develop, consult your physician promptly for guidance.
Mild Adverse Effects
Allergic reactions: skin rash, hives—rare.
Headache, dizziness, inability to concentrate, blurred or double vision, difficult urination—infrequent.
Reduced tolerance for contact lenses—possible.
Nausea, vomiting, diarrhea—possible.
Serious Adverse Effects
Allergic Reaction: Anaphylactic reaction (see Glossary)—case reports.
Idiosyncratic reactions: insomnia, excitement, confusion—case reports.
Hemolytic anemia (see Glossary) or porphyria—case reports.
Reduced white blood cell count: fever, sore throat, infections, or blood platelet destruction (abnormal bleeding or bruising; see Glossary)—case reports.
Movement disorders (dyskinesias)—case reports.

▷ **Possible Effects on Sexual Function:** Shortened menstrual cycle (early arrival of expected menstrual onset).

Natural Diseases or Disorders That May Be Activated by This Drug
Latent epilepsy, glaucoma, prostatism.

Possible Effects on Laboratory Tests
Red blood cell counts and hemoglobin: decreased.
Urine screening tests for drug abuse: *initial* test result may be falsely **positive**; *confirmatory* test result will be **negative**. (Test results depend upon amount of drug taken and testing method used.)

CAUTION
1. Stop this drug 5 days before diagnostic skin testing procedures in order to prevent false negative test results.
2. Do not use if you have active bronchial asthma, bronchitis, or pneumonia.

Precautions for Use

By Infants and Children: This drug should not be used in premature or full-term newborn infants. Doses for children should be small, as the young child is especially sensitive to the effects of antihistamines on the brain and nervous system. For use to decrease coughing (antitussive) in children 6 to 12 years old: 12.5 mg every 4 to 6 hours. The maximum daily dose here is 75 mg/day. Avoid the use of this drug in the child with chicken pox or a flu-like infection—may adversely affect Reye syndrome if it develops.

By Those Over 60 Years of Age: Increased risk of drowsiness, dizziness, and unsteadiness, and impairment of thinking, judgment, and memory. Can increase the degree of impaired urination associated with prostate enlargement (prostatism). Sedative effects may be misinterpreted as senility or emotional depression.

▷ **Advisability of Use During Pregnancy**

Pregnancy Category: C by the manufacturer. See Pregnancy Risk Categories at the back of this book.

Animal studies: No birth defects reported in rats or rabbits.

Human studies: Some case reports of fetal toxicity have been made. Information from studies of pregnant women are not available. A withdrawal syndrome of tremor and diarrhea was reported in a 5-day-old infant whose mother used this drug (150 mg daily) during pregnancy.

Use is a benefit to risk decision. Ask your doctor for help.

Advisability of Use If Breast-Feeding

Presence of this drug in breast milk: Yes.

Avoid drug or refrain from nursing.

Habit-Forming Potential: Combination use of pentazocine and diphenhydramine has become an abused intravenous drug combination. There have been rare reports of a withdrawal syndrome after use of high doses.

Effects of Overdose: Marked drowsiness, confusion, incoordination, muscle tremors, fever, dilated pupils, stupor, coma, seizures.

Possible Effects of Long-Term Use: The development of tolerance (see Glossary) and reduced effectiveness of drug.

Suggested Periodic Examinations While Taking This Drug (at physician's discretion)

Complete blood cell counts.

▷ **While Taking This Drug, Observe the Following**

Foods: No restrictions.

Beverages: No restrictions. May be taken with milk.

▷ *Alcohol:* Use extreme caution. The combination of alcohol and antihistamines can cause rapid and marked sedation.

Tobacco Smoking: No interactions expected, but I advise everyone to quit smoking.

Marijuana Smoking: Increased drowsiness and mouth dryness; accentuation of impaired thinking.

▷ *Other Drugs*
Diphenhydramine may ***increase*** the effects of
- all drugs with a sedative effect such as benzodiazepines, tricyclic antidepressants, and narcotics (see Drug Classes), and cause oversedation.
- amitriptyline (Elavil) and cause increased urinary retention.
- atropine and atropinelike drugs (see ***anticholinergic drugs*** in Drug Classes).
- tramadol (Ultram), leading to increased sedation risk.

The following drugs may ***increase*** the effects of diphenhydramine:
- monoamine oxidase (MAO) type A inhibitor drugs (see Drug Classes)—can delay elimination, exaggerating and prolonging its action.

Diphenhydramine ***taken concurrently*** with
- phenothiazines (see Drug Classes) may result in increased difficulty urinating, intestinal obstruction, or glaucoma, especially in those over 70 years old.
- temazepam (Restoril) in pregnancy may increase risk of death of the fetus.
- tricyclic antidepressants (see Drug Classes) may cause increased risk of urinary retention.

▷ *Driving, Hazardous Activities:* This drug may impair alertness, judgment, coordination, and reaction time. Restrict activities as necessary.

Aviation Note: The use of this drug ***is a disqualification*** for piloting. Consult a designated aviation medical examiner.

Exposure to Sun: Caution—this drug may cause photosensitivity (see Glossary).

Exposure to Environmental Chemicals: The insecticides Aldrin, Dieldrin, and Chlordane may decrease the effectiveness of this drug. Sevin may increase the sedative effects of this drug.

DISOPYRAMIDE (di so PEER a mide)

Introduced: 1969 **Class:** Antiarrhythmic **Prescription:** USA: Yes
Controlled Drug: USA: No Canada: No **Available as Generic:** USA: Yes Canada: No

Brand Names: Napamide, Norpace, Norpace CR, Pisopyramide, ✦Rythmodan, ✦Rythmodan-LA

BENEFITS versus RISKS	
Possible Benefits	*Possible Risks*
EFFECTIVE TREATMENT OF SELECTED HEART RHYTHM DISORDERS	NARROW TREATMENT RANGE LOW BLOOD PRESSURE LOW BLOOD SUGAR— INFREQUENT AGRANULOCYTOSIS—RARE Peripheral neuropathy Liver toxicity Heart conduction and rhythm abnormalities Frequent atropinelike side effects

▷ **Principal Uses**

As a Single Drug Product: Uses currently included in FDA-approved labeling: Treats abnormal rhythms in the heart ventricles (ventricular arrhythmias). It is classified as a Type 1 antiarrhythmic agent, similar to quinidine.

Other (unlabeled) generally accepted uses: (1) Abolishes and prevents recurrence of premature heart beats in the atria (upper chambers) and ventricles (lower heart chambers); (2) treats and prevents abnormally rapid heart rates (tachycardia) beginning in the atria or the ventricles; (3) eases arrhythmias and abnormal heart pressures arising from cardiomyopathy or subaortic stenosis.

How This Drug Works: Slows activity of the heart pacemaker and delays electrical impulses through the conduction system and muscle of the heart. These effects help restore normal heart rate and rhythm.

Available Dose Forms and Strengths
Capsules — 100 mg, 150 mg
Capsules, prolonged action — 100 mg, 150 mg, 250 mg LA (in Canada)
Tablet, controlled release — 150 mg, 250 mg (Canada)

▷ **Usual Adult Dose Range:**   For most adults, 600 mg per day. Immediate-release form: 150 mg every 6 hours. If weight is less than 110 pounds (50 kg) dose is 400 milligrams/day given as 100 milligrams every 6 hours (immediate-release) or 200 milligrams every 12 hours (controlled-release). For refractory cases: 1600 mg every 24 hours. Loading dose (if quick control is critical): for more than 50 kg: 300 mg of immediate-release form. If less than 50 kg: 200 mg (immediate-release form). **Note: Actual dose and schedule must be determined for each patient individually.**

Conditions Requiring Dosing Adjustments
Liver Function: Dose decreased in patients with liver compromise by 25 to 50%.
Kidney Function: Dosing **must** be adjusted in kidney compromise. In moderate to severe kidney failure: immediate-release form is given every 12 to 24 hours. May cause urine retention and should be used with caution in patients with urinary outflow problems.

▷ **Dosing Instructions:**   Regular capsules may be opened, and are best taken on an empty stomach, 1 hour before or 2 hours after eating. May also take with or following food to reduce stomach irritation. Prolonged-action capsules should not be opened, chewed, or crushed.

Usual Duration of Use: Regular use for 2 to 4 days is needed to see effectiveness in correcting or preventing rhythm disorders. Long-term use requires supervision and ongoing evaluation by your doctor.

▷ **This Drug Should Not Be Taken If**
• you have had an allergic reaction to it previously.
• you have second-degree, third-degree or bifasicular heart block.
• you have sick sinus syndrome (talk with your doctor).
• you are in heart (cardiogenic) shock.

▷ **Inform Your Physician Before Taking This Drug If**
• you have had unfavorable reactions to antiarrhythmic drugs.
• you have heart disease, especially "heart block."
• you have a history of atrial fibrillation.
• you have a history of low blood potassium.

- you have a history of low blood pressure.
- you have a history of low white blood cells.
- you have impaired liver or kidney function.
- you have glaucoma, a family history of glaucoma, or myasthenia gravis.
- you have an enlarged prostate gland.
- you are prone to low blood sugars.
- you take digitalis or any diuretic drug that can cause loss of body potassium (ask your doctor).

Possible Side Effects (natural, expected, and unavoidable drug actions)

Drop in blood pressure in susceptible individuals. Dry mouth, constipation, blurred vision, impaired urination—may be frequent.

▷ **Possible Adverse Effects** (unusual, unexpected, and infrequent reactions)

If any of the following develop, consult your physician promptly for guidance.

Mild Adverse Effects

Allergic reactions: Skin rash, itching—case reports.

Headache, nervousness, fatigue, muscular weakness, mild aches—infrequent.

Loss of appetite, indigestion, nausea, vomiting, diarrhea—infrequent to frequent.

Serious Adverse Effects

Idiosyncratic reaction: Acute psychotic behavior—rare.

Severe drop in blood pressure, fainting   possible.

Progressive heart weakness, possible congestive heart failure.

Inability to empty urinary bladder, prostatism (see Glossary).

Abnormal heart rhythms—case reports, usually within first month of treatment.

Low blood sugar (glucose)—infrequent.

Jaundice (see Glossary) or liver toxicity—case reports.

Porphyria—rare.

Abnormally low white blood cell count   case report.

▷ **Possible Effects on Sexual Function:**   Rare impotence (300 mg/day); enlargement and tenderness of male breasts—case reports.

Adverse Effects That May Mimic Natural Diseases or Disorders

Reversible jaundice may suggest viral hepatitis.

Natural Diseases or Disorders That May Be Activated by This Drug

Glaucoma, myasthenia gravis.

Possible Effects on Laboratory Tests

White blood cell counts: decreased.

Liver function tests: increased liver enzymes (ALT/GPT, AST/GOT, and alkaline phosphatase), increased bilirubin.

CAUTION

1. Thorough heart exam (including electrocardiogram) is critical prior to using this drug.
2. Periodic heart exams are needed to follow drug responses. Some people may have heart rhythm or function declines. Close monitoring of heart rate, rhythm, and overall performance is essential.
3. Dose must be individualized. Do not change your dose without your doctor's supervision.

4. Talk with your doctor about signs and symptoms of low blood sugar.
5. Do not take any other antiarrhythmic drug while taking this drug unless directed to do so by your doctor.

Precautions for Use

By Infants and Children: In pediatric patients, disopyramide is given on a mg-per-kg-of-body-mass basis. Dose is then divided into equal doses, given at times determined by patient response. Some patients from 1 to 4 years old will receive 10 to 20 mg per kg of body mass per day, divided into equal doses and given every 6 hours. Initial use of this drug requires hospitalization and supervision by a qualified pediatrician.

By Those Over 60 Years of Age: Reduced kidney function may require dose reductions. This drug can aggravate existing prostatism (see Glossary) and promote constipation. Watch closely for light-headedness, dizziness, unsteadiness, and tendency to fall.

▷ ### Advisability of Use During Pregnancy

Pregnancy Category: C. See Pregnancy Risk Categories at the back of this book.
Animal studies: No birth defects reported in rats and rabbits.
Human studies: Adequate studies of pregnant women are not available. It has been reported that this drug can cause contractions of the pregnant uterus. Use this drug only if clearly needed. Ask your physician for guidance.

Advisability of Use If Breast-Feeding

Presence of this drug in breast milk: Yes.
Avoid drug or refrain from nursing.

Habit-Forming Potential: None.

Effects of Overdose: Dryness of eyes, nose, mouth, and throat; impaired urination; constipation; marked drop in blood pressure; abnormal heart rhythms; congestive heart failure.

Possible Effects of Long-Term Use: None reported.

Suggested Periodic Examinations While Taking This Drug (at physician's discretion)

Electrocardiograms, complete blood counts, potassium blood levels.

▷ ### While Taking This Drug, Observe the Following

Foods: No restrictions. Ask your physician regarding need for salt restriction and advisability of eating potassium-rich foods.
Beverages: No restrictions. May be taken with milk.
▷ *Alcohol:* Use caution. Alcohol can increase the blood-pressure-lowering effects and the blood-sugar-lowering effects of this drug.
Tobacco Smoking: Nicotine can irritate the heart, reducing effectiveness. I advise everyone to quit smoking.
▷ *Other Drugs*

Disopyramide may *increase* the effects of
- antihypertensive drugs, and cause excessive lowering of blood pressure.
- atropinelike drugs (see *anticholinergic drugs* in Drug Classes).
- warfarin (Coumadin, etc.); check INR (prothrombin times) more often, adjust dosing.

Disopyramide may *decrease* the effects of
- ambenonium (Mytelase).
- neostigmine (Prostigmin).
- pyridostigmine (Mestinon).

Benefits of these three drugs in treating myasthenia gravis may be reduced. Disopyramide *taken concurrently* with

- amiodarone (Codarone) may result in an abnormal heart effect (torsade de pointes).
- beta-blockers (see Drug Classes) may result in abnormally low heart rates.
- digoxin (Lanoxin) can cause digoxin toxicity.
- erythromycins (E.E.S., others) can cause increased disopyramide blood concentrations and abnormal heart effects. Caution is advised in combining with azithromycin, clarithromycin, or dirithromycin because they are structurally similar.
- insulin or oral antidiabetic drugs (see Drug Classes) agents may result in abnormally low blood sugars.
- phenobarbital may result in loss of disopyramide's effectiveness.
- phenytoin (Dilantin) can result in decreased disopyramide effectiveness and accumulation of a metabolite of phenytoin, which causes a severe increase in anticholinergic effects.
- potassium supplements may result in elevated potassium levels, which can lead to disopyramide toxicity.
- quinidine can cause increases in disopyramide blood levels and decreases in quinidine levels.
- ritonavir (Norvir) and perhaps other protease inhibitors (see Drug Classes) may increase disopyramide blood levels and lead to toxicity.
- sparfloxacin (Zagam) may result in increased risk of abnormal heart rhythms. DO NOT combine.
- verapamil (Calan, others) can precipitate or worsen congestive heart failure.
- warfarin (Coumadin) may cause increased bleeding risk. INR must be checked more frequently.

The following drugs may *decrease* the effects of disopyramide:

- all diuretics that promote potassium loss.
- rifabutin (Mycobutin).
- rifampin (Rimactane, Rifadin).

▷ *Driving, Hazardous Activities:* May cause dizziness or blurred vision. Limit activities as needed.

Aviation Note: The use of this drug *may be a disqualification* for piloting. Consult a designated aviation medical examiner.

Exposure to Sun: Use caution. This drug causes photosensitivity (see Glossary).

Exposure to Heat: Use caution. The use of this drug in hot environments may increase the risk of heatstroke.

Occurrence of Unrelated Illness: Vomiting, diarrhea, or dehydration can affect this drug's action adversely. Report such developments promptly.

Discontinuation: This drug should not be stopped abruptly after long-term use. Ask your doctor for help regarding gradual dose reduction.

DISULFIRAM (di SULF i ram)

Introduced: 1948   **Class:** Antialcoholism   **Prescription:** USA: Yes
Controlled Drug: USA: No; Canada: No   **Available as Generic:** USA: Yes
Canada: No
Brand Name: Antabuse

```
┌─────────────────────────────────────────────────────────────┐
│                    BENEFITS versus RISKS                      │
│        Possible Benefits              Possible Risks          │
│   EFFECTIVE ADJUNCT IN THE       DANGEROUS REACTIONS WITH     │
│   TREATMENT OF CHRONIC             ALCOHOL INGESTION          │
│   ALCOHOLISM                     Acute psychotic reactions    │
│                                  Drug-induced liver damage    │
│                                  Drug-induced optic and/or    │
│                                    peripheral neuritis        │
│                                  Low blood platelets          │
└─────────────────────────────────────────────────────────────┘
```

▷ **Principal Uses**

As a Single Drug Product: Uses currently included in FDA-approved labeling: Deters abusive drinking of alcoholic beverages. It does not abolish the craving or impulse to drink.

Other (unlabeled) generally accepted uses: (1) Limited use in helping skin problems (dermatitis) caused by nickel exposure; (2) some data showing increase in infection-fighting cells (CD4) in AIDS.

How This Drug Works: This drug blocks normal liver enzyme activity after alcohol is changed to acetaldehyde. This causes accumulation of acetaldehyde, and causes the disulfiram (Antabuse) reaction (see Glossary).

Available Dose Forms and Strengths

Tablets — 250 mg, 500 mg

▷ **Usual Adult Dose Range:** Once all signs of intoxication are gone and no less than 12 hours after the last alcohol drink, therapy begins with 500 mg/day for 1 to 2 weeks, followed by an ongoing dose of 250 mg/day. Range is 125 mg to 500 mg daily and is individually determined. Maximum daily dose is 500 mg. **Note: Actual dose and schedule must be determined for each patient individually.**

Conditions Requiring Dosing Adjustments

Liver Function: This drug is a benefit-to-risk decision in mild liver compromise. Disulfiram is clearly contraindicated in portal hypertension and active hepatitis.

Kidney Function: Dosing adjustments are not indicated.

Diabetes: People with diabetes who take disulfiram can be at increased risk for diabetic blood vessel (micro- and macrovascular) problems. The risk is worsened by potential adverse drug effects such as increased cholesterol levels and peripheral neuropathy.

Lung Disease: Accumulation of a metabolite may occur in severe lung problems. Drug levels or dose reduction will be needed.

▷ **Dosing Instructions:** The tablet may be crushed and taken with or following food to decrease stomach irritation.

Usual Duration of Use: Use on a regular schedule for several months is needed to see effectiveness in deterring alcohol use. If tolerated well, use should continue until self-control and sobriety is ongoing.

▷ **This Drug Should Not Be Taken If**

• you have had a severe allergic reaction to disulfiram. (Note: The interaction of disulfiram and alcohol is *not* an allergic reaction.)

• you have taken any form of alcohol within the past 12 hours.

- you are pregnant.
- you have a history of psychosis.
- you are taking paraldehyde.
- you have significant exposure to ethylene dibromide where you live or work. Disulfiram inhibits the removal of this chemical and enhances the ability of ethylene dibromide to cause cancer.
- you are taking (or have taken recently) metronidazole (Flagyl).
- you have coronary heart disease or a serious heart rhythm disorder.

▷ **Inform Your Physician Before Taking This Drug If**
- you have used disulfiram in the past.
- you do not intend to avoid alcohol completely while taking this drug.
- you do not understand what will happen if you drink alcohol while taking this drug.
- you are planning pregnancy in the near future.
- you have a history of diabetes, epilepsy, or kidney or liver disease.
- you take oral anticoagulants, digitalis, isoniazid, paraldehyde, or phenytoin (Dilantin).
- you have a history of low thyroid function (hypothyroidism).
- you have a history of lung disease.
- you plan to have surgery under general anesthesia while taking this drug.

Possible Side Effects (natural, expected, and unavoidable drug actions)
Drowsiness, lethargy during early use.
Offensive breath and body odor.

▷ **Possible Adverse Effects** (unusual, unexpected, and infrequent reactions)
If any of the following develop, consult your physician promptly for guidance.
Mild Adverse Effects
Allergic reactions: Skin rash, hives—case reports.
Headache, dizziness, restlessness, tremor—infrequent.
Metallic or garliclike taste, indigestion (usually subsides in 2 weeks).
Decreased or increased blood pressure—possible.
Serious Adverse Effects
Allergic reactions: Severe skin rashes, drug-induced hepatitis—rare.
Idiosyncratic reaction: Acute toxic effect on brain, including abnormal movements and psychotic behavior—case reports.
Optic or peripheral neuritis (see Glossary)—case reports.
Seizures—case reports.
Decreased thyroid gland function—possible.
May increase risk for blood vessel problems in people with diabetes or cause low blood platelets—case reports.
Carpal tunnel syndrome, peripheral neuropathy—case reports.

▷ **Possible Effects on Sexual Function:**   Decreased libido and/or impaired erection in users taking recommended doses of 125 to 500 mg daily—case reports.

Adverse Effects That May Mimic Natural Diseases or Disorders
Liver reaction may suggest viral hepatitis.
Brain toxicity may suggest spontaneous psychosis.

Possible Effects on Laboratory Tests

Blood cholesterol level: increased.

INR (prothrombin time): increased (taken concurrently with warfarin).

Liver function tests: liver enzymes increased (ALT/GPT, AST/GOT, and alkaline phosphatase), increased bilirubin.

CAUTION

1. No one intoxicated with alcohol should take this drug.
2. Patients must be fully informed about purpose and actions of this drug *before* treatment is started.
3. Long-term use requires exam for reduced thyroid function.
4. Carry a personal identification card noting you are taking this drug.

Precautions for Use

By Infants and Children: Safety and effectiveness for those under 12 years of age not established.

By Those Over 60 Years of Age: Watch for excessive sedation when the drug is started. *Do not* perform an "alcohol trial" to see the effects of this drug.

▷ Advisability of Use During Pregnancy

Pregnancy Category: C. See Pregnancy Risk Categories at the back of this book.

Animal studies: No defects reported in rats and hamsters.

Human studies: Two reports indicate that four of eight fetuses exposed had serious birth defects. Adequate studies of pregnant women are not available. Avoid this drug completely if possible.

Advisability of Use If Breast-Feeding

Presence of this drug in breast milk: Unknown.

Talk with your doctor, as this is a question of the benefit of the drug versus the risk of adverse effects to the fetus.

Habit-Forming Potential: None.

Effects of Overdose: Marked lethargy, impaired memory, altered behavior, confusion, unsteadiness, weakness, stomach pain, nausea, vomiting, diarrhea.

Possible Effects of Long-Term Use: Decreased function of thyroid gland.

Suggested Periodic Examinations While Taking This Drug (at physician's discretion)

Visual acuity, liver function tests, thyroid function tests.

▷ While Taking This Drug, Observe the Following

Foods: Avoid all foods prepared with alcohol, including sauces, marinades, vinegars, desserts, etc. Ask when dining out about use of alcohol in cooking food. Many herbal medicines such as Ginseng and Echinacea contain alcohol. DO NOT combine them with Disulfiram.

Beverages: Avoid all punches, fruit drinks, etc., that may contain alcohol. This drug may be taken with milk.

▷ *Alcohol: **Avoid completely in all forms*** while taking this drug and for 14 days after the last dose. Disulfiram and alcohol—even in small amounts—produces the disulfiram (Antabuse) reaction. This starts 5 to 10 minutes after alcohol: intense flushing, severe headache, shortness of breath, chest pains, nausea, repeated vomiting, sweating, and weakness. If large amounts of alcohol: reaction may progress to blurred vision, vertigo, confusion, severely low blood pressure, and loss of consciousness. May go on to convulsions and death. Reaction may last from 30 minutes to hours, depending upon amount of alcohol and disulfiram.

Tobacco Smoking: No interactions expected. I advise everyone to quit smoking.

Marijuana Smoking: Possible increase in drowsiness or lethargy.

▷ *Other Drugs*

Disulfiram may *increase* the effects of
- chlordiazepoxide (Librium) and diazepam (Valium), and cause oversedation. Other benzodiazepines such as alprazolam, clonazepam, clorazepate, flurazepam, halazepam, prazepam, or triazolam may also be subject to this interaction.
- oral anticoagulants (warfarin, etc.), and increase the risk of bleeding; dose adjustments may be necessary.
- paraldehyde, and cause excessive depression of brain function.
- phenytoin (Dilantin), and cause toxicity; dose must be decreased.

Disulfiram may *decrease* the effects of
- perphenazine (Trilafon, etc.).

Disulfiram *taken concurrently* with
- bacampicillin (Spectrobid) can theoretically cause a disulfiram reaction, but no cases have been reported.
- cisplatin (Platinol) can increase risk of toxicity of cisplatin.
- cyclosporine (Sandimmune) may result in a disulfiram reaction, as there is alcohol in the intravenous and oral forms of cyclosporine.
- isoniazid (INH, etc.) may cause acute mental problems and incoordination.
- metronidazole (Flagyl) may cause acute mental and behavioral disturbances, making it necessary to stop treatment.
- omeprazole (Prilosec) may result in increased disulfiram levels and toxicity.
- over-the-counter (OTC) cough syrups, tonics, etc., containing alcohol may cause a disulfiram (Antabuse) reaction; avoid concurrent use (see *Over-the-counter-drugs* in Glossary).
- paraldehyde may result in a disulfiram reaction.
- theophylline (Theo-Dur, others) can lead to theophylline toxicity because the metabolism of theophylline is decreased.
- warfarin will result in an increased risk of bleeding. More frequent INR testing is recommended.

The following drugs may *increase* the effects of disulfiram:
- amitriptyline (Elavil), and perhaps other tricyclic antidepressants may enhance the disulfiram + alcohol interaction; avoid concurrent use of these drugs.

▷ *Driving, Hazardous Activities:* This drug may cause drowsiness or dizziness. Limit activities as necessary.

Aviation Note: Alcoholism *is a disqualification* for piloting. Consult a designated aviation medical examiner.

Exposure to Sun: No restrictions.

Exposure to Environmental Chemicals: Thiram, a pesticide, and carbon disulfide, a pesticide and industrial solvent, can have additive toxic effects. Watch for toxic effects on the brain and nervous system.

Discontinuation: This medicine is only part of your program. Do not stop it unless you have talked with your doctor. Even if it is stopped, no alcohol should be ingested for 14 days.

DORNASE ALPHA (DOOR nase AL fa)

Introduced: 1994   **Class:** Anti-cystic-fibrosis agent   **Prescription:** USA:
Yes   **Controlled Drug:**   USA: No; Canada: No   **Available as Generic:**   USA:
No Canada: No
Brand Name: Pulmozyme

BENEFITS versus RISKS	
Possible Benefits	*Possible Risks*
DECREASED MUCOUS VISCOSITY	Hoarseness
IMPROVED LUNG FUNCTION	Antibodies to DNA
DECREASED OCCURRENCE OF	Facial swelling (edema)
RESPIRATORY INFECTIONS	
DECREASED NUMBER OF	
HOSPITALIZATIONS	

▷ **Principal Uses**

As a Single Drug Product: Uses currently included in FDA-approved labeling: Eases symptoms of cystic fibrosis (used with standard therapies).

Other (unlabeled) generally accepted uses: May help treat chronic bronchitis.

How This Drug Works: Large amounts of DNA is found in sputum of people with cystic fibrosis, making it thicker than normal. Dornase breaks the DNA down, making the sputum easier to remove. Other undiscovered mechanisms may also account for its benefits.

Available Dose Forms and Strengths

Solution — 2.5 ml ampules of 1.0 mg/ml dornase alpha (2.5 mg)

▷ **Recommended Dose Ranges** (Actual dose and schedule must be determined for each patient individually.)

Infants and Children: Now approved for patients 3 months to less than 5 years of age. Rashes, cough, and runny nose (rhinitis) may happen at a higher rate in this population than in older patients.

5 to 60 Years of Age: One 2.5-mg dose administered by one of the tested nebulizers each day. Some selected patients may benefit from twice-daily dosing (older patients).

Over 60 Years of Age: Same as 12 to 60 years of age.

Conditions Requiring Dosing Adjustments

Liver Function: Not defined.

Kidney Function: Not defined.

▷ **Dosing Instructions:**   Solution must be refrigerated and protected from strong light. The drug should not be used if it is cloudy or discolored. Do **not** mix dornase with other medicines. Clinical trials have only been conducted with the Hudson T Up-Draft 2, Marquest Acorn ll, and Pulmo-Aide compressor. The reusable PARI LC Jet nebulizer and PARI PRONEB compressor were also tested. Do **not** use with other equipment.

Usual Duration of Use: Regular use for up to 8 days may be needed in cystic fibrosis. Long-term use (up to 12 months has been studied) requires periodic physician evaluation.

Possible Advantages of This Drug
Reduction in number of infections, use of antibiotics, and hospitalizations with minimal side effects.

▷ **This Drug Should Not Be Taken If**
- you have had an allergic reaction to it.
- you have an allergy to Chinese hamster ovary cells.

▷ **Inform Your Physician Before Taking This Drug If**
- you had a rash after the last dose was taken.
- you are uncertain how to use the nebulizer or compressor.
- you are uncertain how much to take or how often to take it.

Possible Side Effects (natural, expected, and unavoidable drug actions)
Hoarseness—may be frequent.

▷ **Possible Adverse Effects** (unusual, unexpected, and infrequent reactions)
If any of the following develop, consult your physician promptly for guidance.
Mild Adverse Effects
Allergic reactions: rash—infrequent (may be more likely in those 3 months to less than 5 years old).
Cough or runny nose—infrequent (may be more likely in those 3 months to less than 5 years old).
Mild pharyngitis or laryngitis—infrequent.
Conjunctivitis—infrequent.
Chest pain—has been reported.
Facial swelling—rare.
Serious Adverse Effects
Allergic reactions: None defined at present.
Antibodies to DNA (2–4%).

▷ **Possible Effects on Sexual Function:** None reported.

Possible Delayed Adverse Effects: None reported.

Possible Effects on Laboratory Tests
Antibodies to DNA.

CAUTION
1. This drug should only be used with one of the studied nebulizers and compressors.
2. Do not use the drug if it is cloudy or discolored.

Precautions for Use
By Infants and Children: Safety and effectiveness for those under 5 years of age not established.
By Those Over 60 Years of Age: No changes or precautions.

▷ **Advisability of Use During Pregnancy**
Pregnancy Category: B. See Pregnancy Risk Categories at the back of this book.
Animal studies: Studies in rats and rabbits at up to 600 times the usual human dose have not revealed any harm to the fetus.
Human studies: Adequate studies of pregnant women are not available.
Ask your doctor for guidance.

Advisability of Use If Breast-Feeding
Presence of this drug in breast milk: Unknown.
Avoid drug or refrain from nursing.

Habit-Forming Potential: None.

Effects of Overdose: Single doses of up to 180 times the usual human dose in rats and monkeys have been well tolerated.

Possible Effects of Long-Term Use: Not defined.

Suggested Periodic Examinations While Taking This Drug (at physician's discretion)

Periodic pulmonary function tests.

▷ **While Taking This Drug, Observe the Following**

Foods: No restrictions.

Nutritional Support: Continued enzyme and nutritional support is still needed.

Beverages: No specific restrictions.

▷ *Alcohol:* Follow your doctor's advice relative to alcohol use.

Tobacco Smoking: No interaction, but smoking irritates airways. I advise everyone to quit smoking.

▷ *Other Drugs:* Clinical studies have revealed that dornase is compatible with medicines typically used to manage cystic fibrosis. Specific drug interactions are not documented at present.

▷ *Driving, Hazardous Activities:* Specific limitations because of drug effects are not defined at present.

Aviation Note: The use of this drug *may be a disqualification* for piloting. Consult a designated aviation medical examiner.

Exposure to Sun: No restrictions.

Discontinuation: This drug's benefits stop soon after its regular use is stopped. It must be continued indefinitely to continue to benefit.

Special Storage Instructions: This drug should be stored at 36–46 degrees F and should be protected from light. Unused ampules should be stored in their protective pouch in the refrigerator.

DOXAZOSIN (dox AY zoh sin)

Introduced: 1986   **Class:** Antihypertensive   **Prescription:** USA: Yes
Controlled Drug: USA: No   **Available as Generic:** No
Brand Name: Cardura

BENEFITS versus RISKS	
Possible Benefits	*Possible Risks*
EFFECTIVE TREATMENT OF MILD TO MODERATE HYPERTENSION when used alone or in combination with other antihypertensive drugs	"First-dose" drop in blood pressure, but without fainting
	Dizziness
	Fluid retention
TREATMENT OF BENIGN PROSTATIC HYPERPLASIA	Rapid heart rate

▷ **Principal Uses**

As a Single Drug Product: Uses currently included in FDA-approved labeling: (1) Once-daily treatment of mild to moderate hypertension; (2) treats benign prostatic hypertrophy/hyperplasia.

Other (unlabeled) generally accepted uses: (1) Used with other drugs to treat congestive heart failure; (2) treats pheochromocytoma.

How This Drug Works: By blocking sympathetic nervous system actions, this drug causes blood vessels to relax, lowering blood pressure. It also lowers peak detrussor muscle pressure, prevents activation of alpha-1 receptors, preventing smooth muscle contractions in the part of the urethra near the prostate and bladder neck, improving urine outflow.

Available Dose Forms and Strengths
Tablets — 1 mg, 2 mg, 4 mg, 8 mg

▷ **Usual Adult Dose Range:** Starts with a "test dose" of 1 mg to check patient's response in the first 2 to 6 hours. If tolerated, dose is increased as needed and tolerated every 2 weeks. Taken as a single dose at bedtime. Doses in excess of 4 mg may be more likely to cause light-headedness or dizziness, and should be avoided. Daily maximum is 16 mg. For benign prostatic hyperplasia (BPH), a similar test dose is used; usual effective doses are from 4 to 8 mg. **Note: Actual dose and schedule must be determined for each patient individually.**

Conditions Requiring Dosing Adjustments
Liver Function: Extreme caution and lower doses **must** be used if the drug is used in patients with liver compromise.
Kidney Function: Doses of 1–16 mg have been used. In one study of kidney compromise, 1 mg decreased the blood pressure for 3 days.

▷ **Dosing Instructions:** The tablet may be crushed and is best taken at bedtime to avoid orthostatic hypotension (see Glossary). May be taken without regard to food.

Usual Duration of Use: Regular use for 6 to 8 weeks needed to see this benefit in controlling hypertension. Long-term use requires supervision by your doctor.

Possible Advantages of This Drug
May be used to start treatment.
Effective with once-a-day dose.
Causes depression or impotence infrequently.
Lowers blood cholesterol and sugar levels.
Does not lose effectiveness with long-term use.

▷ **This Drug Should Not Be Taken If**
• you have had an allergic reaction to this drug or to prazosin (Minipres) or terazosin (Hytrin).
• you have active liver disease.

▷ **Inform Your Physician Before Taking This Drug If**
• you have had orthostatic hypotension (see Glossary) when using other antihypertensive drugs.
• you have a history of mental depression.
• you have impaired circulation to the brain, or a history of stroke.
• you have coronary artery disease.
• you are taking other medicine to help lower your blood pressure.
• you have had a stroke and have high blood pressure.
• you have a history of low white blood cells.
• you have active liver disease or impaired liver function.

- you have impaired kidney function.
- you have angina (active coronary artery disease) and you are not taking a beta-blocking drug (consult your physician).
- you will have surgery with general anesthesia.

Possible Side Effects (natural, expected, and unavoidable drug actions)
Orthostatic hypotension—infrequent; drowsiness, salt and water retention, dry mouth—rare; nasal congestion, constipation—rare.

▷ **Possible Adverse Effects** (unusual, unexpected, and infrequent reactions)
If any of the following develop, consult your physician promptly for guidance.

Mild Adverse Effects
Allergic reaction: Skin rash or itching—rare.
Headache, dizziness, fatigue, nervousness, numbness and tingling, blurred vision—rare to infrequent.
Palpitation, rapid heart rate, or shortness of breath—rare.
Nausea, diarrhea, indigestion—rare to infrequent.
Increased urination—rare.

Serious Adverse Effects
Mental depression—rare.
Arrhythmias—case reports.
Decreased blood sugar (glucose)—case reports.
Low white blood cell counts (has not caused symptoms in patients who had follow-up visits).

▷ **Possible Effects on Sexual Function:**   Impotence—rare.

Natural Diseases or Disorders That May Be Activated by This Drug
Latent coronary artery insufficiency.

Possible Effects on Laboratory Tests
White blood cell counts: rare and mild decreases.
Blood lipid tests: decreased total cholesterol, LDL cholesterol, and cholesterol/HDL ratio; decreased triglycerides; increased HDL.
Blood sugar level: variable decreases.

CAUTION
1. "First-dose" precipitous drop in blood pressure, with or without fainting, is possible and can happen in the first 6 hours. Starting dose is 1 mg taken at bedtime for the first week. Lie down and do not get up after taking these trial doses.
2. Impaired liver function will increase drug level and require smaller than usual doses.
3. Ask your doctor or pharmacist before you take nonprescription products for allergic rhinitis or head colds. These medicines may contain drugs that may interact with doxazosin.

Precautions for Use
By Infants and Children: Safety and effectiveness for those under 12 years of age not established.
By Those Over 60 Years of Age: Starting dose of no more than 1 mg/day for the first week. Later dose increases must be very gradual. Orthostatic hypotension can cause unexpected falls and injury. Sit or lie down promptly if you feel light-headed or dizzy. Report dizziness or chest pain promptly.

▷ **Advisability of Use During Pregnancy**
  Pregnancy Category: C, B by one researcher. See Pregnancy Risk Categories at the back of this book.
  Animal studies: No birth defects found in rat or rabbit studies.
  Human studies: Adequate studies of pregnant women are not available.
  Use this drug only if clearly needed. Ask your doctor for help.

Advisability of Use If Breast-Feeding
  Presence of this drug in breast milk: Unknown.
  Watch nursing infant closely and discontinue drug or nursing if adverse effects develop.

Habit-Forming Potential: None.

Effects of Overdose: Orthostatic hypotension, headache, generalized flushing, rapid heart rate, extreme weakness, irregular heart rhythm, circulatory collapse.

Possible Effects of Long-Term Use: None reported.

Suggested Periodic Examinations While Taking This Drug (at physician's discretion)
  Measurements of blood pressure in lying, sitting, and standing positions.
  Measurements of body weight to check for fluid retention.

▷ **While Taking This Drug, Observe the Following**
  Foods: No restrictions. Avoid excessive salt intake.
  Beverages: No restrictions. May be taken with milk.
▷ *Alcohol:* Use with extreme caution. Alcohol can exaggerate the blood-pressure-lowering actions of this drug and cause excessive reduction.
  Tobacco Smoking: Nicotine can contribute to this drug's ability to intensify coronary insufficiency. All forms of tobacco should be avoided.
▷ *Other Drugs*
  The following drugs may *increase* the effects of doxazosin:
  • beta adrenergic-blocking drugs (see Drug Classes); severity and duration of the "first-dose" response may be increased.
  The following drugs may *decrease* the effects of doxazosin:
  • estrogens.
  • indomethacin (Indocin) and other NSAIDs.
  • Ritonavir (Norvir).
▷ *Driving, Hazardous Activities:* This drug may cause dizziness or drowsiness. Restrict activities as necessary.
  Aviation Note: The use of this drug *is a disqualification* for piloting. Consult a designated aviation medical examiner.
  Exposure to Sun: No restrictions.
  Exposure to Cold: Use caution. Cold environments may increase coronary insufficiency (angina) and hypothermia (see Glossary).
  Heavy Exercise or Exertion: Excessive exertion can augment this drug's ability to induce angina.
  Discontinuation: If you are taking this drug for congestive heart failure, do not stop it abruptly. Ask your physician for guidance.

DOXEPIN (DOX e pin)

Introduced: 1969   **Class:** Antidepressant   **Prescription:** USA: Yes
Controlled Drug: USA: No; Canada: No   **Available as Generic:** USA: Yes;
Canada: No
Brand Names: Adapin, Sinequan, ✦Triadapin, Zonalon

BENEFITS versus RISKS	
Possible Benefits	*Possible Risks*
EFFECTIVE RELIEF OF ENDOGENOUS DEPRESSION	ADVERSE BEHAVIORAL EFFECTS: Confusion, disorientation, hallucinations, delusions
EFFECTIVE RELIEF OF ANXIETY AND NERVOUS TENSION	CONVERSION OF DEPRESSION TO MANIA in manic-depressive (bipolar) disorders
EFFECTIVE RELIEF OF SOME KINDS OF ITCHING (TOPICAL FORM)	Aggravation of schizophrenia and paranoia
Possibly beneficial in other depressive disorders	Rare blood cell disorders
	Rare liver toxicity
	Low blood pressure on standing

▷ **Principal Uses**

As a *Single Drug Product:* Uses currently included in FDA-approved labeling: (1) Relieves symptoms of spontaneous (endogenous) depression, refractory depression, neurotic depression, mixed depression anxiety, and depression and anxiety in alcoholism; (2) helps treat sleep disturbances; (3) treats depression and anxiety associated with alcoholism.

Other (unlabeled) generally accepted uses: (1) Helps decrease frequency of urination at night in people with excessively active detrusor muscles; (2) pain management in cancer patients; (3) can ease the extent of lowered blood glucose (postprandial hypoglycemia) after meals in some patients; (4) management of post-traumatic stress disorder; (5) helps itching and swelling of unknown cause (idiopathic urticaria); (6) may decrease craving when people try to stop smoking.

How This Drug Works: Relieves depression by slowly restoring normal levels of chemicals (norepinephrine and serotonin) that transmit nerve impulses.

Available Dose Forms and Strengths
Capsules — 10 mg, 25 mg, 50 mg, 75 mg, 100 mg, 150 mg
Oral concentrate — 10 mg/ml
Topical cream — 50 mg/g

▷ **Usual Adult Dose Range:**   Initially 25 mg three to four times daily. Dose may be increased cautiously as needed and tolerated by 10 to 25 mg daily at intervals of 1 week. Usual maintenance dose is 75 to 150 mg daily. Usually there is no greater benefit achieved by using more than 300 mg/day. There have been rare uses of 500 mg/day. When the optimal requirement is determined, it may be taken at bedtime as one dose.

Topical cream: The cream is applied four times daily for up to 8 days. **Note: Actual dose and schedule must be determined for each patient individually.**

Conditions Requiring Dosing Adjustments

Liver Function: This drug should be used with caution and in lower doses in people with liver compromise. It is a rare cause of liver problems.

Kidney Function: Use with caution in patients with compromised kidneys and urine outflow problems.

▷ **Dosing Instructions:**   May be taken without regard to meals. Capsule may be opened to take it. The cream may be applied four times a day for up to 8 days. DO NOT cover the area where cream was applied with an occlusive (water-tight) dressing, as this may lead to excessive drug absorption.

Usual Duration of Use: Some benefit may be apparent within to 2 weeks, but adequate response may require continual use for 3 weeks or longer. Long-term use should not exceed 6 months without evaluation by your doctor.

▷ **This Drug Should Not Be Taken If**
- you have had an allergic reaction to it previously.
- you take or took a monoamine oxidase (MAO) type A inhibitor (see Drug Classes) in the past 14 days.
- you are recovering from a recent heart attack.
- you have significant urine retention.
- you have narrow-angle glaucoma.

▷ **Inform Your Physician Before Taking This Drug If**
- you are allergic or sensitive to any other tricyclic antidepressant (see Drug Classes).
- you have a history of diabetes, epilepsy, glaucoma, heart disease, liver compromise, prostate gland enlargement, or overactive thyroid function.
- you are pregnant or are breast-feeding.
- you will have surgery with general anesthesia.

Possible Side Effects (natural, expected, and unavoidable drug actions)

Drowsiness—frequent and may be dose related.

Blurred vision, dry mouth, constipation, impaired urination, low blood pressure on standing—infrequent to frequent.

▷ **Possible Adverse Effects** (unusual, unexpected, and infrequent reactions)

If any of the following develop, consult your physician promptly for guidance.

Mild Adverse Effects

Allergic reactions: skin rash, hives, swelling of face or tongue, drug fever (see Glossary)—possible.

Ringing in the ears—rare.

Stinging or burning of the skin with application of doxepin cream—possible.

Headache, dizziness, drowsiness, weakness, fainting, unsteady gait, tremors—case reports.

Increased appetite, craving for sweets, weight gain—case reports.

Peculiar taste, irritation of tongue or mouth, nausea, indigestion—case reports.

Fluctuation of blood sugar levels—case reports.

Serious Adverse Effects

Allergic reactions: hepatitis, with or without jaundice (see Glossary).

Confusion, hallucinations, agitation, restlessness, delusions—rare with systemic use.

Bone marrow depression (see Glossary): fatigue, weakness, fever, sore throat, abnormal bleeding or bruising—case reports.

Peripheral neuritis (see Glossary): numbness, tingling, pain, loss of strength in arms and legs—case reports.

Elevations in temperature or seizures—case reports.

Kidney or liver damage—case reports.

Parkinson-like disorders (see Glossary)—usually mild and infrequent; more likely to occur in the elderly.

Abnormal heart rhythm or rate—case reports.

▷ **Possible Effects on Sexual Function:** Female breast enlargement with milk production.

Swelling of testicles. Enlargement and tenderness of male breast tissue (gynecomastia). Ejaculation disorder. Painful and persistent erection (priapism)—case reports.

Adverse Effects That May Mimic Natural Diseases or Disorders

Liver toxicity may suggest viral hepatitis.

Natural Diseases or Disorders That May Be Activated by This Drug

Latent diabetes, epilepsy, glaucoma, impaired urination due to prostate gland enlargement (prostatism; see Glossary).

Possible Effects on Laboratory Tests

White blood cell and platelet counts: may be decreased.

Liver function tests: increased.

Blood sugar (glucose): may be increased.

CAUTION

1. Dose must be adjusted for each person individually. Report for follow-up evaluation and laboratory tests as directed by your physician.
2. It is advisable to withhold this drug if electroconvulsive therapy (ECT, "shock" treatment) is to be used to treat your depression.

Precautions for Use

By Infants and Children: Safety and effectiveness for those under 12 years of age not established.

By Those Over 60 Years of Age: During the first 2 weeks, watch for confusion, agitation, forgetfulness, delusions, and hallucinations. Lower doses or stopping the drug may be necessary. Unsteadiness may make falls and injury more likely. Drug may increase the degree of impaired urination seen with prostate gland enlargement (prostatism).

▷ **Advisability of Use During Pregnancy**

Pregnancy Category: C. See Pregnancy Risk Categories at the back of this book.

Animal studies: No birth defects reported in rats, rabbits, dogs, or monkeys.

Human studies: Adequate studies of pregnant women are not available.

Use this drug only if clearly needed. If possible, avoid use during the first 3 months and the last month. Ask your doctor for guidance.

Advisability of Use If Breast-Feeding

Presence of this drug in breast milk: Yes.

Monitor nursing infant very closely and discontinue drug or nursing if adverse effects develop.

Habit-Forming Potential: None.

Effects of Overdose: Confusion, hallucinations, marked drowsiness, heart palpitations, dilated pupils, tremors, stupor, deep sleep, coma, convulsions.

Suggested Periodic Examinations While Taking This Drug (at physician's discretion)

Complete blood cell counts, liver function tests, serial blood pressure readings, and electrocardiograms.

▷ **While Taking This Drug, Observe the Following**

Foods: No restrictions. This drug may increase the appetite and cause excessive weight gain.

Beverages: No restrictions. May be taken with milk.

▷   *Alcohol:* Avoid completely. May markedly increase intoxicating effects of alcohol and accentuate depressant action on brain function.

Tobacco Smoking: May hasten drug removal, requiring higher doses. I advise everyone to quit smoking.

Marijuana Smoking: Possible increase in heart rate.

▷   *Other Drugs*

Doxepin may *increase* the effects of

- albuterol (Ventolin) on blood vessels.
- atropinelike drugs (see *anticholinergic drugs* in Drug Classes).
- dicumarol, and increase the risk of bleeding; dose adjustments may be necessary.
- other drugs with central nervous system effects (narcotics, benzodiazepines, etc.; see Drug Classes).
- phenytoin (Dilantin).
- thyroid hormones.

Doxepin may *decrease* the effects of

- clonidine (Catapres).
- guanethidine (Ismelin).

Doxepin *taken concurrently* with

- bepridil (Vascor) may result in abnormal heart beats. Do not combine.
- carbamazepine (Tegretol) may decrease the effectiveness of doxepin.
- cimetidine (Tagamet) may result in doxepin toxicity (urine retention, dry mouth).
- cholestyramine (Questran) may blunt doxepin levels and benefits.
- diphenhydramine (Benadryl) or other drugs with anticholinergic actions may result in increased risk of urine retention or bowel obstruction.
- epinephrine will result in an exaggerated increase in blood pressure.
- estrogens may change the action of doxepin.
- fluoxetine (Prozac) can result in doxepin toxicity.
- grepafloxacin (Raxar) may result in abnormal heart beats. Do not combine.
- meperidine (Demerol) may result in an increased risk of respiratory depression.
- methylphenidate (Ritalin) can result in doxepin toxicity.
- monoamine oxidase (MAO) type A inhibitor drugs (see Drug Classes) may cause high fever, delirium, and convulsions.
- paroxetine (Paxil) can cause increased doxepin levels and toxicity.
- propoxyphene (Darvon) can result in doxepin toxicity.
- pseudoephedrine will result in abnormal increases in blood pressure and should not be combined in therapy.

- quinidine (Quinaglute) can result in doxepin toxicity.
- ritonavir (Norvir) may result in doxepin toxicity.
- sertraline (Zoloft) can result in increased doxepin levels.
- sparfloxacin (Zagam) may result in abnormal heart beats. Do not combine.
- tramadol (Ultram) may increase seizure risk. Don't combine.
- verapamil (Calan, Verelan, others) may result in increased doxepin levels.
- vitamin C (ascorbic acid) may result in decreased doxepin benefits.
- warfarin (coumadin) will result in prolonged action of the anticoagulant. More frequent INR testing is needed.

▷ *Driving, Hazardous Activities:* This drug may impair mental alertness, judgment, physical coordination, and reaction time. Avoid hazardous activities.

Aviation Note: The use of this drug *is a disqualification* for piloting. Consult a designated aviation medical examiner.

Exposure to Sun: Use caution until sensitivity has been determined. This drug may cause photosensitivity (see Glossary).

Exposure to Heat: This drug can inhibit sweating and impair the body's adaptation to hot environments, increasing the risk of heatstroke. Avoid saunas.

Exposure to Cold: The elderly should use caution and avoid conditions conducive to hypothermia (see Glossary).

Discontinuation: It is advisable to discontinue this drug gradually. Abrupt withdrawal after long-term use can cause headache, malaise, and nausea.

ENALAPRIL (e NAL a pril)

Class: Antihypertensive, ACE inhibitor

Please see the new angiotensin-converting enzyme (ACE) inhibitor combination profile for more information.

EPINEPHRINE (ep i NEF rin)

Other Name: Adrenaline

Introduced: 1900   **Class:** Antiasthmatic, anti-glaucoma, decongestant
Prescription: USA: Varies   **Controlled Drug:** USA: No; Canada: No
Available as Generic: USA: Yes; Canada: No

Brand Names: Adrenalin, Adreno-Mist, Ana-Kit, Asthmahaler, Asthmanephrine, Bronkaid Mist, ✦Bronkaid Mistometer, ✦Citanest Forte, Duranest [CD], ✦Dysne-Inhal, Epifrin, E-Pilo Preparations [CD], Epinal Ophthalmic, EpiPen, Epitrate, Marcaine, Medihaler-Epi Preparations, Micronephrine, Norocaine, Octocaine, P1E1, P2E1, P3E1, P4E1, P6E1, Primatene Mist, Propine Ophthalmic, Sensoricaine, Sus-Phrine, Thalfed [CD], Therex [CD], ✦Ultracaine, Vaponefrin, Xylocaine

---

BENEFITS versus RISKS

Possible Benefits	*Possible Risks*
EFFECTIVE RELIEF OF SEVERE ALLERGIC (ANAPHYLACTIC) REACTIONS	Significant increase in blood pressure (in sensitive people)
TEMPORARY RELIEF OF ACUTE BRONCHIAL ASTHMA	Idiosyncratic reaction: pulmonary edema (fluid formation in lungs)
Reduction of internal eye pressure (treatment of glaucoma)	Heart rhythm disorders (in sensitive people)
Relief of allergic congestion of the nose and sinuses	

▷ **Principal Uses**

As a Single Drug Product: Uses currently included in FDA-approved labeling: (1) Inhalation to relieve acute attacks of bronchial asthma; (2) as a decongestant for symptomatic relief of allergic nasal congestion and as eyedrops in the management of glaucoma; (3) treats anaphylactic shock; (4) emergency treatment of abnormal heart rhythms and in cardiopulmonary resuscitation; (5) increases beneficial effects of topical anesthetics.

Other (unlabeled) generally accepted uses: (1) Septic shock; (2) wheezing in infants; (3) croup; (4) can have a role in easing painful erections (priapism); (5) may be used in cataract surgery.

How This Drug Works: By stimulating some nerve (sympathetic) terminals, this drug
• contracts blood vessel walls, raising blood pressure.
• inhibits histamine release into skin and internal organs.
• dilates constricted bronchial tubes, increasing the size of the airways and improving the ability to breathe.
• decreases fluid formation in the eye, increases its outflow, and reduces internal eye pressure.
• decreases blood flow in the nose, shrinking swelling (decongestion) and expanding nasal airways.

Available Dose Forms and Strengths

Aerosol — 0.2, 0.27, and 0.3 mg per spray
Eyedrops — 0.1%, 0.25%, 0.5%, 1%, 2%
Injection — 0.01, 0.1, 1, and 5 mg/ml
Nose drops — 0.1%
Solution for nebulizer — 1%, 1.25%, 2.25%

▷ **Usual Adult Dose Ranges:** Aerosols: One inhalation, repeated in 1 to 2 minutes if needed; wait 4 hours before next inhalation. Eyedrops: One drop every 12 hours. Dose may vary with product; follow printed instructions and label directions. **Note: Actual dose and schedule must be determined for each patient individually.**

Conditions Requiring Dosing Adjustments

Liver Function: Dose reduction is not needed in liver compromise.
Kidney Function: Dose adjustment is not defined in kidney compromise.

▷ **Dosing Instructions:** Aerosols and inhalation solutions: After first inhalation, wait 1 to 2 minutes to see if a second inhalation is needed. If relief does not occur within 20 minutes of use, stop this drug and seek medical attention **promptly. Avoid prolonged and excessive use**. Eyedrops: During instillation of drops and for 2 minutes after, press finger against the tear sac (inner corner of eye) to prevent rapid absorption of drug into body.

Usual Duration of Use: According to individual needs. Long-term use requires physician supervision.

▷ **This Drug Should Not Be Taken If**
- you have had an allergic reaction to it previously.
- you have narrow-angle glaucoma.
- you are in shock.
- you have organic brain damage.
- you are in labor—it may delay the second stage of labor.
- you are to undergo general anesthesia with cyclopropane or halogenated hydrocarbons.
- your heart is dilated and you have a coronary deficiency.
- you have experienced a recent stroke or heart attack.

▷ **Inform Your Physician Before Taking This Drug If**
- you have any degree of high blood pressure.
- you have any form of heart disease, especially coronary heart disease (with or without angina), or a heart rhythm disorder.
- you have diabetes or overactive thyroid function (hyperthyroidism).
- you have a history of stroke.
- you have a chronic lung disease
- you take monoamine oxidase (MAO) type A inhibitors, phenothiazines, digitalis preparations, or quinidine (see Drug Classes).

Possible Side Effects (natural, expected, and unavoidable drug actions)
In some people—restlessness, anxiety, headache, tremor, palpitation, cold hands and feet, dryness of mouth and throat (with use of aerosol).

▷ **Possible Adverse Effects** (unusual, unexpected, and infrequent reactions)
If any of the following develop, consult your physician promptly for guidance.
Mild Adverse Effects
Allergic reactions: skin rash; eyedrops may cause redness, swelling, and itching of the eyelids.
Weakness, dizziness, pallor.
Serious Adverse Effects
Idiosyncratic reaction: sudden development of excessive fluid in the lungs (pulmonary edema).
In predisposed individuals—excessive rise in blood pressure with risk of stroke (cerebral hemorrhage).
Rapid heart rate and arrhythmias—case reports.
Seizures or porphyria—rare.
Pulmonary edema—case reports.
Pigmentation of the eye—case reports.
Kidney toxicity—rare.

▷ **Possible Effects on Sexual Function:**   May ease painful and abnormally prolonged erections (priapism).

Possible Effects on Laboratory Tests

Complete blood counts: red cells and white cells increased; eosinophils decreased.

Blood glucose level: increased.

Urine sugar tests: false low or negative results with Clinistix; true positive with Benedict's or Fehling's solution.

Acidosis.

Blood platelets: temporarily increased.

CAUTION

1. Medication failure can result from frequent repeat use at short intervals. If this develops, avoid use for 12 hours, and a normal response should return.

2. Excessive use of aerosol preparations in asthmatics has been associated with sudden death.

3. May cause significant irritability of nerve pathways (conduction system) and heart muscle, predisposing to serious heart rhythm disorders. Talk with your doctor about this.

4. This drug can increase blood sugar level. If you have diabetes, test for sugar often to detect significant changes.

5. If this drug no longer works for you and you substitute isoproterenol (Isuprel), allow 4 hours between drugs.

6. Promptly throw this drug away if a pinkish-red to brown coloration or cloudiness (precipitation) occurs.

Precautions for Use

By Infants and Children: Use cautiously in small doses until tolerance is determined. Watch for: weakness, light-headedness, or fainting.

By Those Over 60 Years of Age: Small doses are prudent. Watch for nervousness, headache, tremor, rapid heart rate. If you have hardening of the arteries (arteriosclerosis), heart disease, high blood pressure, Parkinson's disease, or prostatism (see Glossary), this drug may aggravate your disorder. Ask your doctor for help.

▷ **Advisability of Use During Pregnancy**

Pregnancy Category: C. See Pregnancy Risk Categories at the back of this book.

Animal studies: Birth defects reported in rats.

Human studies: Adequate studies of pregnant women are not available.

This drug can cause significant reduction of oxygen supply to the fetus. Use it only if clearly needed and in small, infrequent doses. Avoid during the first 3 months and during labor and delivery.

Advisability of Use If Breast-Feeding

Presence of this drug in breast milk: Yes.

Avoid drug or refrain from nursing.

Habit-Forming Potential: Tolerance to this drug (see Glossary) can develop with frequent use, but dependence does not occur.

Effects of Overdose: Nervousness, throbbing headache, dizziness, tremor, palpitation, disturbance of heart rhythm, difficult breathing, abdominal pain, vomiting of blood.

Possible Effects of Long-Term Use: "Epinephrine fastness": loss of ability to respond to this drug's bronchodilator effect. With long-term treatment of glaucoma: pigment deposits on eyeballs and eyelids, possible damage to retina, impaired vision, blockage of tear ducts.

Suggested Periodic Examinations While Taking This Drug (at physician's discretion)

Blood pressure measurements; blood or urine sugar measurements in diabetics; vision testing and measurement of internal eye pressure in glaucoma.

▷ **While Taking This Drug, Observe the Following**

Foods: No restrictions, except those that cause you to have asthma.

Beverages: No restrictions.

▷ *Alcohol:* Alcoholic beverages can increase the urinary excretion of this drug.

Tobacco Smoking: No interactions expected. I advise everyone to quit smoking.

▷ *Other Drugs*

Epinephrine *taken concurrently* with

- some beta-blockers (carteolol, nadolol, propranolol) may cause increased blood pressure and decreased heart rate.
- chlorpromazine (Thorazine) or other phenothiazines (see Drug Classes) may cause decreased blood pressure and increased heart rate.
- furazolidone (Furoxone) may cause increased blood pressure.
- guanethidine (Esimil, Ismelin) may cause increased blood pressure.
- halothane may cause abnormal heartbeats.
- pilocarpine (Ocusert) may cause increased myopia.
- tricyclic antidepressants (amitriptyline, etc.) may cause increased blood pressure and heart rhythm disturbances.

▷ *Driving, Hazardous Activities:* This drug may cause dizziness or nervousness. Limit activities as necessary.

Aviation Note: The use of this drug *may be a disqualification* for piloting. Consult a designated aviation medical examiner.

Exposure to Sun: No restrictions.

Heavy Exercise or Exertion: No interactions expected. However, exercise can induce asthma in sensitive individuals.

Occurrence of Unrelated Illness: Use caution in severe burns. This drug can increase drainage from burned tissue and cause serious loss of tissue fluids and blood proteins.

Discontinuation: If this drug fails after an adequate trial, stop using it and call your doctor. It is dangerous to increase the dose or frequency.

Special Storage Instructions: Protect drug from exposure to air, light, and heat. Keep in a cool place, preferably in the refrigerator.

ERGOTAMINE (er GOT a meen)

Introduced: 1926   **Class:** Anti-migraine, ergot derivative   **Prescription:** USA: Yes   **Controlled Drug:** USA: No; Canada: No   **Available as Generic:** No

Brand Names: ✦Bellergal [CD], Bellergal-S [CD], ✦Bellergal Spacetabs [CD], Cafergot [CD], Cafergot P-B [CD], Cafetrate [CD], Ercaf [CD], ✦Ergodryl [CD], Ergomar, Ergostat, Genergen, ✦Gravergol [CD], ✦Gynergen, Medihaler Ergotamine (form no longer available in US), ✦Mcgral [CD], Oxoids, Spastrin [CD], Wigraine [CD], ✦Wigraine [CD], Wigrettes

```
┌─────────────────────────────────────────────────────────────────┐
│                    BENEFITS versus RISKS                        │
│      Possible Benefits                    Possible Risks        │
│   PREVENTION AND RELIEF OF        GANGRENE OF THE FINGERS,       │
│     VASCULAR HEADACHES:             TOES, OR INTESTINE           │
│   migraine, migrainelike, and     AGGRAVATION OF CORONARY        │
│   histamine headaches               ARTERY DISEASE (ANGINA)     │
│                                   INCREASED RISK OF ABORTION (if │
│                                     used during pregnancy)      │
└─────────────────────────────────────────────────────────────────┘
```

▷ **Principal Uses**

As a Single Drug Product: Uses currently included in FDA-approved labeling: Treats vascular headaches, especially migraine and "cluster" headaches. Often effective in stopping headache if taken in the first hour following start of pain. Short-term basis use is a valid attempt to prevent or abort "cluster" headaches. The inhalation form provides rapid onset of action.

Other (unlabeled) generally accepted uses: Helps to ease the symptoms of narcolepsy.

As a Combination Drug Product [CD]: Combined with caffeine to enhance its absorption. This makes a smaller dose of ergotamine effective, and reduces risk of adverse effects with repeated use. This drug is also combined with belladonna (atropine) and a barbiturates to help premenstrual tension and the menopausal syndrome—nervousness, nausea, hot flushes, and sweating.

How This Drug Works: It constricts blood vessel walls in the head, preventing or relieving dilation that causes pain of migrainelike headaches.

Available Dose Forms and Strengths

           Aerosol — 9 mg/ml (0.36 mg/inhalation)
    Nasal inhaler (Canada) — 9 mg/ml (360 mcg/dose)
         Suppositories — 2 mg (in combination with 100 mg of caffeine)
    Tablets, sublingual — 2 mg

▷ **Usual Adult Dose Range:** Inhalation: One spray (0.36 mg) when headache starts; repeat one spray after 30 to 60 minutes as needed for relief, up to a maximum of 6 sprays every 24 hours. Do not exceed 15 sprays per week. Sublingual tablets: Dissolve 2 mg under tongue at the start of headache; repeat 2 mg in 30 to 60 minutes as needed, up to a maximum of 6 mg per attack. Do not exceed 6 mg every 24 hours or 10 mg/week. **Note: Actual dose and schedule must be determined for each patient individually.**

Conditions Requiring Dosing Adjustments

Liver Function: Should be used with caution by patients with liver compromise.
Kidney Function: This drug is a rare cause of acute renal failure, and should be used with caution by patients with compromised kidneys.

▷ **Dosing Instructions:** Follow written instructions and doses **carefully**. The regular tablets (combination drug) may be crushed; sustained-release tablets should be taken whole (not crushed). Sublingual tablets should be dissolved under the tongue, not swallowed.

Usual Duration of Use: Regular use for several headache episodes often needed to see effectiveness in aborting or relieving vascular headache. Do not exceed recommended schedules. If headaches are not controlled after several trials of maximal doses, ask your doctor about other treatments.

▷ **This Drug Should Not Be Taken If**
- you have had an allergic reaction to any dose form.
- you are pregnant.
- you have a severe infection.
- you have any of the following conditions:
  angina pectoris (coronary artery disease)
  Buerger's disease
  hardening of the arteries (arteriosclerosis)
  high blood pressure (severe hypertension)
  ischemic heart disease
  peptic ulcer
  kidney disease or impaired kidney function
  liver disease or impaired liver function
  Raynaud's phenomenon
  thrombophlebitis
  severe itching

▷ **Inform Your Physician Before Taking This Drug If**
- you are allergic or overly sensitive to *any* ergot preparation.
- you are planning to have a face-lift (rhytidectomy). This drug may cause serious skin flap problems.

Possible Side Effects (natural, expected, and unavoidable drug actions)
Usually infrequent and mild with recommended doses.
Some people may have cold hands and feet, with mild numbness and tingling.

▷ **Possible Adverse Effects** (unusual, unexpected, and infrequent reactions)
If any of the following develop, consult your physician promptly for guidance.
Mild Adverse Effects
Allergic reactions: localized swellings (angioedema), itching—case reports.
Headache, drowsiness, dizziness, confusion—possible.
Chest pain, abdominal pain, numbness and tingling of fingers and toes, muscle pains in arms or legs—infrequent.
Nausea, vomiting, diarrhea—possible.
Serious Adverse Effects
Gangrene of the extremities: coldness; numbness; pain; dark discoloration; eventual loss of fingers, toes, or feet—possible.
Gangrene of the intestine: severe abdominal pain and swelling; emergency surgery required—case reports.
Retroperitoneal fibrosis—case reports.
Fibrous changes in the lung (pleuropulmonary fibrosis)—case reports.
Pain syndromes (reflex sympathetic dystrophy)—possible.
Insufficient blood flow to the heart (myocardial ischemia) or arrhythmias—case reports.
Fibrous changes in the heart (myocardial fibrosis) or porphyria—case reports.
Lesions of the rectum or anus (anorectal lesions)—case reports.
Kidney failure—case reports.

▷ **Possible Effects on Sexual Function:**   None reported.

Natural Diseases or Disorders That May Be Activated by This Drug
Angina pectoris (coronary artery insufficiency), Buerger's disease, Raynaud's phenomenon.

Possible Effects on Laboratory Tests
None reported.

CAUTION
1. Excessive use of this drug can actually provoke migraines and increase their frequency.
2. Do not exceed a total dose of 6 mg daily or 10 mg/week of the oral form.
3. Individual drug sensitivity varies greatly. Some may have early toxic effects while taking recommended doses. Promptly report numbness in fingers or toes, muscle cramping, chest pain.

Precautions for Use
By Infants and Children: Safety and effectiveness for those under 12 years of age are not established.
By Those Over 60 Years of Age: Natural circulation changes may make you more susceptible to adverse effects of this drug. See the preceding list of disorders that are contraindications for the use of this drug.

▷ **Advisability of Use During Pregnancy**
Pregnancy Category: X. See Pregnancy Risk Categories at the back of this book.
Animal studies: Fetal deaths reported due to this drug.
Human studies: Information from studies of pregnant women indicates that this drug can cause abortion.
This drug should be avoided during the entire pregnancy.

Advisability of Use If Breast-Feeding
Presence of this drug in breast milk: Yes. Avoid drug or refrain from nursing.

Habit-Forming Potential: None.

Effects of Overdose: "Ergotism": cold skin, severe muscle pain, tingling or burning pain in hands and feet, loss of blood supply to extremities resulting in tissue death (gangrene) in fingers and toes. Acute ergot poisoning: nausea, vomiting, diarrhea, cold skin, numbness of extremities, confusion, seizures, coma.

Possible Effects of Long-Term Use: A form of functional dependence (see Glossary) may develop, resulting in withdrawal headaches if the drug is stopped.

Suggested Periodic Examinations While Taking This Drug (at physician's discretion)
Evaluation of circulation (blood flow) to the extremities.

▷ **While Taking This Drug, Observe the Following**
Foods: No interactions expected. Avoid all foods to which you are allergic; some migraine headaches are due to food allergies.
Beverages: No restrictions.
▷ *Alcohol:* Best avoided; alcohol can intensify vascular headache.
Tobacco Smoking: Best avoided; nicotine can further reduce the restricted blood flow produced by this drug.
Marijuana Smoking: Best avoided; additive effects can increase the coldness of hands and feet.
▷ *Other Drugs*
Ergotamine may *decrease* the effects of:

- nitroglycerin, and reduce its effectiveness in preventing or relieving angina pain.

The following drugs may *increase* the effects of ergotamine:
- beta-blockers (see Drug Classes).
- dopamine (Intropin).
- erythromycins: clarithromycin (Biaxin), dirithromycin (Dynabac), or E-Mycin, ERYC, etc. Azithromycin (Zithromax) has not been reported to cause this effect.
- saquinavir (Fortovase).
- sumatriptan (Imitrex); can also result in extended vasospastic reactions.
- troleandomycin (TAO).

▷ *Driving, Hazardous Activities:* This drug may cause drowsiness or dizziness. Restrict activities as necessary.

Aviation Note: Vascular headache *is a disqualification* for piloting. Consult a designated aviation medical examiner.

Exposure to Sun: No restrictions.

Exposure to Cold: Avoid as much as possible. Cold further reduces restricted blood flow to the extremities.

Discontinuation: Following long-term use, it may be necessary to withdraw this drug gradually to prevent withdrawal headache. Ask your doctor for help.

ERYTHROMYCIN (er ith roh MY sin)

See the macrolide antibiotic profile for more information.

ESTROGENS (ES troh jenz)

Other Names: Chlorotrianisene, conjugated estrogens, esterified estrogens, estradiol, estriol, estrone, estropipate, quinestrol

Introduced: 1933   **Class:** Female sex hormones   **Prescription:** USA: Yes   **Controlled Drug:** USA: No; Canada: No   **Available as Generic:** USA: Yes; Canada: No

Brand Names: ✦C.E.S., ✦Climestrone, ✦Congest, Delestrogen, DV, Estinyl, Estrace, Estraderm, Estraguard, Estratab, Estrovis, Feminone, ✦Femogen, ✦Femogex, Gynetone, Gynogen LA, Menest, Menotab, Menotab-M, Menrium [CD], Milprem [CD], ✦Minestrin, ✦Neo-Pause, ✦Oestrilin, Ogen, PMB [CD], PMS-Estradiol, Premarin, Premphase, Prempro, Progynon Pellet, TACE, Valergen-10, Vivelle (transdermal), White Premarin

Author's Note: A generic form (from Duramed) of Premarin is now approved.

BENEFITS versus RISKS	
Possible Benefits	*Possible Risks*
RELIEF OF MENOPAUSAL HOT FLASHES AND NIGHT SWEATS	INCREASED RISK OF CANCER OF THE UTERUS
PREVENTION OR RELIEF OF ATROPHIC VAGINITIS, ATROPHY OF THE VULVA AND URETHRA	INCREASED RISK OF BREAST CANCER
	Increased frequency of gallstones
PREVENTION OF POSTMENOPAUSAL HEART DISEASE	Accelerated growth of preexisting fibroid tumors of the uterus
	Fluid retention
PREVENTION OF POSTMENOPAUSAL OSTEOPOROSIS	Postmenopausal bleeding
	Deep vein thrombophlebitis and thromboembolism (less likely with conjugated estrogens, more likely with synthetic unconjugated hormones)
EARLY DATA APPEARS TO SHOW A BENEFIT IN PREVENTING ALZHEIMER'S	
Prevention of thinning of the skin	Increased blood pressure
Mental tonic effect	Decreased sugar tolerance

▷ **Principal Uses**

As a Single Drug Product: "Replacement" therapy in: (1) ovarian failure or removal; (2) the menopausal syndrome; (3) postmenopausal atrophy of genital tissues; (4) postmenopausal osteoporosis; (5) selected cases of breast cancer and prostate cancer; (6) also treats difficulty having sexual intercourse (dysparunia) caused by vaginal secretion drying.

As a Combination Drug Product [CD]: Estrogen is available in combination with chlordiazepoxide (Librium) and with meprobamate (Equanil, Miltown). These drugs provide a calming effect, easing symptoms in selected cases of menopause. See oral contraceptives profile for a discussion of estrogens and progestins.

How This Drug Works: When used to correct hormonal deficiency states, estrogens restore normal cellular activity by increasing nuclear material and protein synthesis. Frequency and intensity of menopausal symptoms are reduced when normal levels of estrogen are restored.

Available Dose Forms and Strengths

Capsules — 12 mg, 25 mg, 72 mg (TACE)

Tablets — 0.02 mg, 0.05 mg, 0.1 mg, 0.3 mg, 0.5 mg, 0.625 mg, — 0.9 mg, 1.25 mg, 2.5 mg

Transdermal patch — 0.025 mg (2 mg), 0.05 mg (4 mg), 0.1 mg (8 mg) — 2 mg (only in Canada)

Vaginal cream — 0.1, 0.625mg/g, 1.5 mg/g

▷ **Usual Adult Dose Range:** For conjugated and esterified estrogens: 1.25 mg daily for 21 days. Omit for 7 days. Repeat cyclically as needed. Progestin typically added during the final 10 days to avoid effects of estrogen alone (unopposed) on the endometrium. For other forms of estrogen: ask your doctor. **Note: Actual dose and schedule must be determined for each patient individually.**

Conditions Requiring Dosing Adjustments

Liver Function: The dose should be decreased in mild liver disease. Estrogens should not be used in acute or severe liver compromise. This drug can be lithogenic (capable of causing stones) in bile.

Kidney Function: No expected dosing changes in kidney compromise.

▷ **Dosing Instructions:**   The tablets may be crushed and taken without regard to food. The capsules should be taken whole.

Usual Duration of Use: Regular use for 10 to 20 days needed to see effectiveness in easing menopausal symptoms. Long-term use requires periodic evaluation by your doctor (every 6 months).

▷ **This Drug Should Not Be Taken If**
- you have had an allergic reaction to it previously.
- you have a history of thrombophlebitis, embolism, heart attack, or stroke.
- you have seriously impaired liver function or recent onset of liver disease.
- you have abnormal and unexplained vaginal bleeding.
- you have sickle cell disease.
- you have or are suspected to have breast cancer (may be used to treat some kinds of breast cancer).
- you have a known or suspected estrogen-dependent cancer (your doctor will determine this).
- you are pregnant.

▷ **Inform Your Physician Before Taking This Drug If**
- you have had an unfavorable reaction to estrogen therapy previously.
- you have a history of breast or reproductive organ cancer.
- you have fibrocystic breast changes, fibroid tumors of the uterus, endometriosis, migrainelike headaches, epilepsy, asthma, heart disease, high blood pressure, gallbladder disease, diabetes, or porphyria.
- you smoke tobacco on a regular basis.
- you have a history of blood-clotting disorders.
- you plan to have surgery in the near future.

Possible Side Effects (natural, expected, and unavoidable drug actions)

Fluid retention, weight gain, "breakthrough" bleeding (spotting in middle of menstrual cycle), altered menstrual pattern, **resumption of menstrual flow ("periods") after natural cessation (postmenopausal bleeding), increased yeast infection susceptibility of the genitals.**

▷ **Possible Adverse Effects** (unusual, unexpected, and infrequent reactions)

If any of the following develop, consult your physician promptly for guidance.

Mild Adverse Effects

Allergic reactions: skin rash, hives, itching—rare.

Headache, nervous tension, irritability, depression, accentuation of migraine headaches—infrequent.

Nausea, vomiting, bloating, diarrhea—infrequent to frequent.

Tannish pigmentation of the face—possible.

Serious Adverse Effects

Allergic reactions: anaphylaxis—case reports.

Idiosyncratic reaction: cutaneous porphyria—fragility and scarring of the skin.

Can produce or worsen high blood pressure—more likely with higher doses.

Gallbladder disease, benign liver tumors, jaundice, rise in blood sugar—case reports.

Erosion of uterine cervix, enlargement of uterine fibroid tumors—possible.

Thrombophlebitis (inflammation of a vein with formation of blood clot): pain or tenderness in thigh or leg, with or without swelling of foot or leg—low dose has minimal increased risk; higher doses may carry more risk.

Pulmonary embolism (movement of blood clot to lung): sudden shortness of breath, pain in chest, coughing, bloody sputum—case reports.

Benign liver tumors (adenomas)—possible.

Systemic lupus erythematosus or porphyria—rare.

Stroke (blood clot in brain): headaches, blackout, sudden weakness or paralysis of any part of the body, severe dizziness, altered vision, slurred speech, inability to speak—case reports.

Endometrial cancer (how long increased risk continues if the drug is stopped is not clear).

Retinal thrombosis (blood clot in eye vessels): sudden impairment or loss of vision—case reports.

Heart attack (blood clot in coronary artery)—sudden pain in chest, neck, jaw, or arm; weakness; sweating; nausea. Has been associated with women taking higher doses and with men using estrogen to treat prostate cancer; however, this is not clearly decided as yet. Estrogen in lower doses appears to decrease overall risk of heart attack.

Breast cancer—increased risk possible (even if combined with a progesterone), although only a slight increase in risk. Long-term use (more than 5 years) does carry increased risk, particularly if not combined with a progesterone. Conjugated estrogens were not associated with increased overall relative risk of breast cancer in one large study.

▷ **Possible Effects on Sexual Function:** Swelling and tenderness of breasts, milk production.

Increased vaginal secretions.

Possible Delayed Adverse Effects: Estrogens taken during pregnancy may predispose a female child to the later development of cancer of the vagina or cervix following puberty.

▷ **Adverse Effects That May Mimic Natural Diseases or Disorders**

Liver reactions may suggest viral hepatitis.

Natural Diseases or Disorders That May Be Activated by This Drug

Latent hypertension, diabetes mellitus, acute intermittent porphyria.

Possible Effects on Laboratory Tests

Red blood cells, hemoglobin, and platelets: decreased.

Blood calcium level: increased.

Blood total cholesterol level: decreased (treatment effect); increased in postmenopausal women.

Blood LDL cholesterol level: decreased in postmenopausal women.

Blood triglyceride level: no drug effect in postmenopausal women.

Blood glucose level: increased.

Glucose tolerance test (GTT): decreased.

Blood thyroid hormone (T_3 and T_4) levels: increased.

Blood uric acid level: decreased.

Liver function tests: increased liver enzymes (ALT/GPT, AST/GOT, and alkaline phosphatase), increased bilirubin.

CAUTION
1. To avoid prolonged (uninterrupted) stimulation of breast and uterine tissues, estrogen should be taken in cycles of 3 weeks on and 1 week off medication.
2. The estrogen in estrogen vaginal creams is absorbed systemically. It may also be absorbed through the penis during sexual intercourse and can cause enlargement and tenderness of male breast tissue.
3. Usual doses may not suffice to prevent osteoporosis in some women. Bone mineral density tests (DEXA or PDEXA) are prudent to see if a selected dose is working.

Precautions for Use

By Those Over 60 Years of Age: Very limited usefulness after 60. Restricted to women who are at increased risk for osteoporosis. In this age group, it is advisable to attempt relief of hot flushes with nonestrogenic medicines. During use, report promptly any indications of impaired circulation: speech disturbances, altered vision, sudden hearing loss, vertigo, sudden weakness or paralysis, angina, leg pains.

▷ **Advisability of Use During Pregnancy**

Pregnancy Category: X. See Pregnancy Risk Categories at the back of this book.
Animal studies: Genital defects reported in mice and guinea pigs; cleft palate reported in rodents.
Human studies: Information from studies of pregnant women indicates that estrogens can masculinize the female fetus. In addition, limb defects and heart malformations have been reported.
It is now known that estrogens taken during pregnancy can predispose the female child to the development of cancer of the vagina or cervix following puberty. *Avoid estrogens completely during entire pregnancy.*

Advisability of Use If Breast-Feeding

Presence of this drug in breast milk: Yes, in minute amounts.
Estrogens in large doses can suppress milk formation.
Breast-feeding is considered to be safe during the use of estrogens.
Malnourished mothers may have unacceptable decreases in protein and nitrogen in their breast milk if this drug is used while breast-feeding.

Habit-Forming Potential: There has been some suggestion of estrogens having potential for psychological dependence and tolerance because of their mood-elevating properties, but clinical reports have not been presented.

Effects of Overdose: Headache, drowsiness, nausea, vomiting, fluid retention, abnormal vaginal bleeding, breast enlargement and discomfort.

Possible Effects of Long-Term Use: High blood pressure, gallbladder disease with gallstone formation, increased growth of benign fibroid tumors of the uterus. Several reports suggest possible association between the long-term use (3+ years) of estrogens and the development of cancer of the lining of the uterus. Further studies are needed to establish a definite cause-and-effect relationship (see Glossary). Prudence dictates that women with intact uteri should use estrogens only when symptoms justify it and with proper supervision.

Suggested Periodic Examinations While Taking This Drug (at physician's discretion)

Regular (every 6 months) evaluation of the breasts and pelvic organs, including Pap smears.

Liver function tests as indicated.

▷ **While Taking This Drug, Observe the Following**

Foods: Avoid excessive use of salt if fluid retention occurs. Combined use of calcium can be a further step to help avoid osteoporosis.

Beverages: No restrictions. May be taken with milk.

▷ *Alcohol:* No interactions expected.

Tobacco Smoking: Some studies show that heavy smoking (15 or more cigarettes daily) in association with use of estrogen-containing oral contraceptives significantly increases risk of heart attack (coronary thrombosis). I advise everyone to stop smoking.

▷ *Other Drugs*

Estrogens *taken concurrently* with

- alendronate (Fosamax) have not been well studied. One small clinical study suggested the combination was beneficial in preventing postmenopausal osteoporosis.
- oral antidiabetic drugs (see *alpha-glucosidase inhibitors, biguanides, meglitnides, sulfonylureas, and thiazolidinediones* in Drug Classes) or oral blood-sugar-lowering medicines may cause loss of glucose control and high blood sugars.
- thyroid hormones may increase the bound (inactive) drug and require an increase in thyroid dose.
- tricyclic antidepressants (Elavil, Sinequan, etc.) may enhance their adverse effects and reduce their antidepressant effectiveness.
- vitamin C (ascorbic acid, various brands) in higher doses may result in increased estrogen effects. A lower dose of estrogens may be indicated if higher-dose vitamin C will be taken on an ongoing basis.
- warfarin (Coumadin) may cause alterations of prothrombin activity. Increased doses may be needed.

The following drugs may *decrease* the effects of estrogens:

- carbamazepine (Tegretol).
- phenobarbital (Belladenal, others).
- phenytoin (Dilantin).
- primidone (Mysoline).
- rifampin (Rifadin, Rimactane).

▷ *Driving, Hazardous Activities:* Usually no restrictions. Consult your physician for assessment of individual risk and for guidance regarding specific restrictions.

Aviation Note: Usually no restrictions. However, watch for the rare occurrence of disturbed vision and restrict activities accordingly. Consult a designated aviation medical examiner.

Exposure to Sun: Caution—May cause photosensitivity (see Glossary).

Discontinuation: Best to stop estrogens periodically to see if they are still needed. The dose is reduced gradually to prevent acute withdrawal hot flushes. Avoid continual, uninterrupted use of large doses. Stop altogether when a definite need for replacement therapy has ended. Ask your doctor for help.

ETHAMBUTOL (eth AM byu tohl)

Introduced: 1971   **Class:** Anti-infective, antituberculosis drug   **Pre-scription:** USA: Yes   **Controlled Drug:** USA: No; Canada: No   **Available as Generic:** USA: No; Canada: No

Brand Names: ◆Etibi, Myambutol

BENEFITS versus RISKS

Possible Benefits	*Possible Risks*
EFFECTIVE ADJUNCTIVE TREATMENT OF PULMONARY TUBERCULOSIS	RARE OPTIC NEURITIS WITH IMPAIRMENT OR LOSS OF VISION
EFFECTIVE ADJUNCTIVE TREATMENT OF AIDS-RELATED *MYCOBACTERIUM AVIUM-*INTRACELLULARE COMPLEX INFECTIONS	Rare peripheral neuritis (see Glossary)
Possibly effective treatment of tuberculous meningitis	Activation of gout

---

▷ **Principal Uses**

As a Single Drug Product: Uses currently included in FDA-approved labeling: Treats lung (pulmonary) tuberculosis. Used with other antitubercular drugs (currently three other medicines are added to ethambutol).

Other (unlabeled) generally accepted uses: (1) Treatment of tuberculous meningitis; (2) treatment of AIDS-related *Mycobacterium avium-intracellulare* (MAI) *complex* infections, in combination with other anti-mycobacterial drugs.

Available Dose Forms and Strengths

Tablets — 100 mg, 400 mg

▷ **Recommended Dose Ranges (Actual dose and schedule must be determined for each patient individually.)**

Infants and Children: Dose not established. Some authorities recommend that children under 6 years of age not be given this drug.

13 to 60 Years of Age: To start—15 mg per kg of body mass, once daily. Daily maximum is 500–1500 mg.

For retreatment of tuberculosis—25 mg per kg of body mass, once daily for 60 days; then 15 mg per kg of body mass. Total daily dose should not exceed 900–2500 mg.

For tuberculous meningitis or AIDS-related MAI infections—15 to 25 mg per kg of body mass, once daily.

Over 60 Years of Age: Same as 13 to 60 years of age.

▷ **This Drug Should Not Be Taken If**

- you have had an allergic reaction to it previously.
- you currently have optic neuritis or peripheral neuritis.
- you currently have active gout.

Author's note: The information in this profile has been shortened to make room for more widely used medicines.

ETHANOL (ETH an all)

Other Names: Prescription: None
  Nonprescription: Moonshine, alcohol, jack, white lightning, wine, beer, whiskey, vodka, others

Introduced: 1980 (prescription); 6,000 years ago (nonprescription)   **Class:** Antianxiety drug (nonprescription form)   **Prescription:** USA: Yes (IV) **Controlled Drug:**   USA: No; Canada: Yes (IV)   **Available as Generic:**   USA: Yes; Canada: Yes

Brand Names: Prescription: Tuss-Ornade (5%), Vicks Formula 44D, Temaril (5.7%), Nyquil Nightime Cold Medicine, Novahistine DMX Liquid, Eskaphen B, ✦Dilusol (38.7%), Nonprescription: Robert Alison Chardonnay (12% by volume), Bud Dry, Glenlivet, Smirnoff (40% by volume), others

Warning: Clinical use is limited to intravenous treatment of methanol and antifreeze (ethylene glycol) poisoning, and as a preservative. Many products contain alcohol. Ask your pharmacist for help if you must avoid alcohol. Widely used in nonprescription form as an antianxiety agent. Recent data appear to show heart (cardiac) benefit of moderate use—however, other data show increased cancer risks. Some people may not have any mental or physical changes even though a breath or blood alcohol test shows they are "legally drunk."

BENEFITS versus RISKS

Possible Benefits	*Possible Risks*
EFFECTIVE TREATMENT OF POISONING	WITHDRAWAL SYMPTOMS
	SEIZURES
MODERATE use may decrease heart disease/heart attack risk	LIVER DAMAGE (with prolonged use)
	Possible increased cancer risk
	Pancreatitis
	Encephalopathy
	Low white blood cell counts and anemia
	Myopathy

▷ **Principal Uses**

  As a Single Drug Product: Uses currently included in FDA-approved labeling: Intravenously in very specific depletion cases. Other (unlabeled) generally accepted uses: (1) Treatment of methanol or antifreeze (ethylene glycol) poisoning; (2) adjunctive treatment of cancer pain; (3) intravenous treatment of DTs (delirium tremens); (4) used to sclerose esophageal varices and stop bleeding; (5) treatment of hepatocellular cancer where severe liver problems preclude surgery; (6) used to sclerose thyroid cysts; (7) used to destroy nerve tissue (neurolytic block) in chronic pain therapy; (8) widely used in nonprescription form as an antianxiety agent; (9) recent data appear to show that use ranging up to moderate (and NO GREATER than 0.7 mg per kg of body mass for 3 days in a row) may actually help prevent coronary heart disease and heart attacks.
  As a Combination Drug Product [CD]: Uses currently included in FDA-approved

labeling: Widely present in elixirs and other liquid vehicles for drugs as a preservative, and partial drug action enhancer.

How This Drug Works: In antifreeze (ethylene glycol) or methanol poisoning, ethanol prevents ethylene glycol from being changed or prevents methanol from being changed (metabolized) into toxic chemicals, letting the body remove antifreeze or methanol harmlessly. If used in nonprescription form in excess, it depresses nerve function, leading to emotional changes and disturbances of perception, coordination, and intoxication. Nonprescription use of up to moderate amounts appears to decrease risk of heart and blood vessel disease, but how it works is unknown.

Available Dose Forms and Strengths

Intravenous — 5%, 10%, 95%

Nonprescription — Each ounce of 100-proof whiskey has 15 ml of ethanol
— 6 ounces (12%) wine has 22 ml of ethanol
— 12 ounces of beer (4.9%) has 18 ml of ethanol

▷ **Recommended Dose Ranges** (Actual dose and schedule must be determined for each patient individually.)

Infants and Children: Methanol or ethylene glycol poisoning: 40 ml per kg of body mass per day.

18 to 60 Years of Age: Methanol or ethylene glycol poisoning: A loading dose of 0.6 mg per kg of body mass is given, and followed by 109 to 125 mg per kg of body mass per hour to maintain a blood level of 100 mg/dl.

Coronary heart disease or heart attack prevention: It APPEARS THAT use of moderate amounts (up to 0.8 g per kg of body mass per day or no more than 0.7 mg per kg of body mass per day for 3 days in a row) of alcohol may help in preventing risk of this kind of blood vessel disease and myocardial infarctions.

Over 60 Years of Age: Same as 12 to 60 years of age for poisonings. Older people may be less able to tolerate the same amount as a younger person for the nonprescription forms. A smaller dose will generally cause an equal or greater loss of coordination or mental ability. Hypothermia risk is also increased.

Conditions Requiring Dosing Adjustments

Liver Function: Ethanol is extensively metabolized in the liver to acetaldehyde and acetyl Co-A. The drug is also a clear cause of liver toxicity. The dose must be decreased in liver compromise.

Kidney Function: Kidneys are minimally involved. No changes needed.

▷ **Dosing Instructions:**   If methanol or ethylene glycol poisoning is suspected—the nearest poison control center should be contacted. Oral dosing (use vodka mixed in orange juice) may be of benefit, depending on distance from a hospital or freestanding emergency center.

For nonprescription antianxiety use: Dose of this drug and the blood alcohol level varies with many factors. Critical ones are weight, metabolic activity of the liver, how much food is in the stomach, strength of alcohol in the beverage, number of "drinks" consumed over a given period of time, and how well hydrated (whether there has been extreme exercise and fluid loss) you are. Again, although a blood or breath alcohol test may be a marker for mental or physical changes, some people may not have physical or mental changes and will actually have a blood or breath alcohol level in the state-defined range of "legally drunk." Specific levels of blood or breath alcohol do not absolutely predict impairment. Each 10 ml of ethanol increases blood ethanol of an average 150-lb (70-kg) man by 16.6 mg percent (3.6 mmol/L). Legal definition of intoxication is a blood alcohol level of 0.10% or 100 mg/dl. "Under the influence" in Maryland is .07%, or 70 mg/dL. Driving impairment **may** occur at blood levels of 0.05% (50 mg/dl) or lower.

Usual Duration of Use: Use on a regular schedule for 48 hours determines effectiveness in methanol overdose. Long-term excessive use as an antianxiety agent is NOT recommended.

▷ **This Drug Should Not Be Taken If**
- you have had an allergic reaction to any dose form of it previously.
- you have epilepsy.
- you have a history of alcohol addiction.
- you have a urinary tract infection.
- you are pregnant.
- you are in diabetic coma.

▷ **Inform Your Physician Before Taking This Drug If**
- you have liver or kidney compromise.
- you have gout.
- you are prone to low blood sugars.
- you are a diabetic.
- you have congestive heart failure.

Possible Side Effects (natural, expected, and unavoidable drug actions)
Intoxication, perception, coordination, and mood changes.

▷ **Possible Adverse Effects** (unusual, unexpected, and infrequent reactions)
If any of the following develop, consult your physician promptly for guidance.
Mild Adverse Effects
Allergic reactions: itching, rash, hives, and flushing
Headache, "hangover" (nausea, headache, malaise)—dose related.
Sedation—dose dependent.
Disorientation, memory loss—dose dependent.
Color blindness or neuropathy (tingling, burning, or numbness)—with chronic use.
Vitamin deficiency or muscle changes (myopathy)—with chronic use.
Stomach irritation—frequent.
Serious Adverse Effects
Allergic reactions: anaphylaxis (rash, swelling of tongue, breathing problems, flushing)—case reports.
Bronchospasm (asthmatics at increased risk)—case reports.
Respiratory depression—dose related.
Elevated or decreased white blood cell count—possible.
Increased or decreased platelets—case reports.
Heart dysfunction (myopathy) or anemia (megaloblastic)—with chronic use.
High blood pressure—possible to frequent.
Abnormal heart rhythms (atrial and ventricular) or chest pain (angina)—increased risk.
Liver toxicity—cirrhosis with chronic use possible.
Osteoporosis—increased risk with chronic use.

Pancreatitis—increased risk with chronic higher-dose use.

Encephalopathy or cerebrovascular bleeding—increased risk with higher-dose chronic use.

Low blood sugar or ketoacidosis—especially if meals are missed or with chronic use.

Vitamin deficiency (folic acid, vitamins B_1 and B_6) or low magnesium—with chronic use.

Low potassium (especially with acute intoxication in children)—possible.

Gout (precipitated by alcohol use in those with gout)—possible.

Tolerance (with chronic use)—possible.

Withdrawal: nausea, fever, rapid heart rate, hallucinations. May progress to delirium tremens (5%): profound confusion, hallucinations, etc.—possible.

▷ **Possible Effects on Sexual Function:**   Decreased libido, impotence (with excessive chronic use). Difficulty achieving an erection in males and decreased vaginal dilation in females. Chronic alcohol use may lead to tenderness and swelling of male and female breast tissue, testicular atrophy, low sperm counts, decreased menstrual blood flow, and diminished capability for orgasm in females.

Possible Delayed Adverse Effects: Liver toxicity, anemia, low or high platelets, vitamin deficiency.

▷ **Adverse Effects That May Mimic Natural Diseases or Disorders**

Alcoholic cirrhosis may mimic hepatitis.

Natural Diseases or Disorders That May Be Activated by This Drug

Peptic ulcer disease.

Possible Effects on Laboratory Tests

Liver function tests: elevated ALT.

Complete blood count: decreased white blood cells, decreased hemoglobin, increased or decreased platelets.

Amylase: elevated.

Sperm count: decreased with chronic use.

Magnesium: decreased with chronic use.

CAUTION

1. Nonprescription form may cause FATAL increases in blood pressure if combined with cocaine.
2. With high doses (nearly pure "grain" alcohol) or many drinks (frequent dosing) over a short period of time, FATAL blood alcohol levels may be reached with the nonprescription form.

Precautions for Use

By Infants and Children: Safety and effectiveness for those under 12 years of age not established. Accidental and unsupervised drinking of the nonprescription form may result in severe consequences in children. Seriously low blood sugar may happen and be delayed up to 6 hours after drinking. Low potassium may also occur with high ethanol levels. Therapy is guided by blood sugar, potassium, and blood alcohol (ethanol) levels. Fatality caused by low blood sugar was reported in a 4-year-old child who drank 12 ounces of a mouthwash that contained 10% ethanol.

By Those Over 60 Years of Age: Poisoning with methanol or ethylene glycol is an emergency situation, and while there may be an increased sensitivity to effects, dosing is adjusted to blood levels. The nonprescription form dosing (number of drinks) tolerated would be expected to decrease with increasing age.

▷ **Advisability of Use During Pregnancy**

Pregnancy Category: D, X if used for long periods. See Pregnancy Risk Categories at the back of this book.

Human studies: Fetal alcohol syndrome—a collection of limb, neurological, and behavioral defects—occurs with excessive alcohol use.

Avoid use of this drug during your **entire** pregnancy.

Advisability of Use If Breast-Feeding

Presence of this drug in breast milk: Yes.

Avoid drug or refrain from nursing.

Habit-Forming Potential: Clearly defined alcoholism exists and occurs.

Effects of Overdose: Toxic levels result in ataxia, loss of consciousness progressing to coma, anesthesia, respiratory failure, and death. Levels of 150 to 300 mg/dl may result in exaggerated emotional states, confusion, and incoordination. Fatalities most often result with blood concentrations greater than 400 mg/dl. Fatal blood levels vary greatly, however, and death has been reported following levels as low as 260 mg/dl. Once again, some people will not have any mental or physical changes with an alcohol level that is in the "legally drunk" range and even with higher levels.

Possible Effects of Long-Term Use: Liver toxicity, anemia, esophageal varices, low white blood cell counts, compromised heart function, high blood pressure, depression, peripheral neuropathy, seizures, cerebrovascular accident (with acute high levels), water intoxication, vitamin and electrolyte disturbances, gastritis or ulcers, pancreatitis, muscle pain, osteoporosis, tolerance, and withdrawal.

Suggested Periodic Examinations While Taking This Drug (at physician's discretion)

Blood alcohol levels and methanol or ethylene glycol levels guide therapy in poisonings.

Chronic alcohol abuse: complete blood counts, liver function tests, amylase and lipase, electrocardiograms.

▷ **While Taking This Drug, Observe the Following**

Foods: Food may decrease the absorption of ethanol from the stomach.

Nutritional Support: Vitamin support, particularly thiamin (B_1), folic acid, and B_6 are needed with chronic use. Magnesium replacement is also needed. Vitamin C may help eliminate ethanol.

Tobacco Smoking: No interactions expected. I advise everyone to quit smoking.

Marijuana Smoking: Additive central nervous system depression.

▷ *Other Drugs*

Ethanol may *increase* the effects of

- central nervous system depressants such as benzodiazepines, barbiturates, opioids, and anesthetic agents.
- chlorpromazine (Thorazine), and will result in increased sedation.
- cocaine, and result in dangerous increases in blood pressure.
- cyclosporine (Sandimmune) (large amounts of ethanol).
- diphenhydramine (Benadryl, others), and increase sedation.

- venlafaxine (Effexor), and increase CNS effects of both drugs.
- warfarin (Coumadin), and require more frequent INR testing and possible dose changes.

Ethanol may **decrease** the effects of

- phenytoin (Dilantin), by reducing blood phenytoin levels.
- propranolol (Inderal), by increasing propranolol elimination.

Ethanol **taken concurrently** with

- acetaminophen (Tylenol) poses an increased risk of liver damage.
- some antihistamines may increase sedation.
- aspirin may result in increased blood loss from the stomach.
- cefamandole (Mandol), cefotetan (Cefotan), metronidazole (Flagyl), and cefoperazone (Cefobid) may result in disulfiramlike reaction (see Glossary).
- cimetidine (Zantac) may decrease the amount of alcohol that it takes to make you drunk (intoxicated).
- disulfiram (Antabuse) will result in severe vomiting and intolerance.
- griseofulvin (Fulvicin) can increase the effects of alcohol.
- insulin may result in potential severe hypoglycemia.
- isoniazid may result in elevated isoniazid levels.
- ketoconazole (Nizoral) may result in disulfiramlike reactions.
- lithium (Lithobid) may result in worsened impairment of coordination and intoxication.
- methotrexate (especially with long-term ethanol use) may increase risk of liver damage.
- metronidazole (Flagyl) may result in a disulfiramlike reaction.
- nitroglycerin (Nitrostat, others) may result in excessive decreases in blood pressure.
- oral hypoglycemic agents poses an increased risk of seriously low glucose levels.
- tricyclic antidepressants may result in increased antidepressant levels and toxicity.
- verapamil (Calan, others) may increase the amount of time ethanol stays in the body and may pose an increased risk of intoxication.

▷ *Driving, Hazardous Activities:* This drug may cause drowsiness, mental impairment, and coordination problems.

Driving skill may be impaired at very low blood levels with the perception that capabilities are **not** reduced. Drinking and driving is **not** recommended. Restrict activities as necessary.

Aviation Note: The use of this drug *is a disqualification* for piloting. Consult a designated aviation medical examiner.

Exposure to Sun: May result in additive dehydration.

Heavy Exercise or Exertion: May worsen the adverse effects of this drug.

Discontinuation: Abrupt discontinuation after chronic use may result in a serious withdrawal syndrome known as DT, or delirium tremens.

ETHOSUXIMIDE (eth oh SUX i mide)

Introduced: 1960   **Class:** Anticonvulsant   **Prescription:** USA: Yes
Controlled Drug: USA: No; Canada: No   **Available as Generic:**   Yes
Brand Name: Zarontin

BENEFITS versus RISKS	
Possible Benefits	*Possible Risks*
EFFECTIVE CONTROL OF ABSENCE SEIZURES (PETIT MAL EPILEPSY)	RARE APLASTIC ANEMIA (see *aplastic anemia and bone marrow depression* in Glossary)
EFFECTIVE CONTROL OF MYOCLONIC AND AKINETIC EPILEPSY in some individuals	Rare decrease in white blood cells and blood platelets

▷ **Principal Uses**

As a Single Drug Product: Uses currently included in FDA-approved labeling: Used to treat petit mal epilepsy and is a drug of choice in absence seizures. Other (unlabeled) generally accepted uses: None at present.

How This Drug Works: Alters some nerve impulses, suppressing abnormal electrical activity that causes absence seizures (petit mal epilepsy).

Available Dose Forms and Strengths

Capsules — 250 mg
Syrup — 250 mg/5 ml

▷ **Recommended Dose Range:** Dosing starts with 500 mg daily, and can be increased by 250 mg every 4 to 7 days until acceptable control is achieved. Ending dose may be 20 to 30 mg per kg daily. Daily maximum is 1500 mg. IMPORTANT: Blood levels increase more quickly in females than males. For children 3 to 6 years old: Usual starting dose is 250 mg per day. May increase by 250-mg doses every 4 to 7 days as needed. Usually 20–30 mg per kg is the once-daily dose.

More than 6 years old with absence seizures: same as adults.

Note: Actual dose and schedule must be determined for each patient individually.

Conditions Requiring Dosing Adjustments

Liver Function: Blood levels are recommended if the liver is damaged.
Kidney Function: In severe kidney failure, 75% of the usual dose should be given at the usual intervals.

▷ **Dosing Instructions:** Capsule may be opened and taken with food to reduce stomach irritation.

Usual Duration of Use: Regular use for 1 to 2 weeks may be needed to identify the best dose and reduce frequency of absence seizures. Long-term use requires physician supervision.

▷ **This Drug Should Not Be Taken If**

• you are allergic to any succinimide anticonvulsant (see Drug Classes).
• you have active liver disease.
• you currently have a blood cell or bone marrow disorder.

▷ **Inform Your Physician Before Taking This Drug If**

• you have a history of liver or kidney disease.
• you have any type of blood disorder, especially one caused by drugs.
• you have serious depression or mental illness.

Possible Side Effects (natural, expected, and unavoidable drug actions)
Drowsiness, lethargy, fatigue.

▷ **Possible Adverse Effects** (unusual, unexpected, and infrequent reactions)
  If any of the following develop, consult your physician promptly for guidance.

  Mild Adverse Effects
    Allergic reactions: skin rash, hives—case reports.
    Headache, unsteadiness, euphoria, impaired vision, numbness and tingling in extremities—infrequent.
    Loss of appetite, nausea, vomiting, hiccups, stomach pain, diarrhea—infrequent to frequent.
    Thickening and overgrowth of gums—possible.

  Serious Adverse Effects
    Allergic reaction: swelling of tongue—case reports.
    Aggravation of emotional depression and paranoid mental disorders—case reports.
    Severe bone marrow depression: fatigue, fever, sore throat, abnormal bleeding or bruising—case reports.
    Porphyria, myasthenia gravis, or systemic lupus erythematosus—rare.

▷ **Possible Effects on Sexual Function:**   Increased libido (questionable); nonmenstrual vaginal bleeding—case reports.

Natural Diseases or Disorders That May Be Activated by This Drug
  Latent psychosis, systemic lupus erythematosus.

Possible Effects on Laboratory Tests
  Complete blood cell counts: decreased red cells, hemoglobin, white cells, and platelets; increased eosinophils.
  Blood aspartate aminotransferase (AST) level: increased in 33% of users.
  Blood bilirubin level: increased (rare liver damage).
  Blood lupus erythematosus (LE) cells: positive—rare.
  Kidney function tests: increased blood urea nitrogen (BUN) level, increased urine protein content.

CAUTION
  1. May increase the frequency of grand mal seizures in people with mixed seizure disorders.
  2. Periodic blood counts and other tests are mandatory.

Precautions for Use
  By Infants and Children: If a single-daily dose causes nausea or vomiting, give in two or three divided doses 8 to 12 hours apart. Large differences in response occur, and require blood levels. Watch for a lupuslike reaction: fever, rash, arthritis.
  By Those Over 60 Years of Age: Rarely used in this age group.

▷ **Advisability of Use During Pregnancy**
  Pregnancy Category: C. See Pregnancy Risk Categories at the back of this book.
  Animal studies: Bone defects reported in rodents.
  Human studies: Three instances of birth defects have been reported. Adequate studies of pregnant women are not available.
  Avoid during first 3 months. Use only if clearly needed during the final 6 months.

Advisability of Use If Breast-Feeding
  Presence of this drug in breast milk: Yes.

Watch nursing infant closely and discontinue drug or nursing if adverse effects develop. If mother requires high doses, refrain from nursing. Ask your doctor for help.

Habit-Forming Potential: None.

Effects of Overdose: Drowsiness, lethargy, dizziness, nausea, vomiting, stupor progressing to coma.

Possible Effects of Long-Term Use: Systemic lupus erythematosus.

Suggested Periodic Examinations While Taking This Drug (at physician's discretion)

Complete blood counts every 2 weeks during the first months of use, then monthly thereafter; liver and kidney function tests.

▷ **While Taking This Drug, Observe the Following**

Foods: No restrictions.

Beverages: No restrictions. May be taken with milk.

▷ *Alcohol:* Use caution—this drug may increase the sedative effects of alcohol. Excessive alcohol may precipitate seizures.

Tobacco Smoking: No interactions expected. I advise everyone to quit smoking.

▷ *Other Drugs*

Ethosuximide may *increase* the effects of
- phenytoin (Dilantin), by slowing its elimination.

Ethosuximide *taken concurrently* with
- carbamazepine (Tegretol) may change ethosuximide blood levels.
- phenobarbital may decrease seizure control success.
- ritonavir (Norvir) and perhaps other protease inhibitors (see Drug Classes) may lead to toxicity.
- tramadol (Ultram) may increase seizure risk.
- valproic acid (Depakene) may unpredictably alter ethosuximide effects.

The following drug may *increase* the effects of ethosuximide:
- isoniazid (INH, Niconyl, etc.).

▷ *Driving, Hazardous Activities:* This drug may cause drowsiness, dizziness, unsteadiness, and impaired vision. Restrict activities as necessary.

Aviation Note: Seizure disorders and the use of this drug *are disqualifications* for piloting. Consult a designated aviation medical examiner.

Exposure to Sun: No restrictions.

Discontinuation: Do not stop taking this drug abruptly. Ask your physician for help with gradual dose reduction.

ETIDRONATE (e ti DROH nate)

Introduced: 1976   **Class:** Anti-osteoporotic   **Prescription:** USA: Yes
Controlled Drug: USA: No; Canada: No   **Available as Generic:** USA: No; Canada: No
Brand Name: Didronel

BENEFITS versus RISKS

Possible Benefits	*Possible Risks*
PARTIAL RELIEF OF SYMPTOMS OF PAGET'S DISEASE OF BONE	Increased bone pain
	Bone fractures
EFFECTIVE PREVENTION AND TREATMENT OF ABNORMAL CALCIFICATION	Kidney failure
	Focal osteomalacia
Effective adjunctive treatment of abnormally high blood calcium levels (associated with malignant disease)	
Treatment of postmenopausal osteoporosis	

▷ **Principal Uses**

As a Single Drug Product: Uses currently included in FDA-approved labeling: (1) Treatment of symptomatic Paget's disease of bone (excessive bone growth of skull, spine, and long bones); (2) prevention and treatment of abnormal bone formation (ossification) following total hip replacement or spinal cord injury; (3) adjunctive treatment of excessively high blood calcium levels due to malignant bone disease.

Other (unlabeled) generally accepted uses: (1) treatment of Paget's disease of bone that is not yet causing symptoms; (2) treatment of abnormal calcium levels that may result from prolonged immobilization; (3) helps hyperparathyroidism; (4) helps pulmonary alveolar microlithiasis (PAM).

How This Drug Works: This drug attaches to the surface of bone and slows the abnormally accelerated processes of "bone turnover" that occur in Paget's disease. In malignant bone disease, this drug slows bone destruction and reduces excessive transfer of calcium from bone to blood.

Available Dose Forms and Strengths

Injection — 50 mg/ml

Tablets — 200 mg, 400 mg

▷ **Recommended Dose Ranges** (Actual dose and schedule must be determined for each patient individually.)

Infants and Children: Dose not established.

12 to 60 Years of Age: For Paget's disease: Initially 5 mg per kg of body mass daily, as a single dose, for up to 6 months. Discontinue for a drug-free period of 6 months. As needed, repeat, alternating 6-month courses of drug treatment and abstention. Doses above 10 mg per kg of body mass per day are only used if there is a critical need to decrease increased work output of the heart or to quickly slow down increased bone turnover.

For ossification associated with hip replacement: 20 mg per kg of body mass daily for 1 month before and 3 months after surgery.

For ossification associated with spinal cord injury: Initially 20 mg per kg of body mass daily for 2 weeks after injury; then decrease dose to 10 mg per kg of body mass daily for an additional 10 weeks.

For high blood calcium associated with malignant bone disease: 20 mg per kg of body mass daily for 30 days; if needed and tolerated, continue for a maximum of 90 days.

The total daily dose should not exceed 20 mg per kg of body mass.
Over 60 Years of Age: Same as 12 to 60 years of age.
Author's note: The information in this profile has been shortened to allow room for more widely used medicines.

ETODOLAC (E TOE do lak)

See the acetic acids (nonsteroidal anti-inflammatory drugs) profile for further information.

ETRETINATE (e TRET i nayt)

Introduced: 1976   **Class:** Anti-psoriatic
Brand Name: Tegison
Author's note: The manufacturer has stopped marketing this medicine.

FAMCICLOVIR (fam SEYE klo veer)

Introduced: 1994   **Class:** Antiviral   **Prescription:** USA: Yes   **Controlled Drug:** USA: No   **Available as Generic:** USA: No
Brand Name: Famvir

BENEFITS versus RISKS	
Possible Benefits	*Possible Risks*
EFFECTIVE TREATMENT OF HERPES ZOSTER (SHINGLES)	Diarrhea Purpura
TREATS AN INFECTION THAT MAY BE LIFE-THREATENING IN AIDS AND MARROW TRANSPLANT PATIENTS	Paresthesias
TREATS RECURRENT GENITAL HERPES	

▷ **Principal Uses**
  As a Single Drug Product: Uses currently included in FDA-approved labeling: (1) Treats acute herpes zoster (shingles); (2) treats recurrent genital herpes; (3) treats recurrent infections caused by herpes simplex in people also HIV positive (infected with HIV).
  Other (unlabeled) generally accepted uses: (1) May treat hepatitis B and related polyarteritis nodosa; (2) promise in treating Varicella-zoster.
How This Drug Works: Changed in the body to active penciclovir. This inhibits viruses by blocking DNA synthesis and reproduction (replication).
Available Dose Forms and Strengths
  Tablets — 250 mg (Germany), 500 mg
▷ **Recommended Dose Ranges** (Actual dose and schedule must be determined for each patient individually.)

Infants and Children: Safety and efficacy for those under 18 not established.

18 to 60 Years of Age: Shingles (herpes zoster): 500 to 750 mg is given every 8 hours for 7 days. It is important to start this medicine promptly after the diagnosis is made.

Recurrent genital herpes: 125 mg twice a day for 5 days.

Over 60 Years of Age: Same as 18 to 60 years of age, except for those with compromised livers or kidneys.

Conditions Requiring Dosing Adjustments

Liver Function: No dose changes are needed in well-compensated liver impairment.

Kidney Function: In people with mild kidney compromise (creatinine clearance greater than 60 ml/min), 500 mg is given every 8 hours. Mild to moderate compromise (creatinine clearance 40 to 59 ml/min): 500 mg every 12 hours. Moderate to severe (creatinine clearance 20 to 39 ml/min) cases receive 500 mg every 24 hours.

Usual Duration of Use: Regular use for 2 days determines effectiveness in herpes zoster. Then the medicine is typically continued for 7 days. Your doctor should decide when to stop the medicine. For recurrent genital herpes: start at first sign of recurrence and continue dosing for 5 days.

▷ **This Drug Should Not Be Taken If**
- you have had an allergic reaction to any dose form of it previously.

▷ **Inform Your Physician Before Taking This Drug If**
- you are unsure how much to take or how often to take it.
- you have a history of kidney or liver problems.
- your immune system is compromised.

▷ **Possible Adverse Effects** (unusual, unexpected, and infrequent reactions)
   If any of the following develop, consult your physician promptly for guidance.

Mild Adverse Effects
   Allergic reactions: itching.
   Fever, headache, or fatigue—infrequent.
   Nausea or diarrhea—infrequent to frequent.

Serious Adverse Effects
   Allergic reactions: unknown.
   Purpura or paresthesias—case reports.
   Rigors—rare.
   Increased breast cancer in male rats given extremely high doses. Does not appear to increase risk in humans.

▷ **Possible Effects on Sexual Function:**   None reported.

Possible Delayed Adverse Effects: Unknown.

Possible Effects on Laboratory Tests
   Unknown.

CAUTION
   1. The best effect occurs if started very soon after diagnosis. If used for recurrent genital herpes, best started at first signs of recurrence.

Precautions for Use
By Infants and Children: Safety and effectiveness for those under 18 years of age are not established.

By Those Over 60 Years of Age: Specific adjustments or precautions are not defined except for those with compromised livers or kidneys.

▷ **Advisability of Use During Pregnancy**
Pregnancy Category: B. See Pregnancy Risk Categories at the back of this book. Human studies: Adequate studies of pregnant women are not available. Ask your doctor for guidance.

Advisability of Use If Breast-Feeding
Presence of this drug in breast milk: Yes, lab animals; unknown in humans. Stop nursing or discontinue the drug.

Effects of Overdose: Symptomatic management.

▷ **While Taking This Drug, Observe the Following**
Foods: No restrictions.
Tobacco Smoking: No interactions expected. I advise everyone to quit smoking.

▷ *Other Drugs*
Famciclovir **taken concurrently** with
• digoxin (Lanoxin) may increase peak digoxin blood level.

▷ *Driving, Hazardous Activities:* This drug may cause dizziness or fatigue. Restrict activities as necessary.
Aviation Note: The use of this drug **may be a disqualification** for piloting. Consult a designated aviation medical examiner.
Exposure to Sun: No restrictions.

FAMOTIDINE (fa MOH te deen)

See the histamine (H₂) blocking drugs profile for further information.

FELODIPINE (fe LOH di peen)

Introduced: 1986   **Class:** Antihypertensive, calcium channel blocker
Prescription: USA: Yes   **Controlled Drug:** USA: No   **Available as Generic:** No
Brand Name: Plendil, Lexxel [CD]

Controversies in Medicine: Medicines in this class have had many conflicting reports. The FDA has held hearings on the calcium channel blocker (CCB) class. A study called ALLHAT is comparing amlodipine, an ACE inhibitor, a diuretic, and an alpha blocker (see Drug Classes) and should clarify adverse effects, mortality and other issues relating to CCBs. **Amlodipine got the first FDA approval to treat high blood pressure or angina in people with congestive heart failure.** CCBs are currently second line agents for high blood pressure according to the JNC VI (see Glossary).

BENEFITS versus RISKS	
Possible Benefits	*Possible Risks*
EFFECTIVE TREATMENT OF MILD TO MODERATE HYPERTENSION	Peripheral edema (fluid retention in feet and ankles)

▷ **Principal Uses**

As a Single Drug Product: Uses currently included in FDA-approved labeling: Treats mild to moderate hypertension.

Other (unlabeled) generally accepted uses: (1) Treats angina; (2) treats arrhythmias; (3) treats adjunctive treatment of congestive heart failure; (4) may inhibit progression of atherosclerosis; (5) can be used in some cases of premature labor.

As a Combination Drug Product [CD]: Available combined with enalapril (Lexxel) (an ACE inhibitor). The combination puts two different actions to work to lower blood pressure.

How This Drug Works: Blocks normal passage of calcium through some cell walls. This slows spread of electrical activity and reduces contraction of peripheral arterial walls, lowering blood pressure.

Available Dose Forms and Strengths

Tablets, sustained release — 5 mg, 10 mg
   Coated tablet (Lexxel) — 5 mg enalapril and 5 mg felodipine

▷ **Recommended Dose Ranges** (Actual dose and schedule must be determined for each patient individually.)

Infants and Children: 0.18 to 0.56 mg/kg daily have controlled blood pressure after kidney transplants.

12 to 60 Years of Age: High blood pressure: Initially 5 mg, once daily. Increased as needed and tolerated (at 2 week intervals). Usual dose range is 5–10 mg, once daily. Total daily maximum is 10 mg. Lexxel: One tablet daily. Increased to two daily if needed.

Over 65 Years of Age: Starting dose is 2.5 mg daily. Daily maximum is 10 mg.

Conditions Requiring Dosing Adjustments

Liver Function: Starting dose is 2.5 mg daily, with a 10 mg maximum.
Kidney Function: No changes needed.

▷ **Dosing Instructions:**   May take with or following food to reduce stomach upset. Tablet should be swallowed whole; do not crush or chew.

Usual Duration of Use: Regular use for 2 to 4 weeks shows benefits in controlling hypertension. Smallest effective dose should be used in long-term (months to years) therapy. Physician visits are essential.

Possible Advantages of This Drug   Gradual onset and prolonged duration of action, permitting effective once-a-day treatment.

▷ **This Drug Should Not Be Taken If**
  • you had an allergic reaction to it or similar medicines.
  • you have active liver disease.
  • you have severe lowering of the blood pressure.
  • you have severe problems (dysfunction) in the left side of your heart.
  • you have atrioventricular blockade or sick sinus syndrome (talk with your doctor).
  • you have uncorrected congestive heart failure.

▷ **Inform Your Physician Before Taking This Drug If**
  • you have had an unfavorable response to any calcium channel blocker drug.
  • you take digitalis or a beta-blocker (see Drug Classes).
  • you are taking any other drugs that lower blood pressure.
  • you have a history of congestive heart failure, heart attack, or stroke.

- you are subject to disturbances of heart rhythm (such as atrial fibrillation).
- you develop a skin reaction while taking this medicine.
- you have circulatory impairment to the fingers.
- you have muscular dystrophy or myasthenia gravis.
- you have a history of impaired liver or kidney function.

Possible Side Effects (natural, expected, and unavoidable drug actions)
Swelling of feet and ankles, flushing and sensation of warmth.

▷ **Possible Adverse Effects** (unusual, unexpected, and infrequent reactions)
If any of the following develop, consult your physician promptly for guidance.

Mild Adverse Effects
Allergic reactions: skin rash—rare.
Headache—frequent; dizziness, fatigue, or sleep disorders—infrequent.
Indigestion, nausea, stomach pain, constipation, or diarrhea—all rare.
Palpitations or fast heart rate (tachycardia)—infrequent to frequent.
Dose-related flushing—possible.
Impaired sense of smell—possible.
Cough or pharyngitis—infrequent.
Increased urination—possible.
Abnormal growth of the gums (gingival hyperplasia)—rare.

Serious Adverse Effects
Allergic reactions: serious skin reactions.
Idiosyncratic reactions: none reported.
Aggravation of angina—possible.
Decreased hemoglobin, hematocrit, and red blood cell count (reported with other drugs in the same family—case reports.
Stroke—case reports.

▷ **Possible Effects on Sexual Function:** Impotence (0.5–1.5%)—rare.

▷ **Adverse Effects That May Mimic Natural Diseases or Disorders**
An allergic rash and swelling of the legs may resemble erysipelas.

Possible Effects on Laboratory Tests
Liver function tests: minor and short-term increases.

CAUTION
1. Tell your health care providers that you take this drug. Carry a note in your purse or wallet saying you take it.
2. You may use nitroglycerin and other nitrate drugs to ease acute episodes of angina pain. Call your doctor if angina attacks become more frequent or intense.

Precautions for Use

By Those Over 60 Years of Age: You may be more susceptible to the development of weakness, dizziness, fainting, and falling. Take necessary precautions to prevent injury.

▷ **Advisability of Use During Pregnancy**
Pregnancy Category: C. See Pregnancy Risk Categories at the back of this book.
Animal studies: No information available.
Human studies: Adequate studies of pregnant women are not available.
Avoid this drug during the first 3 months. Use during the final 6 months only if clearly needed. Ask your physician for guidance.

Advisability of Use If Breast-Feeding

Presence of this drug in breast milk: Unknown.

Avoid drug or refrain from nursing.

Habit-Forming Potential: None.

Effects of Overdose: Weakness, fainting, fast pulse, low blood pressure, shortness of breath, flushed and warm skin, tremors.

Possible Effects of Long-Term Use: None reported.

Suggested Periodic Examinations While Taking This Drug (at physician's discretion)

Heart function tests (electrocardiograms) and blood pressure checks in supine, sitting, and standing positions.

▷ **While Taking This Drug, Observe the Following**

Foods: Avoid eating grapefruit for 1 hour after taking this medicine. Avoid excessive salt intake. Ginseng may increase blood pressure.

Beverages: Grapefruit juice can cause **a serious increase** in the absorption of this drug—levels may be increased by over 400%. Do **not** take this drug with grapefruit juice. May be taken with milk or water.

▷ *Alcohol:* Use with caution—alcohol may exaggerate the drop in blood pressure experienced by some individuals.

Tobacco Smoking: Nicotine may reduce effectiveness. I advise everyone to quit smoking.

▷ *Other Drugs*

Felodipine *taken concurrently* with

- adenosine may result in an extended slowing of the heart.
- beta-blocker drugs or digitalis preparations (see Drug Classes) may affect heart rate and rhythm adversely. Careful monitoring by your physician is necessary if these drugs are taken concurrently.
- carbamazepine (Tegretol) may decrease felodipine benefits.
- delavirdine (Rescriptor) may lead to felodipine toxicity.
- digoxin (Lanoxin) may increase digoxin levels and result in toxicity.
- itraconazole, fluconazole, or ketoconazole (see *antifungal drugs* in Drug Classes) may lead to felodipine toxicity.
- magnesium (particularly in high doses) may cause low blood pressure (not specifically reported for felodipine, but another drug in the calcium channel blocker class does this).
- phenobarbital can cause decreased felodipine benefits.
- phenytoin (Dilantin) may cause decreased phenytoin levels.
- rifampin (Rifadin) may cause decreased felodipine benefits (reported with other calcium channel blockers).
- ritonavir (Norvir) and perhaps other protease inhibitors (see Drug Classes) may lead to toxicity.

The following drugs may *increase* the effects of felodipine:

- cimetidine (Tagamet).
- erythromycin—may also occur with other macrolide antibiotics (see Drug Classes), since they are structurally similar.

▷ *Driving, Hazardous Activities:* Usually no restrictions. This drug may cause dizziness. Restrict activities as necessary.

Aviation Note: Hypertension *is a disqualification* for piloting. Consult a designated aviation medical examiner.

Exposure to Sun: No restrictions.

Exposure to Heat: Caution is advised. Hot environments can exaggerate the blood-pressure-lowering effects of this drug. Observe for light-headedness or weakness.

Discontinuation: Do not stop this drug abruptly. Ask your physician about gradual withdrawal. Watch for development of rebound hypertension.

FENAMATE (NONSTEROIDAL ANTI-INFLAMMATORY DRUGS) FAMILY

Meclofenamate (MEK low fen a mate)   **Mefenamic Acid** (MEF en amik a sid)
Introduced: 1977, 1966   **Class:** Analgesic, mild; NSAIDs   **Prescription:** USA: Yes   **Controlled Drug:** USA: No; Canada: No   **Available as Generic:** Yes
Brand Names: Meclofenamate: Meclodium, Meclomen; Mefenamic Acid: Ponstel, ✦Ponstan

BENEFITS versus RISKS	
Possible Benefits	*Possible Risks*
EFFECTIVE RELIEF OF MILD TO MODERATE PAIN AND INFLAMMATION	Gastrointestinal pain, ulceration, bleeding
	Kidney damage
	Fluid retention
	Bone marrow depression (mefenamic acid)
	Hemolytic anemia (mefenamic acid)
	Systemic lupus erythematosus (mefenamic acid)
	Pancreatitis (mefenamic acid)

Author's Note: All these risks are rare.

▷ **Principal Uses**

As a Single Drug Product: Uses currently included in FDA-approved labeling: (1) Meclofenamate is used to relieve pain of osteoarthritis and rheumatoid arthritis; (2) mefenamic acid is used to relieve chronic pain, painful menstruation (dysmenorrhea), and general and postoperative pain.

Other (unlabeled) generally accepted uses: (1) Meclofenamate is used to treat temporal arteritis and the nephrotic syndrome; (2) mefenamic acid is used to treat PMS, osteoarthritis (maximum 1 week), and temporal arteritis.

How These Drugs Work: These drugs reduce prostaglandins (and related substances), chemicals involved in producing inflammation and pain.

Available Dose Forms and Strengths:

Meclofenamate (Meclomen):
Capsules — 50 mg, 100 mg
Mefenamic acid (Ponstel):
  Capsule — 250 mg

▷ **Usual Adult Dose Range:** Meclofenamate: For osteoarthritis or rheumatoid arthritis: 200 to 400 mg daily, in three or four divided doses. Total daily dose should not be more than 400 mg.

Mefenamic acid: 500 mg initially, then 250 mg every 6 hours, taken with food. **Note: Actual dose and schedule must be determined for each patient individually.**

Conditions Requiring Dosing Adjustments

Liver Function: Dosing changes not presently recommended.

Kidney Function: Meclofenamate is removed by the kidneys; however, specific dosing guidelines have not been specified. Mefenamic acid **not** to be used by patients with compromised kidneys.

▷ **Dosing Instructions:** Take with food or milk to prevent stomach irritation. Take with a full glass of water and remain upright (do not lie down) for 30 minutes. The capsule may be opened to take it.

Usual Duration of Use: Meclofenamate: Use on a regular schedule for 2 to 3 weeks usually determines its effectiveness in arthritis therapy. Long-term use (months to years) requires physician supervision and periodic evaluation.

Mefenamic acid: Peak levels occur in up to 4 hours. Use beyond 7 days is **not recommended**.

▷ **These Drugs Should Not Be Taken If**
- you have had an allergic reaction to them previously.
- you get asthma or nasal polyps caused by aspirin.
- you have active peptic ulcer disease, regional enteritis, ulcerative colitis, or gastrointestinal bleeding.
- you have a bleeding disorder or a blood cell disorder.
- you have severe impairment of kidney function (mefenamic acid).
- you have systemic lupus erythematosus (mefenamic acid).
- you have recently had pancreatitis (mefenamic acid).

▷ **Inform Your Physician Before Taking These Drugs If**
- you are allergic to aspirin or to other aspirin substitutes.
- you have a history of peptic ulcer disease, regional enteritis, or ulcerative colitis.
- you have a history of any type of bleeding disorder.
- you have impaired liver or kidney function.
- you have high blood pressure or a history of heart failure.
- you take acetaminophen, aspirin, or other aspirin substitutes; anticoagulants; oral antidiabetic drugs; or cortisonelike drugs.

Possible Side Effects (natural, expected, and unavoidable drug actions)

Ringing in ears, fluid retention, or drowsiness.

▷ **Possible Adverse Effects** (unusual, unexpected, and infrequent reactions)

If any of the following develop, consult your physician promptly for guidance.

Mild Adverse Effects

Allergic reactions: skin rash, hives, itching.

Headache, dizziness, altered or blurred vision, depression—possible.

Mouth sores, indigestion, nausea, vomiting, diarrhea (10–33%, sometimes severe).

Serious Adverse Effects

Allergic reactions: severe skin reactions, drug fever (see Glossary)—case reports.

Active peptic ulcer, with or without bleeding—possible.

Kidney damage with painful urination, bloody urine, reduced urine formation—case reports.

Bone marrow depression (see Glossary) (mefenamic acid): fatigue, weakness, fever, sore throat, abnormal bleeding or bruising—case reports.

Mefenamic acid also causes rare hemolytic anemia, seizures, porphyria, liver damage, pancreatitis, and systemic lupus erythematosus.

▷ **Possible Effects on Sexual Function:** None reported.

Possible Delayed Adverse Effects: Mild anemia due to "silent" blood loss from the stomach (less than that caused by aspirin).

Natural Diseases or Disorders That May Be Activated by These Drugs

Peptic ulcer disease, ulcerative colitis.

Possible Effects on Laboratory Tests

Complete blood cell counts: decreased red cells, hemoglobin, white cells, and platelets—all rare. For mefenamic acid, also add SLE test.

CAUTION

1. The smallest dose that offers improvement should be used.
2. May hide early signs of infection. Call your doctor if you think you are developing an infection.
3. Mefenamic acid should be used for a maximum of 7 days.

Precautions for Use

By Infants and Children: Safety and effectiveness for those under 14 years of age have not been established for meclofenamate, and under 18 years of age for mefenamic acid.

By Those Over 60 Years of Age: Small doses are advisable. Watch for indications of liver or kidney toxicity, fluid retention, dizziness, confusion, stomach bleeding, or diarrhea.

▷ **Advisability of Use During Pregnancy**

Pregnancy Category: Meclofenamate: B normally and D in the final 3 months of pregnancy. Mefenamic acid: C. See Pregnancy Risk Categories at the back of this book.

Animal studies: Some minor birth defects reported in rodents for meclofenamate. Increased fetal resorption in rabbits with 2.5 times the human mefenamic acid dose.

Human studies: Adequate studies of pregnant women are not available.

The manufacturer does not recommend the use of meclofenamate during pregnancy.

Use of mefenamic acid in late pregnancy should be avoided. Ask your doctor for help regarding mefenamic acid use during pregnancy.

Advisability of Use If Breast-Feeding

Presence of these drugs in breast milk: Yes.

Avoid drug or refrain from nursing.

Habit-Forming Potential: None.

Effects of Overdose: Drowsiness, nausea, vomiting, diarrhea, marked agitation, irrational behavior, metabolic acidosis, and seizures.

Possible Effects of Long-Term Use: None identified.

Suggested Periodic Examinations While Taking These Drugs (at physician's discretion)

Complete blood cell counts, kidney function tests, complete eye examinations if vision is altered in any way.

▷ **While Taking These Drugs, Observe the Following:**

Foods: No restrictions.

Beverages: No restrictions. May be taken with milk.

▷ *Alcohol:* Use with caution. Alcohol and this drug both irritate the stomach. May increase risk of stomach ulcers or bleeding.

Tobacco Smoking: No interactions expected. I advise everyone to quit smoking.

▷ *Other Drugs*

Meclofenamate *taken concurrently* with the following drugs may increase the risk of bleeding (avoid these combinations):

- aspirin (various).
- dipyridamole (Persantine).
- sulfinpyrazone (Anturane).
- valproic acid (Depakene).

Mefenamic acid *taken concurrently* with

- aspirin, dipyridamole, or sulfinpyrazone may result in increased bleeding risk.
- cyclosporine (Sandimmune) may result in increased cyclosporine levels and toxicity.
- magnesium-containing antacids may result in rapid mefenamic acid toxicity.

Meclofenamate or mefenamic acid *taken concurrently* with

- anticoagulants (Coumadin, etc.) increase the risk of bleeding; monitor INR (prothrombin time), adjust dose accordingly.
- diuretics (see Drug Classes) or other medicines for high blood pressure may result in decreased blood pressure control.
- enoxaparin (Lovenox) may result in increased surgical blood loss if patients receiving this combination undergo surgery.
- lithium (Lithobid, others) will increase blood lithium levels over time and may result in toxicity.
- methotrexate (Mexate) can result in serious methotrexate toxicity.

▷ *Driving, Hazardous Activities:* This drug may cause dizziness or altered vision. Restrict activities as necessary.

Aviation Note: The use of these drugs *may be a disqualification* for piloting. Consult a designated aviation medical examiner.

Exposure to Sun: No restrictions.

FENOPROFEN (fen oh PROH fen)

See the propionic acids (nonsteroidal anti-inflammatory drugs) profile for further information.

FENTANYL (FEN ta nil)

Introduced: 1991   **Class:** Analgesic, strong   **Prescription:** USA: Yes
Controlled Drug: USA: C-II*; Canada: Yes   **Available as Generic:** USA: No;
Canada: No
Brand Names: Duragesic, ✦Innovar, Oralet, Sublimaze

BENEFITS versus RISKS	
Possible Benefits	*Possible Risks*
EFFECTIVE PAIN RELIEF	Habit-forming potential with
SKIN PATCH APPLICATION	prolonged use
NEEDED ONLY ONCE EVERY 3	Impairment of mental function
DAYS	Methemoglobinemia
	Respiratory depression

▷ **Principal Uses**
> *As a Single Drug Product:* Uses currently included in FDA-approved labeling:
> Treatment of chronic pain.
> Other (unlabeled) generally accepted uses: None.

How This Drug Works: Acts at specific pain receptors (Mu agonist) to block
pain.

Available Dose Forms and Strengths

> Transdermal patch — 2.5 mg, 5 mg, 7.5
> mg, 10 mg
> Lozenge on a handle (has been likened to a lollipop) — 200 mcg, 300 mcg,
> 400 mcg

Author's Note: Injectable forms are not presented in this profile.

▷ **Recommended Dose Ranges (Actual dose and schedule must be determined
for each patient individually.)**
> *Infants and Children:* Sucker form: Based on weight for those over 10 kg: 5–15
> mcg/kg range. Those 40 kg or greater are given 400 mcg.
> *18 to 60 Years of Age:* Patch: Not indicated for patients 18 years old who weigh
> less than 50 kg (110 lb).
> In patients who have not been using opioids such as morphine, the 25 mcg per
> hour (2.5-mg) patch should be used. In people who used opioids previously,
> the amount needed to control pain on a 24-hour basis is calculated, con-
> verted to an equal amount of morphine (morphine equianalgesic dose), and
> then converted to fentanyl.
> Lozenge (sucker): Used to treat pain/anxiety before surgery; 400 mcg for those
> with a body mass of 50 kg or more.
> *Over 60 Years of Age:* Should receive 25 mcg per hour (2.5-mg) patch, unless al-
> ready receiving equivalent of 135 mg of oral morphine daily. Intravenous
> fentanyl clears more slowly in patients over 60 than in younger patients.
> Watch carefully for overdose.

Conditions Requiring Dosing Adjustments
> *Liver Function:* The dose **must be decreased** in liver compromise.
> *Kidney Function:* In moderate to severe kidney failure, 75% of the usual dose.

*See Controlled Drug Schedules at the back of this book.

Dose reduced by 50% in severe kidney failure. People in end-stage kidney disease may be more sensitive to this medicine.

▷ **Dosing Instructions:**   Take the patch from pouch. Remove stiff protective liner from sticky side of patch. Do not cut the system. Place sticky side on a non-hairy, dry area (back, chest, side, or upper arm). Avoid burned, irritated, or oily areas. Wash your hands patch is applied. Apply a new patch to a different area after 3 days. Fold the old patch onto itself and flush it down the toilet. Avoid heat such as electric blankets or heating pads. The lozenge or sucker should slowly dissolve in the mouth. Do not bite or chew it.

Usual Duration of Use: Regular use for 1 to 3 days determines benefits in pain control.

Immediate-release morphine or similar drug should be available while this drug reaches peak effect. Long-term use (months) requires evaluation by your doctor.

Possible Advantages of This Drug   Effective pain relief with patch placement once every 3 days and no injections.

▷ **This Drug Should Not Be Taken If**
- you had an allergic reaction to any form of it previously.
- you have had an allergic reaction to the adhesive in the patch before.
- you are less than 12 years old.
- you weigh less than 50 kg and are less than 18 years old.
- you have mild or intermittent pain.
- you have acute or postoperative pain without opportunity for proper dose adjustment.

▷ **Inform Your Physician Before Taking This Drug If**
- you have liver or kidney compromise.
- you have chronic lung disease (such as chronic obstructive pulmonary disease, or COPD).
- you have an abnormally slow heartbeat or other heart disease.
- you develop a high fever.
- you have not taken narcotic pain medicines before and you are given a dose more than 25 mcg per hour.
- you take an MAO inhibitor (see Drug Classes).
- you have a brain tumor.
- you are anemic or have heart disease.
- you have a history of alcoholism or drug abuse.
- you take prescription or nonprescription drugs not discussed with your doctor when fentanyl was prescribed.

Possible Side Effects (natural, expected, and unavoidable drug actions)
Constipation, dry mouth. Sleepiness (somnolence) or euphoria—infrequent.

▷ **Possible Adverse Effects** (unusual, unexpected, and infrequent reactions)
If any of the following develop, consult your physician promptly for guidance.
Mild Adverse Effects
Allergic reactions: skin rash and itching.
Blurred vision or amblyopia—rare to infrequent.
Nausea or vomiting—infrequent.

Urinary retention—infrequent.

Tremor or muscular rigidity—possible.

Serious Adverse Effects

Allergic reactions: exfoliative dermatitis and/or anaphylactic reactions—case reports.

Arrhythmias—rare.

Paranoid reaction, depersonalization, speech problems (aphasia)—rare, dose related.

Seizures or hallucinations—case reports.

Methemoglobinemia or porphyrias—rare.

Paresthesias—rare.

Respiratory depression (this effect may last longer than the pain-relieving effect)—dose related.

▷ **Possible Effects on Sexual Function:** Impotence and blunted orgasm sensation in men. Irregular menstrual periods and blunted orgasm sensation in women.

Possible Delayed Adverse Effects: Dependence and tolerance.

Possible Effects on Laboratory Tests

Methemoglobinemia.

CAUTION

1. Extreme caution should be used if this drug is combined with other opioids, narcotic drugs, benzodiazepines, or alcohol.
2. May cause serious constipation in older patients.
3. Do not expose the patch site to external sources of heat such as heating pads or electric blankets, as an increased rate of drug release may occur.

Precautions for Use

By Infants and Children: Safety and effectiveness for those under 12 years of age are not established.

By Those Over 60 Years of Age: The 2.5-mg patch should **NOT** be used as a starting dose unless you are already taking more than 135 mg of morphine daily. Those with cardiac, respiratory, kidney, or liver compromise should be given low doses and carefully monitored.

▷ **Advisability of Use During Pregnancy**

Pregnancy Category: C, D if used in high doses when the baby is born or for prolonged periods. See Pregnancy Risk Categories at the back of this book.

Animal studies: Some fetal death data with intravenous use in rats.

Human studies: Adequate studies of pregnant women are not available.

Ask your doctor for guidance.

Advisability of Use If Breast-Feeding

Presence of this drug in breast milk: Yes.

Avoid drug or refrain from nursing.

Habit-Forming Potential: Fentanyl is a Schedule II narcotic and can cause dependence resembling morphine dependence. Physical and psychological dependence and tolerance can occur with repeated use.

Effects of Overdose: Dizziness, amnesia, and stupor. Respiratory depression and apnea may occur.

Possible Effects of Long-Term Use: Tolerance and physical or psychological dependence.

Suggested Periodic Examinations While Taking This Drug (at physician's discretion)
    Liver function tests.

▷ **While Taking This Drug, Observe the Following**
    Foods: No restrictions.
    Beverages: No restrictions.
▷   *Alcohol:* **DO NOT DRINK ALCOHOL** while you are taking this drug—leads to additive loss of mental status, respiratory depression, and confusion.
    Tobacco Smoking: No interactions expected. I advise everyone to quit smoking.
    Marijuana Smoking: Additive adverse effects; however, marijuana may block the vomiting effect of fentanyl.
▷   *Other Drugs*
        Fentanyl may *increase* the effects of
        • benzodiazepines such as diazepam (Valium) and alprazolam (Xanax).
        • central nervous system depressants such as opiates, barbiturates, tranquilizers, and tricyclic antidepressants.
        Fentanyl *taken concurrently* with
        • amiodarone (Codarone) may result in heart (cardiac) toxicity.
        • clonidine (Catapres, others) may result in greater than expected fentanyl effects. The fentanyl dose may need to be decreased if these medicines are to be combined.
        • MAO inhibitors (see Drug Classes) may worsen the lowering of blood pressure and depression of breathing seen with fentanyl.
        • ritonavir (Norvir) and perhaps other protease inhibitors (see Drug Classes) can lead to major fentanyl toxicity.
▷   *Driving, Hazardous Activities:* This drug may cause drowsiness, sedation, and respiratory depression. Restrict activities as necessary.
    Aviation Note: The use of this drug *is a disqualification* for piloting. Consult a designated aviation medical examiner.
    Exposure to Sun: No restrictions.
    Discontinuation: Once the patch is removed, fentanyl will still be released from the site for 17 hours or more. If pain medicine is still needed, the alternative should be substituted once the fentanyl level is low enough.

FILGRASTIM (fil GRA stem)

Other Name: Recombinant G-CSF

Introduced: 1991   **Class:** Hematopoietic agent   **Prescription:** USA: Yes   **Controlled Drug:** USA: No; Canada: No   **Available as Generic:** USA: No; Canada: No

Brand Name: Neupogen

```
┌─────────────────────────────────────────────────────────────────────┐
│                      BENEFITS versus RISKS                          │
│        Possible Benefits                    Possible Risks          │
│  PREVENTION OF INFECTIONS      Bone pain                            │
│    DUE TO LOWERED WHITE        Changes in heart waves              │
│    BLOOD CELL COUNTS:                                              │
│  FOLLOWING CHEMOTHERAPY                                            │
│  FOLLOWING BONE MARROW                                             │
│    TRANSPLANT                                                      │
│  IN PATIENTS WITH CHRONIC OR                                       │
│    CYCLIC NEUTROPENIA                                              │
│  INCREASED BLOOD CELLS IN                                          │
│    AIDS PATIENTS                                                   │
│  CORRECTION OF DRUG-INDUCED                                        │
│    LOWERING OF WHITE BLOOD                                         │
│    CELLS                                                           │
└─────────────────────────────────────────────────────────────────────┘
```

▷ **Principal Uses**

As a Single Drug Product: Uses currently included in FDA-approved labeling: (1) Used to help white blood cell counts recover after chemotherapy and bone marrow transplants; (2) used subcutaneously or intravenously to reduce or prevent low white blood cell counts that occur after cancer chemotherapy; (3) treats patients who have an absence of white blood cells at birth; (4) used to help patients with Kostmann syndrome have improved white blood cell counts; (5) used to help patients who have low white blood cell counts (neutropenia) of unknown cause (idiopathic); (6) used to treat low white blood cells (neutropenia) in HIV-positive people or in those with AIDS.

Other (unlabeled) generally accepted uses: (1) Helps patients recover from a particular kind of lack of white blood cells (agranulocytosis) that has been caused by medicines (drug induced); (2) used in AIDS (orphan drug status) patients (taking ganciclovir) to help restore white blood cell counts; (3) used to treat patients with severe long-term (chronic) low white blood cell counts; (4) used to treat patients with abnormally low white blood cell and neutrophil counts (myelodysplastic syndrome).

How This Drug Works: Regulates proliferation and release of early (progenitor) forms of white blood cells. Can tell bone marrow to increase rate that it makes white blood cells. Filgrastim may also work with other factors to increase the production of blood platelets.

Available Dose Forms and Strengths

Solution for injection — 300 mcg/ml (supplied as a 300- or 480-mcg vial)

How to Store

The prepared solution should be stored at 36 to 46 degrees F (2 to 8 degrees C). This medicine **should not** be frozen. Some centers draw up a 7-day supply of syringes that are then stored in a refrigerator.

▷ **Recommended Dose Ranges** (Actual dose and schedule must be determined for each patient individually.)

Infants and Children: Studied doses of 0.6 to 120 mcg per kg of body mass per day for up to 3 years have been well tolerated in children 3 months to 18 years of age. In chronic low white blood cell counts (chronic neutropenia), doses of 5 to 10 mcg per kg of body mass per day have been used.

18 to 60 Years of Age: Patients having bone marrow destroyed (myeloablative treatment) and getting a bone marrow transplant, wait 24 hours after chemo was given and 24 hours after bone marrow transplant, then receive 10 mcg per kg of body mass per day to start. Dosing is adjusted to increase of white blood cells (absolute neutrophil count).

Patients receiving bone marrow suppression should wait until 24 hours after or before the chemotherapy is given. Filgrastim is started with 5 mcg per kg of body mass per day, increased by 5 mcg per kg per day for each cycle of chemotherapy. Dosing is based on severity of white blood cell count decrease (nadir) and how long lowered white cell (absolute neutrophil) count lasts. Drug can be given daily for up to 14 days.

Over 60 Years of Age: Same as 12 to 60 years of age.

Conditions Requiring Dosing Adjustments

Liver Function: Not significantly involved in the elimination of this drug.

Kidney Function: Roughly 90% of a given filgrastim dose is eliminated by the kidneys. Changes in dosing are not defined.

▷ **Dosing Instructions:**   The solution in the reconstituted vial should be colorless and clear. Once your doctor or nurse has taught you how to inject the medicine:

- Make certain the solution has not expired (check the expiration date).
- Make certain you have the correct kind of syringe (insulin syringes are commonly used).
- Follow the provided patient instructions carefully.
- If you are using a syringe, make certain you inject the medicine under the skin, not into a vein.
- This medicine can also be given intravenously over a period of 15 to 30 minutes.

Usual Duration of Use: Ten to 14 days of regular use may be needed to see benefits in correcting low white blood cell (absolute neutrophil) counts after chemotherapy. Bone marrow transplant patients may take still longer to respond. Long-term problems with white blood cells (such as chronic neutropenia) may require years of therapy. Long-term use requires periodic evaluation of response and dose adjustment. Consult your physician on a regular basis.

Possible Advantages of This Drug

Effective recombinant product with few side effects.

▷ **This Drug Should Not Be Taken If**
- you had an allergic reaction to it previously.
- you have a known allergy to products derived from *E. coli* (a bacteria).

▷ **Inform Your Physician Before Taking This Drug If**
- you have a history of gout or psoriasis.
- you have received chemotherapy within the last 24 hours.
- you have a history of heart problems (heart rhythm should be closely monitored).
- you have a history of leukemia (myeloid type). The safety and efficacy of this medicine is not established in that condition.
- you have a history of cancer (with myeloid characteristics). There is a possibility that this drug may act as a growth factor for these tumors. However,

use in a small number of leukemia patients has not resulted in worsening of their leukemia.

- you are unsure how much to take or how often to take it.

Possible Side Effects (natural, expected, and unavoidable drug actions)
Pain on injection.
Bone pain (up to 22% in Phase Three studies).

▷ **Possible Adverse Effects** (unusual, unexpected, and infrequent reactions)
If any of the following develop, consult your physician promptly for guidance.

Mild Adverse Effects
Allergic reactions: skin rash or itching—infrequent.
Mild decreases in blood pressure or increases in uric acid—case reports.
Drug-induced fever—infrequent to frequent.
Nausea and anorexia—rare.
Irritation of the eye (iridocyclitis, conjunctival erythema)—case reports.
Enlargement of the spleen: reported in patients with chronic lowering of the white blood cells (chronic neutropenia)—frequent, though asymptomatic in these patients.

Serious Adverse Effects
Allergic reactions: anaphylaxis—case report.
Depression of part of the heart action (ST depression)—rare to infrequent.
Sweet syndrome (acute neutrophilic dermatosis)—possible.
Worsening of psoriasis—case report.
Low oxygen in the blood (hypoxemia)—very rare.
Potential (though not yet reported) for this medicine to act as a growth factor for certain cancers (malignancies of the myeloid type)—possible.
Potential (though not yet reported) breathing problems (respiratory distress syndrome) in patients with serious (septic) infections, because white blood cells may travel to the infected area—possible.

▷ **Possible Effects on Sexual Function:** None reported.

Possible Delayed Adverse Effects: Increased uric acid.

▷ **Adverse Effects That May Mimic Natural Diseases or Disorders**
None reported.

Natural Diseases or Disorders That May Be Activated by This Drug
Gout.

Possible Effects on Laboratory Tests
Absolute neutrophil count: increased.
Alkaline phosphatase: increased markedly.
Uric acid: increased mildly.
Lactate dehydrogenase (LDH): increased.

CAUTION

1. Bone pain may be prevented by taking acetaminophen (Tylenol, others) before this medicine is injected.
2. Call your doctor if you have chills, fever, or any other sign of infection.
3. Be certain to follow up with your laboratory testing as scheduled.
4. The solution in the vial should be clear. Do **not** inject any discolored or cloudy solution.

5. Make sure you have the correct kind of syringe before you inject this medicine.
6. This medicine can be given intravenously when it is appropriately prepared. If your doctor has instructed you on how to give yourself an injection using a syringe, the medicine should be given under the skin. Be certain you understand the technique.
7. Always change the site in which you inject this medicine, as your doctor instructed.

Precautions for Use

By Infants and Children: This medicine has been used in children with long-term lowering of white blood cell counts (chronic neutropenia) in doses of 5 to 10 mcg per kg of body mass per day.

By Those Over 60 Years of Age: No specific precautions.

▷ **Advisability of Use During Pregnancy**

Pregnancy Category: C. See Pregnancy Risk Categories at the back of this book.

Animal studies: In rabbits given 80 mcg per kg of body mass per day (very high doses), increased abortion and death of embryos were observed.

Human studies: Information from adequate studies of pregnant women is not available. Ask your doctor for help with this benefit-to-risk decision.

Advisability of Use If Breast-Feeding

Presence of this drug in breast milk: Unknown.

Ask your doctor for guidance.

Habit-Forming Potential: None.

Effects of Overdose: No maximum tolerated dose has been identified.

Possible Effects of Long-Term Use: Enlarged spleens (splenomegaly) may occur in up to 25% of patients with severe chronic neutropenia. Skin rashes may occur in up to 6% of patients.

Suggested Periodic Examinations While Taking This Drug (at physician's discretion)

Complete blood cell counts and platelet counts should be obtained prior to chemotherapy and twice weekly during filgrastim therapy.

▷ **While Taking This Drug, Observe the Following**

Foods: No restrictions.

Beverages: No restrictions.

▷ *Alcohol:* No restrictions.

Tobacco Smoking: No interactions expected. I advise everyone to quit smoking.

▷ *Other Drugs*

Filgrastim *taken concurrently* with

• lithium (Lithobid, others) may (in theory) result in additive release of white blood cells.

• topotecan (Hycamtin) may cause extended low white blood cells.

▷ *Driving, Hazardous Activities:* No restrictions presently attributed to this medicine.

Aviation Note: The use of this drug *is probably not a disqualification* for piloting. Consult a designated aviation medical examiner.

Exposure to Sun: SEVERE intolerance of sunlight (photophobia) has been a treatment-limiting factor.

Occurrence of Unrelated Illness: Report development of chills, fever, or other signs or symptoms of infection immediately to your doctor.

Discontinuation: In people taking bone marrow suppressing drugs: Filgrastim is usually stopped when white blood cell (absolute neutrophil count) reaches 10,000 per cubic mm (once the lowest white blood cell count was reached for the chemotherapy given).

In people taking bone marrow destroying medicine who then have a bone marrow transplant: The drug is started as described. If white blood cell count reaches 1,000 per cubic mm, dose is decreased to 5 mcg per kg of body mass per day. Once white cell count reaches 1,000 per cubic mm for 6 consecutive days, filgrastim can be stopped.

Special Storage Instructions: This drug should be stored at 36 to 46 degrees F (2 to 8 degrees C) once it has been reconstituted. Care should be taken **not to shake** the prepared drug, as it may lose activity. Care should also be taken **not to freeze** the prepared medicine, as it will clump and lose therapeutic activity.

Observe the Following Expiration Times: Once the medicine is prepared, it is stable for 1 day (24 hours) if it is refrigerated. If the drug is stored at room temperature, it is stable for 6 hours. Medicine left at room temperature for more than 6 hours should be returned.

FINASTERIDE (fin ES tur ide)

Introduced: 1992   **Class:** 5-alpha reductase inhibitor   **Prescription:** USA: Yes   **Controlled Drug:** USA: No; Canada: No   **Available as Generic:** USA: No; Canada: No

Brand Names: Proscar, Propecia

BENEFITS versus RISKS	
Possible Benefits	*Possible Risks*
NONSURGICAL TREATMENT OF SYMPTOMATIC BENIGN PROSTATIC HYPERPLASIA. Shrinkage of prostatic tissue and increase in urine flow RETENTION OF HAIR OR INCREASED HAIR GROWTH	Impotence (small percentage) Decreased libido (small percentage) Gynecomastia

▷ **Principal Uses**

As a Single Drug Product: Uses currently included in FDA-approved labeling: (1) Treats symptomatic benign prostatic hyperplasia (BPH)—peak decrease in prostate size has occurred after 6 months of therapy; (2) approved to decrease risk of urine retention and need for prostate surgery in BPH; (3) used as Propecia brand (1 mg) to retain or regrow hair.

Other (unlabeled) generally accepted uses: (1) Treats excessive hair in women (hirsutism).

How This Drug Works: Blocks an enzyme (5-alpha reductase) which decreases change of testosterone to dihydrotestosterone (in liver); this causes the prostate to shrink. Symptoms such as urgency and trouble urinating improve. Inhibiting 5-alpha reductase also leads to hair growth.

Available Dose Forms and Strengths

Finasteride (Proscar) tablets — 5 mg

Finasteride (Propecia) tablets — 1 mg

How to Store

Keep at room temperature. Avoid exposure to extreme humidity.

▷ **Recommended Dose Ranges** (Actual dose and schedule must be determined for each patient individually.)

Infants and Children: Not indicated.

12 to 60 Years of Age: Symptomatic benign prostatic hyperplasia often does not occur in the younger end of this adult dosing range; however, the dose for this age range is 5 mg each day, taken by mouth.

Hair-restoring agent: 1 mg daily dose.

Over 60 Years of Age: Same as 12 to 60 years of age, unless liver function has decreased.

Conditions Requiring Dosing Adjustments

Liver Function: People with abnormal liver tests should be closely followed by their doctors.

Kidney Function: No changes needed.

▷ **Dosing Instructions:**   May be taken without regard to food. Food changes time to peak blood concentration only.

Usual Duration of Use: Use on a regular schedule for at least 6 months is needed to see this drug's peak benefit in shrinking the prostate and decreasing symptoms. Use for 1 year may be required to demonstrate hair regrowth.

Possible Advantages of This Drug

May give you symptomatic relief of benign prostatic hyperplasia (BPH) without surgery. May be more effective than other available agents in helping hair regrowth.

▷ **This Drug Should Not Be Taken If**

• you had an allergic reaction to it previously.

▷ **Inform Your Physician Before Taking This Drug If**

• you have impaired liver function or liver disease.

• you are a woman or a child.

• you have kidney problems of any nature.

• your sexual partner is pregnant.

Possible Side Effects (natural, expected, and unavoidable drug actions)

May or may not increase testosterone levels; however, the significance of this effect is not known.

▷ **Possible Adverse Effects** (unusual, unexpected, and infrequent reactions)

If any of the following develop, consult your physician promptly for guidance.

Mild Adverse Effects

Allergic reactions: skin rash, hives—rare.

Plasma testosterone—decreased.

Serious Adverse Effects

Allergic reactions: hypersensitivity reactions—case reports.

▷ **Possible Effects on Sexual Function:**   Gynecomastia (most frequent adverse effect)—rare.

Impotence, decreased libido, or decreased volume of ejaculate—infrequent.

Adverse sexual effects may resolve in more than 60% of patients who continue this medication.

Possible Delayed Adverse Effects: Possible enlargement of male breast tissue (gynecomastia).

Possible Effects on Laboratory Tests

Decreased PSA (prostate specific antigen).

CAUTION

1. A digital rectal exam and other prostate cancer exams are prudent before this medicine is started.
2. If you have a change in liver function, inform your doctor.
3. If your sexual partner is pregnant, avoid exposing your partner to your semen. Exposure to finasteride-containing semen may cause genital abnormalities in male offspring.

Precautions for Use

By Infants and Children: Safety and effectiveness for infants and children are not established.

By Those Over 60 Years of Age: No specific precautions other than changes related to decreased liver function.

▷ **Advisability of Use During Pregnancy**

Pregnancy Category: X. See Pregnancy Risk Categories at the back of this book.

Animal studies: When administered to pregnant rats, the male offspring developed hypospadias. The offspring experienced decreased prostatic and seminal vesicular weight, slow preputial separation, and transient nipple problems.

Human studies: Contraindicated in women who are pregnant or who plan to become pregnant. Women who are pregnant must avoid exposure to crushed tablets and semen of a sexual partner who is on finasteride.

Ask your physician for guidance.

Advisability of Use If Breast-Feeding

Refrain from nursing if you have been exposed to finasteride or finasteride-containing semen.

Habit-Forming Potential: None.

Effects of Overdose: Multiple doses of up to 80 mg per day have been taken without adverse effect.

Possible Effects of Long-Term Use: Adverse effects of long-term use are similar to short-term use effects.

Suggested Periodic Examinations While Taking This Drug (at physician's discretion)

Patients should be monitored for signs and symptoms of hypersensitivity.

Patients should be monitored for improvement in symptoms of BPH.

▷ **While Taking This Drug, Observe the Following**

Foods: This medicine is best taken on an empty stomach.

Beverages: No restrictions.

▷   *Alcohol:* No restrictions.

Tobacco Smoking: No interactions expected. I advise everyone to quit smoking.
Marijuana Smoking: No interactions expected.
▷ *Other Drugs*
   Finasteride may **decrease** the effects of
   • theophylline (Theo-Dur, others).
▷ *Driving, Hazardous Activities:* No restrictions.
Aviation Note: No restrictions.
Exposure to Sun: No restrictions.
Special Storage Instructions: Keep at room temperature. Avoid exposure to extreme humidity.

FLUCONAZOLE (flu KOHN a zohl)

Introduced: 1985   **Class:** Antifungal (triazole)   **Prescription:** USA: Yes
Controlled Drug: USA: No; Canada: No   **Available as Generic:** USA: No;
Canada: No
Brand Name: Diflucan

BENEFITS versus RISKS	
Possible Benefits	*Possible Risks*
EFFECTIVE TREATMENT AND SUPPRESSION OF CRYPTOCOCCAL MENINGITIS	Severe skin reactions Possible liver damage
EFFECTIVE TREATMENT OF *CANDIDA* INFECTIONS OF THE MOUTH, THROAT, AND ESOPHAGUS	
EFFECTIVE TREATMENT OF SYSTEMIC *CANDIDA* INFECTIONS	
EFFECTIVE SINGLE-DOSE TREATMENT OF VAGINAL YEAST INFECTIONS	

▷ **Principal Uses**
   As a Single Drug Product: Uses currently included in FDA-approved labeling: (1) *Candida* (yeast) infections of the mouth, throat, and esophagus (may be AIDS related); (2) systemic *Candida* infections: lungs, peritonitis, urinary tract infections (may be AIDS related); (3) treats vaginal yeast infections.
   Other (unlabeled) generally accepted uses: (1) Prevention of yeast infections in patients with low white blood cell counts or cancer, or those taking steroids; (2) treatment and suppression of cryptococcal meningitis; (3) treatment of some fungal eye infections (endophthalmitis); (4) single-dose treatment of vaginal yeast infections; (5) treatment of *Aspergillus* pneumonia; (6) treatment of candidal urinary tract infections; (7) used to treat some fungal infections that may occur in people who have received transplanted organs.

How This Drug Works: By damaging cell walls and blocking essential cell enzymes, this drug inhibits cell growth and reproduction (with low drug concentrations) and destroys fungal cells (with high drug concentrations).

Available Dose Forms and Strengths

Injection — 200 mg in 100 ml and 400 mg in 200 ml
Tablets — 50 mg, 100 mg, 150 mg, 200 mg
Oral suspension — 50 mg/5 ml
— 200 mg/5 ml

▷ **Recommended Dose Ranges** (Actual dose and schedule must be determined for each patient individually.)

Infants and Children: From 3 to 13 years of age: 3–6 mg per kg of body mass daily, depending on the kind and site of infection.

Cryptococcal meningitis: 12 mg per kg on the first day, then 6 mg per kg daily for 10 to 12 weeks after cerebrospinal fluid (CSF) culture becomes negative.

13 to 60 Years of Age: Cryptococcal meningitis: 400 mg once daily until improvement occurs; then 200 to 400 mg once daily for 10 to 12 weeks after cerebrospinal fluid (CSF) culture becomes negative.

Suppression of cryptococcal meningitis: 200 mg once daily.

Candida infections of mouth and throat: 200 mg first day; then 100 mg once daily for 2 weeks.

Candida infection of the esophagus: 200 mg first day; then 100 mg once daily for at least 3 weeks; treat for 2 weeks after all signs of infection are gone. Doses up to 400 mg daily may be used. Some patients with chronic mucocutaneous *Candida* infections have benefited from 50 mg/day of this medicine.

Systemic *Candida* infections: 400 mg daily for at least 4 weeks; treat for 2 weeks after all symptoms of infection are gone.

Vaginal yeast infections (*Candida*): one 150-mg tablet by mouth.

Over 60 Years of Age: Same as 13 to 60, adjusted if kidneys are impaired.

Conditions Requiring Dosing Adjustments

Liver Function: Caution: rare cause of hepatitis.

Kidney Function: Mild to moderate failure: usual dose every 48 hours. In severe kidney failure: half (50%) of usual dose every 48 hours.

▷ **Dosing Instructions:** The tablet may be crushed; may be taken with or after food to reduce stomach upset.

Usual Duration of Use: Use on a regular schedule for 2 to 4 weeks is usually needed to see this drug's benefit in controlling candidal or cryptococcal infections. Actual cures or long-term suppression often require continual treatment for many months. May be continuous therapy in AIDS patients.

Currently a "Drug of Choice"

For maintenance therapy to prevent relapse following control of AIDS-related candidal esophagitis.

▷ **This Drug Should Not Be Taken If**
- you have had an allergic reaction to it previously.
- you have active liver disease.

▷ **Inform Your Physician Before Taking This Drug If**
- you are allergic to clotrimazole, itraconazole, ketoconazole, or miconazole.
- you have impaired liver or kidney function.
- you are taking any other drugs currently.
- you tend to have low blood potassium.
- you get a skin rash while taking this medicine.

▷ **Possible Adverse Effects** (unusual, unexpected, and infrequent reactions)
If any of the following develop, consult your physician promptly for guidance.
Mild Adverse Effects
Allergic reactions: skin rash—rare.
Hair loss—very rare with usual doses. Reversible hair loss (alopecia) may be more common with high doses of fluconazole given for 2 months or longer.
Headache—rare.
Nausea, vomiting, stomach pain, diarrhea—frequent.
Serious Adverse Effects
Allergic reactions: severe dermatitis (Stevens-Johnson syndrome)—very rare.
Anaphylactic reactions—case reports.
Liver toxicity—rare.
Abnormally low platelet counts: abnormal bruising/bleeding or low white blood cell counts—rare.
Seizures or adrenal suppression—case reports, rare.

▷ **Possible Effects on Sexual Function:**   No conclusive reports.

Possible Delayed Adverse Effects: Liver toxicity.

▷ **Adverse Effects That May Mimic Natural Diseases or Disorders**
Possible liver reaction may suggest viral hepatitis.

Possible Effects on Laboratory Tests
Blood platelet counts: decreased.
Liver function tests: increased liver enzymes (ALT/GPT, AST/GOT, and alkaline phosphatase), increased bilirubin.
Blood potassium: lowered—rare.

Precautions for Use
By Infants and Children: Safety and effectiveness for those under 13 years of age are not established.
By Those Over 60 Years of Age: Age-related decrease in kidney function may require adjustment of dose.

▷ **Advisability of Use During Pregnancy**
Pregnancy Category: C. See Pregnancy Risk Categories at the back of this book.
Animal studies: Rat studies revealed significant abnormalities in bone growth and development.
Human studies: Adequate studies of pregnant women are not available.
Use this drug only if clearly needed. Ask your doctor for help.

Advisability of Use If Breast-Feeding
Presence of this drug in breast milk: Unknown.
Avoid drug or refrain from nursing.

Habit-Forming Potential: None.

Effects of Overdose: Possible nausea, vomiting, diarrhea.

Possible Effects of Long-Term Use: None reported.

Suggested Periodic Examinations While Taking This Drug (at physician's discretion)
Liver and kidney function tests.

▷ **While Taking This Drug, Observe the Following**
Foods: No restrictions.
Beverages: No restrictions. May be taken with milk.

▷ *Alcohol:* No interactions expected.

Tobacco Smoking: No interactions expected. I advise everyone to quit smoking.

▷ *Other Drugs*

Fluconazole may *increase* the effects of

- benzodiazepines (see Drug Classes).
- cyclosporine (Sandimmune).
- oral antidiabetic drugs (chlorpropamide, glipizide, glyburide, tolbutamide, others), and cause hypoglycemia; check sugar levels carefully.
- phenytoin (Dilantin, etc.), and cause phenytoin toxicity; monitor phenytoin blood levels.
- tricyclic antidepressants (see Drug Classes).
- trimetrexate (Neutrexin).
- warfarin (Coumadin), and cause unwanted bleeding; monitor prothrombin times as necessary.
- zidovudine (AZT), and result in toxicity. The zidovudine dose may need to be decreased if this combination is to be continued.

The following drugs may *decrease* the effects of fluconazole:

- cimetidine (Tagamet).
- rifampin (Rifadin, Rimactane, etc.).

Fluconazole *taken concurrently* with

- astemizole (Hismanal) may result in fatal toxicity to the heart.
- atorvastatin (Lipitor) may increase risk of muscle toxicity.
- cisapride (Propulsid) may lead to adverse effects on the heart. DO NOT COMBINE.
- hydrochlorothiazide (Esidrix, others) may increase potassium loss.
- loratadine (Claritin) may result in increased blood levels of loratadine, but to date, toxicity to the heart has not been reported. Since blood levels may be increased if combined use is undertaken, it is prudent to decrease the dose of loratadine.
- oral contraceptives (birth control pills) may blunt contraception and result in pregnancy.
- terfenadine (Seldane) may result in toxicity to the heart.

▷ *Driving, Hazardous Activities:* No restrictions.

Aviation Note: The use of this drug *is probably not a disqualification* for piloting. Consult a designated aviation medical examiner.

Exposure to Sun: No restrictions.

Discontinuation: Take all of the medicine. Ongoing therapy for months may be needed. Ask your doctor when it is okay to stop this medicine.

FLUCYTOSINE (flu SI toh seen)

Other Names: 5-fluorocytosine, 5-FC   **Introduced:** 1977   **Class:** Antifungal   **Prescription:** USA: Yes   **Controlled Drug:** USA: No; Canada: No   **Available as Generic:** USA: No; Canada: No

Brand Names: Ancobon, ✦Ancotil

BENEFITS versus RISKS

Possible Benefits	*Possible Risks*
EFFECTIVE ADJUNCTIVE TREATMENT OF CERTAIN INFECTIONS CAUSED BY *CANDIDA, CRYPTOCOCCUS* FUNGI, and *Aspergillus*	BONE MARROW DEPRESSION DRUG-INDUCED LIVER DAMAGE Peripheral neuritis
Effective adjunctive treatment of chromomycosis infection	

▷ **Principal Uses**

As a Single Drug Product: Uses currently included in FDA-approved labeling: (1) Treats endocarditis, osteomyelitis, arthritis, meningitis, pneumonia, septicemia, and urinary tract infections caused by *Candida;* (2) treats meningitis, pneumonia, septicemia, endocarditis, and urinary tract infections caused by *Cryptococcus*.

Other (unlabeled) generally accepted uses: (1) Treatment of disseminated candidiasis, chromomycosis, and cryptococcosis (these infections may be AIDS related); (2) treatment of general fungal infections.

Note: Flucytosine is usually used together with amphotericin B to treat disseminated fungal infections.

How This Drug Works: This drug goes into fungal cells and blocks production of RNA and DNA, inhibiting fungal development and reproduction.

Available Dose Forms and Strengths

Capsules — 250 mg, 500 mg

▷ **Recommended Dose Ranges** (Actual dose and schedule must be determined for each patient individually.)

Infants and Children: 50 to 150 mg per kg of body mass, divided into four equal doses and given every 6 hours.

12 to 60 Years of Age: 50 to 150 mg per kg of body mass, divided into equal doses and given every 6 hours. In some severe infections, 250 mg per kg of body mass per day have been given.

Over 60 Years of Age: Same as 12 to 60 years of age. If kidney function is impaired, dose reduction is mandatory.

Conditions Requiring Dosing Adjustments

Liver Function: No changes needed in mild to moderate liver compromise. This drug may cause liver toxicity (with blood levels greater than 100 mcg/ml). Used with caution in liver compromise.

Kidney Function: In mild to moderate kidney failure, the usual dose can be given every 12–24 hours. In severe kidney failure, the usual dose can be given every 24–48 hours.

▷ **Dosing Instructions:**   If a single dose requires more than one capsule, space doses over a period of 15 minutes to reduce stomach upset and nausea. The capsule may be opened and taken with or after food.

Usual Duration of Use: Use on a regular schedule for 4 to 6 weeks is needed to see effectiveness in controlling *Candida* or cryptococcal infection. Long-term use (months to years) requires periodic physician evaluation.

▷ **This Drug Should Not Be Taken If**
- you have had an allergic reaction to it previously.
- you have an active blood cell or bone marrow disorder.
- you have active liver disease.

▷ **Inform Your Physician Before Taking This Drug If**
- you have a history of drug-induced bone marrow depression.
- you have a history of peripheral neuritis.
- you have impaired liver or kidney function.

Possible Side Effects (natural, expected, and unavoidable drug actions)
None.

▷ **Possible Adverse Effects** (unusual, unexpected, and infrequent reactions)
If any of the following develop, consult your physician promptly for guidance.
Mild Adverse Effects
Allergic reactions: skin rash, itching.
Headache, dizziness, drowsiness, confusion, hallucinations—infrequent.
Loss of appetite, nausea, vomiting, stomach pain, diarrhea—possible and dose related.
Serious Adverse Effects
Allergic reactions: anaphylactic reactions.
Bone marrow depression (see Glossary): fatigue, weakness, fever, sore throat, abnormal bleeding or bruising—rare.
Liver damage, with or without jaundice (see Glossary)—case reports.
Peripheral neuritis (see Glossary)—possible.
Bowel perforation or kidney damage—rare.

▷ **Possible Effects on Sexual Function:** None reported.

▷ **Adverse Effects That May Mimic Natural Diseases or Disorders**
Drug-induced hepatitis may suggest viral hepatitis.

Natural Diseases or Disorders That May Be Activated by This Drug
Crohn's disease, ulcerative colitis.

Possible Effects on Laboratory Tests
Complete blood counts: decreased red cells, hemoglobin, white cells, and platelets.
Liver function tests: increased liver enzymes (ALT/GPT, AST/GOT, and alkaline phosphatase), increased bilirubin.
Kidney function tests: increased blood urea nitrogen (BUN) and creatinine.
Serum creatinine: may be falsely increased if tested by some methods.

CAUTION
1. When this drug is used alone, resistance can occur rapidly; it is usually used concurrently with amphotericin B (Abelcet) (given intravenously).

Precautions for Use
By Infants and Children: No information available.
By Those Over 60 Years of Age: If necessary, adjust dose for age-related decrease in kidney function.

▷ **Advisability of Use During Pregnancy**
Pregnancy Category: C. See Pregnancy Risk Categories at the back of this book.
Animal studies: Rat studies reveal drug-induced birth defects.

Human studies: Adequate studies of pregnant women are not available. Use this drug only if clearly needed. Ask your physician for guidance.

Advisability of Use If Breast-Feeding
Presence of this drug in breast milk: Yes.
Avoid drug or refrain from nursing.

Habit-Forming Potential: None.

Effects of Overdose: Nausea, vomiting, stomach pain, diarrhea, confusion.

Possible Effects of Long-Term Use: Bone marrow depression, liver or kidney damage.

Suggested Periodic Examinations While Taking This Drug (at physician's discretion)
Measurement of blood levels of flucytosine.
Complete blood cell counts.
Liver and kidney function tests.

▷ **While Taking This Drug, Observe the Following**
Foods: No restrictions.
Beverages: No restrictions. May be taken with milk.
▷ *Alcohol:* No interactions expected.
Tobacco Smoking: No interactions expected. I advise everyone to quit smoking.
▷ *Other Drugs*
The following drugs may ***decrease*** the effects of flucytosine:
• antacids.
• cytarabine (Cytosar).
Flucytosine ***taken concurrently*** with
• amphotericin B may result in increased risk of kidney toxicity; lipid-associated form (Abelcet) may help avoid this.
• zidovudine (AZT) may result in additive and serious blood (hematological) toxicity.
▷ *Driving, Hazardous Activities:* This drug may cause dizziness, drowsiness, or confusion. Limit activities as necessary.
Aviation Note: The use of this drug ***may be a disqualification*** for piloting. Consult a designated aviation medical examiner.
Exposure to Sun: Use caution—may cause photosensitivity (see Glossary).
Discontinuation: This drug may be needed for an extended period. Your doctor must decide when to stop it.

FLUNISOLIDE (flu NIS oh lide)

Introduced: 1980   **Class:**   Antiasthmatic, cortisonelike drugs   **Prescription:** USA: Yes   **Controlled Drug:**   USA: No; Canada: No   **Available as Generic:**   No

Brand Names: AeroBid, AeroBid-M, ✤Bronalide, Nasalide, Nasarel, ✤Rhinalar

```
┌─────────────────────────────────────────────────────────────────┐
│                      BENEFITS versus RISKS                        │
│    Possible Benefits                  Possible Risks              │
│  EFFECTIVE CONTROL OF SEVERE,    Yeast infections of mouth and throat │
│  CHRONIC BRONCHIAL ASTHMA          (inhaler form)                 │
│                                   Increased susceptibility to respiratory │
│                                    tract infections (inhaler form) │
│                                   Localized areas of "allergic"   │
│                                    pneumonia (inhaler form)        │
└─────────────────────────────────────────────────────────────────┘
```

▷ **Principal Uses**

As a Single Drug Product: Uses currently included in FDA-approved labeling: (1) Treats chronic bronchial asthma in people requiring cortisonelike drugs for asthma control; (2) treats various kinds of hay fever (seasonal or perennial allergic rhinitis).

Other (unlabeled) generally accepted uses: (1) Treatment of nasal polyps; (2) treats bronchopulmonary dysplasia; (3) may have a role in acute or chronic sinusitis in combination with an antibiotic (amoxicillin/clavulanate in one study).

How This Drug Works: Increases cyclic AMP, which may increase epinephrine, an effective bronchodilator and antiasthmatic. Also reduces local allergic reaction and inflammation.

Available Dose Forms and Strengths

Inhalation aerosol — 0.25 mg (250 mcg) per metered spray
Nasal solution — 25 mcg per actuation

▷ **Recommended Dose Ranges** (Actual dose and schedule must be determined for each patient individually.)

Infants and Children: Oral inhalation: Up to 6 years old—not recommended. 6–15 years old—two inhalations or 500 mcg twice a day. Maximum daily dose is 1 mg.

Nasal inhalation: Up to 6 years old—not recommended. 6–15 years old—0.25 mcg (one spray in each nostril) three times a day. Once the peak effect is seen, the dose should be reduced to the smallest dose and frequency that works. Maximum is four sprays in each nostril (200 mcg/day).

Aqueous nasal form: Up to 6 years old—not recommended.

6–14 years old—two sprays in each nostril twice daily or one spray in each nostril three times a day. Once the peak effect is seen, the dose should be reduced to the smallest dose and frequency that works.

15 to 60 Years of Age: Oral inhalation: 0.5 to 1 mg (two to four metered sprays) twice a day, morning and evening. Limit total daily dose to 2 mg (four inhalations twice daily). Once the peak effect is seen, the dose should be reduced to the smallest dose and frequency that works.

Nasal inhalation: Two sprays per nostril twice daily. The dose may be increased to two sprays in each nostril three times a day (300 mcg/day). Maximum dose with this route is eight sprays in each nostril (400 mcg) daily. Once the peak effect is seen, the dose should be reduced to the smallest dose and frequency that works.

Aqueous nasal form: Two sprays in each nostril twice daily to start. Maintenance dosing is continued with the lowest dose that is effective. This may be as low as one spray in each nostril daily.

Over 60 Years of Age: Same as 15 to 60 years of age.

Conditions Requiring Dosing Adjustments
Liver Function: Specific guidelines are not available.
Kidney Function: No specific changes needed.

▷ **Dosing Instructions:**   May be used as needed without regard to eating. Shake the container well before using. Carefully follow the printed patient instructions provided with the inhaler; rinse the mouth and throat (gargle) with water thoroughly after each inhalation.

Usual Duration of Use: Use on a regular schedule for 1 to 4 weeks is necessary to see effectiveness in controlling severe, chronic asthma. Long-term use requires physician supervision and guidance.

▷ **This Drug Should Not Be Taken If**
• you have had an allergic reaction to it previously.
• you are having severe acute asthma or status asthmaticus that requires more intense treatment for prompt relief.
• you have a form of nonallergic bronchitis with asthmatic features.

▷ **Inform Your Physician Before Taking This Drug If**
• you are now taking or have recently taken any cortisone-related drug (including ACTH by injection; see *adrenocortical steroids* in Drug Classes) for any reason.
• you have a history of tuberculosis (inhalation form).
• you have herpes simplex infection of the eye.
• you have chicken pox.
• you have had recent surgery of the nose, have ulcers of the nose or nosebleeds—this medicine should be used cautiously until the site has healed.
• you have chronic bronchitis or bronchiectasis.
• you think you may have an active infection of any kind, especially a respiratory infection.

Possible Side Effects (natural, expected, and unavoidable drug actions)
Yeast infections (thrush) of the mouth and throat.
Unpleasant taste. Orally inhaled flunisolide can cause flu-like symptoms occasionally in people taking the drug by oral inhalation.

▷ **Possible Adverse Effects** (unusual, unexpected, and infrequent reactions)
If any of the following develop, consult your physician promptly for guidance.

Mild Adverse Effects
Allergic reactions: skin rash, hives, itching.
Headache, dizziness, nervousness, moodiness, insomnia, loss of smell or taste—rare to infrequent.
Aftertaste (nasal form)—frequent.
Upper respiratory infections, cough—possible.
Heart palpitation, increased blood pressure, swelling of feet and ankles (inhalation form)—possible to infrequent.
Loss of appetite, indigestion, nausea, vomiting, stomach pain, diarrhea—infrequent.
Sore throat, stinging of the nose—infrequent to frequent.

Nasal irritation—infrequent to frequent (less common with the aqueous form).

Impaired sense of smell—possible.

Serious Adverse Effects

Allergic reaction: localized areas of "allergic" pneumonitis (lung inflammation).

Bronchospasm, asthmatic wheezing—rare with the inhalation form.

Tachycardia or hypertension—rare with the inhalation form.

Osteoporosis—possible with long-term use.

▷ **Possible Effects on Sexual Function:** None reported.

Natural Diseases or Disorders That May Be Activated by This Drug

Cortisone-related drugs (used by inhalation) that produce systemic effects can impair immunity and lead to reactivation of "healed" or quiescent tuberculosis. People with a history of tuberculosis should be watched closely during use of cortisonelike drugs by inhalation.

Possible Effects on Laboratory Tests

None reported.

CAUTION

1. Does NOT act primarily as a brochodilator. **Should not be used** for immediate relief of acute asthma.
2. If you were using any cortisone-related drugs for treatment of your asthma *before* changing to this inhaler, the cortisone-related drug may be required if you are injured, have an infection, or require surgery. Tell your doctor about prior use of cortisone-related drugs.
3. If severe asthma returns while using this drug, call your doctor immediately.
4. If you have used cortisone-related drugs in the past year, carry a card that says this has happened.
5. Five to ten minutes should separate the inhalation of bronchodilators such as albuterol, epinephrine, pirbuterol, etc. (which should be used first) and the inhalation of this drug. This lets more flunisolide reach the bronchial tubes and reduces risk of adverse effects from the propellants used in the two inhalers.
6. A decongestant may be a good idea in people with blocked nasal passages. Talk with your doctor or pharmacist.

Precautions for Use

By Infants and Children: Safety and effectiveness for those under 4 years of age are not established. To obtain maximal benefit, the use of a spacer device is recommended for inhalation therapy in children.

By Those Over 60 Years of Age: People with chronic bronchitis or bronchiectasis should be watched closely for the development of lung infections.

▷ **Advisability of Use During Pregnancy**

Pregnancy Category: C. See Pregnancy Risk Categories at the back of this book.

Animal studies: Rat and rabbit studies reveal significant birth defects due to this drug.

Human studies: Adequate studies of pregnant women are not available.

Avoid drug during the first 3 months. Use infrequently and only as clearly needed during the final 6 months.

Advisability of Use If Breast-Feeding
   Presence of this drug in breast milk: Unknown.
   Avoid drug or refrain from nursing.

Habit-Forming Potential: With recommended dose, a state of functional dependence (see Glossary) is not likely to develop.

Effects of Overdose: Indications of cortisone excess (due to systemic absorption)—fluid retention, flushing of the face, stomach irritation, nervousness.

Possible Effects of Long-Term Use: Development of acne, cataracts, altered menstrual pattern. Osteoporosis.

Suggested Periodic Examinations While Taking This Drug (at physician's discretion)
   Inspection of mouth and throat for evidence of yeast infection.
   Check of adrenal function in people who have used cortisone-related drugs for an extended period of time before using this drug. X ray of the lungs of people with a prior history of tuberculosis. Bone mineral density testing (osteoporosis test) with long-term use.

▷ **While Taking This Drug, Observe the Following**
   Foods: No specific restrictions beyond those advised by your physician.
   Beverages: No specific restrictions.
▷   *Alcohol:* No interactions expected.
   Tobacco Smoking: No interactions expected. Smoking can worsen asthma and reduce benefits of flunisolide. I advise everyone to quit smoking.
▷   *Other Drugs*
      The following drugs may ***increase*** the effects of flunisolide:
      • inhalant bronchodilators—albuterol, bitolterol, epinephrine, etc.
      • oral bronchodilators—aminophylline, ephedrine, terbutaline, theophylline, etc.
      Flunisolide ***taken concurrently*** with
      • stanozolol may result in increased risk of acne or edema.
▷   *Driving, Hazardous Activities:* No restrictions.
   Aviation Note: The use of this drug and the disorder for which this drug is prescribed ***may be disqualifications*** for piloting. Consult a designated aviation medical examiner.
   Exposure to Sun: No restrictions.
   Occurrence of Unrelated Illness: Acute infections, serious injuries, or surgical procedures can create an urgent need for cortisone-related drugs given by mouth and/or injection. Call your doctor immediately in the event of new illness or injury.
   Discontinuation: If this drug has made it possible to reduce or discontinue cortisonelike drugs by mouth, ***do not*** stop this drug abruptly. If you must stop this drug, call your doctor promptly. Cortisone preparations and other measures may be necessary.
   Special Storage Instructions: Store at room temperature. Avoid exposure to temperatures above 120 degrees F (49 degrees C). Do not store or use this inhaler near heat or open flame.

FLUOROQUINOLONE ANTIBIOTIC FAMILY

Ciprofloxacin (sip roh FLOX a sin)   **Grepafloxacin** (GREP ah flox a sin)   **Levofloxacin** (leev oh FLOX a sin)   **Lomefloxacin** (loh me FLOX a sin)   **Norfloxacin** (nor FLOX a sin)   **Ofloxacin** (oh FLOX a sin)   **Sparfloxacin** (SPAR flox a sin)   **Trovafloxacin** (TROV ah flox a sin)

Introduced: 1984, 1997, 1996, 1992, 1986, 1984, 1996, 1997.   **Class:** Antiinfective, fluoroquinolone   **Prescription:**   USA: Yes   **Controlled Drug:** USA: No   **Available as Generic:**   USA: No

Brand Names: Ciprofloxacin: Ciloxan, Cipro, Cipro HC [CD]; Grepafloxacin: Raxar; Lomefloxacin: Maxaquin; Norfloxacin: Chibroxin, Noroxin, Noroxin Ophthalmic; Ofloxacin: Floxin, Floxin Otic, Floxin Uropak, Ocuflox; Lomefloxacin: Levaquin; Sparfloxacin: Zagam; Trovafloxacin: Trovan

Warning: Some doctors use "Norflox" to identify norfloxacin. This is not an accepted name in any setting for any reason. This name has resulted in serious medication errors—the dispensing of Norflex, the generic drug or phenadrine, a skeletal muscle relaxant. Check to be sure you get the right drug.

Warning: **Reports are being made for some drugs in this class which find tendon rupture as a rare adverse effect. Ask your doctor about limits on strenuous exercise while you are taking this medicine. A rare idiosyncratic reaction has also been reported which presents as mental confusion and disorientation. Use of these medicines after head trauma may be a risk factor. If you have suffered a fall, ask your doctor if a medicine in a different antibiotic class should be substituted. If you are taking this drug and notice a change in your thinking, call your doctor.**

BENEFITS versus RISKS

Possible Benefits	*Possible Risks*
HIGHLY EFFECTIVE TREATMENT FOR INFECTIONS OF THE LOWER RESPIRATORY TRACT (ciprofloxacin and ofloxacin), URINARY TRACT, BONES, JOINTS, AND SKIN TISSUES due to susceptible organisms	Nausea, indigestion Drug-induced colitis Hallucination or seizure Tendon rupture
EFFECTIVE TREATMENT OF BACTERIAL (EYE) INFECTIONS	
Effective treatment for some forms of bacterial gastroenteritis (diarrhea)	
Effective treatment for some infections of the prostate gland	

▷ **Principal Uses**

As a Single Drug Product: Uses currently included in FDA-approved labeling: Treats responsive infections (in adults) of: (1) the lower respiratory tract (lungs and bronchial tubes); (2) the urinary tract (kidneys, bladder, urethra [including uncomplicated gonorrhea], and prostate gland); (3) the digestive tract (small intestine and colon); (4) bones and joints (ciprofloxacin; ofloxacin—unlabeled); (5) skin and related tissues; (6) used in an ophthalmic preparation to treat bacterial conjunctivitis caused by susceptible organisms; (7) ciprofloxacin has been approved to treat mild to moderate acute sinusitis caused by *Streptococcus pneumoniae, Haemophilus influenzae*, or *Moraxella catarrhalis*; (8) sparfloxacin is very active against strep; (9) ciprofloxacin/hydrocortisone is used for sudden infections of the outside of the ear (acute otitis externa).

Other (unlabeled) generally accepted uses: (1) can have a role in treating cholera where the organisms are resistant to doxycycline (ciprofloxacin); (2) lessens symptoms of or prevents traveler's diarrhea; (3) ciprofloxacin can be of use in treating some unusual organisms such as *Aeromonas*, cat-scratch fever, or chancroid; (4) ofloxacin may help in combination therapy of leprosy. Sparfloxacin also works in leprosy.

How These Drugs Work: These medicines block the bacterial enzyme DNA gyrase (required for DNA synthesis and cell reproduction), and arrests bacterial growth (in low concentrations) and kill bacteria (in high concentrations).

Available Dose Forms and Strengths

Ciprofloxacin:
　　　　Tablets — 250 mg, 500 mg, 750 mg
Ophthalmic solution — 0.3%
Levofloxacin:
　　　　Tablets — 250 mg, 500 mg
Lomefloxacin:
　　　　Tablets — 400 mg
Norfloxacin:
　　　　Tablets — 400 mg
Ophthalmic solution — 3 mg/ml
Ofloxacin:
　　　　Tablets — 200 mg, 300 mg, 400 mg
Ophthalmic solution — 3 mg/ml
Sparfloxacin:
　　　　Tablet — 200 mg

▷ **Usual Adult Dose Ranges:**   Ciprofloxacin: 250 mg to 750 mg every 12 hours (depends on nature and severity of infection). Daily maximum is 1500 mg. Mild to moderate sinusitis (caused by organisms outlined above) treated with 500 mg every 12 hours for 10 days in adults. Ophthalmic: one or two drops instilled in the eye every 2 hours while awake for 2 days, then one or two drops for 5 more days (given every 4 hours while awake).

Levofloxacin: 500 mg every 24 hours.

Norfloxacin: Uncomplicated urinary tract infections—400 mg every 12 hours for 3 days. Complicated urinary tract infections—400 mg every 12 hours for 10 to 21 days. Total daily dose should not exceed 800 mg. Ophthalmic dosing: one to two drops to the affected eye four times daily.

Ofloxacin: 200 mg to 400 mg every 12 hours (for 10 days for lower respiratory infections), depending on nature and severity of infection. Daily maximum is 800 mg. Ophthalmic dosing (conjunctivitis)—one to two drops every 2 to 4 hours for 2 days, then four times a day for 7 to 10 days.

Sparfloxacin: 400 mg now, then 200 mg a day for 10 days for pneumonia.

Infants and Children: None of these medicines are recommended.

18 to 60 Years of Age: Lomefloxacin: For bronchitis—400 mg daily for 10 days. For bladder infections (cystitis)—400 mg daily for 10 days. For complicated urinary tract infections—400 mg daily for 14 days. For preoperative prevention of urinary tract infection—400 mg (single dose) taken 2 to 6 hours before surgery.

Over 60 Years of Age: Same as 18 to 60 years of age unless kidney function is an issue.

Note: Actual dose and schedule for all these medicines must be determined for each patient individually.

Conditions Requiring Dosing Adjustments

Liver Function: Ciprofloxacin, norfloxacin: use with caution in severe liver failure. No changes for ofloxacin or sparfloxacin.

Kidney Function: Ciprofloxacin, levofloxacin, lomefloxacin, norfloxacin, ofloxacin and sparfloxacin **must** be decreased (or time between doses increased) in kidney compromise. For moderate to severe kidney compromise, ofloxacin dose is decreased to 400 mg daily. For patients with moderate kidney failure, the usual ofloxacin dose can be taken every 24 hours. For patients with severe failure, one-half the usual dose should be taken every 24 hours. Since some of these medicines can form crystals in urine, drink adequate quantities of water.

Cystic Fibrosis: A loading dose for ciprofloxacin, as well as ongoing doses of 750 mg every 8 hours, is taken by cystic fibrosis patients. This dosing gives blood levels that are more aggressive versus the bacteria which usually cause infections in these patients. No changes for the other drugs are presented.

▷ **Dosing Instructions:**   Ciprofloxacin, levofloxacin, lomefloxacin, norfloxacin or sparfloxacin may be taken with or without food (NOT dairy products) and all may be crushed. Ofloxacin is best taken 2 hours after eating. Drink large amounts of fluids while taking any of these drugs. Avoid aluminum or magnesium antacids, iron, zinc, or calcium for 2 hours before and after drug doses.

Usual Duration of Use: Regular use for 7 to 14 days is needed to see benefits in eradicating infection. Dosing should be continued for at least 2 days after all indications of infection have disappeared. Bone and joint infections (ciprofloxacin or ofloxacin) or prostate gland infections may be treated for 6 weeks or longer. Long-term use requires periodic evaluation of response.

Possible Advantages of These Drugs

Ciprofloxacin and ofloxacin: very broad spectrums of antibacterial activity of all currently available oral antimicrobial drugs. Highly effective in treating numerous types of infection caused by a wide spectrum of bacteria. Provide effective drug levels in the prostate gland (a difficult place to penetrate). Lomefloxacin has not had significant effects on kidney function. Sparfloxacin has better gram positive (strep and staph) activity than other medicines in this family.

▷ **These Drugs Should Not Be Taken If**
   • you take an antiarrhythmic drug (see Drug Classes) or have a prolonged QTc (heartbeat interval). Talk with your doctor (sparfloxacin only).

- you had an allergic reaction to any quinolone antibiotic.
- you are pregnant or breast-feeding.
- you have a poorly controlled seizure disorder.
- you are less than 18 years of age.

▷ **Inform Your Physician Before Taking These Drugs If**
- you are allergic to cinoxacin (Cinobac), nalidixic acid (NegGram), or other quinolone drugs.
- you have a seizure disorder or a brain circulatory disorder.
- you have impaired liver or kidney function.
- you have a history of mental disorders (psychosis).
- you are taking any form of probenecid or theophylline.
- your work requires heavy manual labor. Several cases of tendon rupture have been reported with fluoroquinolone use. Heavy exercise or work may be contraindicated. Call your doctor immediately if you develop inflammation or pain in a tendon.

Possible Side Effects (natural, expected, and unavoidable drug actions)
Superinfections (see Glossary). Permanent greenish tooth discoloration if used in infants (ciprofloxacin).

▷ **Possible Adverse Effects** (unusual, unexpected, and infrequent reactions)
If any of the following develop, consult your physician promptly for guidance.

Mild Adverse Effects
Allergic reactions: rash, itching, localized swelling—rare.
Dizziness, headache (frequent with lomefloxacin), weakness, migraine, anxiety, abnormal vision—rare.
Nausea, diarrhea, vomiting, indigestion—rare to frequent.
Muscle aches—case reports.
Burning feeling in the eye when the ophthalmic solutions are used—possible.
Decreased vision (with ophthalmic use)—case reports.

Serious Adverse Effects
Allergic reactions: anaphylaxis—case reports. Serious skin rashes—case reports for some, call your doctor immediately.
Idiosyncratic reactions: central nervous system stimulation—restlessness, tremor, confusion, hallucinations, seizures. One medication of this class has had reports of severe neurological compromise. Stop the drug immediately and call your doctor if you become confused or have trouble speaking while taking this drug—case reports.
Kidney disease (interstitial nephritis)—case reports.
Tendon rupture—case reports for some family members.
Abnormal heart beats or palpitations—rare.
Liver toxicity—rare.
Intracranial hypertension (ciprofloxacin or ofloxacin)—case reports.
Worsening of myasthenia gravis—case reports.

▷ **Possible Effects on Sexual Function:** Vaginitis with discharge has been reported. Painful menstruation, excessive menstrual bleeding (ofloxacin only)—case reports. Lomefloxacin has case reports of intermenstrual bleeding.

Natural Diseases or Disorders That May Be Activated by These Drugs
Latent epilepsy, latent gout.

Possible Effects on Laboratory Tests

Kidney function: increased blood creatinine and urea nitrogen (BUN)—rare.

Liver function tests: increased as a sign of liver toxicity—rare.

Red and white blood cell counts: rarely decreased (norfloxacin).

Blood glucose levels: rare fluctuations.

CAUTION

1. With high doses or prolonged use, crystal formation in the kidneys may occur. This can be prevented by drinking large amounts of water, up to 2 quarts daily.
2. These drugs may decrease saliva formation, making dental cavities or gum disease more likely. Consult your dentist if dry mouth persists.
3. Strenuous exercise is NOT recommended while these medicines are being taken.
4. If a sudden change in mental status is noticed, call your doctor immediately.

Precautions for Use

By Infants and Children: Avoid the use of these drugs completely. Impairs normal bone growth and development.

By Those Over 60 Years of Age: Impaired kidney function may require dose reduction.

▷ **Advisability of Use During Pregnancy**

Pregnancy Category: C. See Pregnancy Risk Categories at the back of this book.

Animal studies: No birth defects due to this drug found in mouse or rat studies. Rabbit studies showed maternal weight loss and increased abortions (ciprofloxacin). Ofloxacin: mild skeletal defects due to this drug were found in rat studies; toxic effects on the fetus were shown in rat and rabbit studies. These drugs can impair normal bone development in immature dogs.

Human studies: Adequate studies of pregnant women are not available. However, the potential for adverse effects on fetal bone development contraindicates the use of these drugs during entire pregnancy.

Advisability of Use If Breast-Feeding

Presence of this drug in breast milk: Probably yes; ofloxacin, yes.

Avoid drug or refrain from nursing.

Habit-Forming Potential: None.

Effects of Overdose: Confusion, headache, abdominal pain, diarrhea, liver toxicity, seizures, kidney toxicity, and hallucinations.

Possible Effects of Long-Term Use: Superinfections (see Glossary); crystal formation in kidneys.

Suggested Periodic Examinations While Taking These Drugs (at physician's discretion)

Liver function tests, urine analysis.

While Taking These Drugs, Observe the Following

Foods: Caffeine will remain in your system longer than usual. Use care in the amount of caffeine consumed. Dairy foods will decrease the effectiveness of these drugs by decreasing the amount absorbed.

Beverages: No restrictions (see note on caffeine above).

▷ *Alcohol:* No interactions expected, but since heavy alcohol intake can blunt the immune system, limit alcohol if you are ill enough to require an antibiotic.

Tobacco Smoking: No interactions expected. I advise everyone to quit smoking.

▷ *Other Drugs*

The following drug may ***increase*** the effects of fluoroquinolones:

• probenecid (Benemid).

Fluoroquinolones ***taken concurrently*** with

• azlocillin may result in toxicity.
• caffeine will result in increased caffeine levels.
• cyclosporine (Sandimmune) may result in increased risk of kidney toxicity.
• foscarnet (Foscavir) may result in an increased risk of seizures.
• phenytoin (Dilantin) may result in increased or decreased Dilantin levels.
• theophylline (Theo-Dur, others) (norfloxacin or ciprofloxacin) may lead to theophylline toxicity over time.
• warfarin (Coumadin) can result in increased risk of bleeding. or blunted warfarin (levofloxacin) response. More frequent INR testing is needed.

The following drugs may ***decrease*** the effects of fluoroquinolones:

• antacids containing aluminum or magnesium, which can reduce absorption and lessen effectiveness.
• calcium supplements.
• didanosine (ciprofloxacin only).
• iron salts.
• magnesium—will decrease the therapeutic benefits.
• nitrofurantoin (Macrodantin, etc.)—may antagonize the antibacterial action in the urinary tract. Avoid this combination.
• sucralfate (Carafate).
• zinc salts.

Sparfloxacin ***taken concurrently*** with

• amiodarone (Codarone) may cause abnormal heartbeats.
• astemizole (Hismanal) may cause abnormal heartbeats.
• bepridil (Vascor) may cause abnormal heartbeats.
• beta-blockers (see Drug Classes) may cause abnormal heartbeats.
• chlorpromazine (Thorazine) may cause abnormal heartbeats.
• cisapride (Propulcid) may cause abnormal heartbeats.
• disopyramide (Norpace) may cause abnormal heartbeats.
• macrolide antibiotics (erythromycin, dirithromycin, others) may cause abnormal heartbeats.
• phenothiazines (see Drug Classes) may cause abnormal heartbeats.
• procainamide (Pronestyl) (see Drug Classes) may cause abnormal heartbeats.
• quinidine (Quinaglute, various) may cause abnormal heartbeats.
• tricyclic antidepressants (see Drug Classes) may cause abnormal heartbeats.

▷ *Driving, Hazardous Activities:* May cause dizziness or impair vision. Restrict activities as necessary.

Aviation Note: The use of these drugs ***may be a disqualification*** for piloting. Consult a designated aviation medical examiner.

Exposure to Sun: Some members of this class have caused photosensitivity (see Glossary). Sunglasses are advised if eyes are overly sensitive to bright light. A strong sunblock is advised for your skin.

Heavy Exercise or Exertion: Several reports have surfaced regarding tendon rupture in patients on some of the medicines in this class. It is prudent to avoid heavy exercise or exertion while you are taking a fluoroquinolone.

Discontinuation: If you experience no adverse effects from these drugs, take the full course prescribed for best results. Ask your doctor when to stop treatment.

FLUOXETINE (flu OX e teen)

Introduced: 1978   **Class:** Antidepressant   **Prescription:** USA: Yes
Controlled Drug: USA: No   **Available as Generic:** USA: No
Brand Name: Prozac

BENEFITS versus RISKS	
Possible Benefits	*Possible Risks*
EFFECTIVE TREATMENT OF MAJOR DEPRESSIVE DISORDERS	Serious allergic reactions
	Conversion of depression to mania in manic-depressive (bipolar) disorders
Possibly effective in relieving the symptoms of obsessive-compulsive disorder	

▷ **Principal Uses**

As a Single Drug Product: Uses currently included in FDA-approved labeling: (1) Treats major forms of depression (including depression in HIV positive patients; (2) obsessive-compulsive disorder; (3) treatment of bulimia.

Other (unlabeled) generally accepted uses: (1) refractory diabetic neuropathy; (2) may help control kleptomania; (3) can be of help in treating obesity, especially when obesity is accompanied by depression; (4) eases symptoms of panic attacks; (5) premenstrual syndrome (PMS); (6) used to treat seasonal affective disorder (such as depression limited to winter months); (7) treats some forms of sexual problems.

How This Drug Works: It slowly restores normal levels of a nerve transmitter (serotonin).

Available Dose Forms and Strengths

Capsules — 10 mg, 20 mg
Syrup — 20 mg/5 ml

▷ **Usual Adult Dose Range:**   Starts with 20 mg in the morning; if no improvement after several weeks, dose may be increased by 20 mg/day. Doses over 20 mg/day should be divided into two equal doses and taken twice daily. Maximum daily dose is 80 mg.

Bulimia: 60 mg once daily in the morning.
Obsessive-compulsive disorder: 20 to 80 mg daily.

Note: Actual dose and schedule must be determined for each patient individually.

Conditions Requiring Dosing Adjustments

Liver Function: The dose should be decreased or the dosing interval lengthened for patients with liver compromise. Some clinicians decrease the dose by 50% in compensated cirrhosis. This drug is also a rare cause of liver toxicity, and should be used with caution by this patient population.

Kidney Function: Dosing changes do not appear to be needed. Patients should be closely watched for adverse effects.

▷ **Dosing Instructions:**   The capsule may be opened and the contents mixed with any convenient food. To make smaller doses, the contents may be mixed with orange juice or apple juice (NOT GRAPEFRUIT JUICE) and refrigerated; doses of 5–10 mg may prove effective and better tolerated.

Usual Duration of Use: Use on a regular schedule for 1 to 2 weeks may reveal start of benefits in depression. Up to 4 to 8 weeks may be needed for peak effects in: (1) relieving depression; (2) the pattern of both favorable and unfavorable effects. Since there is an active metabolite and a long half-life, it may take several weeks before the benefits of a change in dose are seen. Long-term use (months to years) requires periodic physician evaluation.

Possible Advantages of This Drug
> Does not cause weight gain, a common side effect of tricyclic antidepressants. May actually cause weight loss.
> Less likely to cause dry mouth, constipation, urinary retention, orthostatic hypotension (see Glossary), and heart rhythm disturbances than tricyclic antidepressants. May be a drug of choice in older depressed patients who also have heart trouble.

▷ **This Drug Should Not Be Taken If**
- you had an allergic reaction to it previously.
- you take or took a monoamine oxidase (MAO) type A inhibitor (see Drug Classes) in the last 14 days.

▷ **Inform Your Physician Before Taking This Drug If**
- you have had any adverse effects from antidepressant drugs.
- you have impaired liver or kidney function.
- you have Parkinson's disease.
- you have a seizure disorder.
- you have a history of psychosis.
- you have a history of SIADH (talk with your doctor).
- you are pregnant or plan a pregnancy while taking this drug.

Possible Side Effects (natural, expected, and unavoidable drug actions)
> Decreased appetite, weight loss. Case reports of orthostatic hypotension (see Glossary).

▷ **Possible Adverse Effects** (unusual, unexpected, and infrequent reactions)
> **If any of the following develop, consult your physician promptly for guidance.**
> *Mild Adverse Effects*
> Allergic reactions: skin rash, hives, itching—rare.
> Headache, nervousness, insomnia, drowsiness, tremor, dizziness, tingling of extremities—rare.
> Altered taste, nausea—frequent; vomiting, diarrhea—possible to rare.
> Hair loss—case reports.
> Fast heart rate (tachycardia) or palpitations—rare.
> Blurred vision—infrequent.
> Excessive sweating—frequent.

Serious Adverse Effects

Allergic reactions: serum-sickness-like syndrome: fever, weakness, joint pain and swelling, swollen lymph glands, fluid retention, skin rash and/or hives.

Drug-induced seizures—rare.

Worsening of Parkinson's disease—possible.

Intense suicidal preoccupation in severe depression that does not respond to this drug (see "Current Controversies in Drug Management," below)—possible.

Mania or hypomania and psychosis or hallucinations—rare.

Abnormal and excessive urination (SIADH)—case reports.

Liver toxicity—rare.

▷ **Possible Effects on Sexual Function:**   Impaired erection (1.9%), inhibition of ejaculation or inhibited orgasm in men and women—case reports. Worsening of fibrocystic breast disease in females—case reports.

Natural Diseases or Disorders That May Be Activated by This Drug

Latent epilepsy.

Possible Effects on Laboratory Tests

Blood glucose level: decreased.

Blood sodium level: decreased.

CAUTION

1. If any skin reaction develops (rash, hives, etc.), stop this drug and inform your physician promptly.
2. If dry mouth develops and persists for more than 2 weeks, consult your dentist for help.
3. Ask your doctor or pharmacist before taking any other prescription or over-the-counter drug while taking fluoxetine.
4. If you must start any monoamine oxidase (MAO) type A inhibitor (see Drug Classes), allow an interval of 4 weeks after stopping this drug before starting the MAO inhibitor.
5. This drug should be withheld if electroconvulsive therapy (ECT, or "shock" treatment) is to be used.

Precautions for Use

By Infants and Children: Safety and effectiveness for those under 12 years of age are not established.

By Those Over 60 Years of Age: Total daily dose should not exceed 60 mg.

▷ **Advisability of Use During Pregnancy**

Pregnancy Category: C. See Pregnancy Risk Categories at the back of this book. Animal studies: No birth defects due to this drug found in rat or rabbit studies.

Human studies: Adequate studies of pregnant women are not available.

Use this drug only if clearly needed.

Advisability of Use If Breast-Feeding

Presence of this drug in breast milk: Yes.

Avoid drug or refrain from nursing.

Habit-Forming Potential: Reports of patients using excess doses of fluoxetine or combining the drug with alcohol have surfaced. It appears possible that a euphoric effect and abuse potential exists.

Effects of Overdose: Agitation, restlessness, excitement, nausea, vomiting, seizures.

Possible Effects of Long-Term Use: None reported.

Suggested Periodic Examinations While Taking This Drug (at physician's discretion)
   None.

▷ **While Taking This Drug, Observe the Following**
   Foods: No restrictions (see "Beverages," below).
   Beverages: Grapefruit juice may lead to increased blood levels. AVOID IT. May be taken with milk.
▷ *Alcohol:* Does not appear to increase the central nervous system effects of fluoxetine or change the metabolism of alcohol.
   Tobacco Smoking: No interactions expected, but I advise everyone to quit smoking.
▷ *Other Drugs*
   Fluoxetine may ***increase*** the effects of
   • beta-blockers (see Drug Classes).
   • diazepam (Valium).
   • digitalis preparations (digitoxin, digoxin).
   • fleccainide (Tambocor).
   • phenytoin (Dilantin) by increasing the drug level.
   • quinidine (Quinaglute).
   • warfarin (Coumadin) and related oral anticoagulants. Test INR more often.
   Fluoxetine ***taken concurrently*** with
   • antidiabetic drugs (insulin, oral hypoglycemics) may increase the risk of hypoglycemic reactions; monitor blood sugar levels carefully.
   • astemizole (Hismanal), terfenadine (Seldane), or similar drugs may result in increased terfenadine levels and risk of heart arrhythmias. **Avoid** combining.
   • buspirone (Buspar) may increase underlying anxiety. **Avoid** the combination.
   • carbamazepine (Tegretol) will increase the carbamazepine level. Drug levels are critical if the drugs are combined.
   • clozapine (Clozaril) may result in increased levels of clozapine. The clozapine dose may need to be decreased if both medicines are to be used at the same time.
   • delavirdine (Rescriptor) may lead to fluoxetine toxicity.
   • dextromethorphan (a cough suppressant in many "DM"-labeled nonprescription cough medicines) may result in visual hallucinations if these drugs are combined. **DO NOT** combine these medicines.
   • haloperidol (Haldol) will increase haloperidol levels. Dose decrease and blood levels are needed.
   • ketorolac (Toradol) may result in hallucinations. **DO NOT** take these medicines at the same time.
   • lithium (Lithobid, etc.) will result in increased lithium levels and increased risk of neurotoxicity. **Avoid** the combination.
   • loratadine (Claritin) may result in increased loratadine levels. It may be prudent to decrease the dose if these medicines are to be combined. Unlike some of the other nonsedating antihistamines (see Drug Classes), loratadine has not (to date) resulted in abnormal heart rhythms.
   • monoamine oxidase (MAO) type A inhibitor drugs may cause confusion, ag-

itation, high fever, seizures, and dangerous elevations of blood pressure. Avoid combining these drugs.

- tryptophan will result in central nervous system toxicity. **Avoid** the combination.
- any tricyclic antidepressant (amitriptyline, nortriptyline, etc.) will result in increased antidepressant drug levels that will persist for weeks. **Avoid** the combination.
- selegiline (Eldepryl) can result in serotonin toxicity syndrome. **Avoid** this combination.
- tramadol (Ultram) may increase seizure risk. DO NOT COMBINE.

▷ *Driving, Hazardous Activities:* This drug may cause drowsiness, dizziness, impaired judgment, and delayed reaction time. Restrict activities as necessary.

Aviation Note: The use of this drug *is a disqualification* for piloting. Consult a designated aviation medical examiner.

Exposure to Sun: No restrictions.

Discontinuation: Slow drug elimination makes withdrawal effects unlikely. However, call your doctor if you plan to stop this drug for any reason.

Current Controversies in Drug Management

In 1990 six patients being treated with fluoxetine experienced intense and violent suicidal preoccupation. All six had severe depression that had not responded to the use of fluoxetine for 2 to 7 weeks. For most of them, suicidal mentality persisted for 2 to 3 months after stopping the drug. Adverse publicity suggested that this may be characteristic of fluoxetine in contrast to other antidepressant drugs. A review of relevant literature on this subject reveals that the development or intensification of suicidal thoughts during treatment (regardless of the severity of depression) has been documented repeatedly for many antidepressant drugs in wide use. Suicidal thinking may emerge during treatment with any antidepressant. Recent reports establish that some patients who become suicidal while taking one antidepressant can be switched to fluoxetine and experience cessation of suicidal thinking and satisfactory relief of depression.

This is another example of the marked variability of individual response to drug therapy. The choice of a drug to treat many serious disorders remains an experiment of trial and error. Successful management requires clinical judgment (based on experience), close monitoring, and appropriate doses.

FLUPHENAZINE (flu FEN a zeen)

Introduced: 1959   **Class:** Strong tranquilizer, phenothiazines   **Prescription:** USA: Yes   **Controlled Drug:** USA: No; Canada: No   **Available as Generic:** USA: Yes; Canada: Yes

Brand Names: ✚Apo-Fluphenazine, ✚Modecate, ✚Moditen, Permitil, PMS-Fluphenazine, Prolixin

BENEFITS versus RISKS	
Possible Benefits	*Possible Risks*
EFFECTIVE CONTROL OF ACUTE MENTAL DISORDERS	SERIOUS TOXIC EFFECTS ON BRAIN with long-term use
Beneficial effects on thinking, mood, and behavior	Liver damage with jaundice
	Blood cell disorders: abnormally low white blood cell counts

▷ **Principal Uses**

As a Single Drug Product: Uses currently included in FDA-approved labeling: Treatment of schizophrenia.

Other (unlabeled) currently accepted uses: (1) Combination treatment of refractory neuropathy; (2) an alternative neuroleptic drug in treating Tourette's syndrome in combination with clonidine; (3) therapy of Alzheimer's disease symptoms; (4) may help control sexual aggressiveness.

How This Drug Works: Inhibits dopamine, correcting an imbalance of nerve impulse transmissions.

Available Dose Forms and Strengths

Concentrate — 5 mg/ml (1% alcohol)
Elixir — 2.5 mg/5 ml (14% alcohol)
Injection — 2.5 mg/ml
Tablets — 1 mg, 2.5 mg, 5 mg, 10 mg

▷ **Usual Adult Dose Range:**   2.5 to 10 mg given three to four times daily. The dose is adjusted as needed and tolerated. Daily maximum is 40 mg.

Note: Actual dose and schedule must be determined for each patient individually.

Conditions Requiring Dosing Adjustments

Liver Function: Use with caution in patients with both liver and kidney compromise.

Kidney Function: Used with caution.

▷ **Dosing Instructions:**   Regular tablets can be crushed and taken with or following meals to reduce stomach irritation. Prolonged-action tablets should be swallowed whole (not crushed). The concentrate must be diluted in 4 to 6 ounces of water, milk, fruit juice, or carbonated beverage.

Usual Duration of Use: Use on a regular schedule for several weeks is needed to determine effectiveness in controlling psychotic disorders. If not of benefit in 6 weeks, it should be stopped. Long-term use (months to years) requires periodic physician evaluation.

▷ **This Drug Should Not Be Taken If**
- you are allergic to this medicine.
- you have a history of brain damage.
- you have active liver disease.
- you have cancer of the breast.
- you have an active blood dyscrasia.
- you are taking large doses of other medicines that can depress the central nervous system.
- you have a current blood cell or bone marrow disorder.

▷ **Inform Your Physician Before Taking This Drug If**
- you are allergic or sensitive to any phenothiazine (see Drug Classes).
- you have impaired liver or kidney function.
- you have any type of seizure disorder.
- you have diabetes, glaucoma, heart disease, or chronic lung disease.
- you have a history of lupus erythematosus.
- you have a history of depressed white blood cell counts of the granulocytic series (agranulocytosis).
- you have a history of neuroleptic malignant syndrome.
- you take any drug with sedative effects or will have surgery under general or spinal anesthesia.

Possible Side Effects (natural, expected, and unavoidable drug actions)
Drowsiness (usually during the first 2 weeks), orthostatic hypotension (see Glossary), blurred vision, dry mouth, nasal congestion, constipation, impaired urination (all mild).

▷ **Possible Adverse Effects** (unusual, unexpected, and infrequent reactions)
If any of the following develop, consult your physician promptly for guidance.
Mild Adverse Effects
Allergic reactions: skin rash, hives, itching.
Lowering of body temperature, especially in the elderly—possible.
Headache, dizziness, weakness, excitement, restlessness, unusual dreaming—infrequent.
Increased appetite and weight gain—possible.
Serious Adverse Effects
Allergic reactions: hepatitis with jaundice (see Glossary), usually between second and fourth week; anaphylactic reaction (see Glossary).
Idiosyncratic reaction: neuroleptic malignant syndrome (see Glossary)—case reports.
Impaired production of white blood cells: fever, sore throat, infections—rare.
Parkinson-like disorders (see Glossary): muscle spasms of face, jaw, neck, back—rare to infrequent and may be dose related.
Liver toxicity—case reports.
Depression or seizures—case reports.
Pituitary tumors or porphyria—case reports.
Abnormal heartbeats—rare.

▷ **Possible Effects on Sexual Function:**   Decreased male libido; increased female libido.
Impaired erection—frequent; complete impotence—case reports. Inhibited male or female orgasm—frequent. Inhibited ejaculation—frequent.
Altered timing and pattern of menstruation—frequent.
Female breast enlargement and milk production (galactorrhea)—possible.
Prolonged and painful erection (priapism)—case reports. Male breast enlargement and tenderness (gynecomastia)—case reports.
May help treat sexual hyperactivity.

▷ **Adverse Effects That May Mimic Natural Diseases or Disorders**
Nervous system reactions may suggest Parkinson's disease.
Liver reactions may suggest viral hepatitis.
Reactions resembling systemic lupus erythematosus may occur.

Natural Diseases or Disorders That May Be Activated by This Drug
Latent epilepsy, glaucoma, prostatism (see Glossary).

Possible Effects on Laboratory Tests
Complete blood counts: decreased red cells, hemoglobin, white cells, and platelets; increased eosinophils (allergic reaction).
Blood sugar (glucose): decreased.
Liver function tests: increased liver enzymes (ALT/GPT, AST/GOT, and alkaline phosphatase), increased bilirubin.
Urine pregnancy tests: false positive results.
Urine screening test for drug abuse: initial test may be falsely *positive* for barbiturates; the confirmatory test will be *negative*.

CAUTION
1. Many over-the-counter (OTC) medicines (see Glossary) for allergies, colds, and coughs can interact unfavorably with this drug. Ask your physician or pharmacist for help.
2. Antacids containing aluminum and/or magnesium can prevent absorption.
3. Obtain prompt evaluation of any change or disturbance of vision.

Precautions for Use
By Infants and Children: Do not use this drug in infants under 6 months of age, or in children of any age with symptoms suggestive of Reye syndrome (see Glossary). Monitor carefully for blood cell changes.
Children with psychosis have been given 0.25 to 0.75 mg from one to four times daily.
By Those Over 60 Years of Age: Small starting doses are advisable. Increased risk of drowsiness, lethargy, constipation, lowering of body temperature (hypothermia), and orthostatic hypotension (see Glossary). This drug can enhance existing prostatism (see Glossary). You may also be more susceptible to the development of Parkinson-like reactions and/or tardive dyskinesia (see discussion of these terms in Glossary).

▷ **Advisability of Use During Pregnancy**
Pregnancy Category: C. See Pregnancy Risk Categories at the back of this book.
Animal studies: Significant birth defects reported in mice.
Human studies: Adequate studies of pregnant women are not available.
Avoid drug during the first 3 months and during the final month because of possible effects on the newborn infant.

Advisability of Use If Breast-Feeding
Presence of this drug in breast milk: Yes.
Does not usually accumulate in high enough concentrations to effect the infant. Watch the infant closely and discuss the situation with your doctor.

Habit-Forming Potential: None.

Effects of Overdose: Marked drowsiness, weakness, tremor, agitation, unsteadiness, deep sleep, coma, convulsions.

Possible Effects of Long-Term Use: Tardive dyskinesia (see Glossary); eye changes—cataracts and pigmentation of retina; gray to violet pigmentation of skin in exposed areas, more common in women.

Suggested Periodic Examinations While Taking This Drug (at physician's discretion)

Complete blood counts.

Liver function tests, electrocardiograms.

Complete eye examinations—eye structures and vision.

Careful tongue exam for evidence of fine, involuntary, wavelike movements that could be the beginning of tardive dyskinesia.

▷ **While Taking This Drug, Observe the Following**

Foods: No restrictions.

Beverages: No restrictions. May be taken with milk.

▷ *Alcohol:* Avoid completely. Alcohol can increase phenothiazine sedation and accentuate depressant effects on brain function and blood pressure. Phenothiazines can increase the intoxicating effects of alcohol.

Tobacco Smoking: Possible increased fluphenazine removal and need for dose increase. I advise everyone to quit smoking.

Marijuana Smoking: Moderate increase in drowsiness; accentuation of orthostatic hypotension; increased risk of precipitating latent psychoses, confusing the interpretation of mental status and drug responses.

▷ *Other Drugs*

Fluphenazine may *increase* the effects of

• all atropinelike drugs, and cause nervous system toxicity.

• all sedative drugs, and cause excessive sedation.

Fluphenazine may *decrease* the effects of

• guanethidine (Ismelin, Esimil), and reduce its effectiveness in lowering blood pressure.

Fluphenazine *taken concurrently* with

• beta-blocker drugs (see Drug Classes) may cause increased effects of both drugs; watch drug effects—may need smaller doses.

• clonidine (Catapres, others) may result in an acute organic brain syndrome (disorientation, agitation, delirium). These medicines should not be combined.

• lithium (Lithobid, others) can cause increase toxicity to the nerves.

• monamine oxidase (MAO) inhibitors (see Drug Classes) can cause very low blood pressure and worsening of the central nervous system and respiratory depression effects.

• oral antidiabetic drugs (see Drug Classes) may result in lower blood sugar levels than expected. Doses of the oral hypoglycemic agents may need to be decreased.

• sparfloxacin (Zagam) may lead to abnormal heart beats.

• tramadol (Ultram) may increase seizure risk. DO NOT COMBINE.

• vitamin C (ascorbic acid) may decrease the therapeutic benefits of fluphenazine:

The following drugs may *decrease* the effects of fluphenazine:

• antacids containing aluminum and/or magnesium.

• benztropine (Cogentin).

• trihexyphenidyl (Artane).

▷ *Driving, Hazardous Activities:* This drug can impair mental alertness, judgment, and physical coordination. Avoid hazardous activities.

Aviation Note: The use of this drug *is a disqualification* for piloting. Consult a designated aviation medical examiner.

Exposure to Sun: Use caution—some phenothiazines can cause photosensitivity (see Glossary).

Exposure to Heat: Use caution and avoid excessive heat. This drug may impair the regulation of body temperature and increase heatstroke risk.

Exposure to Cold: Use caution and dress warmly. Increased risk of hypothermia in the elderly.

Discontinuation: After long-term use, do not stop this drug suddenly. Gradual withdrawal over 2 to 3 weeks under physician supervision is needed. Do not stop this drug without your doctor's knowledge and approval. The relapse rate of schizophrenia after discontinuation is 50–60%.

FLURAZEPAM (flur AZ e pam)

Introduced: 1970   **Class:** Hypnotic, benzodiazepines   **Prescription:** USA: Yes   **Controlled Drug:** USA: C-IV* Canada: No   **Available as Generic:**   USA: Yes Canada: Yes

Brand Names: ✦Apo-Flurazepam, Dalmane, Durapam, ✦Novo-Flupam, ✦Somnol

BENEFITS versus RISKS	
Possible Benefits	*Possible Risks*
EFFECTIVE HYPNOTIC	Habit-forming potential with long-
NO SUPPRESSION OF REM (RAPID	term use
EYE MOVEMENT) SLEEP	Minor impairment of mental
NO REM SLEEP REBOUND after	functions ("hangover" effect)
discontinuation	Jaundice
Wide margin of safety with	Blood cell disorder
therapeutic doses	Suppression of stage-4 sleep with
	reduced "quality" of sleep

▷ **Principal Uses**

As a Single Drug Product: Uses currently included in FDA-approved labeling: Short-term treatment of insomnia consisting of difficulty in falling asleep, frequent nighttime awakenings, and/or early morning awakenings.

Other (unlabeled) generally accepted uses: May be of benefit in patients who have undergone herniorrhaphy, in helping them sleep.

Author's note: Information in this profile has been shortened in order to make room for more widely used medicines.

The National Institute of Mental Health has a new information page on anxiety. It can be found on the World Wide Web at www.nimh .nih.gov/anxiety.

FLURBIPROFEN (flur BI proh fen)

See the propionic acids (nonsteroidal anti-inflammatory drugs) profile for further information.

*See Controlled Drug Schedules at the back of this book.

FLUTAMIDE (FLU ta mide)

Introduced: 1983   **Class:** Anticancer (antineoplastic)   **Prescription:**
USA: Yes   **Controlled Drug:**   USA: No; Canada: No   **Available as Generic:**
USA: No; Canada: No
Brand Names: ✦Euflex, Eulexin, Flutamex (Germany)

BENEFITS versus RISKS	
Possible Benefits	*Possible Risks*
EFFECTIVE ADJUNCTIVE	Rare drug-induced hepatitis
TREATMENT OF PROSTATE	Breast enlargement and tenderness
CANCER	Hot flashes

▷ **Principal Uses**
As a Single Drug Product: Uses currently included in FDA-approved labeling:
Treatment of metastatic prostate cancer, used concurrently with leuprolide
(given by injection).
Other (unlabeled) generally accepted uses: (1) There has been some isolated
use as a 2% alcoholic gel in treating acne; (2) some early data on use in bulimia; (3) can help excessive hair growth in women (hirsutism).

How This Drug Works: Flutamide suppresses effects of testosterone (a male sex
hormone) by blocking uptake and binding target tissues (such as the
prostate gland). Used in conjunction with leuprolide (a drug that suppresses
testosterone from testicles by damping the pituitary gland's testicular stimulation). The combination of these two drug actions—chemical castration
by leuprolide and testosterone blockage by flutamide—significantly reduces
hormonal stimulation of cancerous prostate tissue.

Available Dose Forms and Strengths
Capsules — 125 mg (U.S.)
Tablets — 250 mg (Canada, Germany)

▷ **Recommended Dose Ranges** (Actual dose and schedule must be determined for
each patient individually.)
Infants and Children: Not used in this age group.
12 to 60 Years of Age: 250 mg every 8 hours. Flutamide is to be taken concurrently with leuprolide; the usual dose of leuprolide is 7.5 mg given by injection once a month.
Over 60 Years of Age: Same as 12 to 60 years of age.

Conditions Requiring Dosing Adjustments
Liver Function: Use with caution by patients with liver compromise. It is also a
rare cause of cholestatic jaundice.
Kidney Function: Primarily eliminated by the kidneys. Use with caution in kidney compromise.

▷ **Dosing Instructions:**   May be taken without regard to food. The capsule may be
opened and the tablet may be crushed.

Warning: Since this medicine is an antineoplastic agent, proper disposal (ask
your doctor) of urine or vomit MUST be undertaken.

Usual Duration of Use: Regular use for 2 to 3 months usually needed to see
drug's benefits in controlling prostate cancer. Long-term use (months to
years) requires periodic physician evaluation.

Possible Advantages of This Drug
Ease of use. Less toxicity than chemotherapeutic drugs.

Currently a "Drug of Choice"
For the management of prostate cancer (in combination with leuprolide).

▷ **This Drug Should Not Be Taken If**
• you have had an allergic reaction to it previously.

▷ **Inform Your Physician Before Taking This Drug If**
• you have a history of liver disease or impaired liver function.
• you have high blood pressure (hypertension).
• you have a history of anemia, low white blood cells, or low blood platelets.
• you have a history of lupus erythematosus.

Possible Side Effects (natural, expected, and unavoidable drug actions)
Hot flashes (61%), loss of libido (with combination LHRH therapy), impotence, breast enlargement and tenderness.

▷ **Possible Adverse Effects** (unusual, unexpected, and infrequent reactions)
If any of the following develop, consult your physician promptly for guidance.
Mild Adverse Effects
Allergic reactions: skin rash.
Drowsiness, confusion, nervousness—rare.
Indigestion, nausea/vomiting, diarrhea—infrequent.
Blurred vision—rare.
Fluid retention (edema) of legs—possible.
Serious Adverse Effects
Drug-induced hepatitis with jaundice (see Glossary)—rare.
Low blood platelets, white blood cells, or anemia—rare.
Lupus-erythematosus-like skin rash—case reports.
Heart attack—rare.

▷ **Possible Effects on Sexual Function:**   See "Possible Side Effects" above. Flutamide itself does not presently appear to change libido, sexual performance, or the ability to have an erection. Combination therapy does appear to carry the risks of these adverse effects. Swelling and tenderness of male breast tissue (gynecomastia) may be frequent.

▷ **Adverse Effects That May Mimic Natural Diseases or Disorders**
Drug-induced hepatitis may suggest viral hepatitis.

Possible Effects on Laboratory Tests
Complete blood counts: decreased red and white cells, hemoglobin, and platelets.
Liver function tests: increased liver enzymes (ALT/GPT, AST/GOT, and alkaline phosphatase), increased bilirubin.
Sperm counts and testosterone levels: decreased.

CAUTION
1. For best results, flutamide and leuprolide should be started together and continued for the duration of therapy.
2. During combination therapy with flutamide and leuprolide, symptoms of prostate cancer (difficult urination, bone pain, etc.) may worsen temporarily; these are transient and not significant.

Precautions for Use

By Those Over 60 Years of Age: Drug is more slowly excreted. If digestive symptoms or edema are troublesome, ask your doctor about adjusting dose.

▷ **Advisability of Use During Pregnancy**

Pregnancy Category: D. See Pregnancy Risk Categories at the back of this book.
  Animal studies: Rat studies reveal malformation of bone structures and feminization of male fetuses.
  Human studies: Adequate studies of pregnant women are not available.
  Discuss this benefit-to-risk decision with your doctor.

Advisability of Use If Breast-Feeding

Presence of this drug in breast milk: Unknown.
Stop nursing.

Habit-Forming Potential: None.

Effects of Overdose: Possible drowsiness, unsteadiness, nausea, vomiting.

Possible Effects of Long-Term Use: None reported.

Suggested Periodic Examinations While Taking This Drug (at physician's discretion)

Prostate-specific antigen (PSA) assays.
Complete blood cell counts.
Liver function tests.

▷ **While Taking This Drug, Observe the Following**

Foods: No restrictions.
Beverages: No restrictions. May be taken with milk.
▷ *Alcohol:* No interactions expected.
Tobacco Smoking: No interactions expected, but I advise everyone to quit smoking.
Marijuana Smoking: Animal studies have shown this combination to result in additive suppression of the immune system. The combination therefore is not advisable.
Other Drugs
  Flutamide **taken concurrently** with
  • influenza, pneumococcal, or yellow fever vaccine may result in blunting of immune response to the vaccine.
▷ *Driving, Hazardous Activities:* This drug may cause drowsiness. Restrict activities as necessary.
Aviation Note: The use of this drug **may be a disqualification** for piloting. Consult a designated aviation medical examiner.
Exposure to Sun: This drug may cause photosensitivity (see Glossary).
Discontinuation: To be determined by your physician.

FLUTICASONE (flu TIC a zone)

Introduced: 1994   **Class:** Adrenocortical steroids   **Prescription:** USA: Yes   **Controlled Drug:** USA: No; Canada: No   **Available as Generic:** USA: No; Canada: No

Brand Names: Cutivate, Flonase, Flovent, Flovent Rotadisc

Author's Note: This profile focuses on the aqueous nasal form of this medicine.

Warning: Even though this medicine is a nasal spray, there is still a remote risk of suppression of the hypothalamic pituitary adrenal (HPA) axis.

BENEFITS versus RISKS	
Possible Benefits	*Possible Risks*
EFFECTIVE, ONCE-A-DAY RELIEF OF SEASONAL ALLERGIC RHINITIS EFFECTIVE ONCE-DAILY ECZEMA TREATMENT	Reversible adrenal gland suppression Irritation of the nose

▷ **Principal Uses**

As a Single Drug Product: Uses currently included in FDA-approved labeling: (1) Helps perennial and seasonal (hay fever) allergic or nonallergic rhinitis in adults or children who are 12 years of age or older; (2) the topical form is used for a variety of skin conditions from sunburn to lupus erythematosus; (3) asthma (inhaler form); (4) cream approved for once-daily treatment of eczema.

Other (unlabeled) generally accepted uses: Crohn's disease.

How This Drug Works: Exact mechanism of action of this medicine is not known; however, halomethyl carbothionates have very potent anti-inflammatory and blood-vessel-contracting (vasoconstrictive) activity.

Available Dose Forms and Strengths

Amber glass bottle — 16 g (120 actuations) and 9 g (60 actuations)

Cream (Germany) — 0.05 mg/g

Inhalation powder (Germany) — 50 mcg, 100 mcg, and 250 mcg per actuation

Nasal spray — 0.05%

▷ **Recommended Dose Ranges** (Actual dose and schedule must be determined for each patient individually.)

Infants and Children: Safety and efficacy for those less than 4 have not yet been defined. For those 4 to 12: Nasal dosing: Started with one spray (50 mcg in each spray) in each nostril once a day. If symptoms are severe, the dose can be increased to two sprays in each nostril (50 mcg each spray) or 200 micrograms a day. After a few days, the dose should be reduced to 50 micrograms in each nostril once daily.

12 to 60 Years of Age: Nasal dosing: Started with two sprays (50 mcg in each spray) in each nostril once daily. The same dose can also be given as 100 mcg twice daily (8 A.M. and 8 P.M.). After a few days, the dose can often be decreased to 100 mcg (one spray in each nostril) daily.

Inhalation for asthma: Starting dose is 88 mcg twice a day for patients who were previously treated with bronchodilators alone. Maximum daily dose is 440 mcg. Patients who required an inhaled corticosteroid previously are given 88 to 220 mcg twice daily. Maximum daily dose is 880 mcg.

Over 60 Years of Age: Same as 12 to 60 years of age.

Conditions Requiring Dosing Adjustments

Liver Function: This drug is extensively changed in the liver; however, no specific dosing changes are defined for patients with compromised livers.

Kidney Function: No changes in dosing are needed.

▷ **Dosing Instructions:**   A patient instruction sheet will always accompany this medicine. The instructions should be followed closely. Your doctor should be called if the condition worsens or does not improve.

Usual Duration of Use: Continual use on a regular schedule for several days is usually necessary to determine this drug's effectiveness in treating seasonal and perennial allergic rhinitis. Long-term use (months to years) requires periodic evaluation of response and dose adjustment. Consult your physician on a regular basis.

Possible Advantages of This Drug

Once-a-day dosing.

▷ **This Drug Should Not Be Taken If**
- you have had an allergic reaction to any dose form of it previously.
- you have sudden onset of asthma (fluticasone not effective).

▷ **Inform Your Physician Before Taking This Drug If**
- you are already taking systemic prednisone.
- you are exposed to measles or chicken pox.
- you are unsure how much to take or how often to take it.
- you take prescription or nonprescription medicines not discussed when fluticasone was prescribed.
- you have signs or symptoms of an infection in your nose.
- your skin is shrunken (atrophied) or you have acne, warts, or other skin problems (topical form).
- you have damage from an accident or surgery to your nose while you are taking this medicine.
- your allergic rhinitis does not improve or worsens.

Possible Side Effects (natural, expected, and unavoidable drug actions)

Irritation of the nose. Systemic steroid effects—possible.

▷ **Possible Adverse Effects** (unusual, unexpected, and infrequent reactions)

If any of the following develop, consult your physician promptly for guidance.

Mild Adverse Effects

Allergic reactions: contact dermatitis.

Nosebleeds or nasal burning—case reports to infrequent.

Dizziness or headache—rare to infrequent.

Unpleasant taste, nausea, or vomiting—rare.

Increased heart rate—case reports.

Serious Adverse Effects

Allergic reactions: anaphylaxis—case report.

Suppression of the hypothalamic pituitary adrenal (HPA) axis—rare.

Increased risk from viral infections—possible.

Increased pressure in the head (more likely in children)—possible.

Yeast infections of the nose—rare.

Glaucoma or cataracts—case reports (inhaled form).

Cushing's syndrome (with excessive doses or very sensitive patients)—possible.

Osteoporosis—increased risk with long-term use.

▷ **Possible Effects on Sexual Function:**   None defined.

Possible Delayed Adverse Effects: Yeast infections of the nose—rare. Osteoporosis—increased risk.

▷ **Adverse Effects That May Mimic Natural Diseases or Disorders**
None defined.

Natural Diseases or Disorders That May Be Activated by This Drug
If systemic effects occur, the patient may be more susceptible to infections, or dormant infections may become active.

Possible Effects on Laboratory Tests
Cortisol levels: decreased.

CAUTION
1. Call your doctor if you are exposed to measles or chicken pox.
2. Long-term use requires periodic evaluation for yeast infection of the nose.
3. Call your doctor if your condition does not improve or worsens.

Precautions for Use
By Infants and Children: Safety and effectiveness for use by those under 12 years of age have not been established for the intranasal form. Many adolescents can be started successfully with one spray in each nostril per day (100 mcg). Maximum total daily dose should not exceed 200 mcg.
By Those Over 60 Years of Age: No specific precautions.

▷ **Advisability of Use During Pregnancy**
Pregnancy Category: C. See Pregnancy Risk Categories at the back of this book.
Animal studies: High-dose studies in rats revealed fetal toxicity consistent with changes caused by other steroids.
Human studies: Information from adequate studies of pregnant women is not available. Ask your doctor for guidance.

Advisability of Use If Breast-Feeding
Presence of this drug in breast milk: Unknown.
Monitor nursing infant closely and discontinue drug or nursing if adverse effects develop.

Habit-Forming Potential: Not defined.

Effects of Overdose: Not defined.

Possible Effects of Long-Term Use: Rare nasal yeast infections.

Suggested Periodic Examinations While Taking This Drug (at physician's discretion)
Nasal exams.

▷ **While Taking This Drug, Observe the Following**
Foods: No restrictions.
Beverages: No restrictions.
▷ *Alcohol:* No interactions expected.
Tobacco Smoking: No interactions expected. I advise everyone to quit smoking.
▷ *Other Drugs*
Fluticasone **taken concurrently** with
• ketoconazole (Nizoral) may increase fluticasone blood levels.
• systemic steroids (such as prednisone) may increase the likelihood of suppression of the hypothalamic pituitary adrenal (HPA) axis.

▷ *Driving, Hazardous Activities:* This drug may cause dizziness. Restrict activities as necessary.

Aviation Note: The use of this drug *may be a disqualification* for piloting. Consult a designated aviation medical examiner.

Exposure to Sun: No restrictions.

Discontinuation: This medicine should not be stopped abruptly. Talk with your doctor before stopping this drug.

FLUVASTATIN (flu va STAT in)

Introduced: 1994 **Class:** Cholesterol-reducing drug, HMG-CoA reductase inhibitor **Prescription:** USA: Yes **Controlled Drug:** USA: No; Canada: No **Available as Generic:** USA: No; Canada: No

Brand Name: Lescol

BENEFITS versus RISKS	
Possible Benefits	*Possible Risks*
EFFECTIVE REDUCTION OF TOTAL BLOOD CHOLESTEROL SLOWS PROGRESSION OF CORONARY ATHEROSCLEROSIS	Increased liver enzymes Muscle pain or weakness

▷ **Principal Uses**

As a Single Drug Product: Uses currently included in FDA-approved labeling: (1) Manages abnormally high cholesterol in people with type 2 hypercholesterolemia; (2) slows progression of atherosclerosis in patients with coronary heart disease.

Other (unlabeled) generally accepted uses: Not fully defined at present.

How This Drug Works: This medicine is changed (hydrolyzed) to a beta-hydroxy-acid form. The beta-hydroxy-acid inhibits HMG-CoA reductase. This enzyme is critical for cholesterol formation. Once inhibited, cholesterol formation slows.

Available Dose Forms and Strengths

Tablets — 10 mg, 20 mg, 40 mg

▷ **Recommended Dose Ranges** (Actual dose and schedule must be determined for each patient individually.)

Infants and Children: Safety and efficacy for those less than 12 years of age have not yet been defined.

18 to 60 Years of Age: Dosing is started with 20 mg a day, taken with the evening meal. This dose is increased as needed and tolerated to 80 mg with each evening (24 hours apart) meal. Any needed increases are made at intervals of 4 weeks. Patients who take immunosuppressant medicines are started on 10 mg of lovastatin daily and should not receive more than 20 mg daily with the evening meal.

Over 60 Years of Age: Same as 12 to 60 years of age.

Conditions Requiring Dosing Adjustments

Liver Function: This drug is extensively changed in the liver. Lower doses appear prudent in liver disease.

Kidney Function: Patients with severe failure (creatinine clearance less than 30 ml/min) should be closely followed if given over 20 mg daily.

▷ **Dosing Instructions:**   This medicine is best taken with the evening meal, as it produces the best cholesterol-lowering results or outcomes.

Usual Duration of Use: Continual use on a regular schedule for 3 to 4 weeks may be needed to determine this drug's effectiveness in helping lower low-density lipoprotein (LDL) level. Long-term use (months to years) requires evaluation of response by your doctor.

Possible Advantages of This Drug   Requires once-daily dosing and has a good side-effect profile.

▷ **This Drug Should Not Be Taken If**
• you had an allergic reaction to it previously.
• you have active liver disease.
• you are pregnant or breast-feeding your infant.

▷ **Inform Your Physician Before Taking This Drug If**
• you have previously taken any other drugs in this class: lovastatin (Mevacor), pravastatin (Pravachol).
• you have a history of liver disease or impaired liver function.
• you are not using any method of birth control, or you are planning a pregnancy.
• you regularly consume substantial amounts of alcohol.
• you have cataracts or impaired vision.
• you have any type of chronic muscular disorder.
• you develop muscle pain, weakness, or soreness that is unexplained while taking this medicine.
• you plan to have major surgery in the near future.

Possible Side Effects (natural, expected, and unavoidable drug actions)
Development of abnormal liver function tests without associated symptoms.

▷ **Possible Adverse Effects** (unusual, unexpected, and infrequent reactions)
If any of the following develop, consult your physician promptly for guidance.
Mild Adverse Effects
Allergic reactions: rash.
Headache or insomnia—infrequent.
Indigestion, nausea, excessive gas, constipation, diarrhea—infrequent.
Lowering of the blood pressure—possible.
Serious Adverse Effects
Marked and persistent abnormal liver function tests with focal hepatitis (without jaundice)—case reports.
Acute myositis (muscle pain and tenderness)—occurred rarely during long-term use.
Rhabdomyolysis—rare.
Cataracts (based on animal data, not reported in humans)—possible.
Lichen planus skin rash—rare.

▷ **Possible Effects on Sexual Function:**   None reported.

Possible Delayed Adverse Effects: None reported to date. Doses of 15 to 33 times the human dose of another drug in this class given to rats caused an increase in liver cancers.

Natural Diseases or Disorders That May Be Activated by This Drug
Latent liver disease.

Possible Effects on Laboratory Tests
Blood alanine aminotransferase (ALT) enzyme level: increased (with higher doses of drug).
Blood total cholesterol, LDL cholesterol, and triglyceride levels: decreased.
Blood HDL cholesterol level: increased.

CAUTION
1. If pregnancy occurs while taking this drug, stop taking the drug immediately and consult your physician.
2. Report promptly any development of muscle pain or tenderness, especially if accompanied by fever or weakness (malaise).
3. Report promptly altered or impaired vision so that appropriate evaluation can be made.

Precautions for Use
By Infants and Children: Safety and effectiveness for those under 20 years of age are not established.
By Those Over 60 Years of Age: Inform your physician regarding any personal or family history of cataracts. Comply with all recommendations regarding periodic eye examinations. Report promptly any alterations in vision.

▷ **Advisability of Use During Pregnancy**
Pregnancy Category: X. See Pregnancy Risk Categories at the back of this book.
Animal studies: Mouse and rat studies reveal skeletal birth defects due to a closely related drug of this class.
Human studies: Adequate studies of pregnant women are not available.
This drug should be avoided during entire pregnancy.

Advisability of Use If Breast-Feeding
Presence of this drug in breast milk: Unknown.
Avoid drug or refrain from nursing.

Habit-Forming Potential: None.

Effects of Overdose: Increased indigestion, stomach distress, nausea, diarrhea.

Possible Effects of Long-Term Use: Abnormal liver function with focal hepatitis.

Suggested Periodic Examinations While Taking This Drug (at physician's discretion)
Blood cholesterol studies: total cholesterol, HDL and LDL fractions.
Liver function tests before treatment, every 6 weeks during the first 3 months of use, every 8 weeks for the rest of the first year, and at 6-month intervals thereafter. Complete eye examination at beginning of treatment and at any time that significant change in vision occurs. Ask your physician for guidance.

▷ **While Taking This Drug, Observe the Following**
Foods: Follow a standard low-cholesterol diet.
Beverages: No restrictions. May be taken with milk.
▷ *Alcohol:* No interactions expected. Use sparingly.
Tobacco Smoking: No interactions expected. I advise everyone to quit smoking.
▷ *Other Drugs*
Fluvastatin may *increase* the effects of

- digoxin (Lanoxin).
- warfarin (Coumadin); more frequent testing of INR (prothrombin time) will be needed.

Fluvastatin *taken concurrently* with
- clofibrate (Atromid-S) or other fibrate compounds may result in increased risk of serious muscle toxicity.
- cyclosporine (Sandimmune) can result in kidney failure and myopathy.
- erythromycin and perhaps other macrolide antibiotics (see Drug Classes) may increase risk of muscle damage (myopathy or rhabdomyolysis).
- gemfibrozil (Lopid) may alter the absorption and excretion of fluvastatin; these drugs should not be taken concurrently.
- niacin may cause an increased frequency of muscle problems (myopathy) when combined with a related medicine (lovastatin). Caution is advised.
- omeprazole (Prilosec) may increase fluvastatin levels and lead to toxicity.
- ranitidine (Zantac) may increase peak blood levels of fluvastatin.
- ritonavir (Norvir) may lead to fluvastatin toxicity.

The following drug may *decrease* the effects of fluvastatin:
- cholestyramine (Questran)—may reduce absorption of fluvastatin; take fluvastatin 1 hour before or 4 hours after cholestyramine.

▷ *Driving, Hazardous Activities:* No restrictions.
Aviation Note: No restrictions.
Exposure to Sun: No restrictions.
Discontinuation: Do not stop this drug without your physician's knowledge and guidance. There may be a significant increase in blood cholesterol levels following discontinuation of this drug.

FLUVOXAMINE (FLU vox a meen)

Introduced: 1995   **Class:** Antidepressant, selective serotonin reuptake inhibitor   **Prescription:** USA: Yes   **Controlled Drug:** USA: No; Canada: No
Available as Generic: USA: No; Canada: No

Brand Name: Luvox

Warning: **Do not** combine this medicine with terfenadine (Seldane) or astemizole (Hismanal).

BENEFITS versus RISKS	
Possible Benefits	*Possible Risks*
TREATMENT OF OBSESSIVE-COMPULSIVE DISORDER IN ADULTS TREATMENT OF OBSESSIVE-COMPULSIVE DISORDER IN CHILDREN	Nausea and vomiting (often resolves with time)

▷ **Principal Uses**
As a Single Drug Product: Uses currently included in FDA-approved labeling: Treatment of obsessive-compulsive disorder in adults and children.
Other (unlabeled) generally accepted uses: (1) May have a role in helping compulsive exhibitionism; (2) can have a role in treating depression; (3)

may be useful in eating problems where binge behaviors are a key factor; (4) can help panic attacks; (5) could have a role in long-standing (chronic) tension headaches.

How This Drug Works: Inhibits reuptake of the neurotransmitter 5-HT, easing symptoms of treated behaviors or conditions.

Available Dose Forms and Strengths

Tablets — 50 mg, 100 mg

▷ **Recommended Dose Ranges** (Actual dose and schedule must be determined for each patient individually.)

Infants and Children: Safety and efficacy have been established in pediatrics (children and adolescents): Dosing is started with 25 mg at bedtime for 3 days. The dose is then increased by 25-mg steps every 3 to 4 days until a maximum of 200 mg is reached. If the required dose is larger than 75 mg, the total daily dose is divided into two equal doses and given twice daily.

18 to 60 Years of Age: Therapy is started with 50 mg taken at bedtime. The dose may then be increased as needed and tolerated by 50-mg intervals every 4 to 7 days to a maximum dose of 300 mg daily. The prescriber should remember that the drug may take from 4 to 14 days to begin to work. If a patient needs a daily dose greater than 100 mg, the dose is divided in half and taken twice daily.

Over 60 Years of Age: This medicine is removed half as slowly as in younger patients. Plasma concentrations are also roughly 40% higher than in younger patients. Slower time frames for any increases beyond the starting dose and lower maintenance doses are indicated.

Conditions Requiring Dosing Adjustments

Liver Function: This drug is extensively changed by the liver. If it is used by patients with liver disease, lower starting doses, slow dose increases, and careful patient monitoring is indicated.

Kidney Function: A lower starting dose and careful patient monitoring is needed.

▷ **Dosing Instructions:**   Take this medicine exactly as prescribed and at the same time. This medicine may be taken with or without food. Call your doctor if vomiting (a possible side effect) continues for more than 2 days after you start treatment.

Usual Duration of Use: Continual use on a regular schedule for 4 to 14 days is usually necessary to determine effectiveness in helping obsessive-compulsive disorder. Long-term use (months to years) requires evaluation by your doctor.

Possible Advantages of This Drug

Requires once-daily dosing and has a good side-effect profile.

▷ **This Drug Should Not Be Taken If**
- you had an allergic reaction to it previously.
- you have taken or are taking terfenadine or astemizole.

▷ **Inform Your Physician Before Taking This Drug If**
- you have continued to have a problem with vomiting 2 days after starting this medicine.
- you feel light-headed when you get up from a sitting position.
- you have a history of seizures.
- you are unsure how much to take or how often to take it.

- you have taken a monoamine oxidase (MAO) inhibitor (see Drug Classes) within the last 14 days.
- you have a history of heart problems.
- you take prescription or nonprescription medicines not discussed when fluvoxamine was prescribed.

Possible Side Effects (natural, expected, and unavoidable drug actions)

Nausea and vomiting (usually stops after a few days of treatment). Dose-related orthostatic hypotension.

▷ **Possible Adverse Effects** (unusual, unexpected, and infrequent reactions)

If any of the following develop, consult your physician promptly for guidance.

Mild Adverse Effects

Allergic reactions: skin rash.

Somnolence, headache, agitation, sleep disorders—infrequent to frequent.

Liver toxicity—rare.

Dry mouth, anorexia, or constipation—possible to frequent.

Serious Adverse Effects

Allergic reactions: anaphylactic reaction—case reports.

Serious skin rash—case reports.

Liver toxicity—rare.

Seizures or mania—rare.

Tourette's syndrome—case reports.

Excessive urination—rare.

▷ **Possible Effects on Sexual Function:**   Delayed or absent orgasm, failure to ejaculate—case reports.

Possible Delayed Adverse Effects: Not reported.

▷ **Adverse Effects That May Mimic Natural Diseases or Disorders**

Not reported.

Natural Diseases or Disorders That May Be Activated by This Drug

None defined.

Possible Effects on Laboratory Tests

Liver function tests: increased.

Melatonin level: increased.

CAUTION

1. This medicine has several important drug–drug interactions. Be certain to tell any health care professionals who provide care for you that you take this medicine.
2. If nausea and vomiting continue for more than 2 days after you start this medicine, call your doctor.

Precautions for Use

By Infants and Children: Safety and effectiveness for use by those under 18 years of age have not been established.

By Those Over 60 Years of Age: Lowered starting and maintenance doses are indicated.

▷ **Advisability of Use During Pregnancy**

Pregnancy Category: C. See Pregnancy Risk Categories at the back of this book.

Animal studies: Consistent with category C.

Human studies: Information from adequate studies of pregnant women is not available. Ask your doctor for help.

Advisability of Use If Breast-Feeding
Presence of this drug in breast milk: Yes, in small amounts.
Monitor nursing infant closely and discontinue drug or nursing if adverse effects develop.

Habit-Forming Potential: None, but a withdrawal syndrome has been reported if the medicine is stopped abruptly.

Effects of Overdose: Nausea, vomiting, seizures.

Possible Effects of Long-Term Use: Not defined.

Suggested Periodic Examinations While Taking This Drug (at physician's discretion)
Liver function tests.

▷ **While Taking This Drug, Observe the Following**
Foods: No restrictions.
Beverages: No restrictions.
▷ *Alcohol:* No significant interaction. Ask your doctor for guidance.
Tobacco Smoking: Fluvoxamine stays in the body up to one-quarter less the time than in nonsmokers. I advise everyone to quit smoking.
Marijuana Smoking: Additive somnolence.
▷ *Other Drugs*
Fluvoxamine ***taken concurrently*** with
- amitriptyline (Elavil others) can result in amitriptyline toxicity.
- astemizole (Hismanal) may cause **serious heart arrhythmias**. Do not combine.
- benzodiazepines (see Drug Classes) may result in benzodiazepine toxicity.
- beta-blockers (see Drug Classes) may result in decreased drug clearance and toxicity.
- buspirone (Buspar) may lead to very slow heart rates.
- carbamazepine (Tegretol) may cause toxicity.
- cimetidine (Tagamet) may lead to toxicity.
- cisapride (Propulsid) may cause heart toxicity. Don't combine.
- clomipramine (Anafranil) may cause toxicity.
- clozapine (Clozaril) can result in higher clozapine levels and toxicity.
- dextromethorphan may cause hallucinations (reported with a similar medicines).
- diltiazem (Cardizem) may cause diltiazem toxicity.
- imipramine (Tofranil, others) may result in imipramine toxicity.
- lithium (Lithobid) can cause serotonin syndrome.
- monoamine oxidase (MAO) inhibitors (see Drug Classes) can cause toxicity. Do **not** combine.
- maprotiline can cause maprotiline toxicity.
- methadone may result in increased opioid effects.
- oral antidiabetic drugs (see Drug Classes) may remain in the body longer than expected, requiring a dose decrease. This has not been reported with fluvoxamine, but has been reported with sertraline, a medicine in the same pharmacological family.
- phenytoin (Dilantin) may lead to phenytoin toxicity. Patients should be

watched closely for problems walking (ataxia) or drowsiness (early toxicity signs), and their doctor notified at once if these occur.

- ritonavir (Norvir) may lead to toxicity.
- sumatriptan (Imitrex) may lead to weakness and confusion.
- terfenadine (Seldane) may cause **serious heart arrhythmias**. Do not combine.
- theophylline may result in theophylline toxicity.
- tramadol (Ultram) may increase seizure risk. **DO NOT combine.**
- tricyclic antidepressants (imipramine, others) may lead totricyclic toxicity.
- tryptophan may increase serotonin effects of fluvoxamine and cause severe vomiting.
- warfarin (Coumadin) can result in increased warfarin concentrations and may lead to bleeding. More frequent INR testing is needed.

▷ *Driving, Hazardous Activities:* This drug may cause drowsiness. Restrict activities as necessary.

Aviation Note: The use of this drug *is probably a disqualification* for piloting. Consult a designated aviation medical examiner.

Exposure to Sun: No restrictions.

Discontinuation: A withdrawal syndrome has been reported if this medicine is abruptly stopped. The doses should be slowly tapered.

FOSINOPRIL (FOH sin oh pril)

Introduced: 1986   **Class:** Antihypertensive, ACE inhibitor

Please see the new angiotensin-converting enzyme (ACE) inhibitor combination profile for more information.

FUROSEMIDE (fur OH se mide)

Introduced: 1964   **Class:** Antihypertensive, diuretic   **Prescription:** USA: Yes   **Controlled Drug:** USA: No; Canada: No   **Available as Generic:** USA: Yes; Canada: Yes

Brand Names: ✤Albert Furosemide, ✤Apo-Furosemide, Fumide MD, Furomide MD, Furocot, Furosemide-10, ✤Furoside, Lasaject, Lasimide, Lasix, ✤Lasix Special, Lo-Aqua, Luramide, Myrosemide, Ro-Semide, SK-Furosemide, ✤Uritol

BENEFITS versus RISKS	
Possible Benefits	*Possible Risks*
PROMPT, EFFECTIVE, RELIABLE DIURETIC	WATER AND ELECTROLYTE DEPLETION with excessive use
MODEST ANTIHYPERTENSIVE IN MILD TO MODERATE HYPERTENSION	Excessive potassium and magnesium loss
ENHANCES EFFECTIVENESS OF OTHER ANTIHYPERTENSIVES	Increased blood sugar level
	Decreased blood calcium level
	Liver damage
	Blood cell disorder

▷ **Principal Uses**

As a Single Drug Product: Uses currently included in FDA-approved labeling: (1) Increases urine and remove excessive water (edema), as in congestive heart failure or some forms of liver, lung, and kidney disease; (2) lowers high blood pressure, usually with other drugs.

Other (unlabeled) generally accepted uses: (1) Inhaled furosemide may help protect the lungs in people with asthma; (2) can have a role in helping infants with lung problems (chronic bronchopulmonary dysplasia).

How This Drug Works: By increasing the elimination of salt and water through increased urine production, this drug reduces fluid in the blood and body tissues. These changes also contribute to lowering blood pressure.

Available Dose Forms and Strengths

Injection — 10 mg/ml

Solution — 10 mg/ml

Tablets — 20 mg, 40 mg, 80 mg

▷ **Usual Adult Dose Range:**   As antihypertensive: 40 mg every 12 hours initially; increase dose as needed and tolerated. As diuretic: 20 to 80 mg in a single dose initially; if necessary, increase the dose by 20 to 40 mg every 6 to 8 hours. The smallest effective dose should be used. Daily maximum is 640 mg. In general, other medicines for high blood pressure should be added before daily dose is increased beyond 80 mg per day. **Note: Actual dose and schedule must be determined for each patient individually.**

Conditions Requiring Dosing Adjustments

Liver Function: Larger doses may be needed for patients with liver compromise, and extreme care must be used to maintain critical electrolytes.

Kidney Function: Larger initial doses may be needed before any benefit is seen. Drug may cause kidney stones and protein in urine.

Cystic Fibrosis: Patients with this disease may be more sensitive to the drug, and smaller starting doses are indicated.

▷ **Dosing Instructions:**   The tablet may be crushed and taken with or following meals to reduce stomach irritation. Best taken in the morning to avoid nighttime urination.

Usual Duration of Use: Use on a regular schedule for 2 to 3 weeks is best to see effectiveness in lowering high blood pressure. Long-term use (months to years) requires periodic physician evaluation of response.

▷ **This Drug Should Not Be Taken If**

• you had an allergic reaction to it previously.

• your kidneys are not making urine.

▷ **Inform Your Physician Before Taking This Drug If**

• you are allergic to any form of "sulfa" drug.

• you are pregnant or planning a pregnancy.

• you have a history of kidney or liver disease.

• you have diabetes, gout, or lupus erythematosus.

• you have impaired hearing.

• you have low blood potassium or other electrolytes (talk with your doctor).

• you take cortisone, digitalis, oral antidiabetics, or insulin.

• you will have surgery with general anesthesia.

Possible Side Effects (natural, expected, and unavoidable drug actions)
> Light-headedness on arising from sitting or lying position (see orthostatic hypotension in Glossary).
> Increase in blood sugar level, affecting control of diabetes.
> Increase in blood uric acid level, affecting control of gout.
> Decrease in blood potassium level, causing muscle weakness and cramping.
> Decreased magnesium level.

▷ **Possible Adverse Effects** (unusual, unexpected, and infrequent reactions)
> **If any of the following develop, consult your physician promptly for guidance.**

Mild Adverse Effects
> Allergic reactions: skin rashes, hives, drug fever—case reports.
> Headache, dizziness, blurred or yellow vision, ringing in ears, numbness and tingling—rare to infrequent.
> Reduced appetite, indigestion, nausea, vomiting, diarrhea—possible.
> Metabolic alkalosis—possible.

Serious Adverse Effects
> Allergic reactions: hepatitis with jaundice (see Glossary), anaphylactic reaction (see Glossary), severe skin reactions—case reports.
> Idiosyncratic reaction: fluid in lungs—case reports.
> Temporary hearing loss—case reports.
> Inflammation of the pancreas (severe abdominal pain)—rare.
> Bone marrow depression (see Glossary): fatigue, weakness, fever, sore throat, abnormal bleeding or bruising—case reports.
> Low blood pressure on standing or abnormal heartbeat (arrhythmias)—rare.
> Drug-induced porphyria or excessive parathyroid gland action (hyperparathyroidism)—case reports.
> Low blood potassium or magnesium—possible.
> Vitamin deficiency (thiamine)—possible.
> Kidney stones (calcium containing)—case reports.
> Liver toxicity (cholestatic jaundice)—rare.
> Skin lesions (erythema multiforme or Stevens-Johnson syndrome)—case reports.
> Hip fractures (may increase risk).

▷ **Possible Effects on Sexual Function:**   Impotence using recommended dose of 20 to 80 mg per day—infrequent.

▷ **Adverse Effects That May Mimic Natural Diseases or Disorders**
> Liver reaction may suggest viral hepatitis.

Natural Diseases or Disorders That May Be Activated by This Drug
> Diabetes, gout, systemic lupus erythematosus.

Possible Effects on Laboratory Tests
> Complete blood counts: reduced red cells, hemoglobin, white cells, and platelets.
> Blood amylase and lipase levels: increased (possible pancreatitis).
> Blood sodium and chloride levels: decreased.
> Blood levels of total cholesterol, LDL and VLDL cholesterol, and triglycerides: increased.
> Blood glucose level: increased.
> Glucose tolerance test (GTT): decreased tolerance.

Blood potassium or magnesium level: decreased.

Blood thyroid hormone (T_3 and T_4) levels: decreased.

Blood uric acid level or blood urea nitrogen (BUN): increased.

Urine sugar tests: no drug effect with Tes-Tape; false low results with Clinistix and Diastix.

CAUTION

1. Take exactly the dose that was prescribed. Increased doses can cause serious loss of sodium and potassium, with resultant loss of appetite, nausea, fatigue, weakness, confusion, and tingling in the extremities.

2. If you take a digitalis preparation (digitoxin, digoxin), ensure an adequate intake of high-potassium foods to prevent potassium deficiency. (See Table 13, "High-Potassium Foods," Section Six.)

Precautions for Use

By Infants and Children: Significant potassium loss can occur within the first 2 weeks of drug use.

By Those Over 60 Years of Age: Small starting doses are critical. Increased risk of impaired thinking, orthostatic hypotension, potassium loss, and blood sugar increase. Overdose and extended use of this drug can cause excessive loss of body water, thickening (increased viscosity) of the blood, and an increased tendency for the blood to clot—predisposing to stroke, heart attack, or thrombophlebitis (vein inflammation with blood clot).

▷ **Advisability of Use During Pregnancy**

Pregnancy Category: C. See Pregnancy Risk Categories at the back of this book.

Animal studies: Significant birth defects have been reported.

Human studies: Adequate studies of pregnant women are not available.

This drug should not be used during pregnancy unless a very serious complication occurs for which it is significantly beneficial. Avoid completely during the first 3 months. Ask your physician for guidance.

Advisability of Use If Breast-Feeding

Presence of this drug in breast milk: Yes.

Avoid drug or refrain from nursing.

Habit-Forming Potential: None.

Effects of Overdose: Dry mouth, thirst, lethargy, weakness, muscle cramping, nausea, vomiting, drowsiness progressing to stupor or coma.

Possible Effects of Long-Term Use: Impaired water, salt, and potassium balance; dehydration and increased blood coagulability, with risk of blood clots. Development of diabetes in predisposed individuals.

Suggested Periodic Examinations While Taking This Drug (at physician's discretion)

Complete blood counts, measurements of blood levels of sodium, potassium, chloride, sugar, and uric acid.

Kidney and liver function tests.

▷ **While Taking This Drug, Observe the Following**

Foods: Ask your doctor about eating foods rich in potassium. If so advised, see Table 13, "High-Potassium Foods," Section Six. Follow your physician's advice regarding the use of salt. Food decreases absorption of furosemide by up to 30%. Take this medicine 1 hour before or 2 hours after a meal.

Beverages: No restrictions. This drug may be taken with milk.

▷　*Alcohol:* Use with caution—alcohol may exaggerate the blood-pressure-lowering effects of this drug and cause orthostatic hypotension.

Tobacco Smoking: No interactions expected. I advise everyone to quit smoking.

▷　*Other Drugs*

Furosemide may ***increase*** the effects of
- other antihypertensive drugs; dose adjustments may be necessary to prevent excessive lowering of blood pressure.
- digoxin (Lanoxin), and result in digoxin toxicity.
- lithium (Lithobid, others), and cause lithium toxicity.

Furosemide may ***decrease*** the effects of
- oral antidiabetic drugs (sulfonylureas); dose adjustments may be necessary for proper control of blood sugar.

Furosemide ***taken concurrently*** with
- adrenocortical steroids (see Drug Classes) may cause additive loss of potassium.
- amikacin, gentamicin, tobramycin, or other aminoglycosides may cause hearing toxicity (ototoxicity).
- bepridil (Vascor) may lead to abnormal heart effects if potassium is low.
- cephalosporin antibiotics (see Drug Classes) may increase risk of kidney problems (nephrotoxicity).
- cholestyramine (Questran) may cause loss of furosemide effectiveness.
- clofibrate (Atromid-S) may lead to muscle stiffness and increased diuretic effects.
- colestipol (Colestid) may cause loss of furosemide effectiveness.
- cyclosporine (Sandimmune) may cause elevated uric acid levels (hyperuricemia) and gout.
- digitalis preparations (digitoxin, digoxin) requires blood tests or dose changes to maintain potassium levels and avoid heart rhythm problems.
- lomefloxacin (Maxaquin) may increase lomefloxacin levels and lead to toxicity.
- metformin (Glucophage) may increase metformin and decrease furosemide effects.
- NSAIDs (see ***nonsteroidal anti-inflammatory drugs*** in Drug Classes) may cause loss of diuretic effectiveness.
- phenytoin (Dilantin) may decrease furosemide diuretic effects.

▷　*Driving, Hazardous Activities:* Use caution until the possible occurrence of orthostatic hypotension, dizziness, or impaired vision has been determined.

Aviation Note: The use of this drug ***may be a disqualification*** for piloting. Consult a designated aviation medical examiner.

Exposure to Sun: Use caution—this drug may cause photosensitivity (see Glossary).

Exposure to Heat: Avoid excessive perspiring, which could cause additional loss of salt and water from the body.

Heavy Exercise or Exertion: Avoid exertion that produces light-headedness, excessive fatigue, or muscle cramping. Ask your doctor for help about participation in exercise.

Occurrence of Unrelated Illness: Vomiting or diarrhea can produce a serious imbalance of important body chemistry. Ask your doctor for guidance.

Discontinuation: It may be best to discontinue this drug 5 to 7 days before major surgery. Ask your physician, surgeon, and/or anesthesiologist for guidance regarding dose adjustment or drug withdrawal.

GABAPENTIN (GAB ah pen tin)

Introduced: 1981   **Class:** Anticonvulsant, pain syndrome modifier   **Prescription:** USA: Yes   **Controlled Drug:** USA: No; Canada: No   **Available as Generic:** USA: No; Canada: Yes

Brand Names: Neurontin

BENEFITS versus RISKS

Possible Benefits	*Possible Risks*
ADJUNCTIVE THERAPY OF PARTIAL SEIZURES EFFECTIVE TREATMENT OF A VARIETY OF PAIN SYNDROMES	SLEEPINESS MOVEMENT PROBLEMS

▷ **Principal Uses**

As a Single Drug Product: Uses currently included in FDA-approved labeling: As an antiepileptic drug adjunctive to other medicines to control partial seizures.

Other (unlabeled) generally accepted uses: (1) Used in chronic pain syndromes; (2) may have a role in controlling spasticity.

How This Drug Works: Similar in chemistry to an inhibitory substance called gamma Amino butyric acid (GABA). Gabapentin appears to increase GABA levels in the brain.

Available Dose Forms and Strengths

Capsules — 100 mg, 300, 400 mg

▷ **Usual Adult Dose Range:** Seizures: Initially 100 mg three times a day. Dose may be increased to 900 mg a day by the third day. Doses up to 2400 mg have been well-tolerated, and 3600 mg used in some patients.

Pain syndromes: 100 mg a day, increased as needed and tolerated.

Maximum doses are as those seen in seizure patients.

Note: Actual dose and schedule must be determined for each patient individually.

Conditions Requiring Dosing Adjustments

Liver Function: Not changed by the liver. No dosing changes needed.

Kidney Function: 300 mg twice daily is given to those with a creatinine clearance of 30 to 60 ml/min. For a creatinine clearance of 15 to 30 ml/min, 300 mg is given daily.

▷ **Dosing Instructions:** May be taken with or after food to reduce stomach irritation. The capsule may be opened and the tablet may be crushed.

Usual Duration of Use: Use on a regular schedule for 2 to 3 weeks usually determines benefit in reducing frequency and severity of seizures. Optimal control will require careful dose adjustments. Use in pain syndromes may take a similar time. Long-term use requires ongoing physician supervision.

▷ **This Drug Should Not Be Taken If**
  • you have had an allergic reaction to this drug.

▷ **Inform Your Physician Before Taking This Drug If**
  • you are taking any other drugs at this time.
  • you have a history of kidney disease or impaired kidney function.
  • you have low blood pressure.

Possible Side Effects (natural, expected, and unavoidable drug actions)
  Mild fatigue, sluggishness, and drowsiness—may be frequent.

▷ **Possible Adverse Effects** (unusual, unexpected, and infrequent reactions)
  If any of the following develop, consult your physician promptly for guidance.
  Mild Adverse Effects
  Allergic reactions: skin rashes, hives—possible.
  Weight gain—infrequent.
  Accumulation of fluid in the ankles (edema)—infrequent.
  Nausea, vomiting, constipation—infrequent.
  Vision changes—infrequent.
  Lowering of blood pressure—infrequent.
  Bedwetting—case reports, mild and resolved with ongoing therapy.
  Serious Adverse Effects
  Allergic reactions: none reported.
  Idiosyncratic reactions: none reported.
  Seizures—case reports.
  Movement disorder—possible (case reports).
  Lowered white blood cell counts—rare.

▷ **Possible Effects on Sexual Function:**   Impotence—rare.

▷ **Adverse Effects That May Mimic Natural Diseases or Disorders**
  Drug-induced hepatitis may suggest viral hepatitis.
  Skin reactions may resemble lupus erythematosus.

Natural Diseases or Disorders That May Be Activated by This Drug
  None reported.

Possible Effects on Laboratory Tests
  Complete blood cell counts: decreased white cells—rare.

CAUTION
  1. When used for the treatment of epilepsy, *this drug must not be stopped abruptly.*
  2. Regularity of drug use is essential. Take this drug at the same time each day.
  3. Carry a personal identification card with a notation that you are taking this drug.

Precautions for Use
  By Infants and Children: Not indicated unless 12 or older.
  By Those Over 60 Years of Age: You may be more sensitive to all of the actions of this drug and require smaller doses. Observe closely for any adverse effects: drowsiness, fatigue, confusion, "cogging" of arms, vision changes.

▷ **Advisability of Use During Pregnancy**
  Pregnancy Category: C. See Pregnancy Risk Categories at the back of this book.

Human studies: Information from adequate studies of pregnant women is not available.

Discuss use of this drug during pregnancy with your doctor.

Advisability of Use If Breast-Feeding
Presence of this drug in breast milk: Unknown.
Monitor nursing infant closely and discontinue drug or nursing if adverse effects develop.

Habit-Forming Potential: None.

Effects of Overdose: Drowsiness, slurred speech, double vision, and diarrhea.

Possible Effects of Long-Term Use: None defined.

Suggested Periodic Examinations While Taking This Drug (at physician's discretion)
Checks of seizure control. Check for "cogging" of arms.

▷ **While Taking This Drug, Observe the Following**
Foods: No restrictions.
Nutritional Support: None required.
Beverages: No restrictions. May be taken with milk.

▷ *Alcohol:* Use extreme caution. Alcohol (in large quantities or with continual use) may reduce effectiveness in preventing seizures.
Tobacco Smoking: No interactions expected. I advise everyone to quit smoking.

▷ *Other Drugs*
Gabapentin *taken concurrently* with
- antacids (various) may lower beneficial effects.
- cimetidine (Tagamet) may increase blood levels of gabapentin.
- phenytoin (Dilantin) may lead to phenytoin toxicity.

▷ *Driving, Hazardous Activities:* This drug may impair mental alertness, vision, and coordination. Restrict activities as necessary.
Aviation Note: The use of this drug *is a disqualification* for piloting. Consult a designated aviation medical examiner.
Exposure to Sun: No restrictions at present.
*Discontinuation: **This drug must not be discontinued abruptly.*** Sudden withdrawal can precipitate severe and repeated seizures. If this drug is to be discontinued, gradual reduction in dose should be made. Discuss this with your doctor.

GANCICLOVIR (ganz EYE klo veer)

Introduced: 1995 (tablet)   **Class:** Antiviral   **Prescription:** USA: Yes
Controlled Drug: USA: No; Canada: No   **Available as Generic:** USA: No; Canada: No

Brand Names: Cytovene, Vitrasert

Warning: The oral form of this medicine should only be used by patients who are not candidates for intravenous dosing and where risk of more rapid cytomegalovirus (CMV) retinitis progression is outweighed by benefit of avoiding the intravenous route.

```
                        BENEFITS versus RISKS
        Possible Benefits                    Possible Risks
  Oral, intravenous, or implanted    More rapid progression of CMV
    treatment of cytomegalovirus        disease (capsules)
    (CMV) retinitis                   Bone marrow suppression
  Decreased side effects with the oral
    form
  Transition to an oral form following
    intravenous induction
```

▷ **Principal Uses**

As a Single Drug Product: Uses currently included in FDA-approved labeling: (1) Treatment of cytomegalovirus (CMV) retinitis; (2) prevention of CMV retinitis in a variety of patients, such as liver, kidney, lung, bone marrow, and heart transplant patients; (3) implantation of the ocular implant into the diseased area—this form may work for 5 months or more; (4) prevention of CMV disease in patients with advanced HIV infection.

Other (unlabeled) generally accepted uses: (1) Treatment of pediatric CMV; (2) may have a role in treating Epstein-Barr virus infection; (3) can have a role in treating leukoplakia.

How This Drug Works: Changed to an active (triphosphate) in infected cells. The active form interferes with DNA and the survival of the virus.

Available Dose Forms and Strengths

            Capsules — 250 mg
        Intravenous — 500 mg/10 ml
  Intravitreal insert — 4.5 mg

How to Store

The intravenous solution should be stored at 39 degrees F (4 degrees C) and used within 12 hours after it has been reconstituted.

▷ **Recommended Dose Ranges** (Actual dose and schedule must be determined for each patient individually.)

Infants and Children: **Author's Note: This drug has potential for reproductive toxicity and the risk of causing cancer. It is used in children only after careful evaluation and with extreme caution.**

Induction: 2.5 mg per kg of body mass given intravenously three times daily.

Maintenance: 6.5 mg per kg of body mass given intravenously once daily five to seven times a week.

12 to 60 Years of Age: Induction: 5 mg per kg of body mass intravenously (infused over 1 hour) every 12 hours for 14 to 21 days.

Maintenance dose: 2.1 to 6 mg per kg of body mass infused into a vein over 1 hour each day. Some centers have used 6 mg per kg of body mass given once daily 5 days per week. The maker of this drug suggests 5 mg per kg of body mass intravenously daily. If retinitis progresses, the patient can be restarted on the twice-daily-dosing approach. Maximum dose is 6 mg per kg of body mass infused over 1 hour.

Oral: Once the intravenous induction dosing has been accomplished, oral ganciclovir is given 1000 mg three times daily. Some centers have opted for 500 mg six times per day, given every 3 hours while the patient is awake. If retinitis progresses, intravenous induction therapy should be given.

Intravitreous: This device is surgically implanted and has been effective for 5 or more months.

Over 60 Years of Age: Kidney function must be checked and the dose appropriately adjusted.

Conditions Requiring Dosing Adjustments

Liver Function: The liver is only minimally involved in the elimination of this drug, and dosing changes in liver compromise are not needed.

Kidney Function: The dose **must** be decreased in kidney compromise. This adjustment is accomplished based on creatinine clearance (see Glossary):

Induction—70 ml/min or higher: 5 mg per kg of body mass every 12 hours; 50–69: 2.5 mg per kg of body mass every 12 hours; 25–49: 2.5 mg per kg of body mass every 24 hours; 10–24: 1.25 mg per kg of body mass every 24 hours; less than 10: 1.25 mg per kg of body mass three times per week.

Maintenance—70 ml/min or higher: 5 mg per kg of body mass every 24 hours; 50–69: 2.5 mg per kg of body mass every 24 hours; 25–49: 1.25 mg per kg of body mass every 24 hours; 10–24: 0.625 mg per kg of body mass every 24 hours; less than 10: 0.625 mg per kg of body mass three times per week.

▷ **Dosing Instructions:** This medicine should be taken with food if taken by mouth (orally). It is best to take the medicine at the same time each day. Capsule form should not be opened or crushed, because you may have adverse reactions from the toxic powder. If you are taking the capsule form and your vision declines, call your doctor immediately.

Usual Duration of Use: Continual use on a regular schedule for up to 16 days is usually needed to determine this drug's effectiveness in treating retinitis. Because of a very high frequency of relapse, most centers recommend ongoing maintenance therapy. Long-term use (months to years) requires periodic evaluation of response and dose adjustment. The ocular implant form may work for 5 months or more. Consult your physician on a regular basis.

Possible Advantages of This Drug

Transition from the intravenous form to the oral form (if successful in treatment) offers a clear quality of life advantage.

Currently a "Drug of Choice"

For patients with kidney failure.

▷ **This Drug Should Not Be Taken If**
- you had an allergic reaction to it previously.
- your absolute neutrophil count (a specific kind of white blood cell) is less than 500 per cubic mm.
- your platelet count is less than 25,000 per cubic mm.

▷ **Inform Your Physician Before Taking This Drug If**
- you think you are dehydrated (this drug is primarily removed by the kidneys).
- you have a sore throat or fever.
- you have a history of blood cell disorders.
- you are planning a pregnancy.
- you are male and are planning a pregnancy (attempted conception should be avoided for at least 3 months after ganciclovir therapy).
- you are uncertain of how much ganciclovir to take, how often to take it, or how to handle the intravenous solution.

- you take other prescription or nonprescription medicines that were not discussed with your doctor when ganciclovir was prescribed. This includes natural extracts or herbal remedies and "underground" therapies for AIDS.

Possible Side Effects (natural, expected, and unavoidable drug actions)
Pain at the injection site with the IV form. Possible phlebitis.

▷ **Possible Adverse Effects** (unusual, unexpected, and infrequent reactions)
If any of the following develop, consult your physician promptly for guidance.
Mild Adverse Effects
Allergic reactions: skin rash and itching.
Confusion, headache, nervousness, tremor, somnolence, abnormal dreams, ataxia, "pins-and-needles" sensations of the hands (paresthesias)—infrequent.
Fever—may be frequent with oral therapy.
Decreased blood glucose or potassium—rare.
Nausea, vomiting, or diarrhea—infrequent to frequent.
Serious Adverse Effects
Allergic reactions: anaphylactic reaction—case reports.
Bone marrow suppression—rare.
Lowered white blood cell (neutropenia) counts—frequent.
Lowered blood platelets—infrequent.
Arrhythmias—rare.
Coma, psychosis, or seizures—case reports.
Neuropathy—infrequent to frequent.
Liver toxicity—rare to infrequent.
Retinal detachment—infrequent.
This drug is a potential cancer-causing (carcinogenic) agent—no percentage defined.

▷ **Possible Effects on Sexual Function:**   Reversible infertility in men.

Possible Delayed Adverse Effects: Lowered white blood cell counts or platelets.

▷ **Adverse Effects That May Mimic Natural Diseases or Disorders**
Increased liver enzymes may mimic hepatitis.

Natural Diseases or Disorders That May Be Activated by This Drug
None defined.

Possible Effects on Laboratory Tests
Liver enzymes: increased.
Serum bilirubin or creatinine: increased.
Blood glucose, platelets, or white blood cells: decreased.

CAUTION
1. The oral form may be less effective than the intravenous form. Call your doctor immediately if your vision declines.
2. May cause bone marrow suppression. Call your doctor if you get a sore throat, start to bruise easily, or develop have fever.

Precautions for Use
By Infants and Children: Safety and effectiveness for use by those under 18 years of age have not been established. The drug has been used selectively in patients as young as 36 weeks.

By Those Over 60 Years of Age: Because of the age-related decline in kidney function, a creatinine clearance should be obtained and dosing adjusted appropriately.

▷ **Advisability of Use During Pregnancy**
Pregnancy Category: C. See Pregnancy Risk Categories at the back of this book.
Animal studies: Rabbits have developed cleft palate, exhibited poorly developed organs, and have experienced fetal death.
Human studies: Information from adequate studies of pregnant women is not available. Use of this drug during pregnancy is not recommended.

Advisability of Use If Breast-Feeding
Presence of this drug in breast milk: Unknown.
Avoid drug or refrain from nursing.

Habit-Forming Potential: None.

Effects of Overdose: Nausea and vomiting, excessive salivation, increased liver function tests, bone marrow suppression, and kidney failure.

Possible Effects of Long-Term Use: Not defined.

Suggested Periodic Examinations While Taking This Drug (at physician's discretion)
Platelet counts and complete blood counts: every 2 days during induction and weekly thereafter. Liver function tests: monthly.
Kidney function tests: every 2 weeks.
Eye (ophthalmologic) exams: weekly during induction and every 2 weeks thereafter. These exams may be needed more frequently if the optic nerve or macula of the eye is involved.

▷ **While Taking This Drug, Observe the Following**
Foods: No restrictions—the oral form should be taken with food.
Beverages: No restrictions.
▷ *Alcohol:* No restrictions; however, alcohol may blunt the immune system.
Tobacco Smoking: No interactions expected. I advise everyone to quit smoking.
Marijuana Smoking: May increase somnolence.
▷ *Other Drugs*
Ganciclovir *taken concurrently* with
- amphotericin B (Fungizone, Abelcet) may result in increased bone marrow suppression.
- cancer chemotherapy may result in additive bone marrow suppression.
- cotrimoxazole (Septra) may result in added bone marrow suppression problems.
- cyclosporine (Sandimmune) can result in increased kidney toxicity.
- dapsone is a benefit-to-risk decision, as additive bone marrow suppression may occur.
- flucytosine (Ancobon) can cause additive bone marrow toxicity.
- imipenem/cilastatin (Primaxin) can cause seizures.
- pentamidine may result in additive bone marrow suppression.
- zidovudine (AZT) will cause a serious increase in bone marrow suppression.
The following drug may *increase* the effects of ganciclovir:
- probenecid (Benemid)—by interfering with elimination by the kidney.

▷   *Driving, Hazardous Activities:* This drug may cause somnolence. Restrict activities as necessary.

Aviation Note: The use of this drug *may be a disqualification* for piloting. Consult a designated aviation medical examiner.

Exposure to Sun: Caution is advised. Photosensitivity has been reported.

Discontinuation: Talk with your doctor before stopping this medicine.

Special Storage Instructions: Store the intravenous form at 39 degrees F (4 degrees C).

Observe the Following Expiration Times: The intravenous form will be stamped or labeled with a specific expiration time if this has been provided by a home infusion company; it should be used within 12 hours after it has been reconstituted.

GEMFIBROZIL (jem FI broh zil)

Introduced: 1976   **Class:** Anticholesterol (cholesterol-reducing drug)
Prescription: USA: Yes   **Controlled Drug:** USA: No; Canada: No   **Available as Generic:** USA: Yes; Canada: No
Brand Names: Lopid, Gemcor

BENEFITS versus RISKS	
Possible Benefits	*Possible Risks*
EFFECTIVE REDUCTION OF TRIGLYCERIDE BLOOD LEVELS	Gallstone formation with long-term use
INCREASE IN HIGH-DENSITY LIPOPROTEIN (HDL) BLOOD LEVELS	Decreased white blood cell counts

▷ **Principal Uses**

As a Single Drug Product: Uses currently included in FDA-approved labeling: (1) Reduces abnormally high blood levels of triglycerides in Types II and IV blood lipid (fat) disorders; (2) decreases risk for developing coronary artery heart disease.

Other (unlabeled) generally accepted uses: Used by diabetics as combination therapy with oral hypoglycemic agents to further increase desirable HDLs.

How This Drug Works: Reduces triglycerides by inhibiting the liver from making them. Decreases VLDL and LDL. Increases HDL more than clofibrate.

Available Dose Forms and Strengths

Capsules — 300 mg
Tablets — 600 mg

▷ **Usual Adult Dose Range:**   1200 to 1600 daily in two divided doses. The average dose is 1200 mg daily. Dose increases should be made gradually over a period of 2 to 3 months. **Note: Actual dose and schedule must be determined for each patient individually.**

Conditions Requiring Dosing Adjustments

Liver Function: This drug is contraindicated in primary biliary cirrhosis and severe liver failure.

Kidney Function: For patients with moderate kidney failure, 50% of the usual dose should be taken at the usual interval. Patients with severe kidney failure should take 25% of the usual dose at the usual dosing interval.

▷ **Dosing Instructions:**   The capsule may be opened and taken 30 minutes before the morning and evening meals.

Usual Duration of Use: Regular use for 4 to 8 weeks determines effectiveness in reducing triglycerides. Long-term use (months to years) requires periodic evaluation by your doctor.

▷ **This Drug Should Not Be Taken If**
- you have had an allergic reaction to it previously.
- you have biliary cirrhosis of the liver.
- you have severe kidney compromise.

▷ **Inform Your Physician Before Taking This Drug If**
- you have impaired liver or kidney function.
- you have gallbladder disease or gallstones.
- you are a diabetic.
- you have an underactive thyroid (hypothyroidism).

Possible Side Effects (natural, expected, and unavoidable drug actions)
Moderate increase in blood sugar levels.

▷ **Possible Adverse Effects** (unusual, unexpected, and infrequent reactions)
If any of the following develop, consult your physician promptly for guidance.
Mild Adverse Effects
Allergic reactions: skin rash, hives, itching.
Headache, dizziness, blurred vision, fatigue, muscle aches, and cramps—infrequent.
Indigestion, excessive gas, stomach discomfort, nausea, vomiting, diarrhea—rare to infrequent.
Paresthesias—very rare.
Serious Adverse Effects
Abnormally low white blood cell count: fever, chills, sore throat—rare.
Formation of gallstones with long-term use or low blood potassium—possible.
Raynaud's phenomenon—case report.
Liver toxicity—possible.
Myopathy (muscle weakness) or rhabdomyolysis (inability to walk)—case reports to rare.
Kidney failure with muscle damage—case reports with HMG-CoA reductase inhibitor use.

▷ **Possible Effects on Sexual Function:**   Decreased libido or impotence—rare to infrequent.

Natural Diseases or Disorders That May Be Activated by This Drug
Latent diabetes, latent urinary tract infections.

Possible Effects on Laboratory Tests
Complete blood counts: decreased red cells, hemoglobin, white cells, and platelets.
Blood HDL cholesterol levels: increased.
Blood triglyceride levels: decreased.
Liver function tests: increased liver enzymes (ALT/GPT, AST/GOT, and alkaline phosphatase), increased bilirubin.

CAUTION
1. Gemfibrozil is used only after diet has NOT worked to lower triglyceride levels.
2. If you used the drug clofibrate (Atromid-S) in the past, inform your physician fully regarding your experience.
3. Periodic triglyceride and cholesterol levels are critical.

Precautions for Use
By Infants and Children: Safety and effectiveness for those under 12 years of age are not established.
By Those Over 60 Years of Age: Watch for increased tendency to infection; treat all infections promptly.

▷ **Advisability of Use During Pregnancy**
Pregnancy Category: C. See Pregnancy Risk Categories at the back of this book.
Animal studies: Produces adverse effects in rabbits and rats.
Human studies: Adequate studies of pregnant women are not available.
Ask your physician for guidance.

Advisability of Use If Breast-Feeding
Presence of this drug in breast milk: Yes.
Avoid drug or refrain from nursing.

Habit-Forming Potential: None.

Effects of Overdose: Abdominal pain, nausea, vomiting, diarrhea.

Possible Effects of Long-Term Use: Formation of gallstones.

Suggested Periodic Examinations While Taking This Drug (at physician's discretion)
Complete blood cell counts and liver function tests.
Measurements of blood levels of total cholesterol, HDL and LDL cholesterol fractions, triglycerides, and sugar.

▷ **While Taking This Drug, Observe the Following**
Foods: Follow the diet prescribed by your physician.
Beverages: No restrictions. May be taken with milk.
▷ *Alcohol:* No interactions expected.
Tobacco Smoking: No interactions expected. I advise everyone to quit smoking.
▷ *Other Drugs*
Gemfibrozil *taken concurrently* with
• ritonavir (Norvir) may risk gemfibrozil toxicity.
Gemfibrozil may *increase* the effects of
• glyburide and other oral antidiabetic drugs (see Drug Classes).
• lovastatin and HMG-CoA type drugs (see Drug Classes); may increase muscle damage risk (myopathy) if taken at the same time.
• warfarin (Coumadin), and increase the risk of bleeding. Increased frequency of INR (prothrombin time or protime) measurements and dose changes based on results are critical.
Gemfibrozil may *decrease* the effects of
• chenodiol (Chenix), reducing its benefit in gallstone therapy.
▷ *Driving, Hazardous Activities:* This drug may cause dizziness and blurred vision. Restrict activities as necessary.
Aviation Note: The use of this drug *is usually not a disqualification* for piloting. Consult a designated aviation medical examiner.

Exposure to Sun: No restrictions.

Discontinuation: If triglyceride lowering does not occur after 3 months, this drug should be stopped.

GLIMEPIRIDE (glim EP er ide)

Introduced: 1996   **Class:** Antidiabetic, sulfonylureas   **Prescription:** USA: Yes   **Controlled Drug:** USA: No   **Available as Generic:** No   **Brand Name:** Amaryl

BENEFITS versus RISKS	
Possible Benefits	*Possible Risks*
TIGHTER CONTROL OF BLOOD SUGAR (adjunctive to appropriate diet and weight control) DECREASED RISK OF HEART DISEASE, KIDNEY DISEASE, ETC., BY ATTAINING TIGHTER CONTROL OF BLOOD SUGAR ONCE-A-DAY DOSING DECREASED RISK OF INCREASED INSULIN LEVELS DECREASED RISK OF HYPOGLYCEMIA	Allergic skin reactions Possible increased risk of heart (cardiovascular) mortality

▷ **Principal Uses**

As a Single Drug Product: Uses currently included in FDA-approved labeling: (1) used in type 2 diabetes (adult, maturity-onset) not requiring insulin, but not adequately controlled by diet alone; (2) approved for combination use with insulin if diet and exercise and this drug are not adequate, and in secondary failures.

Other (unlabeled) generally accepted uses: None at present.

How This Drug Works: This drug (1) stimulates insulin secretion; (2) enhances use of insulin by tissues (increased sensitivity); and (3) may bind to a different receptor site than other sulfonylureas.

Available Dose Forms and Strengths

Tablets — 1 mg, 2 mg, 4 mg, 6 mg

▷ **Usual Adult Dose Range (Note: Actual dose and schedule must be determined for each patient individually):** Started with 1 or 2 mg once daily, with breakfast or the first meal. Once a dose of 2 mg is reached, further dose increases should be made at 1- to 2-week intervals in increments of no more than 2 mg; the maximum daily dose is 8 mg. Typical ongoing doses have ranged from 1 to 4 mg a day. Some clinicians say that type 2 patients with secondary failure be considered for combined glimepiride and insulin therapy. If fasting blood sugar (glucose) is greater than 150 mg/dl and this is undertaken, 8 mg given with the first main meal is recommended. Low-dose insulin is started, and increased as needed and tolerated on a weekly basis based on blood sugar testing.

Conditions Requiring Dosing Adjustments

Liver Function: Starting dose is 1 mg daily in mild liver failure. Further dose changes are based on results of blood sugar testing. No data on use in more severe liver compromise.

Kidney Function: Starting dose is 1 mg daily. Further dose changes are based on results of blood sugar testing.

▷ **Dosing Instructions:** The tablet may be crushed. Follow doctor's instructions about dosing and diet closely. If meals are skipped, hypoglycemia may result. Know the signs and symptoms of hypoglycemia.

Usual Duration of Use: Use on a regular schedule for 1 to 2 weeks determines effectiveness in controlling diabetes. Failure to respond to maximal doses within 1 month constitutes a primary failure. Blood sugars must be measured, and your doctor will decide if the drug should be continued.

Possible Advantages of This Drug

Effective with once-daily dosing.

May be less likely to cause excessive lowering of the blood sugar (hypoglycemia).

May cause less excessive insulin in the bloodstream (hyperinsulinemia).

▷ **This Drug Should Not Be Taken If**

- you have had an allergic reaction to it previously.
- you have severe impairment of liver or kidney function.
- you have diabetic ketoacidosis (insulin is the drug of choice).
- you are pregnant or are breast-feeding your infant.

▷ **Inform Your Physician Before Taking This Drug If**

- you are allergic to other sulfonylurea drugs or to "sulfa" drugs.
- you have been experiencing prolonged vomiting.
- you do not know how to recognize or treat hypoglycemia (see Glossary).
- you have a history of congestive heart failure, peptic ulcer disease, cirrhosis of the liver, or hypothyroidism.
- you are malnourished or have a high fever or pituitary or adrenal insufficiency.

Possible Side Effects (natural, expected, and unavoidable drug actions)

Hypoglycemia will occur if drug dose is excessive or if meals are missed or inadequate. The risk of hypoglycemia may be increased if this medicine is combined with insulin.

▷ **Possible Adverse Effects** (unusual, unexpected, and infrequent reactions)

If any of the following develop, consult your physician promptly for guidance.

Mild Adverse Effects

Allergic reactions: skin rash, hives, itching (may subside over time).

Headache, dizziness, or blurred vision—rare.

Nausea—rare.

Serious Adverse Effects

Allergic reactions: none reported.

Lowering of sodium or porphyria reported with other medicines in this class—case reports.

Low blood sugar (hypoglycemia)—possible.

▷ **Possible Effects on Sexual Function:** None reported.

▷ **Adverse Effects That May Mimic Natural Diseases or Disorders**
Increased liver enzymes may suggest viral hepatitis.

Possible Effects on Laboratory Tests
Hemoglobin A1C (glycosylated hemoglobin): trending toward normal if tight control of blood sugar has been achieved.
Blood glucose levels: decreased.
Liver function tests: increased liver enzymes (ALT/GPT, AST/GOT, and alkaline phosphatase), increased bilirubin.

CAUTION
1. This drug is only one part of a diabetes program. It is not a substitute for a proper diet and regular exercise.
2. Over time (usually several months) this drug may not work. Periodic follow-up examinations are necessary.

Precautions for Use
By Infants and Children: Safety and effectiveness in pediatrics have not been established.
By Those Over 60 Years of Age: Use with caution, and start with 1 mg/day. Dose should be increased slowly as needed and tolerated and glucose checked often. Repeated hypoglycemia in the elderly can cause brain damage.

▷ **Advisability of Use During Pregnancy**
Pregnancy Category: C. See Pregnancy Risk Categories at the back of this book.
Human studies: Adequate studies of pregnant women are not available.
Because uncontrolled blood sugar levels during pregnancy are dangerous for the fetus, many experts recommend insulin instead of an oral agent.

Advisability of Use If Breast-Feeding
Presence of this drug in breast milk: Yes, in animal data; unknown in humans.
Avoid drug or refrain from nursing.

Habit-Forming Potential: None.

Effects of Overdose: Symptoms of mild to severe hypoglycemia: headache, light-headedness, faintness, nervousness, confusion, tremor, sweating, heart palpitation, weakness, hunger, nausea, vomiting, stupor progressing to coma.

Possible Effects of Long-Term Use: Increased frequency and severity of heart and blood vessel diseases with long-term use of this class of drugs are highly controversial and inconclusive. A direct cause-and-effect relationship (see Glossary) is tenuous. Ask your physician for help.

Suggested Periodic Examinations While Taking This Drug (at physician's discretion)
Hemoglobin A1C, liver function tests, evaluation of heart and circulatory system, blood sugar levels.

▷ **While Taking This Drug, Observe the Following**
Foods: Follow the diabetic diet prescribed by your physician.
Beverages: As directed in the diabetic diet. May be taken with milk.
▷ *Alcohol:* Use with extreme caution—alcohol can prolong this drug's hypoglycemic effect. Other drugs in this class can also cause a disulfiram-like reaction (see Glossary).
Tobacco Smoking: No interactions expected. I advise everyone to quit smoking.

▷ *Other Drugs*

The following drugs may ***increase*** the effects of glimepiride:
- aspirin and other salicylates.
- cimetidine (Tagamet).
- chloramphenicol.
- clofibrate (Atromid-S).
- fenfluramine (Pondimin).
- miconazole (Lotrimin).
- monoamine oxidase (MAO) type A inhibitors (see Drug Classes).
- NSAIDs (see ***nonsteroidal anti-inflammatory drugs*** in Drug Classes).
- probenecid (SK-Probenecid).
- ranitidine (Zantac).
- sulfa drugs such as Septra.

The following drugs may ***decrease*** the effects of glimepiride:
- beta-blocker drugs (see Drug Classes).
- bumetanide (Bumex).
- conjugated estrogens (Premarin).
- diazoxide (Proglycem).
- ethacrynic acid (Edecrin).
- furosemide (Lasix).
- phenytoin (Dilantin).
- rifampin (Rifadin, others).
- steroids (betamethasone, prednisone, others).
- thiazide diuretics (see Drug Classes).

Glimepiride ***taken concurrently*** with
- antacids (magnesium hydroxide containing) may result in increased risk of excessively lowered blood sugar.
- antifungal agents (such as itraconazole or other azoles) may result in severe lowering of blood sugar.
- calcium channel blockers (see Drug Classes) may cause excessive lowering of blood glucose.
- cyclosporine (Sandimmune) may result in cyclosporine toxicity.
- warfarin (Coumadin) can cause an increased hypoglycemic effect.

▷ *Driving, Hazardous Activities:* Dosing schedule, eating schedule, and physical activities must be coordinated to prevent hypoglycemia. Know the early symptoms of hypoglycemia so you can avoid hazardous activities and take corrective measures.

Aviation Note: Diabetes ***is a disqualification*** for piloting. Consult a designated aviation medical examiner.

Exposure to Sun: Some drugs of this class can cause photosensitivity (see Glossary).

Occurrence of Unrelated Illness: Acute infections, vomiting or diarrhea, serious injuries, and surgical procedures can worsen diabetic control and may require insulin. If any of these conditions occur, call your doctor.

Discontinuation: Because of secondary failures, the continued benefit of this drug should be evaluated every 6 months.

GLIPIZIDE (GLIP i zide)

Introduced: 1972   **Class:** Antidiabetic, sulfonylureas   **Prescription:**
USA: Yes   **Controlled Drug:** USA: No   **Available as Generic:** Yes
Brand Names: Glucotrol, Glucotrol XL

BENEFITS versus RISKS

Possible Benefits	*Possible Risks*
TIGHTER CONTROL OF BLOOD SUGAR (adjunctive to appropriate diet and weight control)	HYPOGLYCEMIA, severe and prolonged
DECREASED RISK OF HEART DISEASE, KIDNEY DISEASE, ETC., BY ATTAINING TIGHTER CONTROL OF BLOOD SUGAR ONCE-A-DAY DOSING	Allergic skin reactions (some severe) Blood cell and bone marrow disorders Possible increased risk of heart (cardiovascular) mortality

---

▷ **Principal Uses**

As a Single Drug Product: Uses currently included in FDA-approved labeling: Type 2 diabetes (adult, maturity-onset) not requiring insulin, but is not adequately controlled by diet alone.

Other (unlabeled) generally accepted uses: Delay of abnormal metabolism and blood vessel disease if given early in diabetes.

How This Drug Works: This drug (1) stimulates the secretion of insulin; and (2) enhances the use of insulin by appropriate tissues.

Available Dose Forms and Strengths

Tablets — 5 mg, 10 mg

Tablets, extended release — 5 mg, 10 mg

▷ **Usual Adult Dose Range:** Starts with 5 mg daily before a meal. At 3- to 7-day intervals dose may be increased (by 2.5 to 5 mg daily) as needed and tolerated. Daily maximum is 40 mg. Extended-release form starts at 5 mg, taken with breakfast. Dose increases are made at 7-day intervals. Most patients have a favorable response to 10 mg daily. Maximum daily extended-release-form dose is 20 mg.

Note: Actual dose and schedule must be determined for each patient individually.

Conditions Requiring Dosing Adjustments

Liver Function: Patients with liver failure should take a starting dose of 2.5 mg, and be closely followed.

Kidney Function: Some clinicians DO NOT recommend use of glipizide in severe renal compromise. Patients should be monitored closely if the drug is used in mild to moderate renal (kidney) compromise. It is a rare cause of kidney stones.

▷ **Dosing Instructions:** If the daily maintenance dose is found to be 15 mg or more, the total dose should be divided into two equal doses—the first taken with the morning meal, the second with the evening meal. The tablet may be crushed.

Usual Duration of Use: Use on a regular schedule for 1 to 2 weeks determines effectiveness in controlling diabetes. Failure to respond to maximal doses within 1 month constitutes a primary failure. Up to 10% of those who respond initially may develop secondary failure. Blood sugars must be measured, and your doctor will decide if the drug should be continued.

Possible Advantages of This Drug
Effective with once-daily dosing.
Onset of action within 30 minutes. Near-normal insulin response to eating.
Well tolerated by the elderly diabetic.

Currently a "Drug of Choice"
For starting therapy in noninsulin-dependent diabetes when diet and weight control fail.

▷ This Drug Should Not Be Taken If
- you have had an allergic reaction to it previously.
- you have severe impairment of liver or kidney function.
- you have diabetic ketoacidosis.
- you are pregnant.

▷ Inform Your Physician Before Taking This Drug If
- you are allergic to other sulfonylurea drugs or to "sulfa" drugs.
- your diabetes has been unstable or "brittle" in the past.
- you do not know how to recognize or treat hypoglycemia (see Glossary).
- you are pregnant.
- you have a history of congestive heart failure, peptic ulcer disease, cirrhosis of the liver, bone marrow depression, hypothyroidism, or porphyria.

Possible Side Effects (natural, expected, and unavoidable drug actions)
If drug dose is excessive or if meals are missed or inadequate, abnormally low blood sugar (hypoglycemia) will occur as a drug effect.

▷ Possible Adverse Effects (unusual, unexpected, and infrequent reactions)
If any of the following develop, consult your physician promptly for guidance.

Mild Adverse Effects
Allergic reactions: skin rash, hives, itching.
Headache, drowsiness, dizziness, fatigue, sweating—rare to infrequent.
Indigestion, nausea, vomiting, diarrhea—rare to infrequent.

Serious Adverse Effects
Allergic reactions: hepatitis with jaundice (see Glossary), severe skin reactions—case reports.
Idiosyncratic reaction: hemolytic anemia (see Glossary).
Disulfiramlike reaction (see Glossary) with concurrent use of alcohol—infrequent.
Low blood sodium or drug-induced urinary stones—possible.
Bone marrow depression (see Glossary): fatigue, weakness, fever, sore throat, abnormal bleeding or bruising—case reports.
Risk of cardiovascular mortality (based on an old study with a different drug)—possible.

▷ Possible Effects on Sexual Function:　None reported.

▷ Adverse Effects That May Mimic Natural Diseases or Disorders
Liver reactions may suggest viral hepatitis.

Possible Effects on Laboratory Tests

Complete blood counts: decreased red cells, hemoglobin, white cells, and platelets.

Blood glucose levels: decreased.

Liver function tests: increased liver enzymes (ALT/GPT, AST/GOT, and alkaline phosphatase), increased bilirubin.

CAUTION

1. This drug is only part of a diabetes program. It is not a substitute for a proper diet and regular exercise.
2. Over time (usually months), this drug may not work. Periodic follow-up examinations are needed.

Precautions for Use

By Infants and Children: This drug does not work in type 1 (juvenile, growth-onset) insulin-dependent diabetes.

By Those Over 60 Years of Age: Use with caution, and start with 2.5 mg/day. Dose should be increased slowly and glucose checked often. Repeated hypoglycemia in the elderly can cause brain damage.

▷ **Advisability of Use During Pregnancy**

Pregnancy Category: C. See Pregnancy Risk Categories at the back of this book.

Animal studies: No birth defects reported in rats and rabbits.

Human studies: Adequate studies of pregnant women are not available.

Because uncontrolled blood sugar levels during pregnancy are associated with a higher incidence of birth defects, many experts recommend that insulin (instead of an oral agent) be used as necessary to control diabetes during the entire pregnancy.

Advisability of Use If Breast-Feeding

Presence of this drug in breast milk: Unknown.

Avoid drug or refrain from nursing.

Habit-Forming Potential: None.

Effects of Overdose: Symptoms of mild to severe hypoglycemia: headache, light-headedness, faintness, nervousness, confusion, tremor, sweating, heart palpitation, weakness, hunger, nausea, vomiting, stupor progressing to coma.

Possible Effects of Long-Term Use: Reduced thyroid function (hypothyroidism). Increased frequency and severity of heart and blood vessel diseases with long-term use of this class of drugs are highly controversial and inconclusive. A direct cause-and-effect relationship (see Glossary) is tenuous. Ask your physician for help.

Suggested Periodic Examinations While Taking This Drug (at physician's discretion)

Complete blood cell counts, liver function tests, thyroid function tests, periodic evaluation of heart and circulatory system.

▷ **While Taking This Drug, Observe the Following**

Foods: Follow the diabetic diet prescribed by your physician.

Beverages: As directed in the diabetic diet. May be taken with milk.

▷   *Alcohol:* Use with extreme caution—alcohol can prolong this drug's hypoglycemic effect. This drug can also cause a disulfiramlike reaction (see Glossary): facial flushing, sweating, palpitation.

Tobacco Smoking: No interactions expected. I advise everyone to quit smoking.

▷ *Other Drugs*

The following drugs may *increase* the effects of glipizide:
- acarbose (Precose); may increase risk of excessive lowering of blood sugar.
- aspirin and other salicylates.
- chloramphenicol (Chloromycetin).
- cimetidine (Tagamet).
- clofibrate (Atromid-S).
- cotrimoxazole (Septra).
- fenfluramine (Pondimin).
- magnesium (increased absorption into the body).
- monoamine oxidase (MAO) type A inhibitors (see Drug Classes).
- NSAIDs (see *nonsteroidal anti-inflammatory drugs* in Drug Classes).
- ranitidine (Zantac).
- sulfa drugs such as trimethoprim/sulfamethoxazole (Septra) or erythromycin/sulfisoxazole (Pediazole).

The following drugs may *decrease* the effects of glipizide:
- beta-blocker drugs (see Drug Classes).
- birth control pills (oral contraceptives).
- bumetanide (Bumex).
- cholestyramine (Questran).
- conjugated estrogens (Premarin).
- diazoxide (Proglycem).
- ethacrynic acid (Edecrin).
- furosemide (Lasix).
- phenytoin (Dilantin).
- rifampin (Rifadin, others).
- ritonavir (Norvir).
- steroids (betamethasone, prednisone, others).
- thiazide diuretics (see Drug Classes).

Glipizide *taken concurrently* with
- antacids (containing magnesium hydroxide) may result in increased risk of excessively lowered blood sugar.
- antifungal agents (such as itraconazole or other azoles) may result in severe lowering of blood sugar.
- calcium channel blockers (see Drug Classes) may cause excessive lowering of blood glucose.
- cyclosporine (Sandimmune) may result in cyclosporine toxicity.
- sildenafil (Viagra) can cause serious interactions. DO NOT combine.
- warfarin (Coumadin) can cause an increased hypoglycemic effect.

▷ *Driving, Hazardous Activities:* Dosing schedule, eating schedule, and physical activities must be coordinated to prevent hypoglycemia. Know the early symptoms of hypoglycemia so you can avoid hazardous activities and take corrective measures.

Aviation Note: Diabetes *is a disqualification* for piloting. Consult a designated aviation medical examiner.

Exposure to Sun: Some drugs of this class can cause photosensitivity (see Glossary).

Occurrence of Unrelated Illness: Acute infections, vomiting or diarrhea, serious injuries, and surgical procedures can worsen diabetic control and may require insulin. If any of these conditions occur, call your doctor.

Discontinuation: Because of secondary failures, the continued benefit of this drug should be evaluated every 6 months.

GLYBURIDE (GLI byoor ide)

Other Name: Glibenclamide **Introduced:** 1970 **Class:** Antidiabetic, sulfonylureas **Prescription:** USA: Yes **Controlled Drug:** USA: No; Canada: No **Available as Generic:** Yes

Brand Names: ✦Albert-Glyburide, ✦Apo-Glyburide, DiaBeta, ✦Euglucon, ✦Gen-Glybe, Glubate, Glynase Prestab, Micronase, ✦Novo-Glyburide

---

BENEFITS versus RISKS

Possible Benefits	*Possible Risks*
Helps in regulating blood sugar in non-insulin-dependent diabetes (adjunctive to appropriate diet and weight control)	HYPOGLYCEMIA, severe and prolonged Liver damage Blood cell and bone marrow disorders Allergic skin reactions (some severe) Possible increased risk of heart (cardiovascular) mortality

---

▷ **Principal Uses**

As a Single Drug Product: Uses currently included in FDA-approved labeling: Type 2 diabetes mellitus (adult, maturity-onset) that does not require insulin, but can't be adequately controlled by diet alone.

Other (unlabeled) generally accepted uses: None.

How This Drug Works: This drug (1) stimulates the secretion of insulin, (2) decreases glucose production in the liver, and (3) enhances insulin use.

Available Dose Forms and Strengths

Tablets — 1.25 mg, 1.5 mg, 2.5 mg, 3 mg, 5 mg, 6 mg

▷ **Usual Adult Dose Range:** Regular-release products: 2.5 to 5 mg daily with breakfast. At 7-day intervals the dose may be increased by increments of 2.5 mg daily as needed and tolerated. Total daily dose should not exceed 20 mg. Some patients respond to 1.25 mg daily.

Micronized products: 1.5 to 3 mg daily taken with breakfast. (Patients more sensitive to oral agents should be started at 0.75 mg daily.) Maximum dose is 12 mg daily.

Note: Actual dose and schedule must be determined for each patient individually.

Conditions Requiring Dosing Adjustments

Liver Function: Glyburide may cause catastrophic hypoglycemia (low blood sugar) if it is used by patients with liver disease. Very low starting doses should be taken and the patient closely followed. It is also a rare cause of hepatitis and cholestatic jaundice.

Kidney Function: Glyburide should be used with caution in mild renal compromise, with low initial doses and careful patient monitoring. The drug

SHOULD NOT be used by patients with moderate kidney failure (creatinine clearances less than 50 ml/min) or in severe kidney failure.

▷ **Dosing Instructions:**   If the daily maintenance dose is 10 mg or more, the total dose should be divided into two equal doses: the first taken with the morning meal, the second with the evening meal. The tablet may be crushed.

Usual Duration of Use: Use on a regular schedule for 1 to 2 weeks determines effectiveness in controlling diabetes. No response to peak doses in 1 month constitutes a primary failure. Up to 10% of those who respond initially may develop secondary failure. The duration of effective use can only be determined by periodic measurement of the blood sugar.

▷ **This Drug Should Not Be Taken If**
- you have had an allergic reaction to it previously.
- you have severe impairment of liver and kidney function.
- you have diabetic ketoacidosis.
- you are pregnant.

▷ **Inform Your Physician Before Taking This Drug If**
- you are allergic to other sulfonylurea drugs or to "sulfa" drugs.
- your diabetes has been unstable or "brittle" in the past.
- you do not know how to recognize or treat hypoglycemia (see Glossary).
- you have a history of problems with blood clotting or have a glucose-6-phosphate dehydrogenase (G6PD) deficiency.
- you have a history of congestive heart failure, peptic ulcer disease, cirrhosis of the liver, hypothyroidism, or porphyria.

Possible Side Effects (natural, expected, and unavoidable drug actions)
If drug dose is excessive or food intake is delayed or inadequate, abnormally low blood sugar (hypoglycemia) will occur as a predictable drug effect.

▷ **Possible Adverse Effects** (unusual, unexpected, and infrequent reactions)
If any of the following develop, consult your physician promptly for guidance.
Mild Adverse Effects
Allergic reactions: skin rash, hives, itching.
Headache, drowsiness, dizziness, fatigue—possible.
Indigestion, heartburn, nausea—rare.
Bed-wetting at night (nocturnal enuresis), especially in young adults—case reports.
Serious Adverse Effects
Allergic reactions: hepatitis with jaundice (see Glossary), severe skin reactions (exfoliative dermatitis)—case reports.
Idiosyncratic reaction: hemolytic anemia (see Glossary).
Disulfiram-like reaction (see Glossary) with concurrent use of alcohol—possible.
Bone marrow depression (see Glossary): fatigue, fever, sore throat, abnormal bleeding—case reports.
Liver toxicity (cholestatic jaundice)—case reports.
Blood clotting defects (coagulation)—rare.
Cardiovascular mortality (based on an old study of a different medicine)—increased risk.

▷ **Possible Effects on Sexual Function:**   None reported.

▷ **Adverse Effects That May Mimic Natural Diseases or Disorders**
   Liver reactions may suggest viral hepatitis.

Possible Effects on Laboratory Tests
   Blood platelet counts: decreased.
   Blood cholesterol and triglyceride levels: decreased.
   Blood glucose levels: decreased.
   Liver function tests: increased liver enzymes (ALT/GPT, AST/GOT, and alkaline phosphatase).

CAUTION
   1. This drug is only part of diabetes management. Much of the damage from diabetes can be delayed or avoided if you keep your blood sugar in the normal range. Ask your doctor about a proper diet and regular exercise.
   2. Over time (usually several months), this drug may not work. Periodic follow-up examinations are necessary.

Precautions for Use
   By Infants and Children: This drug does not work in type 1 (juvenile, growth-onset) insulin-dependent diabetes.
   By Those Over 60 Years of Age: Use with caution and start with 1.25 mg/day of the regular form. Dose should be slowly increased and glucose closely followed. Repeated hypoglycemia in the elderly can cause brain damage.

▷ **Advisability of Use During Pregnancy**
   Pregnancy Category: C. See Pregnancy Risk Categories at the back of this book.
   Animal studies: No birth defects reported in rats and rabbits.
   Human studies: Adequate studies of pregnant women are not available.
   Uncontrolled blood sugar levels during pregnancy are associated with a higher incidence of birth defects, so many experts recommend insulin (instead of an oral agent) to control diabetes during the entire pregnancy.

Advisability of Use If Breast-Feeding
   Presence of this drug in breast milk: Unknown.
   Avoid drug or refrain from nursing.

Habit-Forming Potential: None.

Effects of Overdose: Symptoms of mild to severe hypoglycemia: headache, light-headedness, faintness, nervousness, confusion, tremor, sweating, heart palpitation, weakness, hunger, nausea, vomiting, stupor progressing to coma.

Possible Effects of Long-Term Use: Reduced thyroid gland function (hypothyroidism). Reports of increased frequency and severity of heart and blood vessel diseases associated with long-term use of this class of drugs are highly controversial and inconclusive. A direct cause-and-effect relationship (see Glossary) is tenuous. Ask your physician for guidance.

Suggested Periodic Examinations While Taking This Drug (at physician's discretion)
   Complete blood cell counts, liver function tests, thyroid function tests, periodic evaluation of heart and circulatory system.

▷ **While Taking This Drug, Observe the Following**
   Foods: Follow the diabetic diet prescribed by your physician.
   Beverages: As directed in the diabetic diet. May be taken with milk.
▷   *Alcohol:* Use with extreme caution—alcohol can exaggerate this drug's hypo-

glycemic effect. This drug can cause a disulfiram-like reaction (see Glossary): facial flushing, sweating, palpitation.

Tobacco Smoking: No interactions expected. I advise everyone to quit smoking.

▷ *Other Drugs*

The following drugs may *increase* the effects of glyburide:
- acarbose (Precose).
- aspirin and other salicylates.
- chloramphenicol (Chloromycetin).
- cimetidine (Tagamet).
- clofibrate (Atromid-S).
- fenfluramine (Pondimin).
- gemfibrozil (Lopid).
- monoamine oxidase (MAO) type A inhibitors (see Drug Classes).
- phenylbutazone (Butazolidin).
- ranitidine (Zantac).
- ritonavir (Norvir).
- sulfa drugs such as trimethoprim/sulfamethoxazole (Septra) or erythromycin/sulfisoxazole (Pediazole).

The following drugs may *decrease* the effects of glyburide:
- beta-blocker drugs (see Drug Classes).
- bumetanide (Bumex).
- diazoxide (Proglycem).
- ethacrynic acid (Edecrin).
- furosemide (Lasix).
- phenytoin (Dilantin).
- rifampin (Rifadin, others).
- thiazide diuretics (see Drug Classes).
- thyroid hormones.

Glyburide *taken concurrently* with
- antacids (containing magnesium hydroxide) or magnesium supplements may result in increased risk of excessively lowered blood sugar.
- antifungal agents (such as itraconazole or other azoles) may result in severe lowering of blood sugar.
- enalapril (Vasotec) may enhance blood sugar lowering effect.
- monoamine oxidase (MAO) inhibitors (see Drug Classes) may increase risk of hyperglycemia.
- steroids (betamethasone, prednisone, others) blunts benefits.
- warfarin (Coumadin) may result in bleeding. More frequent INR (prothrombin time) testing is needed.

▷ *Driving, Hazardous Activities:* Regulate dosing, eating, and physical activities carefully to prevent hypoglycemia. Know the early symptoms of hypoglycemia so you can avoid hazardous activities and take corrective measures.

Aviation Note: Diabetes *is a disqualification* for piloting. Consult a designated aviation medical examiner.

Exposure to Sun: Use caution until sensitivity has been determined. Some drugs of this class can cause photosensitivity (see Glossary).

Occurrence of Unrelated Illness: Acute infections, vomiting or diarrhea, serious injuries, and surgical procedures can worsen diabetic control and may require insulin. If any of these conditions occur, consult your physician promptly.

Discontinuation: Because of the possibility of secondary failure, it is advisable to evaluate the continued benefit of this drug every 6 months.

GUANFACINE (GWAHN fa seen)

Introduced: 1980   **Class:** Antihypertensive   **Prescription:** USA: Yes
Controlled Drug: USA: No   **Available as Generic:** USA: Yes
Brand Name: Tenex

BENEFITS versus RISKS	
Possible Benefits	*Possible Risks*
EFFECTIVE ANTIHYPERTENSIVE in mild to moderate high blood pressure	Amnesia
EFFECTIVE in high blood pressure of pregnancy	

▷ **Principal Uses**

As a Single Drug Product: Uses currently included in FDA-approved labeling: (1) Used to treat mild to moderate high blood pressure; (2) used alone or in combination to treat high blood pressure caused by kidney problems.

Other (unlabeled) generally accepted uses: (1) Heroin withdrawal; (2) may be useful in problem pregnancies; (3) could have a role in treating attention deficit hyperactivity disorder (ADHD); (4) may help some sleep disorders.

How This Drug Works: Reduces sympathetic nervous system output (alpha-2-receptors), causing blood vessels to relax and blood pressure to lower.

Available Dose Forms and Strengths

Tablets — 1 mg, 2 mg

▷ **Usual Adult Dose Range:** Starts with 1 mg taken at bedtime. Dose may be increased after 3 to 4 weeks to 2 mg daily, as needed and tolerated. Dose may then be increased after 3 to 4 weeks to 3 mg daily. Total daily dose may be taken in two divided doses if needed. Up to 40 mg daily has been reported, but combination therapy is used before such doses. Usual maximum is 6 mg daily. **Note: Actual dose and schedule must be determined for each patient individually.**

Conditions Requiring Dosing Adjustments

Liver Function: Should be used with caution by patients with liver compromise.
Kidney Function: Used with caution.

▷ **Dosing Instructions:** Tablets may be crushed and taken without regard to eating. Taking daily dose at bedtime reduces daytime drowsiness.

Usual Duration of Use: Regular use for 4 to 6 weeks is usually needed to see drug's effect in controlling high blood pressure. Peak benefit may not be seen for 12 weeks. Long-term use (months to years) requires follow-up by your doctor.

▷ **This Drug Should Not Be Taken If**

• you have had an allergic reaction to it previously.

▷ **Inform Your Physician Before Taking This Drug If**
- you have a circulatory disorder of the brain.
- you have angina or coronary artery disease.
- you have or have had serious emotional depression.
- you have impaired liver or kidney function.
- you are a diabetic.
- you have a history of orthostatic hypotension.
- you are taking any sedative or hypnotic drugs or an antidepressant.
- you will have surgery with general anesthesia.

Possible Side Effects (natural, expected, and unavoidable drug actions)
Drowsiness—frequent; dry nose and mouth—frequent; constipation—infrequent; mild lowering of blood pressure on standing (orthostatic hypotension; see Glossary).

▷ **Possible Adverse Effects** (unusual, unexpected, and infrequent reactions)
If any of the following develop, consult your physician promptly for guidance.
Mild Adverse Effects
Allergic reactions: skin rash, itching.
Headache, dizziness, fatigue, sedation, or insomnia—rare to infrequent.
Indigestion, nausea, diarrhea—infrequent.
Edema or leg cramps—rare.
Serious Adverse Effects
Slow heartbeat (bradycardia)—infrequent.
Liver toxicity—rare.
Amnesia—infrequent.
Rebound hypertension (if abruptly stopped).

▷ **Possible Effects on Sexual Function:**   Dose-related decreased libido, impotence—case reports.

Possible Effects on Laboratory Tests
Liver function tests: increased.
Blood sugar (glucose): increased.

CAUTION
1. ***Do not stop this drug suddenly.*** Sudden withdrawal can produce anxiety, nervousness, tremors, fast or irregular heart action, nausea, stomach cramps, vomiting, and rebound hypertension.
2. Hot weather and fever can reduce blood pressure significantly. Dose adjustments may be necessary.
3. Report the development of any tendency to emotional depression.

Precautions for Use
By Infants and Children: Safety and effectiveness for use by those under 12 years of age have not been established.
*By Those Over 60 Years of Age: **Proceed cautiously**.* Pressure should be reduced without creating the risks associated with excessively low blood pressure. Watch for light-headedness, dizziness, unsteadiness, fainting, and falling. Sedation and dry mouth occur commonly in elderly users. Report promptly any changes in mood or behavior: depression, delusions, hallucinations.

▷ **Advisability of Use During Pregnancy**
Pregnancy Category: B. See Pregnancy Risk Categories at the back of this book.

Animal studies: No birth defects due to this drug reported in rat and rabbit studies.

Human studies: Adequate studies of pregnant women are not available.

Use this drug only if clearly needed. Ask your physician for guidance.

Advisability of Use If Breast-Feeding

Presence of this drug in breast milk: Probably.

Avoid drug or refrain from nursing.

Habit-Forming Potential: None.

Effects of Overdose: Marked drowsiness, dry mouth, slow pulse, low blood pressure, vomiting, stupor progressing to coma.

Possible Effects of Long-Term Use: Development of tolerance (see Glossary) with loss of drug effectiveness.

Suggested Periodic Examinations While Taking This Drug (at physician's discretion)

Blood pressure measurements.

▷ **While Taking This Drug, Observe the Following**

Foods: Avoid excessive salt, and ask your doctor about degree of salt restriction.

Beverages: No restrictions. May be taken with milk.

▷ *Alcohol:* Use with extreme caution—can cause marked drowsiness or exaggerated reduction of blood pressure.

Tobacco Smoking: No interactions expected. I advise everyone to quit smoking.

▷ *Other Drugs*

Guanfacine *taken concurrently* with

- amitriptyline (Elavil) and other tricyclic antidepressants (see Drug Classes) can cause decreased effectiveness as an antihypertensive.
- desipramine and other tricyclic antidepressants can cause loss of therapeutic benefits of guanfacine.
- phenobarbital can lead to loss of therapeutic effect of guanfacine.

▷ *Driving, Hazardous Activities:* Use caution. This drug can cause drowsiness and can impair mental alertness, judgment, and coordination.

Aviation Note: Hypertension (high blood pressure) *is a disqualification* for piloting. Consult a designated aviation medical examiner.

Exposure to Sun: No restrictions.

Exposure to Heat: Use caution. Hot environments may reduce the blood pressure significantly; be alert to the possibility of orthostatic hypotension (see Glossary).

Heavy Exercise or Exertion: Use caution. Isometric exercises can raise blood pressure significantly. This drug may intensify the hypertensive response to isometric exercise. Ask your physician for guidance.

Occurrence of Unrelated Illness: Fever may lower blood pressure significantly. Vomiting may prevent regular use of this drug and result in acute withdrawal reactions. Call your doctor.

Discontinuation: **Do not stop this drug suddenly.** Withdrawal reactions occur within 2 to 7 days after the last dose. It is best to reduce dose gradually (over 3 to 4 days), with periodic monitoring of the blood pressure.

HALOPERIDOL (hal oh PER i dohl)

Introduced: 1958   **Class:** Antipsychotic; tranquilizer, strong   **Prescription:** USA: Yes   **Controlled Drug:** USA: No; Canada: No   **Available as Generic:** USA: Yes; Canada: Yes

Brand Names: ✷Apo-Haloperidol, Haldol, ✷Haldol LA, Halperon, ✷Novo-Peridol, ✷Peridol, ✷PMS-Haloperidol

---

BENEFITS versus RISKS

Possible Benefits	*Possible Risks*
EFFECTIVE CONTROL OF PSYCHOSES	FREQUENT PARKINSON-LIKE side effects
BENEFICIAL EFFECTS ON THINKING, MOOD, AND BEHAVIOR	SERIOUS TOXIC EFFECTS ON BRAIN with long-term use
EFFECTIVE CONTROL OF SOME CASES OF TOURETTEíS SYNDROME	Rare blood cell disorders Abnormally low white blood cell count
Beneficial in management of some hyperactive children	

▷ **Principal Uses**

As a Single Drug Product: Uses currently included in FDA-approved labeling: (1) Helps control psychotic thinking and abnormal behavior in acute psychosis of unknown nature, acute schizophrenia, paranoid states, and the manic phase of manic-depressive disorders; (2) helps control outbursts of aggression and agitation; (3) used to treat Tourette's syndrome.

Other (unlabeled) generally accepted uses: (1) Helps control refractory hiccups; (2) used to lessen delirium in LSD flashbacks and phencyclidine intoxication; (3) used as combination (adjuvant) therapy in chronic pain syndromes; (4) may be helpful in autistic patients; (5) may have a role in refractory vomiting caused by cancer chemotherapy; (6) can ease symptoms in refractory sneezing; (7) may be helpful as adjunctive therapy in stuttering.

How This Drug Works: By interfering with a nerve impulse transmitter (dopamine), this drug reduces anxiety and agitation, improves coherence and thinking, and abolishes delusions and hallucinations.

Available Dose Forms and Strengths

Concentrate — 2 mg/ml
Injection — 5 mg/ml, 50 mg/ml, and 100 mg/ml
Tablets — 0.5 mg, 1 mg, 2 mg, 5 mg, 10 mg, 20 mg

▷ **Usual Adult Dose Range:** Initially 0.5 to 2 mg two or three times daily. Dose may be increased by 0.5 mg/day at 3- to 4-day intervals as needed and tolerated. The usual dose range is 0.5 to 30 mg daily. The total daily dose should not exceed 100 mg. **Note: Actual dose and schedule must be determined for each patient individually.**

Conditions Requiring Dosing Adjustments

Liver Function: The dose, dosing interval, and titration interval (time to adjust the drug to desired effect) should be adjusted for liver compromise.
Kidney Function: High doses used with caution in kidney compromise.

▷ **Dosing Instructions:** The tablet may be crushed and taken with or following food to reduce stomach irritation. The concentrate may be diluted in 2 ounces of water or fruit juice; do not add it to coffee or tea.

Usual Duration of Use: Use on a regular schedule for several weeks determines this drug's effectiveness in controlling psychotic behavior. If it doesn't provide a significant benefit in 6 weeks, it should be stopped. Long-term use requires supervision and periodic physician evaluation.

▷ **This Drug Should Not Be Taken If**
- you had an allergic reaction to it previously.
- you are experiencing severe mental depression.
- you have any form of Parkinson's disease.
- you have cancer of the breast.
- you have severe active liver disease.
- you are presently experiencing central nervous system (CNS) depression due to alcohol or narcotics.
- you currently have a bone marrow or blood cell disorder.

▷ **Inform Your Physician Before Taking This Drug If**
- you are allergic or abnormally sensitive to phenothiazine drugs (see Glossary).
- you have a history of mental depression.
- you have any type of heart disease.
- you have impaired liver or kidney function.
- you have thyroid disease.
- you are allergic to the dye tartrazine.
- you are pregnant or are planning a pregnancy.
- you have a history of neuroleptic malignant syndrome (see Glossary).
- you have low blood pressure, epilepsy, or glaucoma.
- you are taking any drugs with a sedative effect.
- you plan to have surgery and general or spinal anesthesia soon.

Possible Side Effects (natural, expected, and unavoidable drug actions)
Mild drowsiness, low blood pressure, blurred vision, dry mouth, constipation, marked and frequent Parkinson-like reactions (see Glossary).

▷ **Possible Adverse Effects** (unusual, unexpected, and infrequent reactions)
If any of the following develop, consult your physician promptly for guidance.
Mild Adverse Effects
Allergic reactions: skin rash, hives.
Dizziness, weakness, agitation, insomnia—case reports to infrequent.
Loss of appetite, indigestion, nausea, vomiting, diarrhea—case reports.
Serious Adverse Effects
Allergic reactions: rare liver reaction with jaundice, asthma, spasm of vocal cords.
Idiosyncratic reactions: neuroleptic malignant syndrome (see Glossary).
Blood cell disorders: lowered white blood cell count—rare.
Nervous system reactions: rigidity of extremities, tremors, seizures, constant movement, facial grimacing, eye rolling, spasm of neck muscles, tardive dyskinesia (see Glossary)—case reports to infrequent.
Abnormal heartbeat (premature ventricular contractions)—possible with aggressive dosing.

Worsening of psychosis—possible.

Low blood sugar or abnormal and frequent urination (SIADH)—case reports.

Liver toxicity—possible.

Bronchospasm or myasthenia gravis—case reports.

▷ **Possible Effects on Sexual Function:**   Decreased libido; impotence—infrequent to frequent; painful ejaculation; priapism (see Glossary).

Tender and enlarged breast tissue in men (gynecomastia); breast enlargement with milk production in women.

Altered timing and pattern of menstruation—case reports.

▷ **Adverse Effects That May Mimic Natural Diseases or Disorders**

Liver reaction may suggest viral hepatitis. Nervous system reactions may suggest Parkinson's disease or Reye syndrome (see Glossary).

Natural Diseases or Disorders That May Be Activated by This Drug

Latent epilepsy, glaucoma, diabetes.

Possible Effects on Laboratory Tests

Complete blood counts: decreased red cells, hemoglobin, and white cells; increased eosinophils.

INR (prothrombin time): decreased.

Blood cholesterol level: decreased.

Blood glucose level: increased.

Liver function tests: increased liver enzymes (ALT/GPT, AST/GOT, and alkaline phosphatase), increased bilirubin.

CAUTION

1. The smallest effective dose should be used for long-term therapy.
2. Use with extreme caution in epilepsy; can alter seizure patterns.
3. Those with lupus erythematosus or who are taking prednisone have more nervous system reactions.
4. Levodopa should **not** be used to treat Parkinson-like reactions; it can cause agitation and worsening of the psychotic disorder.
5. Obtain prompt evaluation of any change or disturbance in vision.

Precautions for Use

By Infants and Children: This drug should not be used in children under 3 years of age or 15 kg in weight. Avoid this drug in the presence of symptoms suggestive of Reye syndrome. Children are quite susceptible to nervous system reactions induced by this drug.

By Those Over 60 Years of Age: Small doses are indicated when therapy is started. This drug can cause significant changes in mood and behavior; watch for confusion, disorientation, agitation, restlessness, aggression, and paranoia. You may be more susceptible to the development of drowsiness, lethargy, orthostatic hypotension (see Glossary), hypothermia (see Glossary), Parkinson-like reactions, and prostatism (see Glossary).

▷ **Advisability of Use During Pregnancy**

Pregnancy Category: C. See Pregnancy Risk Categories at the back of this book.

Animal studies: Cleft palate reported in mouse studies.

Human studies: No increase in birth defects reported in 100 exposures. Adequate studies of pregnant women are not available.

Avoid during the first 3 months (trimester). Use only if clearly needed. Ask your physician for guidance.

Advisability of Use If Breast-Feeding
> Presence of this drug in breast milk: Yes.
> Monitor nursing infant closely and discontinue drug or nursing if adverse effects develop.

Habit-Forming Potential: Reports of recreational use have been filed. If the drug is stopped suddenly, patient may experience a withdrawal syndrome.

Effects of Overdose: Marked drowsiness, weakness, tremor, unsteadiness, agitation, stupor, coma, convulsions.

Possible Effects of Long-Term Use: Eye damage—deposits in cornea, lens, or retina; tardive dyskinesia (see Glossary).

Suggested Periodic Examinations While Taking This Drug (at physician's discretion)
> Complete blood counts, liver function tests, eye examinations, electrocardiograms.
> The tongue should be watched for fine, involuntary, wavelike movements that could be the beginning of tardive dyskinesia.

▷ **While Taking This Drug, Observe the Following**
> *Foods:* No restrictions.
> *Beverages:* No restrictions. May be taken with milk.
▷ *Alcohol:* Avoid completely. Alcohol can increase the sedative action of haloperidol and accentuate its depressant effects on brain function. Haloperidol can increase the intoxicating effects of alcohol.
> *Tobacco Smoking:* Combination with nicotine actually increased suppression of tics in Tourette's syndrome in one study. I advise everyone to quit smoking.
> *Marijuana Smoking:* Moderate increase in drowsiness; accentuation of orthostatic hypotension; increased risk of precipitating latent psychosis, confusing interpretation of mental status and of drug response.

▷ *Other Drugs*
> Haloperidol may ***increase*** the effects of
> - all drugs with sedative actions, and cause excessive sedation.
> - fluvoxamine (Luvox), and result in toxicity (altered mental status, GI side effects).
> - some antihypertensive drugs, and cause excessive lowering of blood pressure; monitor the combined effects carefully.
>
> Haloperidol may ***decrease*** the effects of
> - guanethidine (Esimil, Ismelin), and reduce its antihypertensive effect.
>
> Haloperidol ***taken concurrently*** with
> - anticholinergic drugs (see Drug Classes) can cause additive anticholinergic effects (dry mouth, constipation, or sedation).
> - beta-blocker drugs (see Glossary) may cause excessive lowering of blood pressure.
> - fluoxetine (Prozac) can result in an increased risk of haloperidol toxicity.
> - lithium (Lithobid, others) may cause toxic effects on the brain and nervous system.
> - monoamine oxidase (MAO) inhibitors (see Drug Classes) may exaggerate low blood pressure and brain (CNS) effects.
> - methyldopa (Aldomet) may cause serious dementia.
> - ritonavir (Norvir) and perhaps other protease inhibitors (see Drug Classes) may lead to toxicity.

- sparfloxacin (Zagam) may lead to abnormal heart beats.
- tacrine (Cognex) may lead to Parkinson-like symptoms.
- tramadol (Ultram) may lead to seizures.
- venlafaxine (Effexor) may lead to haloperidol toxicity.

The following drugs may **_decrease_** the effects of haloperidol:

- antacids containing aluminum and/or magnesium, reducing its absorption.
- barbiturates.
- benztropine (Cogentin).
- carbamazepine (Tegretol).
- phenytoin (Dilantin).
- rifampin (Rifater, others).
- trihexyphenidyl (Artane).

▷ *Driving, Hazardous Activities:* This drug may impair mental alertness, judgment, and physical coordination. Restrict activities as necessary.

Aviation Note: The use of this drug **_is a disqualification_** for piloting. Consult a designated aviation medical examiner.

Exposure to Sun: Use caution—this drug can cause photosensitivity (see Glossary).

Exposure to Heat: Use caution in hot environments. This drug may impair the regulation of body temperature and increase the risk of heatstroke.

Exposure to Cold: This drug can increase the risk of hypothermia (see Glossary) in the elderly.

Discontinuation: This drug should not be stopped abruptly following long-term use. Gradual withdrawal over a period of 2 to 3 weeks is advised. Ask your doctor for help.

HISTAMINE (H₂) BLOCKING DRUG FAMILY

Cimetidine (si MET i deen)   **Ranitidine** (ra NI te deen)   **Famotidine** (fa MOH te deen)   **Nizatidine** (ni ZA te deen)

Introduced: 1977, 1983, 1986, 1988, respectively   **Class:** Histamine (H₂) blocking drugs   **Prescription:** USA: Yes   **Controlled Drug:** USA: No; Canada: No   **Available as Generic:** USA: Yes (prescription forms) Cimetidine and Tagamet HB, Ranitidine; Canada: Yes

Brand Names: Cimetidine: ✦Apo-Cimetidine, ✦Enlon, ✦Novo-Cimetine, ✦Nu-Cimet, ✦Peptol, Tagamet, Tagamet HB 200 (nonprescription form); Ranitidine: ✦Apo-Ranitidine, Novo-Ranidine, Nu-Ranit, Zantac, ✦Zantac-C, Xantac 75 and Zantac 75 EFFERdose (nonprescription forms); Famotidine: Pepcid, Pepcid AC (nonprescription form); Nizatidine: Axid, Axid AR (nonprescription form)

Warning: The brand names Zantac and Xanax are similar and can be mistaken. These are very different drugs, and can lead to serious problems. Check the color chart insert of drugs and verify that you are taking the correct drug.

BENEFITS versus RISKS

Possible Benefits	*Possible Risks*
EFFECTIVE TREATMENT OF PEPTIC ULCER DISEASE: relief of symptoms, acceleration of healing, prevention of recurrence	Drug-induced hepatitis
	Bone marrow depression (lowered white blood cells or hemoglobin)
CONTROL OF HYPERSECRETORY STOMACH DISORDERS	Confusion (particularly in compromised elderly with some of these drugs)
TREATMENT OF REFLUX ESOPHAGITIS	Low blood platelet counts
TREATMENT OF HEARTBURN	(All of the above are case report to rare effects.)
PREVENTION OF HEARTBURN (cimetidine, famotidine, and nizatidine)	

Author's Note: The nonprescription heartburn-preventing or -treating forms of these medicines have, in general because of episodic use and lower doses, side effects or adverse effects that occur even less frequently or not at all when compared to the already well-tolerated prescription forms.

▷ **Principal Uses**

As a Single Drug Product: Uses currently included in FDA-approved labeling: (1) Treatment and prevention of recurrence of peptic ulcer; (2) all are used for both duodenal and gastric ulcers; (3) cimetidine, ranitidine, and famotidine are used in conditions where extreme production (Zollinger-Ellison syndrome) of stomach acid occurs; (4) all four medicines are used to control excess acid moving from the stomach into the lower throat (gastroesophageal reflux disease—GERD); (5) cimetidine is approved for use in preventing upper stomach/intestinal bleeding; (6) all have been used with antibiotics and bismuth compounds (Pepto-Bismol and others) in refractory ulcers where *Helicobacter pylori* has been found; (7) cimetidine is approved to prevent ulcers caused by stress (stress ulcer prophylaxis); (8) all are approved in nonprescription forms for treatment of heartburn. Cimetidine (Tagamet HB 200), famotidine (Pepcid AC), and nizatidine (Axid AR) are also approved for *prevention* of heartburn.

Other (unlabeled) generally accepted uses: (1) Ranitidine, famotidine, and nizatidine have been used in the prevention of upper stomach/intestinal bleeding; (2) cimetidine has been used prior to surgery to prevent aspiration pneumonitis caused by anesthesia, and ranitidine has shown some benefit here as well; (3) ranitidine and famotidine have been used to help prevent ulcers that may occur in acutely and seriously ill patients; (4) cimetidine appears to have a role in helping patients with colorectal cancer live longer, but further research is needed; (5) famotidine may have a role in treating anaphylactic reactions (6) cimetidine also may have a role in helping recurrent and resistant warts in some children.

How These Drugs Work: They block the action of histamine, and by doing this, inhibit the ability of the stomach to make acid. Once acid is decreased, the body is able to heal itself. Ulcers resistant to healing have now been shown to have an infectious component (*Helicobacter pylori*), and antibiotics combined with a histamine (H$_2$) blocking drug can work.

Available Dose Forms and Strengths
Cimetidine:

Injection	— 300 mg/2 ml
	— 300 mg/50 ml (single dose in 0.9% sodium chloride)
Liquid	— 300 mg/5 ml (2.8% alcohol)
Oral solution	— 300 mg/5 ml
Tablets	— 100 mg, 200 mg, 300 mg, 400 mg, 600 mg, 800 mg
Tablets (nonprescription)	— 200 mg

Ranitidine:

Gelcap	— 168 mg and 336 mg (Canada only)
GELdose capsules	— 150 mg, 300 mg
Injection	— 0.5 mg/ml (single dose in 100 ml)
	— 25 mg/ml (in 2-, 10-, and 40-ml vials and 2-ml syringes)
Oral solution (Canada)	— 84 mg/5 ml
Syrup	— 15 mg/ml (7.5% alcohol)
Tablets	— 150 mg, 300 mg (effervescent)
	— 150 mg
Tablets (nonprescription)	— 75 mg

Famotidine:

Injection	— 10 mg/ml (in 2- and 4-ml vials)
Oral suspension	— 40 mg/5 ml
Tablets	— 20 mg, 40 mg
Tablets (nonprescription)	— 10 mg

Nizatidine:

Pulvules (capsules)	— 150 mg, 300 mg
	— 75 mg
Tablets (nonprescription)	— 75 mg

▷ **Recommended Dose Ranges** (Actual dose and schedule must be determined for each patient individually.)

Infants and Children: Cimetidine: Routine use is not recommended in those less than 16 years old. Doses of 20 to 40 mg per kg of body mass per day have been used.

Ranitidine: For those 2 to 18 years old: 1.25 to 2 mg per kg of body mass per dose given every 12 hours, or 37.5 mg per dose.

Famotidine: 0.5 mg per kg of body mass twice a day for 8 weeks in those 6–15 years old.

Nizatidine: No data.

16 to 60 Years of Age:

Peptic ulcer and hypersecretory states:

Cimetidine: 300 mg by mouth four times daily, taken with meals and at bedtime. A maintenance dose of 400 mg at bedtime is useful for some patients.

Ranitidine: 150 mg by mouth twice daily, or 300 mg at bedtime. Maintenance doses of 150 g at bedtime may be of benefit for some patients. Up to 6 g in hypersecretory states.

Famotidine: 40 mg by mouth at bedtime for 4 or up to 8 weeks. Maintenance doses of 20 mg at bedtime have been used. Up to 640 mg daily for hypersecretory states.

Nizatidine: 300 mg by mouth at bedtime, or 150 mg twice a day for up to 8 weeks. A maintenance dose of 150 mg at bedtime is useful for some patients. Not used for hypersecretory states.

Heartburn (nonprescription forms):

Cimetidine: 200 mg by mouth 30 minutes or less before eating foods or drinking liquids that cause you problems. May also be taken once heartburn has started.

Ranitidine: 75 mg by mouth.

Famotidine: 10 mg by mouth before eating foods or drinking liquids that cause you problems or once heartburn has started.

Nizatidine: 75 mg up to twice daily before eating foods or drinking liquids that cause you problems or once heartburn has started.

Over 60 Years of Age: Cimetidine: Half the usual adult dose to start.

Ranitidine, famotidine, and nizatidine: Same dose as 16 to 60 years of age. All pose a risk for formation of masses (phytobezoars) of undigested vegetable fibers. Watch for nervousness, confusion, loss of appetite, stomach fullness, nausea, and vomiting.

Conditions Requiring Dosing Adjustments:

Liver Function: Cimetidine and famotidine are most dependent on the liver for elimination. Dose must be decreased in liver failure.

Kidney Function: All of these H₂ blockers are primarily eliminated by the kidneys. Doses **must** be decreased in moderate kidney failure.

▷ **Dosing Instructions:** Cimetidine and ranitidine should be taken immediately after meals to obtain the longest decrease in stomach acid when treating peptic ulcers. Cimetidine, ranitidine, and famotidine should be taken after meals when used in hypersecretory states.

Usual Duration of Use: Use on a regular schedule for 4 to 6 weeks usually determines effectiveness in healing active peptic ulcer disease. Long-term use (months to years) for prevention requires periodic individualized consideration by your physician. Continual use for 6 to 12 weeks is needed to heal the esophagus when cimetidine, ranitidine, famotidine, or nizatidine is used in gastroesophageal reflux disease (GERD). Since nonprescription forms are available for heartburn, if heartburn relief has not occurred in 2 hours, call your doctor, as there may be another reason for your symptoms.

Possible Advantages of These Drugs

Famotidine, ranitidine, and nizatidine offer effective treatment of peptic ulcer disease with once-daily dosing. Nonprescription forms offer relief of heartburn discomfort. Famotidine is approved for nonprescription *prevention* of heartburn.

▷ **These Drugs Should Not Be Taken If**
- you had an allergic reaction to any form previously.

▷ **Inform Your Physician Before Taking These Drugs If**
- you have impaired liver or kidney function.
- you have a low sperm count (cimetidine).
- you are taking any anticoagulant drug.
- you do not tolerate or should not take phenylalanine (ranitidine EFFERdose tablets or granules).

- you have had low white blood cell counts.
- you have a history of acute porphyria (ranitidine).

Possible Side Effects (natural, expected, and unavoidable drug actions)
None reported.

▷ **Possible Adverse Effects** (unusual, unexpected, and infrequent reactions)
If any of the following develop, consult your physician promptly for guidance.

Mild Adverse Effects
Allergic reactions: skin rash and hives.
Headache: ranitidine—rare, cimetidine—rare, famotidine—infrequent, and nizatidine—frequent.
Abnormal dreams: nizatidine—rare.
Diarrhea: ranitidine, nizatidine, cimetidine, and famotidine—all rare.
Joint pain (arthralgia): cimetidine, ranitidine, and famotidine—all rare.
Depression: cimetidine—case reports.
Muscle pain: cimetidine, nizatidine, and famotidine—rare.

Serious Adverse Effects
Allergic reactions: cimetidine and ranitidine can be rare causes of pancreatitis and anemia. Cimetidine and nizatidine can cause exfoliative dermatitis. There have been some case reports of serious skin rashes with cimetidine, nizatidine, and famotidine.
Anaphylactic reactions: cimetidine, nizatidine—rare.
Idiosyncratic reactions: nervousness, confusion, hallucinations.
Liver damage—case reports.
Abnormal heart rhythm changes (slow heartbeat or atrioventricular block): cimetidine, ranitidine, famotidine, and nizatidine—case reports.
Bone marrow depression: cimetidine, ranitidine, and famotidine—rare.
Decreased platelets: cimetidine, ranitidine, and nizatidine—rare. Famotidine has been in case reports as a questionable cause.
Bronchospasm: cimetidine and ranitidine—rare; famotidine—rare and questionable.

▷ **Possible Effects on Sexual Function:**   Impotence: ranitidine, famotidine, cimetidine, and nizatidine—case reports.
Decreased libido: cimetidine—rare.
Male breast enlargement (gynecomastia): nizatidine and cimetidine—case reports.

Possible Delayed Adverse Effects: Male breast enlargement (nizatidine and cimetidine).

▷ **Adverse Effects That May Mimic Natural Diseases or Disorders**
Liver changes may mimic viral hepatitis.

Possible Effects on Laboratory Tests
Blood platelet counts: may be decreased by all histamine (H$_2$) blockers.
Complete blood counts: rare white blood cell (granulocytes) decrease by cimetidine, ranitidine, and famotidine.
Urine protein tests (Multistix): false positive with ranitidine use.
Urine urobilinogen: false positive with nizatidine.
Thyroid hormones: T$_4$ and free T$_4$ are decreased with ranitidine use.
Liver enzymes (SGPT, OT, etc.): can be increased with liver damage.
Sperm count: decreased with cimetidine.

CAUTION
1. Ulcer rebound/perforation may occur if you stop these drugs abruptly when they are being used to treat ulcers.
2. Once medicines are stopped, call your doctor promptly if symptoms recur.
3. Use of these medicines and symptom relief does not absolutely remove possibility of cancer of the stomach (gastric malignancy).
4. The nonprescription forms of these medicines should NOT be used to treat ulcers.
5. Some of cimetidine is removed by hemodialysis. Redose is needed.

Precautions for Use
By Infants and Children: Cimetidine: Routine use is not recommended in those less than 16 years old. Doses of 20 to 40 mg per kg of body mass per day have been used.
Ranitidine: For those 2 to 18 years old—1.25 to 2 mg per kg of body mass per dose given every 12 hours, or 37.5 mg per dose.
Famotidine: 0.5 mg per kg of body mass twice a day for 8 weeks in those 6–15 years old.
Nizatidine: No data.
By Those Over 60 Years of Age: Increased risk of masses of partially digested vegetable fibers (phytobezoars), especially in people who can't chew well. Watch closely for decreased appetite, stomach fullness, nausea, and vomiting.

▷ **Advisability of Use During Pregnancy**
Pregnancy Category: B for all. See Pregnancy Risk Categories at the back of this book.
Animal studies: No birth defects for cimetidine, ranitidine, and famotidine. Rabbit studies of nizatidine showed abortions, while rat studies showed no effects.
Human studies: Adequate studies of pregnant women are not available.
Use only if clearly needed. Ask your doctor for advice.

Advisability of Use If Breast-Feeding
Presence of these drugs in breast milk: Yes.
Avoid drugs or refrain from nursing.

Habit-Forming Potential: None.

Effects of Overdose: Cimetidine (rarely documented): confusion, tachycardia, sweating, drowsiness, muscle twitching, seizures, respiratory failure, severe CNS symptoms such as coma (after 20–40 g). Nizatidine (rarely documented): increased tearing of the eyes, salivation, vomiting, and diarrhea.
Ranitidine and famotidine: no documentation of overdose changes. Adverse effects of the usual dose. Symptomatic and supportive care would be indicated (nonprescription forms do not have documentation of overdoses).

Possible Effects of Long-Term Use: Rare liver damage with cimetidine, ranitidine, and nizatidine. Swelling and tenderness of breast tissue with cimetidine, ranitidine, and nizatidine.

Suggested Periodic Examinations While Taking This Drug (at physician's discretion)
Complete blood counts, liver and kidney function tests, more frequent tests of

INR (prothrombin times) if an anticoagulant is also taken, and sperm counts (cimetidine).

▷ **While Taking This Drug, Observe the Following**

Foods: Protein-rich foods increase stomach acid secretion. Garlic, onions, citrus fruits, and tomatoes may also increase acid secretion. Many people know the kinds of foods that are likely to result in significant heartburn. Ask your doctor or pharmacist for help in timing the dose of a nonprescription agent for heartburn.

Nutritional Support: Diet as prescribed by your doctor.

Beverages: The caffeine in caffeine-containing beverages such as coffee, tea, and some sodas may stay in the body up to 50% longer than usual with cimetidine (Tagamet) use. Milk may increase acid secretion.

▷ *Alcohol:* Stomach acidity is increased by alcohol—avoid use. Cimetidine may produce a drug interaction with higher than expected levels.

Tobacco Smoking: Smoking is a clear risk factor for peptic ulcer disease. I advise everyone to quit smoking.

Marijuana Smoking: Possible additive reduction in sperm counts with cimetidine use.

▷ *Other Drugs*

Cimetidine may *increase* the effects of

- amiodarone (Codarone).
- amitriptyline (Elavil) and perhaps other tricyclic antidepressants (see Drug Classes). Decreased doses may be needed if the medicines are to be combined.
- benzodiazepines (Librium, etc.—see Drug Classes).
- carbamazepine (Tegretol), with increased toxicity risk. Blood levels are recommended and ongoing carbamazepine doses adjusted to blood levels.
- flecainide (Tambocor), and require dosing changes and more frequent blood level checks.
- loratadine (Claritin), by causing a large increase in blood levels. A study did NOT report any adverse effects on the heart from these levels, but since excessive blood levels of any medicine may be more likely to cause undesirable effects, it appears prudent to lower loratadine doses if these medicines are to be combined.
- meperidine (Demerol, others) and result in toxicity with potential respiratory depression and low blood pressure.
- metformin (Glucophage).
- metoprolol (Lopressor, others, and perhaps other beta-blockers—see Drug Classes), and result in very slow heartbeat and excessively low blood pressure.
- morphine (MS Contin, MSIR, others), and result in central nervous system depression and respiratory depression.
- oral anticoagulants, with increased risk of bleeding. Increased frequency of INR testing is recommended.
- phenytoin (Dilantin).
- procainamide (Procan, Pronestyl).
- propranolol (Inderal).
- quinidine (Quinaglute).
- sertraline (Zoloft).

- sildenafil (Viagra), elevating blood levels of sildenafil by up to 56% (800 mg cimetidine dose). Talk to your doctor about this BEFORE using these medicines together.
- terbinafine (Lamisil).
- theophylline (Theo-Dur, etc.).
- venlafaxine (Effexor).
- warfarin (Coumadin).

Ranitidine may *increase* the effects of
- diazepam (Valium).
- fluvastatin (Lescol).
- glipizide (Glucotrol) and perhaps other oral antidiabetic drugs (see Drug Classes).
- metformin (Glucophage).
- midazolam (Versed).
- procainamide (Procan, Pronestyl).
- theophylline (Theo-Dur, etc.).
- warfarin (Coumadin)—rarely. Increased INR testing is recommended.

Nizatidine, ranitidine, and famotidine (prescription forms) may *increase* the effects of
- amoxicillin.
- high-dose aspirin (may increase level and toxicity risk).
- pentoxifylline (Trental); however, this interaction has only been documented with cimetidine.
- theophylline (Theo-Dur, others). Ongoing theophylline dosing should be based on more frequent blood levels if these medicines are to be taken together.

Cimetidine *taken concurrently* with
- most calcium channel blockers (see Drug Classes) may result in increased blood levels of the calcium channel blockers and potential toxicity. Decreased calcium channel blocker doses may be needed. This may also occur with other H$_2$ blockers and caution is advised.
- carmustine (BiCNU) may cause severe bone marrow depression.
- chloroquine may result in toxicity and may cause cardiac arrest.
- cisapride (Propulsid) may result in increased cisapride levels and a potential serious increase in heart rate.
- clozapine (Clozaril) may result in increased blood levels and clozapine toxicity.
- digoxin (Lanoxin) may result in changes in digoxin levels.
- oral hypoglycemic agents such as glipizide (Glucotrol), glyburide (DiaBeta, Micronase), and tolbutamide (Tolinase, others) may result in severe low blood sugars and seizures.
- paroxetine (Paxil) and perhaps other SSRI antidepressants (see Drug Classes) may result in increased blood levels of the SSRI and require dosing changes.
- pentoxifylline (Trental) may result in increases in blood levels of pentoxifylline. Pentoxifylline dose changes may be needed.
- ritonavir (Norvir) may result in increased cimetidine levels.
- zalcitabine (Hivid) may result in increased blood levels of zalcitabine and result in toxicity. Decreased doses of zalcitabine may be needed.

Cimetidine, ranitidine, famotidine, and nizatidine *taken concurrently* with

- antacids will result in a decreased histamine blocker level. It may be prudent to separate the dosing of these medicines (prescription forms).

Cimetidine *may decrease* the effects of
- indomethacin (Indocin), and perhaps other NSAIDs, by decreasing absorption.
- iron salts, by decreasing absorption.
- ketoconazole, itraconazole, and fluconazole.
- tetracyclines, by decreasing absorption.

Ranitidine, nizatidine, and famotidine may *decrease* the effects of
- indomethacin, by decreasing absorption.
- ketoconazole, itraconazole, and fluconazole.
- sucralfate (Carafate).

▷ *Driving, Hazardous Activities:* Use caution until the degree of confusion, dizziness, or other effect is seen.

Aviation Note: The use of these drugs (prescription forms) *may be a disqualification* for piloting. Consult a designated aviation medical examiner.

Exposure to Sun: Rare and questionable association with ranitidine; use caution with sun exposure when first starting this medicine.

Occurrence of Unrelated Illness: Idiopathic thrombocytopenic purpura (ITP), a rare lowering of blood platelets, is a contraindication for use of any of these medicines. Aplastic anemia, whatever the cause, may be worsened by cimetidine. If symptoms of heartburn get worse, you experience unexplained weight loss, and are over 45 years old, talk with your doctor ... this may be an indication of stomach cancer.

Discontinuation: **Do not** stop these medicines suddenly if they are being taken for peptic ulcer disease. Ask your doctor for withdrawal instructions. Be alert to the recurrence of ulcers any time after these drugs are stopped. Recurrent or refractory ulcers may also represent an infectious disease caused by *Helicobacter pylori*. If this is the case, combination therapy with an antibiotic may be indicated.

HYDRALAZINE (hi DRAL a zeen)

Introduced: 1950   **Class:** Antihypertensive   **Prescription:** USA: Yes
Controlled Drug: USA: No; Canada: No   **Available as Generic:**   USA: Yes;
Canada: No

Brand Names: Alazine, Apo-Hydralazine, Apresazide [CD], Apresoline, Apresoline-Esidrix [CD], Cam-Ap-Es, Dralserp, Dralzine, H-H-R, H.H.R., Hydroserpine [CD], Lo-Ten, Novo-Hylazin, Nu-Hydral, Ser-Ap-Es [CD], Serpasil-Apresoline [CD], Tri-Hydroserpine, Unipres [CD]

BENEFITS versus RISKS	
Possible Benefits	*Possible Risks*
EFFECTIVE ADJUNCT IN MODERATE TO SEVERE HYPERTENSION	DRUG-INDUCED LUPUS-ERYTHEMATOSUS-LIKE SYNDROME
Possibly beneficial in severe congestive heart failure	Intensification of angina pectoris
	Rare blood cell disorders
	Rare liver damage

▷ **Principal Uses**

As a Single Drug Product: Uses currently included in FDA-approved labeling: (1) used with other drugs in moderate to severe high blood pressure or hypertensive crisis; (2) therapy of hypertension caused by abnormal changes in kidney blood vessels.

Other (unlabeled) generally accepted uses: (1) Therapy for aortic or mitral heart valve insufficiency, providing support until surgery can be performed; (2) treatment of acute congestive heart failure in combination with dobutamine; (3) help in anorexia or cachexia; (4) therapy of high blood pressure in pregnancy; (5) painful erections that may occur in sickle cell disease (sickle cell priapism).

As a Combination Drug Product [CD]: Available combined with hydrochlorothiazide (a diuretic) and with reserpine (another type of antihypertensive). When used in combination, several different types of drug action occur at the same time and result in a more beneficial decrease in blood pressure.

How This Drug Works: Causing direct relaxation of arterial walls, lowering blood pressure. Dilation can also help in some cases of heart failure by reducing workload and increasing the output of the heart. Combination with a diuretic reduces sodium and water inthe body, and combination with reserpine reduces the rate and force of contraction of the heart and increases blood vessel expansion.

Available Dose Forms and Strengths

Tablets — 10 mg, 25 mg, 50 mg, 100 mg

▷ **Usual Adult Dose Range:** Hypertension: Initially 10 mg four times daily for 2 to 4 days; then increase to 25 mg four times daily for the balance of the first week. During the second week the dose may be increased to 50 mg four times daily if needed and tolerated. Total daily dose should not exceed 300 mg for fast acetylators or 200 mg for slow acetylators. Ask your doctor for guidance. **Note: Actual dose and schedule must be determined for each patient individually.**

Conditions Requiring Dosing Adjustments

Liver Function: Hydralazine can cause hepatitis, hepatic necrosis, and noncancerous growths. It should be used with caution by patients with liver compromise.

Kidney Function: In cases of mild to moderate kidney failure the usual dose can be taken every 8 hours. In severe kidney failure and for people with slow hydralazine metabolism, the usual dose is taken every 12 to 24 hours and 200 mg per day is a maximum. This medication should be used with caution.

▷ **Dosing Instructions:** The tablet may be crushed and the capsule [CD] may be opened, and is best taken with or following meals to help absorption and reduce stomach upset.

Usual Duration of Use: Use on a regular schedule for several weeks determines effectiveness in lowering blood pressure. Long-term use requires physician supervision.

▷ **This Drug Should Not Be Taken If**
- you have had an allergic reaction to it previously.
- you have rheumatic heart disease.
- you have coronary artery disease.

- you have a dissecting aneurysm of the aorta.
- you have mitral valvular heart disease.

▷ **Inform Your Physician Before Taking This Drug If**
- you have a history of any type of heart disease.
- you have lupus erythematosus.
- you are allergic to aspirin or yellow dyes.
- you have active angina pectoris.
- you have impaired brain circulation, or have had a stroke.
- you are subject to migraine headaches.
- you have impaired kidney function.
- you have systemic lupus erythematosus.
- you have a history of liver sensitivity to other drugs.
- you plan to have surgery under general anesthesia in the near future.

Possible Side Effects (natural, expected, and unavoidable drug actions)

Orthostatic hypotension (see Glossary), nasal congestion, constipation, delayed or impaired urination, increased heart rate of 10 to 25 beats/min, excessive lowering of blood pressure.

▷ **Possible Adverse Effects** (unusual, unexpected, and infrequent reactions)

If any of the following develop, consult your physician promptly for guidance.

Mild Adverse Effects

Allergic reactions: skin rash, hives, itching, drug fever.

Headache, dizziness, flushing of face, palpitation—infrequent.

Loss of appetite, nausea, vomiting, diarrhea—possible.

Taste or smell disorders—rare.

Arthritis, tremors, muscle cramps—infrequent.

Reflex tachycardia—possible.

Serious Adverse Effects

Allergic reactions: liver reaction, with or without jaundice. Serious skin rashes (Stevens-Johnson syndrome)—case reports.

Idiosyncratic reactions: behavioral changes: nervousness, confusion, emotional depression. Asthma, bleeding into lung tissue: densities found on X ray.

Syndrome resembling rheumatoid arthritis or lupus erythematosus (see Glossary)—case reports.

Intensification of coronary artery disease—possible.

Peripheral neuropathy (see Glossary): weakness, numbness, and/or pain—case reports.

Drug-induced periarteritis nodosa, porphyria, gastrointestinal bleeding, gallstones, or congestive heart failure—case reports.

Kidney problems (glomerulonephritis)—infrequent.

Bone marrow depression (see Glossary): fatigue, fever, sore throat, bleeding/bruising—case reports.

▷ **Possible Effects on Sexual Function:**   Impotence and priapism (see Glossary)—case reports.

▷ **Adverse Effects That May Mimic Natural Diseases or Disorders**

Drug fever may suggest systemic infection.

Liver reaction may suggest viral hepatitis.

Skin and joint symptoms may suggest lupus erythematosus.

Natural Diseases or Disorders That May Be Activated by This Drug
Latent coronary artery disease.

Possible Effects on Laboratory Tests
Complete blood cell counts: decreased red cells, hemoglobin, white cells, and platelets.
Blood antinuclear antibodies (ANA): positive.
Blood cholesterol level: decreased.
Blood lupus erythematosus (LE) cells: positive.
Blood urea nitrogen (BUN) level: increased (kidney damage).
Liver function tests: increased liver enzymes (ALT/GPT, AST/GOT, and alkaline phosphatase), increased bilirubin.

CAUTION
1. Increased risk of toxicity with large doses. Follow prescribed doses exactly and keep appointments for follow-up examinations.
2. Report the development of any tendency to emotional depression.
3. May cause salt and water retention if not taken with a diuretic.
4. This drug can provoke migraine headache.
5. Apresoline tablets may have FD & C yellow (tartrazine).

Precautions for Use
By Infants and Children: Dose is based upon age, weight, and kidney function status. For high blood pressure: 0.75 to 1 mg per kg of body mass daily. This dose is divided into two to four equal doses and given every 6 to 12 hours. This is gradually increased as needed and tolerated to a maximum of 200 mg per day. Watch for development of a lupus-erythematosus-like reaction.
By Those Over 60 Years of Age: Low doses are indicated. Unacceptably high blood pressure should be slowly reduced, avoiding the risks associated with excessively low blood pressure. Sudden, rapid, and excessive reduction of blood pressure can predispose to stroke or heart attack. Watch for dizziness, unsteadiness, fainting, or falling. Headache, palpitation, and rapid heart rates are more common in the elderly and can mimic acute anxiety states.

▷ **Advisability of Use During Pregnancy**
Pregnancy Category: C. See Pregnancy Risk Categories at the back of this book.
Animal studies: Birth defects of head and facial bones reported in mice.
Human studies: Adequate studies of pregnant women are not available.
Avoid use during the first and final 3 months; if taken late in pregnancy, this drug can cause low blood platelets (see Glossary) in the newborn.

Advisability of Use If Breast-Feeding
Presence of this drug in breast milk: Yes.
Avoid drug or refrain from nursing.

Habit-Forming Potential: None, but sudden stopping of this medicine may result in congestive heart failure.

Effects of Overdose: Marked light-headedness, dizziness, headache, flushing of skin, nausea, vomiting, collapse of circulation; loss of consciousness, cold and sweaty skin, weak and rapid pulse, irregular heart rhythm.

Possible Effects of Long-Term Use: An acute or subacute syndrome resembling rheumatoid arthritis or lupus erythematosus, usually seen in slow acetylators taking daily doses of over 200 mg. Tolerance to the therapeutic benefits may develop.

Suggested Periodic Examinations While Taking This Drug (at physician's discretion)
> Complete blood counts, liver function tests, blood tests for evidence of lupus erythematosus.

▷ **While Taking This Drug, Observe the Following**
> *Foods:* May decrease hydralazine absorption and lessen its therapeutic effect.
> *Nutritional Support:* Watch for peripheral neuropathy and take pyridoxine (vitamin B_6) as needed. Ask your physician for guidance.
> *Beverages:* No restrictions. May be taken with milk.

▷ *Alcohol:* Use with extreme caution—alcohol can exaggerate the blood-pressure-lowering effect of this drug and cause excessive reduction.
> *Tobacco Smoking:* Avoid completely. Nicotine can contribute significantly to this drug's ability to intensify angina in susceptible patients.

▷ *Other Drugs*
> Hydralazine may *increase* the effects of
> • metoprolol (Lopressor) and other beta-blocking medicines.
> • oxprenolol (Trasicor).
> • propranolol (Inderal).
>
> Hydralazine *taken concurrently* with
> • clonidine (Catapres) may result in additive lowering of blood pressure. This may be used to therapeutic benefit.
> • furosemide (Lasix) can result in decreased furosemide levels and a need to increase the dose in order to get the same therapeutic benefit if these two drugs are combined.
> • nitrates (isosorbide dinitrate, others) may result in increased benefits in patients with heart failure.
> • NSAIDs (see *nonsteroidal anti-inflammatory drugs* in Drug Classes) may blunt hydralazine's benefit in lowering blood pressure.

▷ *Driving, Hazardous Activities:* May cause light-headedness or dizziness. Limit activities as necessary.
> *Aviation Note:* Hypertension and the use of this drug *are disqualifications* for piloting. Consult a designated aviation medical examiner.
> *Exposure to Sun:* No restrictions.
> *Exposure to Heat:* Caution is advised. Hot environments may reduce blood pressure significantly.
> *Exposure to Cold:* Caution is advised. Cold environments may increase this drug's ability to cause angina in susceptible individuals.
> *Heavy Exercise or Exertion:* Caution is advised. Exertion can increase this drug's ability to cause angina. Also, isometric exercises can raise blood pressure significantly.

HYDROCHLOROTHIAZIDE (hi droh klor oh THI a zide)

See the thiazide diuretics profile for further information.

HYDROCODONE (hi droh KOH dohn)

Other Name: Dihydrocodeinone

Introduced: 1951 **Class:** Analgesic, strong; cough suppressant; opioid
Prescription: USA: Yes **Controlled Drug:** USA: C-III*; Canada: Yes
Available as Generic: USA: Yes hydrocodone/APAP; Canada: No

Brand Names: Allay [CD], Anaplex, Anexsia [CD], Anexsia 7.5 [CD], Anolor
DH5, Azdone [CD], Ban-Tuss-HC [CD], ✦Biohisdex DHC [CD], ✦Biohisdine
DHC [CD], Chemdal-HD [CD], Codone, Detussin [CD], DHC Plus, Dicoril,
Dimetane Expectorant-DC [CD], Duocet [CD], Duratuss HD [CD], Enda-
gen HD [CD], Endal-HD, Entuss-D, Histinex-HC [CD], Histussin HC [CD],
✦Hycodan, Hycodan [CD], ✦Hycomine [CD], Hycomine Compound [CD],
Hycomine Pediatric Syrup [CD], ✦Hycomine-S [CD], Hycomine Syrup
[CD], Hycotuss Expectorant [CD], Lorcet-HD [CD], Lorcet Plus [CD],
Lortab [CD], Lortab ASA [CD], Medipain 5, Norcet 7 [CD], ✦Novahistex
DH [CD], ✦Novahistine DH [CD], Polygesic, Protuss, ✦Robidone, T-Gesic
[CD], Triaminic Expectorant DH [CD], ✦Tussaminic Expectorant DH [CD],
Tussend [CD], Tussend Expectorant [CD], Tussionex [CD], Tycolet [CD],
Vanex [CD], Vicodin [CD], Vicodin ES [CD], Zydone [CD]

BENEFITS versus RISKS

Possible Benefits	*Possible Risks*
EFFECTIVE RELIEF OF MILD TO MODERATE PAIN	Mild allergic reactions—infrequent
	Nausea, constipation
EFFECTIVE CONTROL OF COUGH	Small potential for addiction

▷ **Principal Uses**

As a Single Drug Product: Uses currently included in FDA-approved labeling: (1)
Controls cough; (2) relieves mild to moderate pain.

Other (unlabeled) generally accepted uses: May be a benefit for some patients
with chronic obstructive lung disease (COPD).

As a Combination Drug Product [CD]: Often added to cough mixtures containing
antihistamines, decongestants, and expectorants to increase effectiveness in
reducing cough. Also combined with analgesics such as acetaminophen and
aspirin, to enhance pain relief.

How This Drug Works: Decreases pain perception, calming emotional responses to pain, and reducing cough reflex sensitivity.

Available Dose Forms and Strengths
Syrup — 5 mg/5 ml
Tablets — 5 mg
Tablets (combination) — 10 mg hydrocodone, 650 mg acetaminophen

▷ **Usual Adult Dose Range:** As analgesic: 5 to 10 mg every 6 hours to start and
may later be reduced as needed. Maximum for pain is 40 mg. For cough: 5
mg every 6 to 8 hours as needed. Lorcet: one tablet every four to six hours
as directed by your doctor. Total daily dose of hydrocodone should not exceed 40 mg.

*See Controlled Drug Schedules at the back of this book.

Note: Actual dose and schedule must be determined for each patient individually.

Conditions Requiring Dosing Adjustments

Liver Function: Use with caution by patients with severe liver compromise, with decreases in dose or longer time between doses.

Kidney Function: This drug may cause urinary retention, and a benefit-to-risk decision should be made for patients with renal (kidney) outflow problems. Up to 20% of this drug is eliminated by the kidneys. Consideration for reduced doses should be given, especially for longer-term therapy.

▷ **Dosing Instructions:** Tablet may be crushed and taken with or following food to reduce stomach irritation or nausea.

Usual Duration of Use: As required, to control pain or cough. Continual use should not exceed 5 to 7 days without interruption and reassessment of need.

▷ **This Drug Should Not Be Taken If**
- you had an allergic reaction to it previously.
- you have a lesion in your head (intracranial) that causes increased pressure.
- you are having an acute attack of asthma.

▷ **Inform Your Physician Before Taking This Drug If**
- you had an unfavorable reaction to any narcotic drug.
- you have a history of drug abuse or alcoholism.
- you have chronic lung disease with impaired breathing.
- you have impaired liver or kidney function.
- you have gallbladder disease, a seizure disorder, or an underactive thyroid gland.
- you have difficulty emptying the urinary bladder.
- you are prone to constipation.
- you are allergic to sulfites (some preparations contain sulfites).
- you are taking any other drugs that have a sedative effect.
- you will have surgery with general anesthesia.

Possible Side Effects (natural, expected, and unavoidable drug actions)
Drowsiness, light-headedness, dry mouth, urinary retention, constipation—infrequent to frequent.

▷ **Possible Adverse Effects** (unusual, unexpected, and infrequent reactions)
If any of the following develop, consult your physician promptly for guidance.

Mild Adverse Effects
Allergic reactions: skin rash, hives, itching.
Dizziness, impaired concentration, sensation of drunkenness, confusion, depression, blurred or double vision, facial flushing, sweating—infrequent to frequent.
Nausea, vomiting—infrequent to frequent (may also be dose related).
Abnormal constriction of the pupils of the eye (miosis)—possible.

Serious Adverse Effects
Allergic reactions: anaphylaxis, severe skin reactions—case reports.
Idiosyncratic reactions: delirium, hallucinations, excitement, increased sensitivity to pain after the analgesic effect has worn off.

Seizures—possible.

Impaired breathing (respiratory depression)—dose related.

Liver or kidney toxicity—case reports.

Psychological and physical dependence—possible.

▷ **Possible Effects on Sexual Function:** Blunting of sexual response or drive—possible.

▷ **Adverse Effects That May Mimic Natural Diseases or Disorders**

Paradoxical behavioral disturbances may suggest psychotic disorder.

Possible Effects on Laboratory Tests

Blood amylase and lipase levels: increased (natural side effect).

Urine screening tests for drug abuse: *initial* test result may be falsely *positive*; *confirmatory* test result will be *negative*. (Test results depend upon amount of drug taken and testing method used.)

CAUTION

1. People with asthma, chronic bronchitis, or emphysema may have breathing problems with extended use of this drug. The secretions of the bronchi may thicken and cough will be suppressed.
2. Combination of this drug with atropinclike drugs can increase the risk of urinary retention and reduced intestinal function.
3. Do not take this drug following acute head injury.

Precautions for Use

By Infants and Children: Do not use this drug in children under 2 years of age because of their vulnerability to life-threatening respiratory depression.

By Those Over 60 Years of Age: Small doses and short-term treatment are indicated. Patients in this group may have increased susceptibility to drowsiness, dizziness, unsteadiness, falling, urinary retention, and constipation (often leading to fecal impaction).

▷ **Advisability of Use During Pregnancy**

Pregnancy Category: B, D if in high doses or near the time of birth. See Pregnancy Risk Categories at the back of this book.

Animal studies: Birth defects reported in hamster studies.

Human studies: Adequate studies of pregnant women are not available. Hydrocodone taken repeatedly during the final few weeks before delivery may cause withdrawal symptoms in the newborn infant.

Use this drug only if clearly needed and in small, infrequent doses.

Advisability of Use If Breast-Feeding

Presence of this drug in breast milk: Unknown.

Monitor nursing infant closely and discontinue drug or nursing if adverse effects develop. Ask your physician for guidance.

Habit-Forming Potential: Psychological and/or physical dependence can develop with use of large doses for an extended period of time. True dependence is infrequent and unlikely with prudent use.

Effects of Overdose: Drowsiness, restlessness, agitation, nausea, vomiting, dry mouth, vertigo, weakness, lethargy, stupor, coma, seizures.

Possible Effects of Long-Term Use: Psychological and physical dependence, chronic constipation.

Suggested Periodic Examinations While Taking This Drug (at physician's discretion)

Liver function tests.

▷ **While Taking This Drug, Observe the Following**

Foods: No restrictions.

Beverages: No restrictions. May be taken with milk.

▷ *Alcohol:* Use extreme caution. Hydrocodone can intensify the intoxicating effects of alcohol, and alcohol can intensify the depressant effects of hydrocodone on brain function, breathing, and circulation.

Tobacco Smoking: No interactions expected. I advise everyone to quit smoking.

Marijuana Smoking: Increased drowsiness and pain relief; impaired mental and physical status.

▷ *Other Drugs*

Hydrocodone may *increase* the effects of

- other drugs with sedative effects.
- atropinelike drugs, and increase the risk of constipation and urinary retention.

Hydrocodone *taken concurrently* with

- cimetidine (Tagamet) may result in increased risk of breathing problems and central nervous system suppression.
- monoamine oxidase (MAO) inhibitors (see Drug Classes) may result in an increased effect and the need to decrease the dose of hydrocodone.
- ritonavir (Norvir) and perhaps other protease inhibitors (see Drug Classes) can lead to toxicity.
- tramadol (Ultram) may result in increased risk of breathing problems and central nervous system suppression.

▷ *Driving, Hazardous Activities:* This drug can impair mental alertness, judgment, reaction time, and physical coordination. Avoid hazardous activities accordingly.

Aviation Note: The use of this drug *is a disqualification* for piloting. Consult a designated aviation medical examiner.

Exposure to Sun: No restrictions.

Discontinuation: This drug is best limited to short-term use. If used for extended periods, discontinuation should be gradual to minimize withdrawal (usually mild with this drug).

HYDROXYCHLOROQUINE (hi drox ee KLOR oh kwin)

Introduced: 1967 **Class:** Antimalarial, immunosuppressant **Prescription:** USA: Yes **Controlled Drug:** USA: No; Canada: No **Available as Generic:** USA: Yes; Canada: No

Brand Names: ✦Dermoplast, Plaquenil

```
┌──────────────────────────────────────────────────────────────┐
│                    BENEFITS versus RISKS                       │
│      Possible Benefits                    Possible Risks       │
│  EFFECTIVE PREVENTION AND          INFREQUENT DAMAGE OF        │
│    TREATMENT OF CERTAIN               CORNEAL AND RETINAL EYE  │
│    FORMS OF MALARIA                   TISSUES                  │
│  Possibly effective in the management  BONE MARROW DEPRESSION  │
│    of acute and chronic rheumatoid   Heart muscle damage      │
│    arthritis and juvenile arthritis  Ear damage: hearing loss, ringing in │
│  Possibly effective in the management   ears                  │
│    of chronic discoid and systemic                            │
│    lupus erythematosus                                        │
└──────────────────────────────────────────────────────────────┘
```

▷ **Principal Uses**

As a Single Drug Product: Uses currently included in FDA-approved labeling: (1) Prevention and therapy of acute attacks of certain types of malaria; (2) reduces disease activity in rheumatoid arthritis; (3) suppresses disease activity in chronic discoid and systemic lupus erythematosus.

Other (unlabeled) generally accepted uses: (1) Treatment of Sjögren's syndrome; (2) treats refractory Lyme arthritis; (3) therapy of sarcoidosis, polymorphous light eruption, porphyria, solar urticaria, and chronic vasculitis; (4) may help decrease steroid requirements in asthma; (5) can help decrease insulin needs in when an oral hypoglycemic agent is taken with insulin; (6) combination therapy of Weber-Christian disease.

How This Drug Works: In malaria, this drug impairs DNA in the organisms. As an antiarthritic and anti-lupus drug, acts as a mild immunosuppressant. Accumulates in white blood cells and inhibits many enzymes involved in tissue destruction.

Available Dose Forms and Strengths

Tablets — 200 mg

▷ **Usual Adult Dose Range:** For malaria suppression: 400 mg once every 7 days.

For malaria treatment: (1) 800 mg as a single dose; or (2) initially 800 mg, followed by 400 mg in 6 to 8 hours; then 400 mg once a day on the second and third days.

For pediatric malaria treatment: 10 mg per kg of body mass followed in 6 hours by 5 mg per kg of body mass, with 5 mg per kg of body mass given 18 hours after the second dose; then 5 mg per kg of body mass taken 24 hours after the first dose.

For lupus erythematosus: 400 mg once or twice daily. This is used for several weeks or cautiously until remission. Ongoing dose is 200–400 mg daily.

For rheumatoid arthritis: Starting dose of 400 to 600 mg and an ongoing dose of 200–400 mg a day.

Note: Actual dose and schedule must be determined for each patient individually.

Conditions Requiring Dosing Adjustments

Liver Function: Benefit-to-risk decision by patients with liver compromise or who take liver-toxic drugs.

Kidney Function: Use with caution in kidney compromise.

▷ **Dosing Instructions:**   Take with food or milk to reduce stomach irritation. The tablet may be crushed and mixed with jam, jelly, or gelatin. Take it exactly as prescribed.

Note: For malaria prevention, begin medication 2 weeks before entering malarious area; continue medication while in the area and for 4 weeks after leaving the area.

For treating arthritis and lupus, take medication on a regular schedule daily; continual use for 6 months may be necessary to determine maximal benefit.

Usual Duration of Use: Use on a regular schedule for 2 weeks before exposure, during period of exposure, and 4 weeks after exposure determines this drug's effectiveness in preventing attacks of malaria. Use on a regular schedule for up to 6 months may be required to evaluate benefits in reducing rheumatoid arthritis and lupus erythematosus. If significant improvement is not achieved, this drug should be stopped. Long-term use (months to years) requires periodic physician evaluation.

Possible Advantages of This Drug

Considered to have less potential for retinal toxicity than chloroquine.

Currently a "Drug of Choice"

For the treatment of chronic discoid and systemic lupus erythematosus.

▷ **This Drug Should Not Be Taken If**
- you had past allergies to chloroquine or hydroxychloroquine.
- you have an active bone marrow or blood cell disorder.
- should not be used for long-term treatment in children.

▷ **Inform Your Physician Before Taking This Drug If**
- you are pregnant or planning a pregnancy.
- you have had bone marrow depression or a blood cell disorder.
- you have a deficiency of glucose-6-phosphate dehydrogenase (G6PD—talk with your doctor).
- you have any disorder of the eyes, especially disease of the cornea or retina, or visual field changes.
- you have impaired hearing or ringing in the ears.
- you have a seizure disorder of any kind.
- you have a history of peripheral neuritis.
- you have low blood pressure or a heart rhythm disorder.
- you have peptic ulcer disease, Crohn's disease, or ulcerative colitis.
- you have impaired liver or kidney function.
- you have a history of porphyria.
- you have any form of psoriasis.
- you are taking antacids, cimetidine, digoxin, or penicillamine.

Possible Side Effects (natural, expected, and unavoidable drug actions)

Light-headedness (low blood pressure); blue-black discoloration of skin, fingernails, or mouth lining with long-term use.

▷ **Possible Adverse Effects** (unusual, unexpected, and infrequent reactions)

If any of the following develop, consult your physician promptly for guidance.

Mild Adverse Effects

Allergic reactions: skin rash, itching (more common in African-Americans).

Loss of hair color, loss of hair.

Headache, blurring of near vision (reading), ringing in ears—possible to infrequent.

Loss of appetite, nausea, vomiting, stomach cramps, diarrhea—infrequent.

Dizziness—case reports.

Serious Adverse Effects

Allergic reactions: severe skin rash, exfoliative dermatitis.

Idiosyncratic reactions: hemolytic anemia in those with glucose-6-phosphate dehydrogenase (G6PD) deficiency in red blood cells.

Emotional or psychotic mental changes; seizures—case reports.

Loss of hearing, porphyria—case reports.

Eye tissue damage, specifically cornea and retina, with significant impairment of vision—case reports.

Aplastic anemia (see Glossary): abnormally low red blood cell counts (fatigue and weakness); abnormally low white blood cell counts (fever, sore throat, infections); abnormally low platelet counts (abnormal bruising or bleeding)—case reports.

▷ **Possible Effects on Sexual Function:**   None reported.

Possible Delayed Adverse Effects: Irreversible retinal damage has developed 7 years after discontinuation of chloroquine, a closely related drug. Retinal damage is more likely to occur following high-dose and/or long-term use.

▷ **Adverse Effects That May Mimic Natural Diseases or Disorders**

Central nervous system toxicity may suggest unrelated neuropsychiatric disorder. Seizures may suggest the onset of epilepsy.

Natural Diseases or Disorders That May Be Activated by This Drug

Porphyria, psoriasis.

Possible Effects on Laboratory Tests

Complete blood cell counts: decreased red cells, hemoglobin, white cells, and platelets.

Liver function tests: increased liver enzymes (ALT/GPT, AST/GOT, and alkaline phosphatase), increased bilirubin.

Electrocardiogram: conduction abnormalities, prolonged QRS interval, T-wave changes, and heart block have all been reported for chloroquine, a closely related drug.

CAUTION

1. Does not prevent relapses in certain types of malaria.
2. High-dose and/or long-term use of this drug may cause irreversible retinal damage, significant visual impairment, or hearing loss due to nerve damage. Report promptly any changes in vision or hearing so appropriate evaluation can be made.

Precautions for Use

By Infants and Children: This age group is very sensitive to the effects of this drug. Doses should be determined and therapy should be monitored by a qualified pediatrician.

By Those Over 60 Years of Age: Tolerance for this drug may be reduced. Watch for behavioral changes, low blood pressure, heart rhythm disturbances, muscle weakness, and changes in vision or hearing.

▷ **Advisability of Use During Pregnancy**

Pregnancy Category: C. See Pregnancy Risk Categories at the back of this book.

Animal studies: No information available.

Human studies: Adequate studies of pregnant women are not available. However, closely related drugs of this class are known to cause abnormal retinal pigmentation and hemorrhage, and congenital deafness in the fetus.

Avoid use during pregnancy except for the suppression or treatment of malaria. Other use is a benefit to risk decision.

Advisability of Use If Breast-Feeding

Presence of this drug in breast milk: Yes.

Avoid drug or refrain from nursing.

Habit-Forming Potential: None.

Effects of Overdose: Drowsiness, headache, blurred vision, excitability, low blood pressure, seizures, coma.

Possible Effects of Long-Term Use: Irreversible eye damage (cornea and retina), hearing loss, muscle weakness, aplastic anemia.

Suggested Periodic Examinations While Taking This Drug (at physician's discretion)

Complete blood cell counts; liver and kidney function tests.

Serial blood pressure readings and electrocardiograms.

Neurological examinations for significant muscle weakness.

Complete eye examinations before starting high-dose and/or long-term treatment and every 3 to 6 months during drug use.

Hearing tests as indicated.

▷ **While Taking This Drug, Observe the Following**

Foods: No restrictions.

Beverages: No restrictions. May be taken with milk.

▷ *Alcohol:* Use sparingly to minimize stomach irritation.

Tobacco Smoking: No interactions expected, but I advise everyone to quit smoking.

▷ *Other Drugs*

Hydroxychloroquine may ***increase*** the effects of

• aurothioglucose (Solganol), increases risk of blood problems.

• digoxin (Lanoxin), and increase its toxic potential.

• penicillamine (Cuprimine, Depen), and increase its toxic potential.

The following drug may ***increase*** the effects of hydroxychloroquine:

• cimetidine (Tagamet).

The following drugs may ***decrease*** the effects of hydroxychloroquine:

• magnesium salts and antacids.

▷ *Driving, Hazardous Activities:* This drug may cause light-headedness, blurred vision, or impaired hearing. Restrict activities as necessary.

Aviation Note: The use of this drug ***may be a disqualification*** for piloting. Consult a designated aviation medical examiner.

Exposure to Sun: Use caution until sensitivity has been determined. Closely related drugs of this class may cause photosensitivity (see Glossary).

Discontinuation: This drug should be stopped and prompt evaluation should be made if any of the following develop—any changes in vision or hearing, seizures, unusual muscle weakness, indications of infection (fever, sore throat, etc.), abnormal bruising or bleeding.

HYDROXYUREA (hi DROX EE yur ia)

Introduced: 1995 (AIDS or sickle cell)   **Class:**   Anti-AIDS, anticancer, anti-sickle-cell-anemia   **Prescription:**   USA: Yes   **Controlled Drug:**   USA: No; Canada: No   **Available as Generic:**   USA: No; Canada: No

Brand Name: Hydrea, Droxia

Warning: This drug is a cytotoxic agent. Appropriate precautions must be taken as with other chemotherapy.

BENEFITS versus RISKS

Possible Benefits	*Possible Risks*
COMBINATION TREATMENT OF AIDS	BONE MARROW SUPPRESSION
DECREASED SEVERITY AND FREQUENCY OF SICKLE CELL CRISES	Hepatitis
Treatment of chronic myelocytic leukemia, melanoma, and other cancers	Possible cancer causing agent

---

▷ **Principal Uses**

As a Single Drug Product: Uses currently included in FDA-approved labeling: (1) blast crisis; (2) chronic myelogenous leukemia; (3) head, neck, and ovarian cancers; (4) chronic leukemias; (5) cancers of certain cell types (squamous cell); (6) decreases frequency and severity of sickle cell crises.

Other (unlabeled) generally accepted uses: (1) used to treat certain diseases of the red blood cells (polycythemia vera); (2) used in combination with other medicines to treat HIV-positive patients; (3) brain cancer.

How This Drug Works: When used in cancer, this medicine is a cell-cycle-specific drug. It works in the S phase of mitosis. When used in AIDS patients, the exact mechanism of action is not fully understood. When used in sickle cell patients, the specific mechanism has not been identified.

Available Dose Forms and Strengths

Capsule (Hydrea) — 500 mg

Caspules (Droxia) — 200 mg, 300 mg, 400 mg

▷ **Recommended Dose Ranges** (Actual dose and schedule must be determined for each patient individually.)

Infants and Children: Safety and effectiveness have not been defined in this age group.

18 to 60 Years of Age: All doses are decided based on ideal or actual body mass, whichever is less.

Oral dosing: Usual oral doses range from 20 to 30 mg per kg of body mass per day, which is given as a single daily dose. Some centers give 80 mg per kg of body mass every third day. If a patient is in blast crisis, up to 12 g per day has been given to rapidly decrease white blood cell counts.

In the sickle cell studies: Patients were started on 15 mg per kg of body mass and had their dose increased by 5 mg per kg of body mass every 12 weeks unless toxicity occurred or the maximum dose of 35 mg per kg of body mass per day was reached.

In AIDS: The protocols are still changing.

Over 60 Years of Age: Same as 18 to 60 years of age.

Conditions Requiring Dosing Adjustments

Liver Function: No changes in dosing are anticipated.

Kidney Function: The dose must be decreased for patients with kidney compromise. Decreases of up to 80% are needed in severe compromise.

▷ **Dosing Instructions:**   This medicine is best taken on an empty stomach. Call your doctor if you vomit after taking this medicine.

Usual Duration of Use: Continual use on a regular schedule for up to 16 weeks may be needed to treat cancers of the head and neck. Treatment in sickle cell disease is ongoing, using the lowest effective dose. Treatment in AIDS is yet to be defined.

Long-term use (months to years) requires periodic evaluation of response and dose adjustment. Consult your physician on a regular basis.

Currently a "Drug of Choice"

For reducing the frequency and severity of sickle cell crises in patients with sickle cell disease.

▷ **This Drug Should Not Be Taken If**
- you had an allergic reaction to it previously.
- you have severely depressed bone marrow. This is seen in very low white blood cell, platelet, or hemoglobin levels.

▷ **Inform Your Physician Before Taking This Drug If**
- you have signs or symptoms of cancer.
- you are considering pregnancy (males or females).
- you have had chemotherapy or radiation therapy previously.
- you have compromised kidneys.
- you have herpes zoster (shingles).
- you have recently been exposed to chicken pox.
- you are having unusual bruising or bleeding.
- you are unsure how to dispose of urine or vomit.
- you are unsure how much to take or how often to take it.
- you take prescription or nonprescription medicines not discussed when hydroxyurea was prescribed.

Possible Side Effects (natural, expected, and unavoidable drug actions)

Hair loss, painful mouth sores, sensitivity to the sun.

▷ **Possible Adverse Effects** (unusual, unexpected, and infrequent reactions)

If any of the following develop, consult your physician promptly for guidance.

Mild Adverse Effects

Allergic reactions: skin rash and itching.

Dizziness, disorientation, headaches, or fever—rare.

Nausea, vomiting, or diarrhea—frequent (vomiting usually mild).

Difficulty urinating—rare.

Ulceration of the skin—rare.

Serious Adverse Effects
Allergic reactions: skin ulceration—case reports.
Idiosyncratic reactions: none reported.
Bone marrow depression—possible.
Convulsions or hallucinations—rare.
Hepatitis or kidney problems—rare.
Drug-induced lupus erythematosus—case report.
Lung problems (acute interstitial lung disease)—rare.
Squamous cancer (carcinoma) or leukemia—possible increased risk.

▷ **Possible Effects on Sexual Function:** None reported.

Possible Delayed Adverse Effects: Bone marrow suppression.

▷ **Adverse Effects That May Mimic Natural Diseases or Disorders**
Liver toxicity may be similar to acute hepatitis.

Natural Diseases or Disorders That May Be Activated by This Drug
Not defined.

Possible Effects on Laboratory Tests
Liver function tests: increased.
Complete blood counts: decreases in several components.

CAUTION
1. This medicine is toxic to cells. Be certain your doctor has carefully explained how to dispose of urine or vomit.
2. Call your doctor at once if you have a seizure.
3. Both women and men should avoid conception for several months after taking this medicine.
4. Wash your hands after taking this medicine **before** you touch your eyes or your nose.

Precautions for Use
By Infants and Children: Safety and effectiveness for use by those under 18 years of age have not been established.
By Those Over 60 Years of Age: Lower doses are prudent as increased sensitivity to any dose may occur. Natural declines in kidney function may require dose decrease.

▷ **Advisability of Use During Pregnancy**
Pregnancy Category: D. See Pregnancy Risk Categories at the back of this book.
Animal studies: Causes birth defects in animals.
Human studies: Adequate studies of pregnant women are not available.
Talk with your doctor about this benefit-to-risk decision.

Advisability of Use If Breast-Feeding
Presence of this drug in breast milk: Yes.
Avoid drug or refrain from nursing.

Habit-Forming Potential: None.

Effects of Overdose: Bone marrow depression, increased heart rate, liver cell and testicular damage.

Possible Effects of Long-Term Use: Bone marrow depression.

Suggested Periodic Examinations While Taking This Drug (at physician's discretion)
Complete blood cell counts; dental exams.

▷ **While Taking This Drug, Observe the Following**
Foods: No restrictions.
Beverages: No restrictions. May be taken with milk.
▷ *Alcohol:* Do not drink alcohol.
Tobacco Smoking: No interactions expected. I advise everyone to quit smoking.
▷ *Other Drugs*
Hydroxyurea *taken concurrently* with
- amphotericin (Abelcet) may increase risk of kidney toxicity and spasm of bronchi.
- fluorouracil (Efudil) may increase toxicity to nerves.
- other medicines that cause bone marrow depression (see Table 5, Section Six) may lead to additive toxicity to bone marrow.
- vaccines (live virus) may result in undesirable effects if immune system is depressed.
▷ *Driving, Hazardous Activities:* This drug may cause light-headedness, blurred vision, or impaired hearing. Restrict activities as necessary.
Aviation Note: The use of this drug *may be a disqualification* for piloting. Consult a designated aviation medical examiner.
Exposure to Sun: Use caution until sensitivity has been determined. Closely related drugs of this class may cause photosensitivity (see Glossary).
Discontinuation: This drug should be stopped and prompt evaluation should be made if any of the following develop—any changes in vision or hearing, seizures, unusual muscle weakness, indications of infection (fever, sore throat, etc.), abnormal bruising or bleeding.

IBUPROFEN (i byu PROH fen)

See the propionic acids (nonsteroidal anti-inflammatory drugs) profile for further information.

IMIPRAMINE (im IP ra meen)

Introduced: 1955   **Class:** Antidepressant   **Prescription:** USA: Yes
Controlled Drug: USA: No; Canada: No   **Available as Generic:** USA: Yes; Canada: Yes
Brand Names: Antipress, ✦Apo-Imipramine, ✦Impril, Janimine, ✦Novopramine, ✦PMS Imipramine, SK-Pramine, Tipramine, Tofranil, Tofranil-PM

BENEFITS versus RISKS

Possible Benefits	*Possible Risks*
EFFECTIVE RELIEF OF NEUROSES AND PSYCHOTIC DEPRESSION	ADVERSE BEHAVIORAL EFFECTS
EFFECTIVE TREATMENT FOR CHILDHOOD BED-WETTING (enuresis)	CONVERSION OF DEPRESSION TO MANIA in manic-depressive (bipolar) disorders
Helps manage chronic, severe pain	Aggravation of schizophrenia and paranoia
Aids cocaine withdrawal	Induction of serious heart rhythm abnormalities
Relieves symptoms of attention deficit disorder	Abnormally low white blood cell and platelet counts
Helps prevent panic attacks	
Helps control binge eating and purging in bulimia	

▷ **Principal Uses**

As a Single Drug Product: Uses currently included in FDA-approved labeling: (1) Relieves severe emotional depression and initiates gradual restoration of normal mood; (2) helps prevents childhood bed-wetting in children over 6 years of age; (3) used to treat delusions.

Other (unlabeled) generally accepted uses: (1) Helps treat agoraphobia; (2) some case evidence of helping in treating aspermia; (3) can be of help in chronic pain syndromes; (4) eases diabetic neuropathy; (5) inappropriate emotionalism (such as pathological crying) can be controlled by this drug; (6) of use in globus hystericus; (7) may have a role in treating panic disorder; (8) can help post-traumatic stress disorder; (9) may help control retrograde ejaculation; (10) can be of adjunctive benefit in helping control schizophrenia; (11) shows some benefit in patients who fail ENT surgery or weight reduction as treatment of sleep apnea; (12) may be of help as a second-line agent in attention deficit hyperactivity disorder (ADHD).

How This Drug Works: By increasing nerve impulse transmitters (norepinephrine and serotonin), this drug relieves the depression. Beneficial effects in treating bed-wetting are thought to be due partially to this drug's atropine-like action.

Available Dose Forms and Strengths

Capsules — 75 mg, 100 mg, 125 mg, 150 mg

Injection — 25 mg/2 ml

Tablets — 1g, 25 mg, 50 mg, 75 mg

▷ **Usual Adult Dose Range:** Initially 75 mg daily, divided into three doses. Dose may be increased cautiously as needed and tolerated by 10 mg to 25 mg daily at intervals of 1 week. The usual maintenance dose is 50 mg to 150 mg every 24 hours. The total daily dose should not exceed 200 mg for outpatient therapy. (When determined, the optimal daily requirement may be given at bedtime as a single dose.) **Note: Actual dose and schedule must be determined for each patient individually.**

Conditions Requiring Dosing Adjustments

Liver Function: Used with caution and in decreased dose by patients with liver compromise. It is also a rare cause of hepatic necrosis.

Kidney Function: No changes in dosing are anticipated in kidney compromise.

▷ **Dosing Instructions:**   May be taken without regard to meals. If necessary, may be taken with food to reduce stomach irritation. The capsule may be opened and the tablet may be crushed. Note: Tofranil-PM capsules should not be used to treat childhood bed-wetting.

Usual Duration of Use: Continual use on a regular schedule for 3 to 4 weeks is usually necessary to determine this drug's effectiveness in relieving depression; optimal response may require 3 or more months of use. Long-term use (months to years) requires periodic evaluation of response and dose adjustment. Consult your physician on a regular basis.

Possible Advantages of This Drug

Less likely to increase the heart rate than other tricyclic antidepressants.

Less hazardous and more easily managed than monoamine oxidase (MAO) inhibitor antidepressants.

Currently a "Drug of Choice"

For adjunctive use in treating childhood bed-wetting when organic causes for this disorder have been eliminated.

▷ **This Drug Should Not Be Taken If**

- you have had an allergic reaction to it previously.
- you are taking, or have taken within the past 14 days, any monoamine oxidase (MAO) type A inhibitor drug (see Drug Classes).
- you have had a recent heart attack (myocardial infarction).
- you have angina, abnormal heartbeats, or congestive heart failure.
- you are pregnant.

▷ **Inform Your Physician Before Taking This Drug If**

- you have had an adverse reaction to any other antidepressant drug.
- you have any type of seizure disorder.
- you have increased internal eye pressure.
- you have narrow-angle glaucoma.
- you have any type of heart disease, especially coronary artery disease or a heart rhythm disorder.
- you are subject to bronchial asthma.
- you have impaired liver or kidney function.
- you have any type of thyroid disorder or are taking thyroid medication.
- you have diabetes or sugar intolerance.
- you have prostatism (see Glossary).
- you have a history of alcoholism.
- you plan to have surgery under general anesthesia in the near future.

Possible Side Effects (natural, expected, and unavoidable drug actions)

Moderate drowsiness; abnormally low blood pressure on standing (orthostatic hypotension); light-headedness (low blood pressure); blurred vision; dry mouth (xerostomia)—frequent; constipation; impaired urination. Increased appetite, weight gain.

▷ **Possible Adverse Effects** (unusual, unexpected, and infrequent reactions)

If any of the following develop, consult your physician promptly for guidance.

Mild Adverse Effects

Allergic reactions: skin rash, hives, swelling of face or tongue, drug fever (see Glossary).

Headache, dizziness, nervousness, weakness, unsteadiness, tremors, fainting—possible to rare.

Sleep disturbances, ringing in the ears—case reports.

Irritation of tongue or mouth, dental cavities, altered taste, indigestion, nausea—possible.

Fluctuations of blood sugar—case reports.

Serious Adverse Effects

Allergic reactions: drug-induced hepatitis, with or without jaundice; anaphylactic reaction (see these terms in Glossary).

Idiosyncratic reactions: neuroleptic malignant syndrome (see Glossary).

Adverse behavioral effects: delirium, delusions, hallucinations, Tourette's syndrome—case reports to rare.

Porphyria or abnormal urine excretion (SIADH)—rare.

Liver or kidney toxicity—rare.

Drug-induced myasthenia gravis—case reports.

Seizures, reduced control of epilepsy—possible.

Eye changes (glaucoma, ophthalmoplegia)—case reports.

Heart rhythm disturbances or spasm of blood vessels—case reports.

Abnormally low white blood cell and platelet counts: fever, sore throat, infections, abnormal bleeding or bruising—case reports.

▷ **Possible Effects on Sexual Function:**   Decreased libido, increased libido (antidepressant effect)—possible.

Impaired erection or ejaculation—frequent; impotence, inhibited male orgasm—case reports to infrequent; inhibited female orgasm—may be frequent.

Male breast enlargement and tenderness, female breast enlargement with milk production, swelling of testicles—case reports.

▷ **Adverse Effects That May Mimic Natural Diseases or Disorders**

Liver toxicity may suggest viral hepatitis.

Natural Diseases or Disorders That May Be Activated by This Drug

Latent diabetes, epilepsy, glaucoma, prostatism.

Possible Effects on Laboratory Tests

Complete blood cell counts: decreased white cells and platelets; increased eosinophils (allergic reaction).

Blood glucose levels: increased and decreased (fluctuations).

Liver function tests: increased liver enzymes (ALT/GPT, AST/GOT, and alkaline phosphatase), increased bilirubin.

CAUTION

1. Look for early signs of toxicity or overdose: confusion, agitation, rapid heart rate, heart irregularity. Measurement of the drug blood level will clarify the situation.
2. Use with caution in treating depression associated with schizophrenia. Watch for deterioration of thinking or behavior.
3. It is advisable to withhold this drug if electroconvulsive therapy (ECT) is to be used to treat depression.

Precautions for Use

By Infants and Children: Safety and effectiveness for use by those under 6 years of age have not been established. Children (6 to 12 years of age) may be more susceptible than adults to heart toxicity from this or related drugs.

Bed-wetting (enuresis): children 6 or older have been given 25 mg by mouth an hour before bedtime. Dose and management should be supervised by a properly trained pediatrician.

By Those Over 60 Years of Age: Treatment is started with 25 mg at bedtime. Dose may be increased gradually as needed and tolerated to 100 mg daily in divided doses. During the first 2 weeks of treatment, observe for behavioral reactions: restlessness, agitation, forgetfulness, disorientation, delusions, or hallucinations. Also observe for unsteadiness and instability that may predispose to falling. This drug may aggravate prostatism.

▷ **Advisability of Use During Pregnancy**

Pregnancy Category: D. See Pregnancy Risk Categories at the back of this book.

Animal studies: Skeletal defects reported in rabbit studies. No defects reported in mouse, rat, and monkey studies.

Human studies: Information from adequate studies of pregnant women is not available. Case reports of fetal respiratory distress, convulsions.

Ask your doctor for guidance.

Advisability of Use If Breast-Feeding

Presence of this drug in breast milk: Yes, in small amounts.

Monitor nursing infant closely and discontinue drug or nursing if adverse effects develop.

Habit-Forming Potential: Psychological or physical dependence is possible. A withdrawal syndrome has been described.

Effects of Overdose: Confusion, hallucinations, drowsiness, tremors, heart irregularity, seizures, stupor, hypothermia (see Glossary) early, fever later.

Possible Effects of Long-Term Use: Neuroleptic malignant syndrome (see Glossary): fever, fast or irregular heartbeat, fast breathing, sweating, weakness, muscle stiffness, seizures, loss of bladder control.

Suggested Periodic Examinations While Taking This Drug (at physician's discretion)

Monitoring of blood drug levels as appropriate.

Complete blood cell counts; liver and kidney function tests.

Serial blood pressure readings and electrocardiograms.

Measurement of internal eye pressure.

▷ **While Taking This Drug, Observe the Following**

Foods: No specific restrictions. May need to limit food intake to avoid excessive weight gain. Vitamin C in large doses (more than 2 g per day) may require higher imipramine doses.

Beverages: No restrictions. May be taken with milk.

▷ *Alcohol:* Avoid completely. This drug can markedly increase the intoxicating effects of alcohol; the combination can depress brain function significantly.

Tobacco Smoking: May accelerate the elimination of this drug and require increased dose. I advise everyone to quit.

Marijuana Smoking: Increased drowsiness and mouth dryness; possible reduced effectiveness of this drug. Excessive increases in heart rate.

▷ *Other Drugs Imipramine may **increase** the effects of*
- all drugs with atropinelike effects (see **anticholinergic drugs** in Drug Classes).

- all drugs with sedative effects; observe for excessive sedation.
- norepinephrine.
- phenytoin (Dilantin).
- warfarin (Coumadin) and require more frequent INR testing.

Imipramine may *decrease* the effects of
- clonidine (Catapres).
- guanadrel (Hylorel).
- guanethidine (Ismelin, Esimil).
- guanfacine (Tenex).

Imipramine *taken concurrently* with
- anticonvulsants requires careful monitoring for changes in seizure patterns and need to adjust anticonvulsant dose.
- antihistamines (see Drug Classes) may result in urinary retention, acute glaucoma, or excessive anticholinergic actions.
- bepridil (Vascor) may increase risk of abnormal heartbeats.
- ethchlorvynol (Placidyl) may cause delirium; avoid concurrent use.
- grepafloxacin (Raxar) increases risk of abnormal heartbeats.
- meperidine (Demerol) may result in increased meperidine-caused depression of breathing.
- monoamine oxidase (MAO) type A inhibitor drugs (see Drug Classes) may cause high fever, seizures, and excessive rise in blood pressure; avoid concurrent use of these drugs and provide periods of 14 days between dosing of either.
- ritonavir (Norvir) and perhaps other protease inhibitors (see Drug Classes) may lead to toxicity.
- sparfloxacin (Zagam) increases risk of abnormal heart beats.
- stimulant drugs (amphetamine, cocaine, epinephrine, phenylpropanolamine, etc.) may cause severe high blood pressure and/or high fever.
- thyroid preparations may increase the risk of heart rhythm disorders.
- tramadol (Ultram) can increase seizure risk.

The following drugs may *increase* the effects of imipramine:
- cimetidine (Tagamet).
- diltiazem (Cardizem).
- estrogens (various) (birth control pills).
- fluoxetine (Prozac).
- fluvoxamine (Luvox).
- labetalol (Normodyne).
- methylphenidate (Ritalin).
- oral contraceptives.
- phenothiazines (see Drug Classes).
- quinidine (Quinaglute, others).
- ranitidine (Zantac).
- venlafaxine (Effexor); increases imipramine metabolite.

The following drugs may *decrease* the effects of imipramine:
- barbiturates (see Drug Classes).
- carbamazepine (Tegretol).
- chloral hydrate (Noctec, Somnos, etc.).
- lithium (Lithobid, Lithotab, etc.).
- reserpine (Serpasil, Ser-Ap-Es, etc.).
- vitamin C (if more than 2 g per day are taken).

▷ *Driving, Hazardous Activities:* This drug may impair mental alertness, judgment, physical coordination, and reaction time. Restrict activities as necessary.

Aviation Note: The use of this drug *is a disqualification* for piloting. Consult a designated aviation medical examiner.

Exposure to Sun: Use caution until sensitivity has been determined. This drug may cause photosensitivity (see Glossary).

Exposure to Heat: Use caution. This drug can inhibit sweating and impair the body's adaptation to hot environments, increasing the risk of heatstroke. Avoid saunas.

Exposure to Cold: The elderly should use caution and avoid conditions conducive to hypothermia (see Glossary).

Exposure to Environmental Chemicals: This drug may mask the symptoms of poisoning due to handling certain insecticides (organophosphorus types). Read their labels carefully.

Discontinuation: It is advisable to discontinue this drug gradually over a period of 3 to 4 weeks. Abrupt withdrawal after prolonged use may cause nausea, vomiting, diarrhea, headache, malaise, disturbed sleep, and vivid dreaming. When this drug is stopped, it may be necessary to adjust the doses of other drugs taken concurrently.

INDAPAMIDE (in DAP a mide)

Introduced: 1974   **Class:** Antihypertensive, diuretic   **Prescription:** USA: Yes   **Controlled Drug:** USA: No; Canada: No   **Available as Generic:** Yes

Brand Names: ✦Lozide, Lozol

BENEFITS versus RISKS	
Possible Benefits	*Possible Risks*
EFFECTIVE ONCE-A-DAY TREATMENT OF MILD TO MODERATE HYPERTENSION	Excessive loss of blood potassium or magnesium
EFFECTIVE, MILD DIURETIC	Increased blood sugar level
	Increased blood uric acid level

▷ **Principal Uses**

As a Single Drug Product: Uses currently included in FDA-approved labeling: (1) Increases urine output (diuresis) to correct fluid retention seen in congestive heart failure (edema); (2) used as starting therapy in high blood pressure (hypertension).

Other (unlabeled) generally accepted uses: (1) Helps ease the excessive elimination of calcium in the urine (hypercalciuria); (2) may help protect the heart after blood-flow problems (preserves ischemic heart from reperfusion injury).

How This Drug Works: Increases elimination of salt and water (through increased urine production). Relaxes the walls of smaller arteries and decreases pressure reactions (angiotensin II). The combined effects lower blood pressure.

Available Dose Forms and Strengths

Tablets — 1.25 mg, 2.5 mg

▷ **Usual Adult Dose Range:**   Hypertension: 1.25 mg per day, as a single dose in the morning. If needed, the dose may be increased to 2.5 mg/day after 4 weeks. Use in treating edema may require a starting dose of 2.5 mg. Maximum total daily dose is 5 mg. (In Canada, the total daily dose limit is given as 2.5 mg.) **Note: Actual dose and dosing schedule must be determined for each individual patient.**

Conditions Requiring Dosing Adjustments
Liver Function: Should be used with caution and in decreased doses by patients with liver problems. Blood chemistry (electrolytes) should be closely followed.
Kidney Function: Must be stopped if kidney failure progresses after indapamide is started.

▷ **Dosing Instructions:**   The tablet may be crushed and taken with or following food to reduce stomach upset. Take in the morning to avoid nighttime urination.

Usual Duration of Use: Use on a regular schedule for 2 to 4 weeks determines peak effect in lowering blood pressure. Long-term use (months to years) requires periodic physician evaluation.

Possible Advantages of This Drug
Causes no significant increase in blood cholesterol levels.
Less likely to cause significant loss of potassium.

▷ **This Drug Should Not Be Taken If**
- you have had an allergic reaction to it previously.
- your kidneys are not making any urine.

▷ **Inform Your Physician Before Taking This Drug If**
- you are allergic to any form of "sulfa" drug.
- you are pregnant or planning a pregnancy.
- you presently have an excessively low blood potassium.
- you have a history of kidney or liver disease.
- you have diabetes, gout, or lupus erythematosus.
- you take any form of cortisone, digoxin, oral antidiabetic drug, or insulin.
- you have had a sympathectomy.
- you plan to have surgery under general anesthesia in the near future.

Possible Side Effects (natural, expected, and unavoidable drug actions)
Light-headedness on arising from sitting or lying position (see orthostatic hypotension in Glossary).
Increase in blood sugar level, affecting control of diabetes.
Increase in blood uric acid level, affecting control of gout.
Decrease in blood potassium level, causing muscle weakness and cramping.
Low blood sodium and magnesium.

▷ **Possible Adverse Effects** (unusual, unexpected, and infrequent reactions)
If any of the following develop, consult your physician promptly for guidance.
Mild Adverse Effects
Allergic reactions: skin rashes, hives, itching—infrequent.
Headache, dizziness, drowsiness, weakness, lethargy, visual disturbance—case reports.
Reduced appetite, indigestion, nausea, vomiting, diarrhea—rare.

Paresthesias—rare.

Urination at night—possible, especially with evening dosing.

Serious Adverse Effects

Abnormal heartbeat (premature ventricular contractions)—rare.

Liver or kidney toxicity—rare.

Serious skin rashes (Stevens-Johnson syndrome, toxic epidermal necrolysis)—case reports.

▷ **Possible Effects on Sexual Function:**   Decreased libido—infrequent; impotence—rare.

Natural Diseases or Disorders That May Be Activated by This Drug

Diabetes, gout, systemic lupus erythematosus.

Possible Effects on Laboratory Tests

Total cholesterol and LDL cholesterol levels: no effect or slightly increased.

Blood HDL cholesterol level: no effect or slightly decreased.

Blood potassium, magnesium, or sodium level: decreased.

Blood uric acid level or blood sugar (glucose): increased.

CAUTION

1. Take exactly as prescribed—excessive doses can cause excessive sodium and potassium loss (decreased appetite, nausea, fatigue, confusion, or tingling extremities).
2. If you take a digitalis preparation (digitoxin, digoxin), ensure intake of high potassium foods to help avoid digitalis toxicity. (See Table 13, "High-Potassium Foods," Section Six.)

Precautions for Use

By Infants and Children: Safety and effectiveness for those under 12 years of age are not established.

By Those Over 60 Years of Age: It is best to start with small doses. You may be more susceptible to impaired thinking, orthostatic hypotension, potassium loss, and blood sugar increase. Overdose or extended use causes excessive loss of body water, thickening (increased viscosity) of blood, and an increased tendency for the blood to clot—predisposing to stroke, heart attack, or thrombophlebitis (vein inflammation with blood clot).

▷ **Advisability of Use During Pregnancy**

Pregnancy Category: B, D by one researcher. See Pregnancy Risk Categories at the back of this book.

Animal studies: No birth defects reported.

Human studies: Data from studies of pregnant women are not available.

This drug should not be used during pregnancy unless a very serious complication occurs for which it is significantly beneficial. Ask your physician for guidance.

Advisability of Use If Breast-Feeding

Presence of this drug in breast milk: Unknown.

Avoid drug or refrain from nursing.

Habit-Forming Potential: None.

Effects of Overdose: Dry mouth, thirst, lethargy, weakness, muscle cramping, nausea, vomiting, drowsiness progressing to stupor or coma.

Possible Effects of Long-Term Use: Impaired balance of water, salt, and potassium in blood and body tissues. Development of diabetes in predisposed individuals.

Suggested Periodic Examinations While Taking This Drug (at physician's discretion)

Measurements of blood levels of sodium, potassium, chloride, sugar, and uric acid.

▷ **While Taking This Drug, Observe the Following**

Foods: Ask about a high-potassium diet. If so advised, see Table 13, "High-Potassium Foods," in Section Six. Follow your doctor's advice about salt use.

Beverages: No restrictions. This drug may be taken with milk.

▷ *Alcohol:* Alcohol may exaggerate the blood-pressure-lowering effects of this drug and cause orthostatic hypotension.

Tobacco Smoking: No interactions expected. I advise everyone to quit smoking.

▷ *Other Drugs Indapamide may **increase** the effects of*

- other antihypertensive drugs; dose adjustments may be necessary to prevent excessive lowering of blood pressure.
- lithium (Lithobid, others), and cause lithium toxicity.

Indapamide may ***decrease*** the effects of

- oral antidiabetic drugs (sulfonylureas); dose adjustments may be needed for proper control of blood sugar.

Indapamide ***taken concurrently*** with

- digitalis preparations (digitoxin, digoxin) must be followed closely and adjustments made to prevent fluctuations of blood potassium levels and serious disturbances of heart rhythm.
- NSAIDs (see ***nonsteroidal anti-inflammatory drugs*** in Drug Classes) may blunt the therapeutic benefit of indapamide.

The following drugs may ***decrease*** the effects of indapamide:

- cholestyramine (Cuemid, Questran)—may interfere with its absorption.
- colestipol (Colestid)—may interfere with its absorption.

Take cholestyramine and colestipol 1 hour before any oral diuretic.

▷ *Driving, Hazardous Activities:* Use caution until the possible occurrence of orthostatic hypotension, drowsiness, dizziness, or impaired vision has been determined.

Aviation Note: The use of this drug ***may be a disqualification*** for piloting. Consult a designated aviation medical examiner.

Exposure to Sun: No restrictions.

Exposure to Heat: Excessive perspiring could cause additional loss of salt and water.

Heavy Exercise or Exertion: Isometric exercises can raise blood pressure significantly. Ask your physician for help.

Occurrence of Unrelated Illness: Vomiting or diarrhea can produce a serious imbalance of important body chemistry. Consult your physician for guidance.

Discontinuation: It may be advisable to discontinue this drug 5 to 7 days before major surgery. Ask your physician, surgeon, and/or anesthesiologist for guidance.

INDOMETHACIN (in doh METH a sin)

See the acetic acids (nonsteroidal anti-inflammatory drugs) profile for further information.

INFLUENZA VACCINE (IN flu en za VAX ceen)

Other Names: Flu vaccine

Introduced: Specific formulation for each year   **Class:** Antiviral   **Prescription:** USA: Yes   **Controlled Drug:** USA: No; Canada: No   **Available as Generic:** USA: No; Canada: No

Brand Names: Fluogen, Flu-Immune, Flu-Shield, Fluzone

> **Author's Note: For the 1998–1999 flu season the shot (vaccine) will have two new viruses: A/Beijing/262/95 and A/Sidney/5/97. The vaccine will also offer B/Harbin/7/94 as in previous vaccines. An intranasal spray form is being studied.**

Warning: Since the vaccine is formulated to contain the viral strains expected to cause the most serious problems in a given year, the side effects or adverse effects may differ annually.

BENEFITS versus RISKS	
Possible Benefits	*Possible Risks*
PREVENTION OF INFLUENZA CAUSED BY THE MOST SERIOUS OR PREVALENT VIRAL STRAINS IDENTIFIED FOR A GIVEN YEAR	GUILLAIN-BARRÉ SYNDROME (questionable causation) Hypersensitivity
Possible cross protection from other similar virus strains	

▷ **Principal Uses**

As a Single Drug Product: Uses currently included in FDA-approved labeling: Prevention of influenza.

Other (unlabeled) generally accepted uses: (1) Used in patients with compromised immune systems (such as HIV-positive, cancer, and bone marrow transplant patients); (2) can be of use in isolated outbreaks such as in nursing homes or military camps; (3) may decrease the number of middle ear infections in children who attend day-care centers.

How This Drug Works: Vaccine made of purified parts of the virus surface, split virus, or whole virus, which has been inactivated. When injected, it stimulates the immune system to make antibodies. The antibodies (2 weeks after vaccination) act to reduce disease severity or decrease probability of infection by the expected flu viruses.

Available Dose Forms and Strengths

Typical split virus: 15 mcg/0.5 ml of each of the three selected strains.

How To Store   This vaccine is ideally stored in the refrigerator. If this is how storage is accomplished, the outdate specified by the manufacturer is valid. If the vaccine is stored at room temperature, it is stable for up to 7 days.

▷ **Recommended Dose Ranges** (Actual dose and schedule must be determined for each patient and each flu season individually.)

Infants and Children: Those 6 to 35 months old should be given 0.25 ml of a split-dose vaccine. If this is the first vaccination, two doses should be given 1 month apart. Split dose is suggested for children because it tends to cause fewer undesirable effects. For infants and young children, the vaccine is usually given in the thigh muscle.

Children 3 to 8 years old should be given 0.5 ml of the selected split-virus vaccine. Children in this age range who have not been previously vaccinated should be given two vaccinations, 1 month apart.

Children 9 years old or older should be given a single vaccination of 0.5 ml of split-virus vaccine in the deltoid muscle.

13 to 60 Years of Age: Should be given 0.5 ml of whole or split-virus vaccine in the deltoid muscle.

Over 60 Years of Age: Same as 13 to 60 years of age.

Conditions Requiring Dosing Adjustments
Liver Function: Not involved.
Kidney Function: Not involved.

▷ **Dosing Instructions:** Prior vaccination **does not** mean you are immune to the current year's virus strains. Some tenderness at the injection site is possible. Fever and muscular aches or pains are also possible and may be treated with acetaminophen (Tylenol, others).

Usual Duration of Use: Single vaccination confers relative immunity to the expected viral strains in 2 weeks. This does **not** confer immunity to all strains of virus capable of causing an influenzalike (flu-like) syndrome. Annual vaccination is strongly suggested.

Possible Advantages of This Drug
Allows the prevention of a viral syndrome that can cause loss of several weeks of work in younger, otherwise healthy patients or serious illness in older or compromised patients.

Currently a "Drug of Choice"
For prevention of type A influenza due to the viral strains that are of the greatest concern in the current flu season.

▷ **This Drug Should Not Be Taken If**
• you have had an allergic reaction to any dose form of it previously.
• you are allergic to eggs (the virus is grown on eggs).
• you have an acute illness and a fever.

▷ **Inform Your Physician Before Taking This Drug If**
• you are HIV-positive.
• you have a history of blood disorders.
• you have had Guillain-Barré syndrome.
• you have a history of seizures.
• you have been receiving cancer therapy (chemotherapy).

Possible Side Effects (natural, expected, and unavoidable drug actions)
Pain at the vaccination site. Muscle aches, fever, or bothersome tiredness (malaise). This is **not** the flu. The vaccine contains viral fragments or non-infectious virus. These symptoms are a reaction to the components of the vaccine.

▷ **Possible Adverse Effects** (unusual, unexpected, and infrequent reactions)
If any of the following develop, consult your physician promptly for guidance.

Mild Adverse Effects
Allergic reactions: swelling and redness—possible.
Muscle aches or fever—infrequent.
Fatigue, nausea, and headache—infrequent.
Vasculitis (joint pain, weakness, fever, and rash)—rare.

Serious Adverse Effects
Allergic reactions: anaphylactic reactions.
Low blood platelets or pericarditis case reports.
Guillain-Barré syndrome (only reported during the 1976–1977 flu season and of questionable causation).
Kidney toxicity—case report.
Vision changes—case report.

▷ **Possible Effects on Sexual Function:**   None reported.

Possible Delayed Adverse Effects: None reported.

▷ **Adverse Effects That May Mimic Natural Diseases or Disorders**
Reaction to vaccine contents may mimic the flu.

Natural Diseases or Disorders That May Be Activated by This Drug
None reported.

Possible Effects on Laboratory Tests
Hepatitis B test: false positive.
Hepatitis C test: false positive.
HTLV-1 test: false positive.

CAUTION
1. A vaccine in the previous year does **not** confer immunity to the flu in following years.
2. The flu vaccine confers immunity to viruses predicted to cause influenza in a particular flu season. Vaccine does not confer immunity to all strains of virus capable of causing a flu-like syndrome.
3. If muscle aches or fever occur after vaccination, acetaminophen (Tylenol, others) is recommended. **Do not** take aspirin, and especially *do not* give aspirin to children.
4. Call your doctor immediately if you develop hives, facial swelling, or difficulty breathing after the vaccination.
5. It is ALWAYS better to prevent a disease or condition than to have to treat it. Talk with your doctor or pharmacist. If you do not have a medical reason for avoiding a flu shot—get one!

Precautions for Use
By Infants and Children: Safety and effectiveness for use by those under 6 months of age have not been established.
By Those Over 60 Years of Age: The vaccine is especially **valuable** in this age group, as the effects of the flu may be devastating.

▷ **Advisability of Use During Pregnancy**
Pregnancy Category: C. See Pregnancy Risk Categories at the back of this book.
Animal studies: Animal studies have not been conducted.

Human studies: Information from adequate studies of pregnant women is not available. Ask your doctor for guidance.

Advisability of Use If Breast-Feeding

Presence of this drug in breast milk: Not defined.

Monitor nursing infant closely and contact your doctor if adverse effects develop. The CDC has **not** listed breast-feeding as a precaution against receiving this vaccine.

Habit-Forming Potential: None.

Effects of Overdose: No specific cases reported. Treatment would be consistent with any symptoms of the patient.

Possible Effects of Long-Term Use: Not indicated for long-term use.

Suggested Periodic Examinations While Taking This Drug (at physician's discretion)

None indicated.

▷ **While Taking This Drug, Observe the Following**

Foods: No restrictions.

Beverages: No restrictions.

▷ *Alcohol:* No restrictions.

Tobacco Smoking: No interactions expected. I advise everyone to quit smoking.

▷ *Other Drugs*

Influenza vaccine may *increase* the effects of

• carbamazepine (Tegretol), by decreasing the elimination of the drug.

• phenobarbital, by increasing the half-life of the drug.

• theophylline (Theo-Dur, others), by increasing the blood level of the drug.

• warfarin (Coumadin), and pose an increased risk of bleeding. More frequent INR (prothrombin time or protime) testing is suggested.

Influenza vaccine *taken concurrently* with

• cyclosporine (Sandimmune) can cause blunting of the immune response to the vaccine.

• immunosuppressive agents (chemotherapy, corticosteroids) may impair or blunt immune response to the vaccine.

• methotrexate (Rheumatrex) can result in blunting of the immune response to this vaccine.

• phenytoin (Dilantin) has had variable effects on the blood levels of this drug.

▷ *Driving, Hazardous Activities:* This drug may cause excessive tiredness and muscle aches. Restrict activities as necessary.

Aviation Note: The use of this drug *may be a short-term disqualification* for piloting. Consult a designated aviation medical examiner.

Exposure to Sun: No restrictions.

Exposure to Heat: Since this vaccine may cause short-duration fevers, it is wise to avoid hot environments for a day after vaccination.

Heavy Exercise or Exertion: A fever may result and it is wise to avoid strenuous exercise for a day after vaccination.

Special Storage Instructions: This vaccine is ideally stored in the refrigerator. If this is how storage is accomplished, the outdate specified by the manufacturer is valid.

Observe the Following Expiration Times: If the vaccine is stored at room temperature, it is stable for up to 7 days.

Author's Note: There is now a Vaccine Adverse Event Reporting System (VAERS). The toll-free number is 1-800-822-7967.

INSULIN (IN suh lin)

Introduced: 1922   **Class:** Antidiabetic   **Prescription:** USA: No
Controlled Drug: USA: No; Canada: No   **Available as Generic:**   Yes
Brand Names: Humalog, Humulin BR, Humulin L, Humulin N, Humulin R, Humulin U, Humulin U Ultralente, Humulin 70/30, Humulin 30/70, Iletin I NPH, Iletin II Pork, ✦Initard, Insulatard NPH, ✦Insulin Human, ✦Insulin-Toronto, Lente Iletin I, Lente Iletin II Beef, Lente Iletin II Pork, Lente Insulin, Lente Purified Pork, Mixtard, Mixtard Human 70/30, Novolin L, Novolin N, NovolinPen, Novolin R, Novolin 30/70, Novolin 70/30, ✦Novolin-Lente, ✦Novolin-NPH, Novolin-70/30, ✦Novolin-Toronto, ✦Novolin-Ultralente, ✦Novolinset, ✦Novolinset 30/70, ✦Novolinset NPH, ✦Novolinset Toronto, NPH Iletin I, NPH Iletin II Beef, NPH Iletin II Pork, NPH Insulin, NPH Purified Pork, Protamine, Zinc & Iletin I, Protamine, Zinc & Iletin II Beef, Protamine, Zinc & Iletin II Pork, Regular Concentrated Iletin II, Regular Iletin I, Regular Iletin II Beef, Regular Iletin II Pork, Regular Iletin II U-500, Regular Insulin, Regular Purified Pork Insulin, Semilente Iletin I, Semilente Insulin, Semilente Purified Pork, Ultralente Iletin I, Ultralente Insulin, Ultralente Purified Beef, Velosulin, ✦Velosulin Cartridge, Velosulin Human
Author's Note: Lilly will stop making all their mixed beef/pork insulins in 1998 (Iletin I).

BENEFITS versus RISKS	
Possible Benefits	*Possible Risks*
EFFECTIVE CONTROL OF TYPE 1 (INSULIN-DEPENDENT) DIABETES MELLITUS TIGHT CONTROL OF BLOOD SUGAR MAY AVOID OR DELAY DEVELOPMENT OF HIGH BLOOD PRESSURE, KIDNEY, HEART, NERVE, EYE, OR OTHER DAMAGE THAT HAPPENS WHEN BLOOD SUGAR IS OUT OF CONTROL	HYPOGLYCEMIA WITH EXCESSIVE DOSE Infrequent allergic reactions

▷ **Principal Uses**

As a Single Drug Product: Uses currently included in FDA-approved labeling: (1) Used in diabetes mellitus that is insulin-dependent, and by people who have non-insulin-dependent diabetes who are experiencing stress such as illness; (2) used to control blood sugar in critically ill patients who are being fed by intravenous nutrient mixtures.

Other (unlabeled) generally accepted uses: (1) Controls blood sugar in pregnancy (gestational diabetes); (2) insulin in combination with glucagon has been used in alcoholic hepatitis; (3) may have a role in combination therapy with an oral hypoglycemic agent in some diabetics; (4) helps diabetic ketoacidosis; (5) can help diabetic neuropathy and retinopathy; (6) can be of help in critically ill patients with maple syrup urine disease.

How This Drug Works: Insulin helps sugar move through the cell wall to the inside of the cell (action on cell membranes), where it is used for energy.

Available Dose Forms and Strengths
>   Injections — 40, 100, and 500 units per ml
>   PenFil cartridges — 150 units

▷ **Usual Adult Dose Range:**   According to individual requirements for the best regulation of blood sugar on a 24-hour basis. **Note: Actual dose and schedule must be determined for each patient individually.**

Conditions Requiring Dosing Adjustments
Liver Function: Specific adjustment guidelines are not available.
Kidney Function: Caution should be used by patients with compromised kidneys. Requirements become extremely variable.
Thyrotoxicosis: Glucose utilization is typically increased and insulin requirements may actually decrease.

▷ **Dosing Instructions:**   Inject insulin subcutaneously according to the schedule prescribed by your physician. The timing and frequency of injections will vary with the type of insulin prescribed. The following table of insulin actions (according to type) will help you understand the treatment schedule prescribed for you.

Insulin Type	Action Onset	Peak	Duration
Insulin lispro	0.25 hr	0.5–1.5 hrs	3–4 hrs
Regular	0.5–1 hr	2–4 hrs	5–7 hrs
Isophane (NPH)	3–4 hrs	6–12 hrs	18–28 hrs
Regular 30%/NPH 70%	0.5 hr	4–8 hrs	24 hrs
Semilente	1–3 hrs	2–8 hrs	12–16 hrs
Lente	1–3 hrs	8–12 hrs	18–28 hrs
Ultralente	4–6 hrs	18–24 hrs	36 hrs
Protamine Zinc	4–6 hrs	14–24 hrs	36 hrs

Usual Duration of Use: In Type 1 insulin-dependent (juvenile-onset) diabetes mellitus, insulin therapy is usually required for life. Type 2 non-insulin-dependent (maturity-onset) diabetes may be controlled by oral antidiabetic drugs and/or diet, but can require insulin when you have a serious infection, injuries, burns, surgical procedures, and other physical stress. See your doctor on a regular basis.

▷ **This Drug Should Not Be Taken If**
   • the need for insulin and its dose schedule has not been established by a qualified physician.

▷ **Inform Your Physician Before Taking This Drug If**
   • you have an insulin allergy.
   • you do not know how to recognize and treat abnormally low blood sugar (see *hypoglycemia* in Glossary).
   • you are pregnant.
   • you take aspirin, beta-blockers, fenfluramine (Pondimin), monoamine oxidase (MAO) type A inhibitors (see Drug Classes).

Possible Side Effects (natural, expected, and unavoidable drug actions)

In stable diabetes, no side effects occur when insulin dose, diet, and physical activity are correctly balanced and maintained. In unstable ("brittle") diabetes, unexpected drops in blood sugar levels can occur, resulting in hypoglycemia (see Glossary).

Weight gain.

▷ **Possible Adverse Effects** (unusual, unexpected, and infrequent reactions)

If any of the following develop, consult your physician promptly for guidance.

Mild Adverse Effects

Allergic reactions: local redness, swelling, and itching at site of injection, or hives—infrequent.

Taste disorders—possible.

Thinning of subcutaneous tissue at sites of injection—infrequent.

Serious Adverse Effects

Allergic reaction: anaphylactic reactions (see Glossary).

Severe, prolonged hypoglycemia—possible to infrequent.

Inflammation of the parotid (parotitis)—case reports.

Hemolytic anemia or porphyria—case reports.

Arrhythmias (associated with hypoglycemia) or very fast heart rate (with intravenous use)—case reports.

▷ **Possible Effects on Sexual Function:** May resolve sexual dysfunction in patients who have this prior to starting insulin therapy. May also cause decrease in libido and erectile dysfunction—case reports (may also be a result of nerve/blood vessel damage).

▷ **Adverse Effects That May Mimic Natural Diseases or Disorders**

The early signs of hypoglycemia may be mistaken for alcoholic intoxication.

Possible Effects on Laboratory Tests

Blood cholesterol level: decreased.

Blood glucose level: decreased.

Blood potassium level: decreased.

Glycosylated hemoglobin (hemoglobin A1-C): decreased.

CAUTION

1. Carry a card in your purse or wallet with a notation that you have diabetes and are taking insulin.

2. Know how to recognize hypoglycemia and how to treat it. Always carry a readily available form of sugar, such as hard candy or sugar cubes. Report all episodes of hypoglycemia to your doctor.

3. Your vision may improve during the first few weeks of insulin therapy. Postpone eye exams for eyeglasses for 6 weeks after starting insulin.

4. Insulin is absorbed more quickly or slowly depending on where it is injected. Absorption is 80% greater from the abdominal wall than from the leg, and 30% greater than from the arm. It is advisable to rotate the injection site within the same body region than from one site to another.

5. The American Diabetic Association (ADA) now says that a person is considered diabetic if two fasting blood sugars in a row are more than 125 mg/dl. This more conservative approach reflects new information saying that complications start at lower blood sugar levels than previously thought.

Precautions for Use

By Infants and Children: Insulin doses and schedules are modified according to patient's size. Adhere strictly to the physician's prescribed routine.

By Those Over 60 Years of Age: Insulin needs may change with age. Periodic individual evaluation is needed to identify the best dose and schedule. The aging brain adapts well to higher blood sugar levels. Rigid attempts at tight sugar control may result in hypoglycemia that shows as confusion and abnormal behavior. Repeated hypoglycemia (especially if severe) may cause brain damage.

▷ **Advisability of Use During Pregnancy**

Pregnancy Category: B. See Pregnancy Risk Categories at the back of this book. Animal studies: Inconclusive.

Human studies: Adequate studies of pregnant women are not available. Birth defects occur two to four times more frequently in infants of diabetic mothers than in infants of mothers who do not have diabetes. The exact causes of this are not known. Insulin is the drug of choice for managing diabetes during pregnancy. To preserve the health of the mother and fetus, every effort must be made to establish the best dose of insulin necessary for good control and to prevent episodes of hypoglycemia.

Advisability of Use If Breast-Feeding

Presence of this drug in breast milk: No.

Insulin treatment of the mother has no adverse effect on the nursing infant. Breast-feeding may decrease insulin requirements; dose adjustment may be necessary.

Habit-Forming Potential: None; however, cases of surreptitious insulin injection have been reported.

Effects of Overdose: Hypoglycemia: fatigue, weakness, headache, nervousness, irritability, sweating, tremors, hunger, confusion, delirium, abnormal behavior (resembling alcoholic intoxication), loss of consciousness, seizures.

Possible Effects of Long-Term Use: Thinning of subcutaneous fat tissue at sites of insulin injection. Insulin resistance.

Suggested Periodic Examinations While Taking This Drug (at physician's discretion)

Historically, estimates of blood sugar were obtained by checking urine sugar. This method has been replaced by fingerstick testing of blood glucose. Fingerstick testing accurately reflects the blood sugar and helps ensure better control (tighter control) of blood glucose. If you are ill, increased frequency of fingerstick blood glucose testing may be indicated. Routine testing of blood sugar levels at intervals recommended by your physician is prudent.

▷ **While Taking This Drug, Observe the Following**

Foods: Follow your diabetic diet conscientiously. Do not omit snack foods in mid-afternoon or at bedtime if they help prevent hypoglycemia.

Beverages: According to prescribed diabetic diet.

▷ *Alcohol:* Used excessively, alcohol can cause severe hypoglycemia, resulting in brain damage.

Tobacco Smoking: Regular smoking can decrease insulin absorption and increase insulin requirements by 30%. It is advisable to stop smoking altogether.

Marijuana Smoking: Possible increase in blood sugar levels.

▷   *Other Drugs*
The following drugs may ***increase*** the effects of insulin:
- acarbose (Precose)—by decreasing the amount of sugar that insulin has to work on.
- aspirin and other salicylates.
- some beta-blocker drugs (especially the nonselective ones; see Drug Classes)—may prolong insulin-induced hypoglycemia.
- clofibrate (Atromid-S).
- fenfluramine (Pondimin).
- monoamine oxidase (MAO) type A inhibitors (see Drug Classes).
- oral antidiabetic drugs (see Drug Classes)—results in additive hypoglycemia.

The following drugs may ***decrease*** the effects of insulin (by raising blood sugar levels):
- birth control pills (oral contraceptives).
- chlorthalidone (Hygroton).
- cortisonelike drugs (see ***adrenocortical steroids*** in Drug Classes).
- furosemide (Lasix).
- phenytoin (Dilantin, etc.).
- thiazide diuretics (see Drug Classes).
- thyroid preparations (various).

▷   *Driving, Hazardous Activities:* Be prepared to stop and take corrective action if hypoglycemia develops.

Aviation Note: Diabetes and the use of this drug ***are disqualifications*** for piloting. Consult a designated aviation medical examiner.

Exposure to Sun: No restrictions.

Exposure to Heat: Use caution. Sauna baths can significantly increase the rate of insulin absorption and cause hypoglycemia.

Heavy Exercise or Exertion: Use caution. Periods of unusual or unplanned heavy physical activity will use up sugar more quickly and predispose to hypoglycemia.

Occurrence of Unrelated Illness: Omission of meals as a result of nausea, vomiting, or injury may lead to hypoglycemia. Infections can increase insulin needs. Ask your doctor for help.

Discontinuation: Do not stop this drug without asking your doctor. Omission of insulin may result in life-threatening coma.

Special Storage Instructions: Keep in a cool place, preferably in the refrigerator. Protect from freezing. Protect from strong light and high temperatures when not refrigerated.

Observe the Following Expiration Times: Do not use this drug if it is older than the expiration date on the vial. Always use fresh, "within-date" insulin.

INSULIN LISPRO (IN suh lin LIS proh)

Introduced: 1996   **Class:** Antidiabetic   **Prescription:** USA: No
Controlled Drug: USA: No; Canada: No   **Available as Generic:** No
Brand Name: Humalog

```
┌─────────────────────────────────────────────────────────────────────┐
│                      BENEFITS versus RISKS                            │
│        Possible Benefits                    Possible Risks            │
│   EFFECTIVE CONTROL OF TYPE 1        HYPOGLYCEMIA                      │
│     (INSULIN-DEPENDENT)              Infrequent allergic reactions     │
│     DIABETES MELLITUS                                                  │
│   TIGHT CONTROL OF BLOOD                                               │
│     SUGAR MAY AVOID OR DELAY                                           │
│     DEVELOPMENT OF HIGH                                                │
│     BLOOD PRESSURE, KIDNEY,                                            │
│     HEART, NERVE, EYE, OR OTHER                                        │
│     DAMAGE THAT HAPPENS WHEN                                           │
│     BLOOD SUGAR IS OUT OF                                              │
│     CONTROL                                                            │
│   RAPID ABSORPTION ALLOWS                                              │
│     INJECTION JUST BEFORE                                              │
│     MEALS                                                              │
└─────────────────────────────────────────────────────────────────────┘
```

▷ **Principal Uses**

As a Single Drug Product: Uses currently included in FDA approved labeling: Used in diabetes mellitus that is insulin-dependent.

Other (unlabeled) generally accepted uses: May be helpful in some cases of resistance to insulin.

How This Drug Works: Insulin lispro helps sugar enter cells (acting on cell membranes), where sugar can be used for energy.

Available Dose Forms and Strengths

Injections — 100 units per ml

▷ **Usual Adult Dose Range:** According to individual requirements for the best regulation of blood sugar on a 24-hour basis. **Note: Actual dose and schedule must be determined for each patient individually.**

Conditions Requiring Dosing Adjustments

Liver Function: Specific adjustment guidelines are not available.

Kidney Function: Caution should be used by patients with compromised kidneys. Requirements become extremely variable.

Thyrotoxicosis: Glucose utilization is typically increased and insulin requirements may actually decrease.

▷ **Dosing Instructions:** Inject insulin subcutaneously according to the schedule prescribed by your physician. The timing and frequency of injections will vary.

Insulin Lispro acts like this:

Insulin Lispro	Action Onset	Peak	Duration
Insulin lispro	0.4 hr	0.5–1.0 hrs	3–4 hrs

Usual Duration of Use: In Type 1 insulin-dependent (juvenile-onset) diabetes mellitus, insulin therapy is usually required for life. Type 2 non-insulin-dependent (maturity-onset) diabetes may be controlled by oral antidiabetic drugs and/or diet, but can require insulin when you have a serious infection, injuries, burns, surgical procedures, and other physical stress. See your doctor on a regular basis.

Possible Advantages of This Drug
> Goes to work faster and has a shorter half life versus other insulins. More physiologic control of blood sugar.

▷ **This Drug Should Not Be Taken If**
- the need for insulin and its dose schedule has not been established by a qualified physician.

▷ **Inform Your Physician Before Taking This Drug If**
- you have an insulin allergy.
- you do not know how to recognize and treat abnormally low blood sugar (see *hypoglycemia* in Glossary).
- you are pregnant.
- you take aspirin, beta-blockers, fenfluramine (Pondimin), monoamine oxidase (MAO) type A inhibitors (see Drug Classes).

Possible Side Effects (natural, expected, and unavoidable drug actions)
> In stable diabetes, no side effects occur when insulin dose, diet, and physical activity are correctly balanced and maintained. In unstable ("brittle") diabetes, unexpected drops in blood sugar levels can occur, resulting in hypoglycemia (see Glossary).
> Antibodies.
> Weight gain.

▷ **Possible Adverse Effects** (unusual, unexpected, and infrequent reactions)
> **If any of the following develop, consult your physician promptly for guidance.**
> *Mild Adverse Effects*
> Allergic reactions: local redness, swelling, and itching at site of injection, or hives—infrequent (often resolve within days).
> *Serious Adverse Effects*
> Allergic reaction: anaphylactic reactions (see Glossary).
> Hypoglycemia—possible to infrequent (less risk than other insulins).
> Arrhythmias (associated with hypoglycemia) or very fast heart rate (with intravenous use)—reported with other insulins.

▷ **Possible Effects on Sexual Function:**   May resolve sexual dysfunction in patients who have this prior to starting insulin therapy. May also cause decrease in libido and erective dysfunction—reported with insulins (may also be a result of nerve/blood vessel damage).

▷ **Adverse Effects That May Mimic Natural Diseases or Disorders**
> The early signs of hypoglycemia may be mistaken for alcoholic intoxication.

Possible Effects on Laboratory Tests
> Blood cholesterol level: decreased.
> Blood glucose level: decreased.
> Blood potassium level: decreased.
> Glycosylated hemoglobin (hemoglobin A1-C): decreased.

CAUTION
1. Carry a card in your purse or wallet with a notation that you have diabetes and are taking insulin lispro.
2. Know how to recognize hypoglycemia and how to treat it. Always carry a readily available form of sugar, such as hard candy or sugar cubes. Report all episodes of hypoglycemia to your doctor.

3. Your vision may improve during the first few weeks of insulin therapy. Postpone eye exams for eyeglasses for 6 weeks after starting insulin.
4. It is advisable to rotate the injection site within the same body region than from one site to another.
5. The American Diabetic Association (ADA) now says that a person is considered diabetic if two fasting blood sugars in a row are more than 125 mg/dl. This more conservative approach reflects new information saying that complications start at lower blood sugar levels than previously thought.

Precautions for Use

By Infants and Children: Insulin doses and schedules are modified according to patient's size. Adhere strictly to the physician's prescribed routine.

By Those Over 60 Years of Age: Insulin needs may change with age. Periodic individual evaluation is needed to identify the best dose and schedule. The aging brain adapts well to higher blood sugar levels. Rigid attempts at tight sugar control may result in hypoglycemia that shows as confusion and abnormal behavior. Repeated hypoglycemia (especially if severe) may cause brain damage.

▷ **Advisability of Use During Pregnancy**

Pregnancy Category: B. See Pregnancy Risk Categories at the back of this book. Animal studies: Inconclusive.

Human studies: Adequate studies of pregnant women are not available. Birth defects occur two to four times more frequently in infants of diabetic mothers than in infants of mothers who do not have diabetes. The exact causes of this are not known. Insulin is the drug of choice for managing diabetes during pregnancy. To preserve the health of the mother and fetus, every effort must be made to establish the best dose of insulin necessary for good control and to prevent episodes of hypoglycemia.

Advisability of Use If Breast-Feeding

Presence of this drug in breast milk: No data.
Discuss this issue with your doctor.

Habit-Forming Potential: None; however, cases of surreptitious insulin injection have been reported.

Effects of Overdose: Hypoglycemia: fatigue, weakness, headache, nervousness, irritability, sweating, tremors, hunger, confusion, delirium, abnormal behavior (resembling alcoholic intoxication), loss of consciousness, seizures.

Possible Effects of Long-Term Use: Thinning of subcutaneous fat tissue at sites of insulin injection. Insulin resistance.

Suggested Periodic Examinations While Taking This Drug (at physician's discretion)

Historically, estimates of blood sugar were obtained by checking urine sugar. This method has been replaced by fingerstick testing of blood glucose. Fingerstick testing accurately reflects the blood sugar and helps ensure better control (tighter control) of blood glucose. If you are ill, increased frequency of fingerstick blood glucose testing may be indicated. Routine testing of blood sugar levels at intervals recommended by your physician is prudent.

▷ **While Taking This Drug, Observe the Following**

Foods: Follow your diabetic diet conscientiously. Do not omit snack foods in mid-afternoon or at bedtime if they help prevent hypoglycemia.

Beverages: According to prescribed diabetic diet.

▷ *Alcohol:* Used excessively, alcohol can cause severe hypoglycemia, resulting in brain damage.

Tobacco Smoking: Regular smoking can decrease insulin absorption and increase insulin requirements by 30%. It is advisable to stop smoking altogether.

Marijuana Smoking: Possible increase in blood sugar levels.

▷ *Other Drugs*

The following drugs may ***increase*** the effects of insulin lispro:

- acarbose (Precose)—by decreasing the amount of sugar that insulin has to work on.
- aspirin and other salicylates.
- some beta-blocker drugs (especially the nonselective ones; see Drug Classes)—may prolong insulin-induced hypoglycemia.
- clofibrate (Atromid-S).
- fenfluramine (Pondimin).
- monoamine oxidase (MAO) type A inhibitors (see Drug Classes).
- oral antidiabetic drugs (see Drug Classes)—results in additive hypoglycemia.

The following drugs may ***decrease*** the effects of insulin lispro (by raising blood sugar levels):

- birth control pills (oral contraceptives).
- chlorthalidone (Hygroton).
- cortisonelike drugs (see ***adrenocortical steroids*** in Drug Classes).
- furosemide (Lasix).
- phenytoin (Dilantin, etc.).
- thiazide diuretics (see Drug Classes).
- thyroid preparations (various).

▷ *Driving, Hazardous Activities:* Be prepared to stop and take corrective action if hypoglycemia develops.

Aviation Note: Diabetes and the use of this drug ***are disqualifications*** for piloting. Consult a designated aviation medical examiner.

Exposure to Sun: No restrictions.

Exposure to Heat: Use caution. Sauna baths can significantly increase the rate of insulin absorption and cause hypoglycemia.

Heavy Exercise or Exertion: Use caution. Periods of unusual or unplanned heavy physical activity will use up sugar more quickly and predispose to hypoglycemia.

Occurrence of Unrelated Illness: Omission of meals as a result of nausea, vomiting, or injury may lead to hypoglycemia. Infections can increase insulin needs. Ask your doctor for help.

Discontinuation: Do not stop this drug without asking your doctor. Omission of insulin lispro may result in life-threatening coma.

Special Storage Instructions: Keep in a cool place, preferably in the refrigerator. Protect from freezing. Protect from strong light and high temperatures when not refrigerated.

Observe the Following Expiration Times: Do not use this drug if it is older than the expiration date on the vial. Always use fresh, "within-date" medicine.

IPRATROPIUM (i pra TROH pee um)

Introduced: 1975   **Class:** Bronchodilator (antiasthmatic drugs)   **Prescription:** USA: Yes   **Controlled Drug:** USA: No; Canada: No
Available as Generic: USA: No; Canada: No
Brand Names: Atrovent, Atrovent Nasal Spray, Combivent

BENEFITS versus RISKS	
Possible Benefits	*Possible Risks*
EFFECTIVE BRONCHODILATOR FOR TREATMENT OF CHRONIC BRONCHITIS AND EMPHYSEMA	Mild and infrequent adverse effects (see below)
EFFECTIVE TREATMENT OF RUNNY NOSE (RHINORRHEA)	
Effective adjunctive treatment in some bronchial asthma	

▷ **Principal Uses**

As a Single Drug Product: Uses currently included in FDA-approved labeling: (1) Helps prevent or relieve episodes of difficult breathing in chronic bronchitis and emphysema (should not be used to treat acute attacks of asthma because it takes a while to work) (2) used in nasal spray to relieve symptoms of runny nose (rhinorrhea) from allergic or nonallergic perennial rhinitis (including runny nose from colds) in adults and children more than 12 years old.

Other (unlabeled) generally accepted uses: (1) Relief of asthma symptoms; (2) treats lung symptoms of congestive heart failure.

How This Drug Works: Through its atropinelike (anticholinergic) action, it blocks bronchial constriction and opens bronchi. Nasal form keeps acetylcholine from working (antagonizes it) and decreases production and secretion of mucus.

Available Dose Forms and Strengths

Inhalation aerosol — 14-g metered dose inhaler; 18 mcg per inhalation
Nebulizer — 250 mcg/ml solution
Nasal inhaler — 20 mcg per actuation
Nasal spray — 0.03%, 0.06%

▷ **Usual Adult Dose Range:** Initially two inhalations (36 mcg) four times a day, 4 hours apart. If needed, the dose may be increased to four inhalations (80 mcg) at one time to get optimal relief. Maintain 4-hour intervals between doses. Maximum daily dose is 12 inhalations (216 mcg). The nasal spray is used as: 0.03%—two sprays (21 mcg each) in each nostril two to three times a day for up to 4 days; 0.06%—two sprays (42 mcg each) in each nostril three to four times a day for up to 4 days. **Note: Actual dose and dosing schedule must be determined for each patient individually.**

Conditions Requiring Dosing Adjustments

Liver Function: Specific guidelines not developed.

Kidney Function: Used with caution by patients with bladder neck obstructions.

▷ **Dosing Instructions:**   Carefully follow the patient instructions provided with the inhaler. Shake well before using. Many people do NOT take the time to learn the best inhaler technique for them; take the time to do this. The pump of the nasal form must be primed before the unit is used. Read the package insert carefully, and ask your pharmacist for help if you don't understand the directions that come with this medicine.

Usual Duration of Use: Inhalation form: continual use on a regular schedule for 48 to 72 hours is usually necessary to determine this drug's effectiveness. Long-term use (months to years) requires check of response and dose adjustment. See your doctor.

Nasal spray: the nasal form helps some people feel better right away and may take a week for others. The nasal spray may only be used for up to 4 days.

Possible Advantages of This Drug

Inhalation form: produces a greater degree of bronchodilation than theophylline in patients with chronic bronchitis and emphysema. Causes minimal adverse effects. Repeated use does not lead to tolerance and loss of effectiveness. Suitable for long-term maintenance therapy.

Nasal spray: eases a very annoying symptom of the common cold.

Currently a "Drug of Choice"

For difficult breathing associated with chronic bronchitis and emphysema.

▷ **This Drug Should Not Be Taken If**

• you have had an allergic reaction to it previously.
• you are allergic to soybeans or peanuts (inhalation form).
• you are allergic to atropine or to aerosol propellants (fluorocarbons; inhalation form).
• you are allergic to benzalkonium chloride or edetate disodium (nasal spray).

▷ **Inform Your Physician Before Taking This Drug If**

• you have had an adverse effect from any belladonna derivative previously.
• you have a history of glaucoma.
• you have any form of urinary retention or prostatism (see Glossary).

Possible Side Effects (natural, expected, and unavoidable drug actions)

Throat dryness, cough, irritation from aerosol—rare; blurred vision, dry mouth. Bad or bitter taste may be frequent.

▷ **Possible Adverse Effects** (unusual, unexpected, and infrequent reactions)

If any of the following develop, consult your physician promptly for guidance.

Mild Adverse Effects

Allergic reactions: skin rash, hives—rare.

Headache, dizziness, nervousness—rare.

Palpitations—rare.

Nosebleeds (with nasal spray)—infrequent to frequent.

Serious Adverse Effects

Allergic reactions: rare first-dose angioedema or bronchospasm.

Author's Note: Other than the rare allergic reactions, the nasal spray does not have any serious adverse effects.

Abnormal heartbeat (supraventricular tachycardia)—case report.
Intraocular pressure changes—rare.

▷ **Possible Effects on Sexual Function**
None reported.

Natural Diseases or Disorders That May Be Activated by This Drug
Angle-closure glaucoma, prostatism (see Glossary).

Possible Effects on Laboratory Tests
None reported.

CAUTION

1. This drug won't start to work for 5 to 15 minutes. It should **not** be used alone to treat acute attacks of asthma needing a fast result.
2. When used as combination therapy with beta-adrenergic antiasthmatic drugs (albuterol, terbutaline, metaproterenol, etc.), the beta-adrenergic aerosol should be used about 5 minutes before using ipratropium to prevent fluorocarbon toxicity.
3. When used as an adjunct to steroid or cromolyn aerosols (beclomethasone; Intal), ipratropium should be used about 5 minutes before using the steroid or cromolyn aerosol to prevent fluorocarbon toxicity.
4. Contact with the eyes can cause temporary blurring of vision.
5. Call your doctor if you are using the nasal spray and your runny nose (rhinorrhea) continues or gets worse and you develop a fever.

Precautions for Use
By Infants and Children: Nasal spray is now approved for use for those 6 to 11 years old. Dosing is the same as for adults for the 0.03% form.
Safety and effectiveness for those under 6 are not established.
By Those Over 60 Years of Age: Watch for possible development of prostatism and adjust dose as necessary.

▷ **Advisability of Use During Pregnancy**
Pregnancy Category: B. See Pregnancy Risk Categories at the back of this book.
Animal studies: No drug-induced birth defects in mouse, rat, or rabbit studies.
Human studies: Adequate studies of pregnant women are not available.
Use this drug during pregnancy only if clearly needed.

Advisability of Use If Breast-Feeding
Presence of this drug in breast milk: Possibly yes, but in very small amounts.
Watch nursing infant closely and stop drug or nursing if adverse effects start.

Habit-Forming Potential: None.

Effects of Overdose: This drug is not well absorbed into the circulation when it is taken by aerosol inhalation. No systemic effects of overdose are expected.

Possible Effects of Long-Term Use: Drying of the nose.

Suggested Periodic Examinations While Taking This Drug (at physician's discretion)
Internal eye pressure measurements if appropriate.

▷ **While Taking This Drug, Observe the Following**
Foods: No restrictions.
Beverages: No restrictions.
▷   *Alcohol:* No interactions expected.

Tobacco Smoking: No interactions expected. However, smoking should be avoided completely if you have chronic bronchitis or emphysema. I advise everyone to quit smoking.

Marijuana Smoking: Possible excessive increase in heart rate (tachycardia).

▷ *Other Drugs*

Ipratropium may *increase* the effects of
- albuterol (Proventil, others).
- other atropinelike drugs (see *anticholinergic drugs* in Drug Classes).

Ipratropium *taken concurrently* with
- cisapride (Propulsid) may lessen benefits of cisapride.
- tricyclic antidepressants (see Drug Classes) may result in additive anticholinergic effects.

▷ *Driving, Hazardous Activities:* May cause dizziness or blurred vision. Restrict activities as necessary.

Aviation Note: The use of this drug *may be a disqualification* for piloting. Consult a designated aviation medical examiner.

Exposure to Sun: No restrictions.

Exposure to Cold: Inhaling cold air may cause bronchospasm and induce asthmatic breathing and cough; dose adjustment of this drug may be necessary.

Heavy Exercise or Exertion: This drug is not considered to be consistently effective in preventing or treating exercise-induced asthma.

Discontinuation: Ask your doctor for help. Substitute medication may be advisable.

ISONIAZID (i soh NI a zid)

Other Names: Isonicotinic acid hydrazide, INH

Introduced: 1956   **Class:** Antituberculosis   **Prescription:** USA: Yes
Controlled Drug: USA: No; Canada: No   **Available as Generic:**   USA: Yes;
Canada: Yes

Brand Names: INH, ✦Isotamine, Laniazid, Nydrazid, P-I-N Forte [CD], ✦PMS Isoniazid, Rifamate [CD], Rifater [CD], Rimactane/INH Dual Pack [CD], Teebaconin, Teebaconin and Vitamin B-6 [CD]

BENEFITS versus RISKS	
Possible Benefits	*Possible Risks*
EFFECTIVE PREVENTION AND TREATMENT OF ACTIVE TUBERCULOSIS	ALLERGIC LIVER REACTION— RARE
	Peripheral neuritis (see Glossary)
	Bone marrow depression (see Glossary)
	Mental and behavioral disturbances

▷ **Principal Uses**

As a Single Drug Product: Uses currently included in FDA-approved labeling: (1) Used alone to prevent the development of tuberculous infection in people who are at high risk because of exposure to infection or recent conversion of a negative tuberculin skin test to positive; (2) used **in combination** with other drugs to treat tuberculosis in a variety of body sites.

Other (unlabeled) generally accepted uses: May have a role in treating atypical mycobacteria that can be associated with Crohn's disease.

As a Combination Drug Product [CD]: Available in combination with rifampin, another antitubercular drug that works in a different way. This combination is more effective than either drug used alone. Isoniazid can cause low pyridoxine (vitamin B$_6$); for this reason, a combination of the two drugs is available in tablet form.

How This Drug Works: By interfering with metabolism or cell walls, this drug kills (bactericidal) or inhibits (bacteriostatic) susceptible tuberculosis organisms.

Available Dose Forms and Strengths
> Injection — 100 mg/ml
>> Syrup — 50 mg/5 ml
> Tablets — 50 mg, 100 mg, 300 mg

▷ **Usual Adult Dose Range:**   For prevention: 300 mg once daily (usually for 6 to 12 months). For treatment: 5 mg per kg of body mass daily. The total daily dose should not exceed 300 mg. **Note: Actual dose and dosing schedule must be determined on an individual basis.**

Conditions Requiring Dosing Adjustments
Liver Function: This drug should **not** be used in sudden (acute) liver disease. It should be discontinued if the liver function tests become increased to three times the normal value.
Kidney Function: This drug is a rare cause of nephrosis. For severe kidney failure (creatinine clearance less than 10 ml/min) daily dose is lowered by 50%.

▷ **Dosing Instructions:**   The tablet may be crushed and taken with food to prevent stomach irritation.

Usual Duration of Use: Use on a regular schedule for 1 year or more is often necessary, depending upon the nature of the infection. Shorter courses of intermittent high doses may work. See your doctor regularly.

▷ **This Drug Should Not Be Taken If**
- you have had an allergic reaction (especially a liver reaction) to any dose form of it previously.
- you have active liver disease.

▷ **Inform Your Physician Before Taking This Drug If**
- you have serious impairment of liver or kidney function.
- you drink an alcoholic beverage daily.
- you are an alcoholic.
- your are pregnant or are breast-feeding your baby.
- you have a seizure disorder.
- you take other drugs on a long-term basis, especially phenytoin (Dilantin).
- you plan to have surgery under general anesthesia in the near future.

Possible Side Effects (natural, expected, and unavoidable drug actions)
Toxic fever—rare.

▷ **Possible Adverse Effects** (unusual, unexpected, and infrequent reactions)
If any of the following develop, consult your physician promptly for guidance.
Mild Adverse Effects
Allergic reactions: skin rash, fever, swollen glands, painful muscles and joints.

Dizziness, indigestion, nausea, vomiting.

Peripheral neuritis (see Glossary): numbness, tingling, pain, weakness in hands and/or feet—frequent in adults, rare in children (may be prevented with pyridoxine).

Serious Adverse Effects

Allergic reactions: drug-induced hepatitis (see ***hepatitis-like reaction*** in Glossary): loss of appetite, nausea, fatigue, itching, dark-colored urine, yellowing of eyes and skin, hypersensitivity, meningitis—case reports.

Severe skin reactions (Stevens-Johnson syndrome, pellagra)—case reports.

Acute mental/behavioral disturbances, psychosis, impaired vision, increase in epileptic seizures—rare.

High or low blood sugars (hyperglycemia or hypoglycemia)—possible.

Porphyria or kidney toxicity—case reports.

Lupus-erythematosus-like syndrome or abnormal muscle changes (rhabdomyolysis)—case reports.

Pellagra—rare.

Bone marrow depression (see Glossary): fatigue, weakness, fever, sore throat, abnormal bleeding or bruising—case reports.

▷ **Possible Effects on Sexual Function:**   Male breast enlargement and tenderness (gynecomastia)—rare.

Possible Delayed Adverse Effects: Increased frequency of liver cirrhosis has been reported.

▷ **Adverse Effects That May Mimic Natural Diseases or Disorders**

Drug-induced hepatitis may suggest viral hepatitis. Collagen vascular changes may mimic rheumatoid arthritis or systemic lupus erythematosus. Pseudolymphoma may occur.

Natural Diseases or Disorders That May Be Activated by This Drug

Latent epilepsy, systemic lupus erythematosus (questionable).

Possible Effects on Laboratory Tests

Complete blood cell counts: decreased red cells, hemoglobin, white cells, and platelets; increased eosinophils (allergic reaction).

Blood amylase level: increased (possible pancreatitis).

Blood antinuclear antibodies (ANA): positive.

Blood lupus erythematosus (LE) cells: positive.

Blood glucose level: increased (with large doses).

Liver function tests: increased liver enzymes (ALT/GPT, AST/GOT, and alkaline phosphatase), increased bilirubin.

Urine sugar tests: increased; false positive results with Benedict's solution and Clinitest.

CAUTION

1. **The FDA has required a new warning for Laniazid: "A recent report suggests an increased risk of fatal hepatitis associated with isoniazid among women, particularly Black and Hispanic women. The risk may also be increased during the postpartum period."** Increased laboratory testing is also suggested.

2. Ask your doctor about determining if you are a "slow" or "rapid" inactivator (acetylator) of isoniazid. This has a bearing on your predisposition to developing adverse effects.

3. Copper sulfate tests for urine sugar may give a false-positive test result. (Diabetics, please note.)

Precautions for Use

By Infants and Children: Use with caution in children with seizure disorders. "Slow acetylators" are more prone to adverse drug effects. It is advisable to give supplemental pyridoxine (vitamin B_6).

By Those Over 60 Years of Age: There is a greater incidence of liver damage in this age group, and liver status should be closely watched. Observe for any indications of an "acute brain syndrome" consisting of confusion, delirium, and seizures.

▷ **Advisability of Use During Pregnancy**

Pregnancy Category: C. See Pregnancy Risk Categories at the back of this book. Animal studies: No birth defects reported in mice, rats, or rabbits.

Human studies: Data from adequate studies of pregnant women are not available.

If clearly needed, this drug is now used at any time during pregnancy. Ask your physician for guidance.

Advisability of Use If Breast-Feeding

Presence of this drug in breast milk: Yes.

Avoid drug or refrain from nursing.

Habit-Forming Potential: None.

Effects of Overdose: Nausea, vomiting, dizziness, blurred vision, hallucinations, slurred speech, stupor, coma, seizures.

Possible Effects of Long-Term Use: Peripheral neuritis due to a deficiency of pyridoxine (vitamin B_6).

Suggested Periodic Examinations While Taking This Drug (at physician's discretion)

Complete blood cell counts, liver function tests, complete eye examinations.

▷ **While Taking This Drug, Observe the Following**

Foods: Eat the following foods cautiously until your tolerance is determined: Swiss and Cheshire cheeses, tuna fish, skipjack fish, and *Sardinella* species. These may interact with the drug to produce skin rash, itching, sweating, chills, headache, light-headedness, or rapid heart rate. Taking this drug with food also acts to decrease absorption and lessen therapeutic benefits. Some red wines and aged cheeses also contain high levels of tyramine. This may result in an undesirable increase in blood pressure if consumed. Avoid this combination.

Nutritional Support: It is advisable to take a supplement of pyridoxine (vitamin B_6) to prevent peripheral neuritis. Ask your physician for help.

Beverages: No restrictions. May be taken with milk.

▷ *Alcohol:* Alcohol may reduce the effectiveness of this drug and increase the risk of liver toxicity.

Tobacco Smoking: No interactions expected. I advise everyone to quit smoking.

▷ *Other Drugs*

Isoniazid may ***increase*** the effects of
- carbamazepine (Tegretol), and cause toxicity.
- disulfiram (Antabuse) and change behavior.
- phenytoin (Dilantin), and cause toxicity.

The following drugs may *decrease* the effects of isoniazid:
- cortisonelike drugs (see *adrenocortical steroids* in Drug Classes).

Isoniazid *taken concurrently* with
- acetaminophen (Tylenol) may increase the risk of hepatoxicity.
- antacids may decrease the absorption of this medicine. Separate antacid dosing by 2 hours from dosing of this medicine.
- BCG vaccine will result in decreased vaccine effectiveness.
- cyclosporine (Sandimmune) may blunt cyclosporine benefits.
- diazepam, and perhaps other benzodiazepines (see Drug Classes), may result in increased blood levels and toxicity.
- ketoconazole, itraconazole, or related compounds may result in decreased therapeutic benefits of the antifungal.
- meperidine (Demerol) may result in excessive lowering of blood pressure.
- oral antidiabetic drugs (see Drug Classes) may result in loss of control of blood glucose.
- rifampin (Rifadin, others) can result in a serious increased risk of liver toxicity.
- theophylline may result in theophylline toxicity.
- valproic acid (Depakene) can result in isoniazid or valproic acid toxicity.
- warfarin (Coumadin) may result in increased bleeding risk. More frequent INR (prothrombin time or protime) testing is needed.

▷ *Driving, Hazardous Activities:* This drug may cause dizziness. Restrict activities as necessary.

Aviation Note: The use of this drug *may be a disqualification* for piloting. Consult a designated aviation medical examiner.

Exposure to Sun: No restrictions.

Discontinuation: Long-term treatment is required. Do not stop this drug without asking your physician.

ISOSORBIDE DINITRATE (i soh SOHR bide di NI trayt)

Other Name: Sorbide nitrate

Introduced: 1959   **Class:** Anti-anginal, nitrates   **Prescription:** USA: Yes   **Controlled Drug:** USA: No; Canada: No   **Available as Generic:** USA: Yes; Canada: No

Brand Names: ✦Apo-ISDN, ✦Cedocard-SR, ✦Coradur, ✦Coronex, Dilatrate-SR, Iso-BID, Isonate, Isordil, Isordil Tembids, Isordil Titradose, Isotrate Timecelles, ✦Novosorbide, Sorbitrate-SA, Sorbitrate

Warning: The brand names Isordil and Isuprel are similar, which can lead to serious errors. Isordil is isosorbide dinitrate, used to treat angina. Isuprel is isoproterenol, used for asthma. Make sure you are taking the correct drug.

BENEFITS versus RISKS	
Possible Benefits	*Possible Risks*
EFFECTIVE RELIEF AND PREVENTION OF ANGINA	Orthostatic hypotension (see Glossary)
EFFECTIVE ADJUNCTIVE TREATMENT IN SOME CASES OF CONGESTIVE HEART FAILURE	Rare skin reactions (severe peeling)

▷ **Principal Uses**

As a Single Drug Product: Uses currently included in FDA-approved labeling: (1) The sublingual (under-the-tongue) tablets and the chewable tablets are used to prevent and relieve acute attacks of anginal pain; (2) the longer-acting tablets and capsules are used to prevent the development of angina, but are not effective in relieving acute episodes of anginal pain (nitroglycerin is the drug of choice in those cases).

Other (unlabeled) generally accepted uses: This drug (1) is also used to improve heart function in selected cases of congestive heart failure; (2) can help ease the pressure in esophageal varices in alcoholics; (3) can help painful leg cramping (intermittent claudication); (4) is used after a heart attack intravenously to help address congestive heart failure.

How This Drug Works: This drug relaxes and dilates arteries and veins. Benefits treating angina and heart failure are due to: (1) dilation of coronary arteries and (2) dilation of systemic veins. Net effects are improved heart blood flow and reduced workload.

Available Dose Forms and Strengths

Capsules — 40 mg

Capsules, prolonged action — 40 mg

Tablets — 5 mg, 10 mg, 20 mg, 30 mg, 40 mg

Tablets, chewable — 5 mg, 10 mg

Tablets, prolonged action — 20 mg, 40 mg

Tablets, sublingual — 2.5 mg, 5 mg, 10 mg

▷ **Recommended Dose Ranges** (Actual dose and schedule must be determined for each patient individually.)

Infants and Children: Dose not established.

12 to 60 Years of Age: Sublingual tablets: 5 to 10 mg dissolved under tongue every 2 to 3 hours; use for relief of acute attack and for prevention of anticipated attack.

Chewable tablets: initially 5 mg chewed to evaluate tolerance; increase dose to 5 or 10 mg every 2 to 3 hours as needed and tolerated. Use for relief of acute attack and for prevention of anticipated attack.

Tablets: 5 to 20 mg four times daily to prevent acute attack, with at least one 12-hour nitrate-free period.

Prolonged-action capsules and tablets: 40 mg to start, then 40–80 mg every 8 to 12 hours as needed to prevent acute attacks.

The total daily dose should not exceed 120 mg.

Author's note: Dosing for all forms is set up to give a 12-hour nitrate-free period in order to avoid tolerance to the therapeutic benefits of this medicine.

Over 60 Years of Age: Same as 12 to 60 years of age; however, excessive lowering of the blood pressure on standing (postural hypotension) may be more likely in this population.

Conditions Requiring Dosing Adjustments

Liver Function: Used with caution and in decreased doses by patients with liver compromise, as increased blood levels will occur.

Kidney Function: No specific dosing changes are needed for compromised kidneys. This drug can discolor (brown to black) urine.

▷ **Dosing Instructions:**   Capsules and tablets to be swallowed are best taken on an empty stomach to achieve maximal blood levels. Regular tablets may be crushed; prolonged-action capsules and tablets should be taken whole, NOT chewed.

Usual Duration of Use: Use on a regular schedule for 3 to 7 days is needed to (1) identify this drug's peak effect in preventing or relieving acute anginal pain, and (2) to find the optimal dose schedule. Long-term use (months to years) requires physician supervision.

▷ **This Drug Should Not Be Taken If**
- you had an allergic reaction to any form of it previously.
- you have severe anemia.
- you have increased intraocular pressure.
- you have suffered trauma to the head.
- you have an overactive thyroid gland.
- you have abnormal growth of the heart muscle (hypertrophic cardiomyopathy).
- you have had a very recent heart attack (myocardial infarction) and have elevated blood pressure or very rapid heart rate (tachycardia).

▷ **Inform Your Physician Before Taking This Drug If**
- you have had an unfavorable response to other nitrate drugs or vasodilators in the past.
- you have a history of low blood pressure.
- you have any form of glaucoma.
- you have had a cerebral hemorrhage recently.
- you are pregnant or are planning pregnancy.
- you are allergic to the dye tartrazine.
- you have a glucose-6-phosphate dehydrogenase (G6PD) deficiency (ask your doctor).

Possible Side Effects (natural, expected, and unavoidable drug actions)
Flushing of face, throbbing in head, palpitation, rapid heart rate, orthostatic hypotension (see Glossary).

▷ **Possible Adverse Effects** (unusual, unexpected, and infrequent reactions)
If any of the following develop, consult your physician promptly for guidance.
Mild Adverse Effects
Allergic reaction: skin rash.
Headache (may be severe and persistent)—infrequent to frequent; dizziness, fainting—possible.
Nausea, vomiting—possible.
Urine discoloration—possible and not clinically significant.
Serious Adverse Effects
Allergic reaction: severe dermatitis with peeling of skin—case reports.
Transient ischemic attacks (TIAs) in presence of impaired circulation within the brain: dizziness, fainting, impaired vision or speech, localized numbness or weakness—possible.
Anemia (in those with G6PD deficiency)—possible.
Abnormal heart rates or conduction—case reports.
Abnormally low blood pressure on standing (postural hypotension)—possible.
Tolerance—possible with 24-hour use (daily 12-hour drug-free period is used to prevent this).

▷ **Possible Effects on Sexual Function:**   None reported.

▷ **Adverse Effects That May Mimic Natural Diseases or Disorders**

    Spells of low blood pressure (due to this drug) may mimic late-onset epilepsy.

Possible Effects on Laboratory Tests

    None reported.

CAUTION

    1. Tolerance (see Glossary) to long-acting forms of nitrates may cause sublingual tablets of nitroglycerin to be less effective in relieving acute anginal attacks. Anti-anginal effectiveness is restored after 1 week of abstinence from long-acting nitrates. Daily 12-hour periods without use of the drug are needed.

    2. Many over-the-counter (OTC) medicines for allergies, colds, and coughs contain drugs that may counteract the desired drug effects. Ask your physician or pharmacist for help before using such medicines.

Precautions for Use

    By Those Over 60 Years of Age: Small starting doses are advisable. You may be more susceptible to the development of low blood pressure and associated "blackout" spells, fainting, and falling. Throbbing headaches and flushing may be more apparent.

▷ **Advisability of Use During Pregnancy**

    Pregnancy Category: C. See Pregnancy Risk Categories at the back of this book.

    Animal studies: No information available.

    Human studies: Adequate studies of pregnant women are not available.

    Use this drug only if clearly needed.

Advisability of Use If Breast-Feeding

    Presence of this drug in breast milk: Unknown.

    If this drug is thought to be necessary, monitor the nursing infant for low blood pressure and poor feeding.

Habit-Forming Potential: None.

Effects of Overdose: Headache, dizziness, marked flushing of face and skin, vomiting, weakness, fainting, difficult breathing, coma.

Possible Effects of Long-Term Use: Development of tolerance with temporary loss of effectiveness at recommended doses. Development of abnormal hemoglobin (red blood cell pigment).

Suggested Periodic Examinations While Taking This Drug (at physician's discretion)

    Measurement of internal eye pressure. Red cell counts and hemoglobin tests.

▷ **While Taking This Drug, Observe the Following**

    Foods: Oral doses are best taken on an empty stomach to insure quick absorption. Vitamin C may help ease nitrate tolerance. More study is needed.

    Beverages: No restrictions. May be taken with milk.

▷   *Alcohol:* Use extreme caution and avoid alcohol completely in the presence of any side effects or adverse effects of this drug. Alcohol may exaggerate the blood-pressure-lowering effect of this drug.

    Tobacco Smoking: Nicotine can reduce benefits. Avoid all forms of tobacco.

    Marijuana Smoking: Possible reduced effectiveness of this drug; mild to moderate increase in angina; possible changes in electrocardiogram, confusing interpretation.

▷ *Other Drugs*
Isosorbide dinitrate *taken concurrently* with
- antihypertensive drugs may cause excessive lowering of blood pressure; dose adjustments may be necessary.
- hydralazine (Apresoline) may work well to help control angina.
- propranolol (Inderal) can help improve exercise time without angina.
- sildenafil (Viagra) may result in LIFE-THREATENING lowering of blood pressure. NEVER COMBINE.

▷ *Driving, Hazardous Activities:* Usually no restrictions. This drug may cause dizziness or spells of low blood pressure. Restrict activities as necessary.

Aviation Note: Coronary artery disease *is a disqualification* for piloting. Consult a designated aviation medical examiner.

Exposure to Sun: No restrictions.

Exposure to Heat: Use caution. Hot environments can cause significant drop in blood pressure.

Exposure to Cold: Cold environments can increase the need for this drug and limit its benefits.

Heavy Exercise or Exertion: This drug may improve your ability to be more active without anginal pain. Use caution and avoid excessive exertion.

Discontinuation: It is advisable to gradually withdraw this drug after long-term use. Dose and frequency of prolonged-action dose forms should be reduced gradually over a period of 4 to 6 weeks.

ISOSORBIDE MONONITRATE (i soh SOHR bide mon oh NI trayt)

Introduced: 1983   **Class:** Anti-anginal, nitrates   **Prescription:** USA: Yes   **Controlled Drug:** USA: No   **Available as Generic:** USA: No
Brand Names: Elan (Italy), Elantan, Imdur, Ismo, Monoket

BENEFITS versus RISKS	
Possible Benefits	*Possible Risks*
EFFECTIVE PREVENTION OF ANGINA	Orthostatic hypotension (see Glossary) Headache

▷ **Principal Uses**
As a Single Drug Product: Uses currently included in FDA-approved labeling: To reduce the frequency and severity of recurrent angina; not effective in acute anginal pain.
Other (unlabeled) generally accepted uses: (1) May have a role in treating congestive heart failure (intravenous); (2) can help in decreasing the number of attacks and time spent in silent myocardial ischemia; (3) may be of help in heart attacks (myocardial infarction); (4) may help stomach bleeding in people with cirrhosis of the liver.

How This Drug Works: Relaxes and dilates arteries and veins. Benefits in angina are due to (1) dilation of coronary arteries, and (2) dilation of systemic veins. Net effects are improved blood flow to the heart and reduced workload of the heart.

Available Dose Forms and Strengths

Capsules, sustained release — 60 mg; 50 mg (Italy)

Tablets — 10 mg, 20 mg

Tablets, sustained release — 30 mg, 60 mg, 120 mg

▷ **Recommended Dose Ranges** (Actual dose and schedule must be determined for each patient individually.)

Infants and Children: Dose not established.

12 to 60 Years of Age: Regular release: 20 mg (one tablet), taken twice daily. Take the first tablet on arising; take the second tablet 7 hours later. Do not take additional doses during the balance of the day. Total daily dose should not exceed 40 mg.

Author's Note: Dosing is set up to give a 12-hour nitrate-free period in order to avoid tolerance to the therapeutic benefits of this medicine.

Sustained release: 30 mg (one half-tablet) or 60 mg (a whole tablet) once daily, taken in the morning when you get up. Total daily dose should not exceed 240 mg.

Over 60 Years of Age: Same as 12 to 60 years of age.

Conditions Requiring Dosing Adjustments

Liver Function: This drug should be used with caution by patients with liver compromise; however, no specific guidelines for dose reduction are available.

Kidney Function: No dosing changes in kidney compromise. Drug turns urine brown to black in color.

▷ **Dosing Instructions:** The tablet may be crushed and is preferably taken on an empty stomach to achieve the best blood levels. Sustained-release forms should not be chewed or crushed.

Usual Duration of Use: Use on a regular schedule for 3 to 7 days determines this drug's effectiveness in preventing episodes of acute anginal pain. Long-term use (months to years) requires physician supervision.

Possible Advantages of This Drug

Designed to provide the best possible prevention of acute angina with minimal development of tolerance (loss of effectiveness—see Glossary). The nitrate-free interval during the evening and night prevents the development of tolerance.

▷ **This Drug Should Not Be Taken If**
- you have had an allergic reaction to it previously.
- you have had a very recent heart attack (myocardial infarction) and your heart is beating quickly (tachycardia) or your blood pressure is excessively high.
- you currently have congestive heart failure or a severe anemia.
- your thyroid is overactive.
- you have a hypertrophic cardiomyopathy.

▷ **Inform Your Physician Before Taking This Drug If**
- you have had an unfavorable response to other nitrate drugs or vasodilators in the past.
- you have a history of low blood pressure.
- you have had a cerebral hemorrhage recently.

- you are pregnant or are planning pregnancy, or you are breast-feeding your baby.
- you have any form of glaucoma.

Possible Side Effects (natural, expected, and unavoidable drug actions)

Flushing of face, throbbing in head, palpitation, rapid heart rate, orthostatic hypotension (see Glossary).

▷ **Possible Adverse Effects** (unusual, unexpected, and infrequent reactions)

If any of the following develop, consult your physician promptly for guidance.

Mild Adverse Effects

Allergic reactions: skin rash, itching—infrequent.

Headache—frequent, but decreases over time.

Dizziness, fainting, or blurred vision—possible.

Nausea, vomiting, or bad breath (halitosis)—possible.

Urine discoloration—possible and not clinically significant.

Serious Adverse Effects

Transient ischemic attacks (TIAs) in presence of impaired circulation within the brain: dizziness, fainting, impaired vision or speech, localized numbness or weakness—possible.

Bone marrow depression—infrequent and of uncertain relationship.

Anemia (in patients with glucose-6-phosphate dehydrogenase—G6PD—deficiency)—possible.

Abnormally low blood pressure—possible.

Abnormal heartbeat—case reports.

Tolerance—possible with 24-hour use (daily 12-hour drug-free period is used to prevent this).

▷ **Possible Effects on Sexual Function:** Decreased libido and impotence—infrequent.

▷ **Adverse Effects That May Mimic Natural Diseases or Disorders**

Spells of low blood pressure with fainting (due to this drug) may be mistaken for late-onset epilepsy.

Possible Effects on Laboratory Tests

Liver function tests: increased.

CAUTION

1. Take this drug exactly as prescribed. If headaches are frequent or troublesome, call your doctor. Aspirin or acetaminophen may be taken to relieve headaches.
2. Many over-the-counter (OTC) medicines for allergies, colds, and coughs contain drugs that may counteract the desired effects of this drug. Ask your doctor or pharmacist for help before using such medicines.

Precautions for Use

By Those Over 60 Years of Age: Small starting doses are advisable. Increased risk of low blood pressure and associated "blackout" spells, fainting, and falling. Throbbing headaches and flushing may be more apparent.

▷ **Advisability of Use During Pregnancy**

Pregnancy Category: Ismo: C. Imdur: B. See Pregnancy Risk Categories at the back of this book.

Animal studies: Rat and rabbit studies reveal embryo deaths due to large doses of Ismo. Rat and rabbit studies did not reveal embryo deaths from Imdur.

Human studies: Adequate studies of pregnant women are not available. Use this drug only if clearly needed. Ask your physician for guidance.

Advisability of Use If Breast-Feeding
Presence of this drug in breast milk: Unknown.
If this drug is thought to be necessary, watch the nursing infant for low blood pressure and poor feeding.

Habit-Forming Potential: None.

Effects of Overdose: Headache, dizziness, marked flushing of face and skin, vomiting, weakness, fainting, difficult breathing, coma.

Possible Effects of Long-Term Use: Development of abnormal hemoglobin (red blood cell pigment).

Suggested Periodic Examinations While Taking This Drug (at physician's discretion)
Measurement of internal eye pressure.

▷ **While Taking This Drug, Observe the Following**
Foods: No restrictions. Vitamin C may help ease nitrate tolerance. More study is needed.
Beverages: No restrictions. May be taken with milk.
▷ *Alcohol:* Use extreme caution. Avoid alcohol completely in the presence of any side effects or adverse effects of this drug. Alcohol may exaggerate the blood-pressure-lowering effect of this drug.
Tobacco Smoking: Nicotine can reduce effectiveness. Avoid all forms of tobacco.
Marijuana Smoking: Possible reduced effectiveness of this drug; mild to moderate increase in angina; possible changes in electrocardiogram, confusing interpretation.
▷ *Other Drugs*
Isosorbide mononitrate *taken concurrently* with
- antihypertensive drugs may cause excessive lowering of blood pressure; dose adjustments may be necessary.
- calcium channel blocking drugs (see Drug Classes) may cause marked orthostatic hypotension (see Glossary).
- hydralazine (Apresoline) may work well to help control angina.
- propranolol (Inderal) can help improve exercise time without angina.
- sildenafil (Viagra) may result in LIFE-THREATENING lowering of blood pressure. NEVER COMBINE.
▷ *Driving, Hazardous Activities:* Usually no restrictions. This drug may cause dizziness or spells of low blood pressure. Restrict activities as necessary.
Aviation Note: Coronary artery disease *is a disqualification* for piloting. Consult a designated aviation medical examiner.
Exposure to Sun: No restrictions.
Exposure to Heat: Use caution. Hot environments can cause significant drop in blood pressure.
Exposure to Cold: Cold environments can increase the need for this drug and limit its effectiveness.
Heavy Exercise or Exertion: This drug may improve your ability to be more active without anginal pain. Use caution and avoid excessive exertion.

Discontinuation: It is best to withdraw this drug gradually (over a period of 2 to 4 weeks) after long-term use.

ISOTRETINOIN (i soh TRET i noin)

Introduced: 1979   **Class:** Anti-acne   **Prescription:** USA: Yes   **Controlled Drug:** USA: No; Canada: No   **Available as Generic:** Yes
Brand Name: Accutane

BENEFITS versus RISKS	
Possible Benefits	*Possible Risks*
EFFECTIVE TREATMENT OF SEVERE CYSTIC ACNE	DEPRESSION
	MAJOR BIRTH DEFECTS
Treatment of other skin conditions	Initial worsening of acne (transient)
	Inflammation of lips
	Dry skin, nose, and mouth
	Musculoskeletal discomfort
	Corneal opacities

▷ **Principal Uses**

As a Single Drug Product: Uses currently included in FDA-approved labeling: (1) treats severe, disfiguring nodular and cystic acne that has failed to respond to all other forms of therapy. ***It should not be used to treat mild forms of acne.*** (2) It is also used to treat some less common conditions of the skin that are due to disorders of keratin production.

Other (unlabeled) generally accepted uses: (1) May be helpful in refractory hypertrophic lupus erythematosus; (2) can help control resistant oral leukoplakia; (3) used in Apert's syndrome facial treatment; (4) used adjunctively to surgery in some cervical cancers; (5) treats mycosis fungoides; (6) eases symptoms in Darier's disease; (7) may have a role in treating dysplastic nevi; (8) eases symptoms of Grover's disease; (9) can help treat the abnormal gum growth (gingival hyperplasia) that can occur with phenytoin therapy; (10) treats severe and refractory rosacea; (11) has been combined with interferon alpha treatment in squamous cell skin cancer.

How This Drug Works: Reduces the size of sebaceous glands and inhibits sebum (skin oil) production. This helps to correct acne and its complications.

Available Dose Forms and Strengths
Capsules — 10 mg, 20 mg, 40 mg

▷ **Usual Adult Dose Range:** Starting dose is based on the patient's weight and severity of acne; the usual dose is 0.5 to 2 mg per kg of body mass daily, taken in two divided doses for 15 to 20 weeks. After weeks of treatment, the dose should be adjusted according to response of the acne and the development of adverse effects. **Note: Actual dose and schedule must be determined for each patient individually.**

Conditions Requiring Dosing Adjustments
Liver Function: The dose should be decreased when isotretinoin is used by patients with compromised livers.

Kidney Function: Isotretinoin should be used with caution in kidney compromise.

▷ **Dosing Instructions:** Begin treatment only on the second or third day of your next normal menstrual period. Take with meals (morning and evening) to achieve optimal blood levels. The capsule should not be opened for administration.

Usual Duration of Use: Use on a regular schedule for 15 to 20 weeks best determines effectiveness in clearing or improving severe cystic acne. The drug may be stopped earlier if the total cyst count is reduced by more than 70%. If a repeat course of treatment is necessary, it should not be started for 2 months. Long-term use (months to years) requires physician supervision.

▷ **This Drug Should Not Be Taken If**
- you have had an allergic reaction to it previously.
- you are allergic to parabens, preservatives used in this drug product.
- you have mild acne.
- you are not able or willing to follow contraception.
- you have not gotten verbal and written warnings about this medicine and fetal damage.
- you have not had a negative urine or serum pregnancy test (at least 50 mIU/ml sensitivity) 1 week before starting this medicine.
- you are pregnant or planning a pregnancy.
- you are not starting treatment on the second or third day of a subsequent normal menstrual period.

▷ **Inform Your Physician Before Taking This Drug If**
- you have a history of depression or become depressed while taking this medicine.
- you had an allergic reaction to vitamin A in the past.
- you routinely take a nonprescription form of vitamin A.
- you have diabetes mellitus.
- you are considering giving blood (you will NOT be eligible for 1 month after the last isotretinoin dose).
- you have a cholesterol or triglyceride disorder.
- you are considering having a child.
- you wear contact lenses (your tolerance for these may decrease while you take this medicine).
- you have a history of liver or kidney disease.

Possible Side Effects (natural, expected, and unavoidable drug actions)
Frequent dryness of the nose and mouth, inflammation of the lips, dryness of the skin with itching, peeling of the palms and soles. Dose-related increase in triglycerides.

▷ **Possible Adverse Effects** (unusual, unexpected, and infrequent reactions)
If any of the following develop, consult your physician promptly for guidance.
Mild Adverse Effects
Allergic reaction: skin rash—may resemble pityriasis rosea.
Thinning of hair, conjunctivitis, intolerance of contact lenses, decreased night vision, muscular and joint aches, headache, fatigue, indigestion—infrequent.

Serious Adverse Effects

Depression—case reports to infrequent.

Skin infections, worsening of arthritis, inflammatory bowel disorders—case reports.

Abnormal acceleration of bone development in children—possible.

Development of opacities in the cornea of the eye—possible.

Reduced red blood cell and white blood cell counts; increased blood platelet count—infrequent.

Seizures—case reports.

Kidney toxicity, liver toxicity, or pancreatitis—rare.

Abnormal blood glucose control—infrequent.

Increased pressure within the head (headache, visual disturbances, nausea/vomiting)—case reports.

▷ **Possible Effects on Sexual Function:**   Decreased male or female libido—possible.

Ejaculatory failure—case report.

Decreased vaginal secretions—possible.

Altered timing and pattern of menstruation—case reports.

Possible Effects on Laboratory Tests

Complete blood cell counts: infrequently decreased red cells and white cells.

Sedimentation rate: increased.

Blood total cholesterol, LDL cholesterol, VLDL cholesterol, and triglyceride levels: increased.

Blood HDL cholesterol levels: decreased.

Blood thyroid hormones (T_3, T_4, and free T_4 index): decreased.

Liver function tests: infrequently increased liver enzymes (ALT/GPT, AST/GOT, and alkaline phosphatase), increased bilirubin.

Blood calcium level: increased.

Protein in the urine: positive though infrequent.

CAUTION

1. This medicine has caused a number of verified cases of depression. Your physician should ask you about mood changes at each office visit, and you should call if depression starts.
2. This drug should not be used to treat mild forms of acne.
3. Worsening of your acne may occur during the first few weeks of treatment; this will subside with continued use of the drug.
4. Do not take any other form of vitamin A while taking this drug. (Check contents of multiple vitamin preparations.)
5. Women with potential for pregnancy should have a ***blood*** pregnancy test within 2 weeks before taking this drug and should use two effective forms of contraception simultaneously during its use. Contraception should be continued until normal menstruation resumes after discontinuing this drug.
6. This drug may cause increased blood levels of cholesterol and triglycerides.
7. If repeated courses of this drug are prescribed, wait a minimum of 2 months between courses before resuming medication.

Precautions for Use

By Infants and Children: Long-term use (6 to 12 months) may cause abnormal acceleration of bone growth and development. Your physician can monitor this possibility by periodic X-ray examination of long bones.

▷ **Advisability of Use During Pregnancy**

Pregnancy Category: X. See Pregnancy Risk Categories at the back of this book.

Animal studies: Birth defects of skull, brain, and vertebral column found in rats; skeletal birth defects found in rabbits.

Human studies: Adequate studies of pregnant women are not available. However, many serious birth defects (thought to be due to this drug) have been reported. These include major abnormalities of the head, brain, heart, blood vessels, and hormone-producing glands.

Avoid this drug completely during entire pregnancy.

Advisability of Use If Breast-Feeding

Presence of this drug in breast milk: Unknown.

Avoid drug or refrain from nursing.

Habit-Forming Potential: None.

Effects of Overdose: Increased blood pressure, lethargy, nausea, vomiting, mild gastrointestinal bleeding, elevated blood calcium, hallucinations, and psychosis.

Suggested Periodic Examinations While Taking This Drug (at physician's discretion)

Complete blood cell counts, including platelet counts.

Measurements of blood cholesterol and triglyceride levels. Complete eye examinations.

Liver and kidney function tests.

▷ **While Taking This Drug, Observe the Following**

Foods: Increases absorption and may be a good mechanism to maintain blood levels.

Beverages: No restrictions.

▷ *Alcohol:* A disulfiram-like reaction was described in one case report.

Tobacco Smoking: No interactions expected. I advise everyone to quit smoking.

▷ *Other Drugs*

Isotretinoin *taken concurrently* with

• carbamazepine (Tegretol) may cause subtherapeutic carbamazepine levels.
• minocycline may increase risk of severe headache, papilledema, and visual changes.
• tetracyclines may cause increased risk of pseudotumor cerebri.

▷ *Driving, Hazardous Activities:* No restrictions.

Exposure to Sun: Caution: this drug can cause photosensitivity (see Glossary).

ISRADIPINE (is RA di peen)

Introduced: 1984   **Class:** Antihypertensive, calcium channel blocker
Prescription: USA: Yes   **Controlled Drug:** USA: No   **Available as Generic:**   USA: No
Brand Name: DynaCirc, Dynacirc CR

Controversies in Medicine: Medicines in this class have had many conflicting reports. The FDA has held hearings on the calcium channel blocker (CCB) class. A study called ALLHAT is comparing amlodipine, an ACE inhibitor, a diuretic, and an alpha blocker (see Drug Classes) and should clarify adverse effects, mortality and other issues relating to CCBs. **Amlodipine got the first FDA approval to treat high blood pressure or angina in people with congestive heart failure**. CCBs are currently second-line agents for high blood pressure according to the JNC VI (see Glossary).

BENEFITS versus RISKS	
Possible Benefits	*Possible Risks*
EFFECTIVE TREATMENT OF MILD TO MODERATE HYPERTENSION	Headache
	Dizziness
	Fluid retention
	Palpitations

▷ **Principal Uses**
As a Single Drug Product: Uses currently included in FDA-approved labeling: (1) Treats mild to moderate hypertension, alone or in combination; (2) treats hypertension in pregnancy.
Other (unlabeled) generally accepted uses: (1) Treatment of chronic, stable angina; (2) in combination therapy of congestive heart failure; (3) may help prevent progression of early lesions in atherosclerosis; (4) treats premature labor.

How This Drug Works: Blocks passage of calcium through cell walls, inhibiting contraction of coronary arteries and peripheral arterioles. As a result, isradipine
• promotes dilation of the coronary arteries (anti-anginal effect);
• reduces the degree of contraction of peripheral arterial walls, resulting in lowering of blood pressure. This further reduces heart workload and helps prevent angina.

Available Dose Forms and Strengths
Capsules — 2.5 mg, 5 mg
Tablets (timed release) — 5 mg and 10 mg

▷ **Usual Adult Dose Range:**   Hypertension: Initially 2.5 mg twice daily, 12 hours apart, for a trial period of 2 to 4 weeks. If needed, the dose may be increased by 5 mg per day at intervals of 2 to 4 weeks. The usual maintenance dose is 5 to 10 mg daily. The total daily dose should not exceed 20 mg. Sustained release form is started at 5 mg once a day and increased slowly if needed. **Note: Actual dose and dosing schedule must be determined for each patient individually.**

Conditions Requiring Dosing Adjustments
Liver Function: Empiric decreases in dosing are prudent in liver damage.
Kidney Function: Use with caution in kidney compromise. Initial dose should be 2.5 mg twice a day. Five mg once daily (sustained release).

▷ **Dosing Instructions:**   May be taken with or following food to reduce stomach irritation. The capsule may be opened, mixed with food, and swallowed promptly. The sustained release tablets MUST NOT be altered.

Usual Duration of Use: Use on a regular schedule for 2 to 4 weeks determines this drug's effectiveness in controlling hypertension or in reducing the frequency and severity of angina. The smallest effective dose should be used for long-term (months to years) therapy. Periodic physician evaluation is essential.

Possible Advantages of This Drug

Does not cause orthostatic hypotension (see Glossary). No adverse effects on heart or kidney function. No adverse effects on blood cholesterol levels.

▷ **This Drug Should Not Be Taken If**

- you have had an allergic reaction to it previously.
- you have symptomatic low blood pressure (hypotension).
- you have advanced narrowing of the aorta.
- you have severe problems in the left side of your heart (left ventricular dysfunction).

▷ **Inform Your Physician Before Taking This Drug If**

- you have had an unfavorable response to any calcium-channel-blocker drug in the past (see Drug Classes).
- you take any beta-blocker drug (see Drug Classes).
- you are taking any drugs that lower blood pressure.
- you have a history of congestive heart failure, heart attack, or stroke.
- you are subject to disturbances of heart rhythm.
- you have muscular dystrophy or myasthenia gravis.
- you develop a skin reaction while taking this drug.
- you have impaired liver or kidney function.
- you will have surgery with general anesthesia.

Possible Side Effects (natural, expected, and unavoidable drug actions)

Rapid heart rate—rare.

Swelling of the feet and ankles, cough, flushing and sensation of warmth—infrequent.

Small weight loss—possible.

▷ **Possible Adverse Effects** (unusual, unexpected, and infrequent reactions)

If any of the following develop, consult your physician promptly for guidance.

Mild Adverse Effects

Allergic reactions: skin rash, hives, itching—rare.

Headache—frequent; dizziness, weakness—infrequent; nervousness, blurred vision—rare.

Decreased skin sensation—rare.

Palpitation, shortness of breath—infrequent.

Indigestion, nausea, vomiting, constipation—infrequent.

Cramps in legs and feet—rare.

Increased urination—rare.

Abnormal growth of the gums (gingival hyperplasia)—frequent with some drugs in the same class.

Serious Adverse Effects

Allergic reactions: erythema multiforme, exfoliative dermatitis—case reports.

Heart rhythm disturbances—infrequent.

Increased frequency or severity of angina (when therapy is started or dose increased)—possible.

Marked drop in blood pressure with fainting—rare.

Low white blood cell counts—rare.

▷ **Possible Effects on Sexual Function:**   Decreased libido, impotence (less than 1%).

▷ **Adverse Effects That May Mimic Natural Diseases or Disorders**

Flushing and warmth may resemble menopausal "hot flashes."

Possible Effects on Laboratory Tests

White blood cell counts: decreased (less than 1% of users).

Liver function tests: increased enzyme levels—infrequent.

Electrocardiogram: slight increase in QT interval.

CAUTION

1. If you check your blood pressure, check it just before each dose and 2 to 3 hours after each dose. Even though high blood pressure usually has no symptoms, high blood pressure MUST be treated to avoid serious complications.

2. Tell health care professionals who treat you that you take this drug. List this drug on a card in your purse or wallet.

3. Nitroglycerin and other nitrate drugs may be used as needed to relieve acute episodes of angina pain. However, if your angina attacks are becoming more frequent or intense, notify your physician promptly.

Precautions for Use

By Infants and Children: Safety and effectiveness under 18 years of age not established.

By Those Over 60 Years of Age: Usually well tolerated by this age group. However, watch for weakness, dizziness, fainting, and falling. Take necessary precautions to prevent injury.

▷ **Advisability of Use During Pregnancy**

Pregnancy Category: C. See Pregnancy Risk Categories at the back of this book.

Animal studies: Embryo and fetal toxicity reported in small animals, but no birth defects due to this drug.

Human studies: Adequate studies of pregnant women are not available.

Avoid this drug during the first 3 months. Use during the final 6 months only if clearly needed. Ask your physician for guidance.

Advisability of Use If Breast-Feeding

Presence of this drug in breast milk: Unknown.

Avoid drug or refrain from nursing.

Habit-Forming Potential: None.

Effects of Overdose: Weakness, light-headedness, fainting, fast pulse, low blood pressure, shortness of breath, flushed and warm skin, tremors, and abnormal heartbeats.

Possible Effects of Long-Term Use: None reported.

Suggested Periodic Examinations While Taking This Drug (at physician's discretion)

Evaluations of heart function, including electrocardiograms; measurements of blood pressure in supine, sitting, and standing positions.

▷ **While Taking This Drug, Observe the Following**

Foods: DO NOT take this medicine with grapefruit or grapefruit juice.

Avoid excessive salt intake.

Beverages: DO NOT take this medicine with grapefruit or grapefruit juice. May be taken with milk.

▷ *Alcohol:* Use caution. Alcohol may exaggerate the drop in blood pressure in some people.

Tobacco Smoking: Nicotine may reduce the effectiveness of this drug. I advise everyone to quit smoking.

Marijuana Smoking: Possible reduced effectiveness; mild to moderate increase in angina; possible changes in electrocardiogram, confusing interpretation.

▷ *Other Drugs*

Isradipine *taken concurrently* with

- antifungals (triazoles) such as fluconazole, itraconazole, or ketoconazole may lead to toxicity.
- beta-blocker drugs or digitalis preparations (see Drug Classes) may affect heart rate and rhythm adversely. Careful monitoring by your physician is needed if these drugs are taken concurrently.
- carbamazepine (Tegretol) has resulted in decreased blood levels of carbamazepine with calcium channel blockers from the same pharmacological family. Caution is advised.
- delavirdine (Rescriptor) may lead to isradipine toxicity.
- digoxin (Lanoxin) may increase blood levels. Laboratory testing of blood levels should be performed more often if these drugs are combined.
- erythromycin (various) may increase the free (active) form of isradipine, resulting in a larger than expected effect.
- magnesium, especially in doses used in premature labor, can cause very low and abnormal blood pressure.
- phenytoin (Dilantin) may result in loss of isradipine's effectiveness. Caution is advised.
- rifampin (Rifadin, others) may result in a decreased therapeutic benefit from isradipine.
- ritonavir (Norvir) and perhaps other protease inhibitors (see Drug Classes) can lead to toxicity.

▷ *Driving, Hazardous Activities:* Usually no restrictions. This drug may cause drowsiness or dizziness. Restrict activities as necessary.

Aviation Note: Coronary artery disease and hypertension *are disqualifications* for piloting. Consult a designated aviation medical examiner.

Exposure to Sun: No restrictions.

Exposure to Heat: Caution is advised. Hot environments can exaggerate the blood-pressure-lowering effects of this drug. Observe for light-headedness or weakness.

Heavy Exercise or Exertion: This drug may improve your ability to be more active without resulting angina pain. Use caution and avoid excessive exercise that could impair heart function in the absence of warning pain.

Discontinuation: Do not stop this drug abruptly. Ask your doctor about gradual withdrawal. Watch for the development of rebound angina.

KETOCONAZOLE (kee toh KOHN a zohl)

Introduced: 1981   **Class:** Antifungal   **Prescription:** USA: Yes   **Controlled Drug:** USA: No; Canada: No   **Available as Generic:** USA: No; Canada: No
Brand Name: Nizoral

BENEFITS versus RISKS

Possible Benefits	*Possible Risks*
EFFECTIVE TREATMENT OF THE FOLLOWING FUNGUS INFECTIONS: Blastomycosis, candidiasis, chromomycosis, coccidioidomycosis, histoplasmosis, paracoccidioidomycosis, tinea (ringworm)	SERIOUS DRUG-INDUCED LIVER DAMAGE
Beneficial short-term treatment of advanced prostate cancer	Allergic reactions
Beneficial auxiliary treatment of Cushing's syndrome	Low blood platelets and anemia

---

▷ **Principal Uses**

As a Single Drug Product: Uses currently included in FDA-approved labeling: Treatment of (1) lung and systemic blastomycosis; (2) *Candida* (yeast) infections of the skin, mouth, throat, and esophagus (may be AIDS-related); (3) systemic *Candida* infections—pneumonia, peritonitis, urinary tract infections (may be AIDS-related); (4) chromomycosis (auxiliary); (5) lung and systemic coccidioidomycosis; (6) lung and systemic histoplasmosis; (7) paracoccidioidomycosis; (8) tinea infections—groin (jock itch)and feet (athlete's foot); (9) tinea versicolor (pityriasis).

Other (unlabeled) generally accepted uses: Treatment of (1) *Candida* infections of the vulva and vagina; (2) prostate cancer (short-term); (3) Cushing's syndrome (excessive adrenal hormones); (4) systemic sporotrichosis; (5) fungal dandruff (topical); (6) fungal toenail infections; (7) kidney toxicity caused by cyclosporine; (8) visceral leishmaniasis.

How This Drug Works: As an antifungal: By damaging cell walls and impairing critical cell enzymes, this drug inhibits cell growth and reproduction (with low drug levels) and destroys fungal cells (with high drug concentrations).

In treating prostate cancer: Decreases testosterone (male hormone) levels—prostate cancer needs testosterone to grow.

In treating Cushing's syndrome: This drug suppresses the excessive production of adrenal corticosteroid hormones.

Available Dose Forms and Strengths

Cream — 2% (for local application to *Candida* or tinea skin infections)
Shampoo — 2%
Oral suspension — 100 mg/5 ml (Canada)
Tablets — 200 mg (U.S. and Canada)

▷ **Recommended Dose Ranges** (Actual dose and schedule must be determined for each patient individually.)

Infants and Children: Up to 2 years of age: Dose not established.

Over 2 years of age: 3.3 to 6.6 mg per kg of body mass, once daily; the dose depends upon the nature of the infection.

12 to 60 Years of Age: For fungus infections—200 to 400 mg once daily; 800 mg maximum daily dose.

For prostate cancer—400 mg three times daily; 1200 mg maximum daily dose.

For Cushing's syndrome—600 to 1200 mg once daily; total daily dose should not exceed 1200 mg.

Over 60 Years of Age: Same as 12 to 60 years of age.

Conditions Requiring Dosing Adjustments

Liver Function: Dose empirically decreased for patients with liver compromise.

Kidney Function: Decreased doses are not needed in kidney compromise.

Achlorhydria (lack of acid in the stomach): This medicine requires an acid environment in the stomach to be absorbed. Talk with your doctor about making a dilute acid solution to drink prior to taking the tablet form.

▷ **Dosing Instructions:**   The tablet may be crushed and is best taken with or after food to enhance absorption and reduce stomach irritation. Do not take with antacids. Take the full course prescribed.

Usual Duration of Use: Use on a regular schedule for 2 to 4 weeks determines effectiveness in controlling fungal infections. Actual cures or long-term suppression often require continual treatment for many months. Periodic physician evaluation of response and dose adjustment are essential.

▷ **This Drug Should Not Be Taken If**
- you have had an allergic reaction to it previously.
- you have active liver disease.
- you take astemizole or terfenadine.

▷ **Inform Your Physician Before Taking This Drug If**
- you are allergic to related antifungal drugs: clotrimazole, fluconazole, itraconazole, or miconazole.
- you have a liver disease or impaired liver function.
- you take loratadine. Heart problems have not been reported as with other nonsedating antihistamines, but the blood level does increase if the drugs are combined; the dose of loratadine may need to be decreased.
- you have a history of adrenal gland problems (adrenal insufficiency).
- you have a history of low blood platelets or anemia.
- you have a history of alcoholism.
- you have a deficiency of stomach hydrochloric acid.
- you are taking any other drugs currently.

Possible Side Effects (natural, expected, and unavoidable drug actions)

Suppression of testosterone and adrenal corticosteroid hormone production (more pronounced with high drug doses).

▷ **Possible Adverse Effects** (unusual, unexpected, and infrequent reactions)

If any of the following develop, consult your physician promptly for guidance.

Mild Adverse Effects

Allergic reactions: skin rash, hives, itching—rare.

Headache, dizziness, drowsiness, photophobia—infrequent.

Nausea (helped by taking with meals) and vomiting, stomach pain, diarrhea—rare.

Increased blood pressure—possible.

Hair loss or ringing in the ears—case reports.

Muscle and joint aches—infrequent.

Serious Adverse Effects

Allergic reactions: anaphylactic reaction (see Glossary).

Severe liver toxicity: loss of appetite, nausea, yellow skin or eyes, dark urine, light-colored stools (see *jaundice* in Glossary)—rare.

Suppression of the adrenal gland or low thyroid function—case reports.

Mental depression—rare.

Hemolytic anemia or abnormally low platelet counts (abnormal bruising or bleeding)—rare.

▷ **Possible Effects on Sexual Function:**   Decreased testosterone blood levels: reduced sperm counts, decreased libido, impotence, male breast enlargement and tenderness (gynecomastia).

Altered menstrual patterns—case reports.

Possible Delayed Adverse Effects: Deficiency of adrenal corticosteroid hormones (cortisone related); this could be serious during stress resulting from illness or injury.

▷ **Adverse Effects That May Mimic Natural Diseases or Disorders**

Drug-induced liver reaction may suggest viral hepatitis.

Possible Effects on Laboratory Tests

Complete blood cell counts: decreased red cells, white cells, and platelets.

Liver function tests: increased liver enzymes (ALT/GPT, AST/GOT, and alkaline phosphatase), increased bilirubin.

Thyroid function tests: decreased—rare.

Adrenal corticosteroid blood levels: decreased.

Testosterone blood levels: decreased.

Precautions for Use

By Infants and Children: Safety and effectiveness for thoseunder 2 years old not established.

By Those Over 60 Years of Age: This drug requires an acid stomach to enter the body. Talk with your doctor if achlorhydria (gastric) has been diagnosed.

▷ **Advisability of Use During Pregnancy**

Pregnancy Category: C. See Pregnancy Risk Categories at the back of this book.

Animal studies: Rat studies revealed significant embryo toxicity and birth defects due to this drug.

Human studies: Adequate studies of pregnant women are not available.

Use this drug only if clearly needed. Ask your physician for guidance.

Advisability of Use If Breast-Feeding

Presence of this drug in breast milk: Yes.

Avoid drug or refrain from nursing.

Habit-Forming Potential: None.

Effects of Overdose: Possible nausea, vomiting, diarrhea.

Possible Effects of Long-Term Use: Suppression of adrenal corticosteroid hormone production, requiring replacement therapy during periods of stress.

Suggested Periodic Examinations While Taking This Drug (at physician's discretion)

Liver function tests should be obtained BEFORE long-term therapy is started, and checked monthly during treatment.

Sperm counts.

▷ **While Taking This Drug, Observe the Following**

Foods: No restrictions.

Beverages: No restrictions. May be taken with milk.

▷ *Alcohol:* Avoid completely. Alcohol can cause a disulfiramlike reaction (see Glossary). In addition, alcohol may cause liver toxicity.

Tobacco Smoking: No interactions expected. I advise everyone to quit smoking.

▷ *Other Drugs*

Ketoconazole *may increase* the effects of

- alprazolam (Xanax) and other benzodiazepines (see Drug Classes).
- carbamazepine (Tegretol).
- cortisonelike drugs (prednisone, etc.).
- cyclosporine (Sandimmune).
- Delavirdine (Rescriptor).
- HMG-CoA reductase inhibitors (atorvastatin, etc.—see Drug Classes), increasing risk of myopathy.
- loratadine (Claritin)—this is also a nonsedating antihistamine, but **HAS NOT** been associated with heart rhythm problems when combined with ketoconazole. The blood level does appear to increase, and lower doses of loratadine are prudent if these medicines are to be combined.
- oral antidiabetic drugs (see Drug Classes), and result in very low blood sugars.
- nonsedating antihistamines such as astemizole (Hismanal) and terfenadine (Seldane), and may cause large increases in blood levels and result in serious heart rhythm problems. DO NOT COMBINE.
- protease inhibitors (see Drug Classes).
- quinidine (Quinaglute), and cause toxicity. Blood levels are needed.
- ritonavir (Norvir).
- sildenafil (Viagra)—TALK to your doctor BEFORE using these medicines together.
- sucralfate (Carafate) may decrease the blood levels of ketoconazole.
- warfarin (Coumadin), and cause bleeding. Increased testing of INR (prothrombin time or protime) are needed.

Ketoconazole may *decrease* the effects of

- amphotericin B (Abelcet).
- didanosine (Videx).
- theophyllines (aminophylline, Theo-Dur, etc.).

The following drugs may *decrease* the effects of ketoconazole:

- antacids; if needed, take antacids 2 hours after ketoconazole.
- histamine (H_2) blocking drugs: cimetidine, famotidine, nizatidine, ranitidine. If needed, take 2 hours after ketoconazole.
- isoniazid (Laniazid, Nydrazid, etc.).
- lansoprazole (Prevacid).
- omeprazole (Prilosec).
- rifampin (Rifadin, Rifater, Rimactane, etc.).

Ketoconazole *taken concurrently* with
- cisapride (Propulsid) can lead to serious heart toxicity. DO NOT COMBINE.
- miconazole (Monistat) may increase the blood levels of ketoconazole or miconazole.
- phenytoin (Dilantin) may change the levels of both drugs.
- trimexate (Neutrexin) may lead to toxicity.

▷ *Driving, Hazardous Activities:* This drug may cause dizziness or drowsiness. Restrict activities as necessary.

Aviation Note: The use of this drug *may be a disqualification* for piloting. Consult a designated aviation medical examiner.

Exposure to Sun: This drug may cause photophobia; wear sunglasses if appropriate.

Discontinuation: Take the full course prescribed. Continual treatment for several months may be needed. Ask your doctor when the drug should be stopped.

KETOPROFEN (kee toh PROH fen)

See the propionic acids (nonsteroidal anti-inflammatory drugs) profile for further information.

LABETALOL (la BET a lohl)

Introduced: 1978   **Class:** Antihypertensive, alpha- and beta-adrenergic blocker   **Prescription:** USA: Yes   **Controlled Drug:** USA: No; Canada: No   **Available as Generic:** Yes

Brand Names: Normodyne, Normozide [CD], Trandate, Trandate HCT [CD]

BENEFITS versus RISKS	
Possible Benefits	*Possible Risks*
EFFECTIVE, WELL-TOLERATED ANTIHYPERTENSIVE in mild to moderate high blood pressure	CONGESTIVE HEART FAILURE in advanced heart disease
PROLONGS LIFE AFTER A HEART ATTACK	Worsening of angina in coronary heart disease (if drug is abruptly withdrawn)
	Masking of low blood sugar (hypoglycemia) in drug-treated diabetes
	Liver toxicity

▷ **Principal Uses**

As a Single Drug Product: Uses currently included in FDA-approved labeling: (1) Treats mild to moderate high blood pressure; (2) treats hypertension in pregnancy; (3) useful in hypertension and angina.

Other (unlabeled) generally accepted uses: (1) Combination therapy of hypertension in heart attacks (acute MI)—beta-blockers have also been shown to decrease the risk of repeat heart attacks, limit the size of the original heart attack damage, and help control arrhythmias; (2) treatment of cocaine overdose; (3) therapy of phobic anxiety reactions; (4) treatment of

angina; (5) therapy of pheochromocytoma, a tumor that releases compounds that increase blood pressure.

As a Combination Drug Product [CD]: This drug has been combined with hydrochlorothiazide (a thiazide diuretic) to attack high blood pressure
through the combination benefit of two different medicines.

How This Drug Works: By blocking part of the sympathetic nervous system,
this drug
- reduces the rate and contraction force of the heart, thus lowering the ejection pressure of blood leaving the heart.
- reduces the degree of contraction of blood vessel walls, resulting in their expansion and lowering of blood pressure.

Available Dose Forms and Strengths
Injection — 5 mg/ml
Tablets — 100 mg, 200 mg, 300 mg

▷ **Usual Adult Dose Range:**   Initially 100 mg twice daily, 12 hours apart; the dose
may be increased by 100 mg twice daily every 2 to 3 days as needed to reduce blood pressure. The usual ongoing dose is 200 to 400 mg twice daily.
Maximum daily dose is 2400 mg daily, given as 800 mg three times daily.
**Note: Actual dose and dosing schedule must be determined individu-
ally.**

Conditions Requiring Dosing Adjustments
Liver Function: The dose **must** be decreased in liver disease. Average dose for
people with long-standing liver disease is 50% of the usual dose. This drug
is a rare cause of liver injury.
Kidney Function: No changes presently needed.

▷ **Dosing Instructions:**   The tablet may be crushed and is best taken at the same
times daily, ideally following morning and evening meals. Do not abruptly
stop this drug.

Usual Duration of Use: Use on a regular schedule for 10 to 14 days determines
effectiveness in lowering blood pressure. Long-term use (months to years)
is determined by individual response to this drug and an overall treatment
program (weight reduction, salt restriction, smoking cessation, etc.).

Possible Advantages of This Drug
Decreases blood pressure more rapidly than other beta-blocker drugs. Can be
used to treat hypertensive emergencies.

▷ **This Drug Should Not Be Taken If**
- you have had an allergic reaction to it previously.
- you have active bronchial asthma.
- you have congestive heart failure.
- you are in cardiogenic shock.
- you have an abnormally slow heart rate or a serious form of heart block.

▷ **Inform Your Physician Before Taking This Drug If**
- you have had an adverse reaction to any beta-blocker drug (see Drug
Classes).
- you have a history of serious heart disease.
- you have a history of hay fever (allergic rhinitis), asthma, chronic bronchitis, or emphysema.
- you have a history of overactive thyroid function (hyperthyroidism).

- you have a history of low blood sugar (hypoglycemia).
- you have sporadic cramping of the leg muscles (intermittent claudication).
- you have a history of spasms of the bronchi of the lungs.
- you have impaired liver or kidney function.
- you have intermittent claudication.
- you have diabetes or myasthenia gravis.
- you take any form of digitalis, quinidine, or reserpine, or any calcium-channel-blocker drug (see Drug Classes).
- you will have surgery with general anesthesia.

Possible Side Effects (natural, expected, and unavoidable drug actions)
Lethargy and fatigability—frequent; light-headedness in upright position (see *orthostatic hypotension* in Glossary).

▷ **Possible Adverse Effects** (unusual, unexpected, and infrequent reactions)
If any of the following develop, consult your physician promptly for guidance.

Mild Adverse Effects
Allergic reactions: skin rash, itching.
Headache, drowsiness, dizziness—frequent; scalp tingling (during early treatment)—possible.
Vivid dreams, nightmares, depression—infrequent.
Urine retention, difficulty urinating—case reports.
Indigestion, nausea, diarrhea—infrequent.
Joint and muscle discomfort, fluid retention (edema)—rare.

Serious Adverse Effects
Allergic reactions: anaphylaxis—case reports.
Chest pain, shortness of breath, precipitation of congestive heart failure—possible.
Induction of bronchial asthma (in asthmatic individuals)—possible.
Lichen planus—case reports.
Muscle toxicity (toxic myopathy, worsening of intermittent claudication)—possible.
Drug-induced systemic lupus erythematosus—rare.
Aggravation of myasthenia gravis—case reports.
Liver damage with jaundice—rare and often reversible.

▷ **Possible Effects on Sexual Function:**   Impotence, inhibited ejaculation, prolonged erection following orgasm (related to higher doses), Peyronie's disease (see Glossary)—rare to infrequent.
Decreased vaginal secretions (with low doses), inhibited female orgasm (higher doses)—possible.

Possible Effects on Laboratory Tests
Blood potassium or glucose: slight increase.
Liver function tests: rare increases.

CAUTION
1. *Do not stop this drug suddenly* without the knowledge and help of your doctor. Carry a note or wear a labetalol drug-identification bracelet.
2. Ask your physician or pharmacist before using nasal decongestants, which are usually present in over-the-counter cold preparations and nose

drops. These can cause sudden increases in blood pressure if combined with labetalol.

3. Report the development of any tendency to emotional depression.

Precautions for Use

By Infants and Children: Safety and effectiveness for those under 12 years of age are not established. However, if this drug is used, watch for low blood sugar (hypoglycemia) during periods of reduced food intake.

By Those Over 60 Years of Age: Proceed **cautiously** with all antihypertensive drugs. Therapy should be started with small doses, with frequent checks of blood pressure. Sudden, rapid, or excessive lowering of blood pressure can increase stroke or heart attack risk. Watch for dizziness, unsteadiness, tendency to fall, confusion, hallucinations, depression, or urinary frequency.

▷ **Advisability of Use During Pregnancy**

Pregnancy Category: C. See Pregnancy Risk Categories at the back of this book.
Animal studies: No significant increase in birth defects found in rats or rabbits; some increase in fetal deaths reported.
Human studies: Adequate studies of pregnant women are not available.
Use this drug only if clearly needed. Ask your physician for guidance.

Advisability of Use If Breast-Feeding

Presence of this drug in breast milk: Yes, in very small amounts.
Avoid drug or refrain from nursing.

Habit-Forming Potential: None.

Effects of Overdose: Weakness, slow pulse, low blood pressure, fainting, cold and sweaty skin, congestive heart failure, possible coma, and convulsions.

Possible Effects of Long-Term Use: Reduced heart reserve and eventual heart failure in susceptible individuals with advanced heart disease.

Suggested Periodic Examinations While Taking This Drug (at physician's discretion)

Measurements of blood pressure, evaluation of heart function.

▷ **While Taking This Drug, Observe the Following**

Foods: May increase the absorption of labetalol and result in a larger than expected blood level. Patients taking this medicine should also avoid excessive salt intake.

Beverages: No restrictions. May be taken with milk.

▷ *Alcohol:* Use with caution. Alcohol may exaggerate this drug's ability to lower blood pressure and may increase its mild sedative effect.

Tobacco Smoking: Nicotine may reduce this drug's effectiveness. I advise everyone to quit smoking.

▷ *Other Drugs*

Labetalol may **increase** the effects of

• oral antidiabetic drugs (see Drug Classes), and prolong recovery from any hypoglycemia (low blood sugar) that may occur.

• other antihypertensive drugs, and cause excessive lowering of blood pressure. Dose adjustments may be necessary.

Labetalol **taken concurrently** with

• amiodarone (Codarone) may result in extremely slow heart rates and cardiac arrest.

- cimetidine (Tagamet) can cause elevated labetalol levels and low blood pressure or heart rate.
- clonidine (Catapres) must be closely watched for rebound high blood pressure if clonidine is withdrawn while labetalol is still being taken.
- epinephrine may result in severe increases in blood pressure.
- fluoxetine (Prozac) may increase labetalol effects.
- fluvoxamine (Luvox) may result in excessive lowering of blood pressure or excessive slowing of the heart.
- imipramine and other tricyclic antidepressants may result in increases in antidepressant blood levels and toxicity.
- insulin must be watched for development of hypoglycemia (see Glossary).
- NSAIDs (see *nonsteroidal anti-inflammatory drugs* in Drug Classes) may result in blunting of the therapeutic effects of labetalol.
- paroxetine (Paxil) may increase labetalol effects.
- phenothiazines (see Drug Classes) may cause additive lowering of the blood pressure.
- ritodrine (Yutopar) may blunt the beneficial effects of ritodrine.
- venlafaxine (Effexor) may increase labetalol effects.
- zileuton (Zyflo) may increase labetalol effects.

▷ *Driving, Hazardous Activities:* Use caution until the full extent of fatigue, dizziness, and blood pressure change has been determined.

Aviation Note: The use of this drug *is a disqualification* for piloting. Consult a designated aviation medical examiner.

Exposure to Sun: No restrictions.

Exposure to Heat: Caution is advised. Hot environments can lower the blood pressure and exaggerate the effects of this drug.

Exposure to Cold: Caution is advised. Cold environments can increase blood flow problems in the extremities that may occur with beta-blocker drugs. The elderly should take precautions to prevent hypothermia (see Glossary).

Heavy Exercise or Exertion: It is prudent to avoid exertion that produces light-headedness, excessive fatigue, or muscle cramping. Use of this drug may intensify hypertensive response to isometric exercise.

Occurrence of Unrelated Illness: Fever can lower blood pressure and require decreased doses. Nausea or vomiting may interrupt scheduled doses. Ask your doctor for help.

Discontinuation: If possible, gradual reduction of dose over a period of 2 to 3 weeks is recommended—otherwise rebound increases in blood pressure may occur. Ask your doctor for help.

LAMIVUDINE (LAMB iv u deen)

Introduced: 1995   **Class:** Antiviral, antiretroviral, reverse transcriptase inhibitor, nucleoside analog   **Prescription:** USA: Yes   **Controlled Drug:** USA: No   **Available as Generic:** No
Brand Name: Epivir

```
┌─────────────────────────────────────────────────────────────────────┐
│                      BENEFITS versus RISKS                           │
│      Possible Benefits                    Possible Risks             │
│  IMPRESSIVE SUPPRESSION OF         DECREASED WHITE BLOOD CELL        │
│    VIRAL LOAD WHEN USED IN            COUNTS                         │
│    COMBINATION THERAPY             Peripheral neuropathy             │
│    TREATING AIDS                   Pancreatitis                      │
│  DOES NOT LEAD TO SUPPRESSION                                        │
│    OF THE BONE MARROW                                                │
│  EFFECTIVE TREATMENT OF                                              │
│    HEPATITIS B INFECTION                                             │
└─────────────────────────────────────────────────────────────────────┘
```

▷ **Principal Uses**

As a Single Drug Product: Uses currently included in FDA-approved labeling: (1) Used to treat HIV infection. Used in combination because of possible resistance. This medicine was one of the three drugs used together (indinavir—a protease inhibitor—and AZT—a nucleoside analog) that resulted in decrease of HIV virus levels to undetectable amounts. (2) Used with zidovudine (AZT) in reducing the risk of disease progression and death in HIV.

Author's Note: ***The Panel on Clinical Practices for Treatment of HIV Infection Report* says that the preferred regimen is two nucleoside analogs and one potent protease inhibitor. Single-agent therapy was rejected by the panel.**

Other (unlabeled) generally accepted uses: Pending FDA approval for use in treating hepatitis B. One significant study found that single-agent therapy with lamivudine cleared hepatitis B virus from the blood of some of the test patients.

As a Combination Drug Product [CD]: Available in combination with zidovudine, a nucleoside analog. This combination along with a protease inhibitor (indinavir), was one of the first regimens to decrease HIV viral burden to undetectable levels.

How This Drug Works: Potent reverse transcriptase inhibitor—interferes ability of HIV virus to create genetic material. The exact mechanism of action in treating hepatitis B is not clear.

Available Dose Forms and Strengths
Solution — 10 mg/ml
Tablets — 150 mg
Tablets (Combivir) — 150 mg lamivudine and 300 mg zidovudine

▷ **Recommended Dose Ranges:** (Actual dose and schedule must be determined for each patient individually.)

Infants and Children: 3 months to 12 years old: 4 mg per kg of body mass twice daily (300 mg maximum a day).

Combivir: One tablet twice a day for those over 12 years old.

12 to 65 Years of Age: Usual dose is 150 mg twice daily.

Adults weighing less than 110 lb or 50 kg: 2 mg per kg of body mass twice daily.

Combivir: One tablet twice a day.

Over 65 Years of Age: Not studied in those over 65.

Conditions Requiring Dosing Adjustments

Liver Function: No changes expected.

Kidney Function: Up to 70% of a given dose is removed by the kidneys. Those with creatinine clearances (see Glossary) of 5 to 14 ml/min should take a first dose of 150 mg and then 50 mg once daily.

▷ **Dosing Instructions:**   Lamivudine tablets and solution can be taken without regard to meals. A solution is available for patients who can't swallow the tablets.

Usual Duration of Use: Measurement of viral load (burden) and/or CD4 counts are now used to decide the effectiveness of treatment and help in the decision to continue or change medications.

Possible Side Effects (natural, expected, and unavoidable drug actions)

Paresthesias and/or peripheral neuropathy (12% in a study in children taking lamivudine monotherapy).

▷ **Possible Adverse Effects** (unusual, unexpected, and infrequent reactions)

If any of the following develop, consult your physician promptly for guidance.

Mild Adverse Effects

Skin rash—infrequent.

Headache—frequent; dizziness—infrequent.

Sleep disorders—infrequent to frequent.

Nausea, vomiting, or diarrhea—infrequent to frequent.

Cough—frequent.

Muscle aches—infrequent.

Serious Adverse Effects

Lowered white blood cell counts—infrequent in adults, frequent in pediatrics.

Pancreatitis (more common in children receiving lamivudine monotherapy)—infrequent.

Seizures—case reports.

▷ **Possible Effects on Sexual Function:**   None reported.

Possible Delayed Adverse Effects: Anemia or lowering of white blood cell counts. Pancreatitis, peripheral neuropathy.

▷ **Adverse Effects That May Mimic Natural Diseases or Disorders**

Seizures may suggest the possibility of epilepsy.

Possible Effects on Laboratory Tests

Complete blood cell counts: decreased red cells. Increased amylase and lipase (if pancreatitis occurs).

CAUTION

1. This drug is **not** a cure for HIV or AIDS, nor does it protect completely against other infections or complications. Follow your doctor's instructions. Take exactly as prescribed.

2. AIDS can still be spread through sexual contact or blood. Use of an effective condom is mandatory. Don't share needles.

Precautions for Use

By Infants and Children: Patients from 3 months to 12 years old are dosed on a mg-per-kg-of-body-mass basis.

By Those Over 60 Years of Age: Impaired kidney function requires dose reduction.

▷ **Advisability of Use During Pregnancy**
    Pregnancy Category: C. See Pregnancy Risk Categories at the back of this book.
      Animal studies: Rat and rabbit studies reveal no birth defects.
      Human studies: Adequate studies of pregnant women are not available. Your
      physician should call 1-800-722-9292, ext. 38465, if the decision is made to
      use this medicine while you are pregnant.

Advisability of Use If Breast-Feeding
    Presence of this drug in breast milk: Unknown.
    Refrain from nursing (HIV may be transferred via breast milk).

Habit-Forming Potential: None.

Effects of Overdose: Nausea, vomiting, diarrhea, bone marrow depression.

Possible Effects of Long-Term Use: Anemia and loss of white blood cells.
    Pancreatitis or peripheral neuropathy.

Suggested Periodic Examinations While Taking This Drug (at physician's discretion)
    Complete blood counts.
    Periodic CD4 counts or viral load tests are needed. Increasing viral load or decreasing CD4 are indicators that therapy is failing and demand change of antiretroviral therapy.
    Amylase and lipase. Check for peripheral neuropathy.

▷ **While Taking This Drug, Observe the Following**
    Foods: No restrictions.
    Beverages: No restrictions. May be taken with milk.
▷   *Alcohol:* No interactions expected.
    Tobacco Smoking: No interactions expected. I advise everyone to quit smoking.
▷   *Other Drugs*
    Lamivudine *taken concurrently* with
    • cotrimoxazole (Septra, Bactrim) may increase lamivudine blood levels.
    • indinavir (Crixivan) and zidovudine (AZT) resulted in undetectable HIV in some AIDS patients.
    • nelfinavir (Viracept) may increase lamivudine levels.
    • other medicines capable of causing pancreatitis may result in increased pancreatitis risk.
    • other medicines capable of lowering white or red cell counts may cause additive risks.
    • trimexate (Mexate) may cause additive blood (hematological) toxicity.
▷   *Driving, Hazardous Activities:* This drug may cause dizziness or fainting. Restrict activities as necessary.
    Aviation Note: The use of this drug *is a disqualification* for piloting. Consult a designated aviation medical examiner.
    Exposure to Sun: No restrictions.
    Discontinuation: Do not stop this drug without your physician's knowledge and guidance.

LAMOTRIGINE (la MOH tri jean)

Introduced: 1995   **Class:** Anticonvulsant, phenyltriazine   **Prescription:** USA: Yes   **Controlled Drugs:** USA: No; Canada: No   **Available as Generic:** USA: No

Brand Name: Lamictal

BENEFITS versus RISKS	
Possible Benefits	*Possible Risks*
EFFECTIVE MANAGEMENT OF SEIZURES THAT RESIST THERAPY	Rashes Changes in vision Dizziness
INCREASE IN SEIZURE-FREE DAYS	

▷ **Principal Uses**

As a Single Drug Product: Uses currently included in FDA-approved labeling: Adjunctive combination therapy of partial seizures in adults who have not responded to treatment with other medicines.

Other (unlabeled) generally accepted uses: (1) May have a role in treating epilepsy in children that have not responded to more established treatment; (2) could have a role in treating status epilepticus; (3) of use in treating Lennox-Gastaut syndrome.

How This Drug Works: The exact mechanism of action is not known, but animal models appear to show that this medicine blocks voltage-dependent sodium channels. This causes a decreased amount of glutamate and aspartate transmitters, and a decreased likelihood of seizures.

Available Dose Forms and Strengths

Tablets — 25 mg, 100 mg, 150 mg, 200 mg

▷ **Recommended Dose Ranges:** (Actual dose and schedule must be determined for each patient individually.)

Infants and Children: Safety and efficacy in those less than 16 years old have not been established. Some researchers used lamotrigine in treating intractable epilepsy: 2 to 15 mg per kg of body mass divided into two equal doses and given every 12 hours.

16 to 65 Years of Age: In patients receiving medicines known to interact (phenytoin, primidone, carbamazepine, or phenobarbital), the starting dose is 50 mg a day for 2 weeks, and then 50 mg twice a day as needed or tolerated, with increases as needed and tolerated of 100 mg a day every week. Most patients end up taking 300–500 mg a day divided into two equal doses. Some centers have used doses as high as 700 mg a day. Patients only taking valproic acid may need still lower doses, but studies have not been done.

Over 65 Years of Age: Same dosing as 16 to 65 (single-dose pharmacokinetics were similar to younger adults). Few patients over 65 were included during premarketing studies, so specific statements can't presently be made.

Conditions Requiring Dosing Adjustments

Liver Function: This drug is mostly changed in the liver, but guidelines are not available for adjusting the dose.

Kidney Function: Most of this medicine (once changed or glucuronidated) is removed by the kidneys. Used with caution and with blood levels to check appropriateness of dosing.

▷ **Dosing Instructions:** Take this medicine exactly as prescribed. Food does not affect how much medicine gets into your body. Talk with your doctor immediately if you get a rash, swollen lymph glands, and fever.

Usual Duration of Use: Regular use for 3 months in children with resistant seizures may be needed to see peak benefits. Long-term use (months to years) will be determined individual response.

Possible Advantages of This Drug
Generally well-tolerated medicine, effective where single medicines have failed.

▷ **This Drug Should Not Be Taken If**
- you have developed a rash with swollen lymph glands while taking this medicine.
- you are allergic to this medicine or ones similar to it.

▷ **Inform Your Physician Before Taking This Drug If**
- you develop a rash.
- you do not understand how much to take or how often to take it.

Possible Side Effects (natural, expected, and unavoidable drug actions)
Somnolence.
Weight gain.

▷ **Possible Adverse Effects** (unusual, unexpected, and infrequent reactions)
If any of the following develop, consult your physician promptly for guidance.
Mild Adverse Effects
Allergic reactions: skin rash (should be reported to your doctor), itching—infrequent.
Dizziness and headache—most common adverse effects.
Problems coordinating movements (ataxia)—infrequent.
Nausea and vomiting—dose related.
Blurred vision—dose related.
Increased liver enzymes—case reports.
Serious Adverse Effects
Allergic reactions: anaphylaxis—case reports.
Serious rashes (Stevens-Johnson syndrome, toxic epidermal necrolysis)—case reports.
Hostility—rare.
Lowered blood platelets (thrombocytopenia) or sudden (acute) liver (hepatic) failure—case reports
Disseminated intravascular coagulation—rare.
Blood in the urine—infrequent.
Peripheral neuropathy—rare and of questionable cause.
Sudden unexplained death (SUDEP). The rate of SUDEP was similar to that of another agent also tested, and appears to be a population effect—case reports.

▷ **Possible Effects on Sexual Function:** None reported.

Possible Effects on Laboratory Tests
Blood levels of interacting medicines may be changed.

CAUTION
1. **DO NOT** stop this medicine suddenly, as seizures may occur.

Precautions for Use
By *Infants and Children:* This medicine is approved for add-on therapy in children over 16 years of age.
By *Those Over 60 Years of Age:* No specific changes.

▷ **Advisability of Use During Pregnancy**
Pregnancy Category: C. See Pregnancy Risk Categories at the back of this book.
Animal studies: No evidence of drug-related changes were found in mice or rabbits that were given up to 1.2 times the human dose.
Human studies: This medicine has been shown to cause toxicity to the mother and, because of this, toxicity to the fetus. Adequate studies of pregnant women are not available. Discuss the benefits-to-risk balance with your doctor.

Advisability of Use If Breast-Feeding
Presence of this drug in breast milk: Probably yes.
Avoid drug or refrain from nursing.

Habit-Forming Potential: None.

Effects of Overdose: Sleepiness, changes in muscular reflexes, coma. Keep a seizure diary to check for decrease in seizure frequency.

Possible Effects of Long-Term Use: Weight gain.

Suggested Periodic Examinations While Taking This Drug (at physician's discretion)
Examinations for nystagmus, muscular coordination.

▷ **While Taking This Drug, Observe the Following**
Foods: No restrictions.
Beverages: No restrictions. May be taken with milk.
▷   *Alcohol:* Avoid alcohol use, unless you discuss this with your doctor.
Tobacco Smoking: No interactions expected. I advise everyone to quit smoking.
▷   *Other Drugs*
Lamotrigine *taken concurrently* with
- long-standing use of acetaminophen (Tylenol, others) may result in decreases in blood levels of this medicine and a potential decrease in seizure control. Periodic use should not cause problems.
- carbamazepine (Tegretol) may increase the removal of lamotrigine from the body and require dosing adjustments.
- phenobarbital may result in a faster removal of lamotrigine from the body and require dosing changes.
- phenytoin (Dilantin) may result in a faster removal of lamotrigine from the body and require dosing changes.
- primidone (Mysoline) may result in a faster removal of lamotrigine from the body and require dosing changes.
- ritonavir (Norvir) may lead to decreased lamotrigine levels and increased risk of seizure.
- valproic acid (Depakene) may result in slower removal of lamotrigine from the body and require decreases in lamotrigine doses in order to avoid toxicity.

▷ *Driving, Hazardous Activities:* Use caution until the full extent of fatigue, dizziness, or coordination or vision changes have been determined.

Aviation Note: The use of this drug *is a disqualification* for piloting. Consult a designated aviation medical examiner.

Exposure to Sun: No restrictions.

Exposure to Heat: Use caution muscular coordination problems may be worsened by excessive heat.

Discontinuation: DO NOT stop this medicine abruptly without talking with your doctor first. Abrupt discontinuation of lamotrigine without first starting another antiseizure medicine may result in seizures.

LANSOPRAZOLE (lan SO pra sole)

Introduced: 1995   **Class:** Antiulcer, proton pump inhibitor   **Prescription:** USA: Yes   **Controlled Drug:** USA: No; Canada: No   **Available as Generic:** USA: No; Canada: No

Brand Name: Prevacid, Prevpac [CD]

BENEFITS versus RISKS	
Possible Benefits	*Possible Risks*
VERY EFFECTIVE TREATMENT OF CONDITIONS ASSOCIATED WITH EXCESSIVE PRODUCTION OF STOMACH (GASTRIC) ACID: ZOLLINGER-ELLISON SYNDROME, MASTOCYTOSIS, ENDOCRINE ADENOMA	Liver enzyme increases Protein in the urine
VERY EFFECTIVE TREATMENT OF REFLUX ESOPHAGITIS	
VERY EFFECTIVE TREATMENT OF DUODENAL ULCER	
EFFECTIVE MAINTENANCE THERAPY OF HEALED DUODENAL ULCERS	

▷ **Principal Uses**

As a Single Drug Product: Uses currently included in FDA-approved labeling: (1) Used to treat duodenal ulcers; (2) treats erosive esophagitis; (3) used in syndromes (such as Zollinger-Ellison) where excessive amounts of stomach acid are produced; (4) maintains healed duodenal ulcers; (5) treats gastroesophageal reflux disease.

Other (unlabeled) generally accepted uses: Treatment of stomach (gastric) ulcers.

As a Combination Drug Product [CD]: This drug is available in combination with two antibiotics—clarithromycin and amoxicillin. Since refractory ulcers are often actually *Helicobacter pylori* infections, the combination works to kill the bacteria and lower acid production.

How This Drug Works: Inhibits an enzyme system (H/K adenosine triphosphate) in the stomach (parietal cells) lining and stops production of stomach acid. By doing this it eliminates the principal cause of ulcers or esophagitis and creates an environment conducive to healing.

Available Dose Forms and Strengths
Capsules — 15 mg, 30 mg

▷ **Recommended Dose Ranges** (Actual dose and schedule must be determined for each patient individually.)

Infants and Children: Not studied in this age group.

18 to 60 Years of Age: For duodenal ulcer: 15 mg daily, taken before a meal. Some patients require 30 mg daily. Four weeks of therapy needed. For ongoing therapy of healed duodenal ulcers: 15 mg daily.

For erosive esophagitis: 30 mg daily, taken before a meal. Up to 8 weeks of treatment can be given. If healing does not occur, an additional 8 weeks may be considered.

For excessive acid production syndromes: dosing is started at 60 mg daily. The dose is increased as needed and tolerated. Doses up to 90 mg twice daily have been used. Once the condition is under control, dose usually slowly reduced to 30 mg a day.

Helicobacter pylori: 30 mg twice daily days 1–7, colloidal bismuth subcitrate 120 mg four times daily days 4–7, tetracycline 500 mg four times daily days 4–7, and metronidazole 500 mg three times daily days 4–7.

Over 60 Years of Age: Same as 18 to 60 years of age.

Conditions Requiring Dosing Adjustments
Liver Function: The manufacturer strongly suggests a dose of 15 mg daily for people with significant liver problems.
Kidney Function: No dosing changes are needed.

▷ **Dosing Instructions:** The capsules contain enteric-coated granules that protect the medicine in the stomach's acid. Take the capsules whole. Some studies have found that lansoprazole **taken in the morning** worked the best in controlling stomach acid. If swallowing is a problem, some patients have been able to take this drug by opening a capsule and sprinkling the intact granules into applesauce. Take this medicine exactly as prescribed.

Usual Duration of Use: Use on a regular schedule for 7 days resulted in a 90–94% decrease in acid release. Patients with stomach (gastric) or duodenal ulcers had a decrease in symptoms in about 1 week—this DOES NOT mean that the ulcer is gone. Especially with maintenance of healing of duodenal ulcers, therapy may be ongoing. People with reflux esophagitis had decreases in heartburn after 7 to 28 days. Some esophagitis patients needed a second 8-week course to bring symptoms under control. Long-term use requires periodic physician follow-up.

▷ **This Drug Should Not Be Taken If**
• you are allergic to the medicine or any of its components.

▷ **Inform Your Physician Before Taking This Drug If**
• you have a history of liver disease.
• you smoke and expect to continue smoking (worsens acid secretion).

Possible Side Effects (natural, expected, and unavoidable drug actions)
Increased serum gastrin levels (clinical significance is unknown).

▷ **Possible Adverse Effects** (unusual, unexpected, and infrequent reactions)
   If any of the following develop, consult your physician promptly for guidance.
   Mild Adverse Effects
   Allergic reactions: skin rash.
   Headache, dizziness, or tiredness—infrequent.
   Diarrhea or nausea—infrequent.
   Ringing in the ears—rare.
   Serious Adverse Effects
   Allergic Reaction: Not defined.
   Protein in the urine—rare.
   Liver toxicity or low blood platelets—rare and of questionable cause.

▷ **Possible Effects on Sexual Function:**   None reported.

▷ **Adverse Effects That May Mimic Natural Diseases or Disorders**
   Drug-induced liver reaction may suggest viral hepatitis.

Possible Effects on Laboratory Tests
   Liver function tests: increased.

CAUTION
   1. Follow your doctor's advice on how long to take this drug.
   2. This drug effectively treats ulcers, but does not preclude the chance of cancer of the stomach.

Precautions for Use
   By Infants and Children: Not indicated in this age group.
   By Those Over 60 Years of Age: This medicine may cause dizziness. Use caution until you've seen the effects it has on you.

▷ **Advisability of Use During Pregnancy**
   Pregnancy Category: B. See Pregnancy Risk Categories at the back of this book.

Advisability of Use If Breast-Feeding
   Presence of this drug in breast milk: Unknown.
   Avoid drug or refrain from nursing.

Habit-Forming Potential: None.

Effects of Overdose: Possible nausea, vomiting, dizziness, lethargy, and abdominal pain.

Possible Effects of Long-Term Use: Serum gastrin levels are increased by this medicine, but the clinical significance is not known. Presently it is indicated for a maximum of two 8-week courses in erosive esophagitis. Maintenance of healed ulcers will further define effects of longer-term treatment.

Suggested Periodic Examinations While Taking This Drug (at physician's discretion)
   Complete blood counts, liver function tests.

▷ **While Taking This Drug, Observe the Following**
   Foods: Lansoprazole is best taken on an empty stomach. Follow your doctor's instructions regarding the types of foods you eat.
   Beverages: No restrictions.
▷ *Alcohol:* No specific interactions; however, alcohol stimulates the secretion of stomach acid and may lessen the therapeutic benefits of this medicine.

Tobacco Smoking: Smoking can stimulate stomach acid and lessen benefits of this drug. I advise everyone to quit smoking.

▷ *Other Drugs*

Lansoprazole *taken concurrently* with

- itraconazole (Sporonox) or ketoconazole (Nizoral) may lower how much antifungal goes to work in your body.
- sucralfate (Carafate) may decrease lansoprazole absorption. Separate doses by 2 hours.
- theophylline (Theo-Dur, others) may decrease blood theophylline level, requiring dosing adjustments.

▷ *Driving, Hazardous Activities:* Caution: this medicine may cause drowsiness. Limit activities as necessary.

Aviation Note: The use of this drug **may be a disqualification** for piloting. Consult a designated aviation medical examiner.

Exposure to Sun: No restrictions.

Discontinuation: Talk with your doctor before stopping this medicine for any reason. Taking the medicine for a shorter time than needed may result in incomplete ulcer healing and continuation of the original problem.

LATANOPROST (La TAN oh prost)

Introduced: 1996   **Class:** Anti-glaucoma, prostaglandin F-2 analogue
Prescription: USA: Yes   **Controlled Drug:** USA: No; Canada: No   **Available as Generic:** No
Brand Name: Xatalan

BENEFITS versus RISKS	
Possible Benefits	*Possible Risks*
EFFECTIVE REDUCTION OF INTERNAL EYE PRESSURE FOR CONTROL OF ACUTE AND CHRONIC GLAUCOMA CONTROL OF OCULAR HYPERTENSION	Mild side effects with systemic absorption Joint or back pain Minor eye discomfort Altered vision Iris pigmentation

▷ **Principal Uses**

As a Single Drug Product: Uses currently included in FDA-approved labeling: (1) Used to manage glaucoma; (2) lowers increased pressure in the eye (intraocular pressure).

Other (unlabeled) generally accepted uses: None at present.

How This Drug Works: This medicine lowers pressure in the eye by increasing outflow from the uveoscleral area without changing aqueous flow.

Available Dose Forms and Strengths

Eyedrop solutions — 0.005% or 50 mcg/ml

▷ **Usual Adult Dose Range:** For open-angle glaucoma or ocular hypertension: One drop in the eye each evening.

Note: Actual dose and dosing schedule must be determined for each patient individually.

Conditions Requiring Dosing Adjustments
> *Liver Function:* The drug is changed in the liver and then removed by the kidneys.
>> Specific dose changes in liver disease are not defined.
>
> *Kidney Function:* Changed drug (metabolites) removed by the kidney, but dosing changes in kidney failure are not defined.

▷ **Dosing Instructions:** Remove contact lenses and do not replace them for at least 15 minutes after putting this medicine into your eye. To avoid excessive absorption into the body, press finger against inner corner of the eye (to close off the tear duct) during application and for 1 minute after dropping the medicine in. Be careful not to touch the dropper to the eye.

Usual Duration of Use: Use on a regular schedule for a day usually sees an effect in lowering the pressure in the eye. A week may be required for the full benefits of the medicine to be realized. Long-term use (months to years) requires physician supervision.

▷ **This Drug Should Not Be Taken If**
- you have had an allergic reaction to it previously.

▷ **Inform Your Physician Before Taking This Drug If**
- you wear contact lenses.
- you have had an eye infection in the last three months.
- you have sudden (acute) angle closure of the eye.

Possible Side Effects (natural, expected, and unavoidable drug actions)
> Burning of the eyes or irritation—frequent (usually mild).

▷ **Possible Adverse Effects** (unusual, unexpected, and infrequent reactions)
> **If any of the following develop, consult your physician promptly for guidance.**
>
> *Mild Adverse Effects*
> Allergic reactions: itching of the eyes, eyelid itching and/or swelling.
> Headache—infrequent.
> Nausea—case reports.
> Muscle or back pain—rare to infrequent.
>
> *Serious Adverse Effects*
> Pigmentation of the iris—infrequent; frequent (up to 16%) with therapy ongoing for more than a year.)

▷ **Possible Effects on Sexual Function:** None reported.

Possible Effects on Laboratory Tests
> None reported.

Precautions for Use
> *By Those Over 60 Years of Age:* No age-specific changes presently needed.

▷ **Advisability of Use During Pregnancy**
> *Pregnancy Category:* C. See Pregnancy Risk Categories at the back of this book.
> Human studies: Adequate studies of pregnant women are not available.
> Discuss use with your doctor BEFORE using this drug.

Advisability of Use If Breast-Feeding
> Presence of this drug in breast milk: Unknown.
> Monitor nursing infant closely and discontinue drug or nursing if adverse effects develop.

Habit-Forming Potential: None.

Effects of Overdose: Not defined.

Possible Effects of Long-Term Use: Pigmentation of the iris.

Suggested Periodic Examinations While Taking This Drug (at physician's discretion)

Measurement of internal eye pressure on a regular basis. Check for early signs of pigmentation.

▷ **While Taking This Drug, Observe the Following**

Foods: No restrictions.

Beverages: No restrictions.

▷ *Alcohol:* No restrictions except prudence in alcohol use.

Tobacco Smoking: No interactions expected. I advise everyone to quit smoking.

Marijuana Smoking: Sustained additional decrease in internal eye pressure.

▷ *Other Drugs*

Latanoprost *taken concurrently* with

• thimerosal (various) can cause a precipitation. DO NOT combine eyedrops with thimerosal and latanoprost. Separate doses by 5 minutes or more.

▷ *Driving, Hazardous Activities:* This drug may cause blurry vision for a time. Restrict activities as necessary.

Aviation Note: The use of this drug *may be a disqualification* for piloting. Consult a designated aviation medical examiner.

Exposure to Sun: This medicine may make your eyes sensitive to the sun. Wear sunglasses.

Discontinuation: Do not stop regular use of this drug without consulting your physician.

LEVODOPA (lee voh DOH pa)

Introduced: 1967   **Class:** Anti-parkinsonism   **Prescription:** USA: Yes
Controlled Drug: USA: No; Canada: No   **Available as Generic:** USA: Yes;
Canada: No
Brand Names: Bendopa, Dopar, Larodopa, ✦Prolopa [CD], Sinemet [CD],
Sinemet CR [CD]

BENEFITS versus RISKS	
Possible Benefits	*Possible Risks*
EFFECTIVE SYMPTOM RELIEF IN IDIOPATHIC PARKINSON'S DISEASE	Emotional depression, confusion, abnormal thinking and behavior
Helpful in parkinsonism after encephalitis	Abnormal involuntary movements
Roughly 6-month benefit in parkinsonism after manganese poisoning	Heart rhythm disturbance
	Urinary bladder retention
	Induction of peptic ulcer
	Blood abnormalities: hemolytic anemia, reduced white blood cell count

▷ **Principal Uses**

As a Single Drug Product: Uses currently included in FDA-approved labeling: Treats major types of Parkinson's disease: paralysis agitans ("shaking palsy" of unknown cause), the type that follows encephalitis, parkinsonism that develops with aging (associated with hardening of the brain arteries), and the parkinsonism that follows poisoning by carbon monoxide or manganese.

Other (unlabeled) generally accepted uses: (1) May have a limited role in treating catatonic stupor; (2) can improve conscious level in coma caused by liver failure; (3) can help restless leg or periodic limb movements in sleep; (4) could be helpful in treating severe congestive heart failure.

As a Combination Drug Product [CD]: This drug is available in combination with carbidopa, a chemical that prevents the breakdown of levodopa before it reaches its site of action. The addition of carbidopa reduces levodopa requirements by 75%, and also decreases the frequency and severity of adverse effects.

How This Drug Works: Levodopa enters the brain tissue and is converted to dopamine. After sufficient dose, this corrects the dopamine deficiency (thought to be the cause of parkinsonism) and restores a more normal brain chemistry. Carbidopa blocks an enzyme (decarboxylase) that degrades levodopa before it reaches the brain. This allows a lower dose to have a greater benefit. Products containing carbidopa also have fewer adverse effects.

Available Dose Forms and Strengths

Capsules — 100 mg, 250 mg, 500 mg

Tablets — 100 mg, 250 mg, 500 mg

Sinemet tablets — 10–100 mg, 25–100 mg, 25–250 mg

Sinemet CR, sustained-release tablets — 25–100 mg, 50–200 mg

▷ **Usual Adult Dose Range:**   Initially 250 mg two to four times daily. Dose may be increased by increments of 100 to 750 mg at 3- to 7-day intervals as needed and tolerated. Total dose should not exceed 8000 mg daily. If the combination drug Sinemet is used, the total levodopa requirement will be considerably less. For someone who has not taken levodopa before (levodopa naive and using the sustained-release form): one 50–200 tablet twice daily, no more frequently than every 6 hours while awake. The dose is then increased as needed and tolerated by either daily or every-other-day dosing of one tablet, to a maximum of eight tablets daily. **Note: Actual dose and schedule must be determined for each patient individually.**

Conditions Requiring Dosing Adjustments

Liver Function: Dosing changes are not indicated in liver compromise.

Kidney Function: Possible urine retention requires that patients with urine outflow problems should be closely watched. No dose decreases are needed in kidney failure.

Intestinal Parasites: A report of large increases in doses needed by patients with *Strongyloides stercoralis* has been filed. Cure of this intestinal parasite allowed the levodopa dose to be decreased by 33%.

▷ **Dosing Instructions:**   Tablet may be crushed and is best taken with or following carbohydrate foods to reduce stomach upset. When possible, don't take this drug with high-protein foods. Sustained-release tablet (Sinemet CR) may be cut in half, but it should not be crushed or chewed. The last daily dose should be taken before 7 P.M. in order to avoid problems with normal sleeping patterns. "Drug holidays" (periods when no medicine is taken) are controversial, and not all patients benefit from this approach to therapy.

Usual Duration of Use: Use on a regular schedule for 3 to 6 weeks determines effectiveness in relieving the major symptoms of parkinsonism. Peak benefits may require continual use for 6 months. Long-term use (months to years) requires physician supervision.

Possible Advantages of This Drug

The slow-release formulation of Sinemet CR allows a 25 to 50% reduction in dosing frequency. The wearing-off phenomenon and end-of-dose failure seen with standard Sinemet may be reduced or eliminated.

▷ **This Drug Should Not Be Taken If**
- you are allergic to any of the medicines listed.
- you have narrow-angle glaucoma (inadequately controlled).
- you have a history of melanoma.
- you are taking, or have taken within the past 14 days, any monoamine oxidase (MAO) type A inhibitor drug (see Drug Classes).

▷ **Inform Your Physician Before Taking This Drug If**
- you have diabetes, epilepsy, heart disease, high blood pressure, or chronic lung disease.
- you have impaired liver or kidney function.
- you have problems making blood (hematopoiesis).
- you have had a heart attack and have some abnormal heart rhythms.
- you have a history of depression or other mental illness.
- you have a history of peptic ulcer disease or malignant melanoma.
- you will have surgery with general anesthesia.

Possible Side Effects (natural, expected, and unavoidable drug actions)

Fatigue, lethargy.

Altered taste, offensive body odor.

Orthostatic hypotension (see Glossary).

Pink- to red-colored urine, which turns black on exposure to air (of no significance).

Gout.

▷ **Possible Adverse Effects** (unusual, unexpected, and infrequent reactions)

If any of the following develop, consult your physician promptly for guidance.

Mild Adverse Effects

Allergic reactions: skin rash, itching.

Headache, dizziness, numbness, insomnia, nightmares, blurred or double vision—infrequent.

Nausea and vomiting—frequent; dry mouth, difficult swallowing, gas, diarrhea, constipation—infrequent.

Decreased taste sensation—possible.

Loss of hair—case reports.

Serious Adverse Effects

Idiosyncratic reactions: hemolytic anemia (see Glossary). Neuroleptic malignant syndrome (see Glossary), high blood pressure—case reports.

Confusion, hallucinations, paranoia, depression—infrequent to frequent; psychotic episodes, seizures—rare.

Congestive heart failure—rare.

Mania or seizures—rare.

Abnormal involuntary movements of the head, face, and extremities—frequent.

Disturbances of heart rhythm—infrequent; low blood pressure—rare.

Development of peptic ulcer, gastrointestinal bleeding—case reports.

Urinary bladder retention—case reports.

Low white blood cell count: increased infection risk, sore throat (transient, but may require you to stop this medicine until the condition clears), or low blood platelets—case reports to rare.

▷ **Possible Effects on Sexual Function:** Increased male or female libido—infrequent; inhibited ejaculation, priapism (see Glossary), postmenopausal bleeding—all rare.

▷ **Adverse Effects That May Mimic Natural Diseases or Disorders**

Mental reactions may resemble idiopathic psychosis.

Natural Diseases or Disorders That May Be Activated by This Drug

Latent peptic ulcer, gout.

Possible Effects on Laboratory Tests

Complete blood cell counts: occasionally decreased white cells; occasionally increased eosinophils (without symptoms).

Blood thyroxine (T_4) level: increased.

Urine sugar tests: no effect with Tes-Tape; false negative with Clinistix; false positive with Clinitest.

Urine ketone tests: false positive with Ketostix and Phenistix.

Blood uric acid, growth hormone: increased.

Blood potassium or sodium: may be decreased.

CAUTION

1. It is best to begin treatment with small doses, increasing gradually until desired response is achieved.
2. As improvement occurs, avoid excessive and hurried activity (often causes falls and injury).

Precautions for Use

By Infants and Children: This drug can cause precocious puberty in prepubertal boys. Watch for hypersexual behavior and premature growth of genital organs.

By Those Over 60 Years of Age: Therapy should start with half the usual adult dose; dose increases should be made in small increments as needed and tolerated. Watch for significant behavioral changes: depression or inappropriate elation, acute confusion, agitation, paranoia, dementia, nightmares, and hallucinations. Abnormal involuntary movements may also occur.

▷ **Advisability of Use During Pregnancy**

Pregnancy Category: C. See Pregnancy Risk Categories at the back of this book.

Animal studies: Significant birth defects reported in rodent studies.

Human studies: Adequate studies of pregnant women are not available.

Avoid use of drug during the first 3 months. Use only if clearly needed during the final 6 months.

Advisability of Use If Breast-Feeding

Presence of this drug in breast milk: Yes.

Avoid drug or refrain from nursing.

Habit-Forming Potential: None.

Effects of Overdose: Muscle twitching, spastic closure of eyelids, nausea, vomiting, diarrhea, weakness, fainting, confusion, agitation, hallucinations.

Possible Effects of Long-Term Use: Development of abnormal involuntary movements involving the head, face, mouth, and extremities. May be reversible and gradually subside as the drug is withdrawn.

Suggested Periodic Examinations While Taking This Drug (at physician's discretion)
Complete blood cell counts; measurements of internal eye pressure; blood pressure measurements in lying, sitting, and standing positions.

▷ **While Taking This Drug, Observe the Following**
Foods: Insofar as possible, do not take concurrently with protein foods; proteins compete for absorption.
Nutritional Support: If taken alone (without carbidopa), watch for tingling of the extremities (peripheral neuritis). Small (10 mg or less) doses of pyridoxine (vitamin B$_6$) may help. Larger doses can decrease the effectiveness of levodopa. If taking Sinemet, supplemental pyridoxine is not required. Rare reports of vitamin C (ascorbic acid) decreasing nausea and other side effects have been made.
Beverages: No restrictions. May be taken with milk.
▷ *Alcohol:* No interactions expected.
Tobacco Smoking: No interactions expected. I advise everyone to quit smoking.
Marijuana Smoking: Increased fatigue and lethargy; possible accentuation of orthostatic hypotension (see Glossary).
▷ *Other Drugs*
Levodopa *taken concurrently* with
- benzodiazepines (see Drug Classes) may blunt the therapeutic benefit of levodopa.
- bromocriptine (Parlodel) may result in decreased blood levels of bromocriptine.
- bupropion (Wellbutrin) may increase adverse effects.
- cisapride (Propulsid) may increase adverse effects.
- clonidine (Catapres) can result in decreased therapeutic benefit of levodopa. Avoid this combination.
- fentanyl/droperidol (Innovar) can cause muscular rigidity.
- isoniazid (INH) may cause flushing, worsening of symptoms, or increased blood pressure. DO NOT COMBINE.
- monoamine oxidase (MAO) type A inhibitor drugs (see Drug Classes) can cause a dangerous rise in blood pressure and body temperature. Do not combine these drugs.
- phenothiazines (see Drug Classes) may blunt therapeutic benefits of levodopa. DO NOT combine.
- reserpine (Naquival, others) may blunt the therapeutic benefits of levodopa. Avoid this combination.
- risperidone (Risperdal) can blunt the therapeutic benefits of levodopa. Avoid this combination.
- tricyclic antidepressants (see Drug Classes) may decrease the therapeutic effect of levodopa.
The following drugs may *decrease* the effects of levodopa:
- amoxapine (Ascendin).

- chlordiazepoxide (Librium) or other benzodiazepines (see Drug Classes).
- iron salts.
- papaverine (Cerespan, Pavabid, Vasospan, etc.).
- phenytoin (Dilantin, etc.).
- pyridoxine (vitamin B$_6$).
- risperidone (Risperdal).

▷ *Driving, Hazardous Activities:* May cause dizziness, impaired vision, and orthostatic hypotension. Restrict activities as necessary.

Aviation Note: Parkinson's disease *is a disqualification* for piloting. Consult a designated aviation medical examiner.

Exposure to Sun: No restrictions.

Exposure to Heat: Use caution. This drug can cause flushing and excessive sweating and predispose to heat exhaustion.

Occurrence of Unrelated Illness: Dark-colored skin lesions should be evaluated carefully by your doctor, as they may be malignant melanoma. White blood cell counts should be closely followed if you develop an infection.

LEVOTHYROXINE (lee voh thi ROX een)

Other Names: L-thyroxine, thyroxine, T-4

Introduced: 1953   **Class:** Thyroid hormones   **Prescription:** USA: Yes

Controlled Drug: USA: No; Canada: No   **Available as Generic:** USA: Yes; Canada: No

Brand Names: Armour Thyroid, ✦Eltroxin, Euthroid [CD], L-Thyroxine, Levothroid, Levoxine, Levoxyl, Synthroid, Synthrox, Syroxine, Thyroid USP, Thyrolar [CD]

BENEFITS versus RISKS	
Possible Benefits	*Possible Risks*
EFFECTIVE REPLACEMENT THERAPY IN STATES OF THYROID HORMONE DEFICIENCY (HYPOTHYROIDISM) EFFECTIVE TREATMENT OF SIMPLE GOITER, CHRONIC THYROIDITIS, AND THYROID GLAND CANCER	Intensification of angina in presence of coronary artery disease Drug-induced hyperthyroidism (with excessive dose) Spasm of the coronary vessels

▷ **Principal Uses**

As a Single Drug Product: Uses currently included in FDA-approved labeling: (1) Replacement therapy to correct thyroid deficiency (drug induced, hypothyroidism, cretinism, myxedema); (2) treatment of simple (nonendemic) goiter and benign thyroid nodules; (3) treatment of Hashimoto's thyroiditis; (4) adjunctive prevention and treatment of thyroid cancer.

Other (unlabeled) generally accepted uses: (1) Helps amenorrhea caused by (secondary to) low thyroid function; (2) may help fetal lung tissue mature in premature babies; (3) treats Grave's disease.

As a Combination Drug Product [CD]: This thyroid hormone is available in combination with the other principal thyroid hormone, liothyronine, in a preparation (generic name: liotrix) that resembles the natural hormone material produced by the thyroid gland.

How This Drug Works: Alters cellular chemistry, making more energy available and increasing metabolism of all tissues. Thyroid hormones are essential to normal growth and development, especially the development of infant brain and nervous systems.

Available Dose Forms and Strengths

Injections — 100 mcg/ml, 200 mcg/ml, 500 mcg/ml
Tablets — 0.0125 mg, 0.025 mg, 0.037 mg, 0.05 mg, 0.075 mg, 0.088 mg, 0.1 mg, 0.112 mg, 0.125 mg, 0.15 mg, 0.175 mg, 0.2 mg, 0.3 mg

▷ **Recommended Dose Ranges** (Actual dose and schedule must be determined for each patient individually.)

Infants and Children: Up to 6 months of age—8 to 10 mcg per kg of body mass, in a single daily dose.

6 to 12 months of age—6 to 8 mcg per kg of body mass, in a single daily dose.

1 to 5 years of age—5 to 6 mcg per kg of body mass, in a single daily dose.

6 to 12 years of age—4 to 5 mcg per kg of body mass, in a single daily dose.

Over 12 years of age—2 to 3 mcg per kg of body mass, in a single daily dose, until the usual adult daily dose is reached: 150 to 200 mcg.

12 to 60 Years of Age: Start at 0.05 mg as a single daily dose; increase by 0.025 to 0.05 mg at intervals of 2 to 3 weeks as needed and tolerated. Usual maintenance dose is 0.17 mg/day. Total daily dose should not exceed 0.3 mg. If response is not seen at this level, absorption problems or misunderstanding in taking the medicine should be evaluated.

Over 60 Years of Age: Initially 0.0125 to 0.025 mg as a single daily dose; increase gradually at intervals of 3 to 4 weeks, as needed and tolerated. The usual maintenance dose is approximately 0.075 mg daily.

Author's Note: A University of California Medical Center at San Francisco study found the generic to be as effective as the brand name and saving 50% of the cost of brand.

Conditions Requiring Dosing Adjustments

Liver Function: Dosing changes are not needed.

Kidney Function: Dosing changes are not indicated in kidney compromise.

▷ **Dosing Instructions:**   The tablets may be crushed and are best taken in the morning on an empty stomach.

Usual Duration of Use: Use on a regular schedule for 4 to 6 weeks determines effectiveness in correcting the symptoms of thyroid deficiency. Long-term use (months to years, possibly for life) requires physician supervision.

Currently a "Drug of Choice"

for treatment of hypothyroidism.

▷ **This Drug Should Not Be Taken If**

- you have had an allergic reaction to it previously.
- you are recovering from a heart attack; ask your doctor for help.
- you have an adrenal insufficiency that has not been corrected.
- you are using it to lose weight and your thyroid function is normal (no deficiency).

▷ **Inform Your Physician Before Taking This Drug If**
- you have high blood pressure, any form of heart disease, or diabetes.
- you have a history of Addison's disease or adrenal gland deficiency.
- you are taking any antiasthmatic medications.
- you are taking an anticoagulant.

Possible Side Effects (natural, expected, and unavoidable drug actions)
None if dose is adjusted correctly.

▷ **Possible Adverse Effects** (unusual, unexpected, and infrequent reactions)
If any of the following develop, consult your physician promptly for guidance.

Mild Adverse Effects
Allergic reactions: skin rash, hives.
Headache in sensitive people, even with proper dose adjustment—may be frequent.

Serious Adverse Effects
Increased frequency or intensity of angina in people with coronary artery disease—possible.
Spasm of the arteries that supply blood to the heart—rare.
Seizures, pseudotumor cerebri, drug-induced porphyria, or myasthenia gravis—case reports to rare.
Decrease in IgA immune concentration—rare.
May be a part of the development of osteoporosis. Bone mineral density testing is recommended.
Note: Other adverse effects are manifestations of excessive dose. See "Effects of Overdose" below.

▷ **Possible Effects on Sexual Function:**   Altered menstrual pattern during dose adjustments.
Possibly beneficial in treating impaired sexual function that is associated with true hypothyroidism.

Natural Diseases or Disorders That May Be Activated by This Drug
Latent coronary artery insufficiency (angina), diabetes.

Possible Effects on Laboratory Tests
Prothrombin time: increased (when taken concurrently with warfarin).
Blood total cholesterol, HDL and LDL cholesterol levels: decreased.
Blood triglyceride levels: no effect.
Blood glucose level: increased.
Blood thyroid hormone levels: increased T_3, T_4, and free T_4.
Blood thyroid-stimulating hormone (TSH) level: decreased.

CAUTION
1. Careful supervision of individual response is needed to identify correct dose. Do not change dosing without asking your physician.
2. This drug should not be used to treat nonspecific fatigue, obesity, infertility, or slow growth. Such use is inappropriate and could be harmful.

Precautions for Use
By Infants and Children: Thyroid-deficient children often require higher doses than adults. Transient hair loss may occur during the early months of treatment. Follow the child's response to thyroid therapy by periodic measurements of bone age, growth, and mental and physical development.

By Those Over 60 Years of Age: Usually requirements for thyroid hormone replacement are about 25% lower than in younger adults. Watch closely for any indications of toxicity.

▷ **Advisability of Use During Pregnancy**

Pregnancy Category: A. See Pregnancy Risk Categories at the back of this book.

Animal studies: Cataract formation reported in rat studies. Other defects reported in rabbit and guinea pig studies.

Human studies: Thyroid hormones do not reach the fetus (cross the placenta) in significant amounts. Clinical experience has shown that appropriate use of thyroid hormones causes no adverse effects on the fetus.

Use this drug only if clearly needed and with carefully adjusted dose.

Advisability of Use If Breast-Feeding

Presence of this drug in breast milk: Yes, in minimal amounts.

Breast-feeding is considered safe with correctly adjusted dose.

Habit-Forming Potential: None.

Effects of Overdose: Headache, sense of increased body heat, nervousness, increased sweating, hand tremors, insomnia, rapid and irregular heart action, diarrhea, muscle cramping, weight loss, heart attack.

Possible Effects of Long-Term Use: Bone loss (osteoporosis) in the lumbar vertebrae (spine). Worsening of abnormal growth of the left side of the heart.

Suggested Periodic Examinations While Taking This Drug (at physician's discretion)

Measurement of thyroid hormone levels in blood. Bone mineral density testing.

▷ **While Taking This Drug, Observe the Following**

Foods: Enteral formulas for nutrition support that contain soybeans may increase the fecal elimination of thyroxine.

Beverages: No restrictions.

▷ *Alcohol:* No interactions expected.

Tobacco Smoking: No interactions expected. I advise everyone to quit smoking.

▷ *Other Drugs*

Levothyroxine may *increase* the effects of
- warfarin (Coumadin), and increase the risk of bleeding; decreased anticoagulant dose is usually needed. More frequent INR testing (prothrombin time or protime) are needed.

Levothyroxine may *decrease* the effects of
- digoxin (Lanoxin), when correcting hypothyroidism; a larger dose of digoxin may be needed.

Levothyroxine *taken concurrently* with
- antacids may cause decreased levothyroxine absorption and a decreased therapeutic effect.
- all antidiabetic drugs (insulin and oral hypoglycemic agents) may require an increased dose to obtain proper control of blood sugar levels.
- benzodiazepines (Librium and others) can enhance the toxic or therapeutic effects of both drugs.
- conjugated estrogens (Premarin) may require an increased levothyroxine dose.

- tricyclic antidepressants (see Drug Classes) may cause an increase in activity of both drugs.

The following drugs may **decrease** the effects of levothyroxine:

- cholestyramine (Cuemid, Questran)—may reduce its absorption; intake of the two drugs should be separated by 5 hours.
- colestipol (Colestid).
- iron salts—by decreasing absorption.
- lovastatin (Mevacor).
- phenytoin (Dilantin)—can increase levothyroxine clearance.
- sodium polystyrene sulfonate (Kayexalate).
- sucralfate (Carafate).

▷ *Driving, Hazardous Activities:* No restrictions.

Aviation Note: The use of this drug *is probably not a disqualification* for piloting. Consult a designated aviation medical examiner.

Exposure to Sun: No restrictions.

Exposure to Heat: This drug may decrease individual tolerance to warm environments, increasing discomfort due to heat. Consult your physician if you develop symptoms of overdose during the warm months of the year.

Heavy Exercise or Exertion: Use caution if you have angina (coronary artery disease). This drug may increase the frequency or severity of angina during physical activity.

Discontinuation: This drug must be taken continually on a regular schedule to correct thyroid deficiency. Do not stop it without consulting your physician.

LIOTHYRONINE (li oh THI roh neen)

Other Names: Triiodothyronine, T-3

Introduced: 1956 **Class:** Thyroid hormone **Prescription:** USA: Yes
Controlled Drug: USA: No; Canada: No **Available as Generic:** USA: Yes;
Canada: No

Brand Names: Armour Thyroid, Cyronine, Cytomel, Euthroid [CD], Thyroid USP, Thyrolar [CD], Triostat

BENEFITS versus RISKS	
Possible Benefits	*Possible Risks*
EFFECTIVE REPLACEMENT THERAPY IN STATES OF THYROID HORMONE DEFICIENCY (HYPOTHYROIDISM) EFFECTIVE TREATMENT OF SIMPLE GOITER, CHRONIC THYROIDITIS, AND THYROID GLAND CANCER	Intensification of angina in presence of coronary artery disease Drug-induced hyperthyroidism (with excessive dosing) Rapid heartbeat Heart attack

▷ **Principal Uses**

As a Single Drug Product: Uses currently included in FDA-approved labeling: (1) Replacement therapy to correct thyroid deficiency (hypothyroidism); (2)

treatment of simple (nonendemic) goiter and benign thyroid nodules; (3) treatment of Hashimoto's thyroiditis; (4) adjunctive prevention and treatment of thyroid cancer; (5) therapy of cretinism; (6) used to help diagnose different kinds of thyroid problems.

Other (unlabeled) generally accepted uses: (1) Can help infertility caused by low thyroid function; (2) thyroid replacement of choice for thyroid cancer.

As a Combination Drug Product [CD]: This thyroid hormone is available in combination with the other principal thyroid hormone, levothyroxine, in a preparation (generic name: liotrix) that resembles the natural hormone material produced by the thyroid gland.

How This Drug Works: Alters cellular chemistry, making more energy available. Increases cellular metabolism in all tissues. Thyroid hormones are essential to normal growth and development, especially the development of the infant's brain and nervous system.

Available Dose Forms and Strengths

Injection — 10 mcg/ml

Tablets — 5 mcg, 25 mcg, 50 mcg

▷ **Recommended Dose Ranges** (Actual dose and schedule must be determined for each patient individually.)

Infants and Children: Infants several months old may need 20 mcg a day. When they reach 1 year, 50 mcg a day may be needed. Children more than 3 years old may need the full adult dose.

12 to 60 Years of Age: For mild hypothyroidism—initially 25 mcg daily; increase by 12.5 to 25 mcg every 1 to 2 weeks as needed and tolerated. The usual maintenance dose is 20 to 75 mcg daily.

For severe hypothyroidism—initially 2.5 to 5 mcg daily; increase by 5 to 10 mcg at intervals of 1 to 2 weeks. When a dose of 25 mcg is reached, increase by 12.5 to 25 mcg at intervals of 1 to 2 weeks, as needed and tolerated. The usual maintenance dose is 50 to 100 mcg daily.

For simple goiter—initially 5 mcg daily; increase by 5 to 10 mcg at intervals of 1 to 2 weeks. When a dose of 25 mcg is reached, increase by 12.5 to 25 mcg at intervals of 1 week, as needed and tolerated. The usual maintenance dose is 50 to 100 mcg daily.

Over 60 Years of Age: Initially 5 mcg as a single daily dose; increase by 5 mcg at intervals of 1 to 2 weeks, as needed and tolerated. The usual maintenance dose is 12.5 to 37.5 mcg daily.

Conditions Requiring Dosing Adjustments

Liver Function: Dosing changes are not indicated for patients with liver compromise.

Kidney Function: Dosing changes are not indicated in renal compromise. Caution should be used when increasing the dose of this medicine by those with kidney problems.

▷ **Dosing Instructions:** The tablets may be crushed and are preferably taken in the morning on an empty stomach to ensure maximal absorption and uniform results.

Usual Duration of Use: Use on a regular schedule for 2 to 4 days determines effectiveness in correcting the symptoms of thyroid deficiency. Long-term use (months to years, possibly for life) requires physician supervision.

▷ **This Drug Should Not Be Taken If**
- you have had an allergic reaction to it previously.
- you are recovering from a heart attack; ask your doctor for guidance.
- you have an uncorrected adrenal cortical deficiency.
- you are using it to lose weight and your thyroid function is normal (no deficiency).

▷ **Inform Your Physician Before Taking This Drug If**
- you have high blood pressure, any form of heart disease, or diabetes.
- you have a history of Addison's disease or adrenal gland deficiency.
- you are taking any antiasthmatic medications.
- you take digoxin.
- you are taking an anticoagulant.

Possible Side Effects (natural, expected, and unavoidable drug actions)
None if dose is adjusted correctly.

▷ **Possible Adverse Effects** (unusual, unexpected, and infrequent reactions)
If any of the following develop, consult your physician promptly for guidance.
Mild Adverse Effects
Allergic reactions: skin rash, hives.
Headache in sensitive individuals, even with proper dose adjustment—may be frequent.
Rapid heart rate (tachycardia)—possible.
Hair loss—case reports.
Serious Adverse Effects
Allergic reactions: erythema, bullae, and papules.
Increased frequency or intensity of angina or abnormal heartbeat—possible.
Lowering of blood pressure—rare.
Heart attack—rare.
Osteoporosis: bone mineral density testing is recommended—possible increased risk.
Hyperthyroidism—possible with improper dosing.
Drug fever or drug-induced myasthenia gravis—case reports.
Note: Other adverse effects are manifestations of excessive dose. See "Effects of Overdose" below.

▷ **Possible Effects on Sexual Function:**   Altered menstrual pattern during dose adjustments.
Possibly beneficial in treating impaired sexual function that is associated with true hypothyroidism.

Natural Diseases or Disorders That May Be Activated by This Drug
Latent coronary artery insufficiency (angina), diabetes.

Possible Effects on Laboratory Tests
Prothrombin time: increased (when taken concurrently with warfarin).
Blood total cholesterol, HDL and LDL cholesterol levels: decreased.
Blood triglyceride levels: no effect.
Blood glucose level: increased.
Blood thyroid hormone levels: increased T_3.
Blood thyroid-stimulating hormone (TSH) level: decreased.

CAUTION
1. Careful supervision of individual response is needed to identify correct dose. Do not change dosing schedule without asking your doctor.
2. This drug should not be used to treat nonspecific fatigue, obesity, infertility, or slow growth. Such use is inappropriate and could be harmful.

Precautions for Use

By Infants and Children: **Not** recommended for treatment of this age group. It must reach the brain and nervous system, and this drug may not do that. Levothyroxine is the drug of choice to treat thyroid deficiency in infants and children.

By Those Over 60 Years of Age: Requirements for thyroid hormone replacement are usually about 25% lower than in younger adults. Watch closely for any toxicity.

▷ **Advisability of Use During Pregnancy**

Pregnancy Category: A. See Pregnancy Risk Categories at the back of this book.
Animal studies: No information available.
Human studies: Thyroid hormones do not reach the fetus (cross the placenta) in significant amounts. Clinical experience has shown that appropriate use of thyroid hormones causes no adverse effects on the fetus.
Use this drug only if clearly needed and with carefully adjusted dose.

Advisability of Use If Breast-Feeding

Presence of this drug in breast milk: Yes, in minimal amounts.
Breast-feeding is considered safe with correctly adjusted dose.

Habit-Forming Potential: None.

Effects of Overdose: Headache, sense of increased body heat, nervousness, increased sweating, hand tremors, insomnia, rapid and irregular heart action, diarrhea, muscle cramping, weight loss, heart attack.

Possible Effects of Long-Term Use: Bone loss (osteoporosis) in the lumbar vertebrae (spine). Bone mineral density testing is recommended.

Suggested Periodic Examinations While Taking This Drug (at physician's discretion)

Measurement of thyroid hormone levels in blood.

▷ **While Taking This Drug, Observe the Following**

Foods: No restrictions.
Beverages: No restrictions.
▷ *Alcohol:* No interactions expected.
Tobacco Smoking: No interactions expected. I advise everyone to quit smoking.

▷ *Other Drugs*

Liothyronine may *increase* the effects of
• warfarin (Coumadin), and increase the risk of bleeding; more frequent INR (prothrombin time or protime) tests are needed.
Liothyronine may *decrease* the effects of
• digoxin (Lanoxin), when correcting hypothyroidism; a larger dose of digoxin may be needed.
Liothyronine *taken concurrently* with
• all antidiabetic drugs (insulin and oral hypoglycemic agents) may require an increased dose to obtain proper control of blood sugar.

- estrogens (including birth control pills and Premarin) may require increased doses of liothyronine.
- monoamine oxidase (MAO) inhibitors (see Drug Classes) may increase the therapeutic benefits of the antidepressant.
- tricyclic antidepressants (see Drug Classes) may cause an increase in the activity of both drugs; watch for signs of toxicity.

The following drugs may *decrease* the effects of liothyronine:

- cholestyramine (Cuemid, Questran), and perhaps other cholesterol-lowering resins, which may reduce its absorption; intake of the two drugs should be separated by 5 hours.

▷ *Driving, Hazardous Activities:* No restrictions.

Aviation Note: The use of this drug *is probably not a disqualification* for piloting. Consult a designated aviation medical examiner.

Exposure to Sun: No restrictions.

Exposure to Heat: This drug may decrease individual tolerance to warm environments, increasing discomfort due to heat. Consult your physician if you develop symptoms of overdose during the warm months of the year.

Heavy Exercise or Exertion: Use caution if you have angina (coronary artery disease). This drug may increase the frequency or severity of angina during physical activity.

Discontinuation: This drug must be taken continually on a regular schedule to correct thyroid deficiency. Do not stop it without consulting your physician.

LISINOPRIL (li SIN oh pril)

Introduced: 1988 **Class:** Antihypertensive, ACE inhibitor

Please see the new angiotensin-converting enzyme (ACE) inhibitor family profile for more information.

LITHIUM (LITH i um)

Introduced: 1949 **Class:** Antidepressant **Prescription:** USA: Yes
Controlled Drug: USA: No; Canada: No **Available as Generic:** USA: Yes; Canada: No
Brand Names: ✦Carbolith, Cibalith-S, ✦Duralith, Eskalith, Eskalith CR, Lithane, ✦Lithizine, Lithobid, Lithonate, Lithotabs

BENEFITS versus RISKS	
Possible Benefits	*Possible Risks*
RAPID REVERSAL OF ACUTE MANIA	VERY NARROW MARGIN OF TREATMENT
STABILIZATION OF MOOD	POTENTIALLY FATAL TOXICITY with inadequate monitoring
Prevention of recurrent depression in "responders"	Infrequent induction of diabetes mellitus, hypothyroidism
	Diabetes-insipidus-like syndrome (excessive dilute urine)

▷ **Principal Uses**

As a Single Drug Product: Uses currently included in FDA-approved labeling: (1) Used to manage bipolar disorder (promptly corrects acute mania, and also reduces frequency and severity of recurrent manic-depressive mood swings); (2) used to treat mania; (3) helps control mania.

Other (unlabeled) generally accepted uses: (1) May be helpful in chronic hair pulling (trichotillomania); (2) can help prevent cluster headaches; (3) may help control aggressive behavior; (4) can have a role in treating Fanconi's aplastic anemia; (5) could have an adjunctive role in treating AIDS patients who have low platelet and white blood cells; (6) may help patients who have mood problems that also affect their sex drive.

How This Drug Works: Lithium changes the way nerve signals are transmitted and interpreted, influencing emotional status and behavior.

Available Dose Forms and Strengths

Capsules — 150 mg, 300 mg, 600 mg
Syrup — 8 mEq/5 ml
Tablets — 300 mg
Tablets, prolonged action — 300 mg, 450 mg

▷ **Usual Adult Dose Range:**   First day: 900 to 1200 mg per day; this is divided into three equal doses. This dose is then increased as needed and tolerated by 300-mg increments to attain a blood level of 1–1.5 mmol/L. The usual maintenance dose is 1200 to 1800 mg daily taken in three divided doses. The total daily dose should not exceed 3600 mg. **Note: Actual dose and dosing schedule must be determined for each patient individually.**

Conditions Requiring Dosing Adjustments

Liver Function: The liver is minimally involved in the elimination of lithium.

Kidney Function: Frequent and careful monitoring and decreased dosing must be provided. Doses are usually decreased and blood levels obtained more often. In moderate to severe kidney failure (creatinine clearance of 10–50 ml/min), 50–75% of the usual dose is taken. In severe kidney failure, 25–50% of the usual dose is taken.

▷ **Dosing Instructions:**   The capsules may be opened and regular tablets crushed and taken with or after meals to reduce stomach upset. The prolonged-action tablets should be swallowed whole and not altered.

Usual Duration of Use: Use on a regular schedule for 1 to 3 weeks determines effectiveness in correcting acute mania; several months of continual treatment may be required to correct depression. Long-term use (months to years) requires physician supervision and periodic evaluation.

Currently a "Drug of Choice"

For the treatment of acute mania in bipolar manic-depressive disorders.

▷ **This Drug Should Not Be Taken If**

- you had an allergic reaction to it previously.
- you have uncontrolled diabetes or uncorrected hypothyroidism.
- you are breast-feeding your infant.
- you will be unable to comply with the need for regular monitoring of lithium blood levels.
- you have severe kidney failure.

▷ **Inform Your Physician Before Taking This Drug If**
- you have a history of a schizophrenic-like thought disorder.
- you have any type of organic brain disease, or a history of grand mal epilepsy.
- you have diabetes, heart disease, hypothyroidism, or impaired kidney function.
- you are on a salt-restricted diet.
- you are pregnant or planning a pregnancy.
- you are taking any diuretic drug or a cortisonelike steroid preparation.
- you will have surgery with general anesthesia.

Possible Side Effects (natural, expected, and unavoidable drug actions)

Increased thirst and urine volume in 60% of initial users and in 20% of long-term users.

Weight gain in first few months of use.

Drowsiness and lethargy in sensitive individuals. Metallic taste.

Increased white blood cells—**not** a sign of infection, but an effect of lithium.

Tremor (fine)—frequent (may respond to a beta-blocker).

▷ **Possible Adverse Effects** (unusual, unexpected, and infrequent reactions)

If any of the following develop, consult your physician promptly for guidance.

Mild Adverse Effects

Allergic reactions: skin rashes, generalized itching.

Skin dryness, loss of hair—case reports.

Headache, joint pain, dizziness, weakness, blurred vision, ringing in ears, unsteadiness—infrequent.

Nausea, vomiting, diarrhea—frequent.

Metallic taste—possible.

Edema—possible.

Serious Adverse Effects

"Blackout" spells, confusion, stupor, slurred speech, spasmodic movements of extremities, epileptic-like seizures—case reports to rare.

Abnormal fixed eye position (oculogyric crisis)—case reports.

Abnormal changes in heart rate, rhythm, and wave forms—frequent.

Loss of bladder or rectal control—infrequent.

Diabetes-insipidus-like syndrome: excessive dilute urine—infrequent to frequent.

Abnormal movements (may be a sign of toxicity)—rare.

Cerebellar atrophy or neuroleptic malignant syndrome (see Glossary)—case reports.

Inflammation of the heart muscle (myocarditis)—case reports.

Pseudotumor cerebri, myasthenia gravis, or systemic lupus erythematosus—case reports.

Low thyroid function or abnormally high thyroid function—possible to case reports.

Elevated blood calcium or blood sugar—rare.

Porphyria or inflammation of the parotid gland—case reports.

Seizures—case reports and certainly with toxicity.

Drug-induced low potassium—possible.

▷ **Possible Effects on Sexual Function:**   Decreased libido (blood level of 0.7 to 0.9 MEq/L)—case reports; inhibited erection (0.6 to 0.8 MEq/L)—frequent; male infertility; female breast swelling with milk production—case reports.

▷ **Adverse Effects That May Mimic Natural Diseases or Disorders**

Painful discoloration and coldness of the hands and feet may resemble Raynaud's phenomenon.

Natural Diseases or Disorders That May Be Activated by This Drug

Diabetes mellitus may be worsened. Psoriasis may be intensified. Myasthenia gravis may be induced (one case).

Possible Effects on Laboratory Tests

White blood cell and platelet counts: increased.

Blood alkaline phosphatase (bone isoenzyme): markedly increased in 66% of users.

Blood cholesterol level: increased.

Blood parathyroid hormone level: increased.

Blood thyroid-stimulating hormone (TSH) level: increased.

Blood thyroid hormone (T_3 and T_4) levels: decreased.

Blood uric acid level: decreased.

Blood bromide, calcium, or glucose levels: increased.

Blood potassium level: increased or decreased.

CAUTION

1. The blood level required for this drug to work is close to the level that can cause toxic effects. Periodic blood lithium levels are mandatory. Follow instructions about drug dose and periodic blood tests.
2. Lithium should be stopped at the first signs of toxicity: drowsiness, sluggishness, unsteadiness, tremor, muscle twitching, vomiting, or diarrhea.
3. The major causes of lithium toxicity are:
   - accidental overdose (may be due to inadequate blood level checks)
   - impaired kidney function
   - salt restriction
   - inadequate fluid intake, dehydration
   - concurrent use of diuretics
   - intercurrent illness
   - childbirth (rapid decrease in kidney clearance of lithium)
   - initiation of treatment with a new drug
4. Over-the-counter preparations that contain iodides (some cough products and vitamin–mineral supplements) should be avoided because of the added antithyroid effect when taken with lithium.

Precautions for Use

By Infants and Children: Safety and effectiveness for those under 12 years of age are not established. Follow your physician's instructions exactly.

By Those Over 60 Years of Age: Treatment should start with a "test" dose of 75 to 150 mg daily. Observe closely for early indications of toxic effects, especially if on a low-salt diet and using diuretics. Increased risk of parkinsonian reactions (abnormal gait and movements); coma can develop without warning symptoms.

▷ **Advisability of Use During Pregnancy**

Pregnancy Category: D. See Pregnancy Risk Categories at the back of this book.

Animal studies: Cleft palate reported in mice; eye, ear, and palate defects reported in rats.

Human studies: Adequate studies of pregnant women are not available. However, cardiovascular defects and goiter in newborn infants (of mothers using lithium) have been reported. If the infant's blood level of lithium approaches the toxic range before delivery, the newborn may suffer the "floppy infant" syndrome: weakness, lethargy, unresponsiveness, low body temperature, weak cry, and poor feeding ability.

Avoid use of drug during the first 3 months. Use only if clearly necessary during the final 6 months. Monitor mother's blood lithium levels carefully to avoid possible toxicity.

Advisability of Use If Breast-Feeding

Presence of this drug in breast milk: Yes, in significant amounts.

Avoid drug or refrain from nursing.

Habit-Forming Potential: None.

Effects of Overdose: Drowsiness, weakness, lack of coordination, nausea, vomiting, diarrhea, muscle spasms, blurred vision, dizziness, staggering gait, slurred speech, confusion, stupor, coma, cerebellar atrophy, seizures.

Possible Effects of Long-Term Use: Hypothyroidism (5%), goiter, reduced sugar tolerance, diabetes-insipidus-like syndrome, serious kidney damage.

Suggested Periodic Examinations While Taking This Drug (at physician's discretion)

Regular determinations of blood lithium levels are absolutely essential.

Time to sample blood for lithium level: 12 hours after evening dose, or in the morning, just before next dose. Therapeutic range: 0.8 to 1.5 MEq/L (acute) and 0.6 to 1.2 (maintenance).

Periodic evaluation of thyroid gland size and function.

Complete blood cell counts; kidney function tests.

▷   **While Taking This Drug, Observe the Following**

Foods: Maintain a normal diet; **do not** restrict your use of salt.

Beverages: No restrictions. Drink at least 8 to 12 glasses of liquids daily. This drug may be taken with milk.

▷   *Alcohol:* Use with caution. May have an increased intoxicating effect. Avoid alcohol completely if any symptoms of lithium toxicity develop.

Tobacco Smoking: Lithium may increase sensitivity to nicotine. I advise everyone to quit smoking.

Marijuana Smoking: Possible increase in apathy, lethargy, drowsiness, or sluggishness; accentuation of lithium-induced tremor; possible increased risk of precipitating psychotic behavior.

▷   *Other Drugs*

Lithium may *increase* the effects of

• tricyclic antidepressants (see Drug Classes).

Lithium *taken concurrently* with

• ACE inhibitors such as captopril (Capoten) may increase lithium levels by as much as three times the level prior to combination therapy.

• calcium channel blockers (see Drug Classes) such as diltiazem may cause neurotoxicity or psychosis.

• carbamazepine (Tegretol) may result in neurotoxicity.

- chlorpromazine (Thorazine, etc.) and other phenothiazines (see Drug Classes) may result in decreased lithium or phenothiazine therapeutic effects.
- clozapine (Clozaril) may result in serious agranulocytosis, delirium, and neuroleptic malignant syndrome. Do not combine these medicines.
- diazepam (Valium) may cause hypothermia.
- fludrocortisone (Florinef) may result in loss of the mineralocorticoid benefits of fludrocortisone.
- fluoxetine (Prozac) may result in neurotoxicity.
- fluvoxamine (Luvox) may result in increased lithium levels and toxicity.
- haloperidol (Haldol) or with other neuroleptics may result in decreased beneficial effects from both medicines.
- methyldopa (Aldomet, etc.) is usually well tolerated; however, it may cause a severe neurotoxic reaction in susceptible individuals. These combinations should be used very cautiously.
- metronidazole (Flagyl) may lead to lithium toxicity.
- monoamine oxidase (MAO) inhibitors (see Drug Classes) may result in the serotonin syndrome and potential fatality.
- nicotine (Nicorette gum or nicotine patches) may cause supersensitivity to nicotine.
- verapamil (Calan, Isoptin) may cause unpredictable effects; both lithium toxicity and decreased lithium blood levels have been reported.

The following drugs may *increase* the effects of lithium:
- bumetanide (Bumex).
- ethacrynic acid (Edecrin).
- fluoxetine (Prozac).
- furosemide (Lasix, etc.).
- indomethacin (Indocin).
- piroxicam (Feldene) or any nonsteroidal anti-inflammatory drug (NSAID— see Drug Classes).
- thiazide diuretics (see Drug Classes).

The following drugs may *decrease* the effects of lithium:
- acetazolamide (Diamox, etc.).
- sodium bicarbonate.
- theophylline (Theo-Dur, etc.) and related drugs.

▷ *Driving, Hazardous Activities:* This drug may impair mental alertness, judgment, physical coordination, and reaction time. Restrict activities as necessary.

Aviation Note: The use of this drug *is a disqualification* for piloting. Consult a designated aviation medical examiner.

Exposure to Sun: No restrictions.

Exposure to Heat: Excessive sweating can cause significant depletion of salt and water and resultant lithium toxicity. Avoid sauna baths.

Occurrence of Unrelated Illness: Fever, sweating, vomiting, or diarrhea can result in significant alterations of blood and tissue lithium concentrations. Close monitoring of your physical condition and blood lithium levels is needed to prevent serious toxicity.

Discontinuation: Sudden discontinuation does not cause withdrawal symptoms. Avoid premature discontinuation; some individuals may require continual treatment for up to a year to achieve maximal response. Discontinuation by "responders" may result in recurrence of either mania or depression.

Lithium should be discontinued if symptoms of brain toxicity appear or if an uncorrectable diabetes-insipidus-like syndrome develops.

LOMEFLOXACIN (loh me FLOX a sin)

Author's Note: See the fluoroquinolone antibiotics profile for more information.

LOPERAMIDE (loh PER a mide)

Introduced: 1977   **Class:** Antidiarrheal   **Prescription:** USA: Yes
Controlled Drug: USA: No; Canada: No   **Available as Generic:** Yes
Brand Names: Anti-Diarrheal, Imodium, Imodium AD, Kaopectate 1-D, Maalox A/D, Pepto Diarrhea Control

BENEFITS versus RISKS	
Possible Benefits	*Possible Risks*
EFFECTIVE RELIEF OF	Drowsiness
INTESTINAL CRAMPING AND	Constipation
DIARRHEA	Induction of toxic megacolon

▷ **Principal Uses**

As a Single Drug Product: Uses currently included in FDA-approved labeling: (1) Control of cramping and diarrhea associated with acute gastroenteritis and chronic enteritis and colitis; (2) used to reduce the volume of discharge from ileostomies; (3) treatment of irritable bowel syndrome that has failed to respond to dietary supplements.

Other (unlabeled) generally accepted uses: (1) Treats traveler's diarrhea; (2) decreases unformed stools in *Shigella* diarrhea.

How This Drug Works: Acts directly on the nerve supply of the gastrointestinal tract, decreases secretions, and relieves cramping and diarrhea.

Available Dose Forms and Strengths

Capsules — 2 mg
Liquid — 1 mg/5 ml (5.25% alcohol)—0.2 mg/5 ml (4.07% alcohol)
Tablets — 2 mg

▷ **Usual Adult Dose Range:**   For acute diarrhea: 4 mg initially, then 2 mg after each unformed stool until diarrhea is controlled. Chronic diarrhea: 4 to 8 mg daily in divided doses, taken 8 to 12 hours apart. Maximum daily dose is 16 mg.

Pediatric dosing: NOT recommended for children under 2 years old. Children 2 to 5 years old can be given 1 mg three times a day on the first day (13–20 kg); 6 to 8 year olds can have 2 mg twice daily on the first day (20–30 kg); 8 to 12 years old can have 2 mg three times daily (greater than 30 kg). Follow-up doses on the next day are 1 mg per 10 kg of body mass, up to the maximum daily doses on day 1. If diarrhea persists, call your doctor.

Note: Actual dose and schedule must be determined for each patient individually.

Conditions Requiring Dosing Adjustments

Liver Function: Dosing adjustments for patients with liver compromise are not needed. Half of a given dose is removed unchanged in the feces.

Kidney Function: Changes in dosing are not indicated in kidney compromise.

▷ **Dosing Instructions:**   The capsule may be opened and taken on an empty stomach or with food if stomach upset occurs.

Usual Duration of Use: Use on a regular schedule for 48 hours determines effectiveness in controlling acute diarrhea; continual use for 10 days may be needed to evaluate its effectiveness in controlling chronic diarrhea. If diarrhea persists, consult your physician.

▷ **This Drug Should Not Be Taken If**
- you have had an allergic reaction to it previously.
- it is prescribed for a child under 2 years of age.

▷ **Inform Your Physician Before Taking This Drug If**
- you have a history of liver disease or impaired liver function.
- you have regional enteritis or ulcerative colitis.
- you develop swelling (distention) of the abdomen while taking this medicine.
- you have acute dysentery.

Possible Side Effects (natural, expected, and unavoidable drug actions)

Drowsiness, constipation.

▷ **Possible Adverse Effects** (unusual, unexpected, and infrequent reactions)

If any of the following develop, consult your physician promptly for guidance.

Mild Adverse Effects

Allergic Reaction: Skin rash.

Fatigue, dizziness—rare.

Reduced appetite, cramps, dry mouth, nausea, vomiting, stomach pain, bloating—infrequent.

Serious Adverse Effects

"Toxic megacolon" (distended, immobile colon with fluid retention) may develop while treating acute ulcerative colitis—possible.

Necrotizing enterocolitis or paralytic ileus—rare.

▷ **Possible Effects on Sexual Function:**   None reported.

Possible Effects on Laboratory Tests

None reported.

CAUTION

1. Do not exceed recommended doses.
2. If treating chronic diarrhea, promptly report development of bloating, abdominal distention, nausea, vomiting, constipation, or abdominal pain.

Precautions for Use

By Infants and Children: Do not use in those under 2 years of age. Follow your physician's instructions exactly regarding dose. Watch for drowsiness, irritability, personality changes, and altered behavior.

By Those Over 60 Years of Age: Small starting doses are needed, as you may be more sensitive to the sedative and constipating effects of this drug.

▷ **Advisability of Use During Pregnancy**

Pregnancy Category: B. See Pregnancy Risk Categories at the back of this book.

Animal studies: No birth defects found in rat and rabbit studies.

Human studies: Adequate studies of pregnant women are not available.

Use sparingly and only if clearly needed. Ask your physician for guidance.

Advisability of Use If Breast-Feeding

Presence of this drug in breast milk: Small, clinically insignificant amounts.

Talk with your doctor about the benefits versus risks of using this medicine and nursing.

Habit-Forming Potential: Physical dependence has occurred in monkeys, but there have been no reports in humans.

Effects of Overdose: Drowsiness, lethargy, depression, dry mouth.

Possible Effects of Long-Term Use: None identified.

Suggested Periodic Examinations While Taking This Drug (at physician's discretion)

Decreased frequency of stools within 48 hours.

▷ **While Taking This Drug, Observe the Following**

Foods: No restrictions. Follow prescribed diet.

Beverages: No restrictions, other than your doctor's recommendations regarding diet.

▷ *Alcohol:* Use with caution. This drug may increase the depressant action of alcohol on the brain.

Tobacco Smoking: No interactions expected. I advise everyone to quit smoking.

▷ *Other Drugs:* No significant drug interactions reported.

▷ *Driving, Hazardous Activities:* This drug may cause drowsiness or dizziness. Restrict activities as necessary.

Aviation Note: The use of this drug *is a disqualification* for piloting. Consult a designated aviation medical examiner.

Exposure to Sun: No restrictions.

LORATADINE (lor AT a deen)

Introduced: 1992   **Class:** Antihistamines, nonsedating

Author's Note: See the new minimally sedating antihistamines family profile for further information.

LORAZEPAM (lor A za pam)

Introduced: 1977   **Class:** Mild tranquilizer, benzodiazepines   **Prescription:** USA: Yes   **Controlled Drug:** USA: C-IV*; Canada: No   **Available as Generic:** USA: Yes; Canada: Yes

Brand Names: ✦Apo-Lorazepam, Ativan, Lorazepam Intensol, ✦Novo-Lorazepam, ✦Nu-Loraz

*See schedules of Controlled Drugs at the back of this book.

BENEFITS versus RISKS	
Possible Benefits	*Possible Risks*
RELIEF OF ANXIETY AND NERVOUS TENSION	Habit-forming potential with prolonged use
NOT CHANGED SIGNIFICANTLY INTO ACTIVE DRUG FORMS IN THE LIVER	Minor impairment of mental functions
Wide margin of safety with therapeutic doses	Blood cell, movement, or liver disorders
	Dose-related respiratory depression
	Withdrawal symptoms if abruptly stopped

▷ **Principal Uses**

As a Single Drug Product: Uses currently included in FDA-approved labeling: (1) Helps treat anxiety; (2) used to relieve insomnia; (3) used in surgical cases to help in delivering effective anesthesia; (4) used intravenously as a sedative.

Other (unlabeled) generally accepted uses: (1) Used to help prevent the severe symptoms of alcohol detoxification (delirium tremens or DT); (2) used under the tongue to treat serial seizures in children; (3) can be used to promote amnesia in patients who must take chemotherapy and have suffered vomiting.

How This Drug Works: Attaches to a specific site (GABA-A receptor) in the brain and enables gamma-aminobutyric acid to inhibit activity of nervous tissue. Drugs in this class also reduce the time it takes to fall asleep and the number of awakenings during the night.

Available Dose Forms and Strengths

Tablet — 0.5 mg, 1 mg, 2 mg

Sublingual tablet — 0.5 mg, 1 mg, 2 mg

Oral solution — 2 mg/ml

Injection — 2 mg/ml, 4 mg/ml

▷ **Recommended Dose Ranges** (Actual dose and dosing schedule must be determined for each patient individually.)

Infants and Children: Safety and effectiveness in those under 18 years of age are not established. Has been used in 1- to 4-mg doses under the tongue for treatment of serial seizures in children.

18 to 60 Years of Age: Sedation and anxiety: Therapy is started with 1 to 2 mg per day in two to three divided doses. Doses may be increased as needed and tolerated to the usual maintenance dose of 2 to 6 mg daily in divided doses. The maximum dose is 10 mg daily in two to three divided doses.

Insomnia: 2 to 4 mg at bedtime.

Over 60 Years of Age: Sedation and anxiety: Therapy is started with 0.5 to 1 mg in divided doses. The initial dose should **not** exceed 2 mg daily.

Insomnia: 0.5 to 1 mg at bedtime.

Conditions Requiring Dosing Adjustments

Liver Function: The dose **must** be decreased in liver compromise, and the drug should **not** be used in liver failure. Use of the lowest effective dose is recommended in those with mild to moderate liver failure.

Kidney Function: The drug should **not** be used in kidney failure. In mild to moderate kidney compromise, the dose **must** be decreased, and the lowest effective dose is recommended.

▷ **Dosing Instructions:**   The tablet may be crushed and taken on an empty stomach or with milk or food. Do **not** stop this drug abruptly if it has been taken for more than 4 weeks.

Usual Duration of Use: Use on a regular schedule for 3 to 5 days usually determines effectiveness in relieving moderate anxiety or insomnia. Continual use should be limited to 1 to 3 weeks. Consult your physician on a regular basis.

Possible Advantages of This Drug

More direct elimination and lack of active forms may be of benefit in the elderly.

Increased lipid solubility is of benefit when the drug is used to treat acute alcohol withdrawal.

Author's Note: The National Institute of Mental Health has a new information page on anxiety. It can be found on the World Wide Web at www.nimh.nih.gov/anxiety

▷ **This Drug Should Not Be Taken If**

- you have had an allergic reaction to any dose form or any component of the dose previously.
- you have a primary depression or psychosis.
- you have excessively low blood pressure.
- you have narrow-angle glaucoma.

▷ **Inform Your Physician Before Taking This Drug If**

- you are allergic to any benzodiazepine (see Drug Classes).
- you have a history of alcoholism or drug abuse.
- you are prone to respiratory depression.
- you are pregnant or planning a pregnancy.
- you have impaired liver or kidney function.
- you have a history of low white blood cell counts.
- you have asthma, emphysema, epilepsy, or myasthenia gravis.
- you take other prescription or nonprescription medicines that were not discussed with your doctor when lorazepam was prescribed.

Possible Side Effects (natural, expected, and unavoidable drug actions)

Sedation, "hangover" effects on the day following bedtime use.

▷ **Possible Adverse Effects** (unusual, unexpected, and infrequent reactions)

If any of the following develop, consult your physician promptly for guidance.

Mild Adverse Effects

Allergic reactions: rashes, hives—rare.

Dizziness, amnesia, insomnia, fainting, confusion, blurred vision, slurred speech, constipation, and sweating—infrequent.

Ringing in the ears (associated with withdrawal), decreased hearing ability—infrequent.

Serious Adverse Effects

Allergic reactions: liver damage with jaundice (see Glossary)—case reports.

Low white blood cell counts (leukopenia)—rare.

Paradoxical excitement and rage—case reports.

Low blood pressure—rare.

Hallucinations (transient)—rare.

Porphyria, seizures, or abnormal body movements—case reports.

Respiratory depression—dose related.

▷ **Possible Effects on Sexual Function:**   Decreased male libido or impotence—case reports.

Possible Effects on Laboratory Tests

White blood cell counts: decreased.

Liver function tests: increased SGPT, SGOT, and LDH.

CAUTION

1. This drug should **not** be stopped abruptly if it has been taken continually for more than 4 weeks.
2. Over-the-counter medicines with antihistamines can cause excessive sedation if taken with lorazepam.
3. Lorazepam should **not** be combined with alcohol. This combination will worsen adverse mental and coordination decreases, and increase lorazepam levels.

Precautions for Use

By Infants and Children: Safety and effectiveness for those under 18 years of age are not established. Lorazepam has been used under the tongue in children with serial seizures.

By Those Over 60 Years of Age: Small doses are indicated. Watch for lethargy, fatigue, weakness, and paradoxical agitation, anger, hostility, and rage.

▷ **Advisability of Use During Pregnancy**

Pregnancy Category: D. See Pregnancy Risk Categories at the back of this book.

Animal studies: Cleft palate has been reported in mice; skeletal defects in rats with similar drugs in this class.

Human studies: Adequate studies of pregnant women are not available.

Frequent use in late pregnancy can result in "floppy infant" syndrome in the newborn: weakness, lethargy, depressed breathing, and low body temperature.

Avoid use during the entire pregnancy

Advisability of Use If Breast-Feeding

Presence of this drug in breast milk: Yes.

Avoid drug or refrain from nursing.

Habit-Forming Potential: This drug can cause psychological and/or physical dependence (see Glossary).

Effects of Overdose: Marked drowsiness, weakness, feeling of drunkenness, staggering gait, depression of breathing, stupor progressing to coma.

Possible Effects of Long-Term Use: Psychological or physical dependence, rare liver toxicity.

Suggested Periodic Examinations While Taking This Drug (at physician's discretion)

Liver function tests and complete blood cell counts.

▷ **While Taking This Drug, Observe the Following**

Foods: No restrictions.

Beverages: Avoid excessive caffeine-containing beverages: coffee, tea, and cola.

▷   *Alcohol:* Avoid this combination. Alcohol increases depression of mental function, further worsens coordination, and causes increased lorazepam levels.

    Tobacco Smoking: Heavy smoking may reduce the calming action of this drug. I advise everyone to quit smoking.

    Marijuana Smoking: Additive drowsiness, and impaired physical performance.

▷   *Other Drugs*

    Lorazepam **taken concurrently** with

- clozapine (Clozaril) may result in marked sedation and muscular incoordination.
- heparin may result in increased effects of lorazepam (increased free fraction).
- lithium (Lithobid, others) may result in a lowering of body temperature (hypothermic reaction).
- oxycodone (Percocet, others) and other central nervous system depressants may result in additive CNS or respiratory depression.
- phenytoin (Dilantin) may result in altered phenytoin or lorazepam levels.

    The following drugs may **increase** the effects of lorazepam:

- macrolide antibiotics (see Drug Classes).
- probenecid (Benemid)—may result in a 50% increased lorazepam level. Decreased lorazepam doses or an increased time between doses is indicated.
- valproic acid (Depakene). Decreased doses or an increased time between doses may be needed.

    The following drugs may **decrease** the effects of lorazepam:

- birth control pills (oral contraceptives).
- caffeine, amphetamines, or other stimulants.
- theophylline (Theo-Dur, others).

▷   *Driving, Hazardous Activities:* This drug can impair alertness and coordination. Restrict activities as necessary.

    Aviation Note: The use of this drug **is a disqualification** for piloting. Consult a designated aviation medical examiner.

    Exposure to Sun: No restrictions.

    Discontinuation: Do **not** stop this drug suddenly if it has been taken for over 4 weeks. Consult your doctor about a gradual tapering of dose.

LOSARTAN (loh SAR tan)

Introduced: 1995   **Class:** Angiotensin-2 Receptor Antagonists   **Prescription:** USA: Yes   **Controlled Drug:** USA: No; Canada: No   **Available as Generic:** USA: No; Canada: No

Brand Names: Cozaar, Hyzaar

BENEFITS versus RISKS	
Possible Benefits	*Possible Risks*
EFFECTIVE CONTROL OF HIGH BLOOD PRESSURE	Increased liver function tests
DECREASED NUMBER OF DEATHS FROM CONGESTIVE HEART FAILURE	
Decreased cough versus ACE inhibitors	

▷ **Principal Uses**

As a Single Drug Product: Uses currently included in FDA-approved labeling: (1) Treatment of high blood pressure; (2) decreases abnormal size of the left ventricle (left ventricular hypertrophy).

Other (unlabeled) generally accepted uses: **The ELITE study compared losartan to an ACE inhibitor (in patients over 65 with ejection fraction mean of 30%) and found a significant decrease in deaths for any reason (all-cause death) in treating congestive heart failure.**

As a Combination Drug Product [CD]: This drug has been combined with hydrochlorothiazide in a fixed-dose form. The drug is called Hyzaar, and it contains 12.5 mg of hydrochlorothiazide and 50 mg of losartan. These drugs work to complement each other, making the combination a more effective antihypertensive.

How This Drug Works: This drug and its active metabolite block the effects of angiotensin II by binding to a specific site (the AT1) receptor. This helps the blood vessels stay open and lowers blood pressure. This drug and metabolite also block aldosterone.

Available Dose Forms and Strengths

Tablet — 25 mg, 50 mg

Tablet (Hyzaar) — losartan 50 mg and hydrochlorothiazide 12.5 mg

▷ **Recommended Dose Ranges** (Actual dose and schedule must be determined for each patient individually.)

Infants and Children: Not recommended for use in this age group.

18 to 60 Years of Age: A starting dose of 50 mg daily is used. If the blood pressure response is not sufficient, the same dose may be divided into two equal doses and given twice daily. The dose may also be increased as needed and tolerated and taken in two divided doses daily. Peak effects may not be seen for 3 to 6 weeks before dosing changes are made. The maximum daily dose is 100 mg.

Over 60 Years of Age: Patients who are dehydrated or have a decreased intravascular volume should take 25 mg once daily as a starting dose.

Conditions Requiring Dosing Adjustments

Liver Function: This drug is extensively changed (metabolized) in the liver to an active metabolite. The starting dose should be 25 mg. Dosing is then increased as needed and tolerated at weekly intervals. The fixed-dose drug Hyzaar should not be used by patients with liver failure.

Kidney Function: No dosing changes appear to be needed. The fixed-dose combination Hyzaar should not be used by patients with creatinine clearances (see Glossary) less than 30 ml/min.

▷ **Dosing Instructions:**   Food slows the absorption of losartan, but does not decrease the total absorption of this medicine.

Usual Duration of Use: Continual use on a regular schedule for 3 to 6 weeks is usually necessary to determine this drug's effectiveness in controlling high blood pressure. Long-term use (months to years) requires periodic evaluation of response and dose adjustment. Consult your physician on a regular basis.

Possible Advantages of This Drug

A completely new mechanism of action.

Appears to avoid the cough effect typical of ACE inhibitors.

▷ **This Drug Should Not Be Taken If**
- you had an allergic reaction to it previously.
- you are pregnant.

▷ **Inform Your Physician Before Taking This Drug If**
- you have a history of liver or kidney disease.
- you have a history of circulation problems in the brain.
- you are breast-feeding your infant.
- you have a history of aspirin or penicillin allergy.
- you have a history of disease in the blood vessels that supply the heart (coronary artery disease).
- you are uncertain how much to take or how often to take it.

Possible Side Effects (natural, expected, and unavoidable drug actions)
Taste disorders.
First dose excessive lowering of blood pressure.

▷ **Possible Adverse Effects** (unusual, unexpected, and infrequent reactions)
If any of the following develop, consult your physician promptly for guidance.
Mild Adverse Effects
Allergic reactions: skin rash.
Dizziness, headache, or sleep disturbances—infrequent.
Fatigue or muscle cramps—infrequent.
Cough—possible.
Diarrhea—infrequent.
Serious Adverse Effects
Allergic reactions: not defined.
Swelling of the face and lips (angioedema)—case reports.
Taste disturbances—possible.
Migraine headaches—rare.
Gout—rare and of questionable cause.
Liver toxicity—case reports.
Dose-related increase in blood potassium (hyperkalemia).
Anemia—case reports and of minimal clinical significance.

▷ **Possible Effects on Sexual Function:**   Decreased libido, impotence—both rare and of questionable causation.

Possible Delayed Adverse Effects: None reported.

▷ **Adverse Effects That May Mimic Natural Diseases or Disorders**
Increases in liver function tests may mimic infectious hepatitis.

Natural Diseases or Disorders That May Be Activated by This Drug
None reported.

Possible Effects on Laboratory Tests
Liver function tests: increased.
Potassium level: may be increased.

CAUTION
1. This drug should **not** be taken during pregnancy.

Precautions for Use
By Infants and Children: Safety and effectiveness for use by those under 18 years of age have not been established.
By Those Over 60 Years of Age: People in this age group may be more sensitive

to the effects of medicines that lower blood pressure. Lower starting doses are indicated for patients who are dehydrated.

▷ **Advisability of Use During Pregnancy**
Pregnancy Category: C in the first 3 months, D in the fourth month through birth. See Pregnancy Risk Categories at the back of this book.
Animal studies: Rat studies have produced kidney toxicity and death in fetuses.
Human studies: Information from adequate studies of pregnant women is not available. If pregnancy is detected, this medicine should be stopped as soon as possible.

Advisability of Use If Breast-Feeding
Presence of this drug in breast milk: Unknown, but expected.
Avoid drug or refrain from nursing.

Habit-Forming Potential: None.

Effects of Overdose: Severe decreases in blood pressure. Increased heart rate.

Possible Effects of Long-Term Use: Not defined.

Suggested Periodic Examinations While Taking This Drug (at physician's discretion)
Periodic checks of blood pressure and liver function tests.

▷ **While Taking This Drug, Observe the Following**
Foods: Follow the diet that your doctor has prescribed.
Nutritional Support: Specific measures are not indicated.
Beverages: Avoid excessive caffeine intake.
▷ *Alcohol:* Alcohol may intensify the blood-pressure-lowering effects of this medicine. Ask your doctor for guidance.
Tobacco Smoking: No interactions expected. I advise everyone to quit smoking.
Marijuana Smoking: May increase the blood-pressure-lowering effects of this drug.
▷ *Other Drugs*
Losartan *taken concurrently* with
- hydrochlorothiazide (various) may increase clinical benefits.
- moxonidine (Cynt, available in Germany) may result in additive lowering of blood pressure.
- ritonavir (Norvir) may change losartan blood levels.
▷ *Driving, Hazardous Activities:* This drug may cause confusion. Restrict activities as necessary.
Aviation Note: The use of this drug *may be a disqualification* for piloting. Consult a designated aviation medical examiner.
Exposure to Sun: Caution is advised. Isolated cases of photosensitivity have been reported.
Exposure to Heat: Caution: excessive sweating (perspiration) may lead to dehydration and an excessive blood-pressure-lowering effect of this drug.
Discontinuation: Talk with your doctor before stopping this medicine for any reason.

LOVASTATIN (loh vah STA tin)

Introduced: 1987 **Class:** Anticholesterol (cholesterol-reducing drug)
Prescription: USA: Yes **Controlled Drug:** USA: No **Available as Generic:** USA: No; Canada: No
Brand Name: Mevacor

BENEFITS versus RISKS

Possible Benefits	*Possible Risks*
EFFECTIVE REDUCTION OF TOTAL BLOOD CHOLESTEROL	Drug-induced hepatitis (without jaundice)
SLOWS PROGRESSION OF CORONARY ATHEROSCLEROSIS	Drug-induced myositis (muscle inflammation)
May reduce risk of stroke like other medicines in this class	Drug-induced stomach ulceration

---

▷ **Principal Uses**

As a Single Drug Product: Uses currently included in FDA-approved labeling: (1) Reduces abnormally high total blood cholesterol levels in people with type II hypercholesterolemia (should not be used until nondrug methods have proven to be inadequate); (2) used to **slow progression** of coronary (heart) atherosclerosis in people with coronary heart disease. (It also showed a reduction in the number of heart attacks.)

Other (unlabeled) generally accepted uses: (1) May help decrease hypercholesterolemia in cholesterol ester storage disease prior to liver transplant; (2) could have a role in helping blue toe syndrome (peripheral atheroembolism); (3) could help lower cholesterol in secondary hyperlipidemia; (4) may help (low dose) in the nephrotic syndrome; (5) could help hyperlipidemia in transplant recipients; (6) may reduce stroke risk.

How This Drug Works: Converted to mcvinolinic acid, which inhibits the liver enzyme that starts to make cholesterol. It decreases low-density lipoproteins (LDL), the fraction of total blood cholesterol that increases risk of coronary heart disease. Also increases high-density lipoproteins (HDL), the fraction thought to reduce the risk of heart disease.

Available Dose Forms and Strengths
Tablets — 10 mg, 20 mg, 40 mg

▷ **Usual Adult Dose Range:** Initially 20 mg once a day with the evening meal. Dose may be increased up to 40 mg twice a day as needed and tolerated. Dose adjustments should be made at 4-week intervals. Limited data support low-dose therapy, where some patients responded to 20 mg as a single evening dose. Maximum daily dose should not exceed 80 mg. **Note: Actual dose and dosing schedule must be determined for each patient individually.**

Conditions Requiring Dosing Adjustments
Liver Function: This drug should be used with caution by patients with liver compromise. 83% of a dose is removed in the feces.
Kidney Function: Great caution should be used in considering doses above 20 mg per day for patients with severe kidney problems (creatinine clearance less than 30 ml/min).

▷ **Dosing Instructions:**   Take with food, preferably with the evening meal for maximal effectiveness. Highest rates of cholesterol production occur between midnight and 5 A.M. Tablet may be crushed.

Usual Duration of Use: Use on a regular schedule for 4 to 6 weeks determines effectiveness in reducing blood levels of total and LDL cholesterol. Long-term use (months to years) requires periodic physician evaluation of response.

Possible Advantages of This Drug
Better tolerated than some of the other drugs in this class.

▷ **This Drug Should Not Be Taken If**
- you have had an allergic reaction to it previously.
- you have active liver disease.
- you are pregnant or breast-feeding.

▷ **Inform Your Physician Before Taking This Drug If**
- you have liver disease or impaired liver function.
- you have had peptic ulcer disease or upper gastrointestinal bleeding.
- you are not using any method of birth control, or you are planning a pregnancy.
- you have a history of kidney compromise.
- you regularly consume substantial amounts of alcohol.
- you have cataracts or impaired vision.
- you have any type of chronic muscular disorder.

Possible Side Effects (natural, expected, and unavoidable drug actions)
Development of abnormal liver function tests without associated symptoms.

▷ **Possible Adverse Effects** (unusual, unexpected, and infrequent reactions)
If any of the following develop, consult your physician promptly for guidance.
Mild Adverse Effects
Allergic reactions: skin rash, itching.
Headache, insomnia, dizziness, blurred vision, altered taste—rare to infrequent.
Indigestion, stomach pain, nausea, excessive gas, constipation, diarrhea—infrequent.
Muscle cramps or pain—infrequent.
Impaired sense of smell—possible.
Serious Adverse Effects
Marked and persistent abnormal liver function tests with focal hepatitis (without jaundice) after 1 year of use—rare.
Acute myopathy (muscle pain and tenderness) or rhabdomyolysis—case reports.
Cataracts were a concern based on some early data; however, long-term information fails to demonstrate any adverse effect on the lens of the eye.
Neuropathy or systemic-lupus-erythematosus-like syndrome—case reports.

▷ **Possible Effects on Sexual Function:**   None reported.

Possible Delayed Adverse Effects: Myopathy.

Natural Diseases or Disorders That May Be Activated by This Drug   Latent liver disease.

Possible Effects on Laboratory Tests

Blood alanine aminotransferase (ALT) enzyme level: increased (with higher doses of drug).

Blood total cholesterol, LDL cholesterol, and triglyceride levels: decreased.

Blood HDL cholesterol level: increased.

CAUTION

1. Stop the drug immediately and call your doctor if you become pregnant.
2. Promptly report development of unexplained muscle pain or tenderness.
3. Call your doctor right away if altered or impaired vision happens.

Precautions for Use

By Infants and Children: Safety and effectiveness for those under 20 years of age are not established.

By Those Over 60 Years of Age: Tell your doctor about any personal or family history of cataracts. Comply with periodic eye examinations. Promptly report any alterations in vision.

▷ **Advisability of Use During Pregnancy**

Pregnancy Category: X. See Pregnancy Risk Categories at the back of this book.

Animal studies: Mouse and rat studies reveal skeletal birth defects due to this drug.

Human studies: Adequate studies of pregnant women are not available.

This drug should be avoided during entire pregnancy.

Advisability of Use If Breast-Feeding

Presence of this drug in breast milk: Probably yes.

Avoid drug or refrain from nursing.

Habit-Forming Potential: None.

Effects of Overdose: Increased indigestion, stomach distress, nausea, diarrhea.

Possible Effects of Long-Term Use: Abnormal liver function with focal hepatitis. Studies in rats with three to four times the human dose have resulted in increases in hepatocellular carcinoma (cancer). Clinical significance in humans is not known.

Suggested Periodic Examinations While Taking This Drug (at physician's discretion)

Blood cholesterol studies: total cholesterol, HDL and LDL fractions.

Liver function tests every 4 to 6 weeks during the first 15 months of use and periodically thereafter.

Complete eye examination at beginning of treatment and periodically thereafter. Ask your physician for guidance.

▷ **While Taking This Drug, Observe the Following**

Foods: Follow a standard low-cholesterol diet.

Beverages: Grapefruit juice can increase blood levels. Prudent not to combine. No restrictions. May be taken with milk.

▷ *Alcohol:* No interactions expected. Use sparingly.

Tobacco Smoking: No interactions expected, but I advise everyone to quit smoking.

▷ *Other Drugs*

Lovastatin *taken concurrently* with

• clofibrate (Atromid-S, others) may result in a severe rhabdomyolysis.

• cyclosporine (Sandimmune) can cause a severe myopathy.

- erythromycin (E.E.S.) and perhaps other macrolide antibiotics (azithromycin, clarithromycin, or dirithromycin) may result in severe rhabdomyolysis.
- fluconazole (Sporonox) or ketoconazole (Nizoral) may increase risk of muscle damage (rhabdomyolysis).
- gemfibrozil (Lopid) may cause myopathy.
- niacin (various) can cause muscle damage (myopathy).
- ritonavir (Norvir) may lead to lovastatin toxicity.
- warfarin may result in bleeding. Increased frequency of INR (prothrombin time or protime) testing is suggested.

▷ *Driving, Hazardous Activities:* This drug may cause dizziness or impaired vision. Restrict activities as necessary.

Aviation Note: The use of this drug *may be a disqualification* for piloting. Consult a designated aviation medical examiner.

Exposure to Sun: No restrictions.

Discontinuation: Do not stop this drug without your physician's knowledge and guidance.

MACROLIDE ANTIBIOTIC FAMILY (ma KRO lied)

Azithromycin (a zith roh MY sin)   **Clarithromycin** (KLAR ith roh my sin)   **Erythromycin** (er ith roh MY sin)

Introduced: 1991, 1991, 1952, respectively   **Class:** Anti-infective, antibiotic, macrolide antibiotic   **Prescription:** USA: Yes   **Controlled Drugs:** USA: No; Canada: No   **Available as Generic:** Azithromycin: No; clarithromycin: No; erythromycin: Yes

Brand Names: Azithromycin: Zithromax; Clarithromycin: Biaxin, Prevpac [CD]; Erythromycin: AK-Mycin Ophthalmic, Akne-Mycin, ✦Apo-Erythro Base, ✦Apo-Erythro E-C, ✦Apo-Erythro-ES, ✦Apo-Erythro-S, A/T/S, Benzamycin [CD], C-Solve 2, E.E.S., E.E.S. 200, E.E.S. 400, Emgel, E-Mycin, E-Mycin Controlled Release, E-Mycin E, E-Mycin 333, Eramycin, ✦Erybid, ERYC, Erycette, Eryderm, Erygel, Erymax, Eryphar, EryPed, Ery-Tab, Erythrocin, ✦Erythromid, E-Solve 2, ETS-2%, Ilosone, Ilotycin, ✦Novorythro, PCE, Pediamycin, ✦Pediazole [CD], ✦PMS-Erythromycin, Robimycin, Sans-Acne, SK-Erythromycin, Staticin, ✦Stievamycin, T-Stat, Wyamycin E, Wyamycin S

BENEFITS versus RISKS	
Possible Benefits	*Possible Risks*
EFFECTIVE TREATMENT OF INFECTIONS due to susceptible microorganisms	Allergic reactions, mild and infrequent
	Liver reaction (most common with erythromycin estolate)
	Mild gastrointestinal symptoms
	Drug-induced colitis
	Superinfections

▷ **Principal Uses**

As a Single Drug Product: Uses currently included in FDA-approved labeling: Treatment of (1) skin and skin structure infections (such as acne and *Streptococcus*); (2) upper and lower respiratory tract infections, including "strep" throat, diphtheria, and several types of pneumonia; (3) gonorrhea and syphilis; (4) amebic dysentery (erythromycin); (5) Legionnaire's disease (erythromycin); (6) long-term prevention of recurrences of rheumatic fever (erythromycin)—effective use requires the precise identification of the causative organism and determination of its sensitivity to a macrolide antibiotic; (7) treatment of mycoplasma pneumonia; (8) listeriosis; (9) neonatal conjunctivitis (erythromycin); (10) treatment of ear infections (otitis media)—all; (11) treatment of AIDS-related *Mycobacterium aviumintracellulare*—all; (12) azithromycin treats *Chlamydia trachomatis* urethritis; (13) therapy of *Helicobacter pylori* duodenal ulcers in combination with omeprazole (clarithromycin).

Author's Note: An Agency for Health Care Policy and Research (AHCPR) study found that most patients who were 60 years of age or younger obtained the same outcomes and significantly reduced costs when erythromycin was used to treat community-acquired pneumonia.

Other (unlabeled) generally accepted uses: (1) Treatment of early Lyme disease (erythromycin; azithromycin is an alternative drug); (2) erythromycin helps sterilize the bowel before surgical procedures; (3) may help threatened preterm labor if the cause is *Ureaplasma* organisms (erythromycin); (4) helps impetigo (erythromycin); (5) azithromycin or clarithromycin are second choices for Legionnaire's disease; (6) can help some cases of stomach slowness in diabetics (gastroparesis); (7) may treat some heart attacks where *Chlamydia pneumoniae* is present.

As a Combination Drug Product [CD]: Clarithromycin is available in combination with amoxicillin and lansoprazole. Since refractory ulcers are often actually *Helicobacter pylori* infections, the combination works to kill the bacteria and lower acid production.

How These Drugs Work: They prevent growth and multiplication of susceptible organisms by interfering with their formation of essential proteins.

Available Dose Forms and Strengths

Azithromycin:

Capsules — 250 mg
Oral suspension — 100 mg/5 ml, 200 mg/5 ml
Tablet — 600 mg

Clarithromycin:

Tablets — 250 mg, 500 mg
Oral suspension granules — 125 mg/5 ml, 250 mg/5 ml

Erythromycin:

Capsules — 125 mg, 250 mg
Capsules, enteric coated — 125 mg, 250 mg
Drops — 100 mg/ml
Eye ointment — 5 mg/gGel
— 2%
Oral suspension — 125 mg/5 ml, 250 mg/5 ml
Skin ointment — 2%

Tablets — 250 mg, 500 mg
Tablets, chewable — 125 mg, 200 mg, 250 mg
Tablets, delayed release — 250 mg, 333 mg
Tablets, dispersible (Canada) — 500 mg
Tablets, enteric coated — 250 mg, 333 mg, 500 mg
Tablets, film coated — 250 mg, 500 mg
Topical solution — 1.5%, 2%

▷ **Usual Adult Dose Range:**   Erythromycin: 250 to 500 mg every 6 hours, according to nature and severity of infection. Total daily dose should not exceed 4 g. For endocarditis prophylaxis (stearate oral form): 1 g 2 hours before procedure and 500 mg 6 hours later. Pediatrics: oral erythromycin is usually given at a dose of 30 to 50 mg per kg of body mass per day and is divided into three or four doses.

Infants and Children: Azithromycin: Otitis media—10 mg per kg of body mass as a single dose on the first day (up to 500 mg), followed by 5 mg per kg of body mass (up to 250 mg) on days 2–5. Pharyngitis—12 mg per kg of body mass (up to 500 mg) daily for 5 days.

Clarithromycin: Used to treat otitis media (caused by *Haemophilus influenzae*, *M. catarrhalis*, or *Strep. pneumoniae*) in children—the dose is 7.5 mg per kg of body mass twice daily, up to a maximum of 500 mg twice a day for 10 days. For *Mycobacterium avium-intracellulare complex* infections in children—the dose is 7.5 mg per kg of body mass twice daily, to a maximum of 500 mg twice a day. If this dose is successful, therapy is continued for life.

12 to 60 Years of Age: Clarithromycin: For pharyngitis/tonsillitis—250 mg every 12 hours for 10 days. For maxillary sinusitis—500 mg every 12 hours for 14 days. For acute bronchitis—250 to 500 mg every 12 hours for 7 to 14 days. For pneumonia—250 mg every 12 hours for 7 to 14 days. For skin infections—250 mg every 12 hours for 7 to 14 days.

16 to 60 Years of Age: Azithromycin: For pharyngitis/tonsillitis, bronchitis, pneumonia, and skin infections—500 mg as a single dose on the first day, then 250 mg once daily on days 2–4 for a total dose of 1.5 g. For *Helicobacter pylori*—500 mg daily for 7 days. For nongonococcal urethritis and cervicitis—a single 1 g (1000 mg) dose.

Over 60 Years of Age: Azithromycin: Same as 16 to 60 years of age. If liver or kidney function is limited, the dose must be reduced.

Clarithromycin: Same as 12 to 60 years of age. Dose must be reduced in kidney compromise.

Note: Actual dose and schedule must be determined for each patient individually.

Conditions Requiring Dosing Adjustments

Liver Function: These drugs are metabolized in the liver, and will accumulate in patients with liver compromise. Decreased doses may be needed. They should be used with caution by patients with biliary tract disease. Clarithromycin does not need to be adjusted for patients with liver problems if kidney function is normal.

Kidney Function: No dosing changes are needed for azithromycin. The dose of clarithromycin **must be decreased** or **the time between doses (dosing interval) prolonged** for patients with compromised kidneys. Patients with severe kidney failure can take 50–75% of the usual erythromycin dose at the usual time. Azithromycin and erythromycin are rare causes of interstitial nephritis (inflammation of a specific part of the kidney).

▷ **Dosing Instructions:**   Non-enteric-coated preparations should be taken 1 hour before or 2 hours after eating. Enteric-coated preparations may be taken without regard to food. Azithromycin may be better tolerated if taken with food. Do not take azithromycin with antacids containing aluminum or magnesium. Regular uncoated capsules may be opened and tablets may be crushed; coated and prolonged-action preparations should be swallowed whole. Ask your pharmacist for help.

Usual Duration of Use: Use on a regular schedule for 3 to 5 days is necessary to determine these drugs' effectiveness in controlling infections. For streptococcal infections: not less than 10 consecutive (5 consecutive for azithromycin) days (without interruption) to reduce the possibility of developing rheumatic fever or glomerulonephritis. The duration of use should not exceed the time required to eliminate the infection.

Possible Advantages of These Drugs
Azithromycin and clarithromycin: broader spectrum of infectious microorganism coverage; equivalent to erythromycin, some penicillins, and some cephalosporins. Effective with fewer doses (only one dose for azithromycin and two for clarithromycin). Azithromycin and clarithromycin are very well tolerated; infrequent and minor adverse effects.

▷ **These Drugs Should Not Be Taken If**
- you had an allergic reaction to a macrolide previously.
- you have active liver disease (erythromycin estolate form).
- you are pregnant or planning a pregnancy (some forms).
- you are allergic to *para*-aminobenzoic-acid-type anesthetics (intramuscular form of erythromycin).
- you are taking terfenadine (Seldane) or astemizole (Hismanal).

▷ **Inform Your Physician Before Taking These Drugs If**
- you have a history of a previous "reaction" to any macrolide antibiotic.
- you are allergic by nature: hay fever, asthma, hives, eczema.
- you have a blood disorder.
- you have an abnormal heart rhythm.
- you have a history of porphyria.
- you have a history of kidney disorder.
- you have myasthenia gravis.
- you have a hearing disorder.
- you have a history of low blood platelets (some macrolides).
- you have taken the estolate form of erythromycin previously.

Possible Side Effects (natural, expected, and unavoidable drug actions)
Superinfections (see Glossary).

▷ **Possible Adverse Effects** (unusual, unexpected, and infrequent reactions)
If any of the following develop, consult your physician promptly for guidance.
Mild Adverse Effects
Allergic reactions: skin rash, hives, itching—rare.
Nausea, vomiting, diarrhea, abdominal cramping—infrequent.

Headache—rare.

Drug-induced increased liver enzymes (see *jaundice* in Glossary)—rare.

Serious Adverse Effects

Allergic Reaction: Anaphylactic reaction (see Glossary)—rare.

Idiosyncratic reactions: liver reaction: nausea, vomiting, fever, jaundice (usually, but not exclusively, associated with erythromycin estolate).

Decreased white blood cells (erythromycin)—rare.

Lowered blood platelets (clarithromycin)—case report.

Abnormal heart rhythm—rare.

Worsening of myasthenia gravis—case reports.

Low body temperature (hypothermia)—rare.

Pseudomembranous colitis—rare.

Pancreatitis (erythromycin)—rare.

Kidney problems (interstitial nephritis) (azithromycin, erythromycin)—case reports.

Hearing loss (ototoxicity)—case reports.

▷ **Possible Effects on Sexual Function:**   None reported.

▷ **Adverse Effects That May Mimic Natural Diseases or Disorders**

Liver toxicity may resemble acute gallbladder disease or viral hepatitis.

Possible Effects on Laboratory Tests

Complete blood cell counts: white cells may increase or decrease; eosinophils increased (allergic reaction); platelets decreased.

INR (prothrombin time): increased (drug taken concurrently with warfarin).

Liver function tests: liver enzymes increased (ALT/GPT, AST/GOT, and alkaline phosphatase), increased bilirubin.

CAUTION

1. Take the **full dose prescribed** to help prevent resistant bacteria.
2. If you have a history of liver disease or impaired liver function, avoid any form of erythromycin estolate.
3. If diarrhea develops and continues for more than 24 hours, consult your physician promptly.

Precautions for Use

By Infants and Children: Watch allergic children closely for indications of developing allergy to this drug. Observe also for evidence of gastrointestinal irritation. Dosing based on body mass is critical.

By Those Over 60 Years of Age: Watch for itching reactions in the genital and anal regions, often due to yeast superinfections. Observe also for evidence of hearing loss. Report such developments promptly. If liver or kidney function is impaired, dose decreases must be considered.

▷ **Advisability of Use During Pregnancy**

Pregnancy Category: C for clarithromycin; B for others. See Pregnancy Risk Categories at the back of this book.

Animal studies: Studies of rats are inconclusive for erythromycin. Monkey, rabbit, and rat studies have shown problems in pregnancy outcomes and fetal development.

Human studies: Information from adequate studies of pregnant women is not available.

Generally thought to be safe during entire pregnancy, *except for erythromycin estolate*; this form of erythromycin can cause toxic liver reactions during pregnancy and should be avoided. Clarithromycin should be avoided unless no other antibiotic option is available.

Advisability of Use If Breast-Feeding
Presence of this drug in breast milk: Yes, for azithromycin and erythromycin; clarithromycin unknown.
Watch nursing infant closely and discontinue drug or nursing if adverse effects develop.

Habit-Forming Potential: None.

Effects of Overdose: Possible nausea, vomiting, hallucinations (clarithromycin), diarrhea, and abdominal discomfort.

Possible Effects of Long-Term Use: Superinfections (see Glossary).

Suggested Periodic Examinations While Taking This Drug (at physician's discretion)
Liver function tests if the erythromycin estolate form is used. Complete blood counts to measure response of infection.

▷ **While Taking This Drug, Observe the Following**
Foods: New formulation absorption is decreased by more than 70% (especially high-fat meals) and effectiveness may be seriously compromised for erythromycin. Azithromycin and clarithromycin are not affected.
Beverages: Avoid fruit juices and carbonated beverages for 1 hour after taking any non-enteric-coated preparation of erythromycin. May be taken with milk.
▷ *Alcohol:* Avoid if you have impaired liver function or are taking the estolate form of erythromycin.
Tobacco Smoking: No interactions expected. I advise everyone to quit smoking.
▷ *Other Drugs*
These medicines may *increase* the effects of
• benzodiazepines (see Drug Classes).
• carbamazepine (Tegretol), and cause toxicity.
• digoxin (Lanoxin), and cause toxicity.
• ergotamine (Cafergot, Ergostat, etc.), and cause impaired circulation to extremities.
• methylprednisolone (Medrol) and prednisone, and cause excess steroid effects.
• sildenafil (Viagra); reported up to 182% increased blood level.
• tacrolimus (Prograf).
• theophylline (aminophylline, Theo-Dur, etc.), and cause toxicity.
• warfarin (Coumadin), and increase the risk of bleeding.
These medicines may *decrease* the effects of
• clindamycin.
• lincomycin.
• penicillins.
These medicines *taken concurrently* with
• astemizole (Hismanal) may cause serious arrhythmias.
• birth control pills (oral contraceptives) can cause loss of effectiveness and result in pregnancy.
• cisapride (Propulsid) may lead to cisapride toxicity (clarithromycin only).
• cyclosporine (Sandimmune) may result in cyclosporine toxicity.

- dihydroergotamine and other ergot derivatives can lead to increased levels and ergot toxicity.
- disopyramide may cause heart (cardiac) arrhythmias.
- loratadine (Claritin) may result in increased loratadine levels, but they do not appear to cause the serious arrhythmia of some of the other nonsedating antihistamines. Since loratadine levels may be increased, it may be prudent to decrease loratadine doses while taking erythromycin.
- lovastatin can cause rhabdomyolysis (serious muscle damage).
- midazolam (and probably other benzodiazepines; (see Drug Classes) may lead to excessive central nervous system depression.
- nevirapine (Viramune) may lead to nevirapine toxicity.
- ritonavir (Norvir), and perhaps other protease inhibitors (see Drug Classes), may lead to toxicity.
- terfenadine (Seldane) can cause cardiac (heart) arrhythmias.
- triazolam may cause toxicity.
- trimexate (Mexate) decrease trimexate metabolism and can lead to toxicity.
- valproic acid (Depakene, Depakote) can lead to toxic blood levels.
- zidovudine (AZT) may lead to decreased levels and lack of zidovudine effectiveness.

▷ *Driving, Hazardous Activities:* This drug may cause nausea and/or diarrhea. Restrict activities as necessary.

Aviation Note: The use of this drug *may be a disqualification* for piloting. Consult a designated aviation medical examiner.

Exposure to Sun: Use caution; some medicines in this class have caused increased sensitivity to the sun (photosensitivity).

Special Storage Instructions: Keep liquid forms refrigerated.

Observe the Following Expiration Times: Freshly mixed oral suspension (clarithromycin)—14 days (DO NOT refrigerate). Freshly mixed oral suspensions of erythromycin should be refrigerated to preserve taste. These go bad (outdate) in 14 days. Single-dose azithromycin suspension should be mixed with water and taken right away. Ask your pharmacist for help.

MAPROTILINE (ma PROH ti leen)

Introduced: 1974   **Class:** Antidepressant   **Prescription:** USA: Yes
Controlled Drug: USA: No; Canada: No   **Available as Generic:** Yes
Brand Name: Ludiomil

BENEFITS versus RISKS	
Possible Benefits	*Possible Risks*
EFFECTIVE RELIEF OF ALL TYPES OF DEPRESSION	ADVERSE BEHAVIORAL EFFECTS
	CONVERSION OF DEPRESSION TO MANIA in manic-depressive (bipolar) disorders
	Irregular heart rhythms
	Liver toxicity with jaundice
	Seizures with therapeutic doses
	Low white blood cells

Author's Note: Because use of this medicine has declined in favor of newer medicines, the information in this profile has been abbreviated.

MECLOFENAMATE (me kloh fen AM ayt)

See the fenamates (nonsteroidal anti-inflammatory drugs) profile for further information.

MEDROXYPROGESTERONE (me DROX e proh jess te rohn)

Introduced: 1959   **Class:** Female sex hormones, progestins   **Prescription:** USA: Yes   **Controlled Drug:** USA: No; Canada: No   **Available as Generic:** Yes
Brand Names: Amen, Curretab, Cycrin, Depo-Provera, Premphase, Prempro, Provera

---

BENEFITS versus RISKS

Possible Benefits	*Possible Risks*
EFFECTIVE TREATMENT OF ABSENT OR ABNORMAL MENSTRUATION due to hormone imbalance	Thrombophlebitis Pulmonary embolism Liver reaction with jaundice Drug-induced birth defects
EFFECTIVE CONTRACEPTION when given by injection	
Useful adjunctive therapy in selected cases of uterine and kidney cancer	

▷ **Principal Uses**

As a Single Drug Product: Uses currently included in FDA-approved labeling: (1) Used to initiate and regulate menstruation and correct abnormal patterns of menstrual bleeding caused by hormonal imbalance (and not by organic disease); (2) used in combination to treat metastatic, inoperable, or recurrent endometrial carcinoma; (3) treatment of renal cell carcinoma; (4) used as a contraceptive injected into the muscle once every 3 months; (5) helps dysfunctional uterine bleeding.

Other (unlabeled) generally accepted uses: (1) Used as a part of combination therapy in breast, refractory prostate, lung, and ovarian cancers; (2) therapy of endometriosis; (3) used in osteoporosis to help increase bone mineral density; (4) helps abnormal hair growth in women (hirsutism); (5) can help breast pain (mastodynia); (6) used in combination with estrogen to help symptoms of menopause; (7) can be of use in pelvic congestion and pickwickian syndrome; (8) may help severe PMS; (9) can be of use in male hypersexuality.

How This Drug Works: By inducing and maintaining a lining in the uterus that resembles pregnancy, this drug can prevent uterine bleeding until it is withdrawn. By suppressing the release of the pituitary gland hormone that induces ovulation, and by stimulating the secretion of mucus by the uterine cervix (to resist the passage of sperm), this drug can prevent pregnancy.

Available Dose Forms and Strengths
    Injection — 150 mg (single-dose vials)
          — 100 mg/ml, 150 mg/ml, 400 mg/ml
    Tablets — 2.5 mg, 5 mg, 10 mg

▷ **Usual Adult Dose Range:**   To initiate menstruation: 5 to 10 mg daily for 5 to 10 days, started at any time.
    To correct abnormal bleeding: 5 to 10 mg daily for 5 to 10 days, started on the 16th or 21st day of the menstrual cycle. Withdrawal bleeding usually begins within 3 to 7 days after stopping the drug.
    As a contraceptive: Intramuscular injections of 150 mg every 3 months are needed.
    Note: Actual dose and schedule must be determined for each patient individually.

Conditions Requiring Dosing Adjustments
    Liver Function: This drug should be used with caution, and the dose empirically decreased, by patients with liver compromise.
    Kidney Function: No dosing changes thought to be needed.

▷ **Dosing Instructions:**   The tablet may be crushed and taken on an empty stomach or with food to prevent nausea.

Usual Duration of Use: Use on a regular schedule for two or three menstrual cycles determines effectiveness in correcting abnormal patterns of menstrual bleeding. See your doctor on a regular basis.

▷ **This Drug Should Not Be Taken If**
- you have had an allergic reaction to it previously.
- you are pregnant.
- you have experienced a missed abortion.
- you have seriously impaired liver function.
- you have a history of cancer of the breast or reproductive organs.
- you have a history of thrombophlebitis, embolism, or stroke.
- you have abnormal and unexplained vaginal bleeding.

▷ **Inform Your Physician Before Taking This Drug If**
- you have impaired kidney function.
- you have any of the following disorders: asthma, diabetes, emotional depression, epilepsy, heart disease, migraine headaches.

Possible Side Effects (natural, expected, and unavoidable drug actions)
    Fluid retention, weight gain, changes in menstrual timing and flow, spotting between periods.

▷ **Possible Adverse Effects** (unusual, unexpected, and infrequent reactions)
    If any of the following develop, consult your physician promptly for guidance.
    Mild Adverse Effects
    Allergic reactions: skin rash, hives, itching.
    Fatigue, weakness, nausea—infrequent.
    Acne, excessive hair growth—case reports.
    Serious Adverse Effects
    Liver toxicity with jaundice (see Glossary): yellow eyes/skin, dark-colored urine, light-colored stools—possible.
    Thrombophlebitis (inflammation of a vein with blood clot formation): pain or

tenderness in thigh or leg, with or without swelling of the foot, ankle, or leg—case reports.

Pulmonary embolism (movement of blood clot to lung): sudden shortness of breath, chest pain, cough, bloody sputum—case reports.

Stroke (blood clot in the brain): sudden headache, weakness or paralysis of any part of the body—possible.

Retinal thrombosis (blood clot in the eye): sudden impairment or loss of vision—case reports.

Drug-induced pseudotumor cerebri—possible.

Pneumonitis, especially in patients who have received radiation therapy—case reports.

Medroxyprogesterone may act as a co-carcinogen—a compound that does not cause cancer, but can promote the host's neoplastic response to a carcinogen.

▷ **Possible Effects on Sexual Function:** Altered timing and pattern of menstruation. Female breast tenderness and secretion. Decreased vaginal secretions. Infertility—case reports.

▷ **Adverse Effects That May Mimic Natural Diseases or Disorders**
Liver toxicity may suggest viral hepatitis.

Possible Effects on Laboratory Tests
Blood total cholesterol, HDL cholesterol, LDL cholesterol, and triglyceride levels: decreased.
Glucose tolerance test (GTT): decreased.

CAUTION
1. There is an increased risk of birth defects in children whose mothers take this drug during the first 4 months of pregnancy.
2. Inform your physician promptly if you think you may be pregnant.
3. This drug should not be used as a test for pregnancy.

Precautions for Use
By Infants and Children: Not used in this age group.
By Those Over 60 Years of Age: Used as adjunctive therapy in cancer of the breast, uterus, prostate, and kidney. Watch for excessive fluid retention.

▷ **Advisability of Use During Pregnancy**
Pregnancy Category: D. See Pregnancy Risk Categories at the back of this book.
Animal studies: Genital defects reported in rat and rabbit studies; masculinization of the female rodent fetus; various defects in chick embryos and rabbits.
Human studies: In a study of 1,016 pregnancies, oral doses of 80–120 mg daily used from the 5th–7th week of pregnancy up to the 18th week were not associated with teratogenic effects. Other data show masculinization of the female genitals: enlargement of the clitoris, fusion of the labia. Increased risk of heart, nervous system, and limb defects when used in the second and third trimesters of pregnancy.
The drug is used as a benefit-to-risk decision in the first 3 months of pregnancy. Avoid this drug completely during the final 6 months of pregnancy.

Advisability of Use If Breast-Feeding
Presence of this drug in breast milk: Yes.
Avoid drug or refrain from nursing.

Habit-Forming Potential: None.

Effects of Overdose: Nausea, vomiting, fluid retention, breast enlargement and discomfort, abnormal vaginal bleeding.

Possible Effects of Long-Term Use: There has been considerable controversy regarding use of this drug and cancer. The most recent large patient studies do not show an increased relative risk that is statistically significant.

Suggested Periodic Examinations While Taking This Drug (at physician's discretion)

Regular examinations (every 6 to 12 months) of the breasts and reproductive organs (pelvic examination of the uterus and ovaries, including Pap smear).

▷ **While Taking This Drug, Observe the Following**

Foods: No restrictions.

Beverages: No restrictions.

▷ *Alcohol:* No interactions expected.

Tobacco Smoking: I advise everyone to quit smoking.

▷ *Other Drugs*

The following drugs may ***decrease*** the effects of medroxyprogesterone:
* nevirapine (Viramine).
* rifampin (Rifadin, Rimactane, etc.); may hasten its elimination.

Medroxyprogesterone ***taken concurrently*** with
* digitoxin may result in slightly higher than expected digoxin levels.
* ritonavir (Norvir), and perhaps other protease inhibitors (see Drug Classes), may lead to toxicity.
* tamoxifen (Nolvadex) may result in blunting of the therapeutic benefits of tamoxifen.
* warfarin (Coumadin) may increase warfarin effects. Increased lab INR (prothrombin time or protime) testing is needed.

▷ *Driving, Hazardous Activities:* Usually no restrictions. Ask your doctor about your individual risk and for guidance regarding specific restrictions.

Aviation Note: The use of this drug ***may be a disqualification*** for piloting. Consult a designated aviation medical examiner.

Exposure to Sun: No restrictions.

MEFENAMIC ACID (me FEN am ik a sid)

See the fenamates (nonsteroidal anti-inflammatory drugs) profile for further information.

MEPERIDINE (me PER i deen)

Other Name: Pethidine

Introduced: 1939   **Class:** Strong analgesic, opioids   **Prescription:** USA: Yes   **Controlled Drug:** USA: C-II*; Canada: Yes   **Available as Generic:** Yes

Brand Names: Demerol, Demerol APAP [CD], Mepergan, Pethadol

*See schedules of Controlled Drugs at the back of this book.

```
┌─────────────────────────────────────────────────────────────────┐
│                    BENEFITS versus RISKS                         │
│      Possible Benefits              Possible Risks               │
│    EFFECTIVE RELIEF OF          POTENTIAL FOR HABIT              │
│      MODERATE TO SEVERE PAIN       FORMATION (DEPENDENCE)        │
│                                 Weakness, fainting               │
│                                 Disorientation, hallucinations   │
│                                 Interference with urination      │
└─────────────────────────────────────────────────────────────────┘
```

▷ **Principal Uses**

As a Single Drug Product: Uses currently included in FDA-approved labeling: Used by mouth or injection to relieve moderate to severe pain of any cause.

Other (unlabeled) generally accepted uses: (1) Used to treat fevers caused by amphotericin B; (2) can help porphyrias; (3) eases postanesthesia chills; (4) used for sickle cell disease pain.

As a Combination Drug Product [CD]: This drug is available in combination with acetaminophen (Demerol APAP) to create a dose form that utilizes two pain relievers, and also reduces fever.

How This Drug Works: Depresses certain brain functions, suppressing perception of pain and calming the emotional response to pain.

Available Dose Forms and Strengths

Injection — 10 mg/ml, 25 mg/ml, 50 mg/ml, 75 mg/ml, 100 mg/ml

Syrup — 50 mg/5 ml teaspoonful

Tablets — 50 mg, 100 mg

▷ **Usual Adult Dose Range:**   Taken by mouth: 50 to 150 mg every 3 to 4 hours to relieve pain. The usual dose is 100 mg. The total daily dose should not exceed 900 mg. **Note: Actual dose and schedule must be determined for each patient individually.**

Author's Note: The old "as-needed" dosing has been replaced by scheduled (such as every 4 hours) dosing because it can keep pain from happening, rather than trying to treat it after the pain medicine blood level has gotten low enough to allow pain to return.

Conditions Requiring Dosing Adjustments

Liver Function: The initial dose should be the same in liver compromise; however, subsequent doses should be decreased by 50% or the dosing interval doubled. Some clinicians report that doses of 25 to 50 mg have produced acceptable effects in some patients with severe liver disease.

Kidney Function: Patients with mild to moderate kidney failure should take 75% of the usual dose at the usual interval. Patients with severe kidney failure should take 50% of the usual dose at the usual time. **Multiple doses should be avoided** as a toxic (normeperidine) metabolite may accumulate and can cause severe central nervous system reactions.

▷ **Dosing Instructions:**   The tablet may be crushed and taken with or following food to reduce stomach irritation or nausea. The syrup may be diluted in 4 ounces of water to reduce the numbing effect on the tongue and mouth tissues.

Usual Duration of Use: As required to control pain. Current pain therapy often uses timed or scheduled doses to prevent pain rather than treat it. Continual use should not exceed 5 to 7 days without interruption and reassessment of need.

▷ **This Drug Should Not Be Taken If**
  • you had an allergic reaction to it previously.
  • you are having an acute attack of asthma.
  • you have increased intracranial pressure (talk with your doctor).
  • you have an abnormal heart rhythm (atrioventricular flutter).
  • you have a history of convulsions or seizures.
  • you have a history of kidney failure and multiple doses are scheduled.
  • you have significant respiratory depression.
  • you are taking, or have taken within the past 14 days, any monoamine oxidase (MAO) type A inhibitor drug (see Drug Classes).

▷ **Inform Your Physician Before Taking This Drug If**
  • you have a history of drug abuse or alcoholism.
  • you have impaired liver or kidney function.
  • you have a history of asthma, epilepsy, or glaucoma.
  • you are taking any other drugs that have a sedative effect.
  • you will have surgery with general anesthesia.

Possible Side Effects (natural, expected, and unavoidable drug actions)
  Drowsiness, light-headedness, weakness, euphoria, dry mouth, urinary retention, constipation.
  Dose-related respiratory depression.

▷ **Possible Adverse Effects** (unusual, unexpected, and infrequent reactions)
  If any of the following develop, consult your physician promptly for guidance.
  Mild Adverse Effects
  Allergic reactions: skin rash, hives, itching.
  Headache, dizziness, impaired concentration, sensation of drunkenness, confusion, depression, blurred or double vision—infrequent, but can be dose related.
  Facial flushing, sweating, heart palpitation—case reports.
  Nausea, vomiting—infrequent to frequent and can be dose related.
  Serious Adverse Effects
  Allergic reactions: anaphylactic reactions.
  Drop in blood pressure, causing severe weakness and fainting—case reports and dose related.
  Disorientation, hallucinations, unstable gait, tremor, muscle twitching—possible, case reports.
  Drug-induced myasthenia gravis—case reports.
  Urinary retention—possible.
  Kidney failure—rare.
  Seizures, especially in patients with kidney failure who are given multiple doses (normeperidine accumulation)—case reports.

▷ **Possible Effects on Sexual Function:**   Blunting of sexual response. Retrograde ejaculation.

▷ **Adverse Effects That May Mimic Natural Diseases or Disorders**
  Paradoxical behavioral disturbances may suggest psychotic disorder.

Possible Effects on Laboratory Tests
  Blood alanine aminotransferase (ALT) and aspartate aminotransferase (AST) levels: increased (natural side effects).
  Blood amylase and lipase levels: increased (natural side effects).

CAUTION
1. If you have asthma, chronic bronchitis, or emphysema, excessive use of this drug may cause significant respiratory difficulty, thickening of bronchial secretions, and suppression of coughing.
2. The concurrent use of this drug with atropinelike drugs can increase the risk of urinary retention and reduced intestinal function.
3. Do not take this drug following acute head injury.

Precautions for Use
By Infants and Children: Do not use this drug in infants under 1 year of age because of their vulnerability to life-threatening respiratory depression.
By Those Over 60 Years of Age: Small doses initially and slow increases as needed and tolerated. Limit use to short-term treatment only if possible. There may be increased risk of drowsiness, dizziness, unsteadiness, falling, urinary retention, and constipation (often leading to fecal impaction).

▷ **Advisability of Use During Pregnancy**
Pregnancy Category: B; D if used in higher doses or for a longer period of time, especially when the baby is due to be born. See Pregnancy Risk Categories at the back of this book.
Animal studies: Significant birth defects reported in hamster studies.
Human studies: Adequate studies of pregnant women are not available. However, no significant increase in birth defects was found in 1,100 drug exposures.
Avoid during the first 3 months. Use sparingly and in small doses during the final 6 months only if clearly needed, as it has clear effects on the breathing capabilities of the infant.

Advisability of Use If Breast-Feeding
Presence of this drug in breast milk: Yes.
Avoid drug or refrain from nursing.

Habit-Forming Potential: This drug can cause psychological and physical dependence (see Glossary).

Effects of Overdose: Marked drowsiness, confusion, tremors, convulsions, stupor leading to coma.

Possible Effects of Long-Term Use: Psychological and physical dependence, chronic constipation.

Suggested Periodic Examinations While Taking This Drug (at physician's discretion)
Should assess bowel status if prone to constipation.

▷ **While Taking This Drug, Observe the Following**
Foods: No restrictions.
Beverages: No restrictions. May be taken with milk.
▷ *Alcohol:* Opioid analgesics can intensify the intoxicating effects of alcohol, and alcohol can intensify the depressant effects of opioids on brain function, breathing, and circulation. Alcohol is best avoided.
Tobacco Smoking: No interactions expected. I advise everyone to quit smoking.
Marijuana Smoking: Increase in drowsiness and pain relief; impairment of mental and physical performance.
▷ *Other Drugs*
Meperidine may *increase* the effects of

- atropinelike drugs, and increase the risk of constipation and urinary retention.
- other drugs with sedative effects.

Meperidine *taken concurrently* with

- acyclovir (Zovirax) may increase risk of nerve toxicity.
- cimetidine (Tagamet), famotidine (Pepcid), nizatidine (Axid), ranitidine (Zantac), and omeprazole (Prilosec) can increase alkalinity of the stomach and may result in increased meperidine levels and toxicity.
- intravenous acyclovir (Zovirax) can result in kidney and nerve problems.
- monoamine oxidase (MAO) type A inhibitor drugs (see Drug Classes) can cause the equivalent of an acute narcotic overdose: unconsciousness, severe breathing depression, slowed heart action and circulation. Can also cause excitability, convulsions, high fever, and rapid heart action.
- phenothiazines (see Drug Classes) can cause excessive and prolonged depression of brain functions, breathing, and circulation.
- phenytoin (Dilantin) can result in decreased therapeutic effects of meperidine.
- ritonavir (Norvir), and perhaps other protease inhibitors (see Drug Classes), may lead to toxicity.
- tramadol (Ultram) may increase seizure risk.
- tricyclic antidepressants (amitriptyline, others) may result in worsening of meperidine's respiratory depression side effect.

▷ *Driving, Hazardous Activities:* This drug can impair mental alertness, judgment, reaction time, and physical coordination. Avoid hazardous activities.

Aviation Note: The use of this drug *is a disqualification* for piloting. Consult a designated aviation medical examiner.

Exposure to Sun: No restrictions.

Discontinuation: This drug is best limited to short-term use. If used for extended periods of time, discontinuation should be gradual to minimize withdrawal effects.

MERCAPTOPURINE (mer kap toh PYUR een)

Other Names: 6-mercaptopurine, 6-MP
Introduced: 1960   **Class:** Anticancer (antineoplastic), immunosuppressant
Prescription: USA: Yes   **Controlled Drug:** USA: No; Canada: No   **Available as Generic:** USA: No; Canada: No
Brand Name: Purinethol

BENEFITS versus RISKS	
Possible Benefits	*Possible Risks*
EFFECTIVE TREATMENT OF CERTAIN ACUTE AND CHRONIC LEUKEMIAS AND LYMPHOMAS	BONE MARROW DEPRESSION (see Glossary)
Effective treatment of polycythemia vera	DRUG-INDUCED LIVER DAMAGE
Possibly effective treatment of Crohn's disease and ulcerative colitis	Rare gastrointestinal ulceration
Possibly effective treatment of severe psoriatic arthritis	

▷ **Principal Uses**

As a Single Drug Product: Uses currently included in FDA-approved labeling: Combination treatment of (1) acute lymphocytic leukemia; (2) acute non-lymphocytic leukemia.

Other (unlabeled) generally accepted uses: Treatment of (1) inflammatory bowel diseases (Crohn's disease and ulcerative colitis); (2) certain cases of severe psoriatic arthritis; (3) may help in cases of autoimmune hepatitis.

How This Drug Works: This drug interferes with specific stages of cell reproduction (tissue growth) by inhibiting the formation of DNA and RNA.

Available Dose Forms and Strengths

Tablets — 50 mg

▷ **Recommended Dose Ranges** (Actual dose and schedule must be determined for each patient individually.)

Infants and Children: For leukemia: 2.5 mg per kg of body mass (to the nearest 25 mg) daily (roughly 50 mg for the average 5-year-old), in single or divided doses. If the platelets and white blood cell counts do not fall, and clinical improvement is not acceptable after 4 weeks of the induction dosing, the dose may be increased to 5 mg per kg of body mass per day. If there is still no re sponse, some centers give mercaptopurine at 75 mg per square meter on days 29–42. This is combined with vincristine, prednisone, and methotrexate. Maintenance therapy then occurs as in adult dosing.

12 to 60 Years of Age: For leukemia: Induction—initially 2.5 mg per kg of body mass (to the nearest 25 mg) daily, in single or divided doses, for 4 weeks. If the white blood cell or platelet counts do not fall and there is no clinical improvement, the dose may be increased as needed and tolerated to 5 mg per kg of body mass daily. For maintenance, 1.5 to 2.5 mg per kg of body mass daily.

For inflammatory bowel disease: 1.5 mg per kg of body mass daily. The dose is subsequently adjusted to keep the platelet count above 100,000 and the white blood cell count above 4,500.

Over 60 Years of Age: Same as 12 to 60 years of age.

Conditions Requiring Dosing Adjustments

Liver Function: Used with caution and in decreased doses by patients with liver compromise. It is also a rare cause of liver toxicity.

Kidney Function: Dose should be decreased in kidney (renal) compromise. It is a rare cause of drug crystals in urine.

TPMT Negatives: Some patients do not have an enzyme called thiopurine methyltransferase (TPMT). The mercaptopurine dose is decreased by 10% for these patients.

▷ **Dosing Instructions:**   The tablet may be crushed and taken with or following food to reduce stomach upset.

Usual Duration of Use: Use on a regular schedule for 4 to 6 weeks determines effectiveness in inducing remission in leukemia; continual use for 2 to 3 months determines benefit in treating inflammatory bowel disease. Long-term use (months to years) requires periodic physician evaluation.

▷ **This Drug Should Not Be Taken If**

- you have had an allergic reaction to it previously.
- you have a solid tumor or lymphoma (this drug is **not** indicated).
- you have leukemia that has spread to the central nervous system.
- you are pregnant. (Ask your physician for guidance.)

▷ **Inform Your Physician Before Taking This Drug If**
- you have a history of drug-induced bone marrow depression.
- you have impaired liver or kidney function.
- you are not using any contraception.
- you have gout.
- you are taking allopurinol (the mercaptopurine dose must be reduced).
- you have inflammatory bowel disease.
- you do not understand the steps needed to dispose of any vomit or urine.
- you have been exposed recently to chicken pox or herpes zoster (shingles).
- you are taking any of the following drugs: allopurinol, probenecid, sulfin-pyrazone, anticoagulants, immunosuppressants.

Possible Side Effects (natural, expected, and unavoidable drug actions)
Bone marrow depression (see Glossary). Abnormally increased blood uric acid levels; possible urate kidney stones, hyperpigmentation of the skin. Possible drug fever.

▷ **Possible Adverse Effects** (unusual, unexpected, and infrequent reactions)
If any of the following develop, consult your physician promptly for guidance.
Mild Adverse Effects
Allergic reactions: skin rash, itching, joint pain—case reports.
Headache, weakness—infrequent.
Loss of appetite, mouth and lip sores, nausea, vomiting, diarrhea—infrequent.
Serious Adverse Effects
Liver damage with jaundice (see Glossary)—infrequent.
Kidney damage: fever, cloudy or bloody urine—rare.
Pancreatitis (especially in patients taking this medicine for inflammatory bowel disease)—infrequent.
Gastrointestinal ulceration: stomach pain, bloody or black stools.
Increased cancer risk (carcinogen): one case report of cancer in a patient with bowel disease—possible.

▷ **Possible Effects on Sexual Function:**   Suppression of sperm production.
Cessation of menstruation—case reports.

Possible Delayed Adverse Effects: Bone marrow depression may not be apparent during early treatment.

▷ **Adverse Effects That May Mimic Natural Diseases or Disorders**
Drug-induced liver damage may suggest viral hepatitis.

Natural Diseases or Disorders That May Be Activated by This Drug
Latent gout, peptic ulcer disease, inflammatory bowel disease.

Possible Effects on Laboratory Tests
Complete blood cell counts: decreased red cells, hemoglobin, white cells, and platelets.
Blood glucose levels: falsely increased with SMA testing.
Blood uric acid levels: increased.
Liver function tests: increased enzymes (ALT/GPT, AST/GOT, and alkaline phosphatase) or bilirubin.
Kidney function tests: increased blood urea nitrogen (BUN) and creatinine.
Sperm counts: decreased.

CAUTION
1. Make sure you get all laboratory tests ordered.
2. Call your doctor at the first sign of infection or abnormal bleeding or bruising.
3. Inform your physician promptly if you become pregnant.
4. It is best to avoid immunizations while taking this drug, and to avoid contact with people who have recently taken oral poliovirus vaccine.

Precautions for Use
By Infants and Children: No specific problems anticipated.
By Those Over 60 Years of Age: Increased risk of bone marrow depression. Periodic blood counts are mandatory.

▷ **Advisability of Use During Pregnancy**
Pregnancy Category: D. See Pregnancy Risk Categories at the back of this book.
Animal studies: Rat studies reveal toxic effects on the embryo.
Human studies: Adequate studies of pregnant women are not available. Known to cause abortions and premature births.
Avoid drug during entire pregnancy if possible. Use a nonhormonal method of contraception.

Advisability of Use If Breast-Feeding
Presence of this drug in breast milk: Unknown.
Avoid drug or refrain from nursing.

Habit-Forming Potential: None.

Effects of Overdose: Headache, dizziness, abdominal pain, nausea.

Possible Effects of Long-Term Use: Development of new malignant diseases.

Suggested Periodic Examinations While Taking This Drug (at physician's discretion)
Complete blood cell counts.
Blood uric acid levels.
Liver and kidney function tests.

▷ **While Taking This Drug, Observe the Following**
Foods: No restrictions.
Beverages: No restrictions. Drink liquids liberally, up to 2 quarts daily.
▷ *Alcohol:* Avoid completely.
Tobacco Smoking: No interactions expected. I advise everyone to quit smoking.
▷ *Other Drugs*
Mercaptopurine may *decrease* the effects of
• warfarin (Coumadin); the INR (prothrombin time or protime) should be checked more frequently.
The following drug may *increase* the effects of mercaptopurine:
• allopurinol (Zyloprim). Doses must be reduced to 33% or even as low as 25% of the usual dose if these two medicines are to be combined.
Mercaptopurine *taken concurrently* with
• amphotericin B (Abelcet) may increase risk of kidney toxicity or spasm of the bronchi.
• methotrexate (Mexate) can result in mercaptopurine toxicity.
• olsalazine (Dipentum) may increase risk of bone marrow depression.
▷ *Driving, Hazardous Activities:* No restrictions.

Aviation Note: The use of this drug **may be a disqualification** for piloting. Consult a designated aviation medical examiner.
Exposure to Sun: No restrictions.
Discontinuation: To be determined by your physician.

MESALAMINE (me SAL a meen)

Other Names: Mesalazine, 5-aminosalicylic acid, 5-ASA

Introduced: 1982   **Class:** Bowel   anti-inflammatory   **Prescription:**
USA: Yes   **Controlled Drug:**   USA: No; Canada: No   **Available as Generic:**
USA: No; Canada: No

Brand Names: Asacol, Pentasa, Rowasa, ✦Salofalk

BENEFITS versus RISKS	
Possible Benefits	*Possible Risks*
EFFECTIVE SUPPRESSION OF INFLAMMATORY BOWEL DISEASE	Allergic reactions: acute intolerance syndrome, drug-induced kidney damage

▷ **Principal Uses**
   As a Single Drug Product: Uses currently included in FDA-approved labeling: Treatment of active mild to moderate ulcerative colitis, proctosigmoiditis, and proctitis.
      Other (unlabeled) generally accepted uses: (1) May help improve semen quality that had been damaged by prior sulfasalazine treatment; (2) can ease canker sores (aphthous ulcers); (3) has a steroid-sparing effect in Crohn's disease; (4) used to maintain remission in ulcerative colitis.

How This Drug Works: Suppresses formation of prostaglandins (and related compounds), chemicals causing inflammation, tissue destruction, and diarrhea, the main problems in ulcerative colitis and proctitis.

Available Dose Forms and Strengths
      Capsules, controlled release — 250 mg
            Rectal suspension — 4 g per 60-ml unit
                  Suppositories — 250 mg (Canada), 500 mg (U.S. and Canada)
      Tablets, delayed release — 250 mg, 400 mg, 500 mg

▷ **Recommended Dose Ranges** (Actual dose and schedule must be determined for each patient individually.)
   Infants and Children: Dose not established.
   12 to 60 Years of Age: Rectal suspension—4 g (as a retention enema) every night for 3 to 6 weeks. Suppositories—500 mg (placed in rectum) two or three times daily. Tablets—400 to 800 mg (one or two tablets by mouth) three times daily for 6 weeks. Daily maximum is 2400 mg.
   Over 60 Years of Age: Same as 12 to 60 years of age.

Conditions Requiring Dosing Adjustments
   Liver Function: Guidelines for dose adjustment not available. Drug changed by the liver and colon wall to Ac-5-ASA.
   Kidney Function: This drug should be used with caution in kidney compromise.

▷ **Dosing Instructions:**   Rectal suspension—use as a retention enema at bedtime.

If possible, empty the rectum before inserting suspension; try to retain the suspension all night.

Tablets—best taken with 8 ounces of water on an empty stomach, 1 hour before or 2 hours after eating. Also may be taken with or following food to reduce stomach upset. Sustained-release tablet should be swallowed whole without alteration.

Usual Duration of Use: Regular use for 1 to 3 weeks determines benefits controlling ulcerative colitis. Long-term use (months to years) requires periodic physician evaluation.

Possible Advantages of This Drug

Does not cause bone marrow or blood cell disorders.

Does not inhibit sperm production or function.

▷ **This Drug Should Not Be Taken If**
- you have had an allergic reaction to it previously.
- you have severely impaired kidney function.
- you have a known sulfite allergy. (Rectal suspension should NOT be used.)
- you have active ulcer disease.

▷ **Inform Your Physician Before Taking This Drug If**
- you are allergic to aspirin (or other salicylates), olsalazine, or sulfasalazine.
- you are allergic by nature: history of hay fever, asthma, hives, eczema.
- you have impaired liver or kidney function.
- you have a history of a blood clotting (coagulation) disorder.
- you have a history of low white blood cell counts.
- you are taking other medicines that effect the bone marrow. Discuss this with your doctor.
- you are currently taking sulfasalazine (Azulfidine).

Possible Side Effects (natural, expected, and unavoidable drug actions)

Anal irritation (with use of rectal suspension or suppositories). Flu-like syndrome with oral mesalamine use.

▷ **Possible Adverse Effects** (unusual, unexpected, and infrequent reactions)

If any of the following develop, consult your physician promptly for guidance.

Mild Adverse Effects

Allergic reactions: skin rash.

Headache (may be dose related), hair loss—rare.

Blurred vision, ringing in the ears—possible.

Paresthesias, neck and joint pain, dizziness, cough—infrequent.

Nausea, stomach pain, excessive gas—infrequent.

Serious Adverse Effects

Allergic reactions: acute intolerance syndrome: fever, skin rash, severe headache, severe stomach pain, bloody diarrhea.

Kidney damage (nephrosis, interstitial nephritis)—rare.

Peripheral neuropathy—rare.

Pancreatitis, peptic ulcers, or hepatitis—rare.

Low white blood cell or platelet counts or anemia—rare.

Myocarditis, pericarditis, pericardial effusions—case reports.

▷ **Possible Effects on Sexual Function:**   Oligospermia and infertility has been reported with other forms of mesalamine, but NOT with the oral form.

Possible Effects on Laboratory Tests
Increased liver function tests.

CAUTION
1. Report promptly any signs of acute intolerance syndrome. Stop taking drug.
2. Shake the rectal suspension thoroughly before administering.
3. This medicine is a salicylate and as such is a cousin of aspirin. Avoid taking this medicine in combination with other medicines or during other conditions in which aspirin is contraindicated.

Precautions for Use
By Infants and Children: Safety and effectiveness by those under 12 years of age are not established.
By Those Over 60 Years of Age: None.

▷ **Advisability of Use During Pregnancy**
Pregnancy Category: B. See Pregnancy Risk Categories at the back of this book.
Animal studies: No drug-induced birth defects found in rat or rabbit studies.
Human studies: Adequate studies of pregnant women are not available.
Use this drug only if clearly needed. Ask your physician for guidance.

Advisability of Use If Breast-Feeding
Presence of this drug in breast milk: Yes.
Avoid drug or refrain from nursing.

Habit-Forming Potential: None.

Effects of Overdose: Headache, dizziness, nausea, vomiting, abdominal cramping.

Possible Effects of Long-Term Use: None reported.

Suggested Periodic Examinations While Taking This Drug (at physician's discretion)
Kidney function tests, urinalysis.

▷ **While Taking This Drug, Observe the Following**
Foods: Decreased mesalamine levels. Follow prescribed diet.
Beverages: No restrictions. May be taken with milk.
▷ *Alcohol:* No interactions expected.
Tobacco Smoking: No interactions expected. I advise everyone to quit smoking.
▷ *Other Drugs:*
Mercaptopurine *taken concurrently* with
- alendronate (Fosamax) may increase stomach or intestinal upset risks (because of salicylate).
- enoxaparin (Lovenox) may increase risk of hemorrhage.
- varicella vaccine (Varivax) may result in Reye syndrome. Avoid taking this medicine for 6 weeks following varicella vaccine.
▷ *Driving, Hazardous Activities:* No restrictions.
Aviation Note: The use of this drug *is probably not a disqualification* for piloting. Consult a designated aviation medical examiner.
Exposure to Sun: No restrictions.

METAPROTERENOL (met a proh TER e nohl)

Other Name: Orciprenaline

Introduced: 1964 **Class:** Antiasthmatic, bronchodilator **Prescription:**
USA: Yes **Controlled Drug:** USA: No; Canada: No **Available as Generic:**
Yes

Brand Names: Alupent, Arm-a-Med, Dey-Dose, Dey-Lute, Metaprel, Metaprel
nasal inhaler, Prometa

BENEFITS versus RISKS	
Possible Benefits	*Possible Risks*
VERY EFFECTIVE RELIEF OF BRONCHOSPASM	Increased blood pressure
	Fine hand tremor
	Fast heart rate
	Irregular heart rhythm (with excessive use)

▷ **Principal Uses**

As a Single Drug Product: Uses currently included in FDA-approved labeling: (1)
Relieves acute bronchial asthma and reduces the frequency and severity of
chronic, recurrent asthmatic attacks; (2) used to relieve reversible bronchospasm associated with chronic bronchitis and emphysema; (3) eases
symptoms in obstructive bronchial disease.

Other (unlabeled) generally accepted uses: Has been used in threatened abortion.

How This Drug Works: Dilates those bronchial tubes that are in sustained constriction, increasing the size of airways and improving breathing.

Available Dose Forms and Strengths

Nasal inhaler — 0.65 mg per metered dose
Oral suspension — 10 mg/5 ml
Powder for inhalation — 0.65 mg per inhalation
Solution for nebulizer — 0.4%, 0.6%, 5%
Syrup — 10 mg/5 ml
Tablets — 10 mg, 20 mg

▷ **Usual Adult Dose Range:** Inhaler: two or three inhalations as often as every 3
to 4 hours; do not exceed 12 inhalations daily.

Hand nebulizer: 5 to 15 inhalations every 4 hours; do not exceed 40 inhalations daily.

Syrup and tablets: 20 mg up to every 6 to 8 hours.

**Note: Actual dose and schedule must be determined for each patient in-
dividually.**

Conditions Requiring Dosing Adjustments

Liver Function: Specific guidelines for dosing adjustment for patients with liver
compromise are not usually indicated.

Kidney Function: Dosing changes are not indicated in kidney compromise.

▷ **Dosing Instructions:** May be taken on empty stomach or with food or milk.
Tablets should not be crushed. For aerosol and nebulizer, follow the written
instructions carefully. Do not overuse. If symptoms not controlled with
most frequent dosing, call your doctor.

Usual Duration of Use: According to individual requirements. Do not use beyond the time necessary to stop episodes of asthma.

▷ **This Drug Should Not Be Taken If**
- you had an allergic reaction to it previously.
- you currently have an irregular heart rhythm.
- you are taking, or have taken within the past 2 weeks, any monoamine oxidase (MAO) type A inhibitor drug (see Drug Classes).

▷ **Inform Your Physician Before Taking This Drug If**
- you are overly sensitive to other sympathetic stimulant drugs.
- you currently use epinephrine (Adrenalin, Primatene Mist, etc.) to relieve asthmatic breathing.
- you have any type of heart or circulatory disorder, especially high blood pressure or coronary heart disease.
- you have diabetes or an overactive thyroid gland (hyperthyroidism).
- you are taking any form of digitalis or any stimulant drug.

Possible Side Effects (natural, expected, and unavoidable drug actions)
Aerosol—dryness or irritation of mouth or throat, altered taste.
Tablet—nervousness, palpitation.

▷ **Possible Adverse Effects** (unusual, unexpected, and infrequent reactions)
If any of the following develop, consult your physician promptly for guidance.
Mild Adverse Effects
Headache, dizziness, restlessness, insomnia, fine tremor of hands—possible, infrequent.
Increased sweating; muscle cramps in arms and legs—case reports.
Nausea, heartburn, vomiting—possible.
Serious Adverse Effects
Rapid or irregular heart rhythm, intensification of angina, increased blood pressure—possible.
Hallucinations and psychosis—rare.
Paradoxical spasm of the bronchi (bronchospasm)—rare.

▷ **Possible Effects on Sexual Function:**   None reported.

Natural Diseases or Disorders That May Be Activated By This Drug   Latent coronary artery disease, diabetes, high blood pressure.

Possible Effects on Laboratory Tests
Urine sugar tests: positive (unreliable results with Benedict's solution).

CAUTION
1. Combined use of this drug by aerosol inhalation with beclomethasone aerosol (Beclovent, Vanceril) may increase the risk of toxicity due to fluorocarbon propellants. Use this aerosol 20 to 30 minutes *before* beclomethasone aerosol, as this will reduce the risk of toxicity and enhance the penetration of beclomethasone.
2. *Avoid excessive use of aerosol inhalation.* Excessive or prolonged use of this drug by inhalation can reduce its effectiveness and cause serious heart rhythm disturbances, including cardiac arrest.
3. Do not combine this drug with epinephrine. These two drugs may be used alternately if an interval of 4 hours is allowed between doses.
4. If you do not respond to your usually effective dose, ask your doctor for

help. Do not increase the size or frequency of the dose without your physician's approval.

Precautions for Use

By Infants and Children: Safety and effectiveness of the aerosol and nebulized solution are not established for children under 12 years of age. Oral dosing in children less than 6 years old: 1.3 to 2.6 mg per kg of body mass per day, divided into equal doses and given three to four times a day. In children 6 to 9 years old or less than 60 pounds: 10 mg per dose three to four times a day. Children more than 9 years old or over 60 pounds are given 20 mg three or four times a day.

Safety and effectiveness of the syrup and tablet are not established for children under 6 years of age.

By Those Over 60 Years of Age: Avoid excessive and continual use. If acute asthma is not relieved promptly, other drugs will have to be tried. Watch for nervousness, palpitations, irregular heart rhythm, and muscle tremors. Use with extreme caution if you have hardening of the arteries, heart disease, or high blood pressure.

▷ **Advisability of Use During Pregnancy**

Pregnancy Category: C. See Pregnancy Risk Categories at the back of this book.

Animal studies: Significant birth defects reported in rabbit studies.

Human studies: Adequate studies of pregnant women are not available.

Avoid use during first 3 months. Use during the final 6 months only if clearly needed.

Advisability of Use If Breast-Feeding

Presence of this drug in breast milk: Unknown.

Avoid drug or refrain from nursing.

Habit-Forming Potential: None.

Effects of Overdose: Nervousness, palpitation, rapid heart rate, sweating, headache, tremor, vomiting, chest pain.

Possible Effects of Long-Term Use: Loss of effectiveness. See "CAUTION" above.

Suggested Periodic Examinations While Taking This Drug (at physician's discretion)

Blood pressure measurements, evaluation of heart status.

▷ **While Taking This Drug, Observe the Following**

Foods: No restrictions.

Beverages: Avoid excessive use of caffeine-containing beverages: coffee, tea, cola, chocolate.

▷ *Alcohol:* No interactions expected.

Tobacco Smoking: No interactions expected. I advise everyone to quit smoking.

▷ *Other Drugs*

Metaproterenol *taken concurrently* with

- albuterol (Proventil, others) may result in increased heart (cardiovascular) side effects.
- monoamine oxidase (MAO) type A inhibitor drugs (see Glossary) may cause excessive increase in blood pressure and undesirable heart stimulation.
- phenothiazines (see Drug Classes) may blunt the central effects of this medicine.

▷ *Driving, Hazardous Activities:* Usually no restrictions. Use caution if excessive nervousness or dizziness occurs.

Aviation Note: The use of this drug *is a disqualification* for piloting. Consult a designated aviation medical examiner.

Exposure to Sun: No restrictions.

Heavy Exercise or Exertion: Use caution. Excessive exercise can induce asthma in sensitive individuals.

METFORMIN (met FOR min)

Introduced: 1995   **Class:** Antidiabetic drug, oral; biguanide   **Prescription:** USA: Yes   **Controlled Drug:** USA: No; Canada: No   **Available as Generic:** USA: No; Canada: No

Brand Name: Glucophage

Warning: Avoid excessive alcohol. Alcohol can cause lactic acidosis, a condition that metformin can also rarely cause. All oral hypoglycemic agents may carry the risk of increased cardiovascular death, based on a 1975 study of tolbutamide and phenformin.

BENEFITS versus RISKS	
Possible Benefits	*Possible Risks*
EFFECTIVE GLUCOSE CONTROL WITHOUT INSULIN INJECTIONS	LACTIC ACIDOSIS Possible anemia with long-term use
MAY BE USED CONCURRENTLY WITH A SULFONYLUREA	
DOES NOT LEAD TO WEIGHT GAIN	
TAKEN BY MOUTH, VERSUS INJECTION OF INSULIN	
Usually avoids excessive lowering of blood sugar	
Favorable effects on lipids	

▷ **Principal Uses**

As a Single Drug Product: Uses currently included in FDA-approved labeling: (1) Used in combination with diet restrictions to treat non-insulin-dependent diabetes (type 2); (2) can be combined with a sulfonylurea (see Drug Classes) for patients who do not have an adequate response to diet restrictions plus a sulfonylurea.

Other (unlabeled) generally accepted uses: (1) May be used as a single-agent therapy to overcome insulin resistance; (2) could help nondiabetic, obese women with high blood pressure in helping improve blood pressure and lipid profile; (3) may help insulin-dependent (type 1) diabetics decrease insulin requirements.

How This Drug Works: Decreases sugar (glucose) production in the liver. It also increases sensitivity of the body to insulin.

Available Dose Forms and Strengths

Tablets — 500 mg, 850 mg

▷ **Recommended Dose Ranges** (Actual dose and schedule must be determined for each patient individually.)

Infants and Children: Not approved for use in this population.

12 to 60 Years of Age: Dosing is started at 500 mg twice daily. It is best to take this medicine with the morning and evening meal. Typical effective doses are 850 mg twice daily. Maximum dose is 850 mg three times daily.

Over 60 Years of Age: Some patients may have acceptable blood sugar control with as little as 500 mg daily. If this dose is used, take it with the morning meal. Dose may be slowly increased if needed.

Conditions Requiring Dosing Adjustments

Liver Function: This drug should **not** be used by patients with liver compromise. This is a risk factor for lactic acidosis.

Kidney Function: This drug should **not** be used by patients who have kidney problems (renal dysfunction), defined as females with steady-state creatinine levels greater than 1.4 or males with steady-state creatinine levels greater than 1.5.

▷ **Dosing Instructions:** This drug should be taken with morning and evening meals if it has been prescribed on a twice-daily basis.

Usual Duration of Use: Continual use on a regular schedule for a week is usually necessary to determine this drug's effectiveness in establishing tight glucose control. A month of continuous use will be needed before an effect on glycosylated hemoglobin (a measure of past success of glucose control) is seen. Long-term use (months to years) requires periodic evaluation of response and dose adjustment. Consult your physician on a regular basis.

Possible Advantages of This Drug

Does not lead to weight gain.

Can be used (because of its mechanism of action) in combination with a sulfonylurea.

Can be used to overcome insulin resistance.

Does not cause excessive lowering of blood sugar (hypoglycemia) when used as a monotherapy.

Currently a "Drug of Choice"

For treatment of hyperglycemia in the elderly.

▷ **This Drug Should Not Be Taken If**
- you had an allergic reaction to it previously.
- you have impaired kidneys (serum creatinine greater than 1.4 for females or 1.5 for males).
- you have liver disease.
- you have a serious infection (increases risk of lactic acidosis).
- you are an alcoholic.
- you have a heart or lung insufficiency (increased lactic acidosis risk).
- you are going to have a radiology test that uses iodinated contrast media (ask your doctor).
- you have chronic metabolic acidosis or ketoacidosis.
- you are breast-feeding your infant.

▷ **Inform Your Physician Before Taking This Drug If**
- you are planning to have surgery soon.
- you have a history of megaloblastic anemia.
- you have seen another doctor and ketoacidosis was diagnosed.
- you are unsure how much to take or how often to take it.

Possible Side Effects (natural, expected, and unavoidable drug actions)
Lactic acidosis—rare. Low blood sugar (hypoglycemia) if meals are skipped or if you exercise strenuously without eating.

▷ **Possible Adverse Effects** (unusual, unexpected, and infrequent reactions)
If any of the following develop, consult your physician promptly for guidance.
Mild Adverse Effects
Allergic reactions: rash.
Metallic taste—case reports.
Anorexia, nausea, vomiting, or diarrhea—up to 30% when started, then they often subside.
Headache, nervousness, dizziness, or tiredness—infrequent.
Serious Adverse Effects
Allergic reactions: not reported.
Idiosyncratic reactions: none reported.
Lactic acidosis—rare.
Lowered vitamin B_{12} levels and resultant anemia (megaloblastic)—rare.
Drug-induced porphyria—case reports.
All oral hypoglycemic agents carry a label indicating that they may increase risk of cardiovascular death (based on a 1975 study of tolbutamide and phenformin)—possible.

▷ **Possible Effects on Sexual Function:**   None reported.

Possible Delayed Adverse Effects: Low vitamin B_{12} levels and anemia (megaloblastic).

▷ **Adverse Effects That May Mimic Natural Diseases or Disorders**
Acidosis may mimic ketoacidosis, which is seen in diabetics.

Natural Diseases or Disorders That May Be Activated by This Drug
None reported.

Possible Effects on Laboratory Tests
Blood glucose: decreased.

CAUTION
1. This drug may cause lactic acidosis. Ask your doctor for signs or symptoms that may occur.
2. Drugs in this class (phenformin) or tolbutamide were reported to increase risk of cardiovascular death. Although there is no data to support that effect for this medicine, patients should be closely followed.

Precautions for Use
By Infants and Children: Safety and effectiveness for use by those under 18 years of age have not been established.
By Those Over 60 Years of Age: Smaller starting doses (500 mg daily) are indicated. People in this age group tend to have an age-related decline in kidney function as well as a more compromised ability to tolerate lower blood sugar levels.

▷ **Advisability of Use During Pregnancy**
Pregnancy Category: B. See Pregnancy Risk Categories at the back of this book.
Animal studies: No birth defects in rats at two times the typical human dose.
Human studies: Information from adequate studies of pregnant women is not available. The manufacturer does not recommend the use of this drug

in pregnancy. Insulin is still considered the drug of choice to control blood sugar in pregnancy.

Advisability of Use If Breast-Feeding

Presence of this drug in breast milk: Yes.

Avoid drug or refrain from nursing.

Habit-Forming Potential: None.

Effects of Overdose: Nausea and vomiting, pulmonary edema, hemorrhage from the stomach, lactic acidosis, seizures, intractable lowering of the blood pressure, coma.

Possible Effects of Long-Term Use: Lowering of vitamin B_{12} and resultant anemia (megaloblastic). Possible malabsorption of folic acid and amino acids.

Suggested Periodic Examinations While Taking This Drug (at physician's discretion)

Vitamin B_{12} levels, tests of kidney and liver function.

▷ **While Taking This Drug, Observe the Following**

Foods: No restrictions.

Nutritional Support: Diet as prescribed by your doctor.

Beverages: No restrictions.

▷ *Alcohol:* Use with extreme caution. Alcohol worsens the effect of metformin on lactate. Avoid alcohol in excessive amounts.

Tobacco Smoking: No interactions expected, but I advise everyone to quit smoking.

Marijuana Smoking: May worsen dizziness.

▷ *Other Drugs*

Metformin may *increase* the effects of

• insulin in the sense that the lowering of blood sugar will be increased. This may be used to therapeutic advantage in some insulin-dependent diabetics.

Metformin *taken concurrently* with

• ACE inhibitors (see Drug Classes) may increase lowering of blood sugar to an undesirable extent.

• beta-blockers (see Drug Classes) may slow recovery from any hypoglycemia that occurs and can also block symptoms of low blood sugar.

• contrast media for certain X-ray studies may increase risk of lactic acidosis. Metformin should not be combined with these agents. Some clinicians substitute a different agent to control blood sugar, stop the metformin 48 hours before the X ray, then stop the substituted agent and restart metformin once kidney function is tested and found to be normal.

• digoxin (Lanoxin, others) may pose a problem because it is a cationic drug and may lead to excess metformin levels.

• itraconazole or other azole antifungal agents can result in severe lowering of the blood sugar.

• procainamide (Pronestyl) may lead to toxicity.

• quinidine (Quinaglute) may lead to toxicity.

• thyroid hormones (see Drug Classes) can result in blunting of metformin's therapeutic effect.

The following drugs may *increase* the effects of metformin:

• cimetidine (Tagamet)—may result in toxicity.

• morphine (various)—may lead to toxicity.

• nifedipine (Adalat)—may lead to toxicity.

- oral antidiabetic drugs (see Drug Classes). This effect may be used to therapeutic advantage.
- ranitidine (Zantac)—may lead to toxicity.
- trimethoprim (Septra)—may lead to toxicity.
- vancomycin (Vancoled)—may lead to toxicity.

▷ *Driving, Hazardous Activities:* This drug may cause drowsiness or dizziness. Restrict activities as necessary.

Aviation Note: Diabetes *is a disqualification* for piloting. Consult a designated aviation medical examiner.

Exposure to Sun: Use caution. Some medicines that are similar in chemical structure can cause increased sensitivity to the sun.

Heavy Exercise or Exertion: Heavy exercise will tend to use up sugar faster than usual. This drug will have an effect on lowering the blood sugar. Be alert to the symptoms of low blood sugar.

Occurrence of Unrelated Illness: Infections or other illness may still require use of insulin to achieve acceptable blood sugar control.

Discontinuation: Periodic physician evaluations of the continued benefit of this medicine are needed.

METHOTREXATE (meth oh TREX ayt)

Other Names: Amethopterin, MTX

Introduced: 1948   **Class:** Anticancer drug, anti-psoriatic drug   **Prescription:** USA: Yes   **Controlled Drug:** USA: No; Canada: No   **Available as Generic:** Yes

Brand Names: Abitrexate, Folex, Folex PFS, Mexate, Mexate AQ, Rheumatrex Dose Pack

BENEFITS versus RISKS	
Possible Benefits	*Possible Risks*
EFFECTIVE TREATMENT OF SOME CASES OF SEVERE DISABLING PSORIASIS	GASTROINTESTINAL ULCERATION AND BLEEDING
EFFECTIVE TREATMENT OF CERTAIN ADULT AND CHILDHOOD CANCERS	MOUTH AND THROAT ULCERATION
PREVENTION OF REJECTION OF BONE MARROW TRANSPLANTS	SEVERE BONE MARROW DEPRESSION
USEFUL IN RHEUMATOID ARTHRITIS and related disorders	DAMAGE TO LUNGS, LIVER, OR KIDNEYS
	Loss of hair

▷ **Principal Uses**

As a Single Drug Product: Uses currently included in FDA-approved labeling: (1) Combination therapy of acute lymphocytic leukemia; (2) combination therapy of various types of adult and childhood cancer; (3) severe and widespread forms of disabling psoriasis that have failed to respond to all standard treatment procedures; (4) various types of both adult and childhood cancer; (5) used to prevent rejection of transplanted bone marrow; (6) used in the treatment of connective tissue disorders such as rheumatoid arthritis and related conditions. Its use in rheumatoid arthritis is restricted to the treatment of selected adults with severe active disease that has failed to respond to conventional therapy.

Other (unlabeled) generally accepted uses: (1) Used in a variety of neoplastic syndromes in combination therapy; (2) may have a role in helping decrease steroid use in steroid-dependent asthma; (3) helps lessen neutropenia in Felty's syndrome; (4) used in combination with misoprostol to cause abortion; (5) can be of help in chronic granulomatous hepatitis of unknown cause (idiopathic).

How This Drug Works: Blocks normal use of folic acid in cell reproduction, and slowsabnormally rapid tissue growth (as in psoriasis and cancer).

Available Dose Forms and Strengths

Injections — 2.5 mg/ml, 10 mg/ml, 25 mg/ml

Powder, intrathecal cryodessicated — 20 mg, 50 mg, 100 mg

Injections, preservative free — 25 mg/ml, 50 mg/ml, 100 mg/ml, 250 mg/ml

Tablets — 2.5 mg

▷ **Usual Adult Dose Range**

For psoriasis (alternate schedules): (1) 10 to 50 mg once a week; (2) 2.5 to 5 mg every 12 hours for three doses, or every 8 hours for four doses, once a week, up to a maximum of 30 mg/week; (3) 2.5 mg/day for 5 days, followed by 2 days without drug, with gradual increase in dose to a maximum of 6.25 mg/day.

For rheumatoid arthritis (alternate schedules): (1) single oral dose of 7.5 mg once weekly; (2) divided doses of 2.5 mg every 12 hours for three doses per week. Dose may be increased gradually as needed and tolerated. Do not exceed a weekly dose of 20 mg.

For acute lymphocytic leukemia (ALL): Induction: 3.3 mg per square meter in combination with corticosteroid treatment is usually taken daily for 4 to 6 weeks. Maintenance: a total weekly dose of 30 mg per square meter is given as two divided oral or intramuscular injections. Some centers also use 2.5 mg per kg of body mass intravenously every 14 days.

Note: Actual dose and schedule determined for each patient individually.

Conditions Requiring Dosing Adjustments

Liver Function: Used with caution and in decreased dose in liver disease. Some clinicians use laboratory tests as a guide; For example, when dose is due, if bilirubin is less than 3 mg % and AST (SGOT) is less than 180 IU, 100% of the scheduled dose can be given. If bilirubin is greater than 5 mg %, dose SHOULD NOT be given.

Kidney Function: Methotrexate is a benefit-to-risk decision. Increased adverse effects are possible with damaged kidneys. DO **not** take with severe kidney failure (creatinine clearance less than 10 ml/min). For moderate failure, 50% of the usual dose should be taken in the usual dosing interval.

▷ **Dosing Instructions:**   The tablet may be crushed and taken with food to reduce stomach irritation. Drink at least 2 to 3 quarts of liquids daily. Many clinicians who give methotrexate to their patients to treat rheumatoid arthritis also give folic acid in order to minimize methotrexate toxicity.

Usual Duration of Use: Use on a regular schedule for several weeks determines benefit in reducing the severity and extent of psoriasis. Response in rheumatoid arthritis usually begins after 3 to 6 weeks of treatment. Dose should be reduced to smallest amount that will maintain acceptable improvement. Long-term use (months to years) requires physician supervision.

▷ **This Drug Should Not Be Taken If**
- you have had an allergic reaction to it previously.
- you currently have, or have had a recent exposure to, either chicken pox or shingles (herpes zoster).
- you are pregnant or planning a pregnancy in the near future, and you are taking this drug to treat psoriasis or rheumatoid arthritis.
- you are breast-feeding your infant.
- you have alcoholic liver disease.
- you have an immune deficiency.
- you have fluid in the pleura of the lung (pleural effusions).
- you have active liver disease, peptic ulcer, regional enteritis, or ulcerative colitis.
- your white blood cell count is less than 3,000 or your platelet count is less than 100,000.
- you are making very small amounts of urine or your creatinine clearance (see Glossary) is less than 40 ml/min.
- you currently have a blood cell or bone marrow disorder.

▷ **Inform Your Physician Before Taking This Drug If**
- you have a chronic infection of any kind.
- you do not understand how to handle vomit or urine while taking chemotherapy.
- you have impaired liver or kidney function.
- you have a history of bone marrow impairment of any kind, especially drug-induced bone marrow depression.
- you are dehydrated.
- you have a history of gout, peptic ulcer disease, regional enteritis, or ulcerative colitis.

Possible Side Effects (natural, expected, and unavoidable drug actions)
The following are due to the pharmacological actions of this drug. **Report such developments to your physician promptly.**
Sores on the lips or in the mouth or throat; vomiting; intestinal cramping; diarrhea (may be bloody); painful urination; bloody urine. Reduced resistance to infection, fatigue, weakness, fever, abnormal bleeding or bruising (bone marrow depression).

▷ **Possible Adverse Effects** (unusual, unexpected, and infrequent reactions)
If any of the following develop, consult your physician promptly for guidance.
Mild Adverse Effects
Allergic reactions: skin rash, hives, itching.
Headache, drowsiness, blurred vision, conjunctivitis—infrequent.
Loss of appetite, nausea, vomiting—infrequent to frequent.
Muscle pain—rare.
Loss of hair, loss of skin pigmentation, acne—infrequent.
Impaired sense of smell or taste—possible.

Serious Adverse Effects

Allergic reactions: drug-induced pneumonia (cough, chest pain, shortness of breath); anaphylaxis.

Nervous system toxicity: speech disturbances, paralysis, seizures—infrequent.

Liver toxicity with jaundice (see Glossary)—case reports.

Kidney toxicity: reduced urine volume, kidney failure—more likely with higher doses.

Colitis or toxic megacolon—case report.

Tumor lysis syndrome: uric acid nephropathy; very low potassium, magnesium, and calcium—possible.

Fluid buildup in the lung pleura (pleural effusion)—possible.

Immune suppression and subsequent infection with *Pneumocystis carinii* pneumonia—possible.

Severe skin reactions (toxic epidermal necrolysis)—case reports.

Chromosomal damage (from occupational exposure)—possible.

▷ **Possible Effects on Sexual Function:** Altered timing and pattern of menstruation. Swelling and tenderness of the male breast tissue (gynecomastia)—case reports.

Possible Delayed Adverse Effects: Some reports suggest that methotrexate therapy may contribute to the later development of secondary cancers. Other studies have not confirmed this.

Possible Effects on Laboratory Tests

Complete blood cell counts: decreased red cells, hemoglobin, white cells, and platelets.

Blood uric acid level: increased.

Liver function tests: increased liver enzymes (ALT/GPT, AST/GOT, and alkaline phosphatase) or bilirubin.

Kidney function tests: increased blood urea nitrogen (BUN) level; increased urine creatinine.

Fecal occult blood test: positive.

Sperm count: decreased.

CAUTION

1. This drug must be monitored carefully by a qualified physician. Request the Patient Package Insert (Rheumatrex Dose Pack) and read it thoroughly.
2. When methotrexate is used to treat rheumatoid arthritis, folic acid can minimize toxicity.
3. Appropriate laboratory examinations, performed before and during the use of this drug, are mandatory.
4. Women with potential for pregnancy should have a pregnancy test before taking this drug and should use an effective form of contraception during its use and for 8 weeks following its discontinuation.
5. Live-virus vaccines should be avoided during use of this drug. Live-virus vaccines could actually produce infection rather than stimulate an immune response.

Precautions for Use

By Those Over 60 Years of Age: Careful evaluation of kidney function should be made before starting treatment and during the entire course of therapy.

▷ **Advisability of Use During Pregnancy**

Pregnancy Category: X. See Pregnancy Risk Categories at the back of this book.

Animal studies: Skull and facial defects reported in mice.

Human studies: This drug is known to cause fetal deaths and birth defects. Its use during pregnancy to treat psoriasis or rheumatoid arthritis cannot be justified.

Advisability of Use If Breast-Feeding

Presence of this drug in breast milk: Yes.

Avoid drug or refrain from nursing.

Habit-Forming Potential: None.

Effects of Overdose: The side effects and adverse effects listed above develop earlier and with greater severity.

Possible Effects of Long-Term Use: Liver compromise (fibrosis and cirrhosis) occurs in 3–5% of long-term users (35 to 49 months).

Suggested Periodic Examinations While Taking This Drug (at physician's discretion)

Complete blood cell counts, liver and kidney function tests, blood uric acid levels, chest X-ray examinations.

▷ **While Taking This Drug, Observe the Following**

Foods: Avoid highly seasoned foods that could be irritating. Between courses of treatment, eat liberally of the following foods: beef, chicken, lamb and pork liver, asparagus, navy beans, kale, and spinach. Any food will reduce the peak methotrexate level obtained.

Beverages: No restrictions. This drug may be taken with milk.

▷ *Alcohol:* Avoid completely.

Tobacco Smoking: No interactions expected. I advise everyone to quit smoking.

Marijuana Smoking: May cause additional impairment of immunity.

▷ *Other Drugs*

Methotrexate may *decrease* the effects of

• digoxin (Lanoxin).

• phenytoin (Dilantin).

The following drugs may *increase* the effects of methotrexate and enhance its toxicity:

• aspirin and other salicylates.

• NSAIDs (see *nonsteroidal anti-inflammatory drugs* in Drug Classes).

• probenecid (Benemid).

Methotrexate *taken concurrently* with

• bismuth subsalicylate (Pepto-Bismol, others) may result in methotrexate toxicity.

• carbenicillin (Geocillin, others) and other penicillins (see Drug Classes) may lead to methotrexate toxicity.

• cholestyramine (Questran, others) and other cholesterol-lowering resins may result in decreased methotrexate effectiveness.

• cotrimoxazole (Bactrim) may result in lowering of all blood cells (pancytopenia).

• cyclosporine (Sandimmune) can result in increased toxicity from both drugs. This combination should be avoided.

• etretinate (Tegison) results in increased liver toxicity.

• influenzae (flu) vaccine may blunt benefits of the vaccine.

- pneumococcal or smallpox vaccine may result in decreased immune response to the vaccine.
- sulfa drugs such as sulfamethoxazole can result in increased hematological toxicity.
- tamoxifen (Nolvadex) may increase risk of blood clots (thromboembolism)—part of a combination regimen that leads to this.
- thiazide diuretics (see Drug Classes) may increase risk of myelosuppression.
- theophylline (Theo-Dur, others) may result in theophylline toxicity. Decreased theophylline doses may be needed.
- triamterine (Dyazide, others) may increase risk of bone marrow problems (myelosuppression).
- trimethoprim (Septra, others) may increase risk of toxicity.
- yellow fever vaccine can result in blunted response and benefit from the vaccine.

▷ *Driving, Hazardous Activities:* This drug may cause drowsiness, dizziness, or blurred vision. Restrict activities as necessary.

Aviation Note: The use of this drug *is a disqualification* for piloting. Consult a designated aviation medical examiner.

Exposure to Sun: Use caution—this drug can cause photosensitivity. Avoid ultraviolet lamps.

METHYCLOTHIAZIDE (METH i kloh thi a zide)

See the thiazide diuretics profile for further information.

METHYLPHENIDATE (meth il FEN i dayt)

Introduced: 1956   **Class:** Amphetaminelike drug, anti-attention-deficit/-hyperactivity-disorder drug   **Prescription:** USA: Yes   **Controlled Drug:** USA: C-II*; Canada: Yes   **Available as Generic:** USA: Yes; Canada: Yes
Brand Names: ✦PMS-Methylphenidate, Ritalin, Ritalin-SR

BENEFITS versus RISKS	
Possible Benefits	*Possible Risks*
EFFECTIVE CONTROL OF NARCOLEPSY	POTENTIAL FOR SERIOUS PSYCHOLOGICAL DEPENDENCE
USEFUL AS ADJUNCTIVE TREATMENT IN ATTENTION-DEFICIT DISORDERS Adjunctive treatment in ADHD	SUPPRESSION OF GROWTH IN CHILDHOOD (recovers when medicine is stopped)
Useful in treatment of mild to moderate depression	Abnormal behavior
Useful in some cases of emotional withdrawal in the elderly	Rare blood cell disorders

*See schedules of Controlled Drugs at the back of this book.

▷ **Principal Uses**

As a Single Drug Product: Uses currently included in FDA-approved labeling: (1) Treats narcolepsy—recurrent spells of uncontrollable drowsiness and sleep; (2) treats attention-deficit disorders of childhood, formerly known as the hyperactive child syndrome, with minimal brain damage and minimal brain dysfunction.

Other (unlabeled) generally accepted uses: (1) Treats mild to moderate depression; (2) manages apathetic and withdrawal states in the elderly; (3) combination therapy of chronic pain, particularly cancer pain; (4) could have a role in treating autism.

How This Drug Works: Activates the brainstem; improves alertness and concentration.

Increases learning ability and attention span.

Available Dose Forms and Strengths

Tablets — 5 mg, 10 mg, 20 mg
Tablets, prolonged action — 20 mg

▷ **Usual Adult Dose Range:**   Narcolepsy: 10 to 60 mg daily. Divided into equal doses, given two to three times daily. Ideally, given 30 minutes before meals.

Pediatric dosing: Children over 6 years old: 5 mg of regular-release form before breakfast and lunch (twice daily). Dose is increased as needed and tolerated (weekly intervals) to maximum daily dose of 60 mg.

Note: Actual dose and schedule must be determined for each patient individually.

Conditions Requiring Dosing Adjustments

Liver Function: Used with caution and in decreased dose in liver disease.

Kidney Function: No changes currently thought to be needed.

▷ **Dosing Instructions:**   The regular tablet may be crushed and taken 30 to 45 minutes before meals. The prolonged-action tablet should be taken whole, not crushed.

Usual Duration of Use: Regular use for 3 to 4 weeks determines benefits in easing the symptoms of narcolepsy or improving behavior of attention-deficit children. If there is no improvement after this time, the drug should be stopped. Long-term use (months to years) requires supervision by your doctor.

▷ **This Drug Should Not Be Taken If**
   • you have had an allergic reaction to it previously.
   • you have glaucoma (inadequately treated).
   • you have Tourette's syndrome.
   • you are experiencing a period of severe anxiety, nervous tension, or emotional depression.

▷ **Inform Your Physician Before Taking This Drug If**
   • you have a history of mental illness.
   • you have a seizure disorder.
   • you have a history of abnormal heart beats.
   • you have high blood pressure, angina, or epilepsy.
   • you are taking, or took within the past 14 days, a monoamine oxidase (MAO) type A inhibitor (see Drug Classes).

Possible Side Effects (natural, expected, and unavoidable drug actions)
Nervousness, excitement, insomnia.
Reduced appetite.
Growth suppression (stopping the medicine in the summer is used to allow a
growth spurt).
Slight increase in heart rate.

▷ **Possible Adverse Effects** (unusual, unexpected, and infrequent reactions)
**If any of the following develop, consult your physician promptly for
guidance.**
Mild Adverse Effects
Allergic reactions: skin rash, hives, drug fever, joint pains—possible.
Headache, dizziness, rapid and forceful heart palpitations—infrequent.
Nausea, abdominal discomfort—infrequent.
Stuttering and hallucinations—case reports.
Serious Adverse Effects
Allergic reactions: severe skin reactions, extensive bruising (allergic destruc-
tion of platelets)—case reports.
Idiosyncratic reactions: abnormal patterns of behavior.
Porphyria or muscle damage (rhabdomyolysis)—rare.
Liver toxicity—case reports.
Precipitation of Tourette's syndrome—case reports

▷ **Possible Effects on Sexual Function:**   None reported.

Natural Diseases or Disorders That May Be Activated by This Drug   Latent
epilepsy. Increased eye pressure unmasking glaucoma.

Possible Effects on Laboratory Tests
Eosinophils: increased (IV abuse).

CAUTION
1. This drug should be used ONLY AFTER a careful assessment by a qualified specialist is made. True attention deficit disorder requires careful
assessment to differentiate it from behavior problems arising from family tensions or other conditions that do not require Ritalin therapy.
2. Careful dose adjustments on an individual basis are mandatory.
3. Paradoxical reactions (see Glossary) can occur, causing aggravation of
initial symptoms for which this drug was prescribed.

Precautions for Use
By Infants and Children: Safety and effectiveness for those under 6 years of age
are not established. If this drug is not beneficial in managing an attention
deficit disorder after a trial of 1 month, it should be stopped. During long-
term use, monitor the child for normal growth and development.
By Those Over 60 Years of Age: Start with small doses. Those in this group may
be at increased risk for nervousness, agitation, insomnia, high blood pressure, angina, or disturbance of heart rhythm.

▷ **Advisability of Use During Pregnancy**
Pregnancy Category: C. See Pregnancy Risk Categories at the back of this book.
Animal studies: No birth defects found in mouse studies.
Human studies: Adequate studies of pregnant women are not available.
Ask your physician for guidance.

Advisability of Use If Breast-Feeding
Presence of this drug in breast milk: Unknown.
Avoid drug or refrain from nursing.

Habit-Forming Potential: This drug can produce tolerance and cause serious psychological dependence (see Glossary), a potentially dangerous characteristic of amphetamine-like drugs (see Drug Classes).

Effects of Overdose: Headache, vomiting, agitation, tremors, dry mouth, sweating, fever, confusion, hallucinations, seizures, coma.

Possible Effects of Long-Term Use: Suppression of growth (in weight and/or height) occurs. Many patients are taken off the drug during summer vacations.

Suggested Periodic Examinations While Taking This Drug (at physician's discretion)
Complete blood cell counts, blood pressure measurements. Height and weight.

▷ **While Taking This Drug, Observe the Following**
Foods: Avoid foods rich in tyramine (see Glossary); this drug in combination with tyramine may cause an excessive rise in blood pressure.
Beverages: Avoid beverages prepared from meat or meat extracts. This drug may be taken with milk.
▷ *Alcohol:* Avoid beer, Chianti wines, and vermouth (may have high tyramine contents).
Tobacco Smoking: No interactions expected. I advise everyone to quit smoking.
▷ *Other Drugs*
Methylphenidate may *increase* the effects of
- tricyclic antidepressants (see Drug Classes), and enhance their toxic effects.
Methylphenidate may *decrease* the effects of
- guanethidine (Ismelin), and impair its ability to lower blood pressure.
Methylphenidate *taken concurrently* with
- anticonvulsants may cause a significant change in the pattern of epileptic seizures; dose adjustments may be necessary for proper control.
- monoamine oxidase (MAO) type A inhibitor drugs (see Drug Classes) may cause a significant rise in blood pressure. Avoid the concurrent use of these drugs.
- morphine may be used to great therapeutic benefit to increase alertness, especially if high doses of morphine must be used.
- tricyclic antidepressants may result in undesirable increases in blood pressure.
▷ *Driving, Hazardous Activities:* This drug may cause dizziness or drowsiness. Restrict activities as necessary.
Aviation Note: The use of this drug *is a disqualification* for piloting. Consult a designated aviation medical examiner.
Exposure to Sun: No restrictions.
Discontinuation: If the drug has been taken for a long time, do not stop it abruptly. Talk to your doctor about how to slowly decrease doses.

METHYLPREDNISOLONE (meth il pred NIS oh lohn)

Introduced: 1957   **Class:** Cortisonelike drugs (adrenocortical steroids)
Prescription: USA: Yes   **Controlled Drug:** USA: No; Canada: No   **Available as Generic:** USA: Yes; Canada: Yes

Brand Names: A-Methapred, Depmedalone-40, Depmedalone-80, Depo-Medrol, Enpak Refill, Mar-Pred 40, Medrol, ✦Medrol Acne Lotion, Medrol Enpak, ✦Medrol Veriderm Cream, Meprolone, ✦Neo-Medrol Acne Lotion, ✦Neo-Medrol Veriderm, Solu-Medrol

---

BENEFITS versus RISKS

Possible Benefits	*Possible Risks*
EFFECTIVE RELIEF OF SYMPTOMS IN A WIDE VARIETY OF INFLAMMATORY AND ALLERGIC DISORDERS	Use exceeding 2 weeks is associated with many adverse effects:
EFFECTIVE IMMUNOSUPPRESSION in selected benign and malignant disorders	ALTERED MOOD AND PERSONALITY
	CATARACTS, GLAUCOMA
	HYPERTENSION
	OSTEOPOROSIS
	ASEPTIC BONE NECROSIS
	INCREASED SUSCEPTIBILITY TO INFECTIONS
	(See "Possible Adverse Effects" and "Possible Effects of Long-Term Use" below.)

▷ **Principal Uses**

As a Single Drug Product: Uses currently included in FDA approved labeling: (1) Treats a wide variety of allergic and inflammatory conditions—used most commonly in the management of serious skin disorders, asthma, regional enteritis, multiple sclerosis, lupus erythematosus, ulcerative colitis, and all types of major rheumatic disorders including bursitis, tendonitis, and most forms of arthritis; (2) helps treat low platelet counts of unknown cause (idiopathic thrombocytopenic purpura); (3) treats shock due to adrenal gland insufficiency—addisonian shock; (4) adjunctive role in anaphylactic shock.

Other (unlabeled) generally accepted uses: (1) Treatment of refractory anemia; (2) therapy of chronic obstructive pulmonary disease; (3) combination treatment of acute nonlymphoblastic leukemia; (4) combination therapy of severe vomiting caused by chemotherapy; (5) helps prevent rejection of transplanted organs; (6) combination therapy of *Pneumocystis carinii* pneumonia in AIDS patients; (7) helps treat bone cysts in children; (8) has a role in treating croup; (9) can help symptoms in Still's disease; (10) used by intramuscular injection to treat polymyalgia rheumatica; (11) used to help control cancer pain, especially where inflammation is involved.

How This Drug Works: Anti-inflammatory effect is due to its ability to block normal defensive functions of certain white blood cells. Immunosuppressant effect comes from reduced production of lymphocytes (a kind of white blood cell) and antibodies.

Available Dose Forms and Strengths

Injection, solution — 1 g per vial, 40 mg per vial, 125 mg per vial, 500 mg per vial

Injection, suspension — 40 mg/ml, 80 mg/ml

Ointment — 0.25%, 1%

Retention enema — 40 mg per bottle

Tablets — 2 mg, 4 mg, 8 mg, 16 mg, 24 mg, 32 mg

▷ **Usual Adult Dose Range:**   4 to 48 mg daily as a single dose or in divided doses. This dose is adjusted depending on the condition being treated and the individual response. **Note: Actual dose and schedule must be determined for each patient individually.**

Conditions Requiring Dosing Adjustments

Liver Function: Specific dose adjustments in liver compromise are not defined. This drug is a rare cause of liver changes (hepatomegaly).

Kidney Function: This drug can worsen existing kidney compromise. A benefit-to-risk decision must be made regarding the use of methylprednisolone by these patients.

Obesity: The amount of time this medicine stays in the body is extended in obese patients. Dosing should be calculated based on ideal body weight.

▷ **Dosing Instructions:**   The tablet may be crushed and taken with or following food to prevent stomach irritation, preferably in the morning.

Usual Duration of Use: For sudden (acute) disorders: 4 to 10 days. For long-standing (chronic) disorders: according to individual requirements. Duration of use should not exceed the time necessary to obtain adequate symptomatic relief in acute self-limiting conditions, or the time required to stabilize a chronic condition and permit gradual withdrawal. Because of its intermediate duration of action, this drug is appropriate for alternate-day use. See your doctor on a regular basis.

▷ **This Drug Should Not Be Taken If**
- you had an allergic reaction to it previously.
- you have active peptic ulcer disease.
- you have had recent bowel surgery where an anastomosis was performed.
- you have a premature infant and the injection form is ordered (contains benzyl alcohol).
- you have an active eye infection from herpes simplex virus.
- you have active tuberculosis.

▷ **Inform Your Physician Before Taking This Drug If**
- you have had an reaction to any cortisonelike drug.
- you have a history of peptic ulcer disease, thrombophlebitis, or tuberculosis.
- you have diabetes, glaucoma, high blood pressure, deficient thyroid function, or myasthenia gravis.
- you have been exposed to measles or chicken pox.
- you plan to have surgery of any kind in the near future.
- you have liver compromise.

Possible Side Effects (natural, expected, and unavoidable drug actions)

Increased appetite, weight gain, retention of salt and water, excretion of potassium, increased susceptibility to infection. Decreased wound healing. Adrenal gland suppression. Growth retardation with chronic use in children. Increased eye pressure (intraocular). Easy bruising (ecchymosis).

▷ **Possible Adverse Effects** (unusual, unexpected, and infrequent reactions)
If any of the following develop, consult your physician promptly for guidance.

Mild Adverse Effects
Allergic Reaction: Skin rash.
Headache, dizziness, insomnia—infrequent.
Acid indigestion, abdominal distention—infrequent.
Muscle cramping, weakness, and joint pain—possible.
Acne, excessive growth of facial hair—case reports.

Serious Adverse Effects
Allergic reactions: anaphylaxis.
Mental and emotional disturbances—infrequent.
Reactivation of latent tuberculosis, *Pneumocystis carinii* pneumonia—possible (case reports).
Development of peptic ulcer—case reports.
Seizures—possible.
Toxic megacolon—case reports.
Liver or kidney compromise—rare.
Blindness, cataracts—case reports.
Changes in white blood cell counts—possible.
Cushing's syndrome with chronic use (central obesity, buffalo hump, and moon-shaped face)—possible.
Osteoporosis, osteonecrosis—possible with long-term use.
Increased blood sugar (hyperglycemia)—possible and dose related.
Muscle changes (myopathy) or pancreatitis—case reports.
Increased blood pressure—case reports.
Abnormal heartbeat (arrhythmias)—case reports.
Development of inflammation of the pancreas—case reports.
Thrombophlebitis (inflammation of a vein with the formation of blood clot): pain or tenderness in thigh or leg, with or without swelling of the foot, ankle, or leg—case reports.
Pulmonary embolism (movement of a blood clot to the lung): sudden shortness of breath, pain in the chest, coughing, bloody sputum—case reports.

▷ **Possible Effects on Sexual Function:** Altered timing and pattern of menstruation—infrequent.

▷ **Adverse Effects That May Mimic Natural Diseases or Disorders**
Pattern of symptoms and signs resembling Cushing's syndrome.

Natural Diseases or Disorders That May Be Activated by This Drug
Latent diabetes, glaucoma, peptic ulcer disease, tuberculosis.

Possible Effects on Laboratory Tests
Blood amylase and lipase levels: increased (possible pancreatitis).
Glucose tolerance test (GTT): decreased.
Blood potassium or testosterone level: decreased.
Cholesterol and LDL: Increased.
HDL: Decreased.

CAUTION

1. Carry a card in your purse or wallet that says you take this drug, if your treatment will exceed 1 week.
2. You have an increased risk of severe infection from viral illnesses such as measles or chicken pox. Try to avoid being exposed, and call your doctor if exposure occurs.
3. Growth and development of children receiving chronic steroids should be carefully followed.
4. Do not stop this drug abruptly after long-term treatment.
5. If vaccination against measles, rabies, smallpox, or yellow fever is required, stop drug 72 hours before vaccination and do not resume it for at least 14 days.
6. Dermatitis around the mouth may occur. Talk with your doctor if this happens.

Precautions for Use

By Infants and Children: Avoid prolonged use if possible. Watch for growth suppression. Long-term use also increases risk of adrenal gland deficiency during stress (up to 18 months after drug is stopped). Pressure in the brain may increase.

By Those Over 60 Years of Age: Cortisonelike drugs should be used very sparingly after 60 and only when the disorder under treatment is unresponsive to adequate trials of unrelated drugs. Avoid prolonged use of this drug. Continual use (even in small doses) can increase the severity of diabetes, enhance fluid retention, raise blood pressure, weaken resistance to infection, induce stomach ulcer, and accelerate the development of cataract and osteoporosis.

▷ **Advisability of Use During Pregnancy**

Pregnancy Category: C. See Pregnancy Risk Categories at the back of this book.

Animal studies: Birth defects reported in mice, rats, and rabbits.

Human studies: Adequate studies of pregnant women are not available.

Avoid completely during the first 3 months. Limit use during the final 6 months as much as possible. If used, the infant should be examined for possible deficiency of adrenal gland function.

Advisability of Use If Breast-Feeding

Presence of this drug in breast milk: Yes.

Avoid drug or refrain from nursing.

Habit-Forming Potential: Use of this drug over an extended period of time may produce a state of functional dependence (see Glossary). Treating asthma and rheumatoid arthritis, the dose should be kept as small as possible and withdrawal should be attempted after periods of reasonable improvement. Such procedures may reduce "steroid rebound"—return of symptoms as the drug is withdrawn.

Effects of Overdose: Fatigue, muscle weakness, stomach irritation, acid indigestion, excessive sweating, facial flushing, fluid retention, swelling of extremities, increased blood pressure.

Possible Effects of Long-Term Use: Increased blood sugar (possible diabetes), increased fat deposits on the trunk of the body ("buffalo hump"), rounding of the face ("moon face"), thinning and fragility of skin, loss of texture and strength of bones (osteoporosis, aseptic necrosis), cataracts, glaucoma, retarded growth and development in children.

Suggested Periodic Examinations While Taking This Drug (at physician's discretion)

Measurements of blood pressure, blood sugar, and potassium levels.

Complete eye examinations at regular intervals.

Chest Xray if history of tuberculosis.

Determination of the rate of development of the growing child to detect retardation of normal growth.

Bone mineral density testing to assess osteoporosis and fracture risk.

▷ **While Taking This Drug, Observe the Following**

Foods: No interactions expected. Ask your physician regarding need to restrict salt intake or eat potassium-rich foods. During long-term use of this drug, it is advisable to eat a high-protein diet.

Nutritional Support: During long-term use, take a vitamin supplement. During wound repair, take a zinc supplement.

Beverages: No restrictions. Drink all forms of milk liberally.

▷ *Alcohol:* No interactions expected. Use caution if you are prone to peptic ulcer disease.

Tobacco Smoking: Nicotine increases the blood levels of naturally produced cortisone and related hormones. I advise everyone to quit smoking.

Marijuana Smoking: May cause additional impairment of immunity.

▷ *Other Drugs*

Methylprednisolone may *decrease* the effects of

• insulin and require higher doses.

• isoniazid (INH, Niconyl, etc.).

• salicylates (aspirin, sodium salicylate, etc.).

Methylprednisolone *taken concurrently* with

• amphotericin B (Fungizone) may increase the risk of potassium loss.

• carbamazepine (Tegretol) may blunt methylprednisolone benefits.

• cholestyramine (Questran) may decrease the amount of medicine that is absorbed into your body.

• cyclosporine (Sandimmune) can result in increased steroid levels and cyclosporine toxicity.

• ketoconazole (Nizoral) may increase blood levels of methylprednisolone and result in toxicity (abnormal heartbeats or psychiatric reactions).

• loop diuretics such as furosemide (Lasix) or bumetanide (Bumex) may result in increased risk of potassium loss.

• NSAIDs may cause increased risk of ulceration of the stomach or intestine.

• oral anticoagulants (warfarin—Coumadin) may either increase or decrease their effectiveness; consult your physician regarding the need for prothrombin time testing and dose adjustment.

• oral antidiabetic drugs (see Drug Classes) or insulin may result in loss of control of blood sugar and require higher doses or more frequent dosing of oral hypoglycemics or insulin in order to control blood sugar.

• primidone (Mysoline) may lead to increased metabolism of methylprednisolone and decreased therapeutic benefits of methylprednisolone.

• rifampin (Rifadin, others) may lead to increased metabolism of methylprednisolone and decreased therapeutic benefits of methylprednisolone.

- ritonavir (Norvir) and perhaps other protease inhibitors (see Drug Classes) may change therapeutic benefits of methylpredisolone.
- thiazide diuretics (see Drug Classes) can result in additive potassium loss.
- theophylline (Theo-Dur) results in variable changes in blood levels. More frequent theophylline blood levels are indicated.
- vaccines (such as flu or pneumococcal) may result in a blunting of the immune response to the vaccine.

The following drugs may *decrease* the effects of methylprednisolone:

- antacids—may reduce its absorption.
- barbiturates (Amytal, Butisol, phenobarbital, etc.).
- phenytoin (Dilantin, etc.).
- rifampin (Rifadin, Rimactane, etc.).

▷ *Driving, Hazardous Activities:* Usually no restrictions. Be alert to the rare occurrence of dizziness.

Aviation Note: The use of this drug *may be a disqualification* for piloting. Consult a designated aviation medical examiner.

Exposure to Sun: No restrictions.

Occurrence of Unrelated Illness: Decreases resistance to infection. Tell your doctor if you get an infection of any kind. May also reduce ability to respond to stress of acute illness, injury, or surgery. Tell your doctor about any significant changes in your state of health.

Discontinuation: After extended use of this drug, do **not** stop it abruptly. Ask your doctor for help regarding slow withdrawal. For 2 years after stopping this drug, it is essential that you tell medical personnel that you have used this drug if you get sick, are injured, or have surgery. Impaired response to stress after taking cortisonelike drugs may last for 1 to 2 years.

METHYSERGIDE (meth i SER jide)

Introduced: 1961   **Class:** Anti-migraine drug   **Prescription:** USA: Yes
Controlled Drug: USA: No; Canada: No   **Available as Generic:** USA: No; Canada: No

Brand Name: Sansert

BENEFITS versus RISKS	
Possible Benefits	*Possible Risks*
EFFECTIVE PREVENTION OF MIGRAINE AND CLUSTER HEADACHES	FIBROSIS (SCARRING) INSIDE CHEST AND ABDOMINAL CAVITIES, OF HEART AND LUNG TISSUES, ADJACENT TO MAJOR BLOOD VESSELS AND INTERNAL ORGANS (see "Possible Effects of Long-Term Use" below)
	Aggravation of hypertension, coronary artery disease, and peripheral vascular disease

▷ **Principal Uses**
As a Single Drug Product: Uses currently included in FDA-approved labeling: Prevention of frequent and/or disabling vascular headaches (migraine and cluster neuralgia) that have not responded to other conventional treatment.
Other (unlabeled) generally accepted uses: May have a role in therapy of some strokes.

How This Drug Works: Blocks serotonin inflammatory and vasoconstrictor effects, easing blood vessel constriction that causes vascular headaches.

Available Dose Forms and Strengths
Tablets — 2 mg

▷ **Recommended Dose Ranges** (Actual dose and schedule must be determined for each patient individually.)
Infants and Children: Use of this drug is not recommended.
12 to 60 Years of Age: 2 to 6 mg daily, in divided doses with meals. A medication-free period of 3 to 4 weeks is REQUIRED after every 6-month course.
Over 60 Years of Age: 2 to 4 mg daily, in divided doses. Use very cautiously, with frequent monitoring for adverse effects.

Conditions Requiring Dosing Adjustments
Liver Function: This drug should not be used by patients with liver compromise.
Kidney Function: This drug should not be used by patients with renal compromise.

▷ **Dosing Instructions:** The tablet may be crushed and taken with food or milk to reduce stomach irritation. Uninterrupted use is limited to 6 months; avoid drug completely for 4 weeks between courses.

Usual Duration of Use: Use on a regular schedule for 3 weeks usually determines effectiveness in preventing recurrence of vascular headache. If significant benefit does not occur during this trial, this drug should be stopped. Long-term use (months to years) requires periodic physician evaluation.

▷ **This Drug Should Not Be Taken If**
- you have had an allergic reaction to it previously.
- you are pregnant.
- you currently have a severe infection.
- you have any of the following conditions:
  angina pectoris
  Buerger's disease
  cellulitis of the lower legs
  chronic lung disease
  connective tissue (collagen) disease
  coronary artery disease
  hardening of the arteries (arteriosclerosis)
  heart valve disease
  high blood pressure (significant hypertension)
  kidney disease or significantly impaired kidney function
  liver disease or significantly impaired liver function
  active peptic ulcer disease
  peripheral vascular disease
  phlebitis of any kind
  Raynaud's disease or phenomenon

▷ **Inform Your Physician Before Taking This Drug If**
- you had an adverse reaction to *any ergot*.
- you have a history of peptic ulcer disease.

Possible Side Effects (natural, expected, and unavoidable drug actions)
Fluid retention, weight gain. Impaired circulation to the extremities (peripheral ischemia).

▷ **Possible Adverse Effects** (unusual, unexpected, and infrequent reactions)
If any of the following develop, consult your physician promptly for guidance.
Mild Adverse Effects
Allergic reactions: skin rashes, flushing of the face, transient loss of scalp hair.
Dizziness, drowsiness, agitation, unsteadiness, altered vision—infrequent to frequent.
Heartburn, nausea, vomiting, diarrhea—infrequent.
Transient muscle and joint pains—infrequent.
Serious Adverse Effects
Idiosyncratic reactions: nightmares, hallucinations, acute mental disturbances.
Fibrosis (scar tissue formation) involving the chest and/or abdominal cavities, heart valves, lungs, kidneys, major blood vessels—case reports.
Spasm and narrowing of coronary and peripheral arteries: anginal chest pain; cold and painful extremities; leg cramps on walking—case reports.
Hemolytic anemia (see Glossary) or abnormally low white blood cell counts—case reports.
Heart attack (myocardial infarction)—case reports.

▷ **Possible Effects on Sexual Function:**   Fibrosis of penile tissues—case reports.

▷ **Adverse Effects That May Mimic Natural Diseases or Disorders**
Swelling of the hands, lower legs, feet, and ankles (peripheral edema) may suggest heart or kidney dysfunction.

Natural Diseases or Disorders That May Be Activated by This Drug
Latent coronary artery insufficiency (angina), Buerger's disease, Raynaud's disease, peptic ulcer disease.

Possible Effects on Laboratory Tests
Complete blood cell counts: decreased white cells (lymphocytes).
Stomach hydrochloric acid: increased.
Kidney function tests: increased blood urea nitrogen (BUN).

CAUTION
1. Continual use limited to 6 months. Gradual dose reduction is prudent during last 2 to 3 weeks of each course to prevent headache rebound. Omit drug for a period of 4 to 6 weeks before resuming. Mandatory "drug-free" period reduces fibrosis risk.
2. Promptly report fatigue, fever, chest pain, difficult breathing, stomach/flank pain, or urinary changes.
3. Useful only for prevention of recurring vascular headaches. NOT recommended for acute headaches. Not effective for tension headaches.

Precautions for Use
By Infants and Children: Use of this drug is not recommended.

By Those Over 60 Years of Age: The age-related changes in blood vessels, circulatory functions, and kidney function can make you more susceptible to the serious adverse effects of this drug. See the list of diseases and disorders above that are contraindications to the use this drug. Ask your doctor for help.

▷ **Advisability of Use During Pregnancy**

Pregnancy Category: X. See Pregnancy Risk Categories at the back of this book. Animal studies: No information is available.

Human studies: Adequate studies of pregnant women are not available.

The manufacturer states that this drug is contraindicated during entire pregnancy.

Advisability of Use If Breast-Feeding

Presence of this drug in breast milk: Yes.

Avoid drug or refrain from nursing.

Habit-Forming Potential: None.

Effects of Overdose: Nausea, vomiting, stomach pain, diarrhea, dizziness, excitement, cold hands and feet.

Possible Effects of Long-Term Use: Formation of scar tissue (fibrosis) inside chest cavity and/or abdominal cavity, on heart valves, in lung tissues, and surrounding major blood vessels and internal organs. Requires close and continual medical supervision.

Suggested Periodic Examinations While Taking This Drug (at physician's discretion)

Careful examination at regular intervals (6 to 12 months) for scar tissue formation or circulatory complications. Complete blood cell counts. Kidney function tests.

▷ **While Taking This Drug, Observe the Following**

Foods: No restrictions except foods you are allergic to. Some vascular headaches are due to food allergy.

Beverages: No restrictions.

▷ *Alcohol:* No interactions expected. Observe closely to determine if alcoholic beverages can initiate a migrainelike headache.

Tobacco Smoking: Avoid completely.

▷ *Other Drugs*

Methysergide *taken concurrently* with

- beta-blocker drugs (see Drug Classes) may cause hazardous constriction of peripheral arteries. Watch combined effects on circulation in the extremities.
- sumatriptan (Imitrex) may cause prolonged spasm of blood vessels. DO NOT COMBINE.

▷ *Driving, Hazardous Activities:* This drug may cause dizziness, drowsiness, or impaired vision. Restrict activities as necessary.

Aviation Note: The use of this drug *is a disqualification* for piloting. Consult a designated aviation medical examiner.

Exposure to Sun: No restrictions.

Exposure to Cold: Use caution. Cold environments may increase the occurrence of reduced circulation (blood flow) to the extremities.

Discontinuation: Do not stop it abruptly if drug has been taken for a long time.

Slowly lowering the dose over 2 to 3 weeks can prevent rebound vascular headaches.

METOCLOPRAMIDE (met oh KLOH pra mide)

Introduced: 1973 **Class:** Gastrointestinal drug, antinausea (antiemetic)
Prescription: USA: Yes **Controlled Drug:** USA: No; Canada: No **Available as Generic:** Yes
Brand Names: ✦Apo-Metoclop, ✦Clopra, ✦Emex, ✦Maxeran, Maxolon, Octamide, Reclomide, Reglan

BENEFITS versus RISKS	
Possible Benefits	*Possible Risks*
EFFECTIVE STOMACH STIMULANT FOR CORRECTING DELAYED EMPTYING	Sedation and fatigue
	Parkinson-like reactions
	Tardive dyskinesia
Symptomatic relief in reflux esophagitis	
Relief of nausea and vomiting associated with migraine headache	

▷ **Principal Uses**

As a Single Drug Product: Uses currently included in FDA-approved labeling: (1) Helps stomach retention (gastroparesis) associated with diabetes; (2) treats acid reflux from the stomach into the esophagus (esophagitis); (3) treats nausea and vomiting associated with migraine headaches; (4) nausea and vomiting induced by anticancer drugs; (5) helps decrease the time needed to place a tube in the intestine; (6) used prior to cesarean section to decrease postdelivery nausea or vomiting;(7) used in some X-ray (radiologic) tests.

Other (unlabeled) generally accepted uses: (1) Used as a preparatory drug in stomach hemorrhage; (2) may help gastrointestinal symptoms in anorexia nervosa; (3) eases drug-induced slowed functioning of the intestine (adynamic ileus); (4) decreases the frequency of accumulations of food in the stomach (bezoars); (5) can be of benefit in migraine attacks.

How This Drug Works: Inhibits relaxation of stomach muscles and enhances parasympathetic nervous system (responsible for stomach muscle contractions) stimulation. This accelerates emptying of stomach contents into the intestine.

Available Dose Forms and Strengths
Injection — 5 mg/ml, 10 mg/ml
Solution — 10 mg/ml
Syrup — 5 mg/5 ml
Tablets — 5 mg, 10 mg

▷ **Usual Adult Dose Range:** Ten mg taken 30 minutes before breakfast, lunch, and dinner and at bedtime (four times a day) for 2 to 8 weeks. Daily maximum is 0.5 mg per kg of body mass. **Note: Actual dose and schedule must be determined for each patient individually.**

Conditions Requiring Dosing Adjustments
Liver Function: No changes appear to be needed.
Kidney Function: For patients with moderate kidney failure, 75% of the usual dose can be taken at the usual dosing interval. In severe kidney failure, 50% of the usual dose can be taken at the usual dosing interval. A benefit-to-risk decision must be made.

▷ **Dosing Instructions:** Take tablet or syrup 30 minutes before each meal and at bedtime. The tablet may be crushed.

Usual Duration of Use: Use on a regular schedule for 5 to 7 days determines benefit in accelerating stomach emptying and relieving symptoms of heartburn, fullness, and belching. Long-term use (months to years) requires physician supervision.

▷ **This Drug Should Not Be Taken If**
- you have had an allergic reaction to it previously.
- you have a seizure disorder of any kind.
- you have active gastrointestinal bleeding.
- you are taking, or have taken within the last 14 days, a monoamine oxidase (MAO) inhibitor (see Drug Classes).
- you are taking tricyclic antidepressants.
- you have a pheochromocytoma (adrenaline-producing tumor).

▷ **Inform Your Physician Before Taking This Drug If**
- you are allergic or overly sensitive to procaine or procainamide.
- you have impaired liver or kidney function.
- you have Parkinson's disease.
- you have epilepsy.
- you have high blood pressure.
- you have a history of depression.
- you are taking atropinelike (anticholinergic) drugs, antipsychotics, or opioid analgesics (see Drug Classes).

Possible Side Effects (natural, expected, and unavoidable drug actions)
Drowsiness and lethargy, breast tenderness and swelling, milk production.

▷ **Possible Adverse Effects** (unusual, unexpected, and infrequent reactions)
If any of the following develop, consult your physician promptly for guidance.
Mild Adverse Effects
Allergic Reaction: Skin rash. Mild decreases in blood pressure.
Headache, dizziness, restlessness, depression, insomnia—infrequent.
Dry mouth, nausea, diarrhea, constipation—infrequent to frequent.
Urinary retention or incontinence—possible.
Serious Adverse Effects
Idiosyncratic reactions: neuroleptic malignant syndrome (see Glossary), bronchospastic reactions in asthmatics.
Parkinson-like reactions (see Glossary) or tardive dyskinesia (see Glossary)—case reports.
Abnormal fixed positioning of the eyes (oculogyric crisis)—case reports.
Severe decrease in white blood cells (agranulocytosis)—case reports.
Abnormal heartbeat—possible (case reports).

Severe increases in blood pressure (hypertensive crisis)—case reports.
Drug-induced porphyria—case reports.

▷ **Possible Effects on Sexual Function:**   Decreased libido, impaired erection, decreased sperm count, sustained painful erection (priapism).
Altered timing and pattern of menstruation, galactorrhea—case reports to infrequent.

Possible Effects on Laboratory Tests
Blood lithium level: increased.
Blood thyroid-stimulating hormone (TSH) level: increased.

Precautions for Use
By Infants and Children: Watch for development of Parkinson-like reactions soon after starting therapy. Use of the smallest effective dose can minimize such reactions. For diabetic gastroparesis, 0.5 mg per kg of body mass per day, divided into three equal doses given every 8 hours, has been used. Children less than 6 years old should NOT receive single doses more than 0.1 mg per kg of body mass.

By Those Over 60 Years of Age: Parkinson-like reactions and tardive dyskinesias are more likely to occur with the use of high doses over an extended period of time. The smallest effective dose should be identified and used only when clearly needed.

▷ **Advisability of Use During Pregnancy**
Pregnancy Category: B. See Pregnancy Risk Categories at the back of this book.
Animal studies: No birth defects found due to this drug.
Human studies: Adequate studies of pregnant women are not available.
Use this drug only if clearly needed.

Advisability of Use If Breast-Feeding
Presence of this drug in breast milk: Yes.
Avoid drug or refrain from nursing.

Habit-Forming Potential: None.

Effects of Overdose: Marked drowsiness, confusion, muscle spasms, jerking movements of head and face, tremors, shuffling gait.

Possible Effects of Long-Term Use: Parkinson-like reactions may appear within several months of use. Tardive dyskinesias usually occur after a year of continual use; they may persist after this drug is discontinued.

Suggested Periodic Examinations While Taking This Drug (at physician's discretion)
During long-term use, watch for the development of fine, wormlike movements on the surface of the tongue; these may be the first indications of an emerging tardive dyskinesia.

▷ **While Taking This Drug, Observe the Following**
Foods: No restrictions.
Beverages: No restrictions. May be taken with milk.
▷ *Alcohol:* Combined effects can result in excessive sedation and marked intoxication. Alcohol is best avoided.
Tobacco Smoking: No interactions expected. I advise everyone to quit smoking.
▷ *Other Drugs*
Metoclopramide may ***decrease*** the effects of

- cimetidine (Tagamet).
- digoxin (slow-dissolving dose forms), and reduce its effectiveness.

Metoclopramide **taken concurrently** with

- acetaminophen may increase the absorption of this drug. Decreased doses are prudent if chronic acetaminophen use will continue with metoclopramide therapy.
- cyclosporine (Sandimmune) may result in increased cyclosporine levels and toxicity.
- major antipsychotic drugs (phenothiazines, thiothixenes, haloperidol, etc.) may increase the risk of developing Parkinson-like reactions.
- morphine (slow release) may result in faster onset and increased sedation.
- penicillin may result in decreased therapeutic benefits of the antibiotic. Increased doses may be needed.
- quinidine (Quinaglute, others) may result in decreased therapeutic benefits from quinidine. Increased blood level testing and adjustment of dosing to levels is indicated.
- sertraline (Zoloft) may increase risk of movement disorders.
- zalcitabine (Hivid) may blunt zalcitabine levels.

The following drugs may **decrease** the effects of metoclopramide:

- atropinelike (anticholinergic) drugs (see Drug Classes).
- opioid analgesics (see Drug Classes).
- ritonavir (Norvir).

▷ *Driving, Hazardous Activities:* This drug may cause drowsiness and dizziness. Restrict activities as necessary.

Aviation Note: The use of this drug **may be a disqualification** for piloting. Consult a designated aviation medical examiner.

Exposure to Sun: No restrictions.

METOLAZONE (me TOHL a zohn)

See the thiazide diuretics profile for further information.

METOPROLOL (me TOH proh lohl)

Introduced: 1974   **Class:** Antihypertensive, beta-adrenergic blocker
Prescription: USA: Yes   **Controlled Drug:** USA: No; Canada: No   **Available as Generic:** Yes
Brand Names: ✤Apo-Metoprolol, ✤Betaloc, ✤Co-Betaloc [CD], Lopressor, Lopressor Delayed-Release, Lopressor HCT [CD], Lopressor OROS, ✤Novo-Metoprol, ✤Nu-Metop, Toprol, Toprol XL

```
┌─────────────────────────────────────────────────────────────────────┐
│                      BENEFITS versus RISKS                            │
│        Possible Benefits                    Possible Risks            │
│  EFFECTIVE, WELL-TOLERATED          CONGESTIVE HEART FAILURE in       │
│    ANTIHYPERTENSIVE in mild to        advanced heart disease          │
│    moderate high blood pressure     Worsening of angina in coronary   │
│  MAY HELP REDUCE DEATH FROM           heart disease (abrupt withdrawal)│
│    HEART ATTACKS                    Masking of low blood sugar        │
│                                       (hypoglycemia) in drug-treated  │
│                                       diabetes                        │
│                                     Provocation of asthma (with high  │
│                                       doses in asthmatics)            │
└─────────────────────────────────────────────────────────────────────┘
```

▷ **Principal Uses**

As a Single Drug Product: Uses currently included in FDA-approved labeling: (1) Treats mild to moderate high blood pressure, alone or with other drugs; (2) helps reduce the frequency and severity of angina; (3) used to reduce the risk of a second heart attack.

Other (unlabeled) generally accepted uses: (1) Reduces symptoms of heart muscle damage (dilated cardiomyopathy); (2) second-line drug in panic attacks; (3) used to decrease pressure in the eye (intraocular pressure) in open-angle glaucoma.

How This Drug Works: Blocks some actions of the sympathetic nervous system:
- reducing rate, contraction force, and ejection pressure of the heart.
- reducing contraction of blood vessels, resulting in lowering of blood pressure.
- prolonging conduction time of nerve impulses through the heart, managing certain heart rhythm disorders.

Available Dose Forms and Strengths
> Injection — 1 mg/ml
> Tablets — 50 mg, 100 mg
> Tablets, prolonged action — 50 mg, 100 mg, 200 mg

▷ **Usual Adult Dose Range:**   Starts with 50 mg once or twice daily (12 hours apart). Dose may be increased gradually at intervals of 7 to 10 days as needed and tolerated, up to 300 mg/day. For maintenance, 100 mg twice a day. The total daily dose should not exceed 450 mg. **Note: Actual dose and schedule must be determined for each patient individually.**

Conditions Requiring Dosing Adjustments
Liver Function: Used with caution by patients with liver compromise.
Kidney Function: No changes thought to be needed.

▷ **Dosing Instructions:**   The regular tablet may be crushed and taken without regard to eating. Prolonged-action forms should be swallowed whole (not altered). Do not stop this drug abruptly.

Usual Duration of Use: Regular use for 10 to 14 days determines benefits in lowering blood pressure. The long-term use will be determined by your response to a treatment program (weight reduction, restricted salt, smoking cessation, etc.). See your doctor regularly.

Currently a "Drug of Choice"
For starting hypertension therapy with one drug, especially for those with bronchial asthma or diabetes.

▷ **This Drug Should Not Be Taken If**
- you have had an allergic reaction to it previously.
- you have congestive heart failure.
- you have had a heart attack and your heart rate is less than 45 beats/min.
- you have an abnormally slow heart rate or a serious form of heart block.
- you took any monoamine oxidase (MAO) type A drug (see Drug Classes) in the last 14 days.

▷ **Inform Your Physician Before Taking This Drug If**
- you had an adverse reaction to any beta-blocker (see Drug Classes).
- you have a history of serious heart disease.
- you have a history of hay fever (allergic rhinitis), asthma, chronic bronchitis, or emphysema. People with bronchial asthma should generally not take beta-blockers. This drug is somewhat heart selective, and may be used with caution by asthmatics.
- you have a history of overactive thyroid function (hyperthyroidism).
- you have a history of low blood sugar (hypoglycemia).
- you have impaired liver or kidney function.
- you have diabetes or myasthenia gravis.
- you currently take digitalis, quinidine, or reserpine, or any calcium-channel-blocker drug (see Drug Classes).
- you have a history of poor circulation to the extremities (peripheral vascular disease).
- you have a history of periodic cramps of your legs (intermittent claudication).
- you will have surgery with general anesthesia.

Possible Side Effects (natural, expected, and unavoidable drug actions)
Lethargy and fatigability, cold extremities, slow heart rate, light-headedness in upright position (see *orthostatic hypotension* in Glossary). Abnormally slow heartbeat (bradycardia).

▷ **Possible Adverse Effects** (unusual, unexpected, and infrequent reactions)
If any of the following develop, consult your physician promptly for guidance.
Mild Adverse Effects
Allergic reactions: skin rash, itching.
Worsening of psoriasis—case reports.
Headache, fatigue, dizziness, insomnia, abnormal dreams—infrequent.
Indigestion, nausea, vomiting, constipation, diarrhea—infrequent.
Eye and joint pain—case reports.
Joint and muscle discomfort, fluid retention (edema)—possible.
Serious Adverse Effects
Mental depression, hallucinations, anxiety—infrequent.
Chest pain, shortness of breath, precipitation of congestive heart failure—case reports.
Induction of bronchial asthma (in asthmatic patients)—possible.
Rebound hypertension—if the drug is abruptly stopped.
Precipitation of myasthenia gravis—case reports.
Carpal tunnel syndrome—case reports.
Low or high blood sugar (hypoglycemia or hyperglycemia)—possible.
Liver compromise (hepatitis)—case reports.

▷ **Possible Effects on Sexual Function:** Decreased libido (four times more common in men); impaired erection (less common with this drug than with most other beta-blockers); Peyronie's disease (see Glossary)—case reports.

Possible Effects on Laboratory Tests
Blood HDL cholesterol level: decreased.
Blood LDL and VLDL cholesterol level: decreased.
Blood glucose level: increased.
Blood triglyceride levels: increased.

CAUTION
1. ***Do not stop this drug suddenly*** without the knowledge and help of your physician. Carry a note with you that says you take this drug.
2. Ask your doctor or pharmacist before using any nasal decongestants. These are often found in nonprescription cold medicines and nose drops. They may increase blood pressure.
3. Report development of emotional depression.

Precautions for Use
By Infants and Children: Safety and effectiveness for use by those under 12 years of age have not been established. However, if this drug is used, watch for the development of low blood sugar (hypoglycemia) during periods of reduced food intake.
By Those Over 60 Years of Age: Proceed *cautiously* with all antihypertensive drugs. Unacceptably high blood pressure should be reduced slowly, to avoid the risks associated with excessively low blood pressure. Therapy should be started with small doses, and the blood pressure checked often. Sudden, rapid, and excessive reduction of blood pressure can predispose to stroke or heart attack. Watch for dizziness, unsteadiness, tendency to fall, confusion, hallucinations, depression, or urinary frequency.

▷ **Advisability of Use During Pregnancy**
Pregnancy Category: C. See Pregnancy Risk Categories at the back of this book.
Animal studies: No significant increase in birth defects due to this drug.
Human studies: Adequate studies of pregnant women are not available.
Use this drug only if clearly needed. Ask your physician for guidance.

Advisability of Use If Breast-Feeding
Presence of this drug in breast milk: Yes.
Discuss benefits versus risks with your doctor.

Habit-Forming Potential: None.

Effects of Overdose: Weakness, slow pulse, low blood pressure, cold and sweaty skin, congestive heart failure, possible coma, and convulsions.

Possible Effects of Long-Term Use: Reduced heart reserve and eventual heart failure in susceptible individuals with advanced heart disease.

Suggested Periodic Examinations While Taking This Drug (at physician's discretion)
Measurements of blood pressure, evaluation of heart function.

▷ **While Taking This Drug, Observe the Following**
Foods: Peak drug concentration and peak effect will increase if taken with food. Avoid excessive salt intake.

Beverages: No restrictions. May be taken with milk.

▷ *Alcohol:* Use with caution. Alcohol may exaggerate this drug's ability to lower the blood pressure and may increase its mild sedative effect.

Tobacco Smoking: Nicotine may reduce this drug's benefit in treating high blood pressure. I advise everyone to quit smoking.

▷ Other Drugs

Metoprolol may *increase* the effects of

- other antihypertensive drugs, causing excessive lowering of blood pressure. Dose adjustments may be necessary.
- reserpine (Ser-Ap-Es, etc.), and cause sedation, depression, slowing of the heart rate, and lowering of the blood pressure.
- verapamil (Calan, Isoptin), and cause excessive depression of heart function; monitor this combination closely.

Metoprolol *taken concurrently* with

- amiodarone (Codarone) may result in extremely slow heartbeat and cardiac arrest. NOT ADVISED.
- clonidine (Catapres) requires close monitoring for rebound high blood pressure if clonidine is withdrawn while metoprolol is still being taken.
- digoxin (Lanoxin, others) may increase heart slowing.
- fluoxetine (Prozac) may cause metoprolol toxicity.
- fluvoxamine (Luvox) may lead to metoprolol toxicity.
- insulin requires close monitoring to avoid undetected hypoglycemia (see Glossary).
- lidocaine can lead to lidocaine toxicity (cardiac arrest).
- nifedipine (Adalat, Procardia, others) may result in heart failure.
- oral antidiabetic drugs (see Drug Classes) can result in prolonged hypoglycemia if it occurs.
- phenothiazines (see Drug Classes) can result in low blood pressure or toxicity due to the phenothiazine.
- quinidine (Quinaglute, others) can lead to abnormally slow heartbeat and shortness of breath.
- ritonavir (Norvir), and perhaps other protease inhibitors (see Drug Classes), may cause toxicity.
- tocainide (Tonocard) may lead to depressed contraction ability of the heart (myocardial contractility).
- venlafaxine (Effexor) may lead to metabolic changes and toxic blood levels of both medicines.

The following drugs may *increase* the effects of metoprolol:

- birth control pills (oral contraceptives).
- cimetidine (Tagamet).
- ciprofloxacin (Cipro).
- diltiazem (Cardizem).
- monoamine oxidase (MAO) inhibitors (see Drug Classes).
- methimazole (Tapazole).
- propylthiouracil (Propacil).

The following drugs may *decrease* the effects of metoprolol:

- barbiturates (phenobarbital, etc.).
- indomethacin (Indocin), and possibly other aspirin substitutes, or NSAIDs, may impair metoprolol's antihypertensive effect.
- rifampin (Rifadin, Rimactane).

▷   *Driving, Hazardous Activities:* Use caution until the full extent of drowsiness, lethargy, and blood pressure change has been determined.

Aviation Note: The use of this drug ***is a disqualification*** for piloting. Consult a designated aviation medical examiner.

Exposure to Sun: No restrictions.

Exposure to Heat: Caution is advised. Hot environments can lower the blood pressure and exaggerate the effects of this drug.

Exposure to Cold: Caution! Cold environments can increase circulatory deficiency in extremities. The elderly should take care to prevent hypothermia (see Glossary).

Heavy Exercise or Exertion: Best to avoid exertion that produces light-headedness, excessive fatigue, or muscle cramping. This drug may intensify the blood pressure response to isometric exercise.

Occurrence of Unrelated Illness: Fever can lower the blood pressure and require adjustment of dose. Nausea or vomiting may interrupt the regular dose schedule. Ask your doctor for help.

Discontinuation: DO NOT stop this drug suddenly. Gradual dose lowering over 1 to 2 weeks is recommended. Ask your doctor for help.

METRONIDAZOLE (me troh NI da zohl)

Introduced: 1960   **Class:** Anti-infective (amebicide)   **Prescription:** USA: Yes   **Controlled Drug:** USA: No; Canada: No   **Available as Generic:** Yes

Brand Names: ✤Apo-Metronidazole, Femazole, Flagyl, Flagyl ER (extended release form), Flagystatin, Lagyl, Metizol, MetroGel, Metro IV, Metryl, ✤Neo-Tric, ✤Novo-Nidazole, Protostat, SK Metronidazole, ✤Trikacide

---

BENEFITS versus RISKS	
Possible Benefits	*Possible Risks*
EFFECTIVE TREATMENT FOR *TRICHOMONAS* INFECTIONS, AMEBIC DYSENTERY, AND GIARDIASIS, and some anaerobic bacterial infections	Superinfection with yeast organisms
	Peripheral neuritis
	Abnormally low white blood cell count (transient)
	Colitis
Effective local treatment for rosacea	Aggravation of epilepsy
TREATMENT OF BACTERIAL VAGINOSIS (ER FORM)	

▷ **Principal Uses**

As a Single Drug Product: Uses currently included in FDA-approved labeling: (1) Treats *Trichomonas* infections of the vaginal canal and cervix and of the male urethra; (2) also used to treat amebic dysentery and liver abscess, *Giardia* infections of the intestine, and serious infections caused by certain strains of anaerobic bacteria; (3) treats *Gardnerella* infections of the vagina; (4) treatment of rosacea with local application of a gel dose form; (5) used in therapy of pseudomembranous colitis; (6) has a role in treating bed sores (decubitis ulcers); (7) can help prevent infection (prophylaxis) in gynecological, appendectomy, or colorectal surgery; (8) ER form used in bacterial vaginosis.

Other (unlabeled) generally accepted uses: (1) Combination therapy with gentamicin in treating intra-abdominal infections; (2) combination antibiotic treatment of duodenal ulcers caused by *Helicobacter pylori*; (3) can help treat infections caused by *Giardia lamblia*; (4) used to help heal the lesions in Crohn's disease; may help abnormal gum growth (gingival hyperplasia) caused by cyclosporine.

How This Drug Works: Interacts with DNA, destroying essential component (nucleus) that is needed for life and growth of infecting organisms.

Available Dose Forms and Strengths

Capsules — 375 mg
Gel — 0.75%
Injection — 500 mg/100 ml
Tablets — 250 mg, 500 mg
Tablets, extended release — 750 mg
Vaginal cream — 10%

▷ **Usual Adult Dose Range:** For bacterial vaginosis: (ER form): 750 mg once a day for seven days in a row.

For trichomoniasis: 1-day course—2 g as a single dose, or 1 g for two doses 12 hours apart. 7-day course—250 mg three times a day for 7 consecutive days. (The 7-day course is preferred.)

For amebiasis: 500 to 750 mg three times a day for 5 to 10 consecutive days.

For giardiasis: 2 g once daily for 3 days; or 250 to 500 mg three times a day for 5 to 7 days.

The total daily dose should not exceed 4 g (4000 mg).

Note: Actual dose and schedule must be determined for each patient individually.

Conditions Requiring Dosing Adjustments

Liver Function: Dose is decreased by one-third in mild to moderate liver disease. Should not be used in severe liver compromise.

Kidney Function: In severe kidney failure, 50% of the normal dose can be taken at the usual dosing interval. A benefit-to-risk decision must be made for these patients, as there is a risk of systemic lupus erythematosus (SLE) from the metabolites of this drug.

▷ **Dosing Instructions:** The tablet may be crushed and taken with or following food to reduce stomach irritation.

Usual Duration of Use: Use on a regular schedule as outlined is needed to ensure effectiveness. Do not repeat the course of treatment without your physician's approval.

▷ **This Drug Should Not Be Taken If**
- you have had an allergic reaction to it or any the parabens contained in the gel form previously.
- you are pregnant.
- you currently have a bone marrow or blood cell disorder.
- you have any type of central nervous system disorder, including epilepsy.

▷ **Inform Your Physician Before Taking This Drug If**
- you have a history of any type of blood cell disorder, especially one induced by drugs.
- you have a history of seizures or peripheral neuropathy.
- you have impaired liver or kidney function.
- you have a history of alcoholism.
- you are pregnant or breast-feeding.

Possible Side Effects (natural, expected, and unavoidable drug actions)

A sharp, metallic, unpleasant taste. Dark discoloration of the urine (of no clinical significance).

Superinfection (see Glossary) by yeast organisms in the mouth or vagina. Pseudomembranous colitis.

▷ **Possible Adverse Effects** (unusual, unexpected, and infrequent reactions)

If any of the following develop, consult your physician promptly for guidance.

Mild Adverse Effects

Allergic reactions: skin rash, hives, flushing, itching.

Headache, dizziness, incoordination, unsteadiness, incontinence—infrequent.

Loss of appetite, nausea, vomiting, abdominal cramps, diarrhea—infrequent.

Irritation of mouth and tongue, possibly due to yeast infection—possible.

Serious Adverse Effects

Idiosyncratic reactions: abnormal behavior; confusion; depression; Herxheimer's reaction—sweating, diarrhea, vomiting, scalding urination, joint pain, and itching—case reports.

Peripheral neuritis (see Glossary)—case reports.

Abnormally low white blood cell count (transient): fever, sore throat, infections—case reports.

Disulfiram-like reactions (nausea, vomiting) if alcoholic beverages are consumed—possible.

Seizures—case reports.

Drug-induced pneumonitis, porphyria, or pancreatitis—case reports.

Hemolytic-uremic syndrome—case reports.

▷ **Possible Effects on Sexual Function:**   Decreased libido; decreased vaginal secretions (difficult or painful intercourse)—case reports.

Possible Delayed Adverse Effects: Studies have shown that this drug can cause cancer in mice and possibly in rats. Two researchers concluded that the carcinogenic risk is low in doses used to treat episodic vaginitis. High-dose, long-term use may carry increased cancer risk. Follow your doctor's instructions exactly. Avoid unnecessary or prolonged use.

▷ **Adverse Effects That May Mimic Natural Diseases or Disorders**

Behavioral changes may suggest spontaneous psychosis.

Natural Diseases or Disorders That May Be Activated by This Drug

Latent yeast infections.

Possible Effects on Laboratory Tests

White blood cell counts: decreased.

INR (prothrombin time): increased.

Blood theophylline levels: falsely increased by some methods.

CAUTION

1. Troublesome and persistent diarrhea can develop. If diarrhea persists for more than 24 hours, stop this drug and call your physician.
2. Stop this drug immediately if you develop any signs of toxic effects on the brain or nervous system: confusion, irritability, dizziness, incoordination, unsteady stance or gait, muscle jerking or twitching, numbness or weakness in the extremities.

Precautions for Use

By Infants and Children: Avoid use in those with a history of bone marrow or blood cell disorders.

By Those Over 60 Years of Age: Natural changes in the skin may predispose to yeast infections in the genital and anal regions. Report the development of rashes and itching promptly.

▷ **Advisability of Use During Pregnancy**

Pregnancy Category: B. See Pregnancy Risk Categories at the back of this book.

Animal studies: No birth defects reported in rat studies. However, this drug is known to cause cancer in mice and possibly in rats.

Human studies: No increase in birth defects reported in 206 exposures to this drug during the first 3 months. However, information from adequate studies of pregnant women is not available.

The manufacturer advises against the use of this drug during the first 3 months. Use during the final 6 months is not advised unless it is absolutely essential to the mother's health.

Advisability of Use If Breast-Feeding

Presence of this drug in breast milk: Yes.

Avoid drug or refrain from nursing.

Habit-Forming Potential: None.

Effects of Overdose: Weakness, stomach irritation, nausea, vomiting, confusion, disorientation.

Possible Effects of Long-Term Use: None reported. Avoid long-term use.

Suggested Periodic Examinations While Taking This Drug (at physician's discretion)

Complete blood cell counts.

▷ **While Taking This Drug, Observe the Following**

Foods: No restrictions.

Beverages: No restrictions. May be taken with milk.

▷ *Alcohol:* A disulfiram-like reaction (see Glossary) has been reported. It is NOT advisable to drink alcohol while taking metronidazole.

Tobacco Smoking: No interactions expected. I advise everyone to quit smoking.

▷ *Other Drugs*

Metronidazole may *increase* the effects of

- warfarin (Coumadin, etc.), and cause abnormal bleeding. The INR (prothrombin time or protime) should be monitored closely, especially during the first 10 days of concurrent use.

Metronidazole *taken concurrently* with

- antacids may decrease absorption of metronidazole.
- birth control pills (oral contraceptives) may block the effectiveness of contraception and result in pregnancy.

- cholestyramine (Questran) or other cholesterol-lowering resins may decrease metronidazole absorption and lower its therapeutic effect.
- cotrimoxazole or other sulfa drugs may result in a disulfiramlike effect.
- cyclosporine (Sandimmune) can lead to cyclosporine toxicity.
- disulfiram (Antabuse) may cause severe emotional and behavioral disturbances.
- lithium (Lithobid, others) can cause lithium toxicity.
- phenytoin (Dilantin) may result in increased blood levels of phenytoin. More frequent blood level testing is needed, and the phenytoin dose should be adjusted to blood levels.
- ritonavir (Norvir) may increase blood levels of metronidazole.

▷ *Driving, Hazardous Activities:* This drug may cause dizziness or incoordination. Restrict activities as necessary.

Aviation Note: The use of this drug *may be a disqualification* for piloting. Consult a designated aviation medical examiner.

Exposure to Sun: No restrictions.

MEXILETINE (mex IL e teen)

Introduced: 1973   **Class:** Antiarrhythmic   **Prescription:** USA: Yes
Controlled Drug: USA: No; Canada: No   **Available as Generic:** Yes
Brand Name: Mexitil

BENEFITS versus RISKS	
Possible Benefits	*Possible Risks*
EFFECTIVE TREATMENT IN SELECTED HEART RHYTHM DISORDERS	NARROW TREATMENT RANGE FREQUENT ADVERSE EFFECTS WORSENING OF SOME ARRHYTHMIAS Rare seizures, liver injury, and reduced white blood cell count

▷ **Principal Uses**

As a Single Drug Product: Uses currently included in FDA-approved labeling: Helps correct premature beats that arise in the ventricles (lower heart chambers) which are resistant (refractory) to other agents.

Other (unlabeled) generally accepted uses: (1) Eases pain in some pain syndromes (diabetic neuropathy); (2) combination therapy of Wolf-Parkinson-White syndrome.

How This Drug Works: Slows transmission of electrical impulses in the heart, restoring normal heart rate and rhythm in selected types of arrhythmia.

Available Dose Forms and Strengths

Capsules — 150 mg, 200 mg, 250 mg
Gelcap — 100 mg, 200 mg (Canada)

▷ **Usual Adult Dose Range:**   Loading dose of 400 mg is given, then 200 mg every 8 hours. Dose can be increased (every 2 to 3 days), as needed and tolerated in 50- or 100-mg steps. Daily maximum is 1200 mg. Testing blood levels is advised (when available) schedule. **Note: Actual dose and schedule must be determined for each patient individually.**

Conditions Requiring Dosing Adjustments

Liver Function: Dose should be decreased by one-fourth to one-third in liver disease.

Kidney Function: Dose is decreased and blood levels obtained more often.

▷ **Dosing Instructions:**   The capsule may be opened and taken with food or antacid to reduce stomach irritation. Take at same times each day to obtain uniform results.

Usual Duration of Use: Use on a regular schedule for 1 to 2 weeks determines effectiveness in correcting or preventing responsive rhythm disorders. Long-term use requires physician supervision.

▷ **This Drug Should Not Be Taken If**
- you have had an allergic reaction to it previously.
- you have second- or third-degree heart block (determined by electrocardiogram), uncorrected by a pacemaker.

▷ **Inform Your Physician Before Taking This Drug If**
- you had adverse reactions to other antiarrhythmic drugs.
- you have a history of heart disease of any kind, especially "heart block" or heart failure.
- you have impaired liver function.
- you have Parkinson's disease.
- you are prone to low blood pressure or have a seizure disorder of any kind.
- you take digitalis, a potassium supplement, or any diuretic drug that can cause potassium loss (ask your doctor).

Possible Side Effects (natural, expected, and unavoidable drug actions)

Nervousness, light-headedness. Unpleasant taste.

▷ **Possible Adverse Effects** (unusual, unexpected, and infrequent reactions)

If any of the following develop, consult your physician promptly for guidance.

Mild Adverse Effects

Allergic Reaction: Skin rash.

Headache, dizziness, visual disturbance, fatigue, weakness, tremor—infrequent.

Loss of appetite, indigestion, nausea, vomiting, constipation, diarrhea, abdominal pain—rare.

Serious Adverse Effects

Idiosyncratic reactions: depression, confusion, amnesia, hallucinations, seizures—all rare.

Drug-induced heart rhythm disorders: shortness of breath, palpitations, chest pain, swelling—rare.

Myelofibrosis or systemic lupus erythematosus—case reports.

Seizures—case reports.

Ataxia and confusion—may be frequent.

Congestive heart failure and sinus arrest—rare.

Urinary retention—possible.

Liver damage with jaundice (see Glossary)—case reports.

Low white blood cell or platelet counts: fever, sore throat, abnormal bleeding/bruising—case reports.

▷ **Possible Effects on Sexual Function:**   Decreased libido, impotence—rare.

▷ **Adverse Effects That May Mimic Natural Diseases or Disorders**
Liver toxicity may suggest viral hepatitis.

Natural Diseases or Disorders That May Be Activated by This Drug
Latent epilepsy.

Possible Effects on Laboratory Tests
Blood white cell and platelet counts: decreased.
Liver function tests: increased liver enzymes (ALT/GPT, AST/GOT) increased
in less than 1% of users.

CAUTION
1. Thorough evaluation of your heart function (including electrocardiograms) is necessary prior to using this drug.
2. Periodic evaluation of your heart function is needed to determine your response to this drug. Some individuals may experience worsening of their
heart rhythm disorder and/or deterioration of heart function. Close monitoring of heart rate, rhythm, and overall performance is essential.
3. Dose must be adjusted carefully for each person. Do not change your
dose without talking to your doctor.
4. Do not take any other antiarrhythmic drug while taking this drug unless
you are directed to do so by your physician.
5. Carry a card in your purse or wallet saying that you take this drug. Tell
any health care providers that you take it.

Precautions for Use
By Infants and Children: Safety and effectiveness for those under 12 years of age
are not established. Initial use of this drug requires hospitalization and supervision by a qualified cardiologist.
By Those Over 60 Years of Age: Reduced liver function may require reduction in
dose. Watch carefully for light-headedness, dizziness, unsteadiness, and a
tendency to fall.

▷ **Advisability of Use During Pregnancy**
Pregnancy Category: C. See Pregnancy Risk Categories at the back of this book.
Animal studies: No birth defects reported in mice, rats, or rabbits. However,
an increased rate of fetal resorption was found.
Human studies: Adequate studies of pregnant women are not available.
Avoid during first 3 months. Use this drug only if clearly needed. Ask your
physician for guidance.

Advisability of Use If Breast-Feeding
Presence of this drug in breast milk: Yes.
Avoid drug or refrain from nursing.

Habit-Forming Potential: None.

Effects of Overdose: Impaired urination, constipation, marked drop in blood
pressure, abnormal heart rhythms, congestive heart failure, dizziness, incoordination, seizures.

Possible Effects of Long-Term Use: None reported.

Suggested Periodic Examinations While Taking This Drug (at physician's discretion)
Electrocardiograms, complete blood cell counts, liver function tests, mexiletine blood levels.

▷ **While Taking This Drug, Observe the Following**

Foods: No restrictions. Ask your physician regarding need for salt restriction.

Beverages: Caffeine may have an effect on heart rate, and may not be desirable. Talk to your doctor about caffeine. Can take with milk.

▷ *Alcohol:* Use caution. Alcohol can increase the blood-pressure-lowering effects of this drug.

Tobacco Smoking: Nicotine irritates the heart, reducing drug effectiveness. I advise everyone to quit smoking.

▷ *Other Drugs*

Mexiletine may ***increase*** the effects of

- antihypertensive drugs, and cause excessive lowering of blood pressure.
- beta-blocker drugs (see Drug Classes).
- disopyramide (Norpace).
- theophylline (Theo-Dur, others), leading to theophylline toxicity and seizures.

Mexiletine ***taken concurrently*** with

- ritonavir (Norvir) and perhaps other protease inhibitors (see Drug Classes) may lead to toxicity.

The following drugs may ***decrease*** the effects of mexiletine:

- phenytoin (Dilantin, etc.).
- rifampin (Rifadin, Rimactane).

▷ *Driving, Hazardous Activities:* This drug may cause weakness, dizziness, or blurred vision. Restrict activities as necessary.

Aviation Note: The use of this drug ***may be a disqualification*** for piloting. Consult a designated aviation medical examiner.

Exposure to Sun: No restrictions.

Occurrence of Unrelated Illness: Vomiting, diarrhea, or dehydration can affect this drug's action adversely. Report such developments promptly.

Discontinuation: Should not be stopped abruptly after long-term use. Ask your doctor about slowly reducing the dose.

MIBEFRADIL (mi BEF rah dill)

Introduced: 1997   **Class:** Antihypertensive, calcium channel blocker
Author's note: This medicine has been withdrawn from the market.

MINIMALLY SEDATING ANTIHISTAMINE FAMILY

Astemizole (a STEM ah zohl)   **Cetirizine** (sa TEER a zeen)   **Fexofenadine** (fen oh FAX a deen)   **Loratadine** (lor AT a deen)   **Terfenadine** (ter FEN a deen)

Introduced: 1982, 1996, 1996, 1992, 1977, respectively   **Class:** Antihistamines, minimally sedating   **Prescription:** USA: Yes   **Controlled Drugs:** USA: No; Canada: No   **Available as Generic:** USA: Astemizole: Yes; cetirizine: no; fexofenadine: no; loratadine: yes; terfenadine: yes; Canada: Same as USA

Brand Names: Astemizole: Hismanal; Cetirizine: Zyrtec; Fexofenadine: Allegra, Allegra-D; Loratadine: ✢Chlor-Tripolon ND [CD], Claritin, Claritin D [CD], ✢Claritin Extra, Claritin Reditabs [CD]; Terfenadine: Seldane, Seldane-D

Author's Note: Terfenadine has been voluntarily removed from the market. Therefore, terfenadine data has been removed from this profile. Some other drugs in this class have life-threatening drug interactions. Loratadine interacts with some antibiotics and antifungals, but HAS NOT shown the same effect on the heart (in studies of otherwise healthy young and subsequently older subjects), but does undergo an increased blood level if combined with these medicines. It would appear prudent to decrease the dose of loratadine if it is to be combined with these medicines. Current FDA labeling DOES NOT require a warning found in package inserts for some other drugs in this family.

BENEFITS versus RISKS	
Possible Benefits	*Possible Risks*
EFFECTIVE AND LONG-LASTING RELIEF OF ALLERGIC RHINITIS	RARE HEART RHYTHM DISTURBANCES (HAVE OCCURRED AS A DRUG INTERACTION EFFECT OR AS A DRUG EFFECT) (astemizole, fexofenadine, loratadine)
EFFECTIVE RELIEF OF SOME ALLERGIC SKIN DISORDERS	
MINIMAL DROWSINESS	
MINOR TO NO ANTICHOLINERGIC SIDE EFFECTS	Low white blood cell count (leukopenia) (1.4% of fexofenadine patients)
	Slight atropinelike effects (some medicines in this class)
	Mild sedation or fatigue

▷ **Principal Uses**

As a Single Drug Product: Uses currently included in FDA-approved labeling: (1) Used to treat non-nasal and nasal symptoms of seasonal allergic rhinitis (hay fever); (2) helps ease symptoms of rhinitis; (3) used to treat swellings of unknown origin (idiopathic urticaria) (astemizole, cetirizine, loratadine); (4) helps ease symptoms of pollen-induced asthma (astemizole, cetirizine, loratadine.

Other (unlabeled) generally accepted uses: (1) Lichen nitidus lesions (astemizole); (2) can help control chronic vertigo (astemizole); (3) chronic idiopathic urticaria (astemizole, loratadine); (4) food allergies (cetirizine).

How These Drugs Work: These medicines block histamine, stopping symptoms (caused by histamine), such as swelling and itching of the eyes.

Available Dose Forms and Strengths

Astemizole:

Tablets — 10 mg
Oral suspension (Canada only) — 2 mg/ml

Cetirizine:

Tablets — 5 mg, 10 mg

Fexofenadine:

Capsules — 60 mg
Tablets, extended release — 60 mg fexofenadine
— 120 mg pseudoephedrine

Loratadine:

Syrup	— 10 mg/ml
Tablets	— 10 mg
Tablets, repeat action (Claritin-D [CD])	— 5 mg loratadine, 120 mg pseudoephedrine
Tablets, extended release (Claritin-D 24-hour)	— 10 mg loratadine, 240 mg pseudoephedrine

▷ **Recommended Dose Ranges** (Actual dose and schedule must be determined for each patient individually.)

Infants and Children: **Safety and efficacy in those less than 12 years old has only been established for cetirizine, not for the rest of the medicines in this family.** Cetirizine (Zyrtec) is approved for children 2 to 5 years old who have seasonal or perennial allergic rhinitis or hives (idiopathic urticaria) of unknown cause.

12 to 60 Years of Age: Astemizole: 10 mg per day. This is also the maximum daily dose.

Cetirizine: The starting dose is 5 mg (depending on severity, may be 10 mg) and is increased as needed and tolerated to a maximum of 20 mg daily.

Fexofenadine: 60 mg twice daily.

Loratadine: A single 10-mg tablet (of the nonrepeat action, noncombination product) is taken once daily. Loratadine/pseudoephedrine (5 mg/120 mg) (nonrepeat action): One tablet twice daily. Loratadine/pseudoephedrine (10 mg/240 mg) (repeat action): One tablet daily.

Over 60 Years of Age: Fexofenadine, loratadine (Claritin-D and Claritin-D 24-hour forms) are NOT recommended for those over 60. Prudent to decrease cetirizine doses as the drug is slowly removed at this age.

Conditions Requiring Dosing Adjustments

Liver Function: Astemizole: NOT to be used in severe liver disease. Dosing guidelines are not available.

Cetirizine: A 5-mg dose is recommended.

Fexofenadine: Dosing changes do not appear to be needed.

Loratadine: Patients with liver compromise take a dose of 10 mg (of the nonrepeat action, noncombination product) every other day.

Kidney Function: Astemizole: No dosing changes appear to be needed.

Cetirizine: Patients with moderate kidney decline (creatinine clearance 11–31 ml/min) may take 5 mg daily.

Fexofenadine: A dose of 60 mg once daily is recommended.

Loratadine: Patients with moderate kidney failure (creatinine clearance less than 30 ml/min) get a starting dose of 10 mg (of nonrepeat action, noncombination product) every other day.

▷ **Dosing Instructions:** Astemizole and loratadine are best taken on an empty stomach. The other medicines in this class may be taken with food. Extended-release forms of these medicines should never be crushed.

Usual Duration of Use: Although all of these medicines may go to work immediately, regular use for up to 1 day (fexofenadine), up to 2 days (astemizole or cetirizine), and up to 3 days (loratadine) may be needed to see substantial symptom improvement. Long-term use requires evaluation of response by your doctor.

Possible Advantages of These Drugs   Less sedating than previously available antihistamines. Once-daily dosing for some agents in this class. Some medicines in this class do not interact with certain antifungals and macrolide antibiotics (see Drug Classes), or do interact but do not appear to cause side effects on the heart or change the safety profile. Cetirizine has NOT had ANY case reports of QTc prolongation. Tachyphylaxis or tolerance may be less likely to occur to these medicines than with earlier agents. Fexofenadine also appears to avoid the QTc interval problems of other drugs in this family.

Currently "Drugs of Choice"

For patients who must take antihistamine-type medicines and require the best possible balance of symptom relief and minimal sedation.

▷ **These Drugs Should Not Be Taken If**
- you have had an allergic reaction to any dose form of the drug or any of the ingredients in it previously.
- you are presently being tested (using skin tests) for allergies.
- you are taking medicines that prolong the QT interval, such as quinidine, pentamidine, disopyramide, or others (for astemizole, cetirizine, fexofenadine, and terfenadine).
- you have urinary retention, liver disease, severe disease of the arteries of the heart (coronary artery disease), or narrow-angle glaucoma (loratadine combination products that contain pseudoephedrine).

▷ **Inform Your Physician Before Taking These Drugs If**
- you have asthma.
- you are at risk for drowsiness or fainting (syncope).
- you have a history of a heart rhythm disorder.
- you are taking other medicines (especially antifungal or macrolide antibiotics). Blood levels of loratadine or fexofenadine may be increased. Decreases in loratadine and fexofenadine doses may be prudent. Astemizole should NOT be combined with these medicines.
- you have a history of liver or kidney compromise.
- you are pregnant.

Possible Side Effects (natural, expected, and unavoidable drug actions)

Dry nose, mouth, or throat; somnolence (drowsiness): cetirizine—frequent, fexofenadine—rare, loratadine-infrequent.

▷ **Possible Adverse Effects** (unusual, unexpected, and infrequent reactions)

If any of the following develop, consult your physician promptly for guidance.

Mild Adverse Effects

Allergic reactions: skin rash, itching.

Headache, fatigue, or dizziness—infrequent.

Dry mouth—possible to infrequent.

Leg cramps, muscle aches (astemizole or loratadine)—rare.

Fast heart rate (tachycardia) (loratadine)—rare.

Prolonged QTc interval (astemizole)—possible if used in people with existing heart disease.

Lowering of the blood pressure (loratadine)—rare.

Vision changes (loratadine)—rare.

Serious Adverse Effects

Allergic reactions: anaphylaxis (astemizole or loratadine)—rare.

Idiosyncratic reactions: not reported.
Serious heart rhythm disorders: astemizole—rare; loratadine—case report.
Tachycardia—rare.
Lowering of the white blood cell count (fexofenadine)—rare.
Abnormal liver function (loratadine)—case reports.
Depression, confusion, paresthesias—rare.
Passing out (syncope)—rare.

▷ **Possible Effects on Sexual Function:**   Vaginitis, painful menses (dysmenorrhea), breast enlargement or breast pain (loratadine)—case reports. Menstrual disorders (loratadine, fexofenadine)—case reports.
Galactorrhea (loratadine)—case reports.
Impotence (loratadine)—case reports.

Possible Delayed Adverse Effects: None reported.

▷ **Adverse Effects That May Mimic Natural Diseases or Disorders**
Increased liver enzymes may mimic hepatitis of infectious origin.

Natural Diseases or Disorders That May Be Activated by These Drugs
None reported.

Possible Effects on Laboratory Tests
Skin tests for allergies will be blunted and less diagnostic.
Liver function tests: may be increased (loratadine or terfenadine).
White blood cell counts: decreased (leukopenia) (fexofenadine)—rare in clin-
ical trials.

CAUTION
1. Loratadine does interact with some antifungals and some macrolide antibiotics—but appears to be free of the heart (cardiac) effects, even though
blood levels of loratadine may increase if it is taken with these interacting medicines. Talk to your doctor or pharmacist before taking any medicines that were not discussed when loratadine was prescribed.
2. Some of these medicines HAVE LIFE-THREATENING DRUG INTERAC-
TIONS. Talk to your doctor or pharmacist BEFORE combining any prescription, nonprescription, or herbal remedies with medicines in this class.
3. Report dizziness, heart palpitation, or chest pain promptly when using
any of these medicines.
4. Astemizole use should be discussed with your doctor if you have any degree of heart disease.

Precautions for Use
By Infants and Children: Safety and effectiveness for use by those under 12 years
of age have not been established.
By Those Over 60 Years of Age: Smaller starting and maintenance doses are
needed. Longer dosing intervals may be needed as well.

▷ **Advisability of Use During Pregnancy**
Pregnancy Category: B (cetirizine, loratadine); C (astemizole, fexofenadine). See
Pregnancy Risk Categories at the back of this book.
Animal studies: No birth defects reported.
Human studies: Information from adequate studies of pregnant women is
not available.
These medicines should be used during pregnancy only if clearly needed. Dis-
cuss the benefits versus risks with your doctor.

Advisability of Use If Breast-Feeding

Presence of this drug in breast milk: No data (cetirizine, fexofenadine); expected (astemizole); yes (loratadine).

Ask your doctor for guidance regarding stopping the drug or stopping nursing (astemizole, cetirizine, fexofenadine, or loratadine).

Habit-Forming Potential: None.

Effects of Overdose: With overdoses greater than 10 mg (40–80 mg): tachycardia, somnolence, and headache (loratadine).

Usual antihistamine protocols (cetirizine or fexofenadine).

Possible life-threatening heart rhythm problems (astemizole).

Possible Effects of Long-Term Use: None defined.

Suggested Periodic Examinations While Taking These Drugs (at physician's discretion)

Examination for relief of the condition(s) being treated. Electrocardiogram (ECG), especially for those with heart conditions.

▷ **While Taking These Drugs, Observe the Following**

Foods: Astemizole and loratadine are best taken on an empty stomach.

Beverages: Grapefruit juice may lead to increased blood levels of astemizole and lead to toxicity. Water is the best liquid to take with medicines in this class.

▷ *Alcohol:* May cause excessive drowsiness (central nervous system depression).

Tobacco Smoking: No interactions expected. I advise everyone to quit smoking.

Marijuana Smoking: May cause additive drowsiness or lethargy.

▷ *Other Drugs*

These medicines *taken concurrently* with

- cimetidine (Tagamet) may produce a significant increase in loratadine blood levels. No serious drug effects have been reported, but since in general the frequency of adverse effects increases with increasing blood levels, it appears prudent to decrease the dose of loratadine if these medicines are to be taken at the same time because of possible loratadine toxicity. The loratadine dose should certainly be decreased if increased frequency of adverse effects occur if these medicines are combined in usual doses. Astemizole may also react.
- fluoxetine (Prozac) produced a serious heart rhythm problem in a patient taking terfenadine. DO NOT combine these medicines. Caution is advised for the other drugs in this class.
- fluvoxamine (Luvox) may result in increased blood levels of astemizole, cetirizine, or loratadine. Caution is advised.
- grepafloxacin (Raxar) may increase risk of heart rhythm problems (astemizole). DO NOT combine these medicines.
- indinavir (Crixivan), and perhaps ritonavir, saquinavir, or nelfinavir, may decrease metabolism of astemizole, and should NEVER be combined. Loratadine levels may be increased, and doses may need to be lowered. Other drugs in this family may also be affected.
- itraconazole (and perhaps other similarly structured antifungals such as ketoconazole) should NEVER be combined with astemizole. These drugs may cause increased blood levels of loratadine. Although no serious heart

rhythm toxicity has been reported to date with this medicine, caution is advised, and it appears prudent to lower the dose of loratadine.

- macrolide antibiotics such as azithromycin, clarithromycin, or erythromycin **must never be combined with astemizole**. Although no serious heart rhythm toxicity has been reported to date with loratadine, caution is advised as excessive blood levels of any medicine may increase risk of adverse effects. It appears prudent to lower the dose of loratadine.
- medicines that prolong the QT interval (such as disopyramide, ibutilide, quinolones [grepafloxacin, sparfloxacin], and others) should be avoided. Cetirizine is the only medicine in this class without any reports of QTc interval changes.
- mibefradil (Posicor) may increase astemizole levels.
- paroxetine (Paxil) may inhibit the enzymes needed to remove astemizole, cetirizine or loratadine. Caution is advised.
- quinidine (Quinaglute, others) may result in a change in the effect of quinidine and result in undesirable effects on the heart. Caution is advised.
- ritonavir (Norvir), and perhaps other protease inhibitors(see Drug Classes), may increase blood levels and toxicity.
- sotalol (Betapace) may cause additive adverse effects (QT interval prolongation) on the heart by these medicines. This combination is not recommended.
- theophylline (Theo-Dur, others) may decrease cetirizine clearance. This combination should be avoided.
- zafirlukast (Accolate), if combined with terfenadine may decrease zafirlukast levels and blunt the therapeutic benefits of zafirlukast (and perhaps zileuton—Zyflo).

▷ *Driving, Hazardous Activities:* Although these medicines are much less likely than earlier antihistamines to cause drowsiness, caution should be used until your individual reaction to these medicines is determined. Restrict activities as necessary.

Aviation Note: The use of these drugs *are probably not a disqualification* for piloting. Consult a designated aviation medical examiner.

Exposure to Sun: Rare cases of photosensitivity have been reported with some medicines (astemizole, loratadine) in this class. Use caution.

MINOXIDIL (min OX i dil)

Introduced: 1972 **Class:** Antihypertensive, hair growth stimulant **Prescription:** USA: Yes **Controlled Drug:** USA: No; Canada: No **Available as Generic:** Yes

Brand Names: Alostil, Loniten, Minodyl, Minoximen, Rogaine, Rogaine Extra Strength

Author's Note: Rogaine treatment for baldness is available without a prescription.

BENEFITS versus RISKS

Possible Benefits | *Possible Risks*

Possible Benefits	*Possible Risks*
POTENT, LONG-ACTING ANTIHYPERTENSIVE	EXCESSIVE BODY HAIR GROWTH
EFFECTIVE IN CASES OF SEVERE HYPERTENSION, ACCELERATED AND MALIGNANT HYPERTENSION	SALT AND WATER RETENTION
Moderately effective in treating male pattern baldness	Excessively rapid heart rate
	Aggravation of angina
	Local scalp irritation (topical use)

▷ **Principal Uses**

As a Single Drug Product: Uses currently included in FDA-approved labeling: (1) Treats severe high blood pressure not controlled by conventional therapy; (2) treats female androgenic baldness or male pattern baldness; (3) effective in patients with high blood pressure and kidney failure.

Other (unlabeled) generally accepted uses: Supportive therapy in hair transplants.

How This Drug Works: (1) Relaxes constricted muscles in walls of small arteries, and permits expansion of the arteries and lower blood pressure. (2) May act directly on the hair follicle, and also may increase size of previously closed small scalp blood vessels, and restoring small hair follicles to normal size and activity.

Available Dose Forms and Strengths

Tablets — 2.5 mg, 10 mg

Topical solution — 2%, 5% (Extra Strength)

▷ **Usual Adult Dose Range:**   For hypertension: Initially 5 mg once a day. The dose is then gradually increased as needed and tolerated to 10 mg, 20 mg, then 40 mg every 24 hours, taken in one or two divided doses daily. The usual ongoing dose is 10 to 40 mg daily. Daily maximum is 50 mg.

For male pattern baldness: Apply thinly 1 ml of topical solution to the balding area of the scalp twice daily. The total daily dose should not exceed 2 ml.

Note: Actual dose and schedule must be determined for each patient individually.

Conditions Requiring Dosing Adjustments

Liver Function: This drug is metabolized (90%) in the liver. It should be used with caution by patients with liver compromise.

Kidney Function: In moderate kidney failure, the dose should be decreased empirically.

▷ **Dosing Instructions:**   For hypertension: Tablets may be crushed and taken with or following food to prevent nausea. Take at the same time each day.

For baldness: ***The topical solution is for external, local use only; it is not to be swallowed.*** Begin application at the center of the bald area; apply thinly to cover the entire area. The scalp and hair must be dry at the time of application. Follow instructions carefully.

Usual Duration of Use: Use on a regular schedule for 3 to 7 days usually determines effectiveness in controlling severe hypertension. Continual use of the topical solution for at least 4 months is necessary to determine its ability to promote hair growth. Long-term use (months to years) of both dose forms requires physician supervision.

▷ **This Drug Should Not Be Taken If**
- you have had an allergic reaction to it previously.
- you are known to have a pheochromocytoma (an adrenaline-producing tumor).
- you have pulmonary hypertension due to mitral valve stenosis.

▷ **Inform Your Physician Before Taking This Drug If**
- you are pregnant or planning a pregnancy.
- you are breast-feeding your infant.
- you have had a heart attack.
- you have existing blood vessel disease in your head (cerebrovascular disease).
- you have a history of coronary artery disease or impaired heart function.
- you have a history of stroke or impaired brain circulation.
- you have impaired liver or kidney function.

Possible Side Effects (natural, expected, and unavoidable drug actions)
Increased heart rate, fluid retention with weight gain; excessive hair growth on face, arms, legs, and back (frequent).

▷ **Possible Adverse Effects** (unusual, unexpected, and infrequent reactions)
If any of the following develop, consult your physician promptly for guidance.
Mild Adverse Effects
Allergic reactions: skin rash. Localized dermatitis at site of application of topical solution—rare.
Headache, dizziness, fainting—rare.
Nausea, increased thirst—infrequent.
Hair growth, and changes in hair color—case reports.
Weight gain—possible.
Mild increase in liver enzymes—infrequent.
Serious Adverse Effects
Allergic reactions: serious skin rash (Stevens-Johnson syndrome).
Idiosyncratic Reaction: Fluid formation around the heart (pericardial effusion).
Development of angina pectoris; high blood pressure in the lungs (pulmonary hypertension)—case reports.
Systemic lupus erythematosus—case reports.
Low white blood cells or platelets—rare and transient.
Author's Note: Topical use of this medicine for hair growth may avoid most of these adverse effects.

▷ **Possible Effects on Sexual Function:** Male breast tenderness (gynecomastia)—case reports. Some data to support that this drug balances male ability to ejaculate and have a healthy sex drive may have been blunted by other drugs that treat high blood pressure.

Natural Diseases or Disorders That May Be Activated by This Drug
Latent coronary artery disease with symptomatic angina.

Possible Effects on Laboratory Tests
Blood HDL cholesterol level: increased.
Blood LDL cholesterol level: decreased.

CAUTION
1. Long-term use for hypertension usually requires use of a diuretic to counteract salt and water retention.
2. The long-term use of this drug for hypertension may require concurrent use of a beta-blocker drug to control excessive acceleration of the heart.
3. It is best to avoid combining this drug and guanethidine; the combination can cause severe orthostatic hypotension (see Glossary).
4. Consult your physician regarding the advisability of using a "no-salt-added" diet.
5. Little of this drug is absorbed into the general circulation when the topical solution is applied to the scalp. However, some systemic effects have been reported. Inform your physician promptly if you experience any unusual symptoms while using the topical solution.

Precautions for Use
By Infants and Children: Dose schedules should be determined by a qualified pediatrician. In children under 12 years old: starting dose is 0.2 mg per kg of body mass in a single dose. Dose is then increased as needed and tolerated by 0.1 to 0.2 mg per kg per day steps at 3-day intervals. Children over 12 are given the adult dose. Monitor closely for salt and water retention.
By Those Over 60 Years of Age: Treatment with small doses and a limit of total daily dose to 75 mg is indicated. Headache, palpitation, and rapid heart rate due to this drug are more common in this age group and can mimic acute anxiety states. Observe for dizziness, unsteadiness, fainting, and falling.

▷ Advisability of Use During Pregnancy
Pregnancy Category: C. See Pregnancy Risk Categories at the back of this book.
Animal studies: No birth defects reported in rats or rabbits. However, studies did reveal decreased fertility and increased fetal deaths.
Human studies: Adequate studies of pregnant women are not available.
Avoid during the first 3 months. Use only if clearly needed during the final 6 months.

Advisability of Use If Breast-Feeding
Presence of this drug in breast milk: Yes.
Avoid drug or refrain from nursing.

Habit-Forming Potential: None.

Effects of Overdose: Headache, dizziness, weakness, nausea, marked low blood pressure, weak and rapid pulse, loss of consciousness.

Possible Effects of Long-Term Use: Excessive growth of body hair occurs in 80% of users after 1 to 2 months of continual treatment for hypertension. Close to 100% of users will experience this effect after 1 year of continual treatment. This may be accompanied by darkening of the skin and coarsening of facial features.

Suggested Periodic Examinations While Taking This Drug (at physician's discretion)
Body weight measurement for insidious gain due to water retention.
Electrocardiographic and echocardiographic heart examinations.

▷ While Taking This Drug, Observe the Following
Foods: Avoid excessive salt and heavily salted foods.
Beverages: No restrictions. May be taken with milk.

▷ *Alcohol:* Use with extreme caution. Alcohol can exaggerate the blood-pressure-lowering effects of this drug.

Tobacco Smoking: Best avoided. Nicotine can contribute significantly to angina. I advise everyone to quit smoking.

▷ *Other Drugs*

Minoxidil may *increase* the effects of
- all other antihypertensive drugs; careful dose adjustments are mandatory.

Minoxidil *taken concurrently* with
- guanethidine (Ismelin, Esimil) may cause severe orthostatic hypotension; avoid this combination.
- NSAIDs may blunt the therapeutic benefit of minoxidil.
- vitamin E may reverse hair growth.

▷ *Driving, Hazardous Activities:* This drug may cause dizziness and fatigue. Restrict activities as necessary.

Aviation Note: The use of this drug *is a disqualification* for piloting. Consult a designated aviation medical examiner.

Exposure to Sun: No restrictions.

Discontinuation: This drug should not be stopped abruptly. If it is to be discontinued, consult your physician regarding gradual reduction in dose and appropriate replacement with other drugs for the management of hypertension. Following discontinuation of the topical solution, the pretreatment pattern of baldness may return within 3 to 4 months.

MIRTAZAPINE (mur TAZ a peen)

Introduced: 1996   **Class:** Antidepressant, piperazinoazepine, norepinephrine serotonin reuptake inhibitor   **Prescription:** USA: Yes   **Controlled Drug:** USA: No; Canada: No   **Available as Generic:** USA: No; Canada: No   **Brand Name:** Remeron

BENEFITS versus RISKS	
Possible Benefits	*Possible Risks*
EFFECTIVE TREATMENT OF DEPRESSION	Sleepiness
BENEFICIAL ACTION ON TWO NERVE TRANSMITTERS	Weight gain
	Lowering of white blood cells

▷ **Principal Uses**

As a Single Drug Product: Uses currently included in FDA-approved labeling: Treatment of depression.

Other (unlabeled) generally accepted uses: Presurgical insomnia.

How This Drug Works: Increases two nerve transmitters (norepinephrine and serotonin) that are thought to be low or lowered in cases of depression.

Available Dose Forms and Strengths

Tablets — 15 mg, 30 mg

▷ **Recommended Dose Ranges** (Actual dose and schedule must be determined for each patient individually.)

Infants and Children: Dose not established.

18 to 60 Years of Age: For treatment of adult depression: 15 to 45 mg at bedtime.
Over 60 Years of Age: Removed more slowly from the body. Lower doses are prudent.

Conditions Requiring Dosing Adjustments
Liver Function: Lower doses and slow dose increases are needed.
Kidney Function: Lower doses and slow dose increases are needed.

▷ **Dosing Instructions:**   The tablet may be crushed and can be taken with or without food. Take it at the same time daily.

Usual Duration of Use: Use on a regular schedule for 1 week will usually start to show benefits in relieving depression. Peak effect may take several weeks to be seen. Long-term use (months to years) requires follow up by your doctor.

Possible Advantages of This Drug
Less likely to cause dry mouth, constipation, urinary retention, orthostatic hypotension (see Glossary), and heart rhythm disturbances than tricyclic antidepressants.
Does not cause Parkinson-like reactions.

▷ **This Drug Should Not Be Taken If**
• you have had an allergic reaction to it previously.
• you are currently taking, or have taken within the past 14 days, any monoamine oxidase (MAO) type A inhibitor drug (see Drug Classes).

▷ **Inform Your Physician Before Taking This Drug If**
• you have experienced any adverse effects from antidepressant drugs.
• you have impaired liver or kidney function.
• you have Parkinson's disease.
• you have had a recent heart attack.
• you have a seizure disorder.
• you are pregnant or plan a pregnancy while taking this drug.

Possible Side Effects (natural, expected, and unavoidable drug actions)
Increased appetite, weight gain. Lower blood pressure on standing (see orthostatic hypotension in Glossary).

▷ **Possible Adverse Effects** (unusual, unexpected, and infrequent reactions)
If any of the following develop, consult your physician promptly for guidance.
Mild Adverse Effects
Allergic reactions: skin rash, itching—rare.
Headache, nervousness, insomnia—rare to infrequent.
Fatigue and dry mouth—frequent.
Tremor, dizziness, abnormal dreams—rare.
Abnormal vision, numbness, and tingling—rare; confusion—rare; hallucinations—rare.
Chest pain and increased blood pressure—rare.
Increased heart rate—infrequent.
Altered taste, nausea, vomiting, diarrhea—rare to infrequent.
Serious Adverse Effects
Allergic reactions: dermatitis (various forms)—rare.
Drug-induced seizures—case reports.
Increased blood cholesterol (hypercholesterolemia)—infrequent.
Agranulocytosis—case reports.

▷ **Possible Effects on Sexual Function:** Male sexual dysfunction: Delayed ejaculation—infrequent.

Female sexual dysfunction: inhibited orgasm—rare.

Swelling and tenderness of male and female breast tissue—case reports.

Dysmenorrhea—rare.

Natural Diseases or Disorders That May Be Activated by This Drug

Latent epilepsy.

Possible Effects on Laboratory Tests

Blood total cholesterol and triglyceride levels: increased—infrequent.

Liver function tests: increased liver enzymes (ALT/GPT, AST/GOT, and alkaline phosphatase).

Blood cell counts: decreased (aplastic anemia)—case reports.

Blood sodium: decreased (with rare SIADH).

CAUTION

1. If any type of skin reaction develops (rash, hives, etc.), discontinue this drug and inform your physician promptly.
2. If dryness of the mouth develops and persists for more than 2 weeks, consult your dentist for guidance.
3. Ask your doctor or pharmacist before taking any other prescription or over-the-counter drug while taking mirtazapine.
4. If you are advised to take any monoamine oxidase (MAO) type A inhibitor drug (see Drug Classes), allow an interval of 5 weeks after discontinuing this drug before starting the MAO inhibitor.
5. It is advisable to withhold this drug if electroconvulsive therapy (ECT, or "shock" treatment) is to be used to treat your depression.

Precautions for Use

By Infants and Children: Safety and effectiveness for those under 12 years of age are not established.

By Those Over 60 Years of Age: The lowest effective dose should be used for maintenance treatment and adjusted as needed for reduced kidney function.

▷ **Advisability of Use During Pregnancy**

Pregnancy Category: C. See Pregnancy Risk Categories at the back of this book.

Animal studies: Delayed bone development due to this drug found in rat and rabbit studies.

Human studies: Adequate studies of pregnant women are not available.

Use this drug only if clearly needed. Ask your physician for guidance.

Advisability of Use If Breast-Feeding

Presence of this drug in breast milk: Unknown.

Avoid drug or refrain from nursing.

Habit-Forming Potential: None.

Effects of Overdose: Agitation, restlessness, excitement, nausea, vomiting, seizures.

Possible Effects of Long-Term Use: None reported.

Suggested Periodic Examinations While Taking This Drug (at physician's discretion)

None.

▷ **While Taking This Drug, Observe the Following**
    Foods: No restrictions.
    Beverages: No restrictions. May be taken with milk.
▷   *Alcohol:* Avoid completely.
    Tobacco Smoking: No interactions expected. I advise everyone to quit smoking.
▷   *Other Drugs*
    Mirtazapine *taken concurrently* with
- diazepam (Valium), and perhaps other benzodiazepines (see Drug Classes), may increase impaired coordination (psychomotor impairment). Caution is advised.
- monoamine oxidase (MAO) type A inhibitor drugs may cause confusion, agitation, high fever, seizures, and dangerous elevations of blood pressure. Avoid the concurrent use of these drugs.
- ritonavir (Norvir), and perhaps other protease inhibitors (see Drug Classes), may lead to toxicity.

▷ *Driving, Hazardous Activities:* This drug may cause drowsiness, dizziness, impaired judgment, and altered vision. Restrict activities as necessary.
    Aviation Note: The use of this drug *is a disqualification* for piloting. Consult a designated aviation medical examiner.
    Exposure to Sun: Use caution—this drug may (rarely) cause photosensitivity (see Glossary).
    Discontinuation: The slow elimination of this drug from the body makes it unlikely that any withdrawal effects will result from abrupt discontinuation. However, call your doctor if you plan to stop this drug for any reason.

MISOPROSTOL (mi soh PROH stohl)

Introduced: 1987   **Class:** Gastrointestinal drug (ulcer preventive)   **Prescription:** USA: Yes   **Controlled Drug:** USA: No; Canada: No   **Available as Generic:** USA: No; Canada: No
Brand Names: Arthrotec, Cytotec

BENEFITS versus RISKS	
Possible Benefits	*Possible Risks*
EFFECTIVE PREVENTION OF STOMACH ULCERATION WHILE TAKING ANTI-INFLAMMATORY DRUGS	INCREASED RISK OF ABORTION (if used during pregnancy)
	Diarrhea (transient)
Effective treatment of duodenal ulcer	Neuropathy

▷ **Principal Uses**
    As a Single Drug Product: Uses currently included in FDA-approved labeling: Prevents development of stomach ulcers during long-term use of anti-inflammatory drugs as therapy for arthritis and related conditions.
    Other (unlabeled) generally accepted uses: (1) Used (in Canada and other countries) for treatment of active duodenal ulcer unrelated to use of anti-inflammatory drugs; (2) has some use in inducing abortions; (3) used in combination with cyclosporine or prednisone to decrease transplanted

organ rejection; (4) may have a benefit in helping ripen the cervix in preparation for a vaginal delivery.

As a Combination Drug Product [CD]: Available in combination with diclofenac, an NSAID (see *nonsteroidal anti-inflammatory drug* in Drug Classes). The misoprostol is used to prevent stomach (gastric) irritation or ulceration from the NSAID.

How This Drug Works: Protects lining of the stomach and duodenum by: (1) replacing tissue prostaglandins depleted by anti-inflammatory drugs; (2) inhibits secretion of stomach acid; (3) increases local production of bicarbonate (to neutralize acids) and mucus (to protect stomach and duodenal tissues). Combined effects prevent new ulcers and promote healing of existing ulcer(s).

Arthrotec form: This combination uses the above mechanism of misoprostol to protect from possible ulcers caused by the NSAID diclofenac.

Available Dose Forms and Strengths
Tablets — 100 mcg, 200 mcg
Tablets (Arthrotec) — misoprostol 200 mcg and diclofenac 50 mcg

Conditions Requiring Dosing Adjustments
Liver Function: Specific dose adjustments in liver compromise are not defined.
Kidney Function: The dose of misoprostol should be decreased in kidney disease. See the diclofenac profile for info on diclofenac.

▷ **Usual Adult Dose Range**
For prevention of stomach ulcer: 200 mcg four times daily with food, taken concurrently during the use of any anti-inflammatory drug (see *antiarthritic* or *nonsteroidal anti-inflammatory drugs* in Drug Classes).
For treatment of duodenal ulcer: 200 mcg four times daily for 4 to 8 weeks.
Combination abortions: RU-496 600 mg taken once, followed by 400–600 mcg of misoprostol in one dose or two equal doses.
Rheumatoid arthritis (Arthrotec form): One tablet 2 to 4 times daily.
Note: Actual dose and schedule must be determined for each patient individually.

▷ **Dosing Instructions:**   The tablet may be crushed and taken with each of three daily meals; take the last (fourth) dose of the day with food at bedtime. Arthrotec form should be taken right after a meal or with food or milk. DO NOT crush or alter.

Usual Duration of Use: For prevention of stomach ulcer, use is recommended for the entire period of anti-inflammatory drug use. For treatment of duodenal ulcer, continual use on a regular schedule for 4 weeks is recommended; if ulcer healing is not complete, a second course of 4 weeks is advised. Long-term use (months to years) requires periodic physician evaluation of response and dose adjustment.

Possible Advantages of This Drug: Significantly more effective than histamine (H_2) blocking drugs (cimetidine, famotidine, nizatidine, ranitidine) or sucralfate in preventing the development of stomach ulcers. The Arthrotec combination form may help patients take misoprostol as directed.

▷ **This Drug Should Not Be Taken If**
• you have had an allergic reaction to it previously.
• you are allergic to any type of prostaglandin.

- you are pregnant or breast-feeding.
- you are not able or willing to use effective contraception (oral contraceptives or intrauterine device) while taking this drug.

▷ **Inform Your Physician Before Taking This Drug If**
- you have a history of peptic ulcer disease or Crohn's disease.
- you have inflammatory bowel disease.
- you have impaired kidney function.
- you have a seizure disorder.

Possible Side Effects (natural, expected, and unavoidable drug actions)

Diarrhea (14–40% of users), usually beginning after 13 days of use and subsiding spontaneously after 8 days.

Abortion (miscarriage) of pregnancy (11% of users); this is often incomplete and accompanied by serious uterine bleeding that may require hospitalization and urgent treatment.

▷ **Possible Adverse Effects** (unusual, unexpected, and infrequent reactions)

If any of the following develop, consult your physician promptly for guidance.

Mild Adverse Effects

Allergic Reaction: Skin rash.

Headache, dizziness—infrequent.

Ringing in the ears—case reports.

Passing out (syncope)—rare.

Abdominal pain, indigestion, nausea, vomiting, flatulence, constipation—rare to infrequent.

Serious Adverse Effects

Allergic reactions: anaphylaxis—rare.

Anemia and low blood platelets—rare.

Blood in the urine—rare.

Bronchospasm—rare.

Neuropathy—rare.

Autonomic dysreflexia (Arthrotec form)—case reports.

Abortion (if taken while pregnant).

▷ **Possible Effects on Sexual Function:** Menstrual irregularity, menstrual cramps, heavy menstrual flow, spotting between periods—all rare.

Postmenopausal vaginal bleeding; this may require further evaluation.

Reduced libido and impotence—rare and causal relationship not established.

▷ **Natural Diseases or Disorders That May Be Activated by This Drug**

Latent epilepsy.

Possible Effects on Laboratory Tests

Mild increase in liver function enzymes.

CAUTION

1. Do not take this drug if you are pregnant. It can cause abortion.
2. Do not make this drug available to others who may be pregnant or who may become pregnant.
3. If this drug is prescribed, it is advisable that you have a negative serum pregnancy test within 2 weeks before starting treatment.
4. Start taking this drug only on the second or third day of your next normal menstrual period.

5. Initiate effective contraceptive measures when you begin to take this drug. Discuss the use of oral contraceptives or intrauterine devices with your physician.

6. Should you become pregnant, stop the drug immediately and call your doctor.

Precautions for Use

By Infants and Children: Safety and effectiveness for those under 18 years of age not established.

By Those Over 60 Years of Age: This drug is usually well tolerated by this age group. However, some forms of prostaglandins can cause drops in blood pressure; watch for light-headedness or faintness that may indicate low blood pressure. Report any such development to your physician.

▷ **Advisability of Use During Pregnancy**

Pregnancy Category: X. See Pregnancy Risk Categories at the back of this book.

Animal studies: No birth defects due to this drug found in rat or rabbit studies.

Human studies: Information from studies of pregnant women confirms that this drug can cause abortion, sometimes incomplete; unpassed products of conception can cause life-threatening complications.

Avoid this drug completely.

Advisability of Use If Breast-Feeding

Presence of this drug in breast milk: Unknown.

Avoid drug or refrain from nursing.

Habit-Forming Potential: None.

Effects of Overdose: Abdominal pain, diarrhea, fever, drowsiness, weakness, tremor, convulsions, difficult breathing.

Possible Effects of Long-Term Use: Unknown at this time.

Suggested Periodic Examinations While Taking This Drug (at physician's discretion)

Monitoring for accidental pregnancy.

▷ **While Taking This Drug, Observe the Following**

Foods: High-fat meals may reduce peak blood concentration.

Beverages: No restrictions. May be taken with milk.

▷ *Alcohol:* No interactions expected. However, alcohol can promote the development of stomach ulcer and reduce the effectiveness of this drug.

Tobacco Smoking: No interactions expected. Nicotine is conducive to stomach ulcers. I advise everyone to quit smoking.

▷ *Other Drugs*

Misoprostol *taken concurrently* with

- antacids that contain magnesium may increase the risk of diarrhea; avoid this combination. Antacids in general may decrease misoprostol absorption and lessen its therapeutic benefits.
- indomethacin and some other NSAIDs may result in decreased NSAID levels.

▷ *Driving, Hazardous Activities:* This drug may cause dizziness, light-headedness, stomach pain, or diarrhea. Restrict activities as necessary.

Aviation Note: The use of this drug *may be a disqualification* for piloting. Consult a designated aviation medical examiner.

Exposure to Sun: No restrictions.

Discontinuation: This drug should be taken as combination therapy while you are taking antiarthritic/anti-inflammatory drugs that can cause stomach ulceration. Call your doctor if you have reason to stop it prematurely.

MOLINDONE (moh LIN dohn)

Introduced: 1971   **Class:** antipsychotic (strong tranquilizer)   **Prescription:** USA: Yes   **Controlled Drug:** USA: No; Canada: No   **Available as Generic:** No

Brand Name: Moban

BENEFITS versus RISKS	
Possible Benefits	*Possible Risks*
EFFECTIVE TREATMENT OF SOME CASES OF ACUTE AND CHRONIC SCHIZOPHRENIA	NARROW TREATMENT MARGIN SERIOUS TOXIC EFFECTS ON BRAIN:
May be effective in schizophrenia that has not responded to other drugs	Parkinson-like reactions severe restlessness abnormal involuntary movements tardive dyskinesias Liver toxicity, jaundice Atropinelike side effects

▷ **Principal Uses**

As a Single Drug Product: Uses currently included in FDA-approved labeling: (1) Helps manage acute and chronic schizophrenia to control thought disorder, disorientation, hallucinations, perceptual distortions, and hostility.

Other (unlabeled) generally accepted uses: (1) May be of help in children with conduct disorders; (2) may have a small role in helping relieve depression.

How This Drug Works: Acts on nerve transmitters (serotonin and dopamine) to restore the activity in the reticular activating system of the brain, and improve distorted patterns of thinking and behavior.

Available Dose Forms and Strengths

Concentrate — 20 mg/ml

Tablets — 5 mg, 10 mg, 25 mg, 50 mg, 100 mg

▷ **Usual Adult Dose Range:**   Initially 50 to 75 mg daily in three or four divided doses; dose may be increased gradually in 3 days to 100 mg/day as needed and tolerated. For maintenance: mild psychosis—5 to 15 mg, three or four times daily; moderate psychosis—10 to 25 mg three or four times daily; severe psychosis—up to 225 mg/day, in three or four divided doses. Daily maximum is 225 mg. **Note: Actual dose and schedule must be determined for each patient individually.**

Conditions Requiring Dosing Adjustments

Liver Function: Specific dose adjustments in liver compromise are not defined. Used with caution in liver disease—rare cause of liver toxicity (hepatoxicity).

Kidney Function: No dosing changes needed.

▷ **Dosing Instructions:**   The tablet may be crushed and taken with food or milk to reduce stomach irritation. The liquid concentrate may be diluted with water, milk, fruit juice, or carbonated beverages.

Usual Duration of Use: Use on a regular schedule for 3 to 6 weeks is usually necessary to determine this drug's effectiveness in controlling the features of schizophrenia. Long-term use (months to years) requires supervision and periodic evaluation by your physician. Consult your physician on a regular basis.

▷ **This Drug Should Not Be Taken If**
  • you have had an allergic reaction to it previously.
  • you have acute alcoholic intoxication.

▷ **Inform Your Physician Before Taking This Drug If**
  • you are taking any drugs that have sedative effects.
  • you use alcohol excessively.
  • you have any type of seizure disorder.
  • you are pregnant or breast-feeding.
  • you have a history of neuroleptic malignant syndrome.
  • you have any type of glaucoma.
  • you have Parkinson's disease or an enlarged prostate gland.
  • you have impaired liver or kidney function.
  • you have a history of breast cancer.

Possible Side Effects (natural, expected, and unavoidable drug actions)
  Drowsiness, dry mouth, nasal congestion, constipation, impaired urination.
  Parkinson-like reactions (see Glossary). Lowering of blood pressure on standing (orthostatic hypotension), weight gain.

▷ **Possible Adverse Effects** (unusual, unexpected, and infrequent reactions)
  If any of the following develop, consult your physician promptly for guidance.
  Mild Adverse Effects
  Allergic reactions: skin rash.
  Headache, dizziness, blurred vision, lethargy, insomnia, depression, euphoria, ringing in ears—infrequent.
  Rapid heartbeat, low blood pressure, fainting—case reports.
  Loss of appetite, indigestion, nausea—possible.
  Temporary lowering or increase in white blood cells—case reports.
  Serious Adverse Effects
  Allergic reactions: liver reaction with jaundice—rare, questionable.
  Idiosyncratic reactions: neuroleptic malignant syndrome (see Glossary).
  Spasms of face and neck muscles, involuntary movements of extremities, severe restlessness—case reports.
  Development of tardive dyskinesia (see Glossary)—case reports.
  Lowering of the seizure threshold—possible.
  Muscle damage (rhabdomyolysis) or liver toxicity—rare.

▷ **Possible Effects on Sexual Function:**   Increased libido.
  Male breast enlargement and tenderness; painful and extended erections.
  Female breast enlargement with milk formation.
  Altered timing and pattern of menstruation.

▷ **Adverse Effects That May Mimic Natural Diseases or Disorders**

Parkinson-like reactions may be mistaken for naturally occurring Parkinson's disease.

Rare liver reaction may suggest viral hepatitis.

Possible Effects on Laboratory Tests

Liver function enzymes: increased.

Blood urea nitrogen (BUN): increased.

CAUTION

1. This drug may alter the pattern of epileptic seizures and require dose adjustments of anticonvulsant drugs.
2. Obtain prompt evaluation of any change or disturbance of vision.
3. Narrow margin between the dose that works and the dose that can cause Parkinson-like reactions. Call your doctor if symptoms develop.

Precautions for Use

By Infants and Children: Safety and effectiveness for those under 12 not established.

By Those Over 60 Years of Age: Start treatment with small doses. This drug can aggravate existing prostatism (see Glossary). You may be more susceptible to the development of Parkinson-like reactions or tardive dyskinesia. Report any suggestive symptoms promptly.

▷ **Advisability of Use During Pregnancy**

Pregnancy Category: C. See Pregnancy Risk Categories at the back of this book.

Animal studies: No birth defects reported in mice, rats, or rabbits.

Human studies: Adequate studies of pregnant women are not available.

Because of its inherent toxicity for brain tissue, avoid use during pregnancy if possible.

Advisability of Use If Breast-Feeding

Presence of this drug in breast milk: Unknown.

Avoid drug or refrain from nursing.

Habit-Forming Potential: None.

Effects of Overdose: Marked drowsiness, weakness, tremor, agitation, impaired stance and gait, stupor progressing to coma, possible seizures.

Possible Effects of Long-Term Use: Development of tardive dyskinesia.

Suggested Periodic Examinations While Taking This Drug (at physician's discretion)

Complete blood cell counts, liver function tests.

▷ **While Taking This Drug, Observe the Following**

Foods: No restrictions.

Beverages: No restrictions. May be taken with milk.

▷ *Alcohol:* Avoid completely. Alcohol can increase the sedative action of this drug and enhance its depressant effects on brain function. Also, this drug can increase the intoxicating effects of alcohol.

Tobacco Smoking: No interactions expected. I advise everyone to quit smoking.

▷ *Other Drugs*

Molindone may *increase* the effects of

- all drugs containing atropine or having atropinelike effects (see *anticholinergic drugs* in Drug Classes).
- all drugs with sedative effects, and cause excessive sedation.

Molindone *taken concurrently* with
- antiepileptic drugs (anticonvulsants) may require close monitoring for changes in seizure patterns and need for dose adjustments.
- monoamine oxidase (MAO) inhibitors (see Drug Classes) may lead to large increases in temperature or convulsions. Some patients who do not respond to either drug may take both at the same time without this effect, but data are limited.
- tramadol (Ultram) may increase seizure risk.

▷ *Driving, Hazardous Activities:* This drug may cause dizziness and drowsiness. Restrict activities as necessary.

Aviation Note: The use of this drug *is a disqualification* for piloting. Consult a designated aviation medical examiner.

Exposure to Sun: No restrictions as far as photosensitivity.

Exposure to Heat: Use caution and avoid excessive heat as much as possible. This drug may impair the regulation of body temperature and increase the risk of heatstroke.

Discontinuation: Do not stop taking this drug suddenly after long-term use. Ask your doctor for help with gradual dose reduction and withdrawal.

MORPHINE (MOR feen)

Other Name: MS (morphine sulfate)

Introduced: 1806   **Class:** Strong analgesic, opioids   **Prescription:** USA: Yes   **Controlled Drug:** USA: C-II*; Canada: Yes   **Available as Generic:** Yes

Brand Names: Astramorph, Astramorph PF, Duramorph, ✦Epimorph, Kadian, Infumorph, ✦Morphine H.P., ✦Morphitec, ✦M.O.S., ✦M.O.S.-S.R., MS Contin, MS-IR, OMS Concentrate, Opium Tincture, Oramorph SR, Paregoric, RMS Uniserts, Roxanol, Roxanol 100, Roxanol SR, ✦Statex

BENEFITS versus RISKS	
Possible Benefits	*Possible Risks*
EFFECTIVE RELIEF OF MODERATE TO SEVERE PAIN	POTENTIAL FOR HABIT FORMATION (DEPENDENCE)
	Respiratory depression
	Disorientation, hallucinations
	Interference with urination
	Constipation

▷ **Principal Uses**

As a Single Drug Product: Uses currently included in FDA-approved labeling: Given by mouth, suppository, or injection (1) to relieve moderate to severe pain of heart attack, cancer, operations, fluid on the lungs, and other causes; (2) used as an adjunct to anesthesia; (3) used in treatment resistant (intractable) cough.

Other (unlabeled) generally accepted uses: (1) Therapy of pain in sickle cell crisis; (2) used in patient-controlled analgesia pumps to fight pain.

*See schedules of Controlled Drugs at the back of this book.

How This Drug Works: Acting primarily as a depressant of certain brain functions, this drug suppresses the perception of pain and calms the emotional response to pain.

Available Dose Forms and Strengths

Injection —	0.5 mg/ml, 1 mg/ml, 2 mg/ml, 4 mg/ml, 5 mg/ml, 8 mg/ml, 10 mg/ml, 15 mg/ml, 25 mg/ml, 50 mg/ml
Oral solution —	20 mg/ml; 10 mg/5 ml, 20 mg/5 ml, 100 mg/5 ml
Suppositories —	5 mg, 10 mg, 20 mg, 30 mg
Syrup —	1 mg/ml, 5 mg/ml, 10 mg/ml, 20 mg/ml, 50 mg/ml (Canada only)
Tablets —	5 mg, 10 mg, 15 mg, 25 mg, 30 mg, 50 mg
Tablets, soluble —	10 mg, 15 mg, 30 mg
Tablets, sustained release —	15 mg, 30 mg, 60 mg, 100 mg, 200 mg
Tablets, extended sustained release —	20 mg, 50 mg, 100 mg

▷ **Recommended Dose Ranges** (Actual dose and schedule must be determined for each patient individually.)

Infants and Children: 0.1 to 0.2 mg per kg of body mass every 4 hours. Single dose should not exceed 15 mg.

12 to 60 Years of Age: By injection—5 to 20 mg every 4 hours.
By mouth (regular solution, syrup, and tablets)—10 to 30 mg every 4 hours.
By mouth (sustained-release forms)—30 mg every 8 to 12 hours.
By mouth (Kadian brand extended sustained-release form)—once daily.
By suppository—10 to 30 mg every 4 hours.

Over 60 Years of Age: Same as 12 to 60 years of age, using smaller doses to start. Dose is slowly increased if needed. Many clinicians treat constipation in this age group with starting morphine doses.

Author's Note: Current pain treatment theory calls for timed or scheduled dosing. This tends to prevent pain, rather than allowing pain to recur and then having to be treated. Some clinicians will use timed dosing immediately after surgery and then revert to as-needed dosing once the most severe period of pain has passed.

Conditions Requiring Dosing Adjustments

Liver Function: The dose and frequency **must** be adjusted (decreased) with liver compromise.

Kidney Function: The dose and frequency should be adjusted in renal compromise.

▷ **Dosing Instructions:**   The regular tablet may be crushed and taken with or following food to reduce stomach irritation or nausea. Sustained-release forms should be swallowed whole; do not break, crush, or chew them. Oral liquid may be mixed with fruit juice to improve taste.

Usual Duration of Use: As required to control pain. For short-term, self-limiting conditions, continual use should not exceed 5 to 7 days without interruption and reassessment of need. For the long-term management of severe chronic pain, it is advisable to determine an optimal fixed-dose schedule.

▷ **This Drug Should Not Be Taken If**
- you had an allergic reaction to it previously.
- you are having an acute attack of asthma.
- you have acute respiratory depression.

▷ **Inform Your Physician Before Taking This Drug If**
- you took a monoamine oxidase (MAO) type A inhibitor drug (see Drug Classes) in the last 14 days.
- you are taking atropinelike drugs, antihypertensives, metoclopramide (Reglan), or zidovudine (AZT).
- you are taking any other drugs that have a sedative effect.
- you have a history of drug abuse or alcoholism.
- you have impaired liver or kidney function.
- you have prostate gland enlargement (see prostatism in Glossary).
- you have a history of asthma, emphysema, epilepsy, gallbladder disease, or inflammatory bowel disease.
- you have a tendency toward constipation.
- you have a history of head injury.
- you have a history of sickle cell anemia.
- you have a history of low blood pressure.
- you plan to have surgery under general anesthesia in the near future.

Possible Side Effects (natural, expected, and unavoidable drug actions)
Drowsiness, light-headedness, weakness, euphoria, dry mouth, urinary retention, dose-related constipation. Miosis or pinpoint pupils.

▷ **Possible Adverse Effects** (unusual, unexpected, and infrequent reactions)
If any of the following develop, consult your physician promptly for guidance.
Mild Adverse Effects
Allergic reactions: skin rash, hives, itching (especially if the intravenous form is injected too quickly).
Headache, dizziness, impaired concentration, sensation of drunkenness, confusion, depression, blurred or double vision—infrequent to frequent and may be dose related.
Facial flushing, sweating, heart palpitation—possible.
Nausea, vomiting—possible and may be dose related.
Spasm of the biliary tract—possible.
Urine retention—possible.
Serious Adverse Effects
Allergic reactions: swelling of throat or vocal cords, spasm of larynx or bronchial tubes.
Hallucinations, psychosis—infrequent.
Drop in blood pressure, causing severe weakness and fainting—possible.
Disorientation, hallucinations, unstable gait, tremor, muscle twitching—possible.
Drug-induced myasthenia gravis or porphyria—case reports.
Respiratory depression—dose related.
Seizures—possible.

▷ **Possible Effects on Sexual Function:**   Reduced libido and/or potency.
Amenorrhea and disruption of ovulation—case reports.

▷ **Adverse Effects That May Mimic Natural Diseases or Disorders**
Paradoxical behavioral disturbances may suggest psychotic disorder.

Possible Effects on Laboratory Tests
Blood amylase and lipase levels: increased (natural side effects).
Liver function tests: increased liver enzymes (ALT/GPT, AST/GOT, and alkaline phosphatase), increased bilirubin.
Urine screening tests for drug abuse: may be **positive**. (Test results depend upon amount of drug taken and testing method used.)

CAUTION
1. If you have asthma, chronic bronchitis, or emphysema, excessive use of this drug may cause significant respiratory difficulty, thickening of bronchial secretions, and suppression of coughing.
2. Taking this drug with atropinelike drugs can increase the risk of urinary retention and reduced intestinal function.
3. Do not take this drug following acute head injury.

Precautions for Use
By Infants and Children: Use very cautiously in infants under 2 years of age because of their vulnerability to life-threatening respiratory depression. Watch for paradoxical excitement in this age group.
By Those Over 60 Years of Age: Small doses and short-term use are indicated. There may be increased risk of drowsiness, dizziness, unsteadiness, falling, urinary retention, and constipation (often leading to fecal impaction).

▷ **Advisability of Use During Pregnancy**
Pregnancy Category: C; D if used long-term or in high doses at term. See Pregnancy Risk Categories at the back of this book.
Animal studies: Significant skeletal birth defects reported in mouse and hamster studies.
Human studies: Adequate studies of pregnant women are not available. However, no significant increase in birth defects was found in 448 exposures to this drug.
Avoid during the first 3 months. Use sparingly and in small doses during the final 6 months only if clearly needed.

Advisability of Use If Breast-Feeding
Presence of this drug in breast milk: Yes.
Avoid drug or refrain from nursing.

Habit-Forming Potential: This drug can cause psychological and physical dependence (see Glossary).

Effects of Overdose: Marked drowsiness, dizziness, confusion, restlessness, depressed breathing, tremors, convulsions, stupor progressing to coma.

Possible Effects of Long-Term Use: Psychological and physical dependence, chronic constipation.

Suggested Periodic Examinations While Taking This Drug (at physician's discretion)
Ask the patient about his or her bowel habits.

▷ **While Taking This Drug, Observe the Following**
Foods: No restrictions.
Beverages: No restrictions. May be taken with milk.
▷ *Alcohol:* Alcohol is best avoided. Opioid analgesics can intensify the intoxicat-

ing effects of alcohol, and alcohol can intensify the depressant effects of opioids on brain function, breathing, and circulation.

Tobacco Smoking: No interactions expected. I advise everyone to quit smoking.

Marijuana Smoking: Increase in drowsiness and pain relief; impairment of mental and physical performance.

▷ *Other Drugs*

Morphine may ***increase*** the effects of
- antihypertensives, and cause excessive lowering of blood pressure.
- atropinelike drugs, and increase the risk of constipation and urinary retention.
- metformin (Glucophage).
- other drugs with sedative effects.

Morphine may ***decrease*** the effects of
- metoclopramide (Reglan).

Morphine ***taken concurrently*** with
- benzodiazepines (see Drug Classes) may result in increased risk of respiratory depression.
- cimetidine (Tagamet) may result in morphine toxicity.
- fluoxetine (Prozac) may antagonize morphine's pain-relieving effect.
- hydroxyzine (Vistaril) can increase pain relief, but carries the risk of increased respiratory depression.
- monoamine oxidase (MAO) type A inhibitor drugs (see Drug Classes) may
cause the equivalent of an acute narcotic overdose: unconsciousness; severe
depression of breathing, heart rate, and circulation. A variation can be excitability, convulsions, high fever, and rapid heart action.
- phenothiazines (see Drug Classes) may cause excessive and prolonged depression of brain functions, breathing, and circulation.
- ritonavir (Norvir) may lead to lower morphine benefits.
- tramadol (Ultram) may increase CNS side effects.
- zidovudine (AZT) may increase the toxicity of both drugs; avoid concurrent use.

▷ *Driving, Hazardous Activities:* This drug can impair mental alertness, judgment,
reaction time, and physical coordination. Avoid hazardous activities.

Aviation Note: The use of this drug ***is a disqualification*** for piloting. Consult a
designated aviation medical examiner.

Exposure to Sun: No restrictions.

Discontinuation: It is advisable to limit this drug to short-term use. Longer-term
use requires gradual tapering (decreasing) of doses to minimize possible effects of withdrawal: body aches, fever, sweating, nervousness, trembling,
weakness, runny nose, sneezing, rapid heart rate, nausea, vomiting, stomach cramps, diarrhea.

MUPIROCIN (myu PEER oh sin)

Introduced: 1987   **Class:** Antibiotic, topical   **Prescription:** USA: Yes
Controlled Drug: USA: No; Canada: No   **Available as Generic:** USA: No;
Canada: No

Brand Names: Bactroban, Bactroban Nasal

```
┌─────────────────────────────────────────────────────────────────┐
│                      BENEFITS versus RISKS                        │
│        Possible Benefits                    Possible Risks        │
│  EFFECTIVE TOPICAL TREATMENT    Skin irritation                   │
│     OF STAPHYLOCOCCUS AND                                         │
│     STREPTOCOCCUS SKIN                                            │
│     INFECTIONS                                                    │
│  EFFECTIVE ERADICATION OF                                        │
│     STAPHYLOCOCCUS AUREUS                                         │
│     FROM THE NOSE                                                │
└─────────────────────────────────────────────────────────────────┘
```

▷ **Principal Uses**

As a Single Drug Product: Uses currently included in FDA-approved labeling: (1) Used to treat skin infections caused by staphylococcal and streptococcal infections such as ecthyma or impetigo; (2) the intranasal form is specifically formulated to kill *Staphylococcus aureus* bacteria that have colonized the nasal passages; (3) treats secondary skin infections caused by strep or staph; (4) treats skin lesions that are traumatic.

Other (unlabeled) generally accepted uses: (1) Used in burns where resistant *Staphylococcus aureus* is causing infection; (2) helps prevent opportunistic infections of venous access devices such as intravascular cannulas; (3) treats cellulitis caused by Gram-positive organisms; (4) has been used in some specific situations in skin surgery to prevent infections; (5) used to eradicate vaginal *Staphylococcus* infections.

How This Drug Works: Binds to isoleucyl transfer-RNA synthetase, an enzyme, and stops susceptible bacteria from being able to make critical proteins.

Available Dose Forms and Strengths

Intranasal form (Bactroban Nasal) — 2.15%

Topical Cream — 2%

Topical Ointment (Bactroban)—2% — 20 mg/g (Canada)

▷ **Recommended Dose Ranges** (Actual dose and schedule must be determined for each patient individually.)

Infants and Children: Not indicated in infants.

Children 5 to 15 years old: Apply a thin coat of the 2% mupirocin calcium (intranasal form) to the infection three times daily for 3 to 5 consecutive days.

16 to 60 Years of Age: 2% ointment: Apply three times daily for 5 to 14 days. Some more involved or extensive infections have been treated for longer periods. If the infection in question has not resolved after the initial course of the ointment, the site should be evaluated by a physician and systemic antibiotics or other treatment considered.

2% topical cream: Apply (small amount) three times daily for ten days, for traumatic skin infections caused by strep pyogenes or staph aureus.

Intranasal: One-half of the ointment from the single-use tube of mupirocin is applied into one nostril and the other half is applied to the second nostril, twice daily in the morning and evening for 5 consecutive days.

Over 60 Years of Age: Same as 16 to 60 years of age.

Conditions Requiring Dosing Adjustments

Liver Function: Little of this ointment is usually absorbed into the body. No guidelines exist for liver disease adjustments.

Kidney Function: A substance in this formulation (polyethylene glycol) may be toxic to the kidneys if the ointment is applied over an extensive burn or wound area.

▷ **Dosing Instructions:** This medicine should be applied as a thin film or as described by your doctor. Call your doctor if the condition has not improved or worsens during the course of treatment. Do **not** combine this medicine with other ointments or treatments unless your doctor has prescribed this approach.

Usual Duration of Use: Continual use on a regular schedule for several days is usually necessary to determine this drug's effectiveness in treating skin infections. Wounds not responding in three to five days must be evaluated by your doctor. Long-term use of other forms requires periodic physician evaluation. See your doctor.

Possible Advantages of This Drug
Effective topical treatment of skin infections.

▷ **This Drug Should Not Be Taken If**
- you had an allergic reaction to any form of it previously.
- you have extensive burns or open wounds.

▷ **Inform Your Physician Before Taking This Drug If**
- several days have passed since this medicine was started and there has been no change or worsening of the wound.
- pain at the site of the infection increases.
- you are unsure how much to apply or how often to apply it.

Possible Side Effects (natural, expected, and unavoidable drug actions)
Irritation at the site of infection caused by the polyethylene glycol component.

▷ **Possible Adverse Effects** (unusual, unexpected, and infrequent reactions)
If any of the following develop, consult your physician promptly for guidance.
Mild Adverse Effects
Allergic reactions: skin rash and irritation at the infection site.
Soreness, stinging, or pain at the infection site—possible.
Headache or taste changes—infrequent (intranasal only).
Serious Adverse Effects
Allergic reactions: not defined, as the medicine is not appreciably absorbed.
If this medicine is applied to an extensive skin area, polyethylene glycol may be absorbed and cause kidney toxicity—possible.

▷ **Possible Effects on Sexual Function:** Not reported.

Possible Delayed Adverse Effects: This medicine is indicated for short-term use.

▷ **Adverse Effects That May Mimic Natural Diseases or Disorders**
None reported.

Natural Diseases or Disorders That May Be Activated by This Drug
None reported.

Possible Effects on Laboratory Tests
None reported.

CAUTION
1. Do not apply this medicine to an area of skin larger than what your doctor prescribed.

Precautions for Use

By Infants and Children: Safety and effectiveness for use by those under 5 years of age have not been established.

By Those Over 60 Years of Age: No special changes are needed.

▷ **Advisability of Use During Pregnancy**

Pregnancy Category: B. See Pregnancy Risk Categories at the back of this book.

Animal studies: No fetal problems defined.

Human studies: Information from adequate studies of pregnant women is not available.

Advisability of Use If Breast-Feeding

Presence of this drug in breast milk: Unknown.

Avoid drug or refrain from nursing.

Habit-Forming Potential: None.

Effects of Overdose: If this medicine is applied to an extensive area of skin, excessive amounts of polyethylene glycol may be absorbed and cause kidney toxicity.

Possible Effects of Long-Term Use: None defined.

Suggested Periodic Examinations While Taking This Drug (at physician's discretion)

None.

▷ **While Taking This Drug, Observe the Following**

Foods: No restrictions.

Beverages: No restrictions.

▷ *Alcohol:* No restrictions.

Tobacco Smoking: No interactions expected. I advise everyone to quit smoking.

▷ *Other Drugs*

Mupirocin *taken concurrently* with

- other medications that are toxic to the kidneys may result in additive kidney toxicity if mupirocin is applied to a large area of skin.

Aviation Note: The use of this drug *does not appear to be a restriction* for piloting. Consult a designated aviation medical examiner.

Exposure to Sun: No restrictions.

NABUMETONE (na BYU me tohn)

See the acetic acids (nonsteroidal anti-inflammatory drugs) profile for further information.

NADOLOL (NAY doh lohl)

Introduced: 1976 **Class:** Anti-anginal, antihypertensive, beta-blocker
Prescription: USA: Yes **Controlled Drug:** USA: No; Canada: No **Available as Generic:** Yes
Brand Names: ✦Apo-Nadol, Corgard, Corzide [CD], Syn-Nadol

```
┌────────────────────────────────────────────────────────────────┐
│                    BENEFITS versus RISKS                         │
│      Possible Benefits                   Possible Risks          │
│  EFFECTIVE, WELL-TOLERATED       CONGESTIVE HEART FAILURE in     │
│    ANTIHYPERTENSIVE for mild to     advanced heart disease       │
│    moderate high blood pressure   Provocation of asthma (in      │
│  EFFECTIVE ANTI-ANGINAL DRUG        predisposed patients)        │
│    IN CLASSICAL CORONARY          Masking of hypoglycemia in drug-│
│    ARTERY DISEASE with moderate     dependent diabetes           │
│    to severe angina               Worsening of angina following abrupt│
│                                     withdrawal                   │
└────────────────────────────────────────────────────────────────┘
```

▷ **Principal Uses**

As a Single Drug Product: Uses currently included in FDA-approved labeling: (1) Treats moderate high blood pressure; (2) helps prevent attacks of effort-induced angina. Should not be used in Prinzmetal's vasospastic angina.

Other (unlabeled) generally accepted uses: (1) Helps prevent hemorrhage from bulging veins (esophageal varices) in cirrhosis; (2) may have an adjunctive role in helping prevent and reduce migraine severity; (3) may have a role in helping prevent death after a heart attack (myocardial infarction); (4) may help ease tremor in patients taking lithium; (5) helps decrease risk of ruptured blood vessels in the esophagus (esophageal varices) in patients with cirrhosis.

As a Combination Drug Product [CD]: Available in combination with bendroflumethiazide, a diuretic antihypertensive drug. This combination product works better and is more convenient for long-term use.

How This Drug Works: By blocking certain actions of the sympathetic nervous system, this drug:

- reduces the rate and contraction force of the heart, lowering oxygen needs of the heart muscle, and reducing ejection pressure of blood leaving the heart. This reduces frequency of angina and lowers blood pressure.
- reduces contraction of blood vessel walls, lowering blood pressure.
- prolongs conduction time of nerve impulses through the heart, of benefit in the management of certain heart rhythm disorders.

Available Dose Forms and Strengths

Tablets — 20 mg, 40 mg, 80 mg, 120 mg, 160 mg

▷ **Usual Adult Dose Range:**   For hypertension: Starts with 40 mg daily; this may be increased gradually as needed and tolerated, up to 320 mg daily. The usual ongoing dose is 80 to 320 mg daily. Daily maximum is 320 mg. For angina: Initially 40 mg daily; increased gradually at intervals of 3 to 7 days up to 240 mg daily. Usual ongoing dose is 80 to 240 mg/24 hours. Daily maximum is 240 mg. **Note: Actual dose and schedule must be determined for each patient individually.**

Conditions Requiring Dosing Adjustments

Liver Function: No dosing changes needed.

Kidney Function: For patients with moderate kidney failure, the usual dose should be taken every 24 to 36 hours. For patients with severe kidney failure, the dose can be taken every 40 to 60 hours.

▷ **Dosing Instructions:**   The tablet may be crushed and taken without regard to eating. Do not stop this drug abruptly.

Usual Duration of Use: Use on a regular schedule for 10 to 14 days determines this drug's effectiveness in lowering blood pressure and preventing angina. The long-term use of this drug (months to years) will be determined by your response to an overall treatment program (weight reduction, salt restriction, smoking cessation, etc.). Consult your physician on a regular basis.

Possible Advantages of This Drug
Does not reduce blood flow to the kidney.
Can be used with other drugs that may reduce blood flow to the kidney (such as most anti-inflammatory aspirin substitutes).

▷ **This Drug Should Not Be Taken If**
- you have had an allergic reaction to it previously.
- you have congestive heart failure.
- you have an abnormally slow heart rate or a serious form of heart block.
- you are subject to bronchial asthma.
- you are presently experiencing seasonal hay fever.
- you are taking, or have taken within the past 14 days, any monoamine oxidase (MAO) type A inhibitor drug (see Drug Classes).

▷ **Inform Your Physician Before Taking This Drug If**
- you have had an adverse reaction to any beta-blocker (see Drug Classes).
- you have a history of serious heart disease.
- you have a history of hay fever (allergic rhinitis), asthma, chronic bronchitis, or emphysema.
- you have a history of overactive thyroid function (hyperthyroidism).
- you have a history of low blood sugar (hypoglycemia).
- you have impaired liver or kidney function.
- you have diabetes or myasthenia gravis.
- you are pregnant or breast-feeding your infant.
- you have difficulty with blood circulation to the periphery (peripheral vascular disease).
- you are currently taking any form of digitalis, quinidine, or reserpine, or any calcium-channel-blocker drug (see Drug Classes).
- you will have surgery with general anesthesia.

Possible Side Effects (natural, expected, and unavoidable drug actions)
Lethargy and fatigability, cold extremities, slow heart rate, light-headedness in upright position (see *orthostatic hypotension* in Glossary).

▷ **Possible Adverse Effects** (unusual, unexpected, and infrequent reactions)
If any of the following develop, consult your physician promptly for guidance.
Mild Adverse Effects
Allergic reactions: skin rash, itching, drug fever.
Headache, dizziness, vivid dreaming, visual disturbances, ringing in ears, slurred speech, paresthesias—case reports to infrequent.
Hair loss and sweating—case reports to infrequent.
Cough, indigestion, nausea, vomiting, diarrhea, abdominal pain—infrequent.
Increased blood potassium—possible.
Numbness and tingling of extremities—case reports.
Serious Adverse Effects
Allergic reactions: facial swelling, anaphylaxis.

Chest pain, shortness of breath, precipitation of congestive heart failure—possible.

Intensification of heart block or severe slowing of the heart—case reports and may be dose related.

Bronchospasm—rare.

Carpal tunnel syndrome or pancreatitis—case reports.

Induction of bronchial asthma (in asthmatic individuals)—possible and dose related.

Masking of warning indications of acute hypoglycemia in drug-treated diabetes—possible.

May precipitate cramping when walking (intermittent claudication)—possible.

Excessively low blood pressure—possible.

▷ **Possible Effects on Sexual Function:** Decreased libido, impotence, impaired erection—case reports to frequent.

▷ **Adverse Effects That May Mimic Natural Diseases or Disorders**
Impaired circulation to the extremities may resemble Raynaud's phenomenon.

Natural Diseases or Disorders That May Be Activated by This Drug
Bronchial asthma, Prinzmetal's variant (vasospastic) angina, latent Raynaud's disease, myasthenia gravis (questionable).

Possible Effects on Laboratory Tests
Blood HDL cholesterol level: decreased.
Blood VLDL cholesterol level: increased.
Blood triglyceride levels: increased.

CAUTION
1. ***Do not stop this drug suddenly*** without the knowledge and help of your doctor. Carry a note which states that you are taking this drug.
2. Ask your physician or pharmacist **before** using nasal decongestants, which are usually present in over-the-counter cold preparations and nose drops. These can cause rapid blood pressure increases when combined with beta-blocker drugs.
3. Report the development of any tendency to emotional depression.

Precautions for Use
By Infants and Children: Safety and effectiveness for those under 12 years of age are not established. However, if this drug is used, watch for the development of low blood sugar (hypoglycemia) during periods of reduced food intake.
By Those Over 60 Years of Age: Unacceptably high blood pressure should be reduced without creating the risks associated with excessively low blood pressure. Small doses and frequent blood pressure checks are needed. Sudden, rapid, and excessive reduction of blood pressure can predispose to stroke or heart attack. Watch for dizziness, unsteadiness, tendency to fall, confusion, hallucinations, depression, or urinary frequency.

▷ **Advisability of Use During Pregnancy**
Pregnancy Category: C. See Pregnancy Risk Categories at the back of this book.
Animal studies: No significant increase in birth defects due to this drug, but embryotoxicity reported in rabbits.
Human studies: Adequate studies of pregnant women are not available.

Avoid use during the first 3 months if possible. Use this drug only if clearly needed. Ask your physician for guidance.

Advisability of Use If Breast-Feeding
Presence of this drug in breast milk: Yes, in large amounts.
Avoid drug or refrain from nursing.

Habit-Forming Potential: None.

Effects of Overdose: Weakness, slow pulse, low blood pressure, fainting, cold and sweaty skin, congestive heart failure, possible coma, and convulsions.

Possible Effects of Long-Term Use: Reduced heart reserve and eventual heart failure in susceptible individuals with advanced heart disease.

Suggested Periodic Examinations While Taking This Drug (at physician's discretion)
Measurements of blood pressure, evaluation of heart function.

▷ **While Taking This Drug, Observe the Following**
Foods: No restrictions. Avoid excessive salt intake.
Beverages: No restrictions. May be taken with milk.
▷ *Alcohol:* Use with caution. Alcohol may exaggerate this drug's ability to lower blood pressure and may increase its mild sedative effect.
Tobacco Smoking: Nicotine may reduce this drug's effectiveness. I advise everyone to quit smoking.

▷ *Other Drugs*
Nadolol may *increase* the effects of
- other antihypertensive drugs, and cause excessive lowering of blood pressure. Dose adjustments may be necessary.
- reserpine (Ser-Ap-Es, etc.), and cause sedation, depression, slowing of the heart rate, and lowering of blood pressure.
- verapamil (Calan, Isoptin) or other calcium channel blockers (see Drug Classes), and cause excessive depression of heart function; monitor this combination closely.

Nadolol may *decrease* the effects of
- ritodrine (Yutopar).
- theophyllines (Aminophyllin, Theo-Dur, etc.), and reduce their effectiveness in treating asthma.

Nadolol *taken concurrently* with
- amiodarone (Codarone) can cause severe slowing of the heart and potentially stop the heart (cardiac arrest).
- antacids containing aluminum can block absorption of this medicine and lessen therapeutic nadolol effects.
- clonidine (Catapres) requires close monitoring for rebound high blood pressure if clonidine is withdrawn while nadolol is still being taken.
- digoxin (Lanoxin) may result in undesirable heart effects.
- epinephrine can cause serious hypertension and slowing of the heart, and should anaphylaxis occur, epinephrine resistance.
- ergot derivatives (see Drug Classes) can cause decreased blood flow to the extremities (peripheral ischemia).
- insulin requires close monitoring to avoid undetected hypoglycemia (see Glossary).
- lidocaine can lead to lidocaine toxicity (depressed heart function, cardiac arrest).

- oral antidiabetic drugs (see Drug Classes) can cause slowed recovery from any hypoglycemia that may occur.

The following drugs may *decrease* the effects of nadolol:

- indomethacin (Indocin) and possibly other "aspirin substitutes," or NSAIDs; these may impair nadolol's antihypertensive effect.

▷ *Driving, Hazardous Activities:* Use caution until the full extent of drowsiness, lethargy, and blood pressure change has been determined.

Aviation Note: The use of this drug *is a disqualification* for piloting. Consult a designated aviation medical examiner.

Exposure to Sun: No restrictions.

Exposure to Heat: Caution is advised. Hot environments can lower blood pressure and exaggerate the effects of this drug.

Exposure to Cold: Caution is advised. Cold environments can enhance the circulatory deficiency in the extremities that may occur with this drug. The elderly should take precautions to prevent hypothermia (see Glossary).

Heavy Exercise or Exertion: Prudent to avoid exertion that produces light-headedness, excessive fatigue, or muscle cramping.

Occurrence of Unrelated Illness: Fever can lower blood pressure, requiring dose decreases. Nausea or vomiting may interrupt dosing. Ask your doctor for help.

Discontinuation: Best not to stop this drug suddenly. Gradual lowering of doses over 2 to 3 weeks is recommended.

NAFARELIN (NAF a re lin)

Introduced: 1984   **Class:** Hormones,   miscellaneous   **Prescription:**
USA: Yes   **Controlled Drug:**   USA: No; Canada: No   **Available as Generic:**
USA: No

Brand Name: Synarel

BENEFITS versus RISKS	
Possible Benefits	*Possible Risks*
VERY EFFECTIVE TREATMENT OF ENDOMETRIOSIS	Symptoms of estrogen deficiency (during treatment)
	Masculinizing effects (during treatment)
	Loss of bone density
	Lowering of the white blood cell count

▷ **Principal Uses**

As a Single Drug Product: Uses currently included in FDA-approved labeling: (1) Treats endometriosis (reduction in the size and activity of endometrial implants within the pelvis; relief of pelvic pain associated with menstruation); (2) also used to treat precocious puberty due to excessive production of gonadotropic hormones.

Other (unlabeled) generally accepted uses: (1) Intranasal dosing helps control abnormal hair growth in women; (2) can be injected below the skin (subcutaneously) to help benign prostatic hyperplasia; (3) may be used before surgery to help decrease size of some tumors (myomas).

How This Drug Works: Stimulates the pituitary gland to release two additional hormones that regulate production of estrogen by the ovaries. With continued use, estrogen levels suppress (by a feedback mechanism) ovary-stimulating hormones—lowering estrogen levels.

The implants of endometrium (from the lining of the uterus) that are attached to the pelvic wall are stimulated by the rise and fall of estrogen in menstruation. When this drug suppresses estrogen production, the displaced endometrial tissue (endometriosis) becomes dormant, and the premenstrual and menstrual pain no longer occurs.

Available Dose Forms and Strengths
Nasal solution — 2 mg/ml (10-ml bottle)

▷ **Usual Adult Dose Range:** Endometriosis: Pregnancy MUST be excluded prior to starting therapy. Dosing starts with 400 mcg daily. Spray one dose of 200 mcg into one nostril in the morning and one dose of 200 mcg into the other nostril in the evening, 12 hours apart. Start dosing between days 2 and 4 of the menstrual cycle. If menstruation persists after 2 months of treatment, the dose may be increased to 800 mcg daily: one spray into each nostril (a total of two sprays, 400 mcg) in the morning and again in the evening.
Note: Actual dose and schedule must be determined for each patient individually.

Conditions Requiring Dosing Adjustments
Liver Function: No dosing changes needed.
Kidney Function: Specific guidelines are not available for dosing. Decreases may be needed in kidney compromise.

▷ **Dosing Instructions:** Carefully read and follow the patient instructions provided with this drug. The solution is to be sprayed directly into the nostrils; it is not to be swallowed. Time the start of therapy and daily dosing exactly as directed. A nasal decongestant (spray or drops) should not be used for at least 30 minutes after dosing the nafarelin spray; earlier use could impair absorption of nafarelin.

Usual Duration of Use: Regular use for 2 to 3 months usually determines benefits in easing endometriosis symptoms. The standard course of treatment is limited to 6 months. Safety data does not exist for retreatment.
If retreatment is considered, a bone mineral density test is prudent.

Possible Advantages of This Drug
Causes fewer masculinizing effects than danazol.
Less tendency than danazol to increase blood cholesterol levels.
Unlike danazol, this drug does not cause abnormally low HDL cholesterol levels or abnormally high LDL cholesterol levels.

Currently a "Drug of Choice"
For management of symptoms associated with endometriosis.

▷ **This Drug Should Not Be Taken If**
• you have had an allergic reaction to it previously.
• you are pregnant or breast-feeding.
• you have abnormal vaginal bleeding of unknown cause.

▷ **Inform Your Physician Before Taking This Drug If**
• you have used this drug, danazol, or similar drugs previously.
• you are taking any type of estrogen, progesterone, or oral contraceptive.

- you are planning a pregnancy in the near future.
- you have a family history of osteoporosis.
- you use alcohol or tobacco regularly.
- you have a history of low white blood cells.
- you are using anticonvulsants or cortisonelike drugs.
- you are subject to allergic or infectious rhinitis and use nasal decongestants frequently.

Possible Side Effects (natural, expected, and unavoidable drug actions)

Effects due to reduced estrogen production: hot flashes (90%), headaches, emotional lability, insomnia. Masculinizing effects: acne, muscle aches, fluid retention, increased skin oil, weight gain, excessive hair growth—rare.

▷ **Possible Adverse Effects** (unusual, unexpected, and infrequent reactions)

If any of the following develop, consult your physician promptly for guidance.

Mild Adverse Effects

Allergic reactions: skin rash, hives—rare.

Nasal irritation—frequent.

Vaginal dryness—infrequent to frequent.

Depression—rare.

Serious Adverse Effects

Loss of vertebral bone density: at completion of 6 months of treatment, bone density decreases an average of 8.7% and bone mass decreases an average of 4.3%; partial recovery during the post-treatment period restores bone density loss to 4.9% and bone mass loss to 3.3%.

Lowering of the white blood cell count—case reports.

Transient prostate enlargement—possible.

▷ **Possible Effects on Sexual Function:** Decreased libido, vaginal dryness, reduced breast size—infrequent to frequent.

Uterine bleeding—case reports.

Impotence occurred in most men who had used this drug for prostate problems. Hot flashes occurred in all of them.

Galactorrhea—case reports.

Natural Diseases or Disorders That May Be Activated by This Drug

Worsening of or increased progression of osteoporosis.

Possible Effects on Laboratory Tests

Blood testosterone level: decreased in men with benign enlargement of prostate gland.

Blood progesterone: decreased to less than 4 ng/ml.

Alkaline phosphatase: increased.

Serum estrone: decreased.

CAUTION

1. With continual use of this drug, menstruation will stop. If regular menstruation persists, call your doctor. Dose changes may be needed.
2. Use this drug consistently on a regular basis. Missed doses can result in breakthrough bleeding and ovulation.
3. It is advisable to avoid pregnancy during the course of treatment. Use a nonhormonal method of birth control; do not use oral contraceptives. Inform your physician promptly if you think you may be pregnant.

4. If you need to use nasal decongestant sprays or drops, delay their use for at least 30 minutes after the intranasal spray of nafarelin.

Precautions for Use

By Infants and Children: Safety and effectiveness for those under 18 years of age are not established.

By Those Over 60 Years of Age: If used for prostatism, impotence is a common side effect. Depression and hot flashes were also often reported.

▷ **Advisability of Use During Pregnancy**

Pregnancy Category: X. See Pregnancy Risk Categories at the back of this book.

Animal studies: Major fetal abnormalities and increased fetal deaths due to this drug have been demonstrated in rat studies.

Human studies: Adequate studies of pregnant women are not available.

Avoid this drug during entire pregnancy.

Advisability of Use If Breast-Feeding

Presence of this drug in breast milk: Unknown.

Avoid drug or refrain from nursing.

Habit-Forming Potential: None.

Effects of Overdose: No significant effects expected.

Possible Effects of Long-Term Use: Continual use should be limited to 6 months. If repeated courses of treatment are considered, bone mineral density testing is prudent.

Suggested Periodic Examinations While Taking This Drug (at physician's discretion)

Blood cholesterol and triglyceride profiles.

Bone density and mass measurements.

▷ **While Taking This Drug, Observe the Following**

Foods: No restrictions.

Beverages: No restrictions.

▷   *Alcohol:* No interactions expected.

Tobacco Smoking: No interactions expected. I advise everyone to quit smoking.

▷   *Other Drugs:*

The following drugs will ***decrease*** the effects of nafarelin:

• birth control pills (oral contraceptives).

• estrogens.

▷   *Driving, Hazardous Activities:* No restrictions.

Aviation Note: The use of this drug ***is not a disqualification*** for piloting. Consult a designated aviation medical examiner for confirmation.

Exposure to Sun: No restrictions.

Discontinuation: Normal ovarian function (ovulation, menstruation, etc.) is usually restored within 4 to 8 weeks after discontinuation of this drug.

Special Storage Instructions: Store in an upright position at room temperature. Protect from light.

NALTREXONE (nahl TREX ohn)

Introduced: 1995 **Class:** Antialcoholism, opioid antagonist **Prescription:** USA: Yes **Controlled Drug:** USA: No; Canada: No **Available as Generic:** USA: No; Canada: No

Brand Names: Trexan, ReVia

Warning: This medication can cause liver damage if taken in excessive doses. If abdominal pain, white stools, or yellowing of the eyes or skin occurs, call your doctor immediately.

BENEFITS versus RISKS

Possible Benefits	*Possible Risks*
CONTROL OF CRAVING FOR ALCOHOL	LIVER DAMAGE IF EXCESSIVE DOSES TAKEN
PART OF AN EFFECTIVE COMBINATION APPROACH TO ALCOHOLISM	
ONCE-DAILY DOSING	

▷ **Principal Uses**

As a Single Drug Product: Uses currently included in FDA-approved labeling: (1) Used as part of a comprehensive program to help alcohol dependence; (2) used to treat narcotic addiction.

Other (unlabeled) generally accepted uses: (1) May help women with a specific type of cessation of menstruation (hypothalamic amenorrhea); (2) helps itching in hemodialysis patients.

How This Drug Works: In narcotic addiction, this medicine antagonizes the effects of opioid medicines and blocks the perceived benefit of the drug to the addicted patient. In alcohol addiction, it may interfere with the body's own opioids that are released in response to drinking alcoholic beverages. If the effect of the body's own opioids (endogenous) is blocked, the craving for alcohol is thereby thought to be reduced.

Available Dose Forms and Strengths

Tablets — 50 mg

▷ **Recommended Dose Ranges** (Actual dose and schedule must be determined for each patient individually.)

Infants and Children: Not indicated.

18 to 60 Years of Age: 50 mg daily. The best results are gained when this medicine is used as part of a comprehensive approach to curbing alcohol use.

Over 60 Years of Age: Same as 12 to 60 years of age.

Conditions Requiring Dosing Adjustments

Liver Function: This drug is extensively metabolized in the liver and is contraindicated in acute hepatitis or liver failure.

Kidney Function: Metabolites of this drug are removed by the kidneys, but specific guidelines for dosing changes are not available.

▷ **Dosing Instructions:** If there is any question of opioid dependence, a Narcan challenge test must be performed. Naltrexone is almost completely absorbed after oral dosing. This medicine may be taken with or without food.

Usual Duration of Use: Continual use on a regular schedule for 12 weeks is usually necessary to determine this drug's effectiveness in treating alcoholism. This drug should be a part of a comprehensive alcohol treatment program. Long-term use (months to years) requires periodic evaluation of response and dose adjustment. Consult your physician on a regular basis.

Possible Advantages of This Drug
Actually decreases the craving for alcohol.

▷ **This Drug Should Not Be Taken If**
  • you had an allergic reaction to any form of it previously.
  • you have liver failure or acute hepatitis.
  • you are in opioid withdrawal.
  • you are physically dependent on narcotics.

▷ **Inform Your Physician Before Taking This Drug If**
  • you have a history of viral hepatitis.
  • you are planning surgery or a diagnostic procedure requiring anesthesia.
  • you are unsure how much to take or how often to take it.
  • you take prescription or nonprescription medicines not discussed with your doctor when naltrexone was prescribed.

Possible Side Effects (natural, expected, and unavoidable drug actions)
None.

▷ **Possible Adverse Effects** (unusual, unexpected, and infrequent reactions)
If any of the following develop, consult your physician promptly for guidance.
Mild Adverse Effects
  Allergic reactions: rash.
  Oily skin, itching, hair loss—case reports.
  Nosebleeds—possible.
  Joint and muscle pain—infrequent.
  Anorexia, weight loss, fatigue, nervousness—case reports.
  Sleep disturbances—infrequent.
  Depression—case reports.
Serious Adverse Effects
  Allergic reactions: none reported.
  - Idiosyncratic reactions: none reported.
  Liver toxicity (hepatocellular injury)—case reports.
  Precipitation of acute withdrawal syndrome in patients dependent on narcotics.
  Suicidal ideation—case reports.
  Abnormal platelet function (idiopathic thrombocytopenic purpura)—case reports.

▷ **Possible Effects on Sexual Function:**   Delayed ejaculation—infrequent.

Possible Delayed Adverse Effects: None reported.

▷ **Adverse Effects That May Mimic Natural Diseases or Disorders**
Liver problems may mimic acute hepatitis.

Natural Diseases or Disorders That May Be Activated by This Drug
None.

Possible Effects on Laboratory Tests
Liver function tests: increased.

CAUTION
1. The therapeutic dose and doses that can cause liver damage are fairly close. Make certain that you understand how much of this medicine to take and how often to take it.
2. Self-administration of any narcotic drug may be fatal.

Precautions for Use

By Infants and Children: Safety and effectiveness for use by those under 18 years of age have not been established.

By Those Over 60 Years of Age: None.

▷ **Advisability of Use During Pregnancy**

Pregnancy Category: C. See Pregnancy Risk Categories at the back of this book.

Animal studies: This drug has been shown to be embryocidal in rats and rabbits at roughly 140 times the typical human dose.

Human studies: Information from adequate studies of pregnant women is not available. Ask your doctor for help with this benefit-to-risk decision.

Advisability of Use If Breast-Feeding

Presence of this drug in breast milk: Unknown.

Avoid drug or refrain from nursing.

Habit-Forming Potential: None.

Effects of Overdose: Human subjects who received over 800 mg daily for a week showed no adverse effects.

Possible Effects of Long-Term Use: None defined.

Suggested Periodic Examinations While Taking This Drug (at physician's discretion)

Liver function tests.

▷ **While Taking This Drug, Observe the Following**

Foods: No restrictions.

Beverages: No restrictions.

▷ *Alcohol:* Obviously not recommended, as this medication is part of a combination approach to help problem drinkers.

Tobacco Smoking: No interactions expected. I advise everyone to quit smoking.

Marijuana Smoking: Should not be attempted.

▷ *Other Drugs:*

Naltrexone **taken concurrently** with

• narcotic medicines may result in a severe reaction.
• other drugs that are toxic to the liver may result in increased risk of liver toxicity.
• thioridazine (Mellaril) may result in somnolence and lethargy.

▷ *Driving, Hazardous Activities:* This drug may cause fatigue. Restrict activities as necessary.

Aviation Note: Alcoholism **is a disqualification** for piloting. Consult a designated aviation medical examiner.

Exposure to Sun: No restrictions.

Discontinuation: Do not stop this medicine without the knowledge of your doctor.

NAPROXEN (na PROX en)

See the propionic acids (nonsteroidal anti-inflammatory drugs) profile for further information.

NEDOCROMIL (na DOK ra mil)

Introduced: 1992   **Class:** Antiasthmatic, preventive   **Prescription:** USA: Yes   **Controlled Drug:** USA: No; Canada: No   **Available as Generic:** USA: No; Canada: No

Brand Name: Tilade, Tilade Nebulizer Solution

BENEFITS versus RISKS	
Possible Benefits	*Possible Risks*
EFFECTIVE PREVENTION OF RECURRENT ASTHMA	Acute bronchospasm—rare
	Taste disorder
Prevention of exercise-induced asthma	

▷ **Principal Uses**

As a Single Drug Product: Uses currently included in FDA-approved labeling: (1) Ongoing therapy of mild to moderate asthma; (2) steroid-sparing effect that may allow reduction or elimination of oral steroids; (3) helps manage asthmatic bronchitis.

Other (unlabeled) generally accepted uses: (1) May have a role in helping ease allergic rhinitis; (2) can help vernal conjunctivitis when instilled as an eyedrop; (3) may help exercise-induced asthma.

How This Drug Works: Inhibits release of inflammatory chemical mediators such as histamine, prostaglandins, and leukotrienes that constrict the bronchi and cause inflammation seen in acute asthma.

Available Dose Forms and Strengths

Inhaler — 16.2-g canister

Solution for inhalation — 1.75 and 2 mg per actuation

▷ **Recommended Dose Ranges** (Actual dose and schedule must be determined for each patient individually.)

Infants and Children: See dosing below.

6 to 60 Years of Age: Two puffs (inhalations) four times daily, to provide a total of 14 mg per day.

Over 60 Years of Age: Same as 6 to 60 years of age.

Conditions Requiring Dosing Adjustments

Liver Function: Adjustments in dose in liver compromise are not defined.

Kidney Function: Adjustments in dose in kidney compromise are not defined.

▷ **Dosing Instructions:** Follow the instructions on the leaflet provided in the medication box carefully. Nedocromil use must be continued, even when you are symptom-free.

Usual Duration of Use: Use on a regular schedule for a week usually determines effectiveness in helping prevent acute asthma. Long-term use (months to years) requires periodic physician evaluation of response and dose adjustment.

Possible Advantages of This Drug

Usually well tolerated. Rare serious adverse effects.

▷ **This Drug Should Not Be Taken If**
- you had an allergic reaction to it previously.
- you are having an acute asthma attack.

▷ **Inform Your Physician Before Taking This Drug If**
- you have impaired kidney function.
- you have angina or a heart rhythm disorder.
- you are unsure how much to take or how often to take it.

Possible Side Effects (natural, expected, and unavoidable drug actions)

Unpleasant taste. Mild throat irritation or hoarseness. May be lessened by a few swallows of water after each inhalation.

▷ **Possible Adverse Effects** (unusual, unexpected, and infrequent reactions)

If any of the following develop, consult your physician promptly for guidance.

Mild Adverse Effects

Allergic reactions: skin rash, hives.

Headache, dizziness—rare to infrequent.

Unpleasant taste or cough—infrequent to frequent.

Nausea or vomiting—infrequent.

Serious Adverse Effects

Allergic reactions: anaphylactic reaction, allergic pneumonitis (allergic reaction of the lung tissue).

Bronchospasm—case reports.

▷ **Possible Effects on Sexual Function:** None reported.

Possible Delayed Adverse Effects: Pneumonitis—case reports.

Possible Effects on Laboratory Tests

Liver function tests: increased ALT.

CAUTION

1. This drug does **not** act as a bronchodilator and should not be used for immediate relief of acute asthma.
2. If use of this drug has allowed you to stop taking a cortisone-related drug, you may need to resume the cortisone-related drug if you are injured, must stop taking nedocromil, have an infection, or need surgery.
3. If severe asthma returns, contact your doctor promptly.
4. If you use a bronchodilator drug by inhalation, it is best to take it about 5 minutes before inhaling nedocromil.

Precautions for Use

By Infants and Children: Safety and effectiveness for those under 12 years of age are not established.

By Those Over 60 Years of Age: This drug does not work in therapy of chronic bronchitis or emphysema.

▷ **Advisability of Use During Pregnancy**

Pregnancy Category: B. See Pregnancy Risk Categories at the back of this book.

Animal studies: Rat, mouse, and rabbit studies show no impairment of fertility or harm to the fetus.

Human studies: Adequate studies of pregnant women are not available. Ask your doctor for guidance.

Advisability of Use If Breast-Feeding
Presence of this drug in breast milk: Unknown.
Avoid drug or refrain from nursing.

Habit-Forming Potential: None.

Effects of Overdose: Head shaking, tremor, and salivation were seen in dogs given high doses.

Suggested Periodic Examinations While Taking This Drug (at physician's discretion)
Sputum analysis and X ray if pneumonitis suspected.
Liver function tests.

▷ **While Taking This Drug, Observe the Following**
Foods: No restrictions.
Beverages: Avoid all beverages to which you may be allergic.
▷ *Alcohol:* No interaction expected.
Tobacco Smoking: No interaction expected. I advise everyone to quit smoking.
▷ *Other Drugs*
Nedocromil may make it possible to reduce the dose or frequency of use of cortisonelike drugs. Ask your doctor for guidance.
There are no known adverse drug interactions at present.
▷ *Driving, Hazardous Activities:* This drug may cause dizziness. Restrict activities as necessary.
Aviation Note: The use of this drug *may be a disqualification* for piloting. Consult a designated aviation medical examiner.
Exposure to Sun: No restrictions.
Heavy Exercise or Exertion: This drug may enable you to partake in exercise. Ask your doctor for guidance.
Discontinuation: If this drug has made it possible to reduce or stop cortisonelike drugs, and you must stop taking nedocromil, you may have to resume the cortisonelike drug as well as other measures to control asthma.

NEFAZODONE (na FAZ oh dohn)

Introduced: 1994   **Class:** Antidepressant, other   **Prescription:** USA: Yes   **Controlled Drug:** USA: No; Canada: No   **Available as Generic:** USA: No; Canada: No

Brand Name: Serzone

BENEFITS versus RISKS	
Possible Benefits	*Possible Risks*
EFFECTIVE TREATMENT OF DEPRESSION	Dizziness
Fewer cardiovascular side effects than older agents	Mild blood pressure changes on standing
Minimal anticholinergic side effects	
Decreased sedation versus other medicines used for depression	

▷ **Principal Uses**

As a Single Drug Product: Uses currently included in FDA-approved labeling: Treatment of major depression.

Other (unlabeled) generally accepted uses: May have a role in pain management.

How This Drug Works: This antidepressant is unique in that it:
- blocks the reuptake of a specific nerve-transmitting chemical (5-HT).
- acts as a 5-HT$_2$ antagonist.

Because of this unique mechanism of action, this drug has fewer cardiovascular and anticholinergic side effects than previously available agents.

Available Dose Forms and Strengths

Tablets — 100 mg, 150 mg, 200 mg, 250 mg

▷ **Recommended Dose Ranges** (Actual dose and schedule must be determined for each patient individually.)

Infants and Children: Not indicated.

18 to 60 Years of Age: Starting dose is 200 mg daily, taken as 100 mg in the morning and 100 mg in the evening. Dose is increased as needed and tolerated in 100-mg increments (1 week between dose changes). Daily maximum is 600 mg.

Over 60 Years of Age: Dosing in this population starts with 100 mg daily in two divided doses. The medicine is then increased (at a slower rate than in younger patients) as needed and tolerated.

Conditions Requiring Dosing Adjustments

Liver Function: The dose should be decreased for patients with liver compromise.

Kidney Function: No specific dosing changes are presently identified.

▷ **Dosing Instructions:**   Food delays the absorption and decreases total absorption, but this effect is not believed to be clinically significant. Water is expected to be the safest liquid to take this medicine with. Grapefruit juice may have an action on some liver enzymes (cytochrome P450), which help remove (metabolize) this medicine. Avoid taking with grapefruit juice until all data are in.

Usual Duration of Use: Continual use on a regular schedule for 4 to 5 weeks usually determines effectiveness in treating depression. Long-term use (months to years) requires periodic evaluation of response, dose adjustment, and physician follow-up.

Possible Advantages of This Drug

Two different mechanisms of action and decreased side effects versus other available agents.

▷ **This Drug Should Not Be Taken If**
- you had an allergic reaction to it previously.
- you are taking astemizole, cisapride, or terfenadine.
- you are taking an monoamine oxidase (MAO) inhibitor (see Drug Classes).

▷ **Inform Your Physician Before Taking This Drug If**
- you take a triazolobenzodiazepine such as triazolam or alprazolam.
- you have a history of seizure disorder.
- you have a history of heart disease.
- you are unsure how much to take or how often to take it.

- you take other medicines that were not discussed with your doctor when nefazodone was prescribed.

Possible Side Effects (natural, expected, and unavoidable drug actions)
Dry mouth, blurred vision, or constipation. Lowered blood pressure on standing (postural hypotension).

▷ **Possible Adverse Effects** (unusual, unexpected, and infrequent reactions)
If any of the following develop, consult your physician promptly for guidance.
Mild Adverse Effects
Allergic reactions: skin rash.
Nausea—infrequent to frequent.
Ringing in the ears—possible.
Headache, dizziness, and tremor—infrequent.
Insomnia, confusion, and agitation—rare.
Slowed heart rate—case report.
Serious Adverse Effects
Allergic reactions: not defined.
Idiosyncratic reactions: not identified.
Activation of mania—one case report.
Low blood sugar (hypoglycemia)—case reports.
Seizures—rare.

▷ **Possible Effects on Sexual Function:**   Impotence, absence of orgasm, or abnormal ejaculation have all been rarely reported. Priapism has been reported with a structurally similar drug.

Possible Delayed Adverse Effects: None reported.

▷ **Adverse Effects That May Mimic Natural Diseases or Disorders**
None reported.

Natural Diseases or Disorders That May Be Activated by This Drug
None reported.

Possible Effects on Laboratory Tests
None reported.

CAUTION
1. Risk of suicide is present in depressed patients. Small quantities of this medicine should be dispensed at a time when therapy is started. Appropriate suicide precautions should be taken.
2. This medicine **must not** be taken with a monoamine oxidase (MAO) inhibitor; there MUST be an interval of 14 days between when an MAO inhibitor is stopped and before nefazodone is started.

Precautions for Use
By Infants and Children: Safety and effectiveness for use by those under 18 years of age have not been established.
By Those Over 60 Years of Age: Lower starting doses and more gradual increases in dose are indicated.

▷ **Advisability of Use During Pregnancy**
Pregnancy Category: C. See Pregnancy Risk Categories at the back of this book.
Animal studies: Increased rat pup mortality was seen when doses five times the typical human dose were used.

Human studies: Information from adequate studies of pregnant women is not available. Ask your doctor for guidance.

Advisability of Use If Breast-Feeding
Presence of this drug in breast milk: Unknown.
Avoid drug or refrain from nursing.

Habit-Forming Potential: None defined at present, but not expected.

Effects of Overdose: Nausea, vomiting, and somnolence.

Possible Effects of Long-Term Use: None reported.

Suggested Periodic Examinations While Taking This Drug (at physician's discretion)
Periodic checks of heart rate.

▷ **While Taking This Drug, Observe the Following**
Foods: No restrictions.
Beverages: Grapefruit juice may lead to toxicity. DO NOT combine.
▷ *Alcohol:* This combination is not recommended.
Tobacco Smoking: No interactions expected. I advise everyone to quit smoking.
Marijuana Smoking: Increased somnolence.
▷ *Other Drugs:*
Nefazodone may *increase* the effects of
- alprazolam (Xanax) and potentially other benzodiazepines (see Drug Classes).
- carbamazepine (Tegretol).
- cisapride (Propulsid), leading to possible heart toxicity.
- dextromethorphan (many cough medicines), leading to nausea.
- digoxin (Lanoxin). Increased blood level checks are suggested.
- flecainide (Tambocor). Blood level checks are prudent.
- haloperidol (Haldol).
- imipramine (Tofranil).
- triazolam (Halcion).

Nefazodone *taken concurrently* with
- acebutolol (Sectral) and perhaps other beta-blockers (see Drug Classes) may result in decreased acebutolol levels and increased nefazodone metabolites.
- astemizole (Hismanal) can cause serious heart toxicity.
- buspirone (Buspar) resulted in liver enzyme increases with a similar drug (trazodone).
- clozapine (Clozaril) may result in clozapine toxicity since the P450 system in the liver is involved in removing clozapine from the liver.
- dextromethorphan (cough medicines with DM on the label) may result in dextromethorphan toxicity since the P450 system in the liver is involved in removing dextromethorphan from the liver.
- monoamine oxidase (MAO) inhibitors (see Drug Classes) may cause serious toxicity. Do not combine.
- phenytoin (Dilantin) may result in increased phenytoin levels. More frequent phenytoin blood level checks are needed, and dosing should be adjusted to blood level results.
- ritonavir (Norvir).
- terfenadine (Seldane) may cause serious heart rhythm problems.
- tryptophan (various) may lead to toxicity.

- tricyclic antidepressants (see Drug Classes) may result in increased tricyclic antidepressant levels and toxicity.

▷ *Driving, Hazardous Activities:* This drug may cause somnolence. Restrict activities as necessary.

Aviation Note: The use of this drug *is a disqualification* for piloting. Consult a designated aviation medical examiner.

Exposure to Sun: Use caution—photosensitivity is possible.

Discontinuation: Do not stop this medication without discussing this with your doctor.

NEOSTIGMINE (nee oh STIG meen)

Introduced: 1931   **Class:** Anti-myasthenic   **Prescription:** USA: Yes   **Controlled Drug:** USA: No; Canada: No   **Available as Generic:** USA: Yes; Canada: Yes

Brand Names: Prostigmin, ✦PMS-Neostigmine, Viaderm-K.C.

BENEFITS versus RISKS	
Possible Benefits	**Possible Risks**
MODERATELY EFFECTIVE TREATMENT OF OCULAR AND MILD FORMS OF MYASTHENIA GRAVIS (symptomatic relief of muscle weakness)	Cholinergic crisis (overdose): excessive salivation, nausea, vomiting, stomach cramps, diarrhea, shortness of breath (asthmalike wheezing), weakness
Eases postoperative bowel slowing or block (paralytic ileus)	

▷ **Principal Uses**

As a Single Drug Product: Uses currently included in FDA-approved labeling: (1) Treats ocular and milder forms of myasthenia gravis by providing temporary relief of muscle weakness and fatigability; (2) reverses depression of bowel function that may occur after surgery; (3) used to ease symptoms of bladder instability.

Other (unlabeled) generally accepted uses: (1) Used to reverse neuromuscular blockade caused by atracurium; (2) used to ease cancer pain.

How This Drug Works: Inhibits cholinesterase, the enzyme that destroys acetylcholine. This produces higher levels of acetylcholine, the nerve transmitter that generates muscular activity. Net effects are increased muscle strength and endurance.

Available Dose Forms and Strengths

Injection — 0.25 mg/ml, 0.5 mg/ml, 1.0 mg/ml

Tablets — 15 mg

▷ **Usual Adult Dose Range:**   Initially: 15 mg every 3 to 4 hours; adjust dose as needed and tolerated. Ongoing dose: up to 300 mg daily; average dose is 75 to 150 mg daily. **Note: Actual dose and schedule must be determined for each patient individually.**

Conditions Requiring Dosing Adjustments

Liver Function: Used with caution by patients with liver disease.

Kidney Function: Half of a given dose of neostigmine is eliminated unchanged by the kidney; however, specific guidelines for decreasing doses are not available.

▷ **Dosing Instructions:** The tablet may be crushed and taken with food or milk. Larger portions of the daily maintenance dose should be timed according to the pattern of fatigue and weakness.

Usual Duration of Use: Use on a regular schedule (with dose adjustment) for 10 to 14 days determines effectiveness in relieving the symptoms of myasthenia gravis. Long-term use (months to years) requires periodic physician evaluation.

▷ **This Drug Should Not Be Taken If**
- you have had an allergic reaction to it previously.
- you are known to be allergic to bromide compounds.
- you have an obstruction in your urinary tract or intestine.

▷ **Inform Your Physician Before Taking This Drug If**
- you have any type of seizure disorder.
- you are subject to heart rhythm disorders or bronchial asthma.
- you have recurrent urinary tract infections.
- you have prostatism (see Glossary).
- you will have surgery with general anesthesia.

Possible Side Effects (natural, expected, and unavoidable drug actions)
Small pupils, watering of eyes, slow pulse, excessive salivation, nausea, vomiting, stomach cramps, diarrhea, urge to urinate, increased sweating.

▷ **Possible Adverse Effects** (unusual, unexpected, and infrequent reactions)
If any of the following develop, consult your physician promptly for guidance.
Mild Adverse Effects
Allergic reactions: skin rash.
Nervousness, anxiety, unsteadiness, muscle cramps or twitching—infrequent.
Serious Adverse Effects
Confusion, slurred speech, seizures, difficult breathing (asthmatic wheezing)—infrequent.
Increased muscle weakness or paralysis—variable.
Excessive vomiting or diarrhea may induce abnormally low blood potassium levels (hypokalemia). This will accentuate muscle weakness.
Abnormally slow heartbeat (bradycardia)—case report.
Drug-induced porphyria—case reports.

▷ **Possible Effects on Sexual Function:** None reported.
▷ **Adverse Effects That May Mimic Natural Diseases or Disorders**
Seizures may suggest the possibility of epilepsy.

Natural Diseases or Disorders That May Be Activated by This Drug
Latent bronchial asthma.

Possible Effects on Laboratory Tests
None reported.

CAUTION
1. Certain drugs can block the action of this drug and reduce its effectiveness in treating myasthenia gravis (see "Other Drugs" below). Ask your physician before starting any new drug, prescription or over-the-counter.

2. Dosing must be carefully individualized. Variations in response may occur. Because generalized muscle weakness is a major symptom of both myasthenia crisis (underdose) and cholinergic crisis (overdose), it may be difficult to recognize the correct cause. As a rule, weakness that starts an hour after taking this drug probably is overdose; weakness that begins 3 or more hours after taking this drug is probably due to underdose. Watch these time relationships and tell your doctor.
3. In long-term therapy, watch for loss of effectiveness. Ask your doctor if stopping this drug for a few days may cause it to work again.

Precautions for Use

By Infants and Children: Dose and schedule must be modified if kidney function is severely impaired.

By Those Over 60 Years of Age: The natural decline of kidney function with aging may require smaller doses to prevent accumulation of this drug to toxic levels.

▷ **Advisability of Use During Pregnancy**

Pregnancy Category: C. See Pregnancy Risk Categories at the back of this book.
Animal studies: No information available.
Human studies: Adequate studies of pregnant women are not available.
There are no reports of birth defects due to the use of this drug during pregnancy. However, there are reports of significant muscular weakness in 20% of newborn infants whose mothers had taken this drug during pregnancy. Ask your doctor for help.

Advisability of Use If Breast-Feeding

Presence of this drug in breast milk: Probably not.
Monitor nursing infant closely and discontinue drug or nursing if adverse effects develop.

Habit-Forming Potential: None.

Effects of Overdose: Generalized muscular weakness, blurred vision, very small pupils, slow heart rate, difficult breathing, salivation, nausea, vomiting, diarrhea, muscle cramps or twitching. This is a cholinergic crisis.

Possible Effects of Long-Term Use: Development of tolerance (see Glossary) with loss of therapeutic benefit.

Suggested Periodic Examinations While Taking This Drug (at physician's discretion)

Assessment of drug effectiveness and dose schedule for best results.

▷ **While Taking This Drug, Observe the Following**

Foods: No restrictions.
Beverages: No restrictions. May be taken with milk.
▷ *Alcohol:* Use caution. Weakness and unsteadiness may be accentuated.
Tobacco Smoking: No interactions expected. I advise everyone to quit smoking.
▷ *Other Drugs:*
The following drugs may *decrease* the effects of neostigmine:
• atropine (belladonna).
• clindamycin (Cleocin).
• guanadrel (Hylorel).
• guanethidine (Esimil, Ismelin).
• procainamide (Procan SR, Pronestyl).

- quinidine (Cardioquin, Duraquin, etc.).
- quinine (Quinamm).

Neostigmine *taken concurrently* with
- edrophonium may cause cholinergic crisis in patients with myasthenic weakness.
- hydrocortisone or other adrenocortical steroids (see Drug Classes) can cause decreased neostigmine benefits.
- physostigmine can result in additive adverse effects.

▷ *Driving, Hazardous Activities:* This drug may cause blurred vision, confusion, or generalized weakness. Restrict activities as necessary.

Aviation Note: The use of this drug *is a disqualification* for piloting. Consult a designated aviation medical examiner.

Exposure to Sun: No restrictions.

Exposure to Heat: Use caution: this may cause excessive sweating and increased weakness.

Exposure to Environmental Chemicals: Avoid excessive exposure (inhalation, skin contamination) to the insecticides Baygon, Diazinon, and Sevin. These can accentuate potential toxicity of this drug.

Discontinuation: Do not stop this drug abruptly without your doctor's knowledge and help.

NIACIN (NI a sin)

Other Names: Nicotinic acid, vitamin B₃

Introduced: 1937 **Class:** Anticholesterol (cholesterol-reducing drug), vasodilator **Prescription:** USA: Tablets and liquid—no; capsules—yes **Controlled Drug:** USA: No; Canada: No **Available as Generic:** USA: Yes; Canada: Yes

Brand Names: ✦Antivert [CD], Endur-Acin, Niac, Niacels, Niacin TR, Niacor, Nia-Bid, Niaplus, Nicobid, Nico-400, Nicolar, Nicotinex, ✦Novoniacin, SK-Niacin, Slo-Niacin, Span-Niacin-150, Tega-Span, Tri-B3

BENEFITS versus RISKS	
Possible Benefits	*Possible Risks*
EFFECTIVE REDUCTION OF TOTAL CHOLESTEROL, LOW-DENSITY CHOLESTEROL, AND TRIGLYCERIDES IN TYPES II, III, IV, AND V CHOLESTEROL DISORDERS	Activation of peptic ulcer Drug-induced hepatitis Aggravation of diabetes or gout
Specific prevention and treatment of pellagra (niacin-deficiency disease)	

▷ **Principal Uses**

As a Single Drug Product: Uses currently included in FDA-approved labeling: (1) Certain patterns of abnormally high blood levels of cholesterol and triglycerides; (2) pellagra, a niacin (vitamin B₃) deficiency disorder characterized by dementia, dermatitis, and diarrhea; (3) therapy of Hartnup disease.

Other (unlabeled) generally accepted uses: (1) Therapy of certain types of vertigo and tinnitus (ringing in the ears); (2) may help decrease diarrhea in patients with cholera; (3) treatment of chilblains.

As a Combination Drug Product [CD]: In Canada this drug is combined with meclizine to enhance its effectiveness in the treatment of motion sickness and vertigo.

How This Drug Works

May inhibit initial production of triglycerides and impair the conversion of fatty tissue to cholesterol and triglycerides.

This drug corrects the specific deficiency of vitamin B_3 that is responsible for the symptoms of pellagra.

This drug causes direct dilation of peripheral blood vessels in the skin of the face and neck; for this reason it has been used to increase the blood flow to the inner ear in an attempt to relieve some types of vertigo and ringing in the ears. The effectiveness of this application is questionable.

Available Dose Forms and Strengths

Capsules, prolonged action — 125 mg, 250 mg, 300 mg, 400 mg, 500 mg

Oral solution — 50 mg/5 ml

Tablets — 20 mg, 25 mg, 50 mg, 100 mg, 500 mg

Tablets, prolonged action — 150 mg, 250 mg, 500 mg, 750 mg

▷ **Usual Adult Dose Range**

For cholesterol disorders: Initially 100 mg three times daily. Dose may be increased in increments of 300 mg daily at intervals of 4 to 7 days as needed and tolerated. The usual ongoing dose is 1 to 2 g three times daily. Daily maximum is 6 to 9 g.

For niacin deficiency: 10 to 20 mg daily.

For treatment of pellagra: 50 mg 3 to 10 times daily.

Note: Actual dose and schedule must be determined for each patient individually.

Conditions Requiring Dosing Adjustments

Liver Function: This drug is metabolized in the liver and is contraindicated in liver disease.

Kidney Function: Specific guidelines for adjustment of dosing are not available.

▷ **Dosing Instructions:**   Take with or immediately following meals to prevent stomach irritation. Also take one-half of an adult's aspirin tablet or one children's aspirin tablet with each dose of niacin to help prevent facial flushing and itching. Dose should be increased very slowly over 2 to 3 months as needed. The prolonged-action form of niacin is preferable to improve tolerance. The regular tablet may be crushed, but the prolonged-action capsules and tablets should not be altered.

Usual Duration of Use: Use on a regular schedule for 3 to 5 weeks determines benefit in reducing levels of cholesterol and triglycerides. Long-term use (months to years) requires periodic physician evaluation.

Currently a "Drug of Choice"

For starting treatment of elevated LDL cholesterol and VLDL triglycerides.

▷ **This Drug Should Not Be Taken If**

- you have had an allergic reaction to it previously.
- you have active peptic ulcer disease or inflammatory bowel disease.
- you have active liver disease.

▷ **Inform Your Physician Before Taking This Drug If**
- you are prone to low blood pressure.
- you have a heart rhythm disorder of any kind.
- you have a history of peptic ulcer disease, inflammatory bowel disease, liver disease, jaundice, or gallbladder disease.
- you have diabetes or gout.

Possible Side Effects (natural, expected, and unavoidable drug actions)

Flushing, itching, tingling, and feeling of warmth, usually in the face and neck. Sensitive individuals may experience orthostatic hypotension (see Glossary).

▷ **Possible Adverse Effects** (unusual, unexpected, and infrequent reactions)

If any of the following develop, consult your physician promptly for guidance.

Mild Adverse Effects

Allergic reactions: skin rash, itching, hives.

Headache, dizziness, faintness, impaired vision—infrequent.

Indigestion, nausea, vomiting, diarrhea—infrequent.

Flushing and tingling—infrequent to frequent.

Dryness of skin, grayish-black pigmentation of skin folds—infrequent.

Serious Adverse Effects

Drug-induced hepatitis with jaundice (see Glossary): yellow eyes and skin, dark-colored urine, light-colored stools—case reports.

Worsening of diabetes and gout—possible.

Development of heart rhythm disorders—case reports.

Myopathy or peptic ulcers—case reports.

Abnormal blood sugar—possible.

▷ **Possible Effects on Sexual Function:**   None reported.

▷ **Adverse Effects That May Mimic Natural Diseases or Disorders**

Liver reactions may suggest viral hepatitis.

Natural Diseases or Disorders That May Be Activated by This Drug

Latent diabetes, gout, inflammatory bowel disease, or peptic ulcer.

Possible Effects on Laboratory Tests

Complete blood cell counts: decreased eosinophils and lymphocytes.

Blood total cholesterol, LDL cholesterol, and triglyceride levels: decreased.

Blood HDL cholesterol level: increased.

Blood glucose level: increased.

Glucose tolerance test (GTT): decreased.

Blood uric acid level: increased.

Liver function tests: increased enzymes (ALT/GPT, AST/GOT, alkaline phosphatase) or bilirubin.

Urine sugar tests: inaccurate test results with Benedict's solution.

CAUTION

1. Large doses may cause increases in blood levels of sugar and uric acid. Diabetics or gout patients should monitor their status regularly.
2. Periodic measurements of blood cholesterol and triglyceride levels are essential for monitoring response and determining the need for changes in dose or medication.
3. Recent reports indicate that the prolonged-action dose forms of niacin

may be more likely to cause liver damage than the rapidly absorbed (crystalline) forms. Ask your doctor which is the most appropriate dose form and schedule for you.

Precautions for Use

By Infants and Children: Safety and effectiveness for use of large doses by those under 12 years of age have not been established.

By Those Over 60 Years of Age: Observe for the possible development of low blood pressure (light-headedness, dizziness, faintness) and heart rhythm disorders.

▷ **Advisability of Use During Pregnancy**

Pregnancy Category: C. See Pregnancy Risk Categories at the back of this book.
Animal studies: Significant birth defects due to this drug were found in chicks.
Human studies: Adequate studies of pregnant women are not available.
Use this drug only if clearly needed. Avoid completely during the first 3 months.

Advisability of Use If Breast-Feeding

Presence of this drug in breast milk: Yes.
Avoid drug or refrain from nursing.

Habit-Forming Potential: None.

Effects of Overdose: Generalized flushing, nausea, vomiting, stomach cramps, diarrhea, weakness, fainting.

Possible Effects of Long-Term Use: Increased blood levels of sugar and uric acid; liver damage.

Suggested Periodic Examinations While Taking This Drug (at physician's discretion)

Measurements of blood levels of total cholesterol, HDL and LDL cholesterol fractions, triglycerides, sugar, and uric acid.
Liver function tests.

▷ **While Taking This Drug, Observe the Following**

Foods: Follow the low-cholesterol diet prescribed by your physician.
Beverages: No restrictions. May be taken with milk.

▷ *Alcohol:* Use with caution. Alcohol used with large doses of this drug may cause excessive lowering of blood pressure. There has been one case report of delirium.

Tobacco Smoking: May increase risk of flushing and dizziness. I advise everyone to quit smoking.

▷ *Other Drugs*

Niacin may ***increase*** the effects of
• some antihypertensive drugs, and cause excessive lowering of blood pressure.

Niacin may ***decrease*** the effects of
• antidiabetic drugs (insulin and oral antidiabetic drugs; see Drug Classes), by raising the level of blood sugar.
• probenecid (Benemid) and sulfinpyrazone (Anturane), by raising the level of blood uric acid.

Niacin ***taken concurrently*** with
• aspirin (various) may decrease flushing, but may also increase niacin blood levels. Talk to your doctor.

- isoniazid (INH) may result in decreased niacin levels and require increased niacin dosing.
- lovastatin and other HMG-CoA-type cholesterol-lowering drugs may result in reversible muscle problems (myopathy or rhabdomyolysis).
- nicotine (particularly transdermal) may result in increased risk of flushing and dizziness.

▷ *Driving, Hazardous Activities:* This drug may cause dizziness and faintness. Restrict activities as necessary.

Aviation Note: The use of this drug **may be a disqualification** for piloting. Consult a designated aviation medical examiner.

Exposure to Sun: No restrictions.

Discontinuation: Do not stop this drug without your physician's knowledge and guidance. Abrupt withdrawal may be followed by excessive increase in blood cholesterol and triglyceride levels.

NICARDIPINE (ni KAR de peen)

Introduced: 1984 **Class:** Anti-anginal, antihypertensive, calcium channel blocker **Prescription:** USA: Yes **Controlled Drug:** USA: No; Canada: No **Available as Generic:** USA: No

Brand Names: Cardene, Cardene SR

Controversies in Medicine: Medicines in this class have had many conflicting reports. The FDA has held hearings on the calcium channel blocker (CCB) class. A study called ALLHAT is comparing amlodipine, an ACE inhibitor, a diuretic, and an alpha blocker (see Drug Classes), and should clarify adverse effects, mortality, and other issues relating to CCBs. CCBs are currently second-line agents for high blood pressure, according to the JNC VI (see Glossary).

BENEFITS versus RISKS	
Possible Benefits	*Possible Risks*
EFFECTIVE PREVENTION OF CLASSICAL ANGINA OF EFFORT	Increase in angina upon starting treatment
EFFECTIVE TREATMENT OF HYPERTENSION	Water retention, ankle swelling

▷ **Principal Uses**

As a Single Drug Product: Uses currently included in FDA-approved labeling: (1) Treats classical angina (due to atherosclerotic disease or angina caused by coronary artery spasm); (2) helps mild to moderate high blood pressure.

Other (unlabeled) generally accepted uses: (1) Combination therapy in preventing repeat strokes; (2) may help congestive heart failure; (3) treats refractory (not responding to nonsteroidal anti-inflammatory drugs) menstrual pain; (4) decreases frequency and severity of migraine attacks; (5) can halt the progression of atherosclerosis; (6) lowers postoperative hypertension; (7) may prevent vessel spasm in some kinds of blood vessel (vascular) surgery; (8) may treat premature labor; (9) decreases pain after shingles (Herpes Zoster).

How This Drug Works: By blocking passage of calcium through certain cell walls (which is a necessary nerve and muscle function), this drug inhibits the contraction of coronary arteries and peripheral arterioles. As a result, it:

- promotes coronary artery dilation (anti-anginal effect).
- reduces the degree of contraction of peripheral arterial walls, lowering blood pressure. This further reduces heart workload and helps prevent of angina.

Available Dose Forms and Strengths

Capsules — 20 mg, 30 mg

Injection — 2.5 mg/ml

SR Capsules — 30 mg, 45 mg, 60 mg

▷ **Usual Adult Dose Range:**   Initially 20 mg three times daily, 6 to 8 hours apart. Dose may be increased gradually at 3-day intervals (as needed and tolerated) up to 40 mg three times daily. The total daily dose should not exceed 120 mg. The sustained-release form is started at 30 mg twice daily and is increased as needed and tolerated to 60 mg twice daily. **Note: Actual dose and schedule must be determined for each patient individually.**

Conditions Requiring Dosing Adjustments

Liver Function: Starting dose is 20 mg twice a day. If the dose must be increased, it should be slowly advanced and taken twice a day.

Kidney Function: In moderate kidney failure, dosing starts at 20 mg twice daily. If needed, dose may be slowly increased. This drug may cause urine retention, and is a benefit-to-risk in urine outflow problems.

▷ **Dosing Instructions:**   May be taken with or following food to reduce stomach irritation, but not a high-fat meal, as total absorption may be reduced by 20 to 30%. The capsule should be swallowed whole (not altered).

Usual Duration of Use: Use on a regular schedule for 2 to 4 weeks determines this drug's benefit in reducing the frequency and severity of angina or controlling hypertension. For long-term use (months to years), the smallest effective dose should be used. Physician supervision and periodic evaluation are essential.

Possible Advantages of This Drug

Does not impair heart function or cause heart rhythm abnormalities.

Can be used safely with beta-blockers, digoxin, diuretics, and nitrate.

▷ **This Drug Should Not Be Taken If**

- you have had an allergic reaction to it previously.
- you have advanced aortic stenosis.

▷ **Inform Your Physician Before Taking This Drug If**

- you have had an adverse reaction to any calcium channel blocker (see Drug Classes).
- you currently take any form of digitalis or a beta-blocker drug (see Drug Classes).
- you are taking any drugs that lower blood pressure.
- you are taking cimetidine (Tagamet) or cyclosporine (Sandimmune).
- you have a history of congestive heart failure, heart attack, or stroke.
- you have a history of circulation impairment to the fingers.
- you have Duchenne muscular dystrophy.

- you are subject to disturbances of heart rhythm.
- you have impaired liver or kidney function.

Possible Side Effects (natural, expected, and unavoidable drug actions)
Rapid heart rate, swelling of the feet and ankles, flushing and sensation of warmth. Marked drop in blood pressure with fainting—rare.

▷ **Possible Adverse Effects** (unusual, unexpected, and infrequent reactions)
If any of the following develop, consult your physician promptly for guidance.

Mild Adverse Effects
Allergic Reaction: Skin rash—rare.
Headache, dizziness, weakness, nervousness, insomnia, or ringing in the ears (tinnitus); blurred vision, confusion, increased urination—rare to infrequent.
Palpitation, shortness of breath—rare.
Indigestion, nausea, vomiting, constipation—all rare.
Joint and muscle pain, cough—rare.
Abnormal growth (hyperplasia) of the gums—rare.

Serious Adverse Effects
Allergic reactions: none reported.
Increased frequency or severity of angina when starting therapy or after an increase in dose—possible.
Difficult urination—rare.
Liver toxicity—rare.
Decreased white blood cell counts reported with medicines in the same class (agranulocytosis).

▷ **Possible Effects on Sexual Function:**   Impotence—rare.

▷ **Adverse Effects That May Mimic Natural Diseases or Disorders**
Flushing and warmth may resemble menopausal "hot flushes." Increased liver enzymes may resemble infectious hepatitis.

Possible Effects on Laboratory Tests
Liver function tests: elevated (1%).

CAUTION
1. If you are checking your own blood pressure, check it just before each dose and 1 to 2 hours after each dose to obtain an accurate picture of the drug's effect.
2. Be sure to tell all health care providers who provide care for you that you take this drug. Note the use of this drug on a card placed in your purse or wallet.
3. You may use nitroglycerin and other nitrate drugs as needed to relieve acute episodes of angina pain. If your angina attacks are becoming more frequent or intense, call your doctor.

Precautions for Use
By Infants and Children: Safety and effectiveness for those under 18 years of age are not established.
By Those Over 60 Years of Age: Usually well tolerated; however, watch for development of weakness, dizziness, fainting, and falling. Take necessary precautions to prevent injury. Report promptly any changes in your pattern of thirst and urination.

▷ **Advisability of Use During Pregnancy**

Pregnancy Category: C. See Pregnancy Risk Categories at the back of this book.

Animal studies: Embryo and fetal toxicity reported in small animals, but no birth defects due to this drug.

Human studies: Adequate studies of pregnant women are not available.

Avoid this drug during the first 3 months. Use during the final 6 months only if clearly needed. Ask your physician for guidance.

Advisability of Use If Breast-Feeding

Presence of this drug in breast milk: Probably yes.

Avoid drug or refrain from nursing.

Habit-Forming Potential: None.

Effects of Overdose: Weakness, light-headedness, fainting, fast pulse, low blood pressure, shortness of breath, flushed and warm skin, tremors.

Possible Effects of Long-Term Use: None reported.

Suggested Periodic Examinations While Taking This Drug (at physician's discretion)

Evaluations of heart function, including electrocardiograms; measurements of blood pressure in supine, sitting, and standing positions.

▷ **While Taking This Drug, Observe the Following**

Foods: Food decreases the amount of this drug that is absorbed. Do NOT take this medicine with grapefruit or grapefruit juice. It is also prudent to avoid excessive salt intake.

Beverages: Do NOT take this medicine with grapefruit or grapefruit juice.

May be taken with milk.

▷   *Alcohol:* Use with caution until combined effects have been determined. Alcohol may exaggerate the drop in blood pressure experienced by some individuals.

Tobacco Smoking: Nicotine may reduce the effectiveness of this drug. I advise everyone to quit smoking.

Marijuana Smoking: Possible reduced effectiveness of this drug; mild to moderate increase in angina; possible changes in electrocardiogram, confusing interpretation.

▷   *Other Drugs:*

Nicardipine may *increase* the effects of

• cyclosporine (Sandimmune), and cause kidney toxicity.

Nicardipine *taken concurrently* with

• amiodarone (Codarone) may result in cardiac arrest.

• beta-blocker drugs or digitalis preparations (see Drug Classes) may affect heart rate and rhythm adversely. Careful monitoring by your physician is necessary if these drugs are taken concurrently.

• magnesium may cause worsening of neuromuscular blockade and further lowering of blood pressure.

• nonsteroidal anti-inflammatory agents (NSAIDs—see Drug Classes) may blunt the therapeutic effects of nicardipine.

• oral anticoagulants (warfarin, others) increasing bleeding risk.

• phenytoin (Dilantin) may result in phenytoin toxicity or decreased efficacy of nicardipine.

• rifampin (Rifadin, others) has caused loss of control of blood pressure with some other calcium channel blockers. Caution is advised if these medicines are combined.

The following drugs may *increase* the effects of nicardipine:
- cimetidine (Tagamet).
- imidazole antifungals (ketocaonazole—Nizoral) or triazole antifungals (itraconazole—Sporonox or fluconazole—Diflucan).
- ritonavir (Norvir).

▷ *Driving, Hazardous Activities:* Usually no restrictions. This drug may cause drowsiness or dizziness. Restrict activities as necessary.

Aviation Note: Coronary artery disease and hypertension *are disqualifications* for piloting. Consult a designated aviation medical examiner.

Exposure to Sun: No restrictions.

Exposure to Heat: Caution is advised. Hot environments can exaggerate the blood-pressure-lowering effects of this drug. Observe for light-headedness or weakness.

Heavy Exercise or Exertion: This drug may improve your ability to be more active without resulting angina pain. Use caution and avoid excessive exercise that could impair heart function in the absence of warning pain.

Discontinuation: Do not stop this drug abruptly. Ask your doctor about gradual withdrawal. Watch for possible development of rebound angina.

NICOTINE (NIK oh teen)

Introduced: 1992, 1996, 1997   **Class:** Smoking cessation adjunct, nicotine replacement therapy   **Prescription:** USA: Both Nicorettes (2 and 4 mg) are now available without a prescription for those over 18 years old. Nicotine patches are FDA approved for nonprescription use. The nicotine inhaler and nasal spray are **only available with a prescription.**   **Controlled Drug:** USA: No; Canada: No   **Available as Generic:** USA: No; Canada: No

Brand Names: Habitrol, Nicoderm CQ, Nicorette, Nicorette DS, Nicotrol, Nicotrol Inhaler, Nicotrol NS, Prostep

BENEFITS versus RISKS	
Possible Benefits	*Possible Risks*
EFFECTIVE REDUCTION OF NICOTINE CRAVING AND WITHDRAWAL EFFECTS when used adjunctively in smoking-cessation treatment programs	Aggravation of existing angina, heart rhythm disorders, hypertension, insulin-dependent diabetes, peptic ulcer, and vascular diseases
	Increased risk of abortion (if used during pregnancy)

▷ **Principal Uses**

As a Single Drug Product: Uses currently included in FDA-approved labeling: Nicotine chewing gum, nicotine transdermal systems, inhaler, and nasal spray are used adjunctively in behavior modification programs to help cigarette smokers who wish to stop smoking.

Other (unlabeled) generally accepted uses: Gum and nasal spray have been used to increase nicotine levels in the blood and help ease sudden cravings.

How This Drug Works: By providing an alternate source of nicotine (for nicotine-dependent smokers), the appropriate use of these drug products can reduce nicotine craving and lessen smoking withdrawal effects such as irritability, nervousness, headache, fatigue, sleep disturbances, and drowsiness.

Available Dose Forms and Strengths

Nicotine chewing gum tablets (newly nonprescription in the U.S.)

Nicorette — 2 mg (U.S., Canada)

— 4 mg (Canada)

Nicorette DS — 4 mg (U.S., Canada)

Inhaler — 10 mg per cartridge

Nasal spray — 10 mg/ml (10-ml bottle)

Transdermal systems — 16-hour systems (U.S. only): 5 mg, 10 mg, 15 mg; 24-hour systems: 7 mg (U.S., Canada), 11 mg (U.S.), 14 mg (U.S., Canada), 21 mg (U.S., Canada), 22 mg (U.S.)

How to Store

Store nicotine gum at room temperature and protect from light. Store nicotine patches at room temperature and be especially careful to avoid exposing the patches to temperatures greater than 86 degrees F (30 degrees C). Do not store unpouched. Once opened, patches should be used promptly because they may lose their strength.

▷ **Recommended Dose Ranges** (Actual dose and schedule must be determined for each patient individually.)

Infants and Children: Avoid use completely in children. Avoid accidental exposure to patches.

12 to 60 Years of Age: For chewing gum tablets: Initially one piece every hour while awake (10 to 12 pieces daily); supplement with one additional piece if and when needed to control urge to smoke. Total daily dose should not exceed 30 pieces (60 mg).

For inhaler form: Information is pending. Once available, this profile will be updated.

Nasal spray: Two sprays, one in each nostril. Starting dose is usually two to four sprays each hour. Maximum is 5 doses per hour (5 mg) and 40 doses per day (40 mg or 80 sprays). It should be used for a maximum of 3 months.

For transdermal systems: Dose depends upon patient characteristics and product used.

For those weighing 100 lb or more, smoking 10 or more cigarettes daily, and *without* cardiovascular disease:

Using a 16-hour system (Nicotrol)—initially one 15 mg patch applied for 16 hours daily for 4 to 12 weeks. For those who have abstained from smoking, reduce dose to one 10-mg patch applied for 16 hours daily for the next 2 to 4 weeks; then to one 5-mg patch applied for 16 hours daily for the following 2 to 4 weeks. Using a 24-hour system: Habitrol, Nicoderm—initially one 21-mg patch applied daily for 4 to 8 weeks. For those who have abstained from smoking, reduce dose to one 14-mg patch daily for the next 2 to 4 weeks; then to one 7-mg patch daily for the following 2 to 4 weeks. Prostep—initially one 22-mg patch applied daily for 4 to 8 weeks. For those who have abstained from smoking, reduce dose to one 11-mg patch daily for 2 to 4 weeks.

For those weighing less than 100 lb, smoking less than 10 cigarettes daily, or *with* cardiovascular disease:

Using a 24-hour system: Habitrol, Nicoderm—Initially one 14-mg patch applied daily for 4 to 8 weeks. For those who have abstained from smoking, reduce dose to one 7-mg patch daily for the next 2 to 4 weeks. Prostep—Initially one 11-mg patch applied daily for 4 to 8 weeks.

Over 60 Years of Age: Same as 12 to 60 years of age.

Conditions Requiring Dosing Adjustments

Liver Function: Lower starting doses are prudent in liver disease.

Kidney Function: Doses are decreased in severe kidney compromise.

Cardiovascular Disease: See above.

▷ **Dosing Instructions: Carefully follow the manufacturer's directions provided with each product.**

For chewing gum: Limit use to one piece of gum at a time. This product is much harder than typical chewing gum. Chew each piece slowly and intermittently for 30 minutes. A tingling of your gum tissue or peppery taste means the nicotine is being released.

Try to gradually reduce the number of pieces chewed each day by using it only when there is an urge to smoke. When trying to quit smoking, always have the gum available.

For transdermal systems: Apply a new patch at the same time each day. Do not alter the patch in any way. Apply the patch to the upper arm or body where the skin is clean, dry, and free of hair, oil, scars, and irritation of any kind; alternate sites of application. Press the patch firmly in place for 10 seconds; ensure good contact throughout. Wash your hands when you have finished applying the patch. Replace patches that are dislodged by showering, bathing, or swimming.

For spray: DO NOT swallow, inhale, or sniff when spraying the spray.

For the inhaler: Follow the patient package insert exactly. Make sure you understand how to use this product.

Usual Duration of Use: Use on a regular schedule for 2 to 3 months determines effectiveness in achieving lasting cessation of smoking. Nicotine chewing gum should not be used for more than 6 months; transdermal systems should not be used for more than 20 weeks. The nasal spray form should be used no longer than 3 months. The inhaler form should NOT be used for more than 6 months. Long-term use requires periodic physician evaluation of response and dose adjustment.

Possible Advantages of These Drugs

Provides control and flexibility of gradual nicotine withdrawal for use in supervised smoking-cessation programs.

Currently a "Drug of Choice"

For people who are motivated to stop smoking. Since many forms are now available without a prescription, be sure to talk with your doctor or pharmacist about how to best use these medicines. Many pharmacists offer programs to help you quit.

▷ **This Drug Should Not Be Taken If**
- you had an allergic reaction to any form of it previously.
- you have severe or uncontrolled or a pattern of worsening angina (physician's discretion).

- you have uncontrolled, life-threatening heart rhythm disorders (physician's discretion).
- you have had a recent heart attack (physician's discretion).

▷ **Inform Your Physician Before Taking This Drug If**
- you have any form of angina (coronary heart disease).
- you have had a heart attack at any time.
- you are subject to heart rhythm disorders.
- you have insulin-dependent diabetes.
- you have hypertension (high blood pressure).
- you have hyperthyroidism (overactive thyroid function).
- you have a pheochromocytoma (adrenaline-producing tumor).
- you have a history of esophagitis or peptic ulcer disease.
- you have a history of Buerger's disease or Raynaud's phenomenon.
- you currently have any dental problems or skin disorders.
- you have a history of kidney or liver disease.
- you have an increase in cardiovascular effects while you are taking this medicine.
- you have already taken a 3-month course of the patch from another doctor.
- you think you are pregnant or plan to become pregnant.
- you are unsure how much or how often to take this medicine.

Possible Side Effects (natural, expected, and unavoidable drug actions)
For chewing gum: mouth or throat irritation; injury to teeth or dental repairs. For transdermal systems: redness, itching, or burning at site of application (mild and transient). For nasal spray: runny nose, nasal irritation. For inhaler: coughing and nose irritation—frequent.

▷ **Possible Adverse Effects** (unusual, unexpected, and infrequent reactions)
If any of the following develop, consult your physician promptly for guidance.

Mild Adverse Effects
Allergic reactions: skin rash, hives, itching, local or generalized swellings.
Headache, light-headedness, dizziness, drowsiness, irritability, nervousness, insomnia, joint pain, muscle aches, abnormal dreams—possible to infrequent, and some may be dose related.
Rapid heartbeat, palpitation, increased sweating—infrequent to frequent, dose related.
Increased or decreased appetite, nausea, dry mouth, indigestion, constipation, or diarrhea—infrequent.

Serious Adverse Effects
Irregular heart rhythms, chest pain (angina), edema—infrequent.
See "Effects of Overdose" below.
Stroke—case report.

▷ **Possible Effects on Sexual Function:** There are some data questioning an effect on sperm, but a distinct demonstration of an effect is lacking.

Natural Diseases or Disorders That May Be Activated by This Drug
Latent angina, atrial fibrillation, hypertension, peptic ulcer disease, temporomandibular joint (TMJ) disorder (by chewing gum).

Possible Effects on Laboratory Tests
Free fatty acids (FFA blood level): increased.
Blood glucose: increased.

Prothrombin time (INR): decreased.

Urine screening test for drug abuse: no effect.

CAUTION

1. For these drug products to be safe and effective, **it is mandatory that all smoking be stopped immediately at the beginning of drug treatment**.

2. Extended use of chewing gum may cause damage to mouth tissues and teeth, loosen fillings and stick to dentures, and initiate or aggravate temporomandibular joint (TMJ) dysfunction.

3. Smoking cessation and the use of these drug products can result in increased blood levels of insulin (in insulin-dependent diabetics); dose reduction of insulin may be necessary to prevent hypoglycemic reactions.

4. If you are taking any of the following drugs, consult your physician regarding the need to reduce their dose while participating in a smoking cessation program: aminophylline, oxtriphylline, theophylline, beta-blocker drugs, propoxyphene, oxazepam, prazosin, pentazocine, imipramine.

5. If you are taking any of the following drugs, consult your physician regarding the need to increase their dose while participating in a smoking cessation program: isoproterenol, phenylephrine.

6. Used patches should be folded in half with the adhesive sides sealed together; place them in the original pouch or aluminum foil and dispose of them promptly; keep out of reach of children and animals.

7. Use of antacids such as Tums prior to chewing nicotine gum can increase the amount of nicotine absorbed from the gum.

8. Habitrol patches have only been shown to be effective when they are part of a complete smoking cessation program that includes counseling.

9. The Centers for Disease Control (CDC) has many excellent publications available to give you more information on stopping smoking. Call 1-800-232-1311 for more information.

Precautions for Use

By Infants and Children: Safety and effectiveness for those under 12 years of age are not established.

By Those Over 60 Years of Age: Because of the increased possibility of cardiovascular disorders in this age group, treatment should be cautiously started. Watch closely for adverse effects.

▷ Advisability of Use During Pregnancy

Pregnancy Category: For nicotine chewing gum: C. For nicotine transdermal systems, nasal spray, and inhaler: D. See Pregnancy Risk Categories at the back of this book.

Animal studies: Impaired fertility found in mouse, rat, and rabbit studies. Birth defects found in high-dose studies of mice.

Human studies: Adequate studies of pregnant women are not available. However, it is known that cigarette smoking during pregnancy may cause low birth weight, increased risk of abortion, and increased risk of newborn death.

The use of these drug products is not recommended during pregnancy.

Advisability of Use If Breast-Feeding

Presence of this drug in breast milk: Yes.

Avoid drug or refrain from nursing.

Habit-Forming Potential: The prolonged use of these drug products may perpetuate the physical dependence of nicotine-dependent smokers. Patches should have the lowest potential for dependence. Potential exists for abuse of nonprescription forms of this medicine.

Effects of Overdose: Nausea, vomiting, increased salivation, stomach cramps, diarrhea, headache, dizziness, impaired vision and hearing, weakness, confusion, fainting, difficult breathing, seizures.

Possible Effects of Long-Term Use: Perpetuation of nicotine dependence.

Suggested Periodic Examinations While Taking This Drug (at physician's discretion)

Evaluation of patient's ability to abstain from smoking.

Evaluation of patient's blood pressure and heart function.

▷ **While Taking This Drug, Observe the Following**

Foods: No restrictions.

Beverages: No restrictions.

▷ *Alcohol:* May cause an increase in cardiovascular effects.

Tobacco Smoking: Avoid all forms of tobacco completely.

Marijuana Smoking: Avoid completely.

▷ *Other Drugs:*

Nicotine may ***increase*** the effects of

• adenosine.

• niacin (flushing and dizziness).

The following drugs may ***increase*** the effects of nicotine:

• antacids such as Tums used prior to chewing nicotine-containing gum may increase the absorption of nicotine from the gum.

• cimetidine (Tagamet).

• lithium (Lithobid).

• ranitidine (Zantac).

Nicotine *taken concurrently* with

• niacin (Nicobid, others) can cause severe facial flushing.

▷ *Driving, Hazardous Activities:* This drug may cause dizziness or drowsiness. Restrict activities as necessary.

Aviation Note: The use of this drug ***may be a disqualification*** for piloting. Consult a designated aviation medical examiner.

Exposure to Sun: No restrictions.

Exposure to Cold: Use caution until tolerance is determined. Cold environments may enhance the vasospastic action of nicotine.

Heavy Exercise or Exertion: Patients with angina, coronary artery disease, or hypertension should use this drug with caution.

Discontinuation: As soon as a lasting cessation of smoking has been achieved, these drugs should be gradually reduced in dose and then discontinued. Continual use of the chewing gum or inhaler should not exceed 6 months, the nasal spray form no longer than 3 months, and the transdermal system no more than 20 weeks.

Special Storage Instructions: Store nicotine gum at room temperature and protect from light. Store nicotine patches at room temperature and be especially careful to avoid exposing the patches to temperatures greater than 86 degrees F (30 degrees C). Do not store unpouched. Once opened, patches should be used promptly because they may lose their strength.

NIFEDIPINE (ni FED i peen)

Introduced: 1972 **Class:** Anti-anginal, antihypertensive, calcium channel blocker **Prescription:** USA: Yes **Controlled Drug:** USA: No; Canada: No **Available as Generic:** Yes

Brand Names: Adalat, Adalat CC, ✦Adalat P.A., ✦Adalat FT, ✦Apo-Nifed, ✦Gen-Nifedipine, ✦Novo-Nifedin, ✦Nu-Nifed, Procardia, Procardia XL

Controversies in Medicine: Medicines in this class have had many conflicting reports. The FDA has held hearings on the calcium channel blocker (CCB) class. A study called ALLHAT is comparing amlodipine, an ACE inhibitor, a diuretic, and an alpha blocker (see Drug Classes) and should clarify adverse effects, mortality, and other issues relating to CCBs. CCBs are currently second-line agents for high blood pressure, according to the JNC VI (see Glossary).

BENEFITS versus RISKS	
Possible Benefits	*Possible Risks*
EFFECTIVE PREVENTION OF BOTH MAJOR TYPES OF ANGINA	Rare increase in angina upon starting treatment
EFFECTIVE TREATMENT OF HYPERTENSION (sustained-release form only)	Rare precipitation of congestive heart failure
	Rare anemia and low white blood cell counts
	Very rare drug-induced hepatitis
	Fainting

▷ **Principal Uses**

As a Single Drug Product: Uses currently included in FDA-approved labeling: (1) Treats angina pectoris due to coronary artery spasm (Prinzmetal's variant angina) that occurs spontaneously and is not associated with exertion; (2) classical angina of effort (due to atherosclerotic disease of the coronary arteries) in people who have not responded to or cannot tolerate the nitrates and beta-blocker drugs customarily used to treat this disorder (sustained-release form); (3) used to treat mild to moderate hypertension (extended-release forms).

Author's Note: A retrospective chart review has found the immediate-release form of this medicine IS NOT recommended for use in treating hypertension, acute myocardial infarction (heart attack), hypertensive crisis, and some forms of unstable angina.

Other (unlabeled) generally accepted uses: (1) Treats symptoms of Raynaud's phenomenon; (2) may stop progression of atherosclerosis; (3) can have a role in treating congestive heart failure; (4) therapy of pulmonary hypertension; (5) helps decrease risk of heart attack after coronary artery bypass grafting; (6) could have a role in some neurologically based pain disorders; (7) treats tardive dyskinesia; (8) can help itching (urticaria) of unknown cause; (9) therapy of achalasia or esophageal spasm; (10) helps intractable hiccups; (11) helps amaurosis fugax; (12) has a role in helping abnormal reactions to cold (chilblains).

How This Drug Works: Blocks passage of calcium through certain cell walls (needed for nerve and muscle tissue function), slowing electrical activity through the heart and inhibiting contraction of coronary arteries and peripheral arterioles. As a result:

- prevents spontaneous spasm of coronary arteries (Prinzmetal's angina).
- reduces heart rate and force during exertion, decreasing oxygen needs of heart muscle and reducing occurrence of effort-induced angina (classical angina pectoris).
- reduces the degree of contraction of peripheral arterial walls, lowering blood pressure. This further reduces the work of the heart during exertion and helps prevent angina.

Author's Note: One study found that nifedipine restored the function of the lining of blood vessels (endothelium).

Available Dose Forms and Strengths

Capsules — 5 mg (Canada), 10 mg (U.S. and Canada), 20 mg (U.S.)

Tablets — 10 mg, 20 mg (Canada)

Tablets, extended release — 10 mg, 20 mg (Canada), 30 mg, 60 mg, 90 mg (U.S.)

Tablets, sustained release — 30 mg, 60 mg, 90 mg

▷ **Recommended Dose Ranges** (Actual dose and schedule must be determined for each patient individually.)

Infants and Children: Dose not established.

12 to 60 Years of Age: Extended-release form for high blood pressure: Initially 30 mg once daily. Dose may be increased gradually at 7- to 14-day intervals (as needed and tolerated) up to 60 mg. Maximum total daily dose should not exceed 90 mg.

For hypertension: Initially a single 30-mg or 60-mg sustained-release tablet taken once daily. Gradually increased as a single daily dose if needed.

Sublingual for hypertensive crisis: **The immediate-release form of this medicine IS NOT recommended for use in treating hypertension, acute myocardial infarction (heart attack), hypertensive crisis, and some forms of unstable angina.**

Over 60 Years of Age: Same as 12 to 60 years of age. **Nifedipine immediate-release use by those over 71 has been associated with almost a fourfold increase in risk for all-cause death when compared to ACE inhibitors, beta-blockers, or other calcium channel blockers.**

Conditions Requiring Dosing Adjustments

Liver Function: Lower doses are prudent in liver disease. This drug is also a rare cause of liver toxicity (allergic hepatitis), and should be used with caution. Also a potential cause of portal hypertension, and should NOT be used by patients with portal hypertension.

Kidney Function: For patients with compromised kidneys, nifedipine is a benefit-to-risk decision, as it can lead to kidney toxicity.

▷ **Dosing Instructions:** May be taken with or following food to reduce stomach irritation. The capsule should be swallowed whole (not altered). The sustained-release tablet should be taken whole (not altered).

Usual Duration of Use: Use on a regular schedule for 2 to 4 weeks determines effectiveness in reducing the frequency and severity of angina and in controlling hypertension. For long-term use (months to years), the smallest effective dose should be used. Supervision and periodic physician evaluation are essential.

Possible Advantages of This Drug

The sustained-release form of this drug permits effective once-a-day treatment for both angina and hypertension.

▷ **This Drug Should Not Be Taken If**

- you have had an allergic reaction to it previously.
- you have active liver disease.
- you are over 71 and have been prescribed the immediate-release form of nifedipine.
- you have low blood pressure—systolic pressure below 90.
- you have significant narrowing of your aorta (aortic stenosis). Ask your doctor.

▷ **Inform Your Physician Before Taking This Drug If**

- you had an adverse response to any calcium channel blocker.
- you take any form of digitalis or a beta-blocker (see Drug Classes).
- you are taking any drugs that lower blood pressure.
- you have a history of congestive heart failure, heart attack, or stroke.
- you are subject to disturbances of heart rhythm.
- you have cardiomyopathy (nonobstructive) or aortic stenosis.
- you have impaired liver or kidney function.
- you have abnormal circulation to your fingers.
- you have atrial fibrillation.
- you develop a skin condition while taking this medicine.
- you have diabetes or Duchenne muscular dystrophy.
- you have a history of drug-induced liver damage.

Possible Side Effects (natural, expected, and unavoidable drug actions)

Low blood pressure, rapid heart rate, swelling of the feet and ankles, flushing and sensation of warmth, sweating.

▷ **Possible Adverse Effects** (unusual, unexpected, and infrequent reactions)

If any of the following develop, consult your physician promptly for guidance.

Mild Adverse Effects

Allergic reactions: skin rash, hives, itching, fever.

Headache, dizziness, weakness, nervousness, blurred vision, eye pain, or swelling around eyes—infrequent.

Pedal edema—frequent.

Depression—rare.

Abnormal growth of the gums (gingival hyperplasia)—rare.

Taste disturbances—possible.

Ringing in the ears (tinnitus)—case reports.

Sleep disturbances or bed-wetting—case reports.

Increased or decreased blood potassium—possible.

Palpitation, shortness of breath, wheezing, cough—infrequent.

Impaired sense of smell—possible.

Heartburn, nausea, taste disturbances, cramps, diarrhea—rare.

Tremors, muscle cramps—possible.

Serious Adverse Effects

Allergic Reaction: Drug-induced hepatitis—very rare; drug eruptions and erysipelas-like reactions, and exfoliative dermatitis or erythema multi-forme.

Idiosyncratic reactions: joint stiffness and inflammation.

Increased frequency or severity of angina on initiation of treatment or following an increase in dose.

Abnormal muscle movements (myoclonus)—case reports.

Kidney toxicity or pulmonary edema—case reports.

Bezoars—rare (seen with sustained-release forms).

Acute psychosis—case report.

Worsening of circulation to the fingers—possible.

Marked drop in blood pressure with fainting—possible.

Low white blood cells, platelets, and hemoglobin—case reports.

▷ **Possible Effects on Sexual Function:**   Altered timing and pattern of menstruation; excessive menstrual bleeding.

Tenderness and swelling of male breast tissue (gynecomastia)—case reports.

▷ **Adverse Effects That May Mimic Natural Diseases or Disorders**

Allergic rash and swelling of the legs may resemble erysipelas.

Drug-induced hepatitis may suggest viral hepatitis.

Transient increases in liver function tests may suggest infectious hepatitis.

Possible Effects on Laboratory Tests

Bleeding time: increased.

Liver function tests: transient increases.

Blood total cholesterol level: no effect in those under 60 years old; decreased in those over 60 years old.

Blood HDL cholesterol level: no effect, or increased.

Blood LDL and VLDL cholesterol levels: no effect.

Blood triglyceride levels: no effect, or decreased.

CAUTION

1. Tell health care providers who care for you that you take this drug. Note the use of this drug on a card in your purse or wallet.

2. You may use nitroglycerin and other nitrate drugs as needed to relieve acute angina pain. If angina attacks become more frequent or intense, call your doctor.

Precautions for Use

By Infants and Children: Safety and effectiveness for those under 12 years of age are not established.

By Those Over 60 Years of Age: You may be more susceptible to the development of weakness, dizziness, fainting, and falling. Take necessary precautions to prevent injury. Report promptly any changes in your pattern of thirst and urination.

▷ **Advisability of Use During Pregnancy**

Pregnancy Category: C. See Pregnancy Risk Categories at the back of this book.

Animal studies: Embryo and fetal deaths reported in mice, rats, and rabbits; birth defects reported in rats.

Human studies: Adequate studies of pregnant women are not available.

Avoid this drug during the first 3 months. Use during the final 6 months only if clearly needed. Ask your physician for guidance.

Advisability of Use If Breast-Feeding
> Presence of this drug in breast milk: Yes.
> Avoid drug or refrain from nursing.

Habit-Forming Potential: None.

Effects of Overdose: Weakness, light-headedness, fainting, fast pulse, low blood pressure, shortness of breath, flushed and warm skin, tremors.

Possible Effects of Long-Term Use: None reported.

Suggested Periodic Examinations While Taking This Drug (at physician's discretion)
> Evaluations of heart function, including electrocardiograms; measurements of blood pressure in supine, sitting, and standing positions.

▷ **While Taking This Drug, Observe the Following**
> *Foods:* Do not eat grapefruit for an hour after taking this medicine. It is also prudent to avoid excessive salt intake.
>
> *Beverages:* Grapefruit juice may greatly increase the absorption (bioavailability) of nifedipine and result in an exaggerated therapeutic effect. Water is the best liquid to take this medicine with. May be taken with milk.
>
> ▷ *Alcohol:* Use with caution. Alcohol may exaggerate the drop in blood pressure experienced by some people.
>
> *Tobacco Smoking:* Nicotine may reduce the effectiveness of this drug. I advise everyone to quit smoking.
>
> *Marijuana Smoking:* Possible reduced effectiveness of this drug; mild to moderate increase in angina; possible changes in electrocardiogram, confusing interpretation.

▷ *Other Drugs:*
> Nifedipine *taken concurrently* with
> * amiodarone (Codarone) may cause the heart to stop.
> * beta-blocker drugs or digitalis preparations (see Drug Classes) may affect heart rate and rhythm adversely. Careful monitoring by your physician is necessary if these drugs are taken concurrently.
> * cyclosporine (Sandimmune) can lead to nifedipine toxicity.
> * digoxin (Lanoxin) may lead to digoxin toxicity.
> * diltiazem (Cardizem) may lead to nifedipine toxicity.
> * magnesium can cause additive lowering of the blood pressure.
> * oral antidiabetic drugs (see Drug Classes) or insulin may result in loss of glucose control.
> * phenytoin (Dilantin) can cause phenytoin toxicity.
> * rifampin (Rifadin) can decrease nifedipine's effectiveness.
> * theophylline can reduce the therapeutic benefits of nifedipine and may lead to theophylline toxicity as well.
> * vincristine (Oncovin) can cause vincristine toxicity.
>
> The following drugs may *increase* the effects of nifedipine:
> * cimetidine (Tagamet).
> * some antifungals (fluconazole, itraconazole, and ketoconazole) may increase nifedipine blood levels and lead to toxicity.
> * quinidine (Quinaglute, others) can lead to nifedipine toxicity as well as decreased quinidine effectiveness.
> * ranitidine (Zantac).
> * ritonavir (Norvir).

▷ *Driving, Hazardous Activities:* Usually no restrictions. This drug may cause drowsiness or dizziness. Restrict activities as necessary.

Aviation Note: Coronary artery disease *is a disqualification* for piloting. Consult a designated aviation medical examiner.

Exposure to Sun: Caution—rare cases of phototoxicity have been reported.

Exposure to Heat: Caution is advised. Hot environments can exaggerate the blood-pressure-lowering effects of this drug. Observe for light-headedness or weakness.

Heavy Exercise or Exertion: This drug may improve your ability to be more active without resulting angina pain. Use caution and avoid excessive exercise that could impair heart function in the absence of warning pain.

Discontinuation: Do not stop this drug abruptly. Consult your physician regarding gradual withdrawal. Observe for the possible development of rebound angina.

NISOLDIPINE (ni SOLD i peen)

Introduced: 1996   **Class:** Anti-anginal, antihypertensive, calcium channel blocker   **Prescription:** USA: Yes   **Controlled Drug:** USA: No; Canada: No   **Available as Generic:** No

Brand Names: Sular

Author's note: Information in this profile will be broadened in subsequent editions.

NITROGLYCERIN (ni troh GLIS er in)

Introduced: 1847   **Class:** Anti-anginal, nitrates   **Prescription:** USA: Yes   **Controlled Drug:** USA: No; Canada: No   **Available as Generic:** Yes

Brand Names: Deponit, Minitran Transdermal Delivery System, Nitro-Bid, Nitrocap TD, Nitrocine Transdermal, Nitrocine Timecaps, Nitrodisc, Nitro-Dur, Nitro-Dur II, Nitrogard, ✦Nitrogard-SR, Nitroglyn, Nitrol, ✦Nitrol TSAR Kit, Nitrolin, Nitrolingual Spray, Nitrong, ✦Nitrong SR, Nitrospan, ✦Nitrostabilin, Nitrostat, Nitro Transdermal System, NTS Transdermal Patch, Transderm-Nitro✦Tridil

BENEFITS versus RISKS	
Possible Benefits	*Possible Risks*
EFFECTIVE RELIEF AND PREVENTION OF ANGINA	Orthostatic hypotension with and without fainting
EFFECTIVE ADJUNCTIVE TREATMENT IN SELECTED CASES OF CONGESTIVE HEART FAILURE	Skin rash—rare
	Altered hemoglobin with large doses—very rare
	Low blood platelets—rare

▷ **Principal Uses**

As a Single Drug Product: Uses currently included in FDA-approved labeling: (1) Treats symptomatic coronary artery disease—Rapid-action forms are used to relieve acute attacks of anginal pain, sustained-action forms prevent development of angina; (2) helps improve breathing difficulty caused by heart failure (left ventricle); (3) intravenous form used in surgery to control blood pressure; (4) relieves congestive heart failure after heart attacks.

Other (unlabeled) generally accepted uses: (1) May help ease spasms of the Oddi's sphincter; (2) topical use may help in impotence; (3) can help reduce the extent of heart damage if given following a heart attack (myocardial infarction); (4) helps relax cocaine-constricted heart arteries; (5) eases the pain of peripheral neuropathy; (6) may be of help in easing esophageal problems (achalasia); (7) when the anal sphincter does not work correctly, this drug can help reduce the muscle pressure and ease constipation; (8) nitroglycerin in combination with vasopressin may be of use in stopping bleeding esophageal varices; (9) can help loss of vision that has been caused by a clot in the retinal artery; (10) if ergot medications (see Drug Classes) have shut down circulation to the extremities, nitroglycerin can open up the circulation; (11) used to delay contractions in order to rotate an abnormally positioned fetus; (12) may help diabetics with nerve damage (diabetic neuropathy).

How This Drug Works: Relaxes and dilates both arteries and veins. Beneficial effects in angina are due to: (1) dilation of narrowed coronary arteries; (2) dilation of veins in the general circulation, with reduced volume and pressure of blood entering the heart. Net effects are improved blood supply to the heart and reduced work for the heart. Both actions reduce the frequency and severity of angina.

Available Dose Forms and Strengths

Canisters, translingual spray — 13.8 g (200 doses), 0.4 mg per metered dose

Capsules, prolonged action — 2.5 mg, 2.6 mg, 6.5 mg, 9 mg

Ointment — 2%

Tablets, buccal — 1 mg, 2 mg, 3 mg

Tablets, prolonged action — 2.6 mg, 6.5 mg, 9 mg

Tablets, sublingual — 0.15 mg, 0.3 mg, 0.4 mg, 0.6 mg

Transdermal systems — 2.5 mg, 5 mg, 7.5 mg, 10 mg, 15 mg (all per 24 hours)

▷ **Usual Adult Dose Range:**   According to dose form:

Sublingual spray—one metered spray (0.4 mg) under tongue every 3 to 5 minutes, up to three doses within 15 minutes, to relieve acute angina. To prevent angina, one spray taken 5 to 10 minutes before exertion.

Sublingual tablets—0.15 to 0.6 mg dissolved under tongue at 5-minute intervals to relieve acute angina.

Prolonged-action tablets—2.5 mg at 6- to 8-hour intervals to prevent angina.

Ointment—0.5 inch or 7.5 mg applied in a thin, even layer of uniform size to hairless skin at 3- to 4-hour intervals to prevent angina.

Buccal tablets—1 to 2 mg every 4 to 5 hours placed between cheek and gum.

Transdermal patches—5-square-cm to 30-square-cm patch applied to hairless skin once every 24 hours to prevent angina.

Note: Actual dose and schedule must be determined for each patient individually.

Author's Note: In order to avoid tolerance to the therapeutic effects of this medicine, a nitrate-free interval of 12 hours daily is recom-

mended: **24-hour patches are removed after having been applied for 12 hours; dosing of ointment is interrupted for 12 hours a day; oral sustained-release formulations are dosed to give a 6- to 12-hour nitrate-free interval.**

Conditions Requiring Dosing Adjustments

Liver Function: Specific dose adjustments in liver compromise are not defined.

Kidney Function: Specific guidelines for dosing changes are not available. This drug can discolor urine.

▷ **Dosing Instructions:**   Dose forms to be swallowed are best taken when stomach is empty (1 hour before or 2 hours after eating) to obtain maximal blood levels. Tablets should not be crushed. Capsules may be opened, but contents should not be crushed or chewed before swallowing.

Usual Duration of Use: Use on a regular schedule for 3 to 5 days is often needed to determine effectiveness in preventing and relieving acute anginal attacks. Individual dose adjustments will be necessary for optimal results. Long-term use (months to years) requires physician supervision.

▷ **This Drug Should Not Be Taken If**
- you have had an allergic reaction to it previously.
- you are severely anemic.
- you have had recent head trauma.
- you have had a heart attack and have an increased heart rate or increased blood pressure.
- you have hyperthyroidism.
- you have increased intraocular pressure.
- you have abnormal growth of the heart muscle in response to vascular disease (hypertrophic cardiomyopathy).
- you have closed-angle glaucoma (inadequately treated).

▷ **Inform Your Physician Before Taking This Drug If**
- you had an unfavorable response to other nitrates.
- you have low blood pressure.
- you have problems absorbing medicines (malabsorption syndromes) or excessive action of your stomach (gastric hypermotility).
- you have any form of glaucoma.
- you have had recent bleeding in your head.

Possible Side Effects (natural, expected, and unavoidable drug actions)

Flushing of face, headaches (50%), orthostatic hypotension (see Glossary), rapid heart rate, palpitation.

▷ **Possible Adverse Effects** (unusual, unexpected, and infrequent reactions)

If any of the following develop, consult your physician promptly for guidance.

Mild Adverse Effects

Allergic reactions: skin rash.

Throbbing headaches (may be severe and persistent), dizziness, fainting—possible.

Nausea, vomiting, taste disorders—infrequent.

Serious Adverse Effects

Allergic reactions: severe skin reactions with peeling.

Idiosyncratic Reaction: Methemoglobinemia—case reports.

Abnormally slow heartbeat (bradycardia)—rare.

Low blood supply to the head (transient ischemic attacks)—case reports.

Increased intracranial pressure—rare.

▷ **Possible Effects on Sexual Function:**   Correction of impotence (one report following sublingual use). Preventive use of nitroglycerin prior to sexual activity has been recommended to eliminate or reduce the risk of angina. Consult your physician for guidance.

▷ **Adverse Effects That May Mimic Natural Diseases or Disorders**

Hypotensive spells (sudden drops in blood pressure) due to this drug may be mistaken for late-onset epilepsy.

Possible Effects on Laboratory Tests

Blood platelet count: decreased—very rare.

Bleeding time: prolonged.

CAUTION

1. This drug can provoke migraine headaches in susceptible individuals.
2. Patients with impaired brain circulation (cerebral arteriosclerosis) have increased risk of transient ischemic attacks—periods of temporary speech impairment, paralysis, numbness, etc.
3. Tolerance to long-acting forms of nitrates will happen in most patients after 24 hours of continuous use. A nitrate-free interval of 10 hours usually restores effectiveness.
4. Many over-the-counter (OTC) drug products for allergies, colds, and coughs contain drugs that may counteract the desired effects of this drug. Ask your physician or pharmacist for help before using any such medications.

Precautions for Use

By Infants and Children: Limited usefulness and experience in this age group. Dose schedules are not established.

By Those Over 60 Years of Age: Begin treatment with small doses and increase dose cautiously as needed and tolerated. You may be more susceptible to the development of flushing, throbbing headache, dizziness, "blackout" spells, fainting, and falling.

▷ **Advisability of Use During Pregnancy**

Pregnancy Category: C. See Pregnancy Risk Categories at the back of this book.

Animal studies: No information available.

Human studies: Adequate studies of pregnant women are not available.

Use this drug only if clearly needed. Ask your physician for guidance.

Advisability of Use If Breast-Feeding

Presence of this drug in breast milk: Unknown.

Watch nursing infant closely and discontinue drug or nursing if adverse effects develop.

Habit-Forming Potential: None.

Effects of Overdose: Throbbing headache, dizziness, marked flushing, nausea, vomiting, abdominal cramps, confusion, delirium, paralysis, seizures, circulatory collapse.

Possible Effects of Long-Term Use: The development of tolerance (see Glossary) and the temporary loss of effectiveness.

Suggested Periodic Examinations While Taking This Drug (at physician's discretion)

Measurements of blood pressure and internal eye pressures.

Evaluation of hemoglobin.

▷ **While Taking This Drug, Observe the Following**

Foods: No restrictions.

Beverages: No restrictions. May be taken with milk.

▷ *Alcohol:* Avoid alcohol completely. This combination may result in severe lowering of blood pressure. There is a potential for collapse of the circulation and pumping effectiveness of the heart.

Tobacco Smoking: Nicotine can reduce the effectiveness of this drug. I advise everyone to quit smoking.

Marijuana Smoking: Possible reduced effectiveness of this drug; mild to moderate increase in angina; possible changes in the electrocardiogram, confusing interpretation.

▷ *Other Drugs:*

Nitroglycerin *taken concurrently* with

- acetylcysteine (NAC) may reverse tolerance to the intravenous form of this medicine.
- antihypertensive drugs may cause excessive lowering of blood pressure. Careful dose adjustments may be necessary.
- dihydroergotamine or similar ergot medicines (see Drug Classes) may result in ergotamine toxicity.
- diltiazem (Cardizem) can result in abnormally low blood pressure when used with the sustained-release form of nitroglycerin.
- heparin can result in decreased therapeutic benefit of heparin.
- isosorbide dinitrate (Isordil) or mononitrate (Ismo) may result in decreased nitroglycerin therapeutic benefits.
- sildenafil (Viagra) may cause very low blood pressure. DO NOT combine.

The following drugs may *increase* the effects of nitroglycerin:

- aspirin in analgesic doses (500 mg or more), and perhaps other NSAIDs.

▷ *Driving, Hazardous Activities:* Usually no restrictions. This drug may cause dizziness or faintness. Restrict activities as necessary.

Aviation Note: Coronary artery disease *is a disqualification* for piloting. Consult a designated aviation medical examiner.

Exposure to Sun: No restrictions.

Exposure to Heat: Hot environments can cause significant lowering of blood pressure.

Exposure to Cold: Cold environments can increase the need for this drug and limit its effectiveness.

Heavy Exercise or Exertion: This drug can increase your tolerance for exercise. Ask your doctor how much exercise is okay for you.

Discontinuation: Do not stop this drug abruptly after long-term use. Best to lower the dose (of prolonged-action forms) slowly over 4 to 6 weeks. Watch for rebound angina.

Special Storage Instructions: For sublingual tablets, to prevent loss of strength:

- keep tablets in the original glass container.
- do not transfer tablets to a plastic or metallic container (such as a pillbox).

- do not place absorbent cotton, paper (such as the prescription label), or other material inside the container.
- do not store other drugs in the same container.
- close the container tightly immediately after each use.
- store at room temperature.

NIZATIDINE (ni ZA te deen)

See the histamine (H₂) blocking drug family profile for more information.

NORFLOXACIN (nor FLOX a sin)

See the new fluoroquinolone antibiotics family profile for more information.

NORTRIPTYLINE (nor TRIP ti leen)

Introduced: 1963   **Class:** Antidepressant   **Prescription:** USA: Yes
Controlled Drug: USA: No; Canada: No   **Available as Generic:** USA: Yes; Canada: No
Brand Names: Aventyl, Pamelor

BENEFITS versus RISKS	
Possible Benefits	*Possible Risks*
EFFECTIVE RELIEF OF ENDOGENOUS DEPRESSION	ADVERSE BEHAVIORAL EFFECTS: confusion, disorientation, hallucinations, delusions
Possibly beneficial in other depressive disorders	CONVERSION OF DEPRESSION TO MANIA in manic-depressive (bipolar) disorders
Possibly beneficial in the management of some types of chronic, severe pain	Aggravation of schizophrenia
	Irregular heart rhythms
	Rare blood cell abnormalities

▷ **Principal Uses**

As a Single Drug Product Uses currently included in FDA-approved labeling: Relieves symptoms of spontaneous (endogenous) depression. Should not be used to treat symptoms of mild and transient (reactive) depression associated with many life situations.

Other (unlabeled) generally accepted uses: (1) Used in conjunction with other drugs to manage chronic, severe pain associated with such conditions as cancer, migraine headache, severe arthritis, peripheral neuropathy, AIDS, etc.; (2) helps decrease the frequency of bed-wetting; (3) may have a role in helping severe PMS; (4) can help attention deficit hyperactivity disorder (ADHD); (5) may have a role in helping ringing in the ears (tinnitus).

How This Drug Works: Slowly restores normal levels of nerve transmitters (norepinephrine and serotonin).

Available Dose Forms and Strengths
    Capsules — 10 mg, 25 mg, 50 mg, 75 mg
    Oral solution — 10 mg/5 ml (4% alcohol)

▷ **Usual Adult Dose Range:**   Starts with 25 mg three or four times daily. Dose is increased cautiously as needed and tolerated by 10 to 25 mg daily at intervals of 1 week. Usual ongoing dose is 50 to 100 mg daily. Daily maximum is 150 mg daily. When the best dose is found, it may be taken at bedtime as one dose. **Note: Actual dose and schedule must be determined for each patient individually.**

Conditions Requiring Dosing Adjustments
    Liver Function: Patients should be closely followed and drug levels obtained. May also a rare cause of hepatoxicity.
    Kidney Function: Specific dosing changes in renal compromise are not usually needed. Nortriptyline can cause a decrease in urine outflow, and should be a benefit-to-risk decision for patients with urine outflow problems.

▷ **Dosing Instructions:**   The capsule may be opened and may be taken without regard to meals.

Usual Duration of Use: Some benefit may be apparent within 1 to 2 weeks, but adequate response may require continual use for 3 months or longer. Long-term use should not exceed 6 months without physician evaluation regarding the need for continuation of the drug.

Possible Advantages of This Drug
    Causes less daytime sedation.
    Causes fewer atropinelike side effects.
    Causes orthostatic hypotension infrequently (see Glossary).

▷ **This Drug Should Not Be Taken If**
 • you have had an allergic reaction to it previously.
 • you are taking, or have taken within the past 14 days, any monoamine oxidase (MAO) type A inhibitor drug (see Drug Classes).
 • you are recovering from a recent heart attack.
 • you have narrow-angle glaucoma.

▷ **Inform Your Physician Before Taking This Drug If**
 • you are allergic or sensitive to any other tricyclic antidepressant (see Drug Classes).
 • you have a history of diabetes, epilepsy, glaucoma, heart disease, prostate gland enlargement, or overactive thyroid function.
 • you will have surgery with general anesthesia.
 • you have a history of bone marrow suppression.
 • you have a history of low blood pressure.

Possible Side Effects (natural, expected, and unavoidable drug actions)
    Light-headedness, drowsiness, blurred vision, dry mouth, constipation, impaired urination (see ***prostatism*** in Glossary). Fluctuation of blood sugar levels.

▷ **Possible Adverse Effects** (unusual, unexpected, and infrequent reactions)
    If any of the following develop, consult your physician promptly for guidance.

Mild Adverse Effects

Allergic reactions: skin rash, hives, swelling of face or tongue, drug fever (see Glossary).

Headache, dizziness, memory problems, weakness, fainting, unsteady gait, tremors, blurred vision, hearing toxicity—rare to infrequent.

Peculiar taste, weight gain, cavities (dental caries), irritation of mouth, nausea—infrequent.

Serious Adverse Effects

Allergic reactions: hepatitis, with or without jaundice (see Glossary).

Confusion, disorientation, hallucinations, delusions—case reports.

Aggravation of paranoid psychoses and schizophrenia; seizures—possible.

Heart palpitation and irregular rhythm—case reports.

Bone marrow depression (see Glossary): fatigue, weakness, fever, sore throat, abnormal bleeding or bruising—case reports.

Drug-induced porphyria or excessive urination, leading to sodium loss—case reports.

Peripheral neuritis (see Glossary): numbness, tingling, pain, weak arms and legs—case reports.

Parkinson-like disorders (see Glossary)—usually mild and infrequent; more likely to occur in the elderly.

▷ **Possible Effects on Sexual Function:** Decreased libido, increased libido (antidepressant effect), male impotence, inhibited female orgasm, male and female breast enlargement, milk production, swelling of testicles—case reports.

▷ **Adverse Effects That May Mimic Natural Diseases or Disorders**

Liver toxicity may suggest viral hepatitis.

Natural Diseases or Disorders That May Be Activated by This Drug

Latent diabetes, epilepsy, glaucoma, prostatism.

Possible Effects on Laboratory Tests

White blood cell and platelet counts: decreased.

Blood glucose levels: increased and decreased (fluctuations).

Liver function tests: increased liver enzymes (ALT/GPT, AST/GOT, and alkaline phosphatase), increased bilirubin.

CAUTION

1. Dose must be individualized. Report for follow-up evaluation and laboratory tests as directed by your physician.
2. It is advisable to withhold this drug if electroconvulsive therapy (ECT, or "shock" treatment) is to be used to treat your depression.

Precautions for Use

By Infants and Children: The manufacturer's labeling says that safety and effectiveness for children have not been established.

By Those Over 60 Years of Age: Usual dose is 30 to 50 mg daily in divided doses. During the first 2 weeks of treatment, watch for confusion, agitation, forgetfulness, delusions, disorientation, and hallucinations. Reduction of dose or discontinuation may be necessary. Unsteadiness may predispose to falling and injury. This drug can increase the degree of impaired urination associated with prostate gland enlargement (prostatism).

▷ **Advisability of Use During Pregnancy**

Pregnancy Category: D. See Pregnancy Risk Categories at the back of this book.
Animal studies: Results are inconclusive.
Human studies: No defects reported in 21 exposures to amitriptyline, a closely
related drug. Adequate studies of pregnant women are not available for this
drug.
Avoid use of drug during first 3 months. Use during final 6 months only if
clearly needed. Ask your physician for guidance.

Advisability of Use If Breast-Feeding

Presence of this drug in breast milk: Yes, in small amounts.
Monitor nursing infant closely and discontinue drug or nursing if adverse effects develop: excessive drowsiness and failure to feed.

Habit-Forming Potential: Psychological or physical dependence is rare and unexpected.

Effects of Overdose: Confusion, hallucinations, marked drowsiness, heart palpitations, dilated pupils, tremors, stupor, deep sleep, coma, convulsions.

Suggested Periodic Examinations While Taking This Drug (at physician's discretion)
Complete blood cell counts, liver function tests, serial blood pressure readings, and electrocardiograms.

▷ **While Taking This Drug, Observe the Following**

Foods: No restrictions. This drug may increase the appetite and cause excessive
weight gain.
Beverages: No restrictions. May be taken with milk.
▷ *Alcohol:* Avoid completely. This drug can markedly increase the intoxicating ef-
fects of alcohol and accentuate its depressant action on brain function.
Tobacco Smoking: May hasten elimination of drug. Higher doses may be neces-
sary. I advise everyone to quit smoking.
▷ *Other Drugs:*

Nortriptyline may *increase* the effects of
• atropinelike drugs (see *anticholinergic drugs* in Drug Classes).
• dicumarol, and increase the risk of bleeding.
• epinephrine (Adrenalin).
• phenytoin (Dilantin) by increasing blood levels.
• warfarin (Coumadin), and require more frequent INR (prothrombin time or
protime) testing and dosing adjustments based on laboratory results.
Nortriptyline may *decrease* the effects of
• clonidine (Catapres).
• ephedrine (Primatene tablets).
• guanethidine (Ismelin).
Nortriptyline *taken concurrently* with
• activated charcoal will decrease and almost block absorption (useful in
overdose situations).
• bepridil (Vascor) may lead to abnormal heart beats.
• benzodiazepines (see Drug Classes) may result in additive sedation.
• disulfiram (Antabuse) may cause acute dementia: confusion, disorientation, hallucinations.
• fluconazole (Diflucan) may result in large increases in nortriptyline levels
and result in toxic reactions.

- lithium (Lithobid) may pose an increased risk of neurotoxicity in elderly patients.
- monoamine oxidase (MAO) inhibitor drugs (see Drug Classes) may cause high fever, delirium, and convulsions.
- nifedipine (Adalat, others) may result in inhibition of nortriptyline's antidepressant effects.
- norepinephrine can cause a serious increase in blood pressure, abnormal heart rhythms, and fast heart rate. Avoid this combination.
- phenothiazines (see Drug Classes) can result in increased phenothiazine levels and toxicity as well as additive anticholinergic problems.
- sparfloxacin (Zagam) may lead to abnormal heart beats.
- thyroid preparations may impair heart rhythm and function. Ask your physician for guidance regarding adjustment of thyroid dose.
- tramadol (Ultram) may increase seizure risk.
- venlafaxine (Effexor) may result in nortriptyline or venlafaxine toxicity.

The following drugs may *increase* the effects of nortriptyline:
- cimetidine (Tagamet), and cause nortriptyline toxicity.
- fluoxetine (Prozac).
- quinidine (Quinaglute, etc.), and cause nortriptyline toxicity.
- sertraline (Zoloft).

The following drugs may *decrease* the effects of nortriptyline:
- ascorbic acid (vitamin C) in high doses.
- barbiturates (see Drug Classes), and reduce its effectiveness.
- carbamazepine (Tegretol).
- conjugated estrogens.
- rifampin (Rifadin).
- ritonavir (Norvir).

▷ *Driving, Hazardous Activities:* This drug may impair mental alertness, judgment, physical coordination, and reaction time. Avoid hazardous activities.

Aviation Note: The use of this drug *is a disqualification* for piloting. Consult a designated aviation medical examiner.

Exposure to Sun: Use caution—this drug may cause photosensitivity (see Glossary).

Exposure to Heat: This drug can inhibit sweating and impair the body's adaptation to hot environments, increasing the risk of heatstroke. Avoid saunas.

Exposure to Cold: The elderly should use caution and avoid conditions conducive to hypothermia (see Glossary).

Discontinuation: It is best to slowly discontinue this drug. Abrupt withdrawal after long-term use can cause headache, malaise, and nausea.

OFLOXACIN (oh FLOX a sin)

See the new fluoroquinolone antibiotic family profile for more information.

OLANZAPINE (oh LAN za pean)

Introduced: 1996   **Class:** Antipsychotic (tranquilizer, major); thienobenzo-diazepine   **Prescription:** USA: Yes   **Controlled Drug:** USA: No; Canada: No   **Available as Generic:** USA: No; Canada: No
Brand Name: Zyprexa

BENEFITS versus RISKS	
Possible Benefits	*Possible Risks*
EFFECTIVE SHORT-TERM CONTROL OF ACUTE MENTAL DISORDERS: beneficial effects on thinking, mood, and behavior Relief of anxiety, agitation, and tension	POSSIBLE TARDIVE DYSKINESIA (SERIOUS TOXIC BRAIN EFFECT with long-term use) RARE NEUROLEPTIC MALIGNANT SYNDROME (see Glossary) Orthostatic hypotension (see Glossary) Increased liver enzymes

▷ **Principal Uses**

As a Single Drug Product: Uses currently included in FDA-approved labeling: Helps manage thinking problems and other difficulties seen in psychosis. Other (unlabeled) generally accepted uses: None at present.

How This Drug Works: This medicine inhibits the action of two primary nerve transmitters (dopamine and serotonin) in certain brain centers, and acts to correct an imbalance of nerve impulse transmissions thought to be responsible for certain mental disorders. It also works at histamine, muscarinic, GABA, BZD, and adrenergic sites.

Available Dose Forms and Strengths

Tablets — 5 mg, 7.5 mg and 10 mg

▷ **Recommended Dose Ranges** (Actual dose and schedule must be determined for each patient individually.)

Infants and Children: Dose not established.

18 to 60 Years of Age: Dosing is started with 5 to 10 mg daily. If the 5-mg dose is used, the dose may be increased to a maximum of 10 mg as needed and tolerated. Dose changes should only be made after one week at a new dose.

Author's Note: Since *gender* data is now FDA required for new approvals, it must be noted that the drug is removed (cleared) 30% slower in women than in men. Therefore, effects (both desirable and undesirable) caused by the medicine may last longer in women (dose to dose) than in men.

Over 60 Years of Age: 5 mg of olanzapine is taken.

Conditions Requiring Dosing Adjustments

Liver Function: The drug is highly metabolized in the liver, and although the manufacturer does not have recommendations for dosing changes, smaller doses and close patient monitoring appear prudent.

Kidney Function: Dosing changes are not thought to be needed.

Seizure Disorders: Seizures happened in 0.9% of patients during clinical trials of olanzapine. Olanzapine should be used with caution by seizure patients. Dose decreases are not defined at present.

▷ **Dosing Instructions:** The tablet may be crushed and taken with food. It is best to take this medicine at the same time every day.

Usual Duration of Use: Use on a regular schedule for at least 1 week is required to reach steady-state levels, and hence determines effectiveness. Clinical trials that led to FDA approval were conducted for 6 weeks. Use beyond 6 weeks requires physician supervision and was not studied in clinical trials.

Possible Advantages of This Drug
Effective reversal of symptoms of psychosis while acting at different sites than previously available agents.

▷ **This Drug Should Not Be Taken If**
- you have had an allergic reaction to it previously.
- you have had neuroleptic malignant syndrome.

▷ **Inform Your Physician Before Taking This Drug If**
- you have a seizure disorder.
- your liver is compromised.
- you have constitutionally low blood pressure or are taking medicine to treat high blood pressure.
- you have severe liver disease.
- you have a history of breast cancer.
- you are taking any drug with sedative effects.
- you tend to be constipated.
- you plan to have surgery under general or spinal anesthesia in the near future.
- you have problems swallowing.

Possible Side Effects (natural, expected, and unavoidable drug actions)
Orthostatic hypotension (see Glossary), drowsiness.

▷ **Possible Adverse Effects** (unusual, unexpected, and infrequent reactions)
If any of the following develop, consult your physician promptly for guidance.
Mild Adverse Effects
Allergic reactions: skin rash, itching—rare.
Drowsiness, agitation, insomnia, and dizziness—frequent.
Headache, drowsiness—rare; depression—rare; dizziness—rare to infrequent.
Fast heart rate (tachycardia)—infrequent.
Weight gain, constipation, or cough—infrequent.
Serious Adverse Effects
Allergic reactions: hair loss—rare.
Abnormal movements (appears to be dose related)—infrequent.
Drug-induced increased liver enzymes—rare.
Difficulty swallowing (dysphagia)—case reports.
Tardive dyskinesia has been reported with other agents.
Neuroleptic malignant syndrome has been reported with other agents.

▷ **Possible Effects on Sexual Function:** Impotence, abnormal ejaculation, or menstrual changes—infrequent.

▷ **Adverse Effects That May Mimic Natural Diseases or Disorders**
Nervous system reactions may suggest true Parkinson's disease.
Liver reactions may suggest viral hepatitis.

Possible Effects on Laboratory Tests

Prolactin levels: increased.

Liver function tests: increased liver enzymes (ALT/GPT, AST/GOT, and alkaline phosphatase).

CAUTION

1. Other medicines (nonprescription or prescription) that can cause drowsiness or central nervous system effects may react unfavorably with this medicine. Talk with your doctor or pharmacist before combining any medicines.

2. Since this medicine can cause orthostatic hypotension, some high blood pressure (antihypertensive) medicines may have a greater than expected effect if taken with olanzapine.

Precautions for Use

By Infants and Children: Safety and effectiveness for those under 18 years of age are not established.

By Those Over 60 Years of Age: Lower starting doses should be taken; caution is advised regarding drowsiness, dizziness, and orthostatic hypotension, since olanzapine can cause changes in the ability of the body to regulate changes in temperature, and this regulation may be less intact in older patients to begin with. You may also be more susceptible to Parkinson-like reactions and/or tardive dyskinesia (see Glossary). Discuss early indications of these reactions with your doctor, as progression of these reactions may lead to symptoms that are not reversible.

▷ **Advisability of Use During Pregnancy**

Pregnancy Category: C. See Pregnancy Risk Categories at the back of this book.

Animal studies: Rat and mouse studies reveal increased mammary gland adenomas (when the animals were given 0.5 and 2 times the mg-per-square-meter human dose) respectively. Increased numbers of nonviable fetuses were seen in one rat study using nine times the maximum human dose.

Human studies: Adequate studies of pregnant women are not available.

Use of this drug is a benefit-to-risk decision. Ask your doctor for guidance.

Advisability of Use If Breast-Feeding

Presence of this drug in breast milk: Yes in rats; unknown in humans.

Avoid drug or refrain from nursing.

Habit-Forming Potential: None.

Effects of Overdose: Reports of 67 overdoses were made during clinical trials. The patient who took the largest dose had drowsiness and slurred speech.

Possible Effects of Long-Term Use: None defined as yet.

Suggested Periodic Examinations While Taking This Drug (at physician's discretion)

Liver function tests. Careful inspection of the tongue for early evidence of fine, involuntary, wavelike movements that could be the beginning of tardive dyskinesia. Sitting and standing blood pressure checks may be advisable when therapy is started to assess orthostatic hypotension.

▷ **While Taking This Drug, Observe the Following**

Foods: No restrictions. Follow prescribed diet.

Beverages: No restrictions. May be taken with milk.

▷   *Alcohol:* Avoid completely.

Tobacco Smoking: Olanzapine is removed from the body up to 40% faster in people who smoke compared to those who do not. Recommendations for dosing changes are not available. I advise everyone to quit smoking.

Marijuana Smoking: Expected to cause an increase in drowsiness; accentuation of orthostatic hypotension; increased risk of precipitating latent psychoses, confusing the interpretation of mental status and drug responses.

▷ *Other Drugs:*

Olanzapine *taken concurrently* with
- any sedative drugs (prescription and nonprescription) can cause excessive sedation.
- any medicine that has central nervous system activity may result in additive effects.
- any medicine that can cause liver damage may result in additive liver problems.
- activated charcoal will decrease absorption of olanzapine. (May be of use in overdoses.)
- benzodiazepines (see Drug Classes) may magnify the orthostatic hypotension problem caused by olanzapine.
- carbamazepine (Tegretol) causes up to a 50% increase in removal of olanzapine from the body. Dosing increases in olanzapine appear prudent.

The following drugs may *decrease* the effects of olanzapine:
- fluvoxamine (Luvox).
- rifampin (Rifater, others).

▷ *Driving, Hazardous Activities:* This drug may cause drowsiness or dizziness. Restrict activities as necessary.

Aviation Note: The use of this drug *may be a disqualification* for piloting. Consult a designated aviation medical examiner.

Exposure to Sun: No problems reported.

Exposure to Heat: This medicine can cause problems in regulating body temperature (core temperature homeostasis). If you work or are frequently in a hot environment, be careful to replace enough fluids to avoid dehydration.

Heavy Exercise or Exertion: Since this medicine may cause problems in temperature regulation, caution is advised.

Discontinuation: Do not stop taking this medicine without first talking to your doctor.

OLSALAZINE (ohl SAL a zeen)

Introduced: 1987   **Class:** Bowel anti-inflammatory   **Prescription:** USA: Yes   **Controlled Drug:** USA: No; Canada: No   **Available as Generic:** USA: No; Canada: No

Brand Name: Dipentum

BENEFITS versus RISKS	
Possible Benefits	*Possible Risks*
EFFECTIVE SUPPRESSION OF INFLAMMATORY BOWEL DISEASE	RARE BONE MARROW DEPRESSION (see Glossary) Drug-induced hepatitis Occasional aggravation of ulcerative colitis

▷ **Principal Uses**

As a Single Drug Product: Uses currently included in FDA-approved labeling: Used to maintain remission of chronic ulcerative colitis and proctitis.

Other (unlabeled) generally accepted uses: Has a role in treatment of active ulcerative colitis.

How This Drug Works: This drug suppresses the formation of prostaglandins (and related compounds), tissue substances that induce inflammation, tissue destruction, and diarrhea—the main features of ulcerative colitis and proctitis.

Available Dose Forms and Strengths

Capsules — 250 mg

Tablets (in Canada only) — 500 mg

▷ **Recommended Dose Ranges** (Actual dose and schedule must be determined for each patient individually.)

Infants and Children: Dose not established.

12 to 60 Years of Age: 500 mg twice daily, morning and evening.

Over 60 Years of Age: Same as 12 to 60 years of age.

Conditions Requiring Dosing Adjustments

Liver Function: No changes needed in liver disease, but since this drug can be toxic to the liver (granulomatous hepatitis), it should be used with caution by patients with liver problems.

Kidney Function: Some of the metabolites of olsalazine are eliminated by the kidneys. There is potential for kidney damage by one of these compounds, and the drug should be a benefit-to-risk decision by patients with compromised kidneys.

▷ **Dosing Instructions:**   The capsule may be opened and taken with food, preferably with breakfast and dinner.

Usual Duration of Use: Use on a regular schedule for 1 to 3 weeks determines effectiveness in controlling the symptoms of ulcerative colitis. Long-term use (months to years) requires physician supervision.

Possible Advantages of This Drug

Does not inhibit sperm production or cause infertility.

▷ **This Drug Should Not Be Taken If**

• you have had an allergic reaction to it previously.

• you have severely impaired kidney function.

• you are allergic to aspirin.

▷ **Inform Your Physician Before Taking This Drug If**

• you are allergic to aspirin (or other salicylates), mesalamine, or sulfasalazine.

• you are allergic by nature: history of hay fever, asthma, hives, eczema.

• you have impaired kidney function.

• you have severe liver disease.

• you are currently taking sulfasalazine (Azulfidine).

Possible Side Effects (natural, expected, and unavoidable drug actions)

None.

▷ **Possible Adverse Effects** (unusual, unexpected, and infrequent reactions)

If any of the following develop, consult your physician promptly for guidance.

Mild Adverse Effects
  Allergic reactions: skin rash, itching—rare.
  Headache, drowsiness, depression, dizziness—rare.
  Loss of appetite, indigestion, nausea, vomiting, stomach pain, diarrhea—rare to infrequent.
  Paresthesias or blurred vision—rare.
  Joint aches and pains—infrequent.
Serious Adverse Effects
  Allergic reactions: dermatitis, hair loss—rare.
  Bone marrow depression (see Glossary): fatigue, fever, sore throat, abnormal bleeding/bruising—case reports.
  Drug-induced hepatitis-like reactions (see Glossary), pericarditis, pancreatitis, or kidney damage—rare.
  Spasm of the bronchi of the lung—rare.

▷ **Possible Effects on Sexual Function:**   Impotence, excessive menstrual flow—case reports.

Possible Effects on Laboratory Tests
  Complete blood cell counts: decreased red cells, hemoglobin, white cells, and platelets; increased eosinophils.
  Liver function tests: increased liver enzymes (ALT/GPT, AST/GOT, and alkaline phosphatase), increased bilirubin.
  Urinalysis: red blood cells and protein present.

CAUTION
  1. Report promptly any signs of infection or unusual bleeding or bruising.
  2. Report promptly any indications of active or intensified ulcerative colitis: abdominal cramping, bloody diarrhea, fever.

Precautions for Use
  By Infants and Children: Safety and effectiveness for those under 12 years of age are not established.
  By Those Over 60 Years of Age: None.

▷ **Advisability of Use During Pregnancy**
  Pregnancy Category: C. See Pregnancy Risk Categories at the back of this book.
  Animal studies: Rat studies reveal toxic effects on the fetus, retarded bone development, and impaired development of internal organs.
  Human studies: Adequate studies of pregnant women are not available.
  Use this drug only if clearly needed. Ask your physician for guidance.

Advisability of Use If Breast-Feeding
  Presence of this drug in breast milk: Controversial; has caused diarrhea in some infants.
  Avoid drug or refrain from nursing.

Habit-Forming Potential: None.

Effects of Overdose: Headache, dizziness, nausea, vomiting, abdominal cramping.

Possible Effects of Long-Term Use: Bone marrow depression (impaired production of blood cells).

Suggested Periodic Examinations While Taking This Drug (at physician's discretion)
  Complete blood cell counts.

Liver function tests.
Kidney function tests, urinalysis.

▷ **While Taking This Drug, Observe the Following**
Foods: No restrictions. Follow prescribed diet.
Beverages: No restrictions. May be taken with milk.
▷ *Alcohol:* No interactions expected.
Tobacco Smoking: No interactions expected. I advise everyone to quit smoking.
▷ *Other Drugs:*
Olsalazine *taken concurrently* with
- alendronate (Fosamax) may increase risk of GI upset.
- enoxaparin (Lovenox) may increase bleeding risk.
- varicella vaccine (Varivax) may result in an increased risk of Reye syndrome. This drug should be avoided for 6 weeks after the vaccine is given.
▷ *Driving, Hazardous Activities:* This drug may cause drowsiness or dizziness. Restrict activities as necessary.
Aviation Note: The use of this drug *may be a disqualification* for piloting. Consult a designated aviation medical examiner.
Exposure to Sun: Use caution—this drug can cause photosensitivity (see Glossary).

OMEPRAZOLE (oh MEH pra zohl)

Introduced: 1986   **Class:** Proton pump inhibitor   **Prescription:** USA: Yes   **Controlled Drug:** USA: No; Canada: No   **Available as Generic:** USA: No; Canada: No
Brand Names: Prilosec, ✚Losec

BENEFITS versus RISKS	
Possible Benefits	*Possible Risks*
VERY EFFECTIVE TREATMENT OF CONDITIONS ASSOCIATED WITH EXCESSIVE PRODUCTION OF GASTRIC ACID: Zollinger-Ellison syndrome, mastocytosis, endocrine adenoma	Rare aplastic anemia Rare liver failure
VERY EFFECTIVE TREATMENT OF REFLUX ESOPHAGITIS, GASTRIC AND DUODENAL ULCERS	
EFFECTIVE IN COMBINATION WITH CLARITHROMYCIN and AMOXICILLIN in treatment of *Helicobacter pylori* infections	
Prevention of NSAID-induced ulcers	

▷ **Principal Uses**
As a Single Drug Product: Uses currently included in FDA-approved labeling: (1) Inhibits stomach acid formation in acute and chronic gastritis, reflux esophagitis, gastroesophageal reflux disease, Zollinger-Ellison syndrome, mastocytosis, endocrine adenomas, and active duodenal ulcer; (2) approved

for long-term use in erosive esophagitis; (3) approved for combination (with clarithromycin—Biaxin) in patients with positive *Helicobacter pylori* cultures; (4) helps in the short-term treatment of active and benign stomach (gastric) ulcers; (5) part of a three-drug, 10-day regimen (omeprazole, amoxicillin, and clarithromycin) to treat duodenal ulcers.

Other (unlabeled) generally accepted uses: (1) May have a role in treating severe stomach bleeding (hemorrhagic gastritis); (2) possible use in ulcerative colitis; (3) prevention of ulcers caused by NSAIDs.

How This Drug Works: Inhibits a specific enzyme system (proton pump H/K ATPase) in the stomach lining, stopping production of stomach acid and thereby (1) eliminates a principal cause of the condition under treatment, and (2) creates an environment conducive to healing.

Available Dose Forms and Strengths

Capsules, delayed release — 20 mg

▷ **Usual Adult Dose Range:** Reflux esophagitis: 20 mg once daily for 4 to 8 weeks.

Excessive stomach acid conditions: 60 mg once daily for as long as necessary. In extreme cases, doses of 120 mg three times a day have been used.

Gastric and duodenal ulcer: 20 mg once daily for 4 to 8 weeks.

Duodenal ulcer combination therapy: 10-day regimen: Omeprazole 20 mg daily with amoxicillin 1000 mg and clarithromycin 500 mg twice daily.

Note: Actual dose and schedule must be determined for each patient individually.

Conditions Requiring Dosing Adjustments

Liver Function: Patients should be monitored closely.

Kidney Function: Dose adjustments do not appear to be needed.

▷ **Dosing Instructions:** Take immediately before eating, preferably the morning meal. The capsule should be swallowed whole without opening; the contents should not be crushed or chewed. This drug may be taken with antacids if they are needed to relieve stomach pain.

Usual Duration of Use: Use on a regular schedule for 2 to 3 weeks determines benefit in suppressing stomach acid production. Long-term use (months to years) requires periodic physician evaluation of response.

Possible Advantages of This Drug

Effectively inhibits acid secretion at all times: basal conditions (stomach empty and at rest) and following food, alcohol, smoking, or other stimulants. More effective than histamine (H_2) receptor blocking drugs in treating severe reflux esophagitis and refractory duodenal ulcer.

Currently a "Drug of Choice"

For the short-term treatment of severe reflux esophagitis and the long-term treatment of Zollinger-Ellison syndrome and erosive esophagitis. Part of a one-week regimen of choice (comparing outcomes) with clarithromycin and metronidazole for treating *H. pylori*.

▷ **This Drug Should Not Be Taken If**
- you have had an allergic reaction to it previously.
- you have a currently active bone marrow or blood cell disorder.

▷ **Inform Your Physician Before Taking This Drug If**
- you have a history of liver disease or impaired liver function.

- your history includes any bone marrow or blood cell disorder, especially a drug-induced one.
- you take any anticoagulant medication, or diazepam (Valium) or phenytoin (Dilantin, etc.).

Possible Side Effects (natural, expected, and unavoidable drug actions)

Acid in the stomach actually works to protect it from some bacterial infections. Since omeprazole is so effective in decreasing acid, it may increase the likelihood of infection by *Campylobacter*. This organism causes gastroenteritis. Symptoms may include mucousy, loose stools and fever. Talk with your doctor if you start to develop these symptoms while taking omeprazole.

▷ **Possible Adverse Effects** (unusual, unexpected, and infrequent reactions)

If any of the following develop, consult your physician promptly for guidance.

Mild Adverse Effects

Allergic reactions: skin rash—rare; itching.

Headache, dizziness, muscle pain, or ringing in ears; drowsiness, paresthesias, weakness—rare to infrequent.

Indigestion, nausea, vomiting, diarrhea, constipation—rare to infrequent.

Serious Adverse Effects

Allergic reactions: rare allergic kidney damage (interstitial nephritis).

Bone marrow depression: fatigue, fever, sore throat, infections, abnormal bleeding/bruising—case reports.

Liver damage with jaundice (see Glossary)—case reports.

Chest pain or angina—case reports.

Half-facial pain—case reports.

Yeast infection (*Candida*) of the esophagus—possible.

Kidney inflammation (interstitial nephritis)—case reports.

Possible Effects on Sexual Function: Drug-induced male breast enlargement and tenderness (gynecomastia)—case report.

▷ **Adverse Effects That May Mimic Natural Diseases or Disorders**

Persistent infection or bruising may be bone marrow depression; blood counts are advisable.

Liver reactions may suggest viral hepatitis.

Possible Effects on Laboratory Tests

Complete blood cell counts: decreased red cells, hemoglobin, white cells, and platelets.

Blood glucose level: decreased.

Liver function tests: increased liver enzymes (ALT/GPT, AST/GOT, and alkaline phosphatase), increased bilirubin.

CAUTION

1. Take this drug for exactly as long as your doctor prescribed. Do not extend its use without your physician's guidance.
2. Report promptly any indications of infection.
3. Tell your doctor if you plan to take any other medications (prescription or over-the-counter) while taking omeprazole.
4. Acid in the stomach actually works to protect it from some bacterial infections. Since omeprazole is so effective in decreasing acid, it may increase the likelihood of infection by *Campylobacter*. This organism causes

gastroenteritis. Symptoms may include mucousy, loose stools and fever. Talk with your doctor if you start to develop these symptoms while taking omeprazole.

5. Although this drug effectively treats ulcers, it does not preclude the possibility of cancer of the stomach.

Precautions for Use

By Infants and Children: Safety and effectiveness for those under 12 years of age are not established.

By Those Over 60 Years of Age: Slower elimination of this drug makes it possible to achieve satisfactory response with smaller doses; this reduces the risk of adverse effects. Limit the daily dose to 20 mg if possible.

▷ **Advisability of Use During Pregnancy**

Pregnancy Category: C. See Pregnancy Risk Categories at the back of this book. Animal studies: No drug-induced birth defects found in rats; drug-induced embryo and fetal toxicity were demonstrated in rats and rabbits.

Human studies: Adequate studies of pregnant women are not available.

Avoid use if possible. Use only if clearly necessary and for the shortest possible time.

Advisability of Use If Breast-Feeding

Presence of this drug in breast milk: Unknown.

Avoid drug or refrain from nursing.

Habit-Forming Potential: None.

Effects of Overdose: Possible drowsiness, dizziness, lethargy, abdominal pain, nausea.

Possible Effects of Long-Term Use: Some long-term (2-year) studies in rats revealed the development of drug-induced carcinoid tumors in the stomach. To date, long-term use of this drug (more than 5 years) in humans has not revealed any drug-induced tumor potential. Pending more studies of long-term human use, it is advisable to limit the use of this drug to the shortest duration possible.

Suggested Periodic Examinations While Taking This Drug (at physician's discretion)

Complete blood cell counts.

▷ **While Taking This Drug, Observe the Following**

Foods: No restrictions.

Beverages: No restrictions. May be taken with milk.

▷ *Alcohol:* No interactions expected. However, alcohol is best avoided; it stimulates the secretion of stomach acid.

Tobacco Smoking: Smoking may stimulate the secretion of stomach acid. I advise everyone to quit smoking.

▷ *Other Drugs:*

Omeprazole may *increase* the effects of

- anticoagulants (warfarin, etc.), and increase the risk of bleeding.
- carbamazepine (Tegretol).
- clonazepam (Klonopin) and some other benzodiazepines (see Drug Classes), and lead to benzodiazepine toxicity.
- cyclosporine (Sandimmune) by increasing its level (decreased levels also reported).

- diazepam (Valium), and cause excessive sedation.
- digoxin (Lanoxin), and lead to toxicity.
- disulfiram (Antabuse).
- fluvastatin (Lescol).
- phenytoin (Dilantin, etc.), and cause phenytoin toxicity.
- warfarin (Coumadin), and lead to bleeding. More frequent INR (prothrombin time or protime) testing is needed. Warfarin doses should be adjusted according to laboratory results.

Omeprazole may *decrease* the effects of

- amoxicillin (various).
- ampicillin (various).
- iron preparations.
- itraconazole (Sporonox).
- ketoconazole (Nizoral).
- ritonavir (Norvir); may also increase omeprazole effects.

▷ *Driving, Hazardous Activities:* This drug may cause drowsiness and dizziness. Limit activities as necessary.

Aviation Note: The use of this drug *may be a disqualification* for piloting. Consult a designated aviation medical examiner.

Exposure to Sun: No restrictions.

Discontinuation: The duration of use will vary according to the condition under treatment and individual patient response. Premature discontinuation could result in incomplete healing or prompt recurrence of symptoms.

ONDANSETRON (on DAN sa tron)

Introduced: 1993   **Class:** Antiemetic, 5-HT$_3$ antagonist   **Prescription:** USA: Yes   **Controlled Drug:** USA: No; Canada: No   **Available as Generic:** USA: No; Canada: No

Brand Name: Zofran, Zofran Oral Solution

BENEFITS versus RISKS	
Possible Benefits	*Possible Risks*
EFFECTIVE ORAL TREATMENT AND RELIEF OR PREVENTION OF SEVERE VOMITING	Bronchospasm Grand mal seizures Liver toxicity Heart rate and rhythm changes Low potassium (All rare)

▷ **Principal Uses**

As a Single Drug Product: Uses currently included in FDA-approved labeling: (1) Prevention of nausea and vomiting associated with initial and repeat courses of chemotherapy; (2) treatment or prevention of postoperative nausea and vomiting; (3) prevention or treatment of emesis (vomiting) caused by radiation therapy.

Other (unlabeled) generally accepted uses: (1) Helps patients keep from vomiting medicines used to treat drug overdoses; (2) may have a role in treating schizophrenia; (3) some panic attack data; (4) eases some tremor cases.

How This Drug Works: Ondansetron antagonizes 5-HT$_3$ receptors. It appears to block vomiting by blocking serotonin (a chemical causing vomiting) at 5-HT$_3$ receptors.

Available Dose Forms and Strengths
> Intravenous — 2 mg/ml
> Oral solution — 4 mg/5 ml
> > Tablets — 4 mg, 8 mg

How to Store
> Keep at room temperature. Avoid exposing this medicine to extreme humidity.

▷ **Recommended Dose Ranges** (Actual dose and schedule must be determined for each patient individually.)
> *Infants and Children:* Little information is available regarding use in those less than 3 years old.
> *4 to 11 Years of Age:* Vomiting from chemotherapy: one (4-mg) tablet or 5 ml of the oral solution is given three times daily by mouth. The method and frequency is then the same as for adults.
> *12 to 60 Years of Age:* One 8-mg tablet or 10 ml of the oral solution taken three times a day. The first dose should be taken 30 minutes before the start of the emetogenic chemotherapy. Subsequent doses should be taken 8 hours after the first dose. Further doses of 8 mg every 12 hours are taken for 1–2 days after chemotherapy is finished.
> *Over 60 Years of Age:* Same as 12 to 60 years of age.

Conditions Requiring Dosing Adjustments
> *Liver Function:* Maximum dose for people with severe liver failure is 8 mg per day.
> *Kidney Function:* Studies have not been conducted on patients with impaired kidneys. The decision to use ondansetron must be made by your physician. Only 5 to 10% of the drug is removed unchanged by the kidneys. Based on this small involvement of the kidneys, no changes are expected to be needed with short-term use.

▷ **Dosing Instructions:** May be taken on an empty stomach.

Usual Duration of Use: Since chemotherapy can cause vomiting long after it has been given, continual use on a regular schedule for 3 days is usually necessary.

Possible Advantages of This Drug
> Effective oral prevention of severe vomiting caused by some kinds of chemotherapy that have been poorly controlled by earlier agents.

Currently a "Drug of Choice"
> For control of vomiting secondary to emetogenic (likely to cause vomiting) cancer chemotherapy.

▷ **This Drug Should Not Be Taken If**
> • you had an allergic reaction to it previously.

▷ **Inform Your Physician Before Taking This Drug If**
> • you have a history of liver disease.
> • you have a history of kidney disease.
> • you have a history of alcoholism.
> • you are unsure how much to take or how often to take it.

Possible Side Effects (natural, expected, and unavoidable drug actions)
Constipation, sedation.

▷ **Possible Adverse Effects** (unusual, unexpected, and infrequent reactions)
If any of the following develop, consult your physician promptly for guidance.
Mild Adverse Effects
Allergic reactions: skin rash—rare.
Headache—frequent; dizziness and light-headedness, constipation, diarrhea, dry mouth—infrequent.
Serious Adverse Effects
Allergic reactions: anaphylaxis—rare.
Extrapyramidal reactions (abnormal body movements) or seizures—case reports.
Bronchospasm—rare.
Angina, tachycardia, arrhythmias—all rare.
Hypokalemia (low potassium)—rare.

▷ **Possible Effects on Sexual Function:**   None reported.

Possible Delayed Adverse Effects: None reported.

▷ **Adverse Effects That May Mimic Natural Diseases or Disorders**
Changes in liver enzymes may mimic hepatitis; however, specific antibodies will not be present. Bronchospasm may mimic asthma.

Natural Diseases or Disorders That May Be Activated by This Drug
Epilepsy, asthma.

Possible Effects on Laboratory Tests
Liver function tests: Transient increases in SGPT, SGOT, and bilirubin.

CAUTION
1. Even though you do not feel an urge to vomit, continue ondansetron for the prescribed length of therapy. The vomit-causing effect of cancer chemotherapy or radiation therapy continues after the medicine or radiation has been given.

Precautions for Use
By Infants and Children: Safety and effectiveness for those under 3 years of age are not established.
By Those Over 60 Years of Age: Same as for general adult population.

▷ **Advisability of Use During Pregnancy**
Pregnancy Category: B. See Pregnancy Risk Categories at the back of this book.
Animal studies: The drug and its metabolites pass into the milk. No adverse effects on gestation, postnatal development, or reproductive performance has been observed in rats.
Human studies: Adequate studies of pregnant women are not available.
Ask your physician for guidance.

Advisability of Use If Breast-Feeding
Presence of this drug in breast milk: This medicine is excreted in the milk of rats; however, human data is not available. Caution should be used if this medicine is to be used by nursing mothers.

Habit-Forming Potential: None.

Effects of Overdose: Doses 10 times greater than recommended have not resulted in illness.

Possible Effects of Long-Term Use: Not indicated for long-term use.

Suggested Periodic Examinations While Taking This Drug (at physician's discretion)

Watch for vomiting occurrence and frequency.

▷ **While Taking This Drug, Observe the Following**

Foods: No restrictions.

Beverages: No restrictions.

▷   *Alcohol:* Additive sedation and potential additive urge to vomit if alcohol is taken in large doses. Alcohol abuse that has led to liver problems may limit the total dose which can be taken.

Tobacco Smoking: No direct clinical interactions; I advise everyone to quit smoking.

Marijuana Smoking: May induce additive sedation and provide additive antiemetic effects.

▷   *Other Drugs:*

The following drugs may *increase* the effects of ondansetron:

- allopurinol (Zyloprim).
- cimetidine (Tagamet).
- disulfiram (Antabuse).
- fluconazole (Diflucan).
- isoniazid (Nydrazid).
- macrolide antibiotics (erythromycin, azithromycin, clarithromycin, dirithromycin).
- metronidazole (Flagyl).
- monoamine oxidase inhibitor antidepressants (MAO inhibitors)—Nardil).
- ritonavir (Norvir), and perhaps other protease inhibitors (see Drug Classes).

The following drugs may *decrease* the effects of ondansetron:

- barbiturates.
- carbamazepine (Tegretol).
- phenylbutazone (Butazolidin, Azolid).
- phenytoin (Dilantin).
- rifampin (Rifadin) and rifabutin (Mycobutin).
- tolbutamide (Orinase).

▷   *Driving, Hazardous Activities:* This drug may cause drowsiness and dizziness. Restrict activities as necessary.

Aviation Note: The use of this drug *may be a disqualification* for piloting. Consult a designated aviation medical examiner.

Exposure to Sun: No restrictions.

Discontinuation: Ondansetron may be stopped after you've completed the prescribed course (usually 3 days) of therapy.

Special Storage Instructions: Keep at room temperature. Avoid exposing this medicine to extreme humidity.

ORAL CONTRACEPTIVES (OR al kon tra SEP tivs)

Other Names: Estrogens/progestins, OCs, birth control pills
Introduced: 1956   **Class:** Female sex hormones   **Prescription:** USA:
Yes   **Controlled Drug:** USA: No; Canada: No   **Available as Generic:**
USA: Yes, in some forms; Canada: No
Brand Names: Brevicon, Demulen, Desogen, Enovid, Genora, Gestodene, Jen-
est 28, Levlen, Loestrin, Lo/Ovral, Micronor*, ♣Minestrin 1/20, Min-Ovral,
Mircette, Modicon, NEE, Nelova, Nelova 1/50 M, Nelova 10/11, Norcept-E
1/35, Nordette, Norethin 1/35E, Norethin 1/50M, Norinyl, Norlestrin, Nor-
Q.D.*, Ortho Cyclen, Ortho Tri-Cyclen, Ortho-Novum 777, Ovcon, Ovral,
Ovrette*, ♣Synphasic, Tri-Levlen, Tri-Norinyl, Triphasil, Triquilar, Zovia

BENEFITS versus RISKS	
Possible Benefits	*Possible Risks*
HIGHLY EFFECTIVE FOR CONTRACEPTIVE PROTECTION	SERIOUS, LIFE-THREATENING THROMBOEMBOLIC DISORDERS in susceptible individuals
Moderately effective as adjunctive treatment in management of excessive menses and endometriosis	Hypertension
	Fluid retention
	Intensification of migrainelike headaches and fibrocystic breast changes
	Accelerated growth of uterine fibroid tumors
	Drug-induced hepatitis with jaundice
	Benign liver tumors—rare

▷ **Principal Uses**

As a Single Drug Product: Uses currently included in FDA-approved labeling: (1)
Prevention of conception. (The "Mini-Pill" contains only one component, a
progestin; this has been shown to be slightly less effective than the combination of estrogen and progestin in preventing pregnancy); (2) used in cases
where women do not make enough hormones (female hypogonadism); (3)
helps decrease excessive blood flow at menstruation (hypermenorrhea); (4)
of use in endometriosis as the combination mestranol and norethynodrel.
Other (unlabeled) generally accepted uses: (1) May be of benefit in abnormal
hair growth in women (hirsutism); (2) some combination forms can have a
protective effect against osteoporosis.

As a Combination Drug Product [CD]: Uses currently included in FDA-approved
labeling: (1) Most oral contraceptives consist of a combination of an estrogen and a progestin—these products are the most effective form of medicinal contraception available; (2) they are sometimes used to treat menstrual
irregularity, excessively heavy menstrual flow, and endometriosis.
Other (unlabeled) generally accepted uses: (1) Gestodene has been reported to
inhibit certain breast cancer cell lines—clinical studies are needed; (2) may
have a protective effect against osteoporosis; (3) triphasic oral contraceptives can help in the prevention or treatment of menopause symptoms.

*"Mini-Pill" type, contains progestin only.

Author's Note: Recent research linked the number of times a woman ovulates to increased risk of ovarian cancer. This finding was associated with a P-53 gene, which may account for as much as 50% of ovarian cancer. Since birth control pills decrease the number of times that women ovulate, they may have a role in helping prevent cancer in people found to carry the P-53 gene. Further research is required.

How These Drugs Work: When estrogen and progestin are taken in sufficient dose and on a regular basis, the blood and tissue levels of these hormones increase to resemble those that occur during pregnancy. This results in suppression of the two pituitary gland hormones that normally cause ovulation (the formation and release of an egg by the ovary). In addition, these drugs may (1) alter the cervical mucus so that it resists the passage of sperm, and (2) alter the lining of the uterus so that it resists implantation of the egg (if ovulation occurs).

Available Dose Forms and Strengths

Tablets — Several combinations of synthetic estrogens and progestins in varying strengths; see the package label of the brand prescribed.

▷ **Usual Adult Dose Range:**   Start with the first tablet on the fifth day after the onset of menstruation. Follow with one tablet daily (taken at the same time each day) for 21 consecutive days. Resume treatment on the eighth day following the last tablet taken during the preceding cycle. The schedule is to take the drug daily for 3 weeks and to omit it for 1 week. For the Mini-Pill (progestin only), initiate treatment on the first day of menstruation and take one tablet daily, every day, throughout the year (no interruption). The new Mircette brand uses 20 mcg of ethinyl estradiol and 150 mcg of do-gesterel for 21 days. Two days of dummy (placebo) tablets are then taken, then five days of 10 mcg ethinyl estradiol.

Note: Actual dose and schedule must be determined for each patient individually.

Conditions Requiring Dosing Adjustments

Liver Function: Should **NOT** be taken if you have liver disease.
Kidney Function: Oral contraceptives are not significantly eliminated by the kidneys.

▷ **Dosing Instructions:**   The tablets may be crushed and taken with or after food to reduce stomach upset. To ensure regular (every day) use and uniform blood levels, it is best to take the tablet at the same time daily.

Possible Advantages of These Drugs

Effective control of conception.
Mircette form may benefit women who have migraines the second week they are "off the pill."

Usual Duration of Use: According to individual needs and circumstances. Long-term use (months to years) requires physician supervision and evaluation every 6 months.

▷ **These Drugs Should Not Be Taken If**
- you have had an allergic reaction to any dose form.
- you have a history of thrombophlebitis, embolism, heart attack, or stroke.
- you have breast cancer.

- you have active liver disease, seriously impaired liver function, or a history of liver tumor.
- you have diabetes and have developed circulatory disease.
- you have high blood pressure.
- you have not had any periods (amenorrhea).
- you have abnormal and unexplained vaginal bleeding.
- you have sickle cell disease.
- you are pregnant.

▷ **Inform Your Physician Before Taking These Drugs If**
- you have had an adverse reaction to any oral contraceptive.
- you have a history of cancer of the breast or reproductive organs.
- you have fibrocystic breast changes, uterine fibroid tumors, endometriosis, migrainelike headaches, epilepsy, asthma, elevated lipids, prolapse of the mitral valve of the heart, heart disease, high blood pressure, gallbladder disease, diabetes, or porphyria.
- you are over 40. This was an age-related limit previously, but current thinking says that use of these medicines may occur as a benefit-to-risk decision.
- you smoke tobacco on a regular basis.
- you plan to have surgery in the near future.

Possible Side Effects (natural, expected, and unavoidable drug actions)
Fluid retention, weight gain, "breakthrough" bleeding (spotting in middle of menstrual cycle), altered menstrual pattern, lack of menstruation (during and following cessation of drug), increased susceptibility to yeast infection of the genital tissues. Tannish pigmentation of the face.

▷ **Possible Adverse Effects** (unusual, unexpected, and infrequent reactions)
If any of the following develop, consult your physician promptly for guidance.

Mild Adverse Effects
Allergic reactions: skin rash, hives, itching.
Headache, nervous tension, irritability, accentuation of migraine headaches—infrequent to frequent.
Rise in blood pressure (in some people)—possible.
Nausea, perhaps with vomiting—frequent (related to estrogen) and may ease if taken with evening meals.
Reduced tolerance to contact lenses or impaired color vision: blue tinge to objects, blue halo around lights—possible.

Serious Adverse Effects
Allergic reactions: anaphylaxis, erythema multiforme and nodosum (skin reactions), loss of scalp hair.
Idiosyncratic reactions: joint and muscle pains.
Emotional depression—infrequent to frequent.
Eye changes: optic neuritis, retinal thrombosis, altered curvature of the cornea, cataracts—possible.
Gallbladder disease, benign liver tumors, jaundice—case reports.
Enlargement of uterine fibroid tumors—possible.
Abnormal glucose tolerance (hyperglycemia)—frequent in people with pregnancy (gestational) diabetes.
Thrombophlebitis (inflammation of a vein with formation of blood clot): pain

or tenderness in thigh or leg, with or without swelling of foot or leg—increased risk, especially with high estrogen doses.

Drug-induced porphyria or worsening of systemic lupus erythematosus (SLE)—case reports.

Esophageal ulcers (especially if the medicine is taken lying down with no water)—case reports.

Stroke (blood clot in brain): headaches, blackout, sudden weakness or paralysis of any part of the body, severe dizziness, altered vision, slurred speech, inability to speak—possible increased risk (more probable in one study with high dose estrogen formulations).

Heart attack (blood clot in coronary artery): sudden pain in chest, neck, jaw, or arm; weakness; sweating; nausea—increased risk.

Liver cancer—increased risk with long-term use.

▷ **Possible Effects on Sexual Function:** Altered character of menstruation; midcycle spotting—may be frequent.

Increased or decreased libido—possible.

Breast enlargement and tenderness with milk production—possible.

Absent menstruation and infertility (temporary) after discontinuation of drug.

Possible Delayed Adverse Effects: Estrogens taken during pregnancy can predispose the female child to the later development of cancer of the vagina or cervix following puberty. Nonpregnant use does not increase breast cancer.

▷ **Adverse Effects That May Mimic Natural Diseases or Disorders**

Liver reactions may suggest viral hepatitis.

Natural Diseases or Disorders That May Be Activated by These Drugs

Latent hypertension, diabetes mellitus, acute intermittent porphyria, lupus-erythematosus-like syndrome.

Possible Effects on Laboratory Tests

Blood lupus erythematosus (LE) cells: positive.

Blood clotting time or INR: decreased.

Blood amylase and lipase levels: increased (very rare pancreatitis).

Blood total cholesterol, HDL, LDL, and VLDL cholesterol levels: usually no effects; some variability, depending upon estrogen and progestin content of preparation used.

Blood triglyceride levels: no effect to increased, depending upon estrogen and progestin content of preparation used.

Blood glucose level: increased.

Blood thyroid-stimulating hormone (TSH) level: no effect.

Blood thyroid hormone levels: T_3 and T_4—increased; free T_4—either no effect or decreased.

Liver function tests: increased liver enzymes (ALT/GPT, AST/GOT, alkaline phosphatase) and bilirubin.

CAUTION

1. Serious adverse effects due to these drugs are a very low risk. However, any unusual development should be reported and evaluated promptly.
2. Studies indicate that women over 30 years of age who smoke and use oral contraceptives are at significantly greater risk of having a serious cardiovascular event than are nonusers.
3. The risk of thromboembolism increases with the amount of estrogen in

the product and the age of the user. Low-estrogen combinations are advised.

4. It is advisable to discontinue these drugs 1 month prior to elective surgery to reduce the risk of postsurgical thromboembolism.

5. Investigate promptly any alteration or disturbance of vision that occurs during the use of these drugs.

6. Investigate promptly the nature of recurrent, persistent, or severe headaches that develop while taking these drugs.

7. Observe for significant change of mood. Call your doctor if depression develops.

8. Certain commonly used drugs may reduce the effectiveness of oral contraceptives. Some of these are listed in the category of "Other Drugs" below.

9. Diarrhea lasting more than a few hours (and occurring during the days the drug is taken) can prevent adequate absorption of these drugs and impair their effectiveness as contraceptives.

10. If two consecutive menstrual periods are missed, ask your doctor if you should get a pregnancy test. Do not continue to use these drugs until you know whether you are pregnant.

11. **Many antibiotics may stop the effectiveness of birth control pills** (oral contraceptives). If your doctor prescribes an antibiotic, ask whether a different method of birth control is needed.

One researcher used the acronym ACHES (A = abdominal pain, C = chest pain, H = headaches, E = eye problems, S = severe leg pain)—these adverse effects require the patient to contact her doctor immediately.

▷ **Advisability of Use During Pregnancy**

Pregnancy Category: X. See Pregnancy Risk Categories at the back of this book.

Animal studies: Genital defects reported in mice and guinea pigs; cleft palate reported in rodents.

Human studies: Information from studies of pregnant women indicates that estrogens can masculinize the female fetus. In addition, limb defects and heart malformations have been reported.

It is now known that estrogens taken during pregnancy can predispose the female child to the development of cancer of the vagina or cervix following puberty.

Avoid these drugs completely during entire pregnancy.

Advisability of Use If Breast-Feeding

Presence of these drugs in breast milk: Yes, in minute amounts (ethinyl estradiol or norethindrone). These drugs may suppress milk formation if started early after delivery.

Breast-feeding is considered to be safe during the use of oral contraceptives.

Habit-Forming Potential: None.

Effects of Overdose: Headache, drowsiness, nausea, vomiting, fluid retention, abnormal vaginal bleeding, breast enlargement and discomfort.

Possible Effects of Long-Term Use: High blood pressure, gallbladder disease with stones, accelerated growth of uterine fibroid tumors, absent menstruation, and impaired fertility after discontinuation of drug.

Suggested Periodic Examinations While Taking These Drugs (at physician's discretion)

Regular (every 6 months) evaluation of the breasts and pelvic organs, including Pap smears. Liver function tests as indicated.

▷ **While Taking These Drugs, Observe the Following**

Foods: Avoid excessive use of salt if fluid retention occurs. Excessive vitamin C may increase risk of failure.

Beverages: No restrictions. May be taken with milk.

▷ *Alcohol:* No interactions expected.

Tobacco Smoking: Studies indicate that heavy smoking (15 or more cigarettes daily) while taking oral contraceptives significantly increases the risk of heart attack (coronary thrombosis). Heavy smoking should be considered a contraindication to the use of oral contraceptives. I advise everyone to quit smoking.

▷ *Other Drugs:*

Oral contraceptives may *increase* the effects of

- cyclosporine (Sandimmune), and cause toxicity.
- metoprolol (Lopressor), and cause excessive beta-blocker effects.
- prednisolone and prednisone, and cause excessive cortisonelike effects.
- some benzodiazepines (see Drug Classes), and cause excessive sedation.
- theophyllines (Theo-Dur, others), and increase the risk of toxic effects.

Oral contraceptives *taken concurrently* with

- antibiotics (such as amoxicillin or ampicillin) can seriously impair effectiveness and allow pregnancy to occur.
- antidiabetic drugs (oral hypoglycemic agents) may cause unpredictable fluctuations of blood sugar.
- ascorbic acid (vitamin C) may result in increased levels of ethinyl estradiol, and breakthrough bleeding if the vitamin C is stopped.
- tricyclic antidepressants (Elavil, Sinequan, etc.) may enhance their adverse effects and reduce their antidepressant effectiveness.
- troleandomycin (TAO) may increase occurrence of liver toxicity and jaundice.
- warfarin (Coumadin) may cause unpredictable alterations of prothrombin activity. More frequent INR (prothrombin time or protime) testing is needed, and warfarin dosing should be adjusted to laboratory test results.

The following drugs may *decrease* the effects of oral contraceptives (and impair their effectiveness):

- barbiturates (phenobarbital, etc.; see Drug Classes).
- carbamazepine (Tegretol).
- griseofulvin (Fulvicin, etc.).
- fluconazole (Diflucan).
- nevirapine (Viramune).
- penicillins (ampicillin, penicillin V).
- phenytoin (Dilantin).
- primidone (Mysoline).
- rifampin (Rifadin, Rimactane).
- ritonavir (Norvir), and perhaps other protease inhibitors (see Drug Classes).
- tetracyclines (see Drug Classes).

▷   *Driving, Hazardous Activities:* Usually no restrictions. Consult your physician for assessment of individual risk and for guidance regarding specific restrictions.

Aviation Note: Usually no restrictions. However, watch for the rare occurrence of disturbed vision and restrict activities accordingly. Consult a designated aviation medical examiner.

Exposure to Sun: Use caution—these drugs can cause photosensitivity (see Glossary).

Discontinuation: Do not stop these drugs if "breakthrough" bleeding occurs. If spotting or bleeding continues, call your doctor. A higher-estrogen pill may be required. Remember: Omitting this drug for only 1 day may allow pregnancy to occur. It is best to avoid pregnancy for 3 to 6 months after stopping these drugs; aborted fetuses from women who became pregnant within 6 months after discontinuation reveal significantly increased chromosome abnormalities.

OXAPROZIN (OX a proh zin)

See the propionic acids (nonsteroidal anti-inflammatory drugs) profile for further information.

OXICAMS
(Nonsteroidal Anti-Inflammatory Drugs)

Piroxicam (peer OX i kam)

Introduced: 1978   **Class:** Mild analgesic, anti-inflammatory   **Prescription:** USA: Yes   **Controlled Drug:** USA: No; Canada: No   **Available as Generic:** Yes

Brand Names: ✦Apo-Piroxicam, Feldene, ✦Novo-Pirocam, ✦Nu-Pirox

BENEFITS versus RISKS	
Possible Benefits	*Possible Risks*
EFFECTIVE RELIEF OF MILD TO MODERATE PAIN AND INFLAMMATION	Gastrointestinal pain, ulceration, and bleeding
	Drug-induced hepatitis—rare
	Rare kidney damage
	Mild fluid retention
	Reduced white blood cell and platelet counts

▷ **Principal Uses**

As a Single Drug Product: Uses currently included in FDA-approved labeling: Relieves mild to moderately severe pain and inflammation associated with (1) rheumatoid arthritis and (2) osteoarthritis.

Other (unlabeled) generally accepted uses: (1) Treats the morning and evening pain associated with ankylosing spondylitis; (2) helps relieve the pain and inflammation of acute gout; (3) used to treat terminal cancer pain in combination with doxepin; (4) may have a role in easing temporal arteritis; (5)

effective in painful menstruation (primary dysmenorrhea); (6) second-line therapy in acute gout.

How This Drug Works: This drug suppresses the formation of prostaglandins (and related compounds), chemicals involved in the production of inflammation and pain.

Available Dose Forms and Strengths
Capsules — 10 mg, 20 mg
Rectal suppository — 10 mg, 20 mg

▷ **Usual Adult Dose Range:** As antiarthritic: 10 mg twice daily, 12 hours apart; or 20 mg once daily. The total daily dose should not exceed 40 mg, and then for no more than 5 days. **Note: Actual dose and schedule must be determined for each patient individually.**

Conditions Requiring Dosing Adjustments
Liver Function: This drug should be used with caution and in decreased dose by patients with liver compromise.
Kidney Function: Piroxicam should be used with caution in renal compromise, and kidney function followed closely.

▷ **Dosing Instructions:** Take with or following food to prevent stomach irritation. Take with a full glass of water and remain upright (do not lie down) for 30 minutes. The capsule may be opened.

Usual Duration of Use: Use on a regular schedule for 2 weeks usually determines effectiveness in relieving the discomfort of arthritis. Long-term use (months to years) requires physician supervision and periodic evaluation.

▷ **This Drug Should Not Be Taken If**
- you have had an allergic reaction to it previously.
- you are subject to asthma or nasal polyps caused by aspirin.
- you have active peptic ulcer disease or any form of gastrointestinal bleeding.
- you have a bleeding disorder or a blood cell disorder.
- you have active liver disease.
- you have severe impairment of kidney function.

▷ **Inform Your Physician Before Taking This Drug If**
- you are allergic to aspirin or to other aspirin substitutes.
- you have a history of peptic ulcer disease, regional enteritis, or ulcerative colitis.
- you have a history of any type of bleeding disorder.
- you have impaired liver or kidney function.
- you develop signs or symptoms of pancreatitis while taking this medicine (talk with your doctor).
- you have high blood pressure or a history of heart failure.
- you take acetaminophen, aspirin or aspirin substitutes, anticoagulants, or oral antidiabetic drugs.
- you plan to have surgery of any type in the near future.

Possible Side Effects (natural, expected, and unavoidable drug actions)
Fluid retention (weight gain), prolongation of bleeding time.

▷ **Possible Adverse Effects** (unusual, unexpected, and infrequent reactions)
If any of the following develop, consult your physician promptly for guidance.

Mild Adverse Effects
　Allergic reactions: skin rash, itching, spontaneous bruising.
　Headache, dizziness, hair loss, altered or vision, ringing in ears, drowsiness, fatigue, paresthesias, inability to concentrate—rare to infrequent.
　Indigestion, nausea, vomiting, abdominal pain, diarrhea—infrequent to frequent.

Serious Adverse Effects
　Esophagitis or active peptic ulcer, stomach or intestinal bleeding—possible and more likely in elderly.
　Drug-induced liver or kidney damage—rare to infrequent.
　Serious skin damage (toxic epidermal necrolysis)—case reports.
　Pancreatitis—rare.
　Bone marrow depression (see Glossary): abnormal bleeding or bruising—case reports.
　Blood clotting problems—dose and half-life related.
　Increased blood potassium or decreased sodium—case reports.

▷ **Possible Effects on Sexual Function:**   None reported.

Possible Delayed Adverse Effects: Mild anemia due to "silent" blood loss from the stomach.

▷ **Adverse Effects That May Mimic Natural Diseases or Disorders**
　Liver reaction may suggest viral hepatitis.

Natural Diseases or Disorders That May Be Activated by This Drug
　Peptic ulcer disease, ulcerative colitis. This drug may hide symptoms of gout.

Possible Effects on Laboratory Tests
　Red blood cell count and hemoglobin level: decreased.
　Bleeding time: increased.
　Blood uric acid level: increased.
　Liver function tests: increased liver enzymes (ALT/GPT, AST/GOT, and alkaline phosphatase), increased bilirubin.
　Kidney function tests: blood creatinine and urea nitrogen (BUN) levels increased; urine analysis positive for red blood cells, casts, and increased protein content (kidney damage).
　Fecal occult blood test: positive.

CAUTION
　1. The smallest effective dose should always be used.
　2. This drug may hide early signs of infection. Tell your doctor if you think you are developing an infection.

Precautions for Use
　By Infants and Children: Indications and dose recommendations for those under 12 years of age are not established.
　By Those Over 60 Years of Age: Small doses are advisable until tolerance is determined. Observe for any indications of liver or kidney toxicity, fluid retention, dizziness, confusion, impaired memory, stomach bleeding, or constipation.

▷ **Advisability of Use During Pregnancy**
　Pregnancy Category: B; D in the final 3 months of pregnancy. See Pregnancy Risk Categories at the back of this book.
　Animal studies: No birth defects reported due to this drug.

Human studies: Adequate studies of pregnant women are not available. The manufacturer does not recommend the use of this drug during pregnancy.

Advisability of Use If Breast-Feeding
Presence of this drug in breast milk: Yes.
Avoid drug or refrain from nursing.

Habit-Forming Potential: None.

Effects of Overdose: Possible drowsiness, dizziness, ringing in the ears, nausea, vomiting, indigestion.

Possible Effects of Long-Term Use: Development of anemia due to "silent" bleeding from the gastrointestinal tract.

Suggested Periodic Examinations While Taking This Drug (at physician's discretion)
Complete blood cell counts, liver and kidney function tests.
Complete eye examinations if vision is altered in any way.
Hearing examinations if ringing in the ears or hearing loss develops.

▷ **While Taking This Drug, Observe the Following**
Foods: No restrictions.
Beverages: No restrictions. May be taken with milk.
▷ *Alcohol:* Use with caution. Both alcohol and piroxicam can irritate the stomach lining, and can increase the risk of stomach ulceration and/or bleeding.
Tobacco Smoking: No interactions expected. I advise everyone to quit smoking.
▷ *Other Drugs:*
Piroxicam may *increase* the effects of
- acetaminophen (Tylenol, etc.), and increase the risk of kidney damage; avoid prolonged use of this combination.
- adrenocortical steroids (see Drug Classes); may result in additive stomach irritation.
- anticoagulants (Coumadin, etc.), and increase the risk of bleeding; more frequent INR (prothrombin time or protime) testing is needed and dosing should then be adjusted accordingly.
- antihypertensives, such as thiazides (see Drug Classes) and others (ACE inhibitors), will blunt their therapeutic benefits.
- beta-blockers (atenolol and others)—can decrease the effectiveness of the beta-blocker.
- enoxaparin (lovenox); may increase bleeding risk.
- lithium (Lithobid, others); can lead to lithium toxicity.
- methotrexate (Mexate); may lead to methotrexate toxicity.
Piroxicam *taken concurrently* with
- ofloxacin (Floxin) may increase seizure risk.
- oral hypoglycemics (see *sulfonylureas*) may increase risk of low blood sugar.
- ritonavir (Norvir), and perhaps other protease inhibitors (see Drug Classes), can lead to toxicity.
Piroxicam *taken concurrently* with the following drugs may increase bleeding risk—avoid these:
- aspirin.
- cholestyramine (Questran).

- dipyridamole (Persantine).
- indomethacin (Indocin).
- sulfinpyrazone (Anturane).
- valproic acid (Depakene).

▷ *Driving, Hazardous Activities:* This drug may cause drowsiness or dizziness. Restrict activities as necessary.

Aviation Note: The use of this drug **may be a disqualification** for piloting. Consult a designated aviation medical examiner.

Exposure to Sun: This drug may cause photosensitivity (see Glossary). Use caution.

OXTRIPHYLLINE (ox TRY fi lin)

Other Names: Choline theophyllinate, theophylline cholinate

Introduced: 1965   **Class:** Antiasthmatic, bronchodilator, xanthines   **Prescription:** USA: Yes   **Controlled Drug:** USA: No; Canada: No   **Available as Generic:** Yes

Brand Names: ✦Apo-Oxtriphylline, Choledyl, Choledyl Delayed-Release, Choledyl SA, ✦Novotriphyl

   Author's Note: This medicine is converted to 64% theophylline by the body. See the theophylline profile for further information.

OXYCODONE (ox ee KOH dohn)

Introduced: 1950   **Class:** Analgesic, strong; opioids   **Prescription:** USA: Yes   **Controlled Drug:** USA: C-II*; Canada: No   **Available as Generic:** USA: Yes; Canada: No

Brand Names: ✦Endocet [CD], ✦Endodan [CD], ✦Oxycocet [CD], ✦Oxycodan [CD], Oxycontin, Percocet [CD], ✦Percocet-Demi [CD], Percodan [CD], Percodan-Demi [CD], Roxicet, Roxicodone, Roxilox, Roxiprin [CD], SK-Oxycodone, ✦Supeudol, Tylox [CD]

BENEFITS versus RISKS	
Possible Benefits	*Possible Risks*
EFFECTIVE RELIEF OF MODERATE TO SEVERE PAIN	POTENTIAL FOR HABIT FORMATION (DEPENDENCE)
	Sedative effects
	Mild allergic reactions—infrequent
	Nausea, constipation

▷ **Principal Uses**

   As a Single Drug Product: Uses currently included in FDA-approved labeling: Used in tablet and suppository form (Canada) to relieve moderate to severe pain.

   Other (unlabeled) generally accepted uses: None.

   As a Combination Drug Product [CD]: Oxycodone is available in combinations

*See Controlled Drug Schedules at the back of this book.

with acetaminophen and with aspirin. These milder pain relievers are added to enhance the analgesic effect and reduce fever when present.

How This Drug Works: Acting primarily as a depressant of certain brain functions, this drug suppresses pain perception and calms the emotional response to pain.

Available Dose Forms and Strengths

Solution — 5 mg/5 ml
Suppositories — 10 mg, 20 mg (Canada)
Tablets — 5 mg, 10 mg (Canada)
Tablets — 2.44 mg, 4.88 mg (in combination drugs)

▷ **Usual Adult Dose Range:** Percodan is taken as one tablet (5 mg) every 6 hours. Current pain theory says that pain medicines should be scheduled; for example, given every 4 hours. The outdated "wait until it hurts" method tended to result in suffering. May be increased to 10 mg every 4 hours if needed for severe pain. The total daily dose should not exceed 60 mg. Oxycontin is taken every 12 hours and is a sustained-release formulation.

Note: Actual dose and schedule must be determined for each patient individually.

Conditions Requiring Dosing Adjustments

Liver Function: Dose adjustments should be empirically made in liver failure.
Kidney Function: Dose adjustment does not appear to be needed. Some combination products contain aspirin, which may be contraindicated in kidney failure.

▷ **Dosing Instructions:** The tablet may be crushed and taken with or following food to reduce stomach upset or nausea.

Usual Duration of Use: As required to control pain. Continual use should not exceed 5 to 7 days without interruption and reassessment of need.

▷ **This Drug Should Not Be Taken If**
- you had an allergic reaction to it previously.
- you are having an acute attack of asthma.

Note: Patients allergic to aspirin should **not** be given Percodan.

▷ **Inform Your Physician Before Taking This Drug If**
- you had an unfavorable reaction to any narcotic drug.
- you have had a head injury with increased pressure (intracranial) in the head.
- you have a history of drug abuse or alcoholism.
- you have chronic lung disease with impaired breathing.
- you have impaired liver or kidney function.
- you have gallbladder disease, a seizure disorder, or an underactive thyroid gland.
- you have difficulty emptying the urinary bladder.
- you are taking any other drugs that have a sedative effect.
- you plan to have surgery under general anesthesia in the near future.

Possible Side Effects (natural, expected, and unavoidable drug actions)
Drowsiness, light-headedness, dry mouth, urinary retention, constipation.

▷ **Possible Adverse Effects** (unusual, unexpected, and infrequent reactions)
If any of the following develop, consult your physician promptly for guidance.

Mild Adverse Effects
Allergic reactions: skin rash, hives, itching.
Idiosyncratic reactions: skin rash and itching when combined with dairy products (milk or cheese).
Dizziness, sensation of drunkenness, depression, blurred or double vision—dose related.
Nausea, vomiting—may be dose related.

Serious Adverse Effects
Impaired breathing: use with caution in chronic lung disease—variable and can be dose related.
Abnormal body movements, if the drug is abruptly stopped.

▷ **Possible Effects on Sexual Function:**   Blunted sexual responses—case reports.

Possible Effects on Laboratory Tests
Urine screening tests for drug abuse: test result may be falsely **positive**; *confirmatory* test result may be **negative**. (Test results depend upon amount of drug taken and testing method used.)

CAUTION
1. If you have asthma, chronic bronchitis, or emphysema, excessive use of this drug may cause significant respiratory difficulty, thickening of bronchial secretions, and suppression of coughing.
2. The concurrent use of this drug with atropinelike drugs can increase the risk of urinary retention and reduced intestinal function.
3. Do not take this drug following acute head injury.

Precautions for Use
By Infants and Children: Do not use this drug in children under 2 years of age because of their vulnerability to life-threatening respiratory depression.
By Those Over 60 Years of Age: Small starting doses and short-term therapy are indicated. There may be increased susceptibility to the development of drowsiness, dizziness, unsteadiness, falling, urinary retention, and constipation (often leading to fecal impaction).

▷ **Advisability of Use During Pregnancy**
Pregnancy Category: C. See Pregnancy Risk Categories at the back of this book.
Animal studies: No information available.
Human studies: Adequate studies of pregnant women are not available. Oxycodone taken repeatedly during the final few weeks before delivery may cause withdrawal symptoms in the newborn.
Use only if clearly needed and in small, infrequent doses.

Advisability of Use If Breast-Feeding
Presence of this drug in breast milk: Unknown.
Avoid drug or refrain from nursing.

Habit-Forming Potential: Psychological and/or physical dependence can develop.

Effects of Overdose: Drowsiness, restlessness, agitation, nausea, vomiting, dry mouth, vertigo, weakness, lethargy, stupor, coma, seizures.

Possible Effects of Long-Term Use: Psychological and physical dependence, chronic constipation.

Suggested Periodic Examinations While Taking This Drug (at physician's discretion)
None.

▷ **While Taking This Drug, Observe the Following**
Foods: No restrictions.
Beverages: No restrictions. May be taken with milk.
▷ *Alcohol:* Oxycodone can intensify the intoxicating effects of alcohol, and alcohol can intensify the depressant effects of oxycodone on brain function, breathing, and circulation. Combined use is best avoided.
Tobacco Smoking: No interactions expected. I advise everyone to quit smoking.
Marijuana Smoking: Increase in drowsiness and pain relief; impairment of mental and physical performance.
▷ *Other Drugs:*
Oxycodone may ***increase*** the effects of
- atropinelike drugs, and increase the risk of constipation and urinary retention.
- other drugs with sedative effects (see Drug Classes for benzodiazepines, tricyclic antidepressants, antihistamines, monoamine oxidase (MAO) inhibitors, phenothiazines, and opioid drugs—narcotics).

Oxycodone ***taken concurrently*** with
- ritonavir (Norvir), and perhaps other protease inhibitors (see Drug Classes), may lead to toxicity.

Oxycodone ***taken concurrently*** with
- naltrexone (ReVia) may lead to withdrawal symptoms.
- rifabutin (Rifater, others) may blunt oxycodone benefits.
- tramadol (Ultram) may increase risk of adverse effects.
▷ *Driving, Hazardous Activities:* This drug can impair mental alertness, judgment, reaction time, and physical coordination. Avoid hazardous activities accordingly.
Aviation Note: The use of this drug ***is a disqualification*** for piloting. Consult a designated aviation medical examiner.
Exposure to Sun: No restrictions.
Discontinuation: It is best to limit this drug to short-term use. If extended use is needed, discontinuation should be gradual to minimize possible effects of withdrawal.

PAROXETINE (pa ROCKS a teen)

Introduced: 1993   **Class:** Antidepressant, other   **Prescription:** USA: Yes   **Controlled Drug:** USA: No; Canada: No   **Available as Generic:** USA: No; Canada: No
Brand Name: Paxil

BENEFITS versus RISKS	
Possible Benefits	*Possible Risks*
EFFECTIVE CONTROL OF DEPRESSION	Withdrawal symptoms
Fewer adverse effects than tricyclic antidepressants	Abnormal ejaculation in males
Helps control obsessive-compulsive disorder and panic disorder	
May help premature ejaculation	

▷ **Principal Uses**

As a Single Drug Product: Uses currently included in FDA-approved labeling: (1) Treatment of depression; (2) helps control obsessive-compulsive disorder; (3) helps control panic attacks.

Other (unlabeled) generally accepted uses: (1) Can have a role in diabetic nerve pain (neuropathy); (2) helps long-standing (chronic) daily headaches; (3) can help premature ejaculation.

How This Drug Works: Inhibits uptake of serotonin. When more of this chemical is available in the brain, a positive impact on thinking results.

Available Dose Forms and Strengths

Capsules — 20 mg, 30 mg
Oral suspension — 10 mg/5 ml

▷ **Recommended Dose Ranges** (Actual dose and schedule must be determined for each patient individually.)

Infants and Children: Not indicated.

18 to 60 Years of Age: Depression: The usual starting dose is 20 mg, taken in the morning. Dose can then be increased as needed and tolerated in 10-mg intervals to a maximum of 50 mg daily.

Obsessive-compulsive disorder: Started with 20 mg daily with increases as in depression to a usual benefit at 40 mg per day. Maximum here is 60 mg daily.

Over 60 Years of Age: The starting dose in this population is 10 mg daily. The maximum dose is 40 mg daily.

Conditions Requiring Dosing Adjustments

Liver Function: Starting dose is 10 mg and the maximum dose is 40 mg daily. Drug levels may be needed.

Kidney Function: Same starting dose and maximum dose as in liver compromise.

▷ **Dosing Instructions:**   The absorption of this medicine is not changed by food.

Usual Duration of Use: Continual use on a regular schedule for 14 days is usually necessary to determine this drug's effectiveness in treating depression. Long-term use (months to years) requires periodic evaluation of response and dose adjustment by your doctor.

Possible Advantages of This Drug

Fewer side effects than tricyclic antidepressants.
May be a drug of choice in people with heart disease who are also depressed.

▷ **This Drug Should Not Be Taken If**

• you had an allergic reaction to it previously.
• you have taken a monoamine oxidase (MAO) inhibitor (see Drug Classes) in the last 14 days.

▷ **Inform Your Physician Before Taking This Drug If**

• you are pregnant or breast-feeding.
• you have a history of mania or seizures.
• you take diuretics or typically drink little water.
• you have a history of liver or kidney disease.
• you take prescription or nonprescription medicines not discussed with your doctor when paroxetine was prescribed.

Possible Side Effects (natural, expected, and unavoidable drug actions)
Lowered blood pressure and fainting upon standing (postural hypotension). Sedation.

▷ **Possible Adverse Effects** (unusual, unexpected, and infrequent reactions)
If any of the following develop, consult your physician promptly for guidance.

Mild Adverse Effects
Allergic reactions: skin rash and itching.
Headache, nervousness, or insomnia—infrequent to frequent.
Palpitations—infrequent.
Loss of appetite, nausea, taste disorders, or constipation—infrequent to frequent.
Tingling of the hands (paresthesias)—infrequent.
Sweating—frequent.
Dizziness, blurred vision—infrequent to frequent.

Serious Adverse Effects
Allergic reactions: not reported.
Idiosyncratic reactions: none reported.
Abnormal movements or positioning of the mouth or face—infrequent.
Seizures—rare.
Liver toxicity—rare and of questionable causation.

▷ **Possible Effects on Sexual Function:** Galactorrhea. USED TO TREAT premature ejaculation.
Abnormal ejaculation—infrequent to frequent; inability to achieve orgasm, impotence, or sexual dysfunction—infrequent; prolonged and painful erection (priapism)—rare.

Possible Delayed Adverse Effects: None reported.

▷ **Adverse Effects That May Mimic Natural Diseases or Disorders**
Increased liver enzymes may mimic early hepatitis.

Natural Diseases or Disorders That May Be Activated by This Drug
None reported.

Possible Effects on Laboratory Tests
Liver function tests: increased.

CAUTION
1. Take this medicine as prescribed and do not stop taking it without talking with your doctor.

Precautions for Use
By Infants and Children: Safety and effectiveness for use by those under 18 years of age have not been established.
By Those Over 60 Years of Age: Lower starting and maximum doses are indicated.

▷ **Advisability of Use During Pregnancy**
Pregnancy Category: B. See Pregnancy Risk Categories at the back of this book.
Animal studies: Reproduction studies in rabbits or rats using doses of up to 10 times the typical human dose have not revealed any fetal changes.
Human studies: Information from adequate studies of pregnant women is not available.
Ask your doctor for guidance.

Advisability of Use If Breast-Feeding
> Presence of this drug in breast milk: Yes, in small amounts.
> Ask your doctor for guidance.

Habit-Forming Potential: None; however, a withdrawal syndrome characterized by dizziness, confusion, sweating, and tremor has been described.

Effects of Overdose: Confusion, heart rhythm changes, seizures.

Possible Effects of Long-Term Use: Not defined.

Suggested Periodic Examinations While Taking This Drug (at physician's discretion)
> Liver function tests.

▷ **While Taking This Drug, Observe the Following**
> *Foods:* No restrictions.
> *Beverages:* No restrictions.
▷ *Alcohol:* The manufacturer recommends avoiding alcohol while taking this medicine.
> *Tobacco Smoking:* No interactions expected. I advise everyone to quit smoking.
> *Marijuana Smoking:* Additive sedation.
▷ *Other Drugs:*
> Paroxetine may *increase* the effects of
> - benzodiazepines (see Drug Classes).
> - desipramine (and potentially other tricyclic antidepressants; see Drug Classes).
> - haloperidol (Haldol), because paroxetine blocks an enzyme system needed to remove haloperidol.
> - labetalol (Normodyne) and perhaps other beta-blockers (see Drug Classes), because paroxetine inhibits an enzyme system needed to remove labetalol.
> - minimally sedating antihistamines astemizole and terfenadine, because paroxetine may inhibit some liver systems that usually remove them from the body. This effect has not been documented, but is theoretically possible.
>
> Paroxetine *taken concurrently* with
> - activated charcoal will reduce absorption of paroxetine.
> - fenfluramine (Pondimin) may cause toxicity (serotonin syndrome).
> - monoamine oxidase (MAO) inhibitors (see Drug Classes) may result in a fatal serotonin syndrome. **Do not** combine these medicines.
> - phenytoin (Dilantin) may result in decreased paroxetine blood levels and lessening of therapeutic benefits. Dose increases may be needed.
> - quinidine (Quinaglute, others) may result in increased paroxetine levels and toxicity. Decreased paroxetine doses may be needed.
> - ritonavir (Norvir) may lead to paroxetine toxicity.
> - sibutramine (Meridia) increases risk of serotonin syndrome.
> - sumatriptan(Imitrex) can lead to hyperreflexia and poor coordination—do not combine.
> - tramadol (Ultram) may lead to increased risk of seizures. DO NOT combine.
> - tryptophan may result in sweating, nausea, and dizziness.
> - warfarin (Coumadin) may result in bleeding. More frequent INR (prothrombin time or protime) testing is recommended. Warfarin doses should be adjusted based on laboratory results.
>
> The following drug may *increase* the effects of paroxetine:
> - cimetidine (Tagamet).

▷ *Driving, Hazardous Activities:* This drug may frequently cause sedation. Restrict
   activities as necessary.
   Aviation Note: The use of this drug *is a disqualification* for piloting. Consult a
   designated aviation medical examiner.
   Exposure to Sun: No specific restrictions.
   Exposure to Heat: This medicine can cause excessive sweating. If you work or are
   frequently in a hot environment, be careful to replace enough fluids to avoid
   dehydration.
   Heavy Exercise or Exertion: Since this medicine may cause excessive sweating,
   be careful to replace lost fluids.
   Occurrence of Unrelated Illness: Fevers may cause more severe dehydration.
   Discontinuation: Do not stop this medicine without talking with your doctor.

PENBUTOLOL (pen BYU toh lohl)

Introduced: 1976   **Class:** Antihypertensive, beta-adrenergic blocker
Prescription: USA: Yes   **Controlled Drug:** USA: No; Canada: No   **Available as Generic:** No
Brand Name: Levatol

BENEFITS versus RISKS	
Possible Benefits	*Possible Risks*
EFFECTIVE, WELL-TOLERATED ANTIHYPERTENSIVE in mild to moderate high blood pressure	CONGESTIVE HEART FAILURE in advanced heart disease
	Worsening of angina in coronary heart disease (abrupt withdrawal)
	Masking of low blood sugar (hypoglycemia) in drug-treated diabetes
	Provocation of asthma (in asthmatics)

▷ **Principal Uses**
   As a Single Drug Product: Uses currently included in FDA-approved labeling:
   Treats mild to moderate high blood pressure. Used alone or combined with
   other antihypertensive drugs.
   Other (unlabeled) generally accepted uses: (1) May help curb aggressive behavior; (2) can help decrease the frequency and severity of angina attacks;
   (3) may help decrease death from heart attack (myocardial infarction); (4)
   supportive role in panic attacks; (5) limited studies support penbutolol use
   in glaucoma (large studies are needed).

How This Drug Works: Blocks certain actions of the sympathetic nervous system:
   • reducing heart rate and contraction force, lowering the pressure of the
     blood leaving the heart.
   • reduces the degree of blood vessel wall contraction, resulting in lower blood
     pressure.

Available Dose Forms and Strengths
   Tablets — 20 mg

▷ **Usual Adult Dose Range:**   Initially 20 mg once daily. The dose may be increased gradually by 10 mg/day at intervals of 2 weeks as needed and tolerated, up to 80 mg/day. Higher doses have been tolerated, but do not give greater efficacy. 20 to 40 mg daily is a common ongoing dose. Daily maximum is 80 mg.
Note: Actual dose and schedule must be determined for each patient individually.

Conditions Requiring Dosing Adjustments
Liver Function: Dose adjustments should be considered in mild to moderate liver disease; however, specific guidelines are not available.
Kidney Function: No dosing changes are thought to be needed.

▷ **Dosing Instructions:**   The tablet may be crushed and taken without regard to eating. Do not stop this drug abruptly.

Usual Duration of Use: Use on a regular schedule for up to 2 weeks determines the full effect in lowering blood pressure. Long-term use of this drug (months to years) will determine your blood pressure over time and your response to an overall treatment program (weight reduction, salt restriction, smoking cessation, etc.).

Possible Advantages of This Drug
Adequate control of blood pressure with a single daily dose.
Causes less slowing of the heart rate than most other beta-blocker drugs.

▷ **This Drug Should Not Be Taken If**
 • you have had an allergic reaction to it previously.
 • you have heart failure (overt).
 • you have an abnormally slow heart rate or a serious form of heart block.
 • you have abnormal growth of the left side of the heart (left ventricular hypertrophy).
 • you have bronchial asthma.

▷ **Inform Your Physician Before Taking This Drug If**
 • you had problems from any beta-blocker (see Drug Classes).
 • you have a history of serious heart disease.
 • you have a history of hay fever (allergic rhinitis), asthma, chronic bronchitis, or emphysema.
 • you have a history of overactive thyroid function (hyperthyroidism).
 • you have a history of low blood sugar (hypoglycemia).
 • you have impaired liver or kidney function.
 • you have diabetes or myasthenia gravis.
 • you have congestive heart failure.
 • you have impaired circulation in the extremities (Raynaud's phenomenon, claudication pains in legs).
 • you take any form of digitalis, quinidine, or reserpine, or any calcium-channel-blocker drug (see Drug Classes).
 • you plan to have surgery under general anesthesia in the near future.

Possible Side Effects (natural, expected, and unavoidable drug actions)
Lethargy and fatigability, cold extremities, slow heart rate, light-headedness in upright position (see *orthostatic hypotension* in Glossary).

▷ **Possible Adverse Effects** (unusual, unexpected, and infrequent reactions)
If any of the following develop, consult your physician promptly for guidance.

Mild Adverse Effects
Allergic reactions: skin rash, itching, reversible hair loss.
Headache, dizziness, blurred vision, insomnia, abnormal dreams—infrequent.
Indigestion, nausea, vomiting, constipation, diarrhea—infrequent.
Joint and muscle discomfort—infrequent.

Serious Adverse Effects
Allergic reactions: anaphylactic reaction (see Glossary).
Mental depression, anxiety, disorientation, short-term memory loss, hallucinations—possible.
Carpal tunnel syndrome or aggravation of myasthenia gravis—case reports.
High blood sugar or low blood sugar in diabetics—possible.
Worsening of circulatory problems (with preexisting conditions—Raynaud's phenomenon)—possible.
Bronchospasm—rare.
Chest pain, shortness of breath, precipitation of congestive heart failure—possible.
Rebound hypertension—if abruptly stopped.
Induction of bronchial asthma—possible in asthmatics.

▷ **Possible Effects on Sexual Function:** Decreased libido and impotence—rare but dose related; Peyronie's disease (see Glossary)—rare.

▷ **Adverse Effects That May Mimic Natural Diseases or Disorders**
Reduced blood flow to extremities may resemble Raynaud's phenomenon (see Glossary).

Natural Diseases or Disorders That May Be Activated by This Drug
Raynaud's disease, intermittent claudication, myasthenia gravis.

Possible Effects on Laboratory Tests
Uric acid, potassium, or blood sugar: increased.

CAUTION
1. ***Do not stop this drug suddenly*** without calling your doctor. Carry a card saying you take this drug.
2. Ask your doctor or pharmacist **before** using nasal decongestants (cold medicines and nose drops). May cause sudden increases in blood pressure when taken with beta-blockers.
3. Call your doctor if emotional depression starts.

Precautions for Use
By Infants and Children: Safety and effectiveness in infants or children not established.
By Those Over 60 Years of Age: High blood pressure should be reduced, avoiding risks of too low a blood pressure. Small starting doses and frequent blood pressure checks are needed. Sudden, rapid, and excessive reduction of blood pressure can predispose to stroke or heart attack. Observe for dizziness, unsteadiness, tendency to fall, confusion, hallucinations, depression, or urinary frequency.

▷ **Advisability of Use During Pregnancy**
Pregnancy Category: C. See Pregnancy Risk Categories at the back of this book.
Animal studies: No birth defects due to this drug found in rat or rabbit studies.
Human studies: Adequate studies of pregnant women are not available.
Ask your physician for guidance.

Advisability of Use If Breast-Feeding
Presence of this drug in breast milk: Unknown.
Avoid drug or refrain from nursing.

Habit-Forming Potential: None.

Effects of Overdose: Weakness, slow pulse, low blood pressure, fainting, cold and sweaty skin, congestive heart failure, possible coma, and convulsions.

Possible Effects of Long-Term Use: Reduced heart reserve and eventual heart failure in susceptible individuals with advanced heart disease.

Suggested Periodic Examinations While Taking This Drug (at physician's discretion)
Measurements of blood pressure, evaluation of heart function.
Complete blood cell counts.

▷ **While Taking This Drug, Observe the Following**
Foods: No restrictions. Avoid excessive salt intake.
Beverages: No restrictions. May be taken with milk.
▷   *Alcohol:* Alcohol may exaggerate this drug's ability to lower blood pressure and may increase its mild sedative effect.
Tobacco Smoking: Nicotine may reduce this drug's benefit in treating high blood pressure. I advise everyone to quit smoking.
Other Drugs
Penbutolol may *increase* the effects of
- other antihypertensive drugs, and cause excessive lowering of blood pressure. Dose adjustments may be necessary.
- reserpine (Ser-Ap-Es, etc.), and cause sedation, depression, slowing of the heart rate, and lowering of blood pressure. This combination is best avoided.
- verapamil (Calan, Isoptin), and cause excessive depression of heart function; monitor this combination closely.

Penbutolol may *decrease* the effects of
- epinephrine, resulting in decreased benefits when used to correct allergic reactions. Slow heartbeat and elevated blood pressure may also occur.

Penbutolol *taken concurrently* with
- amiodarone (Codarone) may result in sinus arrest or symptomatic bradycardia. DO NOT combine these medicines.
- clonidine (Catapres) requires close monitoring for rebound high blood pressure if clonidine is withdrawn while penbutolol is still being taken.
- digoxin (Lanoxin) increases risk of heart attack or heart block.
- fluoxetine (Prozac) may cause very slow heartbeat (bradycardia) and excessive lowering of blood pressure.
- fluvoxamine (Luvox) may cause very slow heartbeat (bradycardia) and excessive lowering of blood pressure.
- insulin or oral hypoglycemic agents requires close monitoring to avoid undetected hypoglycemia (see Glossary).
- mibefradil (Posicor) may impair heart performance in people with poor left heart function or the elderly.
- venlafaxine (Effexor) may result in increased risk of toxicity from penbutolol.

The following drugs may *increase* the effects of penbutolol:
- birth control pills (oral contraceptives).

- methimazole (Tapazole).
- propylthiouracil (Propacil).
- ritonavir (Norvir), and perhaps other protease inhibitors (see Drug Classes).

The following drugs may *decrease* the effects of penbutolol:

- barbiturates (phenobarbital, etc.).
- indomethacin (Indocin) and possibly other "aspirin substitutes," or NSAIDs—may impair penbutolol's antihypertensive effect.
- rifampin (Rifadin, Rimactane).

▷ *Driving, Hazardous Activities:* Use caution until the full extent of fatigue, dizziness, and blood pressure change have been determined.

Aviation Note: The use of this drug *is a disqualification* for piloting. Consult a designated aviation medical examiner.

Exposure to Sun: No restrictions.

Exposure to Heat: Hot environments can lower blood pressure and exaggerate effects.

Exposure to Cold: Cold environments can worsen low circulation to the extremities. Elderly should be careful to prevent hypothermia (see Glossary).

Heavy Exercise or Exertion: Avoid exertion that produces light-headedness, excessive fatigue, or muscle cramping. The use of this drug may intensify the hypertensive response to isometric exercise.

Occurrence of Unrelated Illness: Fever can lower blood pressure and require lower doses. Vomiting may interrupt the regular dose schedule. Ask your doctor for help.

Discontinuation: Best to avoid stopping this drug suddenly. If possible, slow dose reduction (over 2 to 3 weeks) is recommended.

PENCICLOVIR (pen SI clo veer)

Introduced: 1997   **Class:** Antiviral, (anti-herpetic)   **Prescription:** USA: Yes   **Controlled Drug:** USA: No; Canada: No   **Available as Generic:** USA: No; Canada: No

Brand Name: Denavir

BENEFITS versus RISKS	
Possible Benefits	*Possible Risks*
TREATMENT OF COLD SORES	Skin irritation

▷ **Principal Uses**

As a Single Drug Product: Uses currently included in FDA-approved labeling: Treats skin and mucous membrane (mucocutaneous) infections caused by herpes simplex.

Other (unlabeled) generally accepted uses: May have a role in treatment of varicella (chicken pox).

How This Drug Works: Blocks genetic material formation of herpes simplex viruses, stopping viral multiplication and spread, reducing severity and duration of the herpes infection.

Available Dosage Forms and Strengths

Ointment — 1%

▷ **Recommended Dosage Ranges** (Actual dose and schedule must be determined for each patient individually.)

Infants and Children: Safety and effectiveness in infants and children not established.

18 to 65 Years of Age: Cover all infected areas every 2 hours for a total of six times daily for 4 consecutive days. Start treatment at the **earliest sign** of infection.

Over 65 Years of Age: The dose **must** be adjusted if the kidneys are impaired.

Conditions Requiring Dosing Adjustments

Liver Function: No dosing changes needed.

Kidney Function: The dose may need to be decreased in significant kidney disease.

▷ **Dosing Instructions:**   Use just enough of the cream to thinly cover the itching area you suspect to be a starting herpes infection. Apply to the lesions every 2 hours while you are awake. Start treatment at the **earliest sign** of infection.

Usual Duration of Use: Use on a regular schedule for 4 days usually needed to see this drug's effect in reducing the severity and duration of the infection.

▷ **This Drug Should Not Be Taken If**
- you have had an allergic reaction to it previously.

▷ **Inform Your Physician Before Taking This Drug If**
- your liver, kidney, or nerve function is impaired.
- you are unsure how much to take or how often to take it.

Possible Side Effects (natural, expected, and unavoidable drug actions)

Cream use—mild pain or stinging at site of application.

▷ **Possible Adverse Effects** (unusual, unexpected, and infrequent reactions)

If any of the following develop, consult your physician promptly for guidance.

Mild Adverse Effects

Allergic reaction: skin rash.

Headache—infrequent.

Serious Adverse Effects

None reported.

▷ **Possible Effects on Sexual Function:**   None reported.

Possible Effects on Laboratory Tests

None reported.

CAUTION

1. This drug does **not** eliminate all herpes virus and is **not a cure**. Recurrence is possible. Resume treatment at the earliest sign of infection.
2. Do not exceed the prescribed dose.
3. If severity or frequency of infections don't improve, call your doctor.

Precautions for Use

By Infants and Children: No data.

By Those Over 60 Years of Age: No changes needed, except in severe kidney disease.

▷ **Advisability of Use During Pregnancy**

Pregnancy Category: B. See Pregnancy Risk Categories at the back of this book.

Animal studies: No birth defects found in animals.
Human studies: Studies not available.

Advisability of Use If Breast-Feeding
Presence of this drug in breast milk: Unknown.
Ask your physician for guidance.

Habit-Forming Potential: None.

Effects of Overdose: Not defined.

Possible Effects of Long-Term Use: Development of penciclovir-resistant strains of herpes virus. Treatment will fail if this occurs.

Suggested Periodic Examinations While Taking This Drug (at physician's discretion)
Not defined.

▷ **While Taking This Drug, Observe the Following**
Foods: No restrictions.
Beverages: No restrictions.
▷ *Alcohol:* No restrictions.
Tobacco Smoking: No interactions expected. I advise everyone to quit smoking.
▷ *Other Drugs:*
No significant drug interactions for the cream.
▷ *Driving, Hazardous Activities:* Use caution if excessive headache occurs.
Aviation Note: The use of this drug *is probably not a disqualification* for piloting. Consult a designated aviation medical examiner.
Exposure to Sun: No restrictions; however, some data indicates that sun exposure may trigger release of herpes simplex from its dormant state (from the optic nerve).

PENICILLAMINE (pen i SIL a meen)

Introduced: 1963   **Class:** Antiarthritic   **Prescription:** USA: Yes
Controlled Drug: USA: No; Canada: No   **Available as Generic:** USA: No; Canada: No
Brand Names: Cuprimine, Depen

BENEFITS versus RISKS	
Possible Benefits	*Possible Risks*
EFFECTIVE TREATMENT OF WILSON'S DISEASE (COPPER TOXICITY)	SEVERE ALLERGIC REACTIONS BONE MARROW DEPRESSION
Effective treatment of cystinuria and cystine kidney stones	Drug-induced damage of lungs, liver, pancreas, and kidneys
Partially effective treatment of rheumatoid arthritis and poisoning due to heavy metals: iron, lead, mercury, and zinc	

▷ **Principal Uses**
As a Single Drug Product: Uses currently included in FDA-approved labeling: Treatment of (1) Wilson's disease (copper toxicity of brain, cornea, liver,

and kidneys); (2) severe rheumatoid arthritis that has failed to respond to less hazardous conventional treatment; also helps rheumatoid arthritis that presents with interstitial lung disease; (3) cystinuria and cystine stone formation (excessive amounts of cystine in the urine).

Other (unlabeled) generally accepted uses: (1) Treatment of heavy metal poisoning, especially that due to lead and mercury; (2) may help increase survival in scleroderma; (3) eases progression of systemic sclerosis.

Author's Note: Due to proliferation of new medicines, this profile has been abbreviated in order to make room for more widely used medicines.

PENICILLIN ANTIBIOTIC FAMILY

Amoxicillin (a mox i SIL in)   **Amoxicillin/Clavulanate** (a mox i SIL in/KLAV yu lan ayt)   **Ampicillin** (am pi SIL in)   **Bacampicillin** (bak am pi SIL in) **Cloxacillin** (klox a SIL in)   **Penicillin VK** (pen i SIL in VEE KAY)

Introduced: 1969, 1982, 1961, 1979, 1962, 1953, respectively   **Class:** Antibiotics, penicillins   **Prescription:**   USA: Yes   **Controlled Drug:**   USA: No; Canada: No   **Available as Generic:**   USA: Yes (all but amoxicillin/clavulanate); Canada: Yes

Brand Names: Amoxicillin: Amoxil, ✦Apo-Amoxi, ✦Clavulin, Larotid, ✦Novamoxin, ✦Nu-Amoxi, Polymox, Prevpac [CD], Trimox, Wymox; Amoxicillin/clavulanate: Augmentin, ✦Clavulin; Ampicillin: Amcill, ✦Ampicin, ✦Ampicin PRB [CD], ✦Ampilean, ✦Apo-Ampi, D-Amp, Faspak Ampicillin, 500 Kit [CD], Nu-Ampi, ✦Novo-Ampicillin, Omnipen, Omnipen Pediatric Drops, Pardec Capsules [CD], ✦Penbritin, Polycillin, Polycillin Pediatric Drops, Polycillin-PRB [CD], ✦Pondocillin, Principen, SK-Ampicillin, Totacillin; Bacampicillin: ✦Penglobe, Spectrobid; Cloxacillin: ✦Apo-Cloxi, ✦Bactopen, Cloxapen, ✦Novo-Cloxin, ✦Nu-Cloxi, ✦Orbenin, Tegopen; Penicillin VK: ✦Apo-Pen-VK, Beepen VK, Betapen-VK, Ledercillin VK, ✦Nadopen-V, ✦Novopen-VK, ✦Nu-Pen-VK, Pehapar VK, Pen-V, ✦Pen-Vee, Pen-Vee K, Pfizerpen VK, ✦PVF, ✦PVF K, Robicillin VK, SK-Penicillin VK, Uticillin VK, V-Cillin K, ✦VC-K 500, Veetids

---

BENEFITS versus RISKS

Possible Benefits	*Possible Risks*
EFFECTIVE TREATMENT OF INFECTIONS due to susceptible microorganisms	ALLERGIC REACTIONS, mild to severe
	Superinfections (yeast)
	Drug-induced colitis—possible
	Lowering of white blood cells (amoxicillin/clavulanate, ampicillin, cloxacillin)
	Decreased kidney function

▷ **Principal Uses**

As a Single Drug Product: Uses currently included in FDA-approved labeling: (1) Used to treat responsive infections of the upper and lower respiratory tract, the middle ear (acute otitis media; amoxicillin is a drug of choice), and the skin; (2) helps prevent rheumatic fever and bacterial endocarditis in people with valvular heart disease; (3) some *Haemophilus influenzae* infections (amoxicillin); (4) some genitourinary tract infections (amoxicillin/clavulanate, ampicillin, penicillin VK); (5) treats some cases of sinusitis; (6) ampicillin is used in combination to treat some kinds of septicemia and meningitis.

Other (unlabeled) generally accepted uses: (1) Combined therapy of animal bite wounds; (2) treats stage one Lyme disease in children (amoxicillin or penicillin VK); (3) therapy of Lyme disease in the central nervous system (penicillin VK); (4) can treat some dental abscesses (penicillin VK); (5) typhoid fever (amoxicillin); (6) therapy of *Helicobacter pylori* ulcers combined with other drugs (amoxicillin); prevention of bacterial endocarditis (amoxicillin); (7) biliary tract infections or chancroid (amoxicillin/clavulanate); (8) cloxacillin treats some bone infections if intravenous (IV) drugs not tolerated.

As a Combination Drug Product [CD]: Amoxicillin and clavulanate are combined (Augmentin) to give the benefits of amoxicillin combined with the ability to treat more resistant bacteria (clavulanate).

Amoxicillin is available in combination with two different drugs (clarithromycin and lansoprazole). Since refractory ulcers are often actually *Helicobacter pylori* infections, the combination works to kill the bacteria and lower acid production.

How These Drugs Work: Destroy susceptible infecting bacteria by damaging ability to make protective cell walls as they multiply and grow. Amoxicillin/clavulanate uses clavulanate blockage of enzymes to enable treatment of resistant bacteria. Bacampicillin is converted to ampicillin, giving peak blood levels three times higher than ampicillin. This allows bacampicillin dosing every 12 hours.

Available Dose Forms and Strengths
Amoxicillin:

Capsules —	250 mg, 500 mg
Tablets, chewable —	125 mg, 250 mg
Oral liquid —	3 g
Oral suspension —	50 mg/ml, 125 mg/ml, 250 mg/5 ml
Pediatric drops —	50 mg/ml

Amoxicillin/clavulanate:

Oral suspension —	125 mg (amoxicillin) and 31.25 mg (clavulanate) per 5 ml; 250 mg (amoxicillin) and 62.5 mg (clavulanate) per 5 ml; 250 mg (amoxicillin) and 125 mg (clavulanate); 500 mg (amoxicillin) and 125 mg (clavulanate)
Pediatric formulation, twice daily —	200 mg (amoxicillin) and 28.6 mg (clavulanate) per 5 ml; 400 mg (amoxicillin) and 57.1 (clavulanate) per 5 ml

Tablets, chewable — 125 mg (amoxicillin) and 31.25 mg (clavulanate); 250 mg (amoxicillin) and 62.5 mg (clavulanate)

Tablets, chewable twice-daily formulation — 200 mg (amoxicillin) and 28.6 mg (clavulanate); 400 mg (amoxicillin) and 57.1 (clavulanate)

Ampicillin:

Capsules — 250 mg, 500 mg
Oral suspension — 100 mg/ml, 125 mg/ml, 250 mg/ml, 500 mg/5 ml
Pediatric drops — 100 mg/ml

Bacampicillin:

Oral suspension — 125 mg/5 ml
Tablets — 400 mg, 800 mg (800 mg in Canada only)

Cloxacillin:

Capsules — 250 mg, 500 mg
Oral suspension — 125 mg/5 ml
Oral liquid — 125 mg/5 ml

Penicillin VK:

Oral solution — 125 mg/5 ml, 250 mg/5 ml
Tablets — 125 mg, 250 mg, 500 mg

▷ **Recommended Dose Ranges:** Dose is based on how sensitive the bacteria that are causing the infection, infection severity, and patient response.

Penicillin VK: Dose range is 125 to 500 mg every 6 to 8 hours. For prevention of bacterial endocarditis: 2 g (2000 mg) taken 1 hour before the procedure, followed by 1 g 6 hours later. Daily maximum is 7 g (7000 mg).

Infants and Children: Amoxicillin: Up to 6 kg of body mass—25 to 50 mg every 8 hours. 6 to 8 kg of body mass—50 to 100 mg every 8 hours. 8 to 20 kg of body mass—6.7 to 13.3 mg per kg of body mass every 8 hours. 20 kg of body mass and over—same as 12 to 60 years of age.

Amoxicillin/clavulanate: Up to 40 kg of body mass—6.7 to 13.3 mg (amoxicillin) per kg of body mass, every 8 hours. 40 kg of body mass and over— same as 12 to 60 years of age. 12-hour formula: For severe infections—45 mg amoxicillin per kg of body mass **per day** (divided into two doses given every 12 hours). For less severe infections (as in skin infections)—25 mg per kg of body mass **per day** (divided into two doses given every 12 hours).

Bacampicillin: 25 mg per kg of body mass per day is given, divided into two equal doses every 12 hours, for respiratory infections.

Cloxacillin: For children weighing less than 44 lb (20 kg)—50 to 100 mg per kg of body mass per day, divided into four doses. Children greater than 20 kg get the adult dose. Intravenous dosing may be required for severe infections.

12 to 60 Years of Age: Amoxicillin: Usual dose—250 to 500 mg every 8 hours. Daily maximum is 4.5 g. For gonorrhea—3 g, with 1 g of probenecid, taken as a single dose. For Lyme disease—250 to 500 mg, three or four times a day, for 10 to 30 days; dose and duration depends on severity of infection and response to treatment.

Author's Note: New American Heart Association (AHA) guidelines for prevention of bacterial endocarditis in patients at risk suggest amoxicillin in an initial dose of 2 g in oral or dental procedures. There is no recommendation for follow-up doses of antibiotics.

Amoxicillin/clavulanate: Usual dose—250 to 500 mg (amoxicillin) every 8 hours. Daily maximum (of amoxicillin) is 4.5 g.

Ampicillin: 50 to 100 mg per kg of body mass per day divided into four doses, or 500 to 1000 mg every 6 hours. Usual daily maximum is 6000 mg daily.

Bacampicillin: For those with a body mass of 25 kg or more: 400 to 800 mg every 12 hours.

Cloxacillin: 250 to 500 mg every 6 hours. The maximum dose is 6000 mg (6 g) every 24 hours.

Over 60 Years of Age: Amoxicillin: Same as 12 to 60 years of age.

Amoxicillin/clavulanate: Same as 12 to 60 years of age. Note: The above doses refer to the amoxicillin component of amoxicillin/clavulanate. The 250-mg regular tablet and the 250-mg chewable tablet contain different amounts of clavulanate and are NOT interchangeable. See "Dose Forms" above.

Ampicillin: Drug is removed more slowly by patients in this age group; however, specific dose decreases are not defined.

Bacampicillin: Tests of kidney function should be obtained. Doses of 400 mg per day have been used in moderate kidney disease or decline (age-related decline in kidney function may be moderate).

Cloxacillin: No specific dosing changes are available.

Note: Actual dose and schedule must be determined for each patient individually for all of these medicines.

Conditions Requiring Dosing Adjustments

Liver Function: Dose adjustments do not appear to be needed (amoxicillin, amoxicillin/clavulanate, ampicillin, and penicillin VK). Caution is advised for bacampicillin use by these patients. The dose is decreased or the time between doses is increased for cloxacillin.

Kidney Function: Amoxicillin, amoxicillin/clavulanate, ampicillin: Dosing interval **must** be adjusted in renal compromise.

Bacampicillin: The dose must be decreased to 400 mg per day in moderate kidney failure. In severe kidney failure a dose of 400 mg every 36 hours is used.

Penicillin VK: For patients with severe kidney compromise, the usual dose is taken every 8 hours.

Cloxacillin: Patients should be watched closely for adverse effects in severe kidney compromise.

▷ **Dosing Instructions:**   The tablet (amoxicillin, bacampicillin, penicillin VK) may be crushed (or amoxicillin and amoxicillin/clavulanate chew-tabs chewed), or the capsule (amoxicillin) opened and taken on an empty stomach or with food or milk (amoxicillin). Absorption may be slightly faster if taken when stomach is empty (penicillin VK). Ampicillin, bacampicillin, and cloxacillin are best taken on an empty stomach. Oral suspension forms should be shaken well before measuring each dose.

Usual Duration of Use: For all streptococcal infections—not less than 10 consecutive (uninterrupted) days to reduce risk of rheumatic fever or glomerulonephritis. For all other infections—as long as needed to eradicate the infection. Incomplete treatment may lead to serious resistance and dangerous infections.

▷ **These Drugs Should Not Be Taken If**
- you had an allergic reaction to them previously.
- you are certain you are allergic to *any* form of penicillin.

▷ **Inform Your Physician Before Taking These Drugs If**
- you suspect you may be allergic to penicillin or have a history of a previous "reaction."
- you are allergic to any cephalosporin antibiotic (Ancef, Ceclor, etc.—see Drug Classes).
- you are allergic by nature (hay fever, asthma, hives, eczema).
- you are unsure how much to take or how often to take them.
- you have a history of liver or kidney disease.
- you have a history of low blood counts (amoxicillin/clavulanate, ampicillin, cloxacillin).

Possible Side Effects (natural, expected, and unavoidable drug actions)

Superinfections (see Glossary), often due to yeast organisms or for some penicillins, due to *Clostridium difficile*.

▷ **Possible Adverse Effects** (unusual, unexpected, and infrequent reactions)

If any of the following develop, consult your physician promptly for guidance.

Mild Adverse Effects

Allergic reactions: skin rashes, hives, itching.

Irritations of mouth or tongue, "black tongue," nausea, vomiting, diarrhea, dizziness—rare to infrequent.

Serious Adverse Effects

Allergic reactions: anaphylactic reaction (see Glossary), severe skin reactions, drug fever, swollen painful joints, sore throat, abnormal bleeding or bruising.

Severe skin reactions (Stevens-Johnson syndrome, bullous pemphigoid)—case reports.

Drug-induced colitis—rare.

Hemolytic anemia (penicillin VK)—case reports.

Drug-induced periarteritis nodosa, meningitis, or porphyria—(penicillin VK)—case reports.

Abnormal liver or kidney changes—rare.

Drug-induced abnormal lowering of white blood cells (amoxicillin/clavulanate, ampicillin, cloxacillin, penicillin VK)—rare.

▷ **Possible Effects on Sexual Function:**   None reported except for case reports of a small decrease in sperm counts for ampicillin.

Possible Effects on Laboratory Tests

Complete blood counts: decreased red cells, hemoglobin, white cells (therapeutic effects of each antibiotic), and platelets (penicillin VK); increased eosinophils (allergic reactions).

INR (prothrombin time): occasionally increased (ampicillin, cloxacillin, and penicillin VK).

Liver function tests: increased aspartate aminotransferase (AST/GOT) and bilirubin (cloxacillin and penicillin VK).

Coombs' test: may be positive with ampicillin or penicillin VK therapy.

CAUTION
1. Take the exact dose and the full course prescribed.
2. If these drugs must be used concurrently with antibiotics such as erythromycin or tetracycline, take the penicillin first.

Precautions for Use

By Infants and Children: Watch children with allergies closely for evidence of a developing allergy to penicillin. These drugs (amoxicillin, penicillin VK) may cause diarrhea, which sometimes necessitates discontinuation. Up to 90% of patients with mononucleosis who take amoxicillin, amoxicillin/clavulanate, or ampicillin get a rash.

By Those Over 60 Years of Age: Natural skin changes may predispose to prolonged itching in the genital and anal regions. Report such reactions promptly.

▷ **Advisability of Use During Pregnancy**

Pregnancy Category: B. See Pregnancy Risk Categories at the back of this book.

Animal studies: Birth defects of the limbs reported in mice (penicillin VK only). (Not confirmed in other studies.)

Human studies: Adequate studies of pregnant women indicate no increased risk of birth defects.

Ask your doctor for guidance, but these drugs are generally considered safe for use during any period of pregnancy.

Advisability of Use If Breast-Feeding

Presence of this drug in breast milk: Yes.

The nursing infant may be sensitized to penicillin and be at risk for developing diarrhea or yeast infections.

Avoid drug if possible or refrain from nursing.

Habit-Forming Potential: None.

Effects of Overdose: Possible nausea, vomiting, and/or diarrhea.

Possible Effects of Long-Term Use: Superinfections, often due to yeast organisms or *Clostridium difficile.*

Suggested Periodic Examinations While Taking This Drug (at physician's discretion)

Complete blood cell counts, kidney function tests.

▷ **While Taking This Drug, Observe the Following**

Foods: No restrictions, except for ampicillin, bacampicillin, and cloxacillin, which are best taken on an empty stomach.

Beverages: No restrictions (except as above). May be taken with milk.

▷ *Alcohol:* No interactions expected, but alcohol can blunt the immune response. It is best NOT to drink while you have an infection severe enough to require antibiotics.

Tobacco Smoking: No interactions expected. I advise everyone to quit smoking.

▷ *Other Drugs:*

Penicillins *taken concurrently* with

- disulfiram (Antabuse) can cause a disulfiram-like reaction (see Glossary) (bacampicillin only). Avoid the combination of these drugs.
- methotrexate (Mexate) may increase risk of methotrexate toxicity (especially amoxicillin and oral penicillin).

- probenecid (Benemid) will increase and sustain blood levels. This interaction is often used to therapeutic advantage.

Ampicillin *taken concurrently* with

- allopurinol may increase the risk of rashes.
- atenolol can blunt the therapeutic benefits of atenolol.

Ampicillin, cloxacillin, or penicillin VK *taken concurrently* with

- warfarin (Coumadin) may intensify the anticoagulant effect and increase risk of bleeding. More frequent INR (prothrombin time or protime) testing is needed.

Penicillins may *decrease* the effects of

- birth control pills (oral contraceptives), and impair their effectiveness in preventing pregnancy.

The following drugs may *decrease* the effects of penicillins:

- antacids, histamine (H_2) blockers, or proton pump inhibitors (see Drug Classes); may reduce the absorption of penicillins.
- chloramphenicol (Chloromycetin).
- erythromycin (Erythrocin, E-Mycin, etc.).
- tetracyclines (Achromycin, Declomycin, Minocin, etc.—see Drug Classes).

▷ *Driving, Hazardous Activities:* Usually no restrictions. Be alert to the rare occurrence of dizziness and/or nausea, and restrict activities accordingly.

Aviation Note: The use of these drugs *may be a disqualification* for piloting. Consult a designated aviation medical examiner.

Exposure to Sun: Ampicillin may increase sensitivity to the sun. Use caution.

Special Storage Instructions: Oral solutions and pediatric drops (amoxicillin) should be refrigerated.

Observe the Following Expiration Times: Do not take the oral solution of these drugs if older than 7 days (cloxacillin is good for only 3 days) when kept at room temperature, or 14 days when kept refrigerated.

PENTAZOCINE (pen TAZ oh seen)

Introduced: 1967   **Class:** Analgesic, strong   **Prescription:** USA: Yes
Controlled Drug: USA: C-IV*; Canada: No   **Available as Generic:** USA: No; Canada: No

Brand Names: Talacen [CD], Talwin, Talwin Compound [CD], ✤Talwin Compound-50 [CD], Talwin Nx [CD]

BENEFITS versus RISKS	
Possible Benefits	*Possible Risks*
EFFECTIVE RELIEF OF MODERATE TO SEVERE PAIN	POTENTIAL FOR HABIT FORMATION (DEPENDENCE)
	Respiratory depression
	Sedative effects
	Mental and behavioral disturbances
	Low blood pressure, fainting
	Nausea, constipation

*See Controlled Drug Schedules at the back of this book.

▷ **Principal Uses**

As a Single Drug Product: Uses currently included in FDA-approved labeling: Relieves acute or chronic pain of moderate to severe degree from any cause. Other (unlabeled) generally accepted uses: None.

As a Combination Drug Product [CD]: Pentazocine is available in combinations with acetaminophen and with aspirin. These milder pain relievers are added to enhance the analgesic effect and reduce fever when present. In the United States the tablet form of pentazocine also contains naloxone (Talwin Nx), a narcotic antagonist that renders the drug ineffective if abused.

How This Drug Works: Acting primarily as a depressant of certain brain functions, this drug suppresses the perception of pain and calms the emotional response to pain.

Available Dose Forms and Strengths

Caplet — 25 mg pentazocine and 650 mg acetaminophen
Injection — 30 mg/ml
Tablets — 50 mg (Canada)
Tablets — 50 mg with 0.5 mg of naloxone (U.S.)

▷ **Usual Adult Dose Range:** Oral dosing: 50 mg every 3 to 4 hours. May be increased to 100 mg every 4 hours for severe pain. The total daily dose should not exceed 600 mg. Many clinicians now use timed or scheduled dosing of pain medicines (analgesics), particularly early in acute pain, as this tends to prevent pain rather than treat it. Others revert to as-needed dosing once the acute pain is controlled. **Note: Actual dose and schedule must be determined for each patient individually.**

Conditions Requiring Dosing Adjustments

Liver Function: Doses should be decreased or the time between doses lengthened, otherwise increased adverse effects may occur.

Kidney Function: For moderate to severe kidney failure, the dose should be reduced by 25–50%.

▷ **Dosing Instructions:** The tablet may be crushed and taken with or following food to reduce stomach irritation or nausea.

Usual Duration of Use: As required to control pain. Continual use should not exceed 5 to 7 days without interruption and reassessment of need.

▷ **This Drug Should Not Be Taken If**
- you had an allergic reaction to it previously.
- you are having an acute attack of asthma.
- you have increased intracranial pressure or brain damage.

▷ **Inform Your Physician Before Taking This Drug If**
- you have had an unfavorable reaction to any narcotic drug in the past.
- you have a history of drug abuse or alcoholism.
- you have chronic lung disease with impaired breathing.
- you have impaired liver or kidney function.
- you have a history of confusion or hallucinations.
- you have gallbladder disease, a seizure disorder, or an underactive thyroid gland.
- you have difficulty emptying the urinary bladder.
- you are taking any other drugs that have a sedative effect.
- you plan to have surgery under general anesthesia in the near future.

Possible Side Effects (natural, expected, and unavoidable drug actions)
Drowsiness, light-headedness, weakness, urinary retention, constipation.

▷ **Possible Adverse Effects** (unusual, unexpected, and infrequent reactions)
If any of the following develop, consult your physician promptly for guidance.

Mild Adverse Effects
Allergic reactions: skin rash, hives, itching, swelling of face.
Headache, dizziness, sensation of drunkenness, blurred or double vision, flushing, sweating—infrequent and can be dose related.
Increased or decreased blood pressure—infrequent.
Drug fever—rare.
Nausea, vomiting, indigestion, diarrhea—infrequent to frequent.

Serious Adverse Effects
Marked drop in blood pressure, possible fainting—case reports and dose related.
Impaired breathing (respiratory depression)—possible and dose related.
Mental and behavioral disturbances, hallucinations, psychosis—case reports.
Drug-induced seizure, porphyria, or toxic epidermal necrolysis—rare.
Fibrous muscle replacement (with injection form)—rare.
Kidney problems—rare.
Fixed positioning of the eyes (oculogyric crisis)—case report.
Bone marrow depression (see Glossary) of a mild and reversible nature—rare.
Aggravation of prostatism (see Glossary)—possible.

▷ **Possible Effects on Sexual Function:**   Blunting of sexual response—possible.

Natural Diseases or Disorders That May Be Activated by This Drug
Porphyria (see Glossary).

Possible Effects on Laboratory Tests
White blood cell count: rarely decreased.
Blood amylase and lipase levels: increased (natural side effects).

CAUTION
1. Use of this drug with atropinelike drugs may increase the risk of urinary retention and reduced intestinal function.
2. Do not take this drug following acute head injury.

Precautions for Use
By Infants and Children: Safety and effectiveness for those under 12 years of age are not established.
By Those Over 60 Years of Age: Use small doses initially and increase dose as needed and tolerated. Limit use to short-term treatment only. There may be increased susceptibility to development of drowsiness, dizziness, unsteadiness, falling, urinary retention, and constipation.

▷ **Advisability of Use During Pregnancy**
Pregnancy Category: C (B or D in high doses at term or extended use). See Pregnancy Risk Categories at the back of this book.
Animal studies: Significant birth defects reported in hamsters.
Human studies: Adequate studies of pregnant women are not available. Pentazocine taken repeatedly during the final few weeks before delivery may cause withdrawal symptoms in the newborn infant.

Avoid this drug during the first 3 months. Use only if clearly needed and in small, infrequent doses during the final 6 months.

Advisability of Use If Breast-Feeding
Presence of this drug in breast milk: Expected.
Avoid drug or refrain from nursing.

Habit-Forming Potential: Psychological and/or physical dependence can develop.

Effects of Overdose: Anxiety, disturbed thoughts, hallucinations, progressive drowsiness, stupor, depressed breathing.

Possible Effects of Long-Term Use: Psychological and physical dependence, chronic constipation.

Suggested Periodic Examinations While Taking This Drug (at physician's discretion)
Complete blood cell counts, if used for an extended period of time.

▷ **While Taking This Drug, Observe the Following**
Foods: No restrictions.
Beverages: No restrictions. May be taken with milk.
▷ *Alcohol:* Pentazocine can intensify the intoxicating effects of alcohol, and alcohol can intensify the depressant effects of pentazocine on brain function, breathing, and circulation. It is best to avoid this combination.
Tobacco Smoking: Heavy smoking may reduce the drug's effectiveness. I advise everyone to quit smoking.
Marijuana Smoking: Increase in drowsiness and pain relief; impairment of mental and physical performance.
▷ *Other Drugs:*
Pentazocine may *increase* the effects of
• atropinelike drugs, and increase the risk of constipation and urinary retention.
• cyclosporine (Sandimmune) and cause toxicity.
• monoamine oxidase(MAO) inhibitors (see Drug Classes)—may result in muscle rigidity.
• sibutramine (Meridia) by increasing risk of serotoninsyndrome.
• other drugs with sedative effects (see Drug Classes on benzodiazepines, phenothiazines, and opioids).
▷ *Driving, Hazardous Activities:* This drug can impair mental alertness, judgment, reaction time, and physical coordination. Avoid hazardous activities accordingly.
Aviation Note: The use of this drug *is a disqualification* for piloting. Consult a designated aviation medical examiner.
Exposure to Sun: No restrictions.
Discontinuation: It is advisable to limit this drug to short-term use. If it is necessary to use it for extended periods of time, discontinuation should be gradual to minimize possible effects of withdrawal.

PENTOXIFYLLINE (pen tox I fi leen)

Other Name: Oxpentifylline

Introduced: 1972   **Class:** Blood flow agent, xanthines   **Prescription:**
USA: Yes   **Controlled Drug:** USA: No; Canada: No   **Available as Generic:**
No

Brand Name: Trental

BENEFITS versus RISKS

Possible Benefits	*Possible Risks*
IMPROVED BLOOD FLOW IN PERIPHERAL ARTERIAL DISEASE	Reduced blood pressure, angina, abnormal heart rhythms
REDUCTION OF INTERMITTENT CLAUDICATION PAIN	Rare low blood counts and aplastic anemia
May help in some AIDS-related pain	Indigestion, nausea, vomiting
	Dizziness, flushing

▷ **Principal Uses**

As a Single Drug Product: Uses currently included in FDA-approved labeling: Adjunctive treatment in the management of peripheral obstructive arterial disease to improve arterial blood flow and reduce frequency and severity of muscle pain due to intermittent claudication.

Other (unlabeled) generally accepted uses: (1) Decreases hemodialysis shunt clots (thrombosis); (2) may have a role in treating impotence that is caused by blood vessel problems (vascular impotence); (3) can increase the motility of sperm; (4) helps decrease interleukin and tumor necrosis factor in patients with cerebral malaria; (5) has had variable results in AIDS patients in attempting to halt weight loss that may be caused by tumor necrosis factor; (6) may ease skin tightening in some cases; (7) has been used to relieve symptoms of septic shock; (8) has been used to help heal refractory ulcers in diabetics; (9) may decrease insulin requirements in some diabetics and help retinopathy and neuropathy.

How This Drug Works: Improves blood flow and increases oxygen supply to working muscles by way of three mechanisms: (1) lowers blood viscosity due to decreased levels of blood fibrinogen; (2) increased flexibility of red blood cells (carrying oxygen) due to increased cyclic AMP (enzyme) in red blood cells—this permits easier movement in small blood vessels; and (3) prevents red blood cell and platelet clumping. Inhibits interleukins and tumor necrosis factor (seen in diabetes, heart attacks, and other conditions).

Available Dose Forms and Strengths

Tablets, prolonged action — 400 mg

▷ **Usual Adult Dose Range:**   400 mg three times a day. If adverse nervous system or gastrointestinal effects occur, reduce the dose to 400 mg twice daily. **Note: Actual dose and schedule must be determined for each patient individually.**

Conditions Requiring Dosing Adjustments

Liver Function: Dosing changes do not appear to be needed in liver compromise.

Kidney Function: The dose should be decreased. 400 mg twice daily to start has been suggested.

▷ **Dosing Instructions:**   Take with or following food to reduce stomach irritation. Swallow the tablet whole without breaking, crushing, or chewing.

Usual Duration of Use: Regular use for 2 to 4 weeks shows benefits in preventing or delaying intermittent claudication pain when walking. Full effect may take a minimum of 3 months. Long-term use (months to years) requires follow-up with your doctor.

Possible Advantages of This Drug
Reduces blood viscosity, improving blood flow.
Increases supply of oxygen to working muscles.

▷ **This Drug Should Not Be Taken If**
• you have had an allergic reaction to it previously.
• you have had a recent brain or eye (retinal) hemorrhage.

▷ **Inform Your Physician Before Taking This Drug If**
• you are allergic to other xanthine drugs: caffeine, theophylline, theobromine.
• you have impaired kidney function.
• you have low blood pressure, impaired brain circulation, or coronary artery disease.
• you are a diabetic.
• you have an ulcer of the stomach or intestine.
• you smoke tobacco.
• you are taking any antihypertensive drugs.

Possible Side Effects (natural, expected, and unavoidable drug actions)
Lowering of blood pressure (usually mild).

▷ **Possible Adverse Effects** (unusual, unexpected, and infrequent reactions)
If any of the following develop, consult your physician promptly for guidance.
Mild Adverse Effects
Allergic Reaction: Skin rash.
Headache, blurred vision and scotoma, dizziness, tremor—rare.
May worsen glucose control in diabetics—possible.
Nosebleeds—rare.
Flu-like syndrome: indigestion, nausea, vomiting—rare to infrequent.
Blood sugar changes—possible.
Serious Adverse Effects
Development of angina or heart rhythm disorders—rare.
Liver toxicity—rare.
Low platelets, white blood cells, or all cells-case reports.
Auditory hallucinations—case report.
Retinal bleeding—case reports.
Bleeding from ulcers of stomach or intestine—case reports and questionable association.

▷ **Possible Effects on Sexual Function:**   May help reverse impotence caused by circulatory problems.

Possible Effects on Laboratory Tests
Complete blood cell counts: rarely lowers red cells, hemoglobin, white cells, and platelets. Liver enzymes—rare increases.

CAUTION
1. Use this drug with caution in the presence of impaired circulation within the brain (cerebral arteriosclerosis) or coronary artery disease. If any related symptoms develop, consult your physician for prompt evaluation.

Precautions for Use

By Infants and Children: Safety and effectiveness for those under 18 years of age are not established. Use by this age group is not anticipated.

By Those Over 60 Years of Age: You may be more susceptible to the adverse effects listed above. Watch closely for any indications of dizziness or chest pain and report these promptly.

▷ **Advisability of Use During Pregnancy**

Pregnancy Category: C. See Pregnancy Risk Categories at the back of this book.

Animal studies: Increased fetal resorptions reported in rats, but no birth defects found in rats or rabbits.

Human studies: Adequate studies of pregnant women are not available.

Avoid use during the first 3 months. Use otherwise only if clearly needed.

Advisability of Use If Breast-Feeding

Presence of this drug in breast milk: Yes.

Avoid drug or refrain from nursing.

Habit-Forming Potential: None.

Effects of Overdose: Drowsiness, flushing, faintness, excitement, seizures.

Possible Effects of Long-Term Use: None reported.

Suggested Periodic Examinations While Taking This Drug (at physician's discretion)

Blood pressure measurements, evaluation of heart status.

▷ **While Taking This Drug, Observe the Following**

Foods: No restrictions.

Beverages: No restrictions. May be taken with milk.

▷ *Alcohol:* Alcohol may increase the blood-pressure-lowering effect of this drug.

Tobacco Smoking: Nicotine constricts arteries and impairs pentoxifylline effectiveness significantly. Avoid tobacco.

▷ *Other Drugs:*

Pentoxifylline may *increase* the effects of
- antihypertensive drugs, and cause excessive lowering of blood pressure.
- warfarin (Coumadin, etc.), and increase the possibility of unwanted bleeding; monitor INR (prothrombin time or protime) more frequently. Dosing should be adjusted to laboratory values.

Pentoxifylline *taken concurrently* with
- cimetidine (Tagamet), nizatidine (Axid), famotidine (Pepcid), or ranitidine (Zantac) may result in pentoxifylline toxicity (increases drug absorption).
- ritonavir (Norvir) may lead to pentoxifylline toxicity.
- theophylline (Theo-Dur, others) may result in theophylline toxicity.

▷ *Driving, Hazardous Activities:* This drug may cause drowsiness or dizziness. Restrict activities as necessary.

Aviation Note: The use of this drug *may be a disqualification* for piloting. Consult a designated aviation medical examiner.

Exposure to Sun: No restrictions.

PERGOLIDE (PER go lide)

Introduced: 1980   **Class:** Anti-parkinsonism, ergot derivative   **Prescription:** USA: Yes   **Controlled Drug:** USA: No; Canada: No   **Available as Generic:** USA: No
Brand Name: Permax

BENEFITS versus RISKS	
Possible Benefits	*Possible Risks*
ADDITIVE RELIEF OF SYMPTOMS OF PARKINSON'S DISEASE when used concurrently with levodopa/carbidopa PERMITS A REDUCTION IN SINEMET DOSE	ABNORMAL INVOLUNTARY MOVEMENTS HALLUCINATIONS INITIAL FALL IN BLOOD PRESSURE/ORTHOSTATIC HYPOTENSION Premature heart contractions (ventricular)

▷ **Principal Uses**

As a Single Drug Product: Uses currently included in FDA-approved labeling: As an adjunct to levodopa/carbidopa treatment of Parkinson's disease for people who experience intolerable abnormal movements (dyskinesia) and/or increasing "on–off" episodes due to levodopa. The addition of pergolide (1) permits reduction of the daily dose of levodopa with consequent lessening of dyskinesia and erratic drug response, and (2) provides additional relief of parkinsonian symptoms.

Other (unlabeled) generally accepted uses: (1) May have a role in helping reduce drug craving in cocaine withdrawal; (2) helps in some conditions where excess prolactin is made; (3) may be of use in acromegaly.

How This Drug Works: By directly stimulating part of the brain (dopamine receptor sites in the corpus striatum), this drug helps to compensate for the deficiency of dopamine that is responsible for the rigidity, tremor, and sluggish movement characteristic of Parkinson's disease.

Available Dose Forms and Strengths

Tablets — 0.05 mg, 0.25 mg, 1 mg

▷ **Usual Adult Dose Range**   Parkinson's (in conjunction with levodopa plus carbidopa): Starts at 0.05 mg daily (first 2 days); slowly increased by 0.1 mg daily or 0.15 mg every third day over next 12 days. If 0.2 needed and tolerated, daily dose may be increased by 0.25 to 0.3 mg every third day until best response. Total daily dose should be divided into three equal portions taken at 6- to 8-hour intervals. Usual ongoing dose is 3 mg every 24 hours; do not exceed 5 mg every 24 hours.

During gradual start of pergolide, dose of levodopa/carbidopa (Sinemet) may be lowered by your doctor.

Note: Actual dose and schedule must be determined for each patient individually.

Conditions Requiring Dosing Adjustments

Liver Function: Used with caution in liver disease.
Kidney Function: Consideration should be given to empirical decreases in dose.

▷ **Dosing Instructions:** The tablet may be crushed and taken with food or milk to reduce stomach irritation.

Usual Duration of Use: Regular use for 4 to 6 weeks reveals benefits controlling Parkinson's symptoms and permitting lower levodopa/carbidopa dose. Long-term use requires follow-up with your doctor.

Possible Advantages of This Drug: May give more effective and uniform control of parkinsonian symptoms, and fewer adverse effects from levodopa therapy.

▷ **This Drug Should Not Be Taken If**
- you have had an allergic reaction to it previously.
- you have had a serious adverse effect from any ergot preparation.
- you have severe coronary artery disease or peripheral vascular disease.

▷ **Inform Your Physician Before Taking This Drug If**
- you have constitutionally low blood pressure.
- you are pregnant or breast-feeding your infant.
- you are taking any antihypertensive drugs or antipsychotic drugs (see Drug Classes).
- you have any degree of coronary artery disease, especially angina or a history of heart attack.
- you have any type of heart rhythm disorder.
- you have impaired liver or kidney function.
- you have a seizure disorder.

Possible Side Effects (natural, expected, and unavoidable drug actions)
Weakness; chest pain—possibly anginal; peripheral edema; orthostatic hypotension (see Glossary)—infrequent.

▷ **Possible Adverse Effects** (unusual, unexpected, and infrequent reactions)
If any of the following develop, consult your physician promptly for guidance.
Mild Adverse Effects
Allergic reactions: skin rash, facial swelling—rare.
Headache, dizziness, hallucinations, drowsiness, insomnia, anxiety, double vision—rare to infrequent.
Nasal congestion, shortness of breath, palpitation, fainting—rare to infrequent.
Altered taste, dry mouth, indigestion, nausea, vomiting, constipation, diarrhea—infrequent.
Serious Adverse Effects
Allergic reactions: none reported.
Idiosyncratic reactions: flu-like symptoms.
Abnormal involuntary movements (dyskinesia)—frequent; psychotic behavior—case reports.
Hallucinations (accounted for 7.8% of patient withdrawals from therapy; 13.8% occurrence).
Abnormal heartbeat (ventricular arrhythmias)—infrequent to frequent.
Anemia—rare.

▷ **Possible Effects on Sexual Function:** Infrequent reports of altered libido (increased or decreased), impotence, breast pain, priapism (see Glossary).

▷ **Adverse Effects That May Mimic Natural Diseases or Disorders**
Effects on mental function and behavior may resemble psychotic disorders.

Natural Diseases or Disorders That May Be Activated by This Drug
Coronary artery disease with anginal syndrome, heart rhythm disorders, Raynaud's phenomenon (see Glossary), seizure disorders.

Possible Effects on Laboratory Tests
Blood prolactin level: decreased (marked reduction).

CAUTION
1. May cause abnormal movements (dyskinesias), or intensify existing dyskinesias. Watch for tremors, twitching, or abnormal, involuntary movements of any kind. Report these promptly.
2. Low starting doses help prevent possibility of excessive drop in blood pressure. See dose routine outlined above.
3. Inform your physician promptly if you become pregnant or plan a pregnancy. This drug has been reported (rarely) to cause abortion and birth defects.

Precautions for Use
By Infants and Children: This drug is not utilized by this age group.
By Those Over 60 Years of Age: Small initial doses are mandatory. Watch closely for any tendency to light-headedness or faintness, especially on arising from a lying or sitting position. You may be more susceptible to the development of impaired thinking, confusion, agitation, nightmares, or hallucinations.

▷ **Advisability of Use During Pregnancy**
Pregnancy Category: B. See Pregnancy Risk Categories at the back of this book.
Animal studies: No birth defects due to this drug were found in mouse or rabbit studies.
Human studies: Adequate studies of pregnant women are not available. However, there are four reports of birth defects associated with the use of this drug and infrequent reports of abortion. Causal relationships have not been established, but prudence advises against the use of this drug during pregnancy. Consult your physician for guidance.

Advisability of Use If Breast-Feeding
Presence of this drug in breast milk: Unknown.
Avoid drug or refrain from nursing.

Habit-Forming Potential: None.

Effects of Overdose: Nausea, vomiting, palpitations, low blood pressure, agitation, severe involuntary movements, hallucinations, seizures.

Possible Effects of Long-Term Use: Increased risk of developing dyskinesias.

Suggested Periodic Examinations While Taking This Drug (at physician's discretion)
Regular evaluation of drug response, heart function, and blood pressure status.

▷ **While Taking This Drug, Observe the Following**
Foods: No restrictions.
Beverages: No restrictions. May be taken with milk.
▷ *Alcohol:* Alcohol can exaggerate the blood-pressure-lowering and sedative effects of this drug.
Tobacco Smoking: No interactions expected. I advise everyone to quit smoking.

▷ *Other Drugs:*

Pergolide *taken concurrently* with

- antihypertensive drugs (and other drugs that can lower blood pressure) requires careful monitoring for excessive drops in pressure. (Lisinopril case report) Dose changes may be needed.

The following drugs may *decrease* the effects of pergolide and diminish its effectiveness:

- chlorprothixene (Taractan).
- haloperidol (Haldol).
- metoclopramide (Reglan).
- phenothiazines (see Drug Classes).
- thiothixene (Navane).

▷ *Driving, Hazardous Activities:* This drug may cause dizziness, drowsiness, impaired coordination, or fainting. Restrict activities as necessary.

Aviation Note: The use of this drug *is a disqualification* for piloting. Consult a designated aviation medical examiner.

Exposure to Sun: No restrictions.

Exposure to Heat: Use caution until the combined effects have been determined. Hot environments can cause lowering of blood pressure.

Discontinuation: Do not stop this drug abruptly. Sudden withdrawal can cause confusion, paranoid thinking, and severe hallucinations. Consult your physician regarding a schedule for gradual withdrawal.

PERPHENAZINE (per FEN a zeen)

Introduced: 1957   **Class:** Tranquilizer, major (antipsychotic drug); phenothiazines   **Prescription:** USA: Yes   **Controlled Drug:** USA: No; Canada: No   **Available as Generic:** USA: Yes; Canada: Yes

Brand Names: ✦Apo-Perphenazine, ✦Elavil Plus [CD], ✦Entrafon, Etrafon [CD], Etrafon-A [CD], Etrafon Forte [CD], ✦Phenazine, ✦PMS-Levazine, ✦PMS-Perphenazine, Triavil [CD], Trilafon

BENEFITS versus RISKS	
Possible Benefits	*Possible Risks*
EFFECTIVE CONTROL OF ACUTE MENTAL DISORDERS	SERIOUS TOXIC EFFECTS ON BRAIN with long-term use
Beneficial effects on thinking, mood, and behavior	Liver damage with jaundice
Relief of anxiety and tension	Blood cell disorders: hemolytic anemia, abnormally low white
Moderately effective control of nausea and vomiting	blood cell and platelet counts

▷ **Principal Uses**

As a Single Drug Product: Uses currently included in FDA-approved labeling: (1) Treats acute and chronic psychotic disorders: agitated depression, schizophrenia, and similar mental dysfunction; (2) used as a tranquilizer to help agitated and disruptive behavior; (3) severe nausea and vomiting treatment. Other (unlabeled) generally accepted uses: Can ease tremors caused by tricyclic antidepressants.

As a Combination Drug Product [CD]: Available combined with amitriptyline. In some severe agitated depression, combining an antipsychotic drug and an antidepressant will be more effective than either drug used alone.

How This Drug Works: Inhibits dopamine, correcting an imbalance of nerve impulses in mental disorders.

Available Dose Forms and Strengths

Concentrate — 16 mg/5 ml

Injection — 5 mg/ml

Tablets — 2 mg, 4 mg, 8 mg, 16 mg

Tablets, prolonged action — 8 mg

▷ **Usual Adult Dose Range:**   Psychotic symptoms (patients not hospitalized): Starts at 4 to 8 mg three times daily. Increased by 4 mg at 3- to 4-day intervals as needed and tolerated. Daily maximum is 64 mg. **Note: Actual dose and schedule must be determined for each patient individually.**

Conditions Requiring Dosing Adjustments

Liver Function: Dose is lowered in liver disease. NOT to be used in moderate to severe liver disease.

Kidney Function: No changes thought to be needed in kidney disease.

▷ **Dosing Instructions:**   May be taken with or after meals to reduce stomach irritation. Regular tablets may be crushed; the prolonged-action tablets should be taken whole, not broken, crushed, or chewed.

Usual Duration of Use: Regular use for several weeks reveals benefits in controlling psychotic disorders. If it does not help in 6 weeks, it should be stopped. Long-term use (months to years) requires periodic physician follow-up.

▷ **This Drug Should Not Be Taken If**
• you are allergic to any form of this medicine.
• you have active liver disease.
• you have brain damage in the subcortical area.
• you have cancer of the breast.
• you have a current blood cell or bone marrow disorder.

▷ **Inform Your Physician Before Taking This Drug If**
• you are allergic or abnormally sensitive to any phenothiazine (see Drug Classes).
• you have impaired liver or kidney function.
• you have any type of seizure disorder.
• you have diabetes, glaucoma, lupus erythematosus, or heart disease.
• you are pregnant or breast-feeding your infant.
• you have an allergy to sulfites.
• you have a history of neuroleptic malignant syndrome (see Glossary).
• you are taking any drug with sedative effects.
• you will have surgery with general or spinal anesthesia.

Possible Side Effects (natural, expected, and unavoidable drug actions)

Drowsiness (usually during the first 2 weeks), orthostatic hypotension (see Glossary), blurred vision, dry mouth, nasal congestion, constipation, impaired urination.

Pink or purple coloration of urine, of no significance.

▷ **Possible Adverse Effects** (unusual, unexpected, and infrequent reactions)
If any of the following develop, consult your physician promptly for guidance.

Mild Adverse Effects

Allergic reactions: skin rash, hives, low-grade fever.

Lowering of body temperature, especially in the elderly (see ***hypothermia*** in Glossary)—possible.

Increased appetite and weight gain—possible.

Dizziness, weakness, agitation, insomnia, impaired day and night vision—frequent.

Chronic constipation, fecal impaction—possible.

Serious Adverse Effects

Allergic reactions: hepatitis with jaundice (see Glossary), severe skin reactions (systemic lupus erythematosus, Stevens-Johnson syndrome), anaphylaxis—case reports.

Idiosyncratic reactions: neuroleptic malignant syndrome (see Glossary).

Depression; disorientation; seizures; deposits in cornea, lens, and retina—possible to infrequent.

Rapid heart rate, heart rhythm disorders—case reports.

Blood cell disorders: hemolytic anemia, reduced white blood cell or platelet counts—case reports.

Nervous system reactions: Parkinson-like disorders (see Glossary), severe restlessness, muscle spasms involving the face and neck, tardive dyskinesia (see Glossary)—case reports.

▷ **Possible Effects on Sexual Function:**   Altered timing and pattern of menstruation.

Female breast enlargement with milk production.

False-positive pregnancy test results.

Male breast enlargement and tenderness (gynecomastia).

Painful and extended duration of erection (priapism) or inhibited ejaculation—case reports.

▷ **Adverse Effects That May Mimic Natural Diseases or Disorders**

Nervous system reactions may suggest true Parkinson's disease.

Liver reactions may suggest viral hepatitis.

Reactions resembling systemic lupus erythematosus can occur.

Natural Diseases or Disorders That May Be Activated by This Drug

Latent epilepsy, glaucoma, diabetes mellitus, prostatism (see Glossary).

Possible Effects on Laboratory Tests

White blood cell counts: decreased.

Blood bilirubin level: increased (jaundice—see Glossary).

Blood glucose level: increased.

Glucose tolerance test (GTT): decreased in 35% of those taking this drug.

CAUTION

1. Many over-the-counter medications (see Glossary) for allergies, colds, and coughs contain drugs that can interact unfavorably with this drug. Ask your physician or pharmacist for help **before** using any such medications.
2. Antacids that contain aluminum and/or magnesium can prevent the absorption of this drug and reduce its effectiveness.
3. Obtain prompt evaluation of any vision change.

Precautions for Use

By Infants and Children: Use of this drug is not recommended in children under 12 years of age. Do not use this drug in the presence of symptoms suggestive of Reye syndrome (see Glossary). Children with acute infectious diseases (flu-like infections, chicken pox, measles, etc.) are more prone to develop spasms of the face, back, and extremities if this drug is used to control nausea or vomiting.

By Those Over 60 Years of Age: Small starting doses are advisable. Increased susceptibility to development of drowsiness, lethargy, constipation, lowering of body temperature (hypothermia), and orthostatic hypotension (see Glossary). This drug can enhance existing prostatism (see Glossary). You may also be more susceptible to the development of Parkinson-like reactions and/or tardive dyskinesia (see Glossary). These reactions must be recognized early, as they may become unresponsive to treatment and irreversible.

▷ **Advisability of Use During Pregnancy**

Pregnancy Category: C. See Pregnancy Risk Categories at the back of this book.

Animal studies: Cleft palate reported in mouse and rat studies.

Human studies: No increase in birth defects reported in 166 exposures. Information from adequate studies of pregnant women is not available.

Avoid drug during the first 3 months; avoid during the final month because of possible effects on the newborn infant.

Advisability of Use If Breast-Feeding

Presence of this drug in breast milk: Yes, in minute amounts.

Monitor nursing infant closely and discontinue drug or nursing if adverse effects develop.

Habit-Forming Potential: None.

Effects of Overdose: Marked drowsiness, weakness, tremor, agitation, unsteadiness, deep sleep, coma, convulsions.

Possible Effects of Long-Term Use: Opacities in the cornea or lens of the eye, pigmentation of the retina.

Tardive dyskinesia (see Glossary).

Suggested Periodic Examinations While Taking This Drug (at physician's discretion)

Complete blood cell counts, especially between the 4th and 10th weeks of treatment.

Liver function tests, electrocardiograms.

Complete eye examinations—eye structures and vision.

Careful inspection of the tongue for early evidence of fine, involuntary, wave-like movements that could indicate the beginning of tardive dyskinesia.

▷ **While Taking This Drug, Observe the Following**

Foods: No restrictions.

Nutritional Support: A riboflavin (vitamin B_2) supplement should be taken with long-term use.

Beverages: No restrictions. May be taken with milk.

▷ *Alcohol:* Avoid completely. Alcohol can increase the sedative action of phenothiazines and accentuate their depressant effects on brain function and blood pressure. Phenothiazines can increase the intoxicating effects of alcohol.

Tobacco Smoking: Possible reduction of drowsiness from drug. I advise everyone to quit smoking.

Marijuana Smoking: Moderate increase in drowsiness; accentuation of orthostatic hypotension; increased risk of precipitating latent psychoses, confusing the interpretation of mental status and drug responses.

▷ *Other Drugs:*

Perphenazine may ***increase*** the effects of
- all atropinelike drugs, and cause nervous system toxicity.
- all sedative drugs, especially meperidine (Demerol), and cause excessive sedation.

Perphenazine may ***decrease*** the effects of
- guanethidine (Ismelin, Esimil), and reduce its effectiveness in lowering blood pressure.
- oral antidiabetic drugs (see Drug Classes), and cause loss of glucose control.

Perphenazine ***taken concurrently*** with
- ascorbic acid may blunt the therapeutic effect of perphenazine.
- grepafloxacin (Raxar) may lead to abnormal heart beats.
- lithium (Lithobid, Lithotabs) may impair the effectiveness of lithium and cause nervous system toxicity.
- monoamine oxidase (MAO) inhibitor drugs (see Drug Classes) may result in increased extrapyramidal reactions.
- ritonavir (Norvir), and perhaps other protease inhibitors (see Drug Classes), may lead to toxicity.
- sparfloxacin (Zagam) may lead to abnormal heart beats.
- tramadol (Ultram) may increase seizure risk.

The following drugs may ***decrease*** the effects of perphenazine:
- antacids containing aluminum and/or magnesium.
- barbiturates (see Drug Classes).
- benztropine (Cogentin).
- disulfiram (Antabuse).
- trihexyphenidyl (Artane).

▷ *Driving, Hazardous Activities:* This drug can impair mental alertness, judgment, and physical coordination. Avoid hazardous activities.

Aviation Note: The use of this drug ***is a disqualification*** for piloting. Consult a designated aviation medical examiner.

Exposure to Sun: Use caution—some phenothiazines can cause photosensitivity (see Glossary).

Exposure to Heat: Use caution and avoid excessive heat as much as possible. This drug may impair the regulation of body temperature and increase the risk of heatstroke.

Exposure to Cold: Use caution and dress warmly. This drug can increase the risk of hypothermia in the elderly.

Discontinuation: After a period of long-term use, do not stop this drug suddenly. Gradual withdrawal over 2 to 3 weeks under physician supervision is recommended. Schizophrenia relapse is 50–60%.

PHENELZINE (FEN el zeen)

Introduced: 1961 **Class:** Antidepressant, MAO type A inhibitor **Prescription:** USA: Yes **Controlled Drug:** USA: No; Canada: No **Available as Generic:** No
Brand Name: Nardil

BENEFITS versus RISKS	
Possible Benefits	*Possible Risks*
EFFECTIVE RELIEF OF REACTIVE, NEUROTIC, ATYPICAL DEPRESSIONS with associated anxiety or phobia	DANGEROUS INTERACTIONS WITH MANY DRUGS AND FOODS CONDUCIVE TO HYPERTENSIVE CRISIS
Beneficial in some depressions that are not responsive to other treatments	DISORDERED HEART RATE AND RHYTHM
	Drug-induced hepatitis—rare
	Mental changes: agitation, confusion, impaired memory, hypomania

▷ **Principal Uses**

As a Single Drug Product: Uses currently included in FDA-approved labeling: Used to treat severe situational (reactive or neurotic) depression, atypical depression, and (though less effective) severe endogenous depression. Because of the supervision required during its use and its potential for serious adverse effects, this drug is usually reserved to treat depressions that have not responded satisfactorily to other antidepressant therapy.

Other (unlabeled) generally accepted uses: (1) Helps control binge eating in bulimia; (2) may be useful in treating chronic headache patients who also suffer from depression or anxiety; (3) a long-term study found phenelzine beneficial in treating social phobia; (4) rare use in intractable narcolepsy; (5) may be of benefit in post-traumatic stress disorder.

▷ **Usual Adult Dose Range:** Initially 15 mg three times a day (or 1 mg per kg of body mass, divided into three equal doses and taken three times daily); increase rapidly up to 60 mg/day, as needed and tolerated, until improvement is apparent. For maintenance, reduce dose gradually over several weeks to the smallest dose that will maintain improvement; this may be as low as 15 mg daily or every other day. The total daily dose should not exceed 90 mg. **Note: Actual dose and dosing schedule must be individually determined.**

▷ **While Taking This Drug, Observe the Following**

Foods: Use of this drug with ginseng has worsened depression and caused tremor and insomnia.

▷ *Other Drugs:*

Phenelzine may *increase* the effects of

- all drugs with stimulant effects on the nervous system, and cause excessive rise in blood pressure.
- all drugs with sedative effects, and cause excessive sedation.
- amphetamine and related drugs.
- appetite suppressants.
- insulin.
- sulfonylureas (see Drug Classes) or other oral hypoglycemic agents.

Phenelzine *taken concurrently* with
- antihistamines (see Drug Classes) can worsen the anticholinergic side effects of antihistamines.
- buspirone (Buspar) may result in undesirable increases in blood pressure.
- carbamazepine (Tegretol) may cause severe toxic reactions.
- dextromethorphan (nonprescription cough medicine with a "DM") can cause severe toxic reactions.
- dopamine (Intropin) may cause severe toxic reactions.
- fluoxetine (Prozac) has resulted in fatal reactions with another MAO inhibitor (tranylcypromine). This combination is to be avoided.
- fluvoxamine (Luvox) or other serotonin reuptake inhibitors may result in neuroleptic malignant syndrome and other serious reactions. This combination is not recommended.
- levodopa (Dopar, Sinemet) may cause a dangerous rise in blood pressure.
- meperidine (Demerol) may cause high fever, seizures, and coma. These drugs are NOT to be combined.
- methyldopa (Aldomet) may cause a dangerous rise in blood pressure.
- methylphenidate (Ritalin) may cause severe headache, weakness, and numbness in the extremities.
- mirtazipine (Remeron) increases seizure risk.
- nadolol (Corgard) and metoprolol (Lopressor) or other beta-blockers (see Drug Classes) may result in significant decreases in heart rate.
- nefazodone (Serzone) may result in serious adverse effects. DO NOT combine these drugs.
- paroxetine (Paxil) may result in serious adverse effects. DO NOT combine these drugs.
- phenothiazines (see Drug Classes) or other antipsychotics may cause exaggeration of the central nervous system and depression of breathing effects.
- phenylephrine (various) may result in serious increases in blood pressure. DO NOT combine.
- phenylpropanolamine (various) may result in serious increases in blood pressure. DO NOT combine.
- propoxyphene (Darvon) may result in coma, heart problems, or severe increases in temperature. DO NOT combine.
- pseudoephedrine (various) may result in serious adverse effects. DO NOT combine these drugs.
- sertraline (Zoloft) may result in muscle rigidity, Central Nervous System toxicity, and chills. DO NOT combine these medicines.
- sibutramine (Meridia) increases central nervous system problem or serotonin syndrome risk.
- sumatriptan (Imitrex) may increase central nervous system problem or serotonin syndrome risk.
- tramadol (Ultram) may increase seizure risk.
- tryptophan (L-Tryptophan) can cause toxic reactions.
- tricyclic antidepressants (see Drug Classes) may cause severe toxic reactions including high fever, delirium, tremor, seizures, and coma.
- venlafaxine (Effexor) may result in serious adverse reactions. DO NOT combine these medicines.

Note: Consult your physician before taking *any other drugs* while taking phenelzine.

▷ *Driving, Hazardous Activities:* This drug may cause dizziness, drowsiness, and blurred vision. Restrict activities as necessary.

Aviation Note: The use of this drug *is a disqualification* for piloting. Consult a designated aviation medical examiner.

Occurrence of Unrelated Illness: Because of the very serious and life-threatening interactions that can occur between this drug and many others, you **must** tell each health care provider you consult that you are taking this drug.

Discontinuation: If this drug is not effective after 4 weeks of continual use, it should be stopped. If it is effective, continue to take it in the proper dose until advised to stop. Do not stop it abruptly. If another antidepressant is to be tried, a drug-free waiting period of 14 days must pass between stopping this drug and starting the new one. Avoid tyramine-rich foods and other interacting drugs during this 14-day period.

Author's Note: Since other medicines are more widely used, the information in this profile has been shortened.

PHENOBARBITAL (fee noh BAR bi tawl)

Other Name: Phenobarbitone

Introduced: 1912 **Class:** Hypnotic drug (sedative), anticonvulsant, barbiturate **Prescription:** USA: Yes **Controlled Drug:** USA: C-IV*; Canada: Yes **Available as Generic:** Yes

Brand Names: Alubelap [CD], Aminodrox-Forte, Antispasmodic [CD], Azpan, Barbidonna [CD], Barbidonna Elixir [CD], Barbita, Belap, Belladenal [CD], Belladenal-S [CD], ✦Belladenal Spacetabs [CD], ✦Bellergal [CD], Bellergal-S [CD], ✦Bellergal Spacetabs [CD], Bronchotabs [CD], Bronkolixir [CD], ✦Cafergot-PB, Chardonna-2 [CD], Daricon PB, ✦Diclophen [CD], Dilantin w/Phenobarbital [CD], Donphen, Donna-Sed, Donnatal [CD], Ergobel [CD], Eskabarb, Eskaphen B [CD], Floramine, ✦Gardenal, Hybephen [CD], Hypnaldyne [CD], Isuprel Compound [CD], Kinesed [CD], Luminal, Mudrane GG Elixir & Tablets [CD], Mudrane Tablets [CD], Neospect, ✦Neuro-Spasex [CD], ✦Neuro-Trasentin [CD], ✦Neuro-Trasentin Forte [CD], Novalene, Phedral [CD], ✦Phenaphen Capsules [CD], ✦Phenaphen No. 2, 3, 4 [CD], Phenergan w/Codeine [CD], Phyldrox, Quadrinal [CD], Relaxadron, SBP [CD], Scodonnar [CD], Sedacord [CD], SK-Phenobarbital, Solfoton, Spasquid [CD], Spazcaps, Tedral Preparations [CD], T.E.P. [CD], Thalfed [CD], Theocardone, Theocord [CD], Theolixer, Vitaphen

BENEFITS versus RISKS	
Possible Benefits	*Possible Risks*
EFFECTIVE CONTROL OF TONIC-CLONIC SEIZURES AND ALL TYPES OF PARTIAL SEIZURES	POTENTIAL FOR DEPENDENCE LIFE-THREATENING TOXICITY WITH OVERDOSE
EFFECTIVE CONTROL OF FEBRILE SEIZURES OF CHILDHOOD	Drug-induced hepatitis or decreased kidney function
Effective relief of anxiety and nervous tension	Blood cell disorders: abnormally low red cell, white cell, and platelet counts

*See Controlled Drug Schedules at the back of this book.

▷ **Principal Uses**

As a Single Drug Product: Uses currently included in FDA-approved labeling: (1) Used as a mild sedative; (2) used as an anticonvulsant to control grand mal epilepsy and all types of partial seizures including febrile seizures of childhood; (3) used as a sedative, yet newer agents carry fewer drug interactions or effects on sleep cycles.

Other (unlabeled) generally accepted uses: (1) May be helpful in detoxification of sedative-hypnotic addiction; (2) can help control seizures found in cerebral malaria; (3) eases neonatal seizures; (4) may have a role in treating pain syndromes.

As a Combination Drug Product [CD]: This drug is available in many combinations with derivatives of belladonna, an antispasmodic commonly used to treat functional disorders of the gastrointestinal tract. It is also available in combination with bronchodilators for the treatment of asthma, and with ergotamine for the treatment of headaches.

How This Drug Works: Impedes transfer of sodium and potassium across cells, and selectively blocks nerve impulses. This can give a sedative effect or suppress nerve impulses causing seizures.

Available Dose Forms and Strengths

Capsules — 16 mg
Elixir — 15 mg/5 ml, 20 mg/5 ml
Tablets — 8 mg, 16 mg, 32 mg, 65 mg, 100 mg

▷ **Usual Adult Dose Range:**   As sedative: 15 to 30 mg two to three times a day. As hypnotic: 100 to 200 mg at bedtime. As anticonvulsant: 60 to 250 mg taken as a single dose at bedtime. Some clinicians give 2 to 3 mg per kg of body mass in order to achieve and maintain a blood level between 15 to 40 mcg/ml. **Note: Actual dose and dosing schedule must be determined for each patient individually.**

Conditions Requiring Dosing Adjustments

Liver Function: Used with caution in decreased doses (with more frequent blood levels) in liver disease.

Kidney Function: Used with caution and in decreased doses in kidney disease. Blood levels should be obtained. One clinician suggests that patients with severe kidney failure (creatinine clearance less than 10 ml/min) can take typical doses every 12 to 16 hours.

▷ **Dosing Instructions:**   Regular tablets may be crushed, and capsules opened and taken with or after food to reduce stomach irritation. Prolonged-action dose forms should be swallowed whole without alteration.

Usual Duration of Use: Regular use for 3 to 5 days shows benefits in relieving anxiety and tension, and 4 to 6 weeks determines ability to control seizures. If used for anxiety-tension, use should not exceed 4 weeks without reappraisal of continued need. Long-term use for seizure control requires follow-up with your doctor.

▷ **This Drug Should Not Be Taken If**

• you have had an allergic reaction to it previously.
• you have severe liver impairment.
• you get acute intermittent porphyria (see Glossary).
• you have a respiratory disease that makes it difficult to breathe.

▷ **Inform Your Physician Before Taking This Drug If**
- you are allergic or overly sensitive to any barbiturate (see Drug Classes).
- you are pregnant or planning a pregnancy.
- you have a history of alcohol or drug abuse.
- you are taking any drugs with sedative effects.
- you have a history of depression.
- you have any type of seizure disorder.
- you have myasthenia gravis.
- you have impaired liver, kidney, or thyroid gland function.
- you plan to have surgery under general anesthesia in the near future.

Possible Side Effects (natural, expected, and unavoidable drug actions)
Drowsiness, impaired concentration, mental and physical sluggishness.

▷ **Possible Adverse Effects** (unusual, unexpected, and infrequent reactions)
If any of the following develop, consult your physician promptly for guidance.

Mild Adverse Effects

Allergic reactions: skin rashes, hives, localized swellings of face, drug fever (see Glossary).

Dizziness, unsteadiness, impaired vision, double vision—possible and may be dose related.

Nausea, vomiting, diarrhea—infrequent.

Abnormal growth of the gums—case reports.

Shoulder-hand syndrome: pain and stiffness in the shoulder, pain/swelling in the hand—case reports.

Serious Adverse Effects

Allergic reactions: drug-induced hepatitis with jaundice (see Glossary), severe skin disorders (Stevens-Johnson syndrome or toxic epidermal necrolysis)—case reports.

Osteoporosis—possible with long-term use.

Idiosyncratic reactions: paradoxical excitement and delirium (instead of sedation).

Drug-induced myasthenia gravis, liver or kidney disease—case reports.

Respiratory depression—dose related.

Mental depression, abnormal involuntary movements—case reports.

Blood cell disorders: lowering of all blood cells (weakness, fever, sore throat, bleeding/bruising)—rare.

Blood clotting disorders in neonates—case reports.

Optic neuropathy—rare.

Drug-induced seizures—possible.

Low blood calcium—case reports.

▷ **Possible Effects on Sexual Function:**   Decreased libido and/or impotence—occasional.

Decreased effectiveness of oral contraceptives taken concurrently—frequent.

▷ **Adverse Effects That May Mimic Natural Diseases or Disorders**
Liver reactions may suggest viral hepatitis.

Natural Diseases or Disorders That May Be Activated by This Drug
Acute intermittent and/or cutaneous porphyria. Systemic lupus erythematosus (SLE) has been reported with primidone which has phenobarbital as one of its metabolites. The way (mechanism) that this occurs is by in-

creased antinuclear antibodies (ANA). Causality is questionable, but of concern.

Possible Effects on Laboratory Tests

Complete blood cell counts: decreased red cells, hemoglobin, white cells, and platelets.

Blood lupus erythematosus (LE) cells: positive—possible.

INR (prothrombin time): decreased (when taken concurrently with warfarin).

Blood calcium level: decreased (with long-term use).

Blood thyroxine (T_4) level: decreased.

Liver function tests: increased liver enzymes (ALT/GPT, AST/GOT, alkaline phosphatase) and bilirubin.

Urine sugar tests: no effect with Tes-Tape; false low results with Clinistix and Diastix.

Urine screening tests for drug abuse: may be **positive**. (Test results depend upon amount of drug taken and testing method used.)

CAUTION

1. Accurate diagnosis and seizure classification are essential for selection of the most appropriate drug therapy.
2. Emotional stress or physical trauma (including surgery) may require increased anticonvulsant dose to control seizures.
3. Prolonged-action dose forms of this drug are not appropriate for the treatment of seizures.

Precautions for Use

By Infants and Children: This drug should not be given to the hyperkinetic child. Possible paradoxical stimulation/hyperactivity can occur in 10 to 40% of children. Changes associated with puberty slow metabolism of this drug and permit its gradual accumulation. Blood levels in adolescents should be checked every 3 months to detect rising concentrations and early toxicity.

By Those Over 60 Years of Age: It is advisable for the elderly to avoid all barbiturates. If use of this drug is attempted, small starting doses are indicated. Watch for confusion, delirium, agitation, and excitement. Do not use this drug concurrently with other drugs for mental disorders. This drug is conducive to the development of hypothermia (see Glossary).

▷ **Advisability of Use During Pregnancy**

Pregnancy Category: D. See Pregnancy Risk Categories at the back of this book.

Animal studies: Conflicting reports of cleft palate and skeletal defects in mouse, rat, and rabbit studies.

Human studies: Information from studies of pregnant women indicates no increase in birth defects in 8,037 exposures to this drug. However, it is reported that barbiturates can cause fetal damage when taken during pregnancy.

Avoid use of drug during entire pregnancy if possible. If it is clearly needed to control seizures, the mother should receive vitamin K prior to delivery and the infant should receive it at birth.

Advisability of Use If Breast-Feeding

Presence of this drug in breast milk: Yes, in small amounts.

Monitor nursing infant closely and discontinue drug or nursing if adverse effects develop.

Habit-Forming Potential: Psychological and physical dependence can occur with prolonged use of excessive doses—300 to 700 mg/day for 1 to 2 months. Dependence is not likely to occur with usual sedative or anticonvulsant doses.

Effects of Overdose: Behavior similar to alcoholic intoxication—confusion, slurred speech, physical incoordination, staggering gait, drowsiness, stupor leading to coma.

Possible Effects of Long-Term Use: Psychological and/or physical dependence; syndrome of chronic intoxication—headache, depression, impaired vision, dizziness, slurred speech, incoordination. Megaloblastic anemia due to folic acid deficiency. Rickets or osteomalacia due to deficiencies of vitamin D and calcium.

Suggested Periodic Examinations While Taking This Drug (at physician's discretion)

Phenobarbital blood levels are needed for seizure control. Time to take blood for phenobarbital level: just before next dose.

Recommended therapeutic range—for adults: 15–40 mcg/ml; for children: 15–30 mcg/ml.

Complete blood cell counts, liver function tests.

During long-term use: blood levels of folic acid, vitamin B_{12}, calcium, and phosphorus; densitometry (DEXA) studies for demineralization/osteoporosis of bone.

▷ **While Taking This Drug, Observe the Following**

Foods: No restrictions. Eat liberally of foods rich in folic acid—fortified breakfast cereals, liver, legumes, green leafy vegetables.

Beverages: No restrictions. May be taken with milk or fruit juices.

▷ *Alcohol:* Avoid completely. Alcohol can increase greatly the sedative and depressant actions of this drug on brain functions.

Tobacco Smoking: May enhance the sedative effects of this drug and increase drowsiness. I advise everyone to quit smoking.

Marijuana Smoking: Increased drowsiness, unsteadiness; significantly impaired mental and physical performance.

▷ *Other Drugs:*

Phenobarbital may *increase* the effects of
- all other drugs with sedative effects, and cause excessive sedation.

Phenobarbital may *decrease* the effects of
- anticoagulants (Coumadin, etc.), and require dose adjustments based on more frequent INR (prothrombin time or protime) testing.
- birth control pills (oral contraceptives), and reduce their effectiveness in preventing pregnancy.
- certain beta-blockers (Inderal, Lopressor), and reduce their effectiveness.
- cortisonelike drugs (see *adrenocortical steroids* in Drug Classes).
- cyclosporine (Sandimmune).
- diltiazem (Cardizem).
- disopyramide (Norpace).
- doxycycline (Vibramycin).
- felodipine (Plendil).
- griseofulvin (Fulvicin, etc.).

- indinavir (Crixivan), and perhaps other protease inhibitors (see Drug Classes).
- lamotrigine (Lamictal).
- metoprolol (Lopressor, others).
- montelukast (Singulair).
- nimodipine (Nimotop).
- quinidine (Quinaglute, etc.), and reduce its effectiveness.
- propranolol (Inderal).
- ritonavir (Norvir).
- theophyllines (Aminophyllin, Theo-Dur, etc.), and reduce their antiasthmatic effectiveness.
- tricyclic antidepressants (see Drug Classes).
- verapamil (Calan), and reduce its effectiveness.
- venlafaxine (Effexor).
- warfarin (Coumadin), and increase risk of clots.

Phenobarbital *taken concurrently* with

- chloramphenicol (Chloromycetin) may result in decreased chloramphenicol benefits and phenobarbital toxicity. These drugs are NOT to be combined.
- colestipol (Colestid) and other cholesterol-lowering resins may bind phenobarbital and limit absorption.
- influenza vaccine may cause phenobarbital toxicity.
- itraconazole (and perhaps other antifungals) may decrease the antifungal effect of itraconazole.
- phenytoin (Dilantin) may alter phenytoin blood levels: a high phenobarbital level will increase the phenytoin level; a low phenobarbital level will decrease the phenytoin level. Periodic determination of blood levels of both drugs is advised.
- primidone (Mysoline) may lead to phenobarbital toxicity.

The following drugs may *increase* the effects of phenobarbital:

- ascorbic acid (vitamin C).
- felbamate (Felbatol).
- valproic acid (Depakene).

▷ *Driving, Hazardous Activities:* This drug may cause drowsiness and may impair mental alertness, judgment, physical coordination, and reaction time. Restrict activities as necessary.

Aviation Note: The use of this drug *is a disqualification* for piloting. Consult a designated aviation medical examiner.

Exposure to Sun: Use caution—this drug may cause photosensitivity.

Exposure to Cold: Observe the elderly for possible hypothermia (see Glossary) while taking this drug.

Discontinuation: If used as an anticonvulsant, this drug must not be stopped abruptly. Sudden withdrawal can precipitate status epilepticus (repetitive seizures). Gradual reduction in dose should be made over a period of 3 months. Total drug withdrawal may be attempted after a period of 3 to 5 years without a seizure. However, seizures are likely to recur in 40% of adults and in 20–30% of children.

PHENYTOIN (FEN i toh in)

Other Name: Diphenylhydantoin

Introduced: 1938   **Class:** Anticonvulsant, hydantoins; pain syndrome modifier **Prescription:** USA: Yes   **Controlled Drug:** USA: No; Canada: No
Available as Generic: USA: Yes; Canada: Yes

Brand Names: Dilantin, Dilantin Infatabs, Dilantin w/Phenobarbital [CD], Di-Phen, Diphenylan, Ekko JR, Ekko SR, Ekko Three, ✦Mebroin [CD], Phelantin

BENEFITS versus RISKS	
Possible Benefits	*Possible Risks*
EFFECTIVE CONTROL OF TONIC-CLONIC (GRAND MAL), PSYCHOMOTOR (TEMPORAL LOBE), MYOCLONIC, AND FOCAL SEIZURES	VERY NARROW TREATMENT MARGIN
	POSSIBLE BIRTH DEFECTS
	Overgrowth of gums
	Excessive hair growth
	Blood cell disorders: impaired production of all blood cells
	Drug-induced hepatitis or nephritis

▷ **Principal Uses**

As a Single Drug Product: Uses currently included in FDA-approved labeling: As an antiepileptic drug to control grand mal, psychomotor, myoclonic, and focal seizures. It can also be used to control seizures following brain surgery.

Other (unlabeled) generally accepted uses: (1) Used to initiate treatment of trigeminal neuralgia (it is sometimes effective in relieving the severe facial pain of this disorder); (2) used in chronic pain syndromes; (3) may have a role (as an applied powder) in helping heal wounds.

As a Combination Drug Product [CD]: This drug is available in combination with phenobarbital, another effective anticonvulsant. Some seizure disorders require the combined actions of these two drugs for effective control.

How This Drug Works: By promoting the loss of sodium from nerve fibers, this drug lowers and stabilizes their excitability and thereby inhibits the repetitious spread of electrical impulses along nerve pathways. This action may prevent seizures altogether, or it may reduce their frequency and severity.

Available Dose Forms and Strengths

Capsules, extended — 30 mg, 100 mg
Capsules, prompt — 30 mg, 100 mg
Injection — 50 mg/ml
Kapseals — 30 mg, 100 mg
Oral suspension — 30 mg/5 ml, 125 mg/5 ml
Tablets, chewable — 50 mg

▷ **Usual Adult Dose Range:** Seizures: Initially (prompt or extended form) 100 mg three times a day. Dose may be increased cautiously by 100 mg/week as needed and tolerated. Once the optimal maintenance dose has been identified, the total daily dose may be taken as a single dose every 24 hours if Dilantin capsules are used. No other formulation is approved for once-a-day use. The total daily dose should not exceed 600 mg. **Note: Actual dose and schedule must be determined for each patient individually.**

Conditions Requiring Dosing Adjustments

Liver Function: The ongoing dose should be decreased based on blood levels.

Kidney Function: The dose or dosing interval must be decreased in moderate kidney failure.

Obesity: The way this medicine is distributed (volume of distribution) changes with increasing body fat. Loading doses must be calculated based on ideal body weight. The product of 1.33 times actual weight divided by the ideal weight is then added to the original number to decide the final loading dose.

▷ **Dosing Instructions:** May be taken with or after food to reduce stomach irritation. The capsule may be opened and the tablet may be crushed.

Usual Duration of Use: Use on a regular schedule for 2 to 3 weeks usually determines benefit in reducing frequency and severity of seizures. Optimal control will require careful dose adjustments over a period of several months. Long-term use (months to years) requires ongoing physician supervision.

▷ **This Drug Should Not Be Taken If**
- you have had an allergic reaction to this drug or other hydantoin drugs previously.
- you have sinus bradycardia or serious heart block.

▷ **Inform Your Physician Before Taking This Drug If**
- you are taking any other drugs at this time.
- you have a history of liver disease or impaired liver function.
- you have low blood pressure, diabetes, or any type of heart disease.
- you are pregnant or planning a pregnancy.
- you plan to have surgery under general anesthesia in the near future.

Possible Side Effects (natural, expected, and unavoidable drug actions)
Mild fatigue, sluggishness, and drowsiness (in sensitive individuals).
Pink to red to brown coloration of urine (of no significance).

▷ **Possible Adverse Effects** (unusual, unexpected, and infrequent reactions)
If any of the following develop, consult your physician promptly for guidance.

Mild Adverse Effects
Allergic reactions: skin rashes, hives, drug fever (see Glossary).
Headache, dizziness, nervousness, insomnia, muscle twitching—infrequent.
Nausea, vomiting, constipation—infrequent.
Bed-wetting—case reports.
Abnormal eye movements—dose related.
Low blood calcium (and potential osteoporosis) and elevated blood sugar—possible.
Overgrowth of gum tissues—most common in children.
Excessive growth of body hair—most common in young girls.

Serious Adverse Effects
Allergic reactions: drug-induced hepatitis, with or without jaundice (see Glossary). Drug-induced nephritis, with acute kidney failure. Severe skin reactions (toxic epidermal necrolysis, Stevens-Johnson syndrome, or erythema

multiforme). Myocarditis, generalized enlargement of lymph glands (pseudolymphoma)—case reports.

Idiosyncratic reactions: hemolytic anemia (see Glossary).

Acute psychotic episodes—case reports.

Mental confusion, unsteadiness, double vision, jerky eye movements, slurred speech—possible.

Drug-induced seizures—possible.

Blood clotting disorders in infants of mothers maintained on phenytoin— rare.

Bone marrow depression (see Glossary): weakness, fever, sore throat, bleeding or bruising—case reports.

Drug-induced periarteritis nodosa, low thyroid function, or myasthenia gravis—case reports.

Tardive dyskinesia or porphyria—case reports.

Abnormal IgA (increased risk of respiratory infections)—possible.

Peripheral nerve damage (neuropathy) or muscle damage (myopathy)—case reports.

Serious heart rhythm problems—with rapid intravenous use.

Elevated blood sugar, due to inhibition of insulin release—possible.

▷ **Possible Effects on Sexual Function:**   Decreased libido and/or impotence— infrequent.

Swelling and tenderness of male breast tissue (gynecomastia) or Peyronie's disease (see Glossary)—rare.

Decreased effectiveness of oral contraceptives.

▷ **Adverse Effects That May Mimic Natural Diseases or Disorders**

Drug-induced hepatitis may suggest viral hepatitis. Skin reactions may resemble lupus erythematosus.

Natural Diseases or Disorders That May Be Activated by This Drug

Latent diabetes, porphyria, systemic lupus erythematosus, low bone mineral density predisposing to osteoporosis.

Possible Effects on Laboratory Tests

Complete blood cell counts: decreased red cells, hemoglobin, white cells, and platelets; increased eosinophils (allergic reaction).

Blood lupus erythematosus (LE) cells: positive.

Prothrombin time: increased (when phenytoin is taken concurrently with warfarin).

Blood calcium level: decreased.

Blood total cholesterol, LDL and VLDL cholesterol levels: no effects.

Blood HDL cholesterol level: increased.

Blood triglyceride levels: no effect.

Blood glucose level: increased.

Blood thyroid hormone levels: T_3, T_4, and free T_4 increased.

Liver function tests: increased liver enzymes (ALT/GPT, AST/GOT, alkaline phosphatase) and bilirubin.

CAUTION

1. Some brand-name capsules of this drug have a significantly longer duration of action than generic name capsules of the same strength. To assure a correct dosing schedule, it is necessary to distinguish between

"prompt"-action and "extended"-action capsules. Do not substitute one for the other without your physician's knowledge and guidance.

2. When used for the treatment of epilepsy, *this drug must not be stopped abruptly.*
3. Periodic measurements of blood levels of this drug are essential in determining appropriate dose (see "Therapeutic Drug Monitoring," chapter 2).
4. Regularity of drug use is essential. Take this drug at the same time each day.
5. Shake the suspension form of this drug thoroughly before measuring the dose. Use a standard measuring device to assure that the dose is accurate.
6. Side effects and mild adverse effects are usually most apparent during the first several days of treatment, and often subside with continued use.
7. It may be necessary to take folic acid to prevent anemia. Talk with your doctor about this.
8. This medicine has an unusual pathway for removal that can fill up (become saturated) and stop working. This means that a small change in dose may give a huge change in blood levels. Make certain you know exactly how much phenytoin your doctor wants you to take.
9. Carry a personal identification card with a notation that you are taking this drug.

Precautions for Use

By Infants and Children: Elimination of this drug varies widely with age. Periodic measurement of blood levels is essential for all ages. Some children will require more than one dose daily for good control. Observe for early indications of drug toxicity: jerky eye movements, unsteadiness in stance and gait, slurred speech, abnormal involuntary movements of the extremities, and odd behavior.

By Those Over 60 Years of Age: You may be more sensitive to all of the actions of this drug and require smaller doses. Watch closely for any indications of early toxicity: drowsiness, fatigue, confusion, unsteadiness, disturbances of vision, slurred speech, muscle twitching.

▷ ## Advisability of Use During Pregnancy

Pregnancy Category: D. See Pregnancy Risk Categories at the back of this book. Animal studies: Cleft lip and palate, skeletal and visceral defects in mice and rats.

Human studies: Available information is conflicting. Some studies suggest a small but significant increase in birth defects. The incidence of birth defects in children of epileptics not taking anticonvulsant drugs is 3.2%; incidence increases to 6.4% with anticonvulsant use in pregnancy. The "fetal hydantoin syndrome" in infants exposed to phenytoin during pregnancy shows birth defects of skull, face, and limbs; deficient growth and development; and subnormal intelligence. Other effects on the infant include reduction in blood clotting factors that predispose it to severe bruising and hemorrhage.

Discuss the benefits and risks of using this drug during pregnancy with your doctor. It is advisable to use the smallest maintenance dose that will control seizures. In addition, you should take vitamin K during the final month of pregnancy to prevent a deficiency of fetal blood clotting factors.

Advisability of Use If Breast-Feeding

Presence of this drug in breast milk: Yes, in trace amounts.

Monitor nursing infant closely and discontinue drug or nursing if adverse effects develop.

Habit-Forming Potential: None.

Effects of Overdose: Drowsiness, jerky eye movements, hand tremor, unsteadiness, slurred speech, hallucinations, delusions, nausea, vomiting, stupor progressing to coma.

Possible Effects of Long-Term Use: Low blood calcium resulting in rickets or osteomalacia; megaloblastic anemia; peripheral neuritis (see Glossary); schizophrenic-like psychosis. Lymphosarcoma, malignant lymphoma, and leukemia have been associated with long-term use; a cause-and-effect relationship (see Glossary) has not been established.

Suggested Periodic Examinations While Taking This Drug (at physician's discretion)

Monitoring of blood phenytoin levels to guide dose.

Time to sample blood for phenytoin level: just before next dose.

Recommended therapeutic range: 10 to 20 ng/ml.

Complete blood cell counts, liver function tests.

Measurements of the following blood levels: glucose, calcium, phosphorus, folic acid, vitamin B$_{12}$.

Bone mineral density testing (DEXA) to check risk for osteoporosis and fracture.

▷ **While Taking This Drug, Observe the Following**

Foods: No restrictions.

Nutritional Support: Supplements of folic acid, calcium, vitamin D, and vitamin K may be necessary.

Beverages: No restrictions. May be taken with milk.

▷   *Alcohol:* Use extreme caution. Alcohol (in large quantities or with continual use) may reduce this drug's effectiveness in preventing seizures.

Tobacco Smoking: No interactions expected. I advise everyone to quit smoking.

▷   *Other Drugs:*

Phenytoin may *decrease* the effects of

- acetaminophen (Tylenol, others).
- bupropion (Wellbutrin).
- clofibrate (Atromid-S).
- conjugated estrogens (Premarin).
- cortisonelike drugs (see *adrenocortical steroids* in Drug Classes).
- cyclosporine (Sandimmune).
- disopyramide (Norpace).
- doxycycline (Vibramycin, etc.).
- itraconazole (Sporanox).
- levodopa (Larodopa, Sinemet).
- levothyroxine (Synthroid, others).
- meperidine (Demerol).
- methadone (Dolophine).
- mexiletine (Mexitil).
- miconazole (Monistat, Micatin, others).
- oral antidiabetic drugs (see Drug Classes).
- oral contraceptives (birth control pills).
- paroxetine (Paxil).

- quinidine (Quinaglute, etc.).
- ritonavir (Norvir), and perhaps other protease inhibitors (see Drug Classes).

Phenytoin *taken concurrently* with

- carbamazepine (Tegretol) may result in increased or decreased levels of phenytoin.
- chlordiazepoxide (Librium—and perhaps other benzodiazepines) may increase or decrease phenytoin levels. Levels should be obtained more frequently if these drugs are combined.
- ciprofloxacin (Cipro) may increase or decrease phenytoin levels.
- dopamine will result in very low blood pressure.
- flu shots (influenza vaccine) may change phenytoin levels.
- ketorolac (Toradol) may result in seizures. DO NOT combine these medicines.
- oral anticoagulants (Coumadin, etc.) can either increase or decrease the anticoagulant effect; monitor this combination very closely with INR (serial prothrombin) testing.
- primidone (Mysoline) may alter primidone actions and enhance its toxicity.
- theophyllines (Aminophyllin, Theo-Dur, etc.) may cause a decrease in the effectiveness of both drugs.
- valproic acid (Depakene) may result in altered phenytoin or valproic acid levels. Increased blood level testing of both medicines is needed if these medicines are to be combined.
- warfarin (Coumadin) may lead to initial increased bleeding risk and subsequent decrease in anticoagulation. More frequent INR (prothrombin time or protime) testing is needed. Warfarin doses should be adjusted to results.

The following drugs may *increase* the effects of phenytoin:

- amiodarone (Codarone).
- chloramphenicol (Chloromycetin).
- chlorpheniramine.
- cimetidine (Tagamet).
- cotrimoxazole (Bactrim).
- diltiazem (Cardizem).
- disulfiram (Antabuse).
- felbamate (Felbatol).
- fluconazole (Diflucan).
- fluoxetine (Prozac).
- fluvoxamine (Luvox).
- gabapentin (Neurontin).
- ibuprofen, and perhaps other NSAIDs.
- isoniazid (INH, Niconyl, etc.).
- nifedipine (Adalat).
- omeprazole (Prilosec).
- phenacemide (Phenurone).
- sulfonamides (see Drug Classes).
- tricyclic antidepressants (see Drug Classes).
- trimethoprim (Proloprim, Trimpex).
- valproic acid (Depakene).
- venlafaxine (Effexor).

The following drugs may *decrease* the effects of phenytoin:

- bleomycin (Blenoxane).

- carmustine (BiCNU).
- cisplatin (Platinol).
- diazoxide (Proglycem, Hyperstat).
- folic acid (various).
- methotrexate (Mexate).
- rifampin (Rifadin).
- vinblastine (Velban).

▷ *Driving, Hazardous Activities:* This drug may impair mental alertness, vision, and coordination. Restrict activities as necessary.

Aviation Note: The use of this drug *is a disqualification* for piloting. Consult a designated aviation medical examiner.

Exposure to Sun: Use caution—this drug may cause photosensitivity (see Glossary).

Occurrence of Unrelated Illness: Intercurrent infections may slow the elimination of this drug and increase the risk of toxicity, due to higher blood levels.

*Discontinuation: **This drug must not be discontinued abruptly.*** Sudden withdrawal can precipitate severe and repeated seizures. If this drug is to be discontinued, gradual reduction in dose should be made over a period of 3 months. Total drug withdrawal may be attempted after a period of 3 to 4 years without a seizure. However, seizures are likely to recur in 40% of adults and in 20–30% of children.

PILOCARPINE (pi loh KAR peen)

Introduced: 1875   **Class:** Anti-glaucoma   **Prescription:** USA: Yes
Controlled Drug: USA: No; Canada: No   **Available as Generic:** Yes
Brand Names: Adsorbocarpine, Akarpine, Almocarpine, E-Pilo Preparations [CD], I-Pilopine, Isopto Carpine, ✦Minims, ✦Miocarpine, Ocusert Pilo-20, -40, PE Preparations [CD], Pilagan, Pilocar, Pilopine HS, Piloptic-1, -2, Pilosyst 20/40, Salagen, ✦Spersacarpine

BENEFITS versus RISKS	
Possible Benefits	*Possible Risks*
EFFECTIVE REDUCTION OF INTERNAL EYE PRESSURE FOR CONTROL OF ACUTE AND CHRONIC GLAUCOMA	Mild side effects with systemic absorption
	Minor eye discomfort
	Altered vision

▷ **Principal Uses**

As a Single Drug Product: Uses currently included in FDA-approved labeling: (1) Used exclusively for the management of all types of glaucoma (selection of the appropriate dose form and strength must be carefully individualized); (2) can help in dry mouth (xerostomia).

Other (unlabeled) generally accepted uses: (1) Treatment of Adie syndrome; (2) can help before laser surgery in order to prevent excessive increases in eye (intraocular) pressure after surgery.

As a Combination Drug Product [CD]: This drug is combined with epinephrine (in eyedrop solutions) to utilize the actions of both drugs in lowering internal eye pressure. The opposite effects of these two drugs on the size of the pupil (pilocarpine constricts, epinephrine dilates) provides a balance that prevents excessive constriction or dilation.

How This Drug Works: By directly stimulating constriction of the pupil, this drug enlarges the outflow canal in the anterior chamber of the eye and promotes the drainage of excess fluid (aqueous humor), thus lowering the internal eye pressure.

Available Dose Forms and Strengths

> Eyedrop solutions — 0.25%, 0.5%, 1%, 2%, 3%, 4%, 5%, 6%
>
> Gel — 4%
>
> Ocuserts — 20 mcg, 40 mcg
>
> Tablets — 5 mg

▷ **Usual Adult Dose Range:**   For open-angle glaucoma: Eyedrop solutions—one drop of a 1 to 2% solution three to four times daily. Eye gel—apply 0.5-inch strip of gel into the eye once daily at bedtime. Ocusert—insert one into affected eye and replace every 7 days with a new one.

Note: Actual dose and dosing schedule must be determined for each patient individually.

Conditions Requiring Dosing Adjustments

Liver Function: The specific elimination of this drug is unclear.

Kidney Function: The elimination of this drug has yet to be defined.

▷ **Dosing Instructions:**   To avoid excessive absorption into the body, press finger against inner corner of the eye (to close off the tear duct) during and for 2 minutes following instillation of the eyedrop. Place the gel and the Ocusert in the eye at bedtime.

Usual Duration of Use: Use on a regular schedule for 1 to 2 weeks usually determines this drug's effectiveness in controlling internal eye pressure. Long-term use (months to years) requires physician supervision.

▷ **This Drug Should Not Be Taken If**

- you have had an allergic reaction to it previously.
- you have acute iritis.
- you have active bronchial asthma and are using the tablet form.

▷ **Inform Your Physician Before Taking This Drug If**

- you have a history of bronchial asthma.
- you have a history of acute iritis.
- you have significant heart disease.
- you have chronic obstructive pulmonary disease.
- you have gallstones.

Possible Side Effects (natural, expected, and unavoidable drug actions)

Temporary impairment of vision, usually lasting 2 to 3 hours following instillation of drops. Burning of the eyes and trouble seeing at night—frequent.

▷ **Possible Adverse Effects** (unusual, unexpected, and infrequent reactions)

If any of the following develop, consult your physician promptly for guidance.

Mild Adverse Effects

Allergic reactions: itching of the eyes, eyelid itching and/or swelling.

Headache, heart palpitation, tremors—infrequent.

Sweating—frequent.

Nausea—case reports.

Serious Adverse Effects
    Provocation of acute asthma in susceptible individuals.
    Mental status changes (memory loss, confusion)—case reports.
    Atrioventricular block (abnormal heart conduction)—case reports.
    Retinal detachment—possible.

▷ **Possible Effects on Sexual Function:** None reported.

Possible Effects on Laboratory Tests
    Red blood cell and white blood cell counts: increased.

Precautions for Use
    By Those Over 60 Years of Age: Maintain personal cleanliness to prevent eye infections. Report promptly any indication of eye infection.

▷ **Advisability of Use During Pregnancy**
    Pregnancy Category: C. See Pregnancy Risk Categories at the back of this book.
    Animal studies: Significant birth defects due to this drug reported in rats.
    Human studies: Adequate studies of pregnant women are not available.
    Limit use to the smallest effective dose. Minimize systemic absorption (see "Dosing Instructions" above).

Advisability of Use If Breast-Feeding
    Presence of this drug in breast milk: May be present in small amounts.
    Monitor nursing infant closely and discontinue drug or nursing if adverse effects develop.

Habit-Forming Potential: None.

Effects of Overdose: Flushing of face, increased flow of saliva, sweating. If solution is swallowed: nausea, vomiting, diarrhea, profuse sweating, rapid pulse, difficult breathing, loss of consciousness.

Possible Effects of Long-Term Use: Development of tolerance (see Glossary), temporary loss of effectiveness.

Suggested Periodic Examinations While Taking This Drug (at physician's discretion)
    Measurement of internal eye pressure on a regular basis.
    Examination of eyes for development of cataracts.

▷ **While Taking This Drug, Observe the Following**
    Foods: No restrictions.
    Beverages: No restrictions.
▷   *Alcohol:* Use caution. If this drug is absorbed, it may prolong the effect of alcohol on the brain.
    Tobacco Smoking: No interactions expected. I advise everyone to quit smoking.
    Marijuana Smoking: Sustained additional decrease in internal eye pressure.
▷   *Other Drugs:*
    The following drugs may *decrease* the effects of pilocarpine:
    • atropine and drugs with atropinelike actions (see *anticholinergic drugs* in Drug Classes).
    Pilocarpine *taken concurrently* with
    • epinephrine will result in increased myopia.
    • sulfacetamide (Sulamyd).
    • timolol can produce additive effects in treating glaucoma.
▷   *Driving, Hazardous Activities:* This drug may impair your ability to focus your vision properly. Restrict activities as necessary.

Aviation Note: The use of this drug **may be a disqualification** for piloting. Consult a designated aviation medical examiner.

Exposure to Sun: This medicine may make you very sensitive to the sun. Wear sunglasses.

Discontinuation: Do not stop regular use of this drug without consulting your physician. Periodic discontinuation and temporary substitution of another drug may be necessary to preserve its effectiveness in treating glaucoma.

PINDOLOL (PIN doh lohl)

Introduced: 1972   **Class:** Antihypertensive, beta-adrenergic blocker
Prescription: USA: Yes   **Controlled Drug:** USA: No; Canada: No   **Available as Generic:** Yes
Brand Names: ✦Apo-Pindol, ✦Novo-Pindol, ✦Nu-Pindol, ✦Syn-Pindolol, ✦Viskazide [CD], Visken

BENEFITS versus RISKS	
Possible Benefits	*Possible Risks*
EFFECTIVE, WELL-TOLERATED ANTIHYPERTENSIVE in mild to moderate high blood pressure	CONGESTIVE HEART FAILURE in advanced heart disease
	Worsening of angina in coronary heart disease (abrupt withdrawal)
	Masking of low blood sugar (hypoglycemia) in drug-treated diabetes
	Provocation of asthma (with high doses)

▷ **Principal Uses**

As a Single Drug Product: Uses currently included in FDA-approved labeling: Treats mild to moderate high blood pressure, alone or with other drugs.

Other (unlabeled) generally accepted uses: (1) May be of benefit in helping control aggressive behavior; (2) can help prevent migraine headaches; (3) combination therapy with digoxin may be effective in limiting some abnormal heart rhythms (atrial fibrillation); (4) can be of benefit in some kinds of anxiety; (5) decreases sympathetic output in hyperthyroidism.

As a Combination Drug Product [CD]: This drug is available in combination with hydrochlorothiazide (in Canada). The addition of a thiazide diuretic to this beta-blocker drug enhances its effectiveness as an antihypertensive.

How This Drug Works: Blocks certain actions of the sympathetic nervous system, reducing rate and contraction force of the heart, thus lowering ejection pressure of blood leaving the heart; reduces degree of contraction of blood vessel walls, lowering blood pressure.

Available Dose Forms and Strengths

Tablets — 5 mg, 10 mg, 15 mg (Canada)

▷ **Usual Adult Dose Range:**   Hypertension: Initially 5 mg twice daily (12 hours apart). The dose may be increased gradually by 10 mg/day at intervals of 3 to 4 weeks as needed and tolerated, up to 60 mg/day. For maintenance, 5 to

10 mg two or three times daily is often effective. The total daily dose should not exceed 60 mg. **Note: Actual dose and schedule must be determined for each patient individually.**

Conditions Requiring Dosing Adjustments
Liver Function: Dose should be decreased for patients with severe liver disease and for those with combined liver and kidney disease.
Kidney Function: Dose should be decreased if urine output is seriously lowered.

▷ **Dosing Instructions:** The tablet may be crushed and taken without regard to eating. Do not stop this drug abruptly.

Usual Duration of Use: Use on a regular schedule for 2 to 3 weeks usually determines effectiveness in lowering blood pressure. The long-term use of this drug (months to years) will be determined by the course of your blood pressure over time and your response to an overall treatment program (weight reduction, salt restriction, smoking cessation, etc.). See your doctor on a regular basis.

Possible Advantages of This Drug
Causes less slowing of the heart rate than most other beta-blocker drugs.

Currently a "Drug of Choice"
For initiating treatment of hypertension with a single drug.

▷ **This Drug Should Not Be Taken If**
• you have bronchial asthma.
• you have had an allergic reaction to it previously.
• you have congestive heart failure.
• you have an abnormally slow heart rate or a serious form of heart block.
• you are taking, or have taken within the past 14 days, any monoamine oxidase (MAO) type A inhibitor drug (see Drug Classes).

▷ **Inform Your Physician Before Taking This Drug If**
• you had an adverse reaction to any beta-blocker (see Drug Classes).
• you have a history of serious heart disease.
• you have a history of hay fever (allergic rhinitis), asthma, chronic bronchitis, or emphysema.
• you have a history of overactive thyroid function (hyperthyroidism).
• you have a history of low blood sugar (hypoglycemia) or diabetes.
• you have impaired liver or kidney function.
• you have diabetes or myasthenia gravis.
• you take digitalis, quinidine, or reserpine, or any calcium-channel-blocker drug (see Drug Classes).
• you have bad circulation to your legs or arms (peripheral vascular disease).
• you plan to have surgery under general anesthesia in the near future.

Possible Side Effects (natural, expected, and unavoidable drug actions)
Lethargy and fatigability, cold extremities, slow heart rate, light-headedness in upright position (see *orthostatic hypotension* in Glossary).

▷ **Possible Adverse Effects** (unusual, unexpected, and infrequent reactions)
If any of the following develop, consult your physician promptly for guidance.
Mild Adverse Effects
Allergic reactions: skin rash, itching.
Headache, dizziness, insomnia, abnormal dreams, fainting—infrequent.

Indigestion, nausea, vomiting, constipation, diarrhea—infrequent.

Joint and muscle discomfort, tremor, fluid retention (edema)—infrequent.

Serious Adverse Effects

Mental depression, anxiety—infrequent.

Chest pain, shortness of breath—possible.

Induction of bronchial asthma—in asthmatic individuals.

Abnormally slow heartbeat or congestive heart failure—possible to infrequent.

Drug-induced systemic lupus erythematosus or myasthenia gravis—case reports.

Worsening of poor circulation to the arms or legs (intermittent claudication)—possible.

Carpal tunnel syndrome—reported with other beta-blockers.

▷ **Possible Effects on Sexual Function:**   Decreased libido or impaired erection—infrequent.

Possible Effects on Laboratory Tests

Blood lupus erythematosus (LE) cells: positive (one case of drug-induced LE).

Blood total cholesterol level: decreased (with long-term use).

Blood HDL cholesterol level: increased.

Blood LDL and VLDL cholesterol levels: no effects.

Blood triglyceride levels: no effects.

Glucose tolerance test (GTT): decreased or increased.

Liver function tests: slightly increased liver enzymes (ALT/GPT and AST/GOT) possible.

CAUTION

1. ***Do not stop this drug suddenly*** without the knowledge and help of your doctor. Carry a card that says you are taking this drug.
2. Ask your doctor or pharmacist before using nasal decongestants, which are usually present in over-the-counter cold preparations and nose drops. These can cause sudden increases in blood pressure when taken concurrently with beta-blocker drugs.
3. Report the development of any tendency to emotional depression.

Precautions for Use

By Infants and Children: Safety and effectiveness for those under 12 years of age are not established. However, if this drug is used, watch for the development of low blood sugar (hypoglycemia) during periods of reduced food intake.

By Those Over 60 Years of Age: Unacceptably high blood pressure should be reduced without creating the risks associated with excessively low blood pressure. Small starting doses and frequent blood pressure checks are indicated. Sudden, rapid, and excessive reduction of blood pressure can predispose to stroke or heart attack. Watch for dizziness, unsteadiness, tendency to fall, confusion, hallucinations, depression, or urinary frequency.

▷ **Advisability of Use During Pregnancy**

Pregnancy Category: C. See Pregnancy Risk Categories at the back of this book.

Animal studies: No significant increase in birth defects due to this drug.

Human studies: Adequate studies of pregnant women not available, but reports of lower growth and fetal problems reported.

Ask your physician for guidance.

Advisability of Use If Breast-Feeding
 Presence of this drug in breast milk: Yes.
 Avoid drug or refrain from nursing.

Habit-Forming Potential: None.

Effects of Overdose: Weakness, slow pulse, low blood pressure, fainting, cold and sweaty skin, congestive heart failure, possible coma, and convulsions.

Possible Effects of Long-Term Use: Reduced heart reserve and eventual heart failure in susceptible individuals with advanced heart disease.

Suggested Periodic Examinations While Taking This Drug (at physician's discretion)
 Measurements of blood pressure, evaluation of heart function.

▷ **While Taking This Drug, Observe the Following**
 Foods: No restrictions. Avoid excessive salt intake.
 Beverages: No restrictions. May be taken with milk.
▷ *Alcohol:* Use with caution. Alcohol may exaggerate lowering of blood pressure or increase mild sedative effect.
 Tobacco Smoking: Nicotine may reduce this drug's effectiveness. I advise everyone to quit smoking.
▷ *Other Drugs:*
 Pindolol may *increase* the effects of
 • digoxin (Lanoxin) on the heart conduction system, leading to AV block and possible digoxin toxicity as well.
 • other antihypertensive drugs, and cause excessive lowering of blood pressure. Dose adjustments may be necessary.
 • reserpine (Ser-Ap-Es, etc.), and cause sedation, depression, slowing of the heart rate, and lowering of blood pressure.
 • verapamil (Calan, Isoptin), and cause excessive depression of heart function; monitor this combination closely.
 Pindolol *taken concurrently* with
 • amiodarone (Codarone) may cause extremely slow heartbeats and risk of sinus arrest.
 • clonidine (Catapres) requires close monitoring for rebound high blood pressure if clonidine is withdrawn while pindolol is still being taken.
 • epinephrine (various) will result in a large increase in blood pressure and reflex increase in heart rate (tachycardia).
 • fluoxetine (Prozac) may result in increased risk of pindolol toxicity.
 • fluvoxamine (Luvox) may result in increased risk of pindolol toxicity.
 • insulin requires close monitoring to avoid undetected hypoglycemia (see Glossary).
 • oral antidiabetic drugs (see Drug Classes) can result in slowed recovery from low blood sugar.
 • phenylpropanolamine (various) may result in severe increases in blood pressure. Avoid this combination.
 • venlafaxine (Effexor) may result in beta-blocker or venlafaxine toxicity. Avoid this combination if possible, or use decreased doses of both medicines.
 The following drugs may *increase* the effects of pindolol:
 • cimetidine (Tagamet).
 • methimazole (Tapazole).

- oral contraceptives.
- propylthiouracil (Propacil).
- ritonavir (Norvir), and perhaps other protease inhibitors (see Drug Classes).
- Zileuton (Zyflo).

The following drugs may **decrease** the effects of pindolol:

- barbiturates (phenobarbital, etc.).
- indomethacin (Indocin), and possibly other NSAIDs—may impair pindolol's antihypertensive effect.
- rifampin (Rifadin, Rimactane).
- theophylline (Theo-Dur, others).

▷ *Driving, Hazardous Activities:* Use caution until the full extent of fatigue, dizziness, and blood pressure change have been determined.

Aviation Note: The use of this drug *is a disqualification* for piloting. Consult a designated aviation medical examiner.

Exposure to Sun: No restrictions.

Exposure to Heat: Caution is advised. Hot environments can lower blood pressure and exaggerate the effects of this drug.

Exposure to Cold: Caution is advised. Cold environments can enhance the circulatory deficiency in the extremities that may occur with this drug. The elderly should take precautions to prevent hypothermia (see Glossary).

Heavy Exercise or Exertion: It is advisable to avoid exertion that produces lightheadedness, excessive fatigue, or muscle cramping. The use of this drug may intensify the hypertensive response to isometric exercise.

Occurrence of Unrelated Illness: Fever can lower blood pressure and require adjustment of dose. Nausea or vomiting may interrupt regular doses. Ask your doctor for help.

Discontinuation: It is advisable to avoid sudden discontinuation of this drug in all situations. If possible, gradual reduction of dose over a period of 2 to 3 weeks is recommended. Ask your physician for specific guidance.

PIRBUTEROL (peer BYU ter ohl)

Introduced: 1983 **Class:** Antiasthmatic, bronchodilator **Prescription:** USA: Yes **Controlled Drug:** USA: No; Canada: No **Available as Generic:** No

Brand Name: Maxair

BENEFITS versus RISKS	
Possible Benefits	*Possible Risks*
VERY EFFECTIVE RELIEF OF BRONCHOSPASM	Increased blood pressure Nervousness Fine hand tremor Irregular heart rhythm (with excessive use)

▷ **Principal Uses**

As a Single Drug Product: Uses currently included in FDA-approved labeling: (1) Relieves acute attacks of bronchial asthma; (2) reduces the frequency and severity of chronic, recurrent asthmatic attacks (prevention); (3) relieves reversible bronchospasm seen in chronic bronchitis, bronchiectasis, and emphysema.

Other (unlabeled) generally accepted uses: May help congestive heart failure.

How This Drug Works: By increasing the production of cyclic AMP, this drug relaxes constricted bronchial muscles to relieve asthmatic wheezing.

Available Dose Forms and Strengths

Aerosol — 200 mcg per actuation (in canisters of 300 inhalations)

▷ **Usual Adult Dose Range:**   Inhaler: Two inhalations (400 mcg) every 4 to 6 hours. **Do not exceed** 12 inhalations (2400 mcg) every 24 hours. Oral dosing: 10 to 15 mg three to four times a day. Maximum dose is 60 mg daily. **Note: Actual dose and schedule must be determined for each patient individually.**

Conditions Requiring Dosing Adjustments

Liver Function: Used with caution by patients with liver disease who use it often.
Kidney Function: No dose adjustments thought to be needed.

▷ **Dosing Instructions:**   Carefully follow the "Patient's Instructions for Use" provided with the inhaler. Do not overuse.

Usual Duration of Use: According to individual requirements. Do not use beyond the time necessary to terminate episodes of asthma.

Possible Advantages of This Drug

Has a more rapid onset of action and a longer duration of effect than most other drugs of this class.

▷ **This Drug Should Not Be Taken If**

- you have had an allergic reaction to it previously.
- you currently have an irregular heart rhythm.
- you are taking, or have taken within the past 2 weeks, any monoamine oxidase (MAO) type A inhibitor drug (see Drug Classes).

▷ **Inform Your Physician Before Taking This Drug If**

- you have any type of heart or circulatory disorder, especially high blood pressure, coronary heart disease, or heart rhythm abnormality.
- you have diabetes or an excessively active thyroid gland (hyperthyroidism).
- you have any type of seizure disorder.
- you are taking any form of digitalis or any stimulant drug.

Possible Side Effects (natural, expected, and unavoidable drug actions)

Aerosol—dryness or irritation of mouth or throat, altered taste.

▷ **Possible Adverse Effects** (unusual, unexpected, and infrequent reactions)

If any of the following develop, consult your physician promptly for guidance.

Mild Adverse Effects

Allergic reactions: skin rash, itching—rare.

Headache, dizziness, nervousness, fine tremor of hands—infrequent.

Palpitations, rapid heart rate, chest pain, cough—rare to infrequent.

Nausea, diarrhea, taste disorders—rare.

Serious Adverse Effects

Irregular heart rhythm, increased blood pressure-possible.

▷ **Possible Effects on Sexual Function:**   None reported.

Natural Diseases or Disorders That May Be Activated by This Drug

Latent coronary artery disease, diabetes, epilepsy, or high blood pressure.

Possible Effects on Laboratory Tests

None reported.

CAUTION

1. Combined use of this drug by inhalation with beclomethasone aerosol (Beclovent, Vanceril) may increase the risk of toxicity due to fluorocarbon propellants. It is advisable to use pirbuterol aerosol 20 to 30 minutes **before** beclomethasone aerosol. This will reduce the risk of toxicity and help beclomethasone reach the lung.

2. Excessive or prolonged use of this drug by inhalation can reduce its effectiveness and cause serious heart rhythm disturbances, including cardiac arrest.

Precautions for Use

By Infants and Children: Safety and effectiveness of use in children under 12 years of age have not been established.

By Those Over 60 Years of Age: Avoid excessive and continual use. If acute asthma is not relieved promptly, other drugs may be needed. Watch for nervousness, palpitations, irregular heart rhythm, and muscle tremors.

▷ **Advisability of Use During Pregnancy**

Pregnancy Category: C. See Pregnancy Risk Categories at the back of this book.
Animal studies: High-dose studies in rabbits revealed abortion and increased fetal deaths. Studies in rats and rabbits found no drug-associated birth defects.
Human studies: Adequate studies of pregnant women are not available.
Avoid use during first 3 months if possible.

Advisability of Use If Breast-Feeding

Presence of this drug in breast milk: Unknown.
Avoid drug or refrain from nursing.

Habit-Forming Potential: None. Tolerance to beneficial effects has been reported.

Effects of Overdose: Nervousness, palpitation, rapid heart rate, sweating, headache, tremor, vomiting, chest pain.

Possible Effects of Long-Term Use: Loss of effectiveness (tolerance).

Suggested Periodic Examinations While Taking This Drug (at physician's discretion)

Blood pressure measurements, evaluation of heart status.

▷ **While Taking This Drug, Observe the Following**

Foods: No restrictions.

Beverages: Avoid excessive use of caffeine-containing beverages—coffee, tea, cola, chocolate.

▷ *Alcohol:* No interactions expected.

Tobacco Smoking: No interactions expected. I advise everyone to quit smoking.

▷ *Other Drugs:*

Pirbuterol *taken concurrently* with

- albuterol (Proventil, Ventolin) may result in adverse effects on the heart.
- monoamine oxidase (MAO) type A inhibitors (see Glossary) may cause excessive increase in blood pressure and undesirable heart stimulation.
- phenothiazines (see Drug Classes) may result in blunting of the therapeutic effects of pirbuterol.

▷ *Driving, Hazardous Activities:* Use caution if excessive nervousness or dizziness occurs.

Aviation Note: The use of this drug *is a disqualification* for piloting. Consult a designated aviation medical examiner.

Exposure to Sun: No restrictions.

Heavy Exercise or Exertion: Use caution—excessive exercise can induce asthma in sensitive individuals.

PIROXICAM (peer OX i kam)

See the oxicams (nonsteroidal anti-inflammatory drugs) profile for further information.

PRAVASTATIN (pra vah STA tin)

Introduced: 1986 **Class:** Cholesterol reducing drug, HMG-CoA reductase inhibitor **Prescription:** USA: Yes **Controlled Drug:** USA: No; Canada: No **Available as Generic:** USA: No; Canada: No

Brand Name: Pravachol

BENEFITS versus RISKS	
Possible Benefits	*Possible Risks*
PREVENTS STROKES	Drug-induced hepatitis
EFFECTIVE REDUCTION OF TOTAL BLOOD CHOLESTEROL AND LDL CHOLESTEROL	Drug-induced myositis (muscle inflammation)
EFFECTIVE REDUCTION IN THE NUMBER OF FIRST-TIME HEART ATTACKS	
REDUCTION IN THE NUMBER OF PATIENT DEATHS	
SLOWS PROGRESSION OF ATHEROSCLEROSIS	
REDUCES RISK OF TRANSIENT ISCHEMIC ATTACKS (TIAs)	

▷ **Principal Uses**

As a Single Drug Product: Uses currently included in FDA-approved labeling: (1) Treats abnormally high total blood cholesterol levels (in people with types IIa and IIb hypercholesterolemia) due to increased low-density lipoprotein (LDL) cholesterol (used with a cholesterol-lowering diet after an adequate trial of nondrug methods have failed); (2) helps prevent a first heart attack and reduces death from cardiovascular disease in people with increased blood cholesterol levels at risk of a first heart attack; (3) slows progression and in some cases makes small reversals in coronary artery disease; (4) used to decrease triglycerides in mixed lipidemias; (5) reduces risk of strokes or transient ischemic attacks (TIAs).

Other (unlabeled) generally accepted uses: Reduces temporary blood flow (to the heart) problems (myocardial ischemia) when combined with other therapies.

How This Drug Works: This drug blocks the liver enzyme that starts production of cholesterol. Its principal action is the reduction of low-density lipoproteins (LDL), the fraction of total blood cholesterol that is thought to increase the risk of coronary heart disease. This drug may also increase the level of high-density lipoproteins (HDL), the cholesterol fraction that is thought to reduce the risk of heart disease.

Available Dose Forms and Strengths
Tablets — 10 mg, 20 mg, 40 mg

▷ **Recommended Dose Ranges** (Actual dose and schedule must be determined for each patient individually.)

Infants and Children: Under 2 years of age—do not use this drug.
2 to 18 years of age—dose not established.

18 to 60 Years of Age: Initially 10 to 20 mg daily, taken at bedtime. Maintenance dose is 10 to 20 mg daily, and is adjusted as needed and tolerated at intervals of 4 weeks.

Over 60 Years of Age: Starting dose for those with kidney or liver compromise is 10 mg daily.

Conditions Requiring Dosing Adjustments

Liver Function: Used with caution by patients with liver disease. Starting dose is decreased to 10 mg per day. Pravastatin should not be used in sudden (acute) liver disease.

Kidney Function: Those with significant kidney disease take a starting dose of 10 mg per day. Used with caution in kidney compromise.

▷ **Dosing Instructions:**   The tablet may be crushed and can be taken without regard to eating. It is preferably taken at bedtime. (Highest rates of cholesterol production occur between midnight and 5 A.M.)

Usual Duration of Use: Use on a regular schedule for 4 to 6 weeks usually determines effectiveness in reducing blood levels of total and LDL-C cholesterol. Long-term use (months to years) requires periodic physician evaluation.

Possible Advantages of This Drug
Recent studies indicate that drugs of this class (HMG-CoA reductase inhibitors) are more effective and better tolerated than other drugs currently available for reducing total and LDL-C cholesterol.

▷ **This Drug Should Not Be Taken If**
• you have had an allergic reaction to it previously.
• you have active liver disease.
• you are pregnant or breast-feeding your infant.

▷ **Inform Your Physician Before Taking This Drug If**
• you have previously taken any other drugs in this class: lovastatin (Mevacor), simvastatin (Zocor).
• you have a history of liver disease or impaired liver function.
• you are not using any method of birth control, or you are a planning pregnancy.
• you regularly consume substantial amounts of alcohol.
• you have kidney disease.

- you have cataracts or impaired vision.
- you get unexplained muscle weakness, pain, or tenderness.
- you have any type of chronic muscular disorder.
- you plan to have major surgery in the near future.

Possible Side Effects (natural, expected, and unavoidable drug actions)
Development of abnormal liver tests without symptoms.

▷ **Possible Adverse Effects** (unusual, unexpected, and infrequent reactions)
If any of the following develop, consult your physician promptly for guidance.

Mild Adverse Effects
Allergic reactions: skin rash, itching—rare.
Headache, dizziness, depression—case reports, rare.
Flu-like syndrome, cough—case reports.
Indigestion, stomach pain, nausea, excessive gas, constipation, diarrhea—rare to infrequent.
Muscle cramps and/or pain—rare.

Serious Adverse Effects
Marked and persistent abnormal liver function tests with focal hepatitis (without jaundice)—rare.
Acute myositis (muscle pain and tenderness) during long-term use—case reports.
Rhabdomyolysis—rare and more likely if combined with fibrates.
Low white blood cells (leukopenia)—rare.
Neuropathy—case report.

▷ **Possible Effects on Sexual Function:** Impotence—questionable causation.

Possible Delayed Adverse Effects: Increased liver enzymes.

Natural Diseases or Disorders That May Be Activated by This Drug
Latent liver disease.

Possible Effects on Laboratory Tests
Blood alanine aminotransferase (ALT) enzyme level: increased (with higher doses of drug).
Blood total cholesterol, LDL cholesterol, and triglyceride levels: decreased.
Blood HDL cholesterol level: increased.

CAUTION
1. If pregnancy occurs while taking pravastatin, discontinue the drug immediately and consult your physician.
2. Report promptly any development of muscle pain or tenderness, especially if accompanied by fever or malaise.
3. Report promptly the development of altered or impaired vision so that appropriate evaluation can be made.
4. If CPK levels become markedly elevated, this medicine should be stopped.

Precautions for Use
By Infants and Children: Safety and effectiveness for those under 18 years of age are not established.
By Those Over 60 Years of Age: Tell your doctor about any personal or family history of cataracts. Comply with all recommendations regarding periodic eye examinations. Report promptly any alterations in vision.

▷ **Advisability of Use During Pregnancy**
  Pregnancy Category: X. See Pregnancy Risk Categories at the back of this book.
    Animal studies: Mouse and rat studies reveal skeletal birth defects due to a closely related drug of this class.
    Human studies: Adequate studies of pregnant women are not available.
    This drug should be avoided during entire pregnancy.

Advisability of Use If Breast-Feeding
  Presence of this drug in breast milk: Yes, in small amounts.
  Avoid drug or refrain from nursing.

Habit-Forming Potential: None.

Effects of Overdose: Increased indigestion, stomach distress, nausea, diarrhea.

Possible Effects of Long-Term Use: Abnormal liver function with focal hepatitis.

Suggested Periodic Examinations While Taking This Drug (at physician's discretion)
  Blood cholesterol studies: total cholesterol, HDL and LDL fractions.
  Liver function tests before treatment, at 12 weeks of treatment, and every 6 months if the 12-week tests are normal. **This is new labeling, and pravastatin was the first HMG-CoA reductase inhibitor to receive labeling from the FDA for less-frequent liver testing.** Complete eye examination at beginning of treatment and at any time that significant change in vision occurs. Ask your doctor for guidance.

▷ **While Taking This Drug, Observe the Following**
  Foods: Follow a standard low-cholesterol diet.
  Beverages: No restrictions. May be taken with milk.
▷ *Alcohol:* No interactions expected. Use sparingly.
  Tobacco Smoking: No interactions expected. I advise everyone to quit smoking.
▷ *Other Drugs:*
  Pravastatin *taken concurrently* with
  • clofibrate (Atromid-S) has been associated with muscle damage (rhabdomyolysis).
  • cyclosporine (Sandimmune) increases the risk for myopathy.
  • erythromycin (various) increases muscle damage risk.
  • gemfibrozil (Lopid) may alter the absorption and excretion of pravastatin; these drugs should not be taken concurrently.
  • niacin (various) increases muscle damage risk.
  • ritonavir (Norvir), and perhaps other protease inhibitors (see Drug Classes), increases toxicity risk.
  • warfarin (Coumadin) can increase the risk of bleeding. More frequent INR (prothrombin time or protime) testing is indicated. Ongoing warfarin doses should be based on laboratory results.
  The following drug may *decrease* the effects of pravastatin:
  • cholestyramine (Questran)—may reduce absorption of pravastatin; take pravastatin 1 hour before or 4 hours after cholestyramine.
▷ *Driving, Hazardous Activities:* This drug may cause dizziness. Restrict activities as necessary.
  Aviation Note: The use of this drug *may be a disqualification* for piloting. Consult a designated aviation medical examiner.

Exposure to Sun: No restrictions.

Discontinuation: Do not stop this drug without your doctor's knowledge and help. There may be a significant increase in blood cholesterol levels following discontinuation of this drug.

PRAZOSIN (PRA zoh sin)

Introduced: 1970 **Class:** Antihypertensive **Prescription:** USA: Yes
Controlled Drug: USA: No; Canada: No **Available as Generic:** Yes
Brand Names: ✦Apo-Prazo, Minipres, Minizide [CD], ✦Novo-Prazin, ✦Nu-Prazo

BENEFITS versus RISKS	
Possible Benefits	*Possible Risks*
EFFECTIVE INITIAL THERAPY FOR MILD TO MODERATE HYPERTENSION	"First-dose" drop in blood pressure with fainting
EFFECTIVE ANTIHYPERTENSIVE IN MODERATE TO SEVERE HYPERTENSION	May cause increased heart rate (paroxysmal tachycardia)
EFFECTIVE CONTROL OF HYPERTENSION IN PHEOCHROMOCYTOMA	
May help urine flow in benign prostatic hyperplasia	
Effective in presence of impaired kidney function	

▷ **Principal Uses**

As a Single Drug Product: Uses currently included in FDA-approved labeling: (1) Used to start treatment in mild to moderate hypertension; (2) also used in conjunction with other drugs to treat moderate to severe hypertension.

Other (unlabeled) generally accepted uses: (1) Combination therapy of congestive heart failure; (2) helps control high blood pressure with a rare tumor (pheochromocytoma); (3) may have an adjunctive role in controlling urine outflow problems caused by prostatic obstruction; (4) may help relieve the symptoms of Raynaud's phenomenon; (5) can ease symptoms of angina; (6) has a role in reducing benign prostatic hyperplasia.

As a Combination Drug Product [CD]: This drug is available in combination with polythiazide, a diuretic of the thiazide class of drugs. By utilizing two different methods of drug action, this combination product is more effective and more convenient for long-term use.

How This Drug Works: By blocking certain actions of the sympathetic nervous system, this drug causes direct relaxation and expansion of blood vessel walls, thus lowering the pressure of the blood within the vessels.

Available Dose Forms and Strengths

Capsules — 1 mg, 2 mg, 5 mg

▷ **Usual Adult Dose Range:** Hypertension: A "test dose" of 1 mg is given to determine the patient's response within the first 2 hours. Patients at risk for first-dose excessive lowering in blood pressure include those with pheochromocytoma and those who have recently suffered a stroke (cerebral vascular accident). If tolerated satisfactorily, dose is increased cautiously up to 15 mg every 24 hours in two or three divided doses. The total daily dose should not exceed 20 mg.

Benign prostatic hyperplasia (BPH): Starting dose is 0.5 mg to 1 mg twice a day. This dose is increased (titrated) as needed and tolerated to 2 mg twice daily.

Note: Actual dose and dosing schedule must be determined for each patient individually.

Conditions Requiring Dosing Adjustments

Liver Function: This drug should be used with caution and in lower doses by patients with liver compromise. The drug is 97% protein bound. Dose adjustments and more frequent blood pressure checks are needed.

Kidney Function: Patients with kidney failure may have adequate response to smaller doses.

The information in this profile has been shortened to make room for more widely used medicines.

PREDNISOLONE (pred NIS oh lohn)

Introduced: 1955   **Class:** Adrenocortical steroid (cortisonelike drug)
Prescription: USA: Yes   **Controlled Drug:** USA: No; Canada: No   **Available as Generic:** USA: Yes; Canada: Yes

Brand Names: ✦Ak-Cide [CD], A & D with Prednisolone [CD], ✦Ak-Pred, ✦Ak-Tate, Blephamide, Cortalone, Delta-Cortef, Duapred, Econopred Ophthalmic, Fernisolone-P, Hydelta-TBA, Hydeltrasol, ✦Inflamase, ✦Inflamase Forte, Isopto Cetapred [CD], Key-Pred, Meticortelone, Menti-Derm, Metimyd [CD], Metreton, ✦Minims Prednisolone, Mydrapred, Niscort, Nor-Pred, ✦Nova-Pred, ✦Novoprednisolone, Ophtho-Tate, Optimyd [CD], Otobione [CD], Pediapred, Pediaject, Polypred, Predcor, ✦Pred Forte, Pred-G [CD], ✦Pred Mild, Prelone, PSP-IV, Savacort, Sterane, TBA Pred, ✦Vasocidin [CD]

BENEFITS versus RISKS	
Possible Benefits	*Possible Risks*
EFFECTIVE RELIEF OF SYMPTOMS IN A WIDE VARIETY OF INFLAMMATORY AND ALLERGIC DISORDERS	Use exceeding 2 weeks is associated with many possible adverse effects:
EFFECTIVE IMMUNOSUPPRESSION in selected benign and malignant disorders	ALTERED MOOD AND PERSONALITY
	CATARACTS, GLAUCOMA
	HYPERTENSION
	OSTEOPOROSIS
Prevention of rejection in organ transplantation	ASEPTIC BONE NECROSIS
	INCREASED SUSCEPTIBILITY TO INFECTIONS

Author's Note: Adverse effects from ophthalmic use are much more limited and more rare than those from systemic use.

▷ **Principal Uses**

    As a Single Drug Product: Uses currently included in FDA-approved labeling: (1) Used in the treatment of a wide variety of allergic and inflammatory conditions; most commonly in the management of serious skin disorders, asthma, regional enteritis, ulcerative colitis, and all types of major rheumatic disorders including bursitis, tendonitis, most forms of arthritis, and inflammatory eye conditions; (2) used as part of combination therapy in lymphoma; (3) used in some kinds of adrenal insufficiencies; (4) used to help tuberculosis patients who also have inflammation around the heart without fluid buildup; (5) eases symptoms in ulcerative colitis.

    Other (unlabeled) generally accepted uses: (1) Used as part of combination therapy in acute leukemias (lymphoblastic, lymphocytic, and myelogenous); (2) may have a role in combination therapy of breast cancer; (3) can help relieve the muscle pain of familial Mediterranean fever; (4) part of a combination therapy in treating abnormal liver tumors (hemangiomas); (5) can help subfertile men decrease seminal antibodies and become fertile; (6) helps people who have drug-induced lowering of white blood cells to recover; (7) treats anaphylactic reactions of unknown cause; (8) treats thrombocytopenic purpura of unknown cause; (9) eases symptoms in myasthenia gravis; (10) can help reflex sympathetic dystrophy.

How This Drug Works: Not fully established. It is thought that this drug's anti-inflammatory effect is due to its ability to inhibit the normal defensive functions of certain white blood cells. Its immunosuppressant effect is attributed to a reduced production of lymphocytes and antibodies.

Available Dose Forms and Strengths

    Eye ointment — 0.6%

    Eye suspension — 0.5%, 1%

        Oral liquid — 6.7 mg/5 ml

           Syrup — 15 mg/5 ml

        Tablets — 5 mg

▷ **Usual Adult Dose Range:** 5 to 60 mg daily as a single dose or in divided doses (some patients are put on alternate-day schedules). Once an adequate response is achieved, the dose should be decreased to the lowest effective dose. Ophthalmic drops: One to two drops is instilled into the eye sac (conjunctival sac) every 3 to 12 hours. Dosing may be increased to every hour in severe cases. **Note: Actual dose and schedule must be determined for each patient individually.**

Conditions Requiring Dosing Adjustments

    Liver Function: Dosing adjustments do not appear to be needed in liver compromise.

    Kidney Function: Dosing adjustments in renal compromise do not appear to be needed. This drug can cause proteinuria. It is a benefit-to-risk decision for kidney compromise (nephropathy) patients who tend to lose protein.

▷ **Dosing Instructions:** The tablet may be crushed and taken with or following food to prevent stomach irritation, preferably in the morning. Suspensions should be gently mixed before using.

Usual Duration of Use: For acute disorders: 4 to 10 days. For chronic disorders: according to individual requirements. Use only for time needed to relieve symptoms in acute self-limiting conditions, or the time required to stabilize

a chronic condition and permit gradual withdrawal. Because of its intermediate duration of action, this drug is appropriate for alternate-day dosing for many forms. See your doctor regularly.

**Author's Note: The information categories provided in this profile are
appropriate for prednisolone. For specific information that is normally found in those categories that have been omitted from this profile, the reader is referred to the profile of prednisone, which follows.
Prednisolone is a derivative of prednisone; all significant actions and
effects are shared by both drugs.**

PREDNISONE (PRED ni sohn)

Introduced: 1955   **Class:** Adrenocortical steroid (cortisonelike) drug
Prescription: USA: Yes   **Controlled Drug:** USA: No; Canada: No   **Available as Generic:** USA: Yes; Canada: Yes

Brand Names: ✦Apo-Prednisone, Aspred-C [CD], Deltasone, Liquid Pred, Meti-
corten, ✦Metreton [CD], ✦Novoprednisone, Orasone, Panasol-S, Paracort,
Prednicen-M, Prednisone Intensol, SK-Prednisone, Sterapred, Sterapred-
DS, ✦Winpred

BENEFITS versus RISKS	
Possible Benefits	*Possible Risks*
EFFECTIVE RELIEF OF SYMPTOMS IN A WIDE VARIETY OF INFLAMMATORY AND ALLERGIC DISORDERS	Use exceeding 2 weeks is associated with many possible adverse effects: ALTERED MOOD AND PERSONALITY
EFFECTIVE IMMUNOSUPPRESSION in selected benign and malignant disorders	CATARACTS, GLAUCOMA HYPERTENSION OSTEOPOROSIS ASEPTIC BONE NECROSIS
Prevention of rejection in organ transplantation	INCREASED SUSCEPTIBILITY TO INFECTIONS

▷ **Principal Uses**

As a Single Drug Product: Uses currently included in FDA-approved labeling: (1)
Treats a wide variety of allergic and inflammatory conditions (it is used
most commonly in the management of serious skin disorders, asthma,
gout, lupus erythematosus, regional enteritis, ulcerative colitis, nephrotic
syndrome, and all types of major rheumatic disorders including bursitis,
tendonitis, and most forms of arthritis); (2) used as part of combination
therapy of lymphoma; (3) helps address adrenal insufficiency; (4) used as
part of combination therapy of several kinds of leukemia; (5) used in kidney transplant patients; (6) helps patients recover from symptoms of multiple sclerosis.

Other (unlabeled) generally accepted uses: (1) Used in combination therapy
of acute (lymphoblastic, lymphocytic, and myelogenous) leukemias; (2)
combination therapy of breast cancer; (3) may be helpful in therapy of
familial Mediterranean fever; (4) used with other medications to treat liver
tumors (hemangiomas); (5) may help subfertile men decrease seminal anti-

bodies and become fertile; (6) helps prevent early lung deterioration in children with AIDS; (7) eases symptoms in alcoholics who have hepatitis and encephalopathy; (8) used in some chronic pain syndromes.

How This Drug Works: Anti-inflammatory effect is due to its ability to inhibit normal defensive functions of certain white blood cells. Its immunosuppressant effect is from a reduced production of lymphocytes and antibodies.

Available Dose Forms and Strengths
Oral solution — 5 mg/5 ml
  Syrup — 5 mg/5 ml (5% alcohol)
  Tablets — 1 mg, 2.5 mg, 5 mg, 10 mg, 20 mg, 25 mg, 50 mg

▷ **Usual Adult Dose Range:**   Five to 60 mg daily as a single dose or in divided doses. With myasthenia gravis, patients not responding to 100 mg will not respond to higher doses. Once initial inflammation has eased, the dose should be gradually lowered to the lowest effective dose for the condition being treated.
  Note: Actual dose and schedule must be determined for each patient individually.

Conditions Requiring Dosing Adjustments
Liver Function: No dosing changes needed.
Kidney Function: Dosing adjustments in kidney disease do not appear to be needed. May cause proteinuria. Use is a benefit-to-risk decision for patients with protein-losing kidney disease (nephropathy).

▷ **Dosing Instructions:**   The tablet may be crushed and taken with or following food to prevent stomach irritation, preferably in the morning.

Usual Duration of Use: For acute disorders: 4 to 10 days. For chronic disorders: according to individual requirements. Use should not exceed time needed for symptomatic relief in acute self-limiting conditions, or time required to stabilize a chronic condition and permit gradual withdrawal. Intermediate duration of action allows alternate-day dosing. See your doctor regularly.

▷ **This Drug Should Not Be Taken If**
  • you had an allergic reaction to it previously.
  • you have active peptic ulcer disease.
  • you have an active herpes simplex virus eye infection.
  • you have active tuberculosis.
  • you have a fungal infection in a large area inside your body (systemic fungal infection).

▷ **Inform Your Physician Before Taking This Drug If**
  • you have had an adverse reaction to any cortisonelike drug.
  • you have a history of peptic ulcer disease, thrombophlebitis, or tuberculosis.
  • you have diabetes, kidney failure, glaucoma, high blood pressure, deficient thyroid function, or myasthenia gravis.
  • you have osteoporosis.
  • you have been exposed to any viral illness such as measles or chicken pox. (Cases may be severe if you are taking this medicine.)
  • you are prone to depression.
  • you have diverticulitis.
  • you plan to have surgery of any kind in the near future.

Possible Side Effects (natural, expected, and unavoidable drug actions)
Increased appetite, weight gain, retention of salt and water leading to increased blood pressure, excretion of potassium, increased susceptibility to infection. Mild euphoria.

▷ **Possible Adverse Effects** (unusual, unexpected, and infrequent reactions)
If any of the following develop, consult your physician promptly for guidance.

Mild Adverse Effects
Allergic Reaction: Skin rash.
Headache, dizziness, insomnia—infrequent.
Acid indigestion, abdominal distention—infrequent.
Patchy blue areas on the great toe (blue toe syndrome)—case reports.
Muscle cramping and weakness—possible.
Elevated intracranial pressure (pseudotumor cerebri)—infrequent.
Acne, excessive growth of facial hair—frequent.

Serious Adverse Effects
Serious mental or emotional disturbances—case reports.
Reactivation of latent tuberculosis—possible in those with past tuberculosis.
Development of peptic ulcer—possible and more likely in those with previous ulcers.
Development of inflammation of the pancreas—rare.
Thrombophlebitis (inflammation of a vein with the formation of blood clot): pain or tenderness in thigh or leg, with or without swelling of the foot, ankle, or leg—rare.
Increased intraocular (inner eye) pressure, glaucoma, or cataracts—infrequent.
Kaposi's sarcoma—case reports.
Growth retardation—possible in children with long-term use.
Cushing's syndrome—possible with long-term use.
Necrosis of bone—case reports.
Osteoporosis—possible with long-term use.
Superinfections—possible.
Inflammation or wasting of muscle (myositis or myopathy)—infrequent.
Increased blood sugar—possible and may be dose related.
Drug-induced porphyria or seizures—case reports.
Pulmonary embolism (movement of a blood clot to the lung)—sudden shortness of breath, pain in the chest, coughing, bloody sputum—increased risk.

▷ **Possible Effects on Sexual Function:**   Altered timing and pattern of menstruation.
Correction of male infertility when due to autoantibodies that suppress sperm activity.

▷ **Adverse Effects That May Mimic Natural Diseases or Disorders**
Pattern of symptoms and signs resembling Cushing's syndrome.

Natural Diseases or Disorders That May Be Activated by This Drug
Latent diabetes, glaucoma, peptic ulcer disease, tuberculosis.

Possible Effects on Laboratory Tests
Complete blood cell counts: decreased eosinophils, lymphocytes, and platelets.
Blood amylase level: increased (possible pancreatitis).

Blood total cholesterol and HDL cholesterol levels: increased.

Blood LDL cholesterol level: no effect.

Blood triglyceride levels: no significant effect.

Blood glucose level: increased.

Glucose tolerance test (GTT): decreased.

Blood potassium or testosterone level: decreased.

Blood thyroid hormone (T_3): decreased.

Blood uric acid level: increased.

Urine sugar tests: no effect with Tes-Tape; false low result with Clinistix and Diastix.

Fecal occult blood test: positive (if gastrointestinal bleeding).

CAUTION

1. If therapy exceeds 1 week, carry an identification card noting that you are taking this drug.
2. Do not stop this drug abruptly after long-term use.
3. If vaccination against measles, rabies, smallpox, or yellow fever is required, discontinue this drug 72 hours before vaccination and do not resume it for at least 14 days after vaccination.

Precautions for Use

By Infants and Children: Avoid prolonged use if possible. During long-term use, observe for suppression of normal growth and the possibility of increased intracranial pressure. Following long-term use, the child may be at risk for adrenal gland deficiency during stress for as long as 18 months after cessation of this drug.

By Those Over 60 Years of Age: Cortisonelike drugs should only be used when the disorder under treatment is unresponsive to adequate trials of unrelated drugs. Avoid the prolonged use of this drug. Continual use (even in small doses) can increase severity of diabetes, enhance fluid retention, raise blood pressure, weaken resistance to infection, induce stomach ulcer, and accelerate development of cataract and osteoporosis.

▷ Advisability of Use During Pregnancy

Pregnancy Category: B or C. See Pregnancy Risk Categories at the back of this book.

Animal studies: Birth defects reported in mice, rats, and rabbits.

Human studies: Adequate studies of pregnant women are not available.

Avoid completely during the first 3 months. Limit use during the final 6 months as much as possible. If used, examine infant for possible deficiency of adrenal gland function.

Advisability of Use If Breast-Feeding

Presence of this drug in breast milk: Yes.

Avoid drug or refrain from nursing.

Habit-Forming Potential: Long-term use of this drug may produce a state of functional dependence (see Glossary). In therapy of asthma and rheumatoid arthritis, it is advisable to keep the dose as small as possible and attempt drug withdrawal after periods of reasonable improvement. Such procedures may reduce the degree of "steroid rebound"—the return of symptoms as the drug is withdrawn.

Effects of Overdose: Fatigue, muscle weakness, stomach irritation, acid indigestion, excessive sweating, facial flushing, fluid retention, swelling of extremities, increased blood pressure.

Possible Effects of Long-Term Use: Increased blood sugar (possible diabetes), increased fat deposits on the trunk of the body ("buffalo hump"), rounding of the face ("moon face"), thinning and fragility of skin, loss of texture and strength of bones (osteoporosis, aseptic necrosis), cataracts, glaucoma, retarded growth and development in children.

Suggested Periodic Examinations While Taking This Drug (at physician's discretion)

Measurements of blood pressure, blood sugar and potassium levels.

Complete eye examinations at regular intervals.

Chest X ray if history of tuberculosis.

Bone mineral density testing (DEXA) to check for osteoporosis.

Determination of the rate of development of the growing child to detect retardation of normal growth.

▷ **While Taking This Drug, Observe the Following**

Foods: No interactions expected. Ask your doctor about restricting salt or eating potassium-rich foods. During long-term use, it is best to eat a high-protein diet.

Nutritional Support: During long-term use, take a vitamin D supplement. During wound repair, take a zinc supplement. Potassium loss may need to be replaced.

Beverages: No restrictions. Drink all forms of milk liberally.

▷ *Alcohol:* No interactions expected. Use caution if you are prone to peptic ulcers.

Tobacco Smoking: Nicotine increases the blood levels of naturally produced cortisone. I advise everyone to quit smoking.

Marijuana Smoking: May cause additional impairment of immunity.

▷ *Other Drugs:*

Prednisone may *decrease* the effects of

- isoniazid (INH, Niconyl, etc.).
- salicylates (aspirin, sodium salicylate, etc.).

Prednisone *taken concurrently* with

- amphotericin B (Abelcet, Fungizone) may result in additive potassium loss.
- birth control pills (oral contraceptives) will prolong the prednisone effect.
- cyclosporine (Sandimmune) can cause increased cyclosporine levels and increased prednisone levels. Dose decreases may be needed for both drugs.
- foscarnet (Foscavir) may result in additive potassium loss.
- ketoconazole (Nizoral) will lessen the therapeutic benefits of ketoconazole.
- loop diuretics (furosemide—Lasix); bumetanide—Bumex) may have blunt their effects.
- macrolide antibiotics (erythromycin, troleandomycin, and perhaps others) can lead to prednisone toxicity.
- NSAIDs may result in additive stomach and intestinal irritation.
- oral anticoagulants may either increase or decrease their effectiveness; consult your physician regarding the need for prothrombin time testing and dose adjustment.
- oral antidiabetic drugs (see Drug Classes) or insulin may result in loss of glucose control.

- ritonavir (Norvir), and perhaps other protease inhibitors (see Drug Classes) may lead to toxicity.
- theophylline (Theo-Dur, others) may result in variable responses to this medicine. Increased frequency of theophylline levels are recommended.
- thiazide diuretics (see Drug Classes) or loop diuretics may result in additive potassium loss.
- vaccines (flu, pneumococcal, varicella, and others) may result in blunted response to the vaccine and decreased preventive benefits.

The following drugs may *decrease* the effects of prednisone:

- antacids—may reduce its absorption.
- barbiturates (Amytal, Butisol, phenobarbital, etc.).
- carbamazepine (Tegretol).
- phenytoin (Dilantin, etc.).
- primidone (Mysoline).
- rifampin (Rifadin, Rimactane, etc.).

▷ *Driving, Hazardous Activities:* Usually no restrictions. Be alert to the rare occurrence of dizziness.

Aviation Note: The use of this drug *may be a disqualification* for piloting. Consult a designated aviation medical examiner.

Exposure to Sun: No restrictions.

Occurrence of Unrelated Illness: This drug may decrease resistance to infection. Tell your doctor if you develop an infection of any kind. It may also reduce your ability to respond to the stress of acute illness, injury, or surgery. Keep your doctor informed of any changes in health.

Discontinuation: After long-term use, do not stop prednisone abruptly. For 2 years after stopping this drug, it is essential in the event of illness, injury, or surgery that you tell medical personnel that you have used this drug.

PRIMIDONE (PRI mi dohn)

Introduced: 1953   **Class:** Anticonvulsant   **Prescription:** USA: Yes
Controlled Drug: USA: No; Canada: No   **Available as Generic:** USA: Yes; Canada: Yes
Brand Names: ✦Apo-Primidone, Myidone, Mysoline, ✦PMS-Primidone

BENEFITS versus RISKS	
Possible Benefits	*Possible Risks*
EFFECTIVE CONTROL OF TONIC-CLONIC (GRAND MAL) AND ALL TYPES OF PARTIAL SEIZURES	Allergic skin reactions Rare blood cell disorders: megaloblastic anemia, deficient white blood cells and platelets

▷ **Principal Uses**

As a Single Drug Product: Uses currently included in FDA-approved labeling: This drug is used exclusively to control generalized grand mal seizures and all types of partial seizures. It can be used to supplement the anticonvulsant action of phenytoin.

Other (unlabeled) generally accepted uses: (1) May have a minor role in helping in therapy of orthostatic tremor; (2) can help ringing in the ears.

How This Drug Works: Reduces and stabilizes the excitability of nerve fibers and inhibits the repetitious spread of electrical impulses along nerve pathways. This action may prevent seizures altogether, or it may reduce their frequency and severity. (Part of this drug's action is attributable to phenobarbital, one of its conversion products in the body.)

Available Dose Forms and Strengths

    Oral suspensions — 250 mg/5 ml

               Tablets — 50 mg, 125 mg, 250 mg

    Tablets, chewable — 125 mg

▷ **Usual Adult Dose Range:**   Initially 100 mg every 24 hours as a single dose at bedtime for 3 days; 100 to 125 mg twice a day for days 4–6, 100 to 125 mg three times a day for days 7–9, and an ongoing (maintenance) dose of 250 mg three or four times a day, 6 to 8 hours apart. Daily maximum is 2000 mg. **Note: Actual dose and schedule must be determined for each patient individually.**

Conditions Requiring Dosing Adjustments

Liver Function: The dose **must** be decreased and blood levels obtained more frequently for patients with liver compromise.

Kidney Function: For patients with mild to moderate kidney failure, the usual dose can be taken every 8 hours. Patients with moderate to severe kidney failure can take the usual dose every 8–12 hours. Patients with severe kidney failure should take the usual dose every 12–24 hours. Primidone should be used with caution in renal compromise, as it can be a cause of crystalluria.

▷ **Dosing Instructions:**   The tablet may be crushed and taken with or following food to reduce stomach irritation. Shake the suspension well before measuring the dose.

Usual Duration of Use: Use on a regular schedule for 2 to 4 weeks usually determines effectiveness in reducing the frequency and severity of seizures. Long-term use (months to years) requires physician supervision.

▷ **This Drug Should Not Be Taken If**

- you have had an allergic reaction to it previously.
- you are allergic to phenobarbital.
- you have a history of porphyria.

▷ **Inform Your Physician Before Taking This Drug If**

- you have had an allergic or idiosyncratic reaction to any barbiturate drug in the past.
- you have a family history of intermittent porphyria.
- you have impaired liver, kidney, or thyroid gland function.
- you have asthma, emphysema, or myasthenia gravis.
- you are pregnant or planning a pregnancy.
- you plan to have surgery under general anesthesia in the near future.

Possible Side Effects (natural, expected, and unavoidable drug actions)

Drowsiness, impaired concentration, mental and physical sluggishness.

▷ **Possible Adverse Effects** (unusual, unexpected, and infrequent reactions)

If any of the following develop, consult your physician promptly for guidance.

Mild Adverse Effects

Allergic reactions: skin rashes, hives, localized swellings. "Hangover" effect, dizziness, unsteadiness, impaired vision, double vision, fatigue, emotional disturbances—more likely during first 3 months, may ease with time.

Low blood pressure, faintness—possible.

Shoulder pain, joint pain—possible with longer-term therapy.

Nausea, vomiting, thirst, increased urine volume—rare to infrequent.

Serious Adverse Effects

Allergic reactions: swelling of lymph glands.

Idiosyncratic reactions: paradoxical anxiety, seizures, agitation, restlessness, rage.

Visual or auditory hallucinations—rare.

Drug-induced porphyria, systemic lupus erythematosus, or low thyroid gland function (hypothyroidism)—case reports.

Blood cell disorders: megaloblastic anemia; low white blood cells or platelets—case reports.

Drug-induced kidney problems (crystalluria)—case reports.

▷ **Possible Effects on Sexual Function:** Decreased libido and/or impotence— case reports.

Decreased effectiveness of oral contraceptives.

▷ **Adverse Effects That May Mimic Natural Diseases or Disorders**

Allergic swelling of lymph glands may suggest a naturally occurring lymphoma.

Natural Diseases or Disorders That May Be Activated by This Drug

Acute intermittent and/or cutaneous porphyria (see Glossary).

Systemic lupus erythematosus.

Possible Effects on Laboratory Tests

Complete blood cell counts: decreased red cells, hemoglobin, white cells, and platelets; increased eosinophils.

Blood lupus erythematosus (LE) cells: positive.

Prothrombin time: decreased (when taken concurrently with warfarin).

Urine screening tests for drug abuse: may be **positive** for phenobarbital (a normal derivative of this drug). (Test results depend upon amount of drug taken and testing method.)

CAUTION

1. This drug must not be stopped abruptly.
2. A wide variation of drug action from person to person requires careful individualization of dose.
3. Regularity of drug use is essential for the successful management of seizure disorders. Take your medication at the same time each day.
4. Side effects and mild adverse effects are usually most apparent during the first several weeks of treatment, and often subside with continued use.
5. It may be necessary to take folic acid to prevent anemia while taking this drug. Consult your physician.
6. It is advisable to carry a personal identification card with a notation that you are taking this drug.

Precautions for Use

By Infants and Children: This drug should be used with caution in the hyperkinetic (overactive) child. Paradoxical hyperactivity is possible. Puberty changes characteristically slow phenobarbital metabolism, permitting gradual accumulation. Measurements of blood levels in young adolescents can detect rising concentrations of this drug that could lead to toxicity (see "Therapeutic Drug Monitoring," in chapter 2).

By Those Over 60 Years of Age: It is advisable for the elderly to avoid all barbiturates. If use of this drug is attempted, small starting doses are indicated. Watch for confusion, delirium, agitation, or paradoxical excitement. This drug may be conducive to hypothermia (see Glossary).

▷ **Advisability of Use During Pregnancy**

Pregnancy Category: D. See Pregnancy Risk Categories at the back of this book. Animal studies: Birth defects due to this drug reported in mice.

Human studies: Adequate studies of pregnant women are not available. However, recent reports suggest a possible association between the use of this drug during the first 3 months of pregnancy and the development of birth defects in the fetus. Discuss with your physician the advantages and possible disadvantages of using this drug during pregnancy. If it is used, determine the smallest maintenance dose that will prevent seizures.

The newborn infants of mothers who take this drug during pregnancy may develop abnormal bleeding or bruising due to the deficiency of certain clotting factors in the blood. Consult your physician regarding the need to take vitamin K during the final month of pregnancy.

Advisability of Use If Breast-Feeding

Presence of this drug in breast milk: Yes.

Monitor nursing infant closely and discontinue drug or nursing if adverse effects develop.

Habit-Forming Potential: None.

Effects of Overdose: Drowsiness, jerky eye movements, blurred vision, staggering gait, incoordination, slurred speech, stupor progressing to coma.

Possible Effects of Long-Term Use: Enlargement of lymph glands; enlargement of thyroid gland. Megaloblastic anemia due to folic acid deficiency. Reduced blood levels of calcium and phosphorus, leading to rickets in children and loss of bone texture (osteomalacia) in adults.

Suggested Periodic Examinations While Taking This Drug (at physician's discretion)

Complete blood cell counts. Measurements of blood levels of calcium and phosphorus. Evaluation of lymph and thyroid glands. Skeletal X-ray examinations for bone demineralization during long-term use.

▷ **While Taking This Drug, Observe the Following**

Foods: No restrictions.

Nutritional Support: Talk with your doctor about calcium, vitamins D and K, and folic acid supplements.

Beverages: No restrictions. May be taken with milk or fruit juice.

▷ *Alcohol:* Avoid completely. Alcohol can increase greatly the sedative and depressant effects of this drug on brain function.

Tobacco Smoking: May enhance the sedative effects of this drug. I advise everyone to quit smoking.

▷ *Other Drugs:*

Note: 15% of primidone is converted to phenobarbital in the body. See the phenobarbital profile for possible interactions with other drugs.

▷ *Driving, Hazardous Activities:* This drug may cause drowsiness and dizziness; it can also impair mental alertness, vision, and physical coordination. Restrict activities as necessary.

Aviation Note: The use of this drug ***is a disqualification*** for piloting. Consult a designated aviation medical examiner.

Exposure to Sun: No restrictions.

Occurrence of Unrelated Illness: Notify your physician of any illness or injury that prevents the use of this drug according to your regular dose schedule.

Discontinuation: Do not stop this drug without your physician's knowledge and approval. Sudden withdrawal of any anticonvulsant drug can cause severe and repeated seizures.

PROBENECID (proh BEN e sid)

Introduced: 1951 **Class:** Anti-gout **Prescription:** USA: Yes **Controlled Drug:** USA: No; Canada: No **Available as Generic:** USA: Yes; Canada: No

Brand Names: ✦Ampicin PRB [CD], Benemid, ✦Benuryl, Colabid [CD], Col-Benemid [CD], Polycillin-PRB [CD], Probalan, Probampacin [CD], Proben-C [CD], ✦Pro-Biosan 500 Kit [CD], SK-Probenecid

BENEFITS versus RISKS	
Possible Benefits	*Possible Risks*
EFFECTIVE LONG-TERM PREVENTION OF ACUTE ATTACKS OF GOUT	Formation of uric acid kidney stones
	Bone marrow depression (aplastic anemia)
Useful adjunct to penicillin therapy (to achieve high blood and tissue levels of penicillin)	Drug-induced liver and kidney damage

▷ **Principal Uses**

As a Single Drug Product: Uses currently included in FDA-approved labeling: (1) Used in helping maintain penicillin levels in therapy of gonorrhea; (2) helps decrease elevated uric acid levels caused by thiazide diuretics; (3) helps prevent gout.

Other (unlabeled) generally accepted uses: (1) May have a role in preventing kidney toxicity in cisplatin chemotherapy; (2) adjunctive use in maintaining effective antibiotic levels in treatment of syphilis; (3) helps decrease uric acid in gout patients.

As a Combination Drug Product [CD]: This drug is available in combination with colchicine, a drug often used for the treatment of acute gout. Each drug works in a different way; when used in combination they provide both relief of the acute gout and some measure of protection from recurrence of acute attacks.

How This Drug Works: Works in the kidney (tubular systems) to increase uric acid excretion in the urine; this drug reduces the levels of uric acid in the blood and body tissues. It also works in the kidney to decrease the amount of penicillin excreted in the urine, and prolongs the presence of penicillin in the blood and helps achieve higher concentrations in body tissues.

Available Dose Forms and Strengths
Tablets — 500 mg

▷ **Usual Adult Dose Range:**   Anti-gout: Initially 250 mg twice a day for 1 week; then 500 mg twice a day. Adjunct to penicillin therapy: 500 mg four times a day. **Note: Actual dose and schedule must be determined for each patient individually.**

Conditions Requiring Dosing Adjustments
Liver Function: Specific guidelines for dose adjustment in liver compromise are not available. This drug should be used with caution.

Kidney Function: Patients with kidney failure (creatinine clearance less than 30 ml/min) should **not** use this drug, as the effectiveness is questionable. Those with moderate kidney failure may still benefit from this medicine, and dose increases (as needed and tolerated) in 500-mg steps up to 2000 mg a day in equally divided doses may be required.

▷ **Dosing Instructions:**   The tablet may be crushed and taken with or following food to reduce stomach irritation. Drink 2.5 to 3 quarts of liquids daily.

Usual Duration of Use: Use on a regular schedule for several months usually determines effectiveness in preventing acute attacks of gout. Long-term use (months to years) requires supervision and periodic evaluation by your physician.

▷ **This Drug Should Not Be Taken If**
- you have had an allergic reaction to it previously.
- you have active liver disease.
- you have acute kidney failure or kidney stones made of uric acid.
- you have an active blood cell or bone marrow disorder.
- you are experiencing an attack of acute gout at the present time.

▷ **Inform Your Physician Before Taking This Drug If**
- you have a history of kidney disease or kidney stones.
- you have a history of liver disease or impaired liver function.
- you have a history of peptic ulcer disease.
- you have a history of a blood cell or bone marrow disorder.
- you are taking any drug product that contains aspirin or aspirinlike drugs.

Possible Side Effects (natural, expected, and unavoidable drug actions)
Development of kidney stones (composed of uric acid); this is preventable. Consult your physician regarding the use of sodium bicarbonate (or other urine alkalizer) to prevent stone formation.

▷ **Possible Adverse Effects** (unusual, unexpected, and infrequent reactions)
If any of the following develop, consult your physician promptly for guidance.

Mild Adverse Effects
Allergic reactions: skin rash, itching, drug fever (see Glossary).
Headache, dizziness, flushing of face—infrequent.
Reduced appetite, sore gums, nausea, vomiting—possible to infrequent.

Serious Adverse Effects
Allergic reactions: anaphylactic reaction (see Glossary).
Idiosyncratic reactions: hemolytic anemia (see Glossary).
Bone marrow depression (see Glossary): fatigue, sore throat, bleeding/bruising—case reports.

Drug-induced liver damage with jaundice (see Glossary) or porphyria (see Glossary)—case reports.

Fluid in the retina (retinal edema)—case reports.

Drug-induced kidney damage: marked fluid retention, reduced urine formation—case reports.

▷ **Possible Effects on Sexual Function:**   None reported.

▷ **Adverse Effects That May Mimic Natural Diseases or Disorders**

Liver reactions may suggest viral hepatitis. Kidney reactions may suggest nephrosis.

Possible Effects on Laboratory Tests

Complete blood cell counts: decreased red cells, hemoglobin, white cells, and platelets.

INR (prothrombin time): increased (when taken concurrently with warfarin).

Blood glucose level and uric acid level: decreased.

Blood urea nitrogen (BUN) level: increased (kidney damage).

Liver function tests: increased enzymes (ALT/GPT, AST/GOT, alkaline phosphatase), or bilirubin.

Urine sugar tests: false positive with Benedict's solution and Clinitest.

CAUTION

1. This drug should not be started until 2 to 3 weeks after an acute attack of gout has subsided.
2. This drug may increase the frequency of acute attacks of gout during the first few months of treatment. Concurrent use of colchicine is advised to prevent acute attacks.
3. Aspirin (and aspirin-containing drug products) can reduce the effectiveness of this drug. Use acetaminophen or a nonaspirin analgesic for pain relief as needed.

Precautions for Use

By Infants and Children: Safety and effectiveness for those under 2 years of age are not established.

By Those Over 60 Years of Age: The natural decline in kidney function that occurs after 60 may require adjustment of your dose. You may be more susceptible to the serious adverse effects of this drug. Report any unusual symptoms promptly for evaluation.

▷ **Advisability of Use During Pregnancy**

Pregnancy Category: B. See Pregnancy Risk Categories at the back of this book.

Animal studies: No information available.

Human studies: Adequate studies of pregnant women are not available.

This drug has been used during pregnancy with no reports of birth defects or adverse effects on the fetus. Ask your physician for guidance.

Advisability of Use If Breast-Feeding

Presence of this drug in breast milk: Unknown.

Avoid drug or refrain from nursing.

Habit-Forming Potential: None.

Effects of Overdose: Stomach irritation, nausea, vomiting, nervous agitation, delirium, seizures, coma.

Possible Effects of Long-Term Use: Formation of kidney stones. Kidney damage in sensitive individuals.

Suggested Periodic Examinations While Taking This Drug (at physician's discretion)

Complete blood cell counts, blood uric acid, liver and kidney function tests.

▷ **While Taking This Drug, Observe the Following**

Foods: Follow your physician's advice regarding the need for a low-purine diet.

Beverages: A large intake of coffee, tea, or cola beverages may reduce the effectiveness of treatment.

▷ *Alcohol:* No interactions expected. However, large amounts of alcohol can raise the blood uric acid level and reduce the effectiveness of treatment.

Tobacco Smoking: No interactions expected. I advise everyone to quit smoking.

▷ *Other Drugs:*

Probenecid may *increase* the effects of

- acetaminophen (Tylenol), increasing risk of toxicity.
- acyclovir (Zovirax), and result in toxicity unless doses are reduced.
- ciprofloxacin (Cipro), increasing toxicity risk.
- clofibrate (Atromid-S).
- dyphylline (Neothylline).
- ketoprofen, and perhaps other NSAIDs (see *nonsteroidal anti-inflammatory drugs* in Drug Classes).
- methotrexate (Mexate), and increase its toxicity.
- midazolam (Versed) and increase CNS depression.
- oral antidiabetic agents (see Drug Classes).
- thiopental (Pentothal), and prolong its anesthetic effect.
- valacyclovir (Valtrex), and result in toxicity unless doses are reduced.
- zalcitabine (Hivid).
- zidovudine (Retrovir), and increase toxicity risk.

Probenecid *taken concurrently* with

- allopurinol (Zyloprim) may result in extended allopurinol half-life.
- cephalosporins (see Drug Classes) may cause a doubling of antibiotic levels. Caution must be used to avoid toxicity.
- dapsone may cause up to a 50% increased dapsone level and result in toxicity unless dapsone doses are decreased.
- penicillins (see Drug Classes) may cause a threefold to fivefold increase in penicillin blood levels, greatly increasing the effectiveness of each penicillin dose.
- rifampin (Rifadin, others) may result in increased blood levels of rifampin.
- ritonavir (Norvir) may lead to changes in probenecid blood levels.

The following drugs may *decrease* the effects of probenecid:

- aspirin and other salicylates—may reduce its effectiveness in promoting the excretion of uric acid.
- bismuth subsalicylate (Pepto-Bismol, others).

▷ *Driving, Hazardous Activities:* This drug may cause dizziness. Restrict activities as necessary.

Aviation Note: The use of this drug *may be a disqualification* for piloting. Consult a designated aviation medical examiner.

Exposure to Sun: No restrictions.

Discontinuation: Do not stop this drug without consulting your physician.

PROCAINAMIDE (proh KAYN a mide)

Introduced: 1950 **Class:** Antiarrhythmic **Prescription:** USA: Yes
Controlled Drug: USA: No; Canada: No **Available as Generic:** USA: Yes;
Canada: No
Brand Names: ✦Apo-Procainamide, Procamide SR, Procanbid, Procan SR,
Promine, Pronestyl, Pronestyl-SR, Rhythmin

BENEFITS versus RISKS

Possible Benefits	*Possible Risks*
EFFECTIVE TREATMENT OF SELECTED HEART RHYTHM DISORDERS	NARROW TREATMENT RANGE INDUCTION OF SYSTEMIC LUPUS ERYTHEMATOSUS SYNDROME Provocation of abnormal heart rhythms Blood cell disorders: insufficient white blood cells and platelets

---

▷ **Principal Uses**

As a Single Drug Product: Uses currently included in FDA-approved labeling:
Used to abolish and prevent the recurrence of premature beats arising in the
ventricles (lower chambers) of the heart.

Other (unlabeled) generally accepted uses: (1) Used to treat and prevent atrial
fibrillation, atrial flutter, and abnormally rapid heart rates (tachycardia)
that originate in the atria or the ventricles; (2) helps treat myotonia and improve breathing in myotonic dystrophy.

How This Drug Works: By slowing the activity of the pacemaker and delaying
the transmission of electrical impulses through the conduction system and
muscle of the heart, this drug assists in restoring normal heart rate and
rhythm.

Available Dose Forms and Strengths

Capsules — 250 mg, 375 mg, 500 mg
Injections — 100 mg/ml, 500 mg/ml
Tablets — 250 mg, 375 mg, 500 mg
Tablets, prolonged action — 250 mg, 500 mg, 750 mg, 1000 mg

▷ **Usual Adult Dose Range:** Dose varies according to indication: Starting dose is
up to 50 mg per kg of body mass per day of the immediate-release form.
This calculated dose is then divided into equal doses and is taken every 3,
4, or 6 hours. The ongoing daily dose should be adjusted to individual
patient response and blood levels. People over 50 years old may get an acceptable clinical response and blood level from a lower dose. The sustained-
release form is usually started in younger patients who do not have kidney
problems at 50 mg per kg of body mass per day. This calculated dose is divided into equal doses and is taken every 6 to 12 hours, depending on patient response and blood levels. **Note: Actual dose and schedule must be
determined for each patient individually.**

Conditions Requiring Dosing Adjustments

Liver Function: This drug should be used with caution by patients with liver
compromise, and blood levels appropriately obtained. Lower ongoing doses

are generally used. Procainamide should be a benefit-to-risk decision for patients with compromised livers, as it may be more likely to cause liver problems in this patient population.

Kidney Function: Patients with moderate to severe kidney failure can be given the usual doses every 6–12 hours. Patients with severe kidney failure can be given the usual dose every 8–24 hours. The drug should be used with caution in renal compromise, and appropriate blood levels obtained.

▷ **Dosing Instructions:** Preferably taken on an empty stomach, 1 hour before or 2 hours after eating. However, it may be taken with or following food to reduce stomach irritation. The regular capsules may be opened and the regular tablets may be crushed; prolonged-action tablets should be swallowed whole without alteration.

Usual Duration of Use: Use on a regular schedule for 24 to 48 hours usually determines effectiveness in correcting or preventing responsive rhythm disorders. Long-term use requires supervision and periodic evaluation by your physician.

▷ **This Drug Should Not Be Taken If**
• you have had an allergic reaction to it previously.
• you have systemic lupus erythematosus.
• you have second- or third-degree heart block (determined by electrocardiogram).
• you have myasthenia gravis.

▷ **Inform Your Physician Before Taking This Drug If**
• you are allergic to procaine (Novocain) or other local anesthetics of the "-cain" drug class, such as those commonly used for glaucoma testing and dental procedures.
• you have had any adverse reactions to other antiarrhythmic drugs.
• you have a history of heart disease of any kind, especially "heart block."
• you have a history of low blood pressure.
• you have a history of lupus erythematosus or myasthenia gravis.
• you have a history of abnormally low blood platelet counts.
• you have impaired liver or kidney function.
• you have an enlarged prostate gland.
• you are taking any form of digitalis or any diuretic drug that can cause excessive loss of body potassium (ask your physician).
• you plan to have surgery under general anesthesia in the near future.

Possible Side Effects (natural, expected, and unavoidable drug actions)
Drop in blood pressure in susceptible individuals.

▷ **Possible Adverse Effects** (unusual, unexpected, and infrequent reactions)
If any of the following develop, consult your physician promptly for guidance.

Mild Adverse Effects
Allergic reactions: skin rash, hives, itching, drug fever (see Glossary).
Weakness, light-headedness—case reports.
Loss of appetite, bitter taste, indigestion, nausea, vomiting, diarrhea—infrequent.

Serious Adverse Effects
Allergic reactions: systemic lupus-erythematosus-like syndrome: joint and

muscle pains, fever, skin eruptions, pleurisy. **This is reported to occur in up to 30% of users.**

Idiosyncratic reactions: mental depression, hallucinations, psychotic behavior, hemolytic anemia (see Glossary).

Severe drop in blood pressure, fainting—possible.

Drug-induced pancreatitis, liver toxicity, or myopathy—case reports.

Drug-induced myasthenia gravis, pancreatitis, or peripheral neuropathy—case reports.

Pericardial effusions—rare.

Asthma-like breathing difficulties—case reports.

Induction of new heart rhythm disturbances—possible.

Inability to empty urinary bladder, prostatism (see Glossary).

Anticholinergic syndrome—rare.

Blood cell disorders: abnormally low white blood cell or platelet count—case reports.

Author's note: The information in this profile has been shortened to make room for more widely used medicines.

PROCHLORPERAZINE (proh klor PER a zeen)

Introduced: 1956   **Class:** Antipsychotic, antiemetic, phenothiazines
Prescription: USA: Yes   **Controlled Drug:** USA: No; Canada: No   **Available as Generic:** USA: Yes; Canada: Yes

Brand Names: ✦Combid [CD], Compazine, Eskatrol, ✦PMS-Prochlorperazine, Pro-Iso, ✦Stemetil, Ultrazine [CD]

BENEFITS versus RISKS	
Possible Benefits	*Possible Risks*
EFFECTIVE CONTROL OF ACUTE MENTAL DISORDERS, NAUSEA, AND VOMITING	SERIOUS TOXIC EFFECTS ON BRAIN with long-term use
Relief of anxiety and nervous tension	Liver damage with jaundice
	Blood cell disorders: abnormally low white cell and platelet counts

▷ **Principal Uses**

As a Single Drug Product: Uses currently included in FDA-approved labeling: (1) Relieves severe nausea and vomiting; (2) may be used to treat schizophrenia; (3) helps prevent motion sickness.

Other (unlabeled) generally accepted uses: (1) Sometimes used to increase the effects of anesthesia; (2) may be of use in treating Ménière's disease (for nausea and vomiting).

How This Drug Works: By inhibiting the action of dopamine, this drug acts to correct an imbalance of nerve impulse transmissions that is thought to be responsible for certain mental disorders. By blocking dopamine in the brain's chemoreceptor trigger zone, this drug prevents stimulation of the vomiting center.

Available Dose Forms and Strengths

Capsules, prolonged action — 10 mg, 15 mg, 30 mg
Injection — 5 mg/ml

Suppositories — 2.5 mg, 5 mg, 25 mg
Syrup — 5 mg/5 ml
Tablets — 5 mg, 10 mg, 25 mg

▷ **Usual Adult Dose Range:**   Initially 5 mg of the immediate-release form every 6 to 8 hours. If needed and tolerated, dose may be increased by 5 mg at intervals of 3 to 4 days. Usual range is 50 to 75 mg daily. The total daily dose should not exceed 150 mg.

Nausea and vomiting: 5 to 10 mg three or four times daily. The sustained-release form can be taken as 15 mg when you wake up in the morning, or 10 mg of the sustained-release form every 12 hours.

Note: Actual dose and dosing schedule must be determined for each patient individually.

Conditions Requiring Dosing Adjustments

Liver Function: This drug should be used with caution by patients with liver compromise. Specific guidelines for dose adjustment are not available.

Kidney Function: Specific guidelines for adjustment of doses are not available.

▷ **Dosing Instructions:**   The tablets may be crushed and taken with or following food to reduce stomach irritation. Prolonged-action capsules should be swallowed whole without alteration.

Usual Duration of Use: Use on a regular schedule for 12 to 24 hours usually determines effectiveness in controlling nausea and vomiting. If used for severe anxiety-tension states or acute psychotic behavior, a trial of several weeks is usually necessary to determine effectiveness. If not significantly beneficial within 6 weeks, it should be stopped. Consult your physician on a regular basis.

▷ **This Drug Should Not Be Taken If**
- you have had an allergic reaction to it previously.
- you have active liver disease.
- you have signs that are indicative of Reye syndrome.
- you have extremely low blood pressure.
- you have cancer of the breast.
- this drug was prescribed for a child who is less than 2 years old or who weighs less than 20 lb.
- you have a current blood cell or bone marrow disorder.

▷ **Inform Your Physician Before Taking This Drug If**
- you are allergic or abnormally sensitive to any phenothiazine drug (see Drug Classes).
- you have impaired liver or kidney function.
- you have any type of seizure disorder.
- you have bone marrow depression or a history of blood diseases.
- you have diabetes, glaucoma, or heart disease.
- you have prostate trouble (prostatic hypertrophy).
- you are pregnant.
- you have had neuroleptic malignant syndrome or lupus erythematosus.
- you are taking any drug with sedative effects.
- you plan to have surgery under general or spinal anesthesia in the near future.

Possible Side Effects (natural, expected, and unavoidable drug actions)

Drowsiness (usually during the first 2 weeks), orthostatic hypotension (see

Glossary), blurred vision, dry mouth, nasal congestion, constipation, impaired urination.

Pink or purple coloration of urine, of no significance.

▷ **Possible Adverse Effects** (unusual, unexpected, and infrequent reactions)

If any of the following develop, consult your physician promptly for guidance.

Mild Adverse Effects

Allergic reactions: skin rash, hives, low-grade fever.

Lowering of body temperature, especially in the elderly (see *hypothermia* in Glossary)—possible.

Increased appetite and weight gain—possible.

Increased blood pressure—infrequent.

Dizziness, weakness—frequent; agitation, insomnia, impaired day and night vision—infrequent.

Chronic constipation, fecal impaction, incontinence—infrequent.

Serious Adverse Effects

Allergic reactions: hepatitis with jaundice (see Glossary), usually between second and fourth week; high fever; asthma; anaphylactic reaction (see Glossary).

Idiosyncratic reactions: toxic dermatitis, Stevens-Johnson syndrome. Neuroleptic malignant syndrome (see Glossary).

Liver toxicity or porphyria (see Glossary)—case reports.

Abnormal eye positioning (oculogyric crisis)—case reports.

Depression, disorientation, seizures—case reports.

Abnormally high blood pressure—rare.

Disturbances of heart rhythm, rapid heart rate—rare.

Bone marrow depression (see Glossary)—case reports.

Parkinson-like disorders (see Glossary); muscle spasms of face, jaw, neck, back, extremities; slowed movements, muscle rigidity, tremors; tardive dyskinesias (see Glossary)—case reports.

▷ **Possible Effects on Sexual Function:** Altered timing and pattern of menstruation.

Female breast enlargement with milk production—case reports. Causes false-positive pregnancy test result.

Male breast enlargement and tenderness (gynecomastia), inhibited ejaculation or priapism (see Glossary)—case reports.

▷ **Adverse Effects That May Mimic Natural Diseases or Disorders**

Nervous system reactions may suggest Parkinson's disease.

Liver reactions may suggest viral hepatitis.

Reactions resembling systemic lupus erythematosus can occur.

Natural Diseases or Disorders That May Be Activated by This Drug

Latent epilepsy, glaucoma, diabetes mellitus, prostatism (see Glossary).

Possible Effects on Laboratory Tests

White blood cell count: decreased.

Liver function tests: increased enzymes (ALT/GPT, AST/GOT, alkaline phosphatase), or bilirubin.

CAUTION

1. Many over-the-counter medications (see Glossary) for allergies, colds, and coughs contain drugs that can interact unfavorably with this drug.

Ask your doctor or pharmacist for help before using any such medications.

2. Antacids containing aluminum or magnesium can limit absorption of this drug and reduce its effectiveness.

3. Obtain prompt evaluation of any change or disturbance of vision.

Precautions for Use

By Infants and Children: Do not use this drug in infants under 2 years of age, or in children of any age with symptoms suggestive of Reye syndrome (see Glossary). Children with acute illnesses ("flu-like" infections, measles, chicken pox, etc.) are very susceptible to adverse effects when this drug is given to control nausea and vomiting.

By Those Over 60 Years of Age: Small starting doses are advisable. You may be more susceptible to drowsiness, lethargy, constipation, lowering of body temperature (hypothermia), and orthostatic hypotension (see Glossary). This drug can worsen existing prostatism (see Glossary). You may also be more susceptible to the development of Parkinson-like reactions and/or tardive dyskinesia (see discussion of these terms in Glossary). These reactions must be recognized early since they may become unresponsive to treatment and irreversible.

▷ **Advisability of Use During Pregnancy**

Pregnancy Category: C. See Pregnancy Risk Categories at the back of this book.
Animal studies: Cleft palate reported in mouse and rat studies.
Human studies: No increase in birth defects reported in 2,023 exposures. Information from adequate studies of pregnant women is not available.
Limit use to small and infrequent doses. Avoid drug during the final month because of possible effects on the newborn infant.

Advisability of Use If Breast-Feeding

Presence of this drug in breast milk: Yes, in small amounts.
Monitor nursing infant closely and discontinue drug or nursing if adverse effects develop.

Habit-Forming Potential: None, but it has been used in combination with pentazocine as a heroin substitute by drug abusers.

Effects of Overdose: Marked drowsiness, weakness, tremor, agitation, unsteadiness, deep sleep, coma, convulsions.

Possible Effects of Long-Term Use: Tardive dyskinesias. Eye changes: opacities in cornea or lens, retinal pigmentation.

Suggested Periodic Examinations While Taking This Drug (at physician's discretion)

Complete blood cell counts, especially between the 4th and 10th weeks of treatment.
Liver function tests, electrocardiograms.
Complete eye examinations—eye structures and vision.
Careful inspection of the tongue for early evidence of fine, involuntary, wave-like movements that could indicate the beginning of tardive dyskinesia.

▷ **While Taking This Drug, Observe the Following**

Foods: No restrictions. Vitamin C in high doses may lower therapeutic benefits.
Nutritional Support: A riboflavin (vitamin B_2) supplement should be taken with long-term use.

Beverages: No restrictions. May be taken with milk.

▷   *Alcohol:* Avoid completely. Alcohol can increase phenothiazine sedation and accentuate depressant effects on brain function and blood pressure. Phenothiazines can increase intoxicating effects of alcohol.

Tobacco Smoking: Possible reduction of drowsiness from drug. I advise everyone to quit smoking.

Marijuana Smoking: Moderate increase in drowsiness; accentuation of orthostatic hypotension; increased risk of precipitating latent psychoses, confusing the interpretation of mental status and drug responses.

▷   *Other Drugs:*

Prochlorperazine may *increase* the effects of
- all atropinelike drugs, and cause nervous system toxicity.
- all sedative drugs, especially meperidine (Demerol), and cause excessive sedation.
- grepafloxacin (Raxar), increasing risk of abnormal heartbeats.

Prochlorperazine may *decrease* the effects of
- guanethidine (Ismelin, Esimil), and reduce its effectiveness in lowering blood pressure.
- sparfloxacin (Zagam), increasing risk of abnormal heartbeats.
- tramadol (Ultram), increasing risk of seizures.

Prochlorperazine *taken concurrently* with
- monoamine oxidase (MAO) inhibitors (see Drug Classes) may result in increased risk of abnormal body movements (extrapyramidal reactions).
- oral antidiabetic drugs (see Drug Classes) agents may blunt their therapeutic benefits.
- propranolol (Inderal) may cause increased effects of both drugs; monitor drug effects closely and adjust doses as necessary.

The following drugs may *decrease* the effects of prochlorperazine:
- antacids containing aluminum and/or magnesium.
- benztropine (Cogentin).
- trihexyphenidyl (Artane).

▷   *Driving, Hazardous Activities:* This drug can impair mental alertness, judgment, and physical coordination. Avoid hazardous activities.

Aviation Note: The use of this drug *is a disqualification* for piloting. Consult a designated aviation medical examiner.

Exposure to Sun: Use caution until sensitivity has been determined. Some phenothiazines can cause photosensitivity (see Glossary).

Exposure to Heat: Use caution and avoid excessive heat as much as possible. This drug may impair the regulation of body temperature and increase the risk of heatstroke.

Exposure to Cold: Use caution and dress warmly. This drug can increase the risk of hypothermia in the elderly.

Discontinuation: After long-term use, do not stop this drug suddenly. Gradual withdrawal over 2 to 3 weeks under physician supervision is recommended.

PROPIONIC ACIDS (NONSTEROIDAL ANTI-INFLAMMATORY DRUG) FAMILY

Ibuprofen (i BYU proh fen)   **Fenoprofen** (FEN oh proh fen)   **Flurbiprofen** (flur BI proh fen)   **Ketoprofen** (kee toh PROH fen)   **Naproxen** (na PROX in) **Oxaprozin** (OX a proh zin)

Introduced: 1974, 1976, 1977, 1973, 1974, 1992, respectively   **Class:** Analgesic, mild; NSAIDs   **Prescription:** USA: Varies   **Controlled Drug:** USA: No; Canada: No   **Available as Generic:** Yes

Brand Names: Ibuprofen: Aches-N-Pain, Actiprofen, Advil, ✦Amersol, ✦Apo-Ibuprofen, Arthritis Foundation Pain Reliever/Fever Reducer, Bayer Select, Children's Advil, Children's Motrin, Children's Motrin Drops (nonprescription), Children's Motrin Suspension (nonprescription), CoAdvil [CD], Dimetapp Sinus [CD], Dologesic, Dristan Sinus, Excedrin IB, Genpril, Guildprofen, Haltran, Ibuprohm, Ibu, Junior Strength Motrin Caplets (nonprescription), Medipren, Medi-Profen, Midol IB, Motrin, Motrin IB, ✦Novo-Profen, Nuprin, PediaProfen, Profen-IB, Rufen, Superior Pain Medicine, Supreme Pain Medicine, Tab-Profen; Fenoprofen: Nalfon; Flurbiprofen: Ansaid, ✦Apo-Flurbiprofen, ✦Froben, ✦Froben-SR, Ocufen; Ketoprofen: Actron (12.5-mg nonprescription), ✦Apo-Keto, ✦Apo-Keto E, Orudis, Orudis E-50, Orudis E-100, Orudis KT (nonprescription), Orudis SR, Oruvail, Oruvail ER, ✦Oruvail SR, ✦Rhodis, ✦Rhodis EC, ✦Rhodis EC Suppository; Naproxen: Aleve (nonprescription), Anaprox, Anaprox DS, ✦Apo-Naproxen, Naprelan, Naprelan Once Daily, Naprosyn, ✦Naxen, Neo-Prox, ✦Novo-Naprox, ✦Nu-Naprox, ✦Synflex; Oxaprozin: Daypro

BENEFITS versus RISKS	
Possible Benefits	*Possible Risks*
EFFECTIVE RELIEF OF MILD TO MODERATE PAIN AND INFLAMMATION	Gastrointestinal pain, ulceration, bleeding
EFFECTIVE RELIEF OF FEVER	Kidney damage
	Fluid retention
	Bone marrow depression (except oxaprozin)
	Liver toxicity (naproxen, oxaprozin, ketoprofen, and flurbiprofen)
	(All rare)

▷ **Principal Uses**

As a Single Drug Product: Uses currently included in FDA-approved labeling: (1) All six agents in this class treat rheumatoid and osteoarthritis; (2) naproxen is useful in treating bursitis, gout, dysmenorrhea (ketoprofen and ibuprofen are also approved for use in primary dysmenorrhea), pain, juvenile rheumatoid arthritis, and tendonitis; (3) fenoprofen is the only agent approved to treat tennis elbow.

Other (unlabeled) generally accepted uses: (1) Naproxen has been used to treat migraine and colds caused by rhinoviruses; (2) oxaprozin is useful in gout and tendonitis; (3) ketoprofen may have a role in temporal arteritis; (4) flurbiprofen has some support for therapy of periodontal disease and miosis inhibition; (5) fenoprofen has been used successfully in therapy of migraine; (6) ibuprofen treats interleukin-2 toxicity, and chronic urticaria, and can decrease IUD-associated bleeding. All of the agents have been used for a variety of pains and fever.

How These Drugs Work: Reduce levels of prostaglandins (and related compounds), chemicals involved in inflammation and pain.

Available Dose Forms and Strengths

Ibuprofen:

Caplets	— 200 mg
Tablets, chewable	— 50 mg, 100 mg
Oral suspension	— 100 mg/5 ml
Tablets	— 40 mg, 200 mg, 300 mg, 400 mg, 600 mg, 800 mg

Fenoprofen:

Capsules	— 200 mg, 300 mg, 600 mg
Tablets	— 600 mg

Flurbiprofen:

Ophthalmic drops	— 0.03%
Tablets	— 50 mg, 100 mg

Ketoprofen:

Capsules	— 50 mg, 75 mg, 100 mg, 150 mg
Suppositories	— 100 mg (in Canada)
Tablets (nonprescription)	— 12.5 mg
Tablets, enteric	— 50 mg (in Canada)

Naproxen:

Caplets	— 220 mg
Oral suspension	— 125 mg/5 ml
Rectal suppository	— 500 mg (Canada)
Tablets	— 125 mg, 250 mg, 275 mg, 375 mg, 500 mg, 550 mg
Tablets, controlled release	— 375 mg, 500 mg
Naprelan Once Daily	— 375 mg, 500 mg

Oxaprozin:

Caplets	— 600 mg

▷ **Usual Adult Dose Range:**   Ibuprofen: 200 to 800 mg three or four times daily. Total daily dose should not exceed 3200 mg.

Fenoprofen: 300 to 600 mg three or four times daily. Daily maximum is 3200 mg.

Flurbiprofen: 100 to 300 mg daily in two to four divided doses. The lowest effective dose should be used. Daily maximum is 300 mg.

Ketoprofen: 75 mg three times daily or 50 mg four times daily. Usual daily dose is 100 to 300 mg, divided into three or four doses. Daily maximum is 300 mg.

Naproxen: Gout—750 mg initially, then 250 mg every 8 hours until attack is relieved. Arthritis—250 mg, 375 mg, or 500 mg twice daily, 12 hours apart.

The sustained-release form (Naprelan) offers an intestinal-protective drug absorption system (IPDAS) and once-daily (two tablets once a day) dosing. Menstrual pain—500 mg initially, then 250 mg every 6 to 8 hours as needed. Maximum dose for pain is 1375 mg.

Oxaprozin: 1200 mg as a single daily dose in the morning. Daily maximum is 1800 mg (or 26 mg per kg of body mass for patients with normal liver and kidney function).

Author's Note: Medicines in this class with available nonprescription forms usually have lower daily maximum doses. For example: Children's Motrin—approved for nonprescription use as temporary relief of minor aches and pains or reduction of fever in children 2 years of age and older. Adverse effects are also less common and fewer in number. Less than 11 kg of body mass and under 2 years old: consult your doctor; 2 to 3 years old and 11 to 15.9 kg of body mass: 100 mg every 6 to 8 hours. Up to four doses may be given a day. Use should NOT go on for longer than 3 days. Please consult individual package labels or ask your pharmacist or doctor for dosing advice.

Note: Actual dose and dosing schedule must be determined for each patient individually.

Conditions Requiring Dosing Adjustments

Liver Function: All of these drugs are metabolized in the liver and therefore should be used with caution, and consideration given to lower doses, by patients with liver compromise.

Kidney Function: These drugs share the risks common to most nonsteroidal anti-inflammatory drugs (NSAIDs). Some patients with kidney compromise are dependent on prostaglandins for kidney function. A benefit-to-risk decision must be made regarding the use of NSAIDs by these patients.

▷ **Dosing Instructions:**   Take either on an empty stomach or with food or milk to prevent stomach irritation. Take with a full glass of water and remain upright (do not lie down) for 30 minutes. The tablets may be crushed and the capsules opened, except for ketoprofen tablets (should not be crushed or altered).

Usual Duration of Use: Use on a regular schedule for 1 to 2 weeks usually determines effectiveness. Peak oxaprozin effect may take 6 weeks. Long-term use requires supervision and periodic physician evaluation.

▷ **These Drugs Should Not Be Taken If**
- you have had an allergic reaction to them previously.
- you are subject to asthma or nasal polyps caused by aspirin.
- you have a bleeding disorder or a blood cell disorder.
- flurbiprofen ophthalmic drops should NOT be used by people with herpes simplex keratitis.
- you have severe impairment of kidney function (some cases).

▷ **Inform Your Physician Before Taking These Drugs If**
- you are allergic to aspirin or other aspirin substitutes.
- you have active peptic ulcer disease or any form of gastrointestinal bleeding.
- you have a history of peptic ulcer disease or any type of bleeding disorder.
- you have impaired liver or kidney function.
- you have high blood pressure or a history of heart failure.
- you are taking acetaminophen, aspirin, or other aspirin substitutes or anticoagulants.

Possible Side Effects (natural, expected, and unavoidable drug actions)

Fluid retention (weight gain); pink, red, purple, or rust coloration of urine (ibuprofen only). Ringing in the ears.

▷ **Possible Adverse Effects** (unusual, unexpected, and infrequent reactions)
If any of the following develop, consult your physician promptly for guidance.

Mild Adverse Effects

Allergic reactions: skin rash, hives, itching.

Headache, dizziness, altered or blurred vision, ringing in the ears, depression—infrequent.

Stinging or burning of the eyes with ophthalmic flurbiprofen drops—possible.

Sleep disturbances (oxaprozin)—infrequent.

Mouth sores, indigestion, nausea, vomiting, constipation, diarrhea—infrequent.

Palpitations (fenoprofen)—rare.

Serious Adverse Effects

Allergic reactions: anaphylactic reaction (see Glossary), severe skin reactions—rare; lung inflammation (naproxen—pneumonitis)—rare.

Idiosyncratic reactions: drug-induced meningitis with fever and coma (ibuprofen and naproxen)—rare.

Active peptic ulcer, with or without bleeding—rare with 6 months use, infrequent after 1 year of use.

Inflammation of the colon—rare.

Porphyria (some drugs in this class)—case reports.

Pancreatitis or lupus erythematosus—two case reports with naproxen.

Some medicines in this class may cause Parkinson-like symptoms in susceptible patients—case reports.

Inflammation of the esophagus—probable if patients lie down soon after taking these medicines.

Liver damage with jaundice (see Glossary)—case reports.

Kidney damage with painful urination, bloody urine, reduced urine formation—possible.

Bone marrow depression (see Glossary): fatigue, sore throat, abnormal bleeding/bruising—case reports.

▷ **Possible Effects on Sexual Function:**   Altered timing and pattern of menstruation (ibuprofen, ketoprofen, and naproxen), and excessive menstrual bleeding (ibuprofen and ketoprofen)—case reports.

Male breast enlargement and tenderness (ibuprofen)—rare.

Naproxen may rarely inhibit ejaculation.

Ketoprofen may rarely decrease libido.

Possible Delayed Adverse Effects: Mild anemia due to "silent" blood loss from the stomach (less than that caused by aspirin).

▷ **Adverse Effects That May Mimic Natural Diseases or Disorders**

Liver reaction may suggest viral hepatitis.

Natural Diseases or Disorders That May Be Activated by These Drugs

Peptic ulcer disease, ulcerative colitis.

Possible Effects on Laboratory Tests

Complete blood cell counts: decreased red cells, hemoglobin, white cells, and platelets.

Blood cholesterol or uric acid levels: increased.

Blood lithium level: increased.

Liver function tests: increased enzymes (ALT/GPT, AST/GOT, alkaline phosphatase) or bilirubin.

Kidney function tests: increased blood creatinine and blood urea nitrogen (BUN) levels.

Fecal occult blood test: positive.

CAUTION

1. Dose should always be limited to the smallest amount that produces reasonable improvement.
2. These drugs may mask early indications of infection. Inform your physician if you think you are developing an infection of any kind.

Precautions for Use

By Infants and Children: Safety and effectiveness for those under 12 years of age are not established.

By Those Over 60 Years of Age: Small doses are prudent until tolerance is determined. Watch for signs of liver or kidney toxicity, fluid retention, dizziness, confusion, impaired memory, stomach bleeding, or constipation.

▷ **Advisability of Use During Pregnancy**

Pregnancy Category: B for ibuprofen, fenoprofen, flurbiprofen, ketoprofen, and naproxen; C for oxaprozin. Ibuprofen and fenoprofen are FDA category D if used in the final 3 months (trimester) of pregnancy. The manufacturers of ketoprofen and flurbiprofen say that both medicines should be avoided in late pregnancy. See Pregnancy Risk Categories at the back of this book.

Animal studies: No birth defects reported in rats or rabbits.

Human studies: Adequate studies of pregnant women are not available.

Avoid these drugs during the final 3 months. Use during the first 6 months only if clearly needed. Ask your physician for guidance.

Advisability of Use If Breast-Feeding

Presence of these drugs in breast milk: Yes, or expected.

Avoid drugs or refrain from nursing.

Habit-Forming Potential: None.

Effects of Overdose: Drowsiness, dizziness, ringing in the ears, nausea, vomiting, diarrhea, confusion, unsteadiness, stupor progressing to coma.

Possible Effects of Long-Term Use: Fluid retention.

Suggested Periodic Examinations While Taking These Drugs (at physician's discretion)

Complete blood cell counts, liver and kidney function tests, complete eye examinations if vision is altered in any way.

▷ **While Taking These Drugs, Observe the Following**

Foods: No restrictions.

Beverages: No restrictions. May be taken with milk.

▷   *Alcohol:* Use with caution. The irritant action of alcohol on the stomach lining, added to the irritant action of these drugs, can increase the risk of stomach ulceration and/or bleeding.

Tobacco Smoking: No interactions expected. I advise everyone to quit smoking.

▷   *Other Drugs:*

These medicines may ***increase*** the effects of
- acetaminophen (Tylenol, etc.), and increase the risk of kidney damage; avoid prolonged use of this combination.
- anticoagulants (Coumadin, etc.), and increase the risk of bleeding. More frequent INR (prothrombin time or protime) tests are needed, and ongoing doses should be adjusted to the laboratory test results.

- enoxaparin (Lovenox) if NSAIDs are used before hip replacement surgery, and enoxaparin is used after surgery.
- lithium (Lithobid, others) by causing toxic lithium levels.
- methotrexate (Mexate, others), and result in major methotrexate toxicity with possible anemia, hemorrhage, and blood infections.

These medicines may *decrease* the effects of

- beta-blockers (see Drug Classes) such as carteolol (Cartrol).
- diuretics (see Drug Classes) such as hydrochlorothiazide (Esidrix) and furosemide (Lasix).

These medicines *taken concurrently* with the following drugs may increase the risk of bleeding; avoid these combinations:

- ACE inhibitors (see Drug Classes)—can worsen kidney diseases.
- aspirin.
- dipyridamole (Persantine).
- enoxaparin (Lovenox).
- histamine (H$_2$) blockers (see Drug Classes)—may increase toxicity from NSAIDs.
- indomethacin (Indocin).
- sulfinpyrazone (Anturane).
- valproic acid (Depakene).
- warfarin (Coumadin).

▷ *Driving, Hazardous Activities:* These drugs may cause drowsiness or dizziness. Restrict activities as necessary.

Aviation Note: The use of these drugs *may be a disqualification* for piloting. Consult a designated aviation medical examiner.

Exposure to Sun: Use caution until sensitivity is determined. Ibuprofen, ketoprofen, flurbiprofen, and naproxen cause photosensitivity (see Glossary).

PROPRANOLOL (proh PRAN oh lohl)

Introduced: 1966   **Class:** Anti-anginal, antiarrhythmic, antihypertensive, anti-migraine drug, beta-blocker   **Prescription:** USA: Yes   **Controlled Drug:** USA: No; Canada: No   **Available as Generic:** Yes

Brand Names: ✚Apo-Propranolol, ✚Detensol, Inderal, Inderal-LA, Inderide [CD], Inderide LA [CD], Ipran, ✚Novo-Pranol, ✚PMS Propranolol

---

BENEFITS versus RISKS

Possible Benefits	*Possible Risks*
EFFECTIVE, WELL-TOLERATED AS: ANTI-ANGINAL DRUG in effort-induced angina; ANTIARRHYTHMIC DRUG in certain heart rhythm disorders; ANTIHYPERTENSIVE DRUG in mild to moderate hypertension EFFECTIVE PREVENTION OF MIGRAINE HEADACHES Effective adjunct in the prevention of recurrent heart attack and the management of pheochromocytoma	CONGESTIVE HEART FAILURE in advanced heart disease Worsening of angina in coronary heart disease (if drug is abruptly withdrawn) Masking of low blood sugar (hypoglycemia) in drug-treated diabetes Provocation of asthma (in asthmatics) Depression Blood cell disorders: low white cell and platelet counts

▷ **Principal Uses**

As a Single Drug Product: Uses currently included in FDA-approved labeling: (1) Treats several cardiovascular disorders—classical effort-induced angina, certain types of heart rhythm disturbance, and high blood pressure—and also helps prevent repeat heart attacks (myocardial infarction); (2) reduces frequency and severity of migraine headaches; (3) decreases tremors in essential tremor.

Other (unlabeled) generally accepted uses: (1) Control of physical signs of anxiety and nervous tension (as in stage fright); (2) helps control familial tremors and symptoms seen with markedly overactive thyroid function (thyrotoxicosis); (3) decreases abnormal abdominal fluid accumulation (ascites) in people with cirrhosis of the liver; (4) may have a role in combination therapy with metronidazole in resistant *Giardia* infections; (5) helps control headaches caused by cyclosporine (Sandimmune); (6) may be useful in certain kinds of pain, especially after amputations; (7) can help control panic attacks; (8) useful in helping decrease bleeding in patients with esophageal varices and liver cirrhosis; (9) helps fight symptoms in narcotic withdrawal cases.

As a Combination Drug Product [CD]: This drug is available in combination with hydrochlorothiazide for the treatment of hypertension. This combination product includes two drugs with different mechanisms of action; it is intended to provide greater effectiveness and convenience for long-term use.

How This Drug Works: Blocks certain actions of the sympathetic nervous system:
- reducing rate and contraction force of the heart, lowering the ejection pressure of the blood leaving the heart and reducing the oxygen requirement for heart function.
- reduces degree of contraction of blood vessel walls, lowering blood pressure.
- prolongs conduction time of nerve impulses through the heart, helping manage certain heart rhythm disorders.

Available Dose Forms and Strengths

Capsules, prolonged action — 60 mg, 80 mg, 120 mg, 160 mg

Concentrate — 80 mg/ml

Injection — 1 mg/ml

Oral solution — 4 mg/ml, 8 mg/ml

Tablets — 10 mg, 20 mg, 40 mg, 60 mg, 80 mg, 90 mg, 120 mg

▷ **Usual Adult Dose Range:**   Anti-anginal: Initially 10 mg three or four times a day; increase dose gradually every 3 to 7 days as needed and tolerated. The total daily dose should not exceed 400 mg.

Antiarrhythmic: 10 to 30 mg three or four times a day as needed and tolerated.

Antihypertensive: Initially 40 mg twice a day; increase dose gradually as needed and tolerated. The total daily dose should not exceed 640 mg.

Migraine headache prevention: Initially 20 mg four times a day; increase dose gradually as needed and tolerated. The total daily dose should not exceed 480 mg. Long-acting formulations offer the advantage of once-daily dosing for many patients.

Note: Actual dose and schedule must be determined for each patient individually.

Conditions Requiring Dosing Adjustments

Liver Function: Used with caution by patients with liver disease. In general, lower starting doses and slower dose increases are indicated.

Kidney Function: This drug should be used with caution by people with combined kidney and liver compromise. Dose adjustments are not needed for people with compromised kidneys.

▷ **Dosing Instructions:**   This drug is preferably taken 1 hour before eating to maximize absorption. The tablet may be crushed; to prevent harmless numbing effect, mix with soft food and swallow promptly. The prolonged-action capsules should be swallowed whole. Do not stop this drug abruptly.

Usual Duration of Use: Use on a regular schedule for 10 to 14 days usually determines effectiveness in preventing angina, controlling heart rhythm disorders, and lowering blood pressure. Peak benefits may be seen in 6 to 8 weeks. Long-term use is determined by your symptoms over time and response to the overall treatment program (weight reduction, salt restriction, smoking cessation, etc.). See your physician on a regular basis.

▷ **This Drug Should Not Be Taken If**
- you have bronchial asthma.
- you have had an allergic reaction to it previously.
- you have Prinzmetal's variant angina (coronary artery spasm).
- you have heart failure (overt).
- you have Raynaud's disease.
- you have an abnormally slow heart rate or a serious form of heart block.
- you are taking, or have taken within the past 14 days, any monoamine oxidase (MAO) type A inhibitor drug (see Drug Classes).

▷ **Inform Your Physician Before Taking This Drug If**
- you had an adverse reaction to a beta-blocker (see Drug Classes).
- you have a history of serious heart disease.
- you have a history of hay fever (allergic rhinitis), asthma, chronic bronchitis, or emphysema.
- you have a history of overactive thyroid function (hyperthyroidism).
- you have a history of low blood sugar (hypoglycemia).
- you have impaired liver or kidney function.
- you are allergic to bee stings.
- you have diabetes or myasthenia gravis.
- you take digitalis, quinidine, or reserpine, or any calcium-channel-blocker drug (see Drug Classes).
- you plan to have surgery under general anesthesia in the near future.

Possible Side Effects (natural, expected, and unavoidable drug actions)

Lethargy and fatigability, cold extremities, slow heart rate, light-headedness in upright position (see *orthostatic hypotension* in Glossary). Increased bowel movements.

▷ **Possible Adverse Effects** (unusual, unexpected, and infrequent reactions)

If any of the following develop, consult your physician promptly for guidance.

Mild Adverse Effects

Allergic reactions: skin rash, temporary loss of hair, drug fever (see Glossary). Joint pain—case reports.

Headache, dizziness, insomnia, vivid dreams—infrequent.

Indigestion, taste disorder, nausea, vomiting, diarrhea—infrequent.

Weight gain—possible.

Serious Adverse Effects

Allergic reactions: anaphylaxis.

Idiosyncratic reactions: acute behavioral disturbances: disorientation, confusion, hallucinations, amnesia.

Paradoxical hypertension—case reports.

Mental depression, anxiety—case reports and dose related.

Chest pain, shortness of breath, precipitation of congestive heart failure—possible.

Peripheral neuropathy or hyperthyroidism—rare.

Drug-induced systemic lupus erythematosus, myasthenia gravis, or porphyria—case reports.

Kidney problems (interstitial nephritis)—rare.

Induction of bronchial asthma—in asthmatics.

May precipitate problems walking (intermittent claudication)—possible.

Blood cell disorders: abnormally low white blood cell or platelet counts—case reports.

Carpal tunnel syndrome—case reports.

▷ **Possible Effects on Sexual Function:**   Decreased libido; impaired erection; impotence—infrequent. Has the highest incidence of libido reduction and erectile impairment of all beta-blocker drugs.

Male infertility (inhibited sperm motility); Peyronie's disease (see Glossary)—possible.

▷ **Adverse Effects That May Mimic Natural Diseases or Disorders**

Reduced blood flow to extremities may resemble Raynaud's phenomenon (see Glossary).

Natural Diseases or Disorders That May Be Activated by This Drug

Prinzmetal's variant angina, Raynaud's disease, intermittent claudication, myasthenia gravis (questionable).

Possible Effects on Laboratory Tests

White blood cell count: occasionally decreased.

Blood platelet count: increased or decreased.

Bleeding time: increased.

Blood total cholesterol, triglycerides or VLDL level: no effect in some; increased in others.

Blood HDL cholesterol level: no effect in some; decreased in others.

Blood LDL cholesterol level: no effect in some; increased and decreased in others.

Blood glucose level: no effect in some; increased or decreased in others.

Glucose tolerance test (GTT): decreased.

Blood thyroid hormone levels: T_3—no effect in some, decreased in others; T_4—increased; free T_4—increased.

Blood uric acid level: no effect in some; increased in others.

Liver function tests: increased liver enzymes (ALT/GPT, AST/GOT, and alkaline phosphatase); effects probably not due to liver damage.

CAUTION

1. ***Do not stop this drug suddenly*** without the knowledge and help of your doctor. Carry a personal identification card that states you are taking this drug.

2. Ask your physician or pharmacist before using nasal decongestants, which are usually present in over-the-counter cold preparations and nose drops. These can cause sudden increases in blood pressure when taken concurrently with beta-blocker drugs.
3. Report the development of any tendency to emotional depression.

Precautions for Use

By Infants and Children: Safety and effectiveness for those under 12 years of age are not established. However, if this drug is used, observe for the development of low blood sugar (hypoglycemia) during periods of reduced food intake.

By Those Over 60 Years of Age: Unacceptably high blood pressure should be reduced without creating the risks associated with excessively low blood pressure. Therapy is started with small doses, and blood pressure checked frequently. Sudden, rapid, and excessive reduction of blood pressure can predispose to stroke or heart attack. Observe for dizziness, unsteadiness, tendency to fall, confusion, hallucinations, depression, or urinary frequency.

▷ Advisability of Use During Pregnancy

Pregnancy Category: C. See Pregnancy Risk Categories at the back of this book.
Animal studies: No significant increase in birth defects due to this drug. Some toxic effects on embryo reported.
Human studies: Adequate studies of pregnant women are not available.
Avoid use of drug during the first 3 months if possible. Ask your physician for guidance.

Advisability of Use If Breast-Feeding

Presence of this drug in breast milk: Yes.
Monitor nursing infant closely and discontinue drug or nursing if adverse effects develop.

Habit-Forming Potential: None.

Effects of Overdose: Weakness, slow pulse, low blood pressure, fainting, cold and sweaty skin, congestive heart failure, possible coma, and convulsions.

Possible Effects of Long-Term Use: Reduced heart reserve and eventual heart failure in susceptible patients with advanced heart disease.

Suggested Periodic Examinations While Taking This Drug (at physician's discretion)

Complete blood cell counts.
Measurements of blood pressure, evaluation of heart function.
Liver function tests.

▷ While Taking This Drug, Observe the Following

Foods: No restrictions. Avoid excessive salt intake.
Beverages: No restrictions. May be taken with milk.
▷ *Alcohol:* Use with caution. Alcohol may exaggerate this drug's ability to lower blood pressure and may increase its mild sedative effect.
Tobacco Smoking: Nicotine may reduce this drug's effectiveness in treating angina, heart rhythm disorders, and high blood pressure. Smoking increases the rate of elimination of this drug. I advise everyone to quit smoking.
▷ *Other Drugs:*
Propranolol may *increase* the effects of
• other antihypertensive drugs, and cause excessive lowering of blood pressure. Dose adjustments may be necessary.

- lidocaine (Xylocaine, etc.).
- reserpine (Ser-Ap-Es, etc.), and cause sedation, depression, slowing of the heart rate, and lowering of blood pressure.
- verapamil (Calan, Isoptin), and cause excessive depression of heart function; monitor this combination closely.
- warfarin (Coumadin), and increase bleeding risk. More frequent INR (prothrombin time or protime) testing are needed. Warfarin dosing should be adjusted to laboratory results.

Propranolol may *decrease* the effects of

- albuterol (Proventil).
- theophyllines (Aminophyllin, Theo-Dur, etc.), and reduce their antiasthmatic effectiveness.

Propranolol *taken concurrently* with

- amiodarone (Codarone) may result in abnormal heart rhythms and low pulse. These agents should not be combined.
- clonidine (Catapres) requires close monitoring for rebound high blood pressure if clonidine is withdrawn while propranolol is still being taken.
- digoxin (Lanoxin) can result in severe slowing of the heart (bradycardia).
- epinephrine (Adrenalin, etc.) may cause marked rise in blood pressure and slowing of the heart rate.
- fluoxetine (Prozac) may increase the risk of slow heartbeat and sedation.
- fluvoxamine (Luvox) may increase the risk of slow heartbeat and sedation.
- insulin requires close monitoring to avoid undetected hypoglycemia (see Glossary).
- oral antidiabetic drugs (see Drug Classes) may cause slow recovery from any low blood sugar that may occur.
- quinidine (Quinaglute) can increase adverse effects without increased therapeutic benefits.
- venlafaxine (Effexor) may result in increased risk of propranolol toxicity.
- X-ray contrast media such as diatrizoate results in up to an eightfold increase in risk of severe allergic (anaphylactic) drug reactions.

The following drugs may *increase* the effects of propranolol:

- chlorpromazine (Thorazine, etc.).
- cimetidine (Tagamet).
- diltiazem (Cardizem).
- disopyramide (Norpace).
- furosemide or other diuretics.
- methimazole (Tapazole).
- nicardipine (Cardene).
- propylthiouracil (Propacil).
- ritonavir (Norvir), and perhaps other protease inhibitors (see Drug Classes).
- zileuton (Zyflo).

The following drugs may *decrease* the effects of propranolol:

- antacids.
- barbiturates (phenobarbital, etc.).
- indomethacin (Indocin) and possibly other "aspirin substitutes," or NSAIDs—may impair propranolol's antihypertensive effect.
- rifampin (Rifadin, Rimactane).
- sertraline (Zoloft), possibly increasing the risk of chest pain.

▷ *Driving, Hazardous Activities:* Use caution until the full extent of drowsiness, lethargy, and blood pressure change have been determined.

Aviation Note: The use of this drug *may be a disqualification* for piloting. Consult a designated aviation medical examiner.

Exposure to Sun: No restrictions.

Exposure to Heat: Caution is advised. Hot environments can lower blood pressure and exaggerate the effects of this drug.

Exposure to Cold: Caution is advised. Cold environments can enhance the circulatory deficiency in the extremities that may occur with this drug. The elderly should take precautions to prevent hypothermia (see Glossary).

Heavy Exercise or Exertion: It is advisable to avoid exertion that produces light-headedness, excessive fatigue, or muscle cramping. The use of this drug may intensify the hypertensive response to isometric exercise.

Occurrence of Unrelated Illness: Fever can lower blood pressure and require adjustment of dose. Nausea or vomiting may interrupt the regular dose schedule. Ask your physician for guidance.

Discontinuation: Best to avoid sudden stopping of this drug, especially in coronary artery disease. If possible, a gradual reduction of dose over a period of 2 to 3 weeks is recommended. Ask your physician for specific guidance.

PROTEASE INHIBITOR FAMILY

Indinavir (in DIN a veer) **Nelfinavir** (nel FIN a veer) **Ritonavir** (ri TOHN a veer) **Saquinavir** (sa KWIN a veer)

Introduced: 1996, 1997, 1996, 1995, respectively **Class:** Protease inhibitor, antiviral, anti-AIDS drug **Prescription:** USA: Yes **Controlled Drug:** USA: No; Canada: Yes **Available as Generic:** USA: No; Canada: No

Brand Names: Indinavir: Crixivan; Nelfinavir: Viracept; Ritonavir: Norvir; Saquinavir: Invirase, Fortovase

BENEFITS versus RISKS	
Possible Benefits	*Possible Risks*
INCREASED CD4 COUNTS	SERIOUS CHANGES IN INSULIN
DECREASED OPPORTUNISTIC	LEVELS TO KETOACIDOSIS
INFECTIONS	SERIOUS INCREASES IN
EFFECTIVE COMBINATION	CHOLESTEROL
THERAPY OF HIV	Increased liver function tests
DECREASES HIV TO	Kidney stones (indinavir)
UNDETECTABLE LEVELS WITH	
EARLY THERAPY	

▷ **Principal Uses**

As a Single Drug Product: Uses currently included in FDA-approved labeling: Treatment of HIV infection when antiretroviral therapy is indicated.

Author's Note: *The Panel on Clinical Practices for Treatment of HIV Infection Report* says that the preferred regimen is two nucleoside analogs and one potent protease inhibitor. Single-agent therapy is not recommended. Indinavir received traditional FDA approval in 1998.

Other (unlabeled) generally accepted uses: (1) Combination therapy of HIV infection; (2) use in making HIV infection undetectable with combination therapy.

How These Drugs Work: They inhibit HIV reproduction (replication) by inhibiting an HIV enzyme (protease), which blocks the ability of the virus to make mature, infectious virus particles.

Available Dose Forms and Strengths

Indinvair:

Capsules — 200 mg, 400 mg

Nelfinavir:

Oral powder — 50 mg per gram

Tablet — 250 mg

Ritonavir:

Capsule — 100 mg

Oral solution — 80 mg per ml

Saquinavir:

(Invirase) Gelcap — 200 mg

(Fortovase) Gelcap — 200 mg

Author's Note: This profile will give Fortovase data.

▷ **Recommended Dose Ranges** (Actual dose and schedule must be determined for each patient individually.)

Infants and Children: Safety and efficacy are not established.

18 to 60 Years of Age: Indinavir: 800 mg by mouth every 8 hours (12-hour dosing is investigational).

Nelfinavir: 750 mg every 8 hours (12-hour dosing is being studied).

Ritonavir: 600 mg twice daily.

Saquinavir: 1200 mg three times daily.

Over 65 Years of Age: These drugs have **not** been specifically studied in those over 65.

Conditions Requiring Dosing Adjustments

Liver Function: Indinavir: The dose should be decreased to 600 mg by mouth every 8 hours in mild to moderate liver failure.

Nelfinavir, ritonavir, and saquinavir: Have not been studied in liver disease, but caution is advised as much of the drug is removed by the liver.

Kidney Function: Indinavir, nelfinavir, ritonavir and saquinavir: Dosing changes are not thought to be needed.

▷ **Dosing Instructions:** Indinavir: This drug is best taken on an empty stomach, but may be taken with a light meal, such as dry toast with jelly, apple juice, or coffee. Nelfinavir, ritonavir and saquinavir should be taken with a meal or light snack. IT IS CRITICAL THAT PROTEASE INHIBITORS DOSES NOT BE MISSED, as resistance may develop. Since case reports of altered blood sugar have been made, knowledge of signs and symptoms of high blood sugar or ketoacidosis and periodic checks of blood sugar appear prudent.

Usual Duration of Use: Use on a regular schedule for several months usually determines effectiveness in lowering the viral burden to nondetectable levels. The lowest level of viral burden, the 12-week level of viral burden, and adherence are key factors in long-term results. Long-term use (months to years) requires periodic physician evaluation of response (viral burden and CD4).

Possible Advantages of These Drugs
> May have a role in eradicating HIV.
>
> Part of a combination regimen (AZT, lamivudine, and indinavir) that lowered viral burden to nondetectable levels in many patients in one study. Favorable profile for combination therapy (except ritonavir because its many adverse drug interactions).

▷ **These Drugs Should Not Be Taken If**
- you had an allergic reaction to any dose form.

▷ **Inform Your Physician Before Taking These Drugs If**
- you have diabetes or a history of blood sugar regulation problems.
- you have elevated cholesterol or lipids.
- you have had kidney stones previously.
- you have kidney or liver compromise.
- You have phenylketonuria (nelfinavir powder has 11.2 mg of phenylalanine in each gram).
- you have had adverse reactions to other protease inhibitors.
- you are unsure how much to take or how often to take them.

Possible Side Effects (natural, expected, and unavoidable drug actions)
> Rare kidney stones (indinavir). Increased liver function tests.

▷ **Possible Adverse Effects** (unusual, unexpected, and infrequent reactions)
> **If any of the following develop, consult your physician promptly for guidance.**
>
> *Mild Adverse Effects*
> Allergic reactions: skin rash.
> Headache or dizziness—rare to infrequent.
> Weakness—infrequent.
> Blurred vision—rare.
> Chills, fever, or sweating—rare to infrequent.
> Nausea and vomiting or abdominal pain—infrequent to frequent.
> Palpitations—rare.
> Joint pain—rare.
> Tingling around the mouth (paresthesias)—frequent for ritonavir.
> Diarrhea—infrequent to frequent.
>
> *Serious Adverse Effects*
> Allergic reactions: not reported.
> Anemia or spleen disorder—rare (indinavir, ritonavir and saquinavir).
> Kidney stones—infrequent (indinavir).
> Changes in insulin levels (increased blood sugar [hyperglycemia]—or ketoacidosis)—84 case reports for the protease inhibitors.
> Increased cholesterol—many case reports.
> Increased bleeding risk (nelfinavir).

▷ **Possible Effects on Sexual Function:** Rare reports of premenstrual syndrome in some early studies.

Possible Delayed Adverse Effects: Kidney stones (indinavir). Blood sugar problems (low blood sugar or ketoacidosis) or cholesterol changes.

▷ **Adverse Effects That May Mimic Natural Diseases or Disorders**
> Increased liver function tests may mimic hepatitis. Changes in insulin levels may mimic diabetes.

Possible Effects on Laboratory Tests

Liver function tests: increased.

Complete blood counts: decreased red blood cells and hematocrit.

Insulin levels: lowered.

Blood sugar (glucose): increased.

Cholesterol: significantly increased.

CAUTION

1. Serious increases in cholesterol (lipids) have been reported.
2. Serious increases in blood sugar has been reported in 84 case reports to date for protease inhibitors. This effect has been seen on average after 76 days of therapy, but has also been reported after as little as 4 days of treatment with protease inhibitors.
3. Make certain you know high blood sugar (hyperglycemia) and ketoacidosis signs and symptoms if you are taking this medicine. Blood sugar problems have been reported for protease inhibitors.
4. These medicines may decrease the amount of virus in your body, but the virus can still be spread to others through sexual contact or blood contamination.
5. Promptly report flank pain or blood in the urine; this could indicate a kidney stone.
6. Periodic measures of viral load and CD4 are critical to make certain therapy is still working.
7. IT IS CRITICAL to take these medicines exactly as directed to get the best results.
8. Ritonavir (Norvir) has MANY drug interactions. Ask your pharmacist to check the most current list.

Precautions for Use

By Infants and Children: Safety and effectiveness not fully established.

By Those Over 65 Years of Age: Not been studied in this age group.

▷ **Advisability of Use During Pregnancy**

Pregnancy Category: Nelfinavir, ritonavir and saquinavir—B, Indinavir—C. See Pregnancy Risk Categories at the back of this book.

Animal studies: Clinical doses in rats and rabbits have not revealed teratogenicity.

Human studies: Adequate studies of pregnant women are not available. Ask your doctor for help.

Advisability of Use If Breast-Feeding

Presence of this drug in breast milk: Yes, in rats (indinavir). Unknown: nelfinavir, ritonavir, and saquinavir.

Refrain from nursing if you are HIV-positive or are taking this drug. Breast milk may also transfer the AIDS virus from mother to infant.

Habit-Forming Potential: None.

Effects of Overdose: Indinavir: No human data are available. Doses of 20 times the human dose in rats and 10 times the human dose in mice were not lethal for indinavir.

Possible Effects of Long-Term Use: Resistance may develop.

Suggested Periodic Examinations While Taking These Drugs (at physician's discretion)

Liver function tests, complete blood counts.

CD4 or viral load measurement.

Measurement of blood sugar (glucose), especially for those with prior blood sugar problems or patients who show signs or symptoms of hyperglycemia or ketoacidosis.

Measurement of cholesterol and fractions before starting therapy and periodically while taking these medicines.

▷ **While Taking These Drugs, Observe the Following**

Foods: If indinavir is taken with a meal high in fat, calories, or protein, a 77–91% decrease in the total amount of drug absorbed has been reported. The other medicines in this class are better absorbed if taken with food.

Beverages: No restrictions.

▷ *Alcohol:* No interactions expected.

Tobacco Smoking: No interactions expected. I advise everyone to quit smoking.

▷ *Other Drugs:*

These medicines *taken concurrently* with

- amiodarone (Codarone) increases heart toxicity risk.
- astemizole (Hismanal) may cause serious toxicity. DO NOT COMBINE.
- bupropion (Wellbutrin) increases seizure risk with ritonavir.
- carbamazepine (Tegretol) decreases protease inhibitor levels.
- diltiazem (Cardizem) may lead to diltiazem toxicity (ritonavir only).
- cimetidine (Tagamet) may lead to cimetidine toxicity (ritonavir) only.
- cisapride (Propulsid) may cause serious toxicity. DO NOT COMBINE.
- didanosine (Videx) may blunt therapeutic benefits. Separate doses by 1 hour.
- ergot derivatives (see Drug Classes) may lead to toxicity with nelfinavir or saquinavir.
- felodipine (Plendil) combined with ritonavir or saquinavir may lead to felodipine toxicity.
- fluvastatin (Lescol) and other HMG-CoA reductase inhibitors removed by the liver may lead to HMG-CoA toxicity (ritonavir only).
- fluvoxamine (Luvox) may lead to fluvoxamine toxicity (ritonavir only).
- ibuprofen (Motrin, others) and other NSAIDS may lead to ibuprofen or other NSAID toxicity (ritonavir only).
- itraconazole (Sporonox) or ketoconazole (Nizoral) may cause indinavir toxicity. Doses of indinavir may need to be reduced.

Combination with ritonavir may lead to itraconazole or ketoconazole toxicity.

- midazolam (Versed) may cause serious toxicity. DO NOT COMBINE.
- narcotics such as morphine (MS Contin) or methadone (Dolophine) may lead to toxic narcotic levels.
- nevirapine (Viramune) may blunt therapeutic indinavir. DO NOT COMBINE.
- birth control pills (oral contraceptives) may lead to low birth control levels and pregnancy.
- oral antidiabetics may lead to excessive lowering of blood sugar (ritonavir only).
- other antiretrovirals may reduce viral load to nondetectable levels and may also interact badly (ritonavir lowers nelfinavir levels while indinavir increases nelfinavir or saquinavir levels).

- other drugs that are toxic to the liver may result in additive toxicity.
- other drugs that can lead to kidney stones may result in additive risk with indinavir.
- phenytoin (Dilantin) may lower protease benefits.
- rifabutin (Mycobutin) may increase rifabutin and decrease indinavir levels. Half the usual dose of rifabutin is used if these drugs are combined.
- rifampin (Rifater, others) may cause loss of indinavir's benefits. DO NOT COMBINE.
- terfenadine (Seldane) may cause serious toxicity. DO NOT COMBINE.
- triazolam (Halcion) and perhaps other benzodiazepines may cause serious toxicity.
- warfarin (Coumadin) may increase risk of bleeding.
- zolpidem (Ambien) may reach toxic levels if combined with ritonavir.

▷ *Driving, Hazardous Activities:* These drugs may rarely cause sleepiness. Restrict activities as necessary.

Aviation Note: The use of these drugs *may be a disqualification* for piloting. Consult a designated aviation medical examiner.

Exposure to Sun: No restrictions.

Discontinuation: Do not stop these drugs without your doctor's knowledge and guidance.

PROTRIPTYLINE (proh TRIP ti leen)

Introduced: 1966   **Class:** Antidepressant   **Prescription:** USA: Yes
Controlled Drug: USA: No; Canada: No   **Available as Generic:** USA: Yes; Canada: No
Brand Names: ✦Triptil, Vivactil

BENEFITS versus RISKS	
Possible Benefits	*Possible Risks*
EFFECTIVE RELIEF OF MAJOR ENDOGENOUS DEPRESSIONS	ADVERSE BEHAVIORAL EFFECTS: confusion, disorientation, hallucinations, delusions
HELPS MANAGE OTHER DEPRESSIVE DISORDERS	CONVERSION OF DEPRESSION TO MANIA in manic-depressive (bipolar) disorders
Possibly beneficial in the management of attention deficit disorder and of narcolepsy/cataplexy syndrome	Aggravation of schizophrenia
	Irregular heart rhythms
	Blood cell abnormalities

▷ **Principal Uses**

As a Single Drug Product: Uses currently included in FDA-approved labeling: Relieves symptoms associated with major spontaneous (endogenous) depression, depressed bipolar disorder, and mixed bipolar disorder.

Other (unlabeled) generally accepted uses: (1) Treatment of sleep disorders such as apnea, hypersomnia, and impaired morning arousal; (2) may have a role in treating glaucoma; (3) used in combination with methylphenidate or amphetamines in treating narcolepsy.

How This Drug Works: It is thought that this drug relieves depression by slowly restoring to normal levels certain constituents of brain tissue (norepinephrine and serotonin) that transmit nerve impulses.

Available Dose Forms and Strengths
>   Tablets — 5 mg, 10 mg

▷ **Recommended Dose Ranges (Actual dose and schedule must be determined for each patient individually.)**
Infants and Children: Dose not established.
12 to 60 Years of Age: For depression: Initially 5 to 10 mg, three or four times daily. The dose is increased cautiously as needed and tolerated by 5 mg daily at intervals of 1 week. The usual maintenance dose is 15 to 40 mg a day, divided into three or four doses. The total daily dose should not exceed 60 mg.
Over 60 Years of Age: Initially 5 mg, two or three times daily to evaluate tolerance. Increase dose cautiously as needed and tolerated by 5 mg daily at intervals of 1 week. Doses above 20 mg daily require careful monitoring of heart function and blood pressure. The total daily dose should not exceed 40 mg.

Conditions Requiring Dosing Adjustments
Liver Function: The dose should be empirically decreased, and blood levels obtained at appropriate intervals. Protriptyline is a rare cause of hepatotoxicity.
Kidney Function: The kidney plays a minor role in the elimination of this drug.

▷ **Dosing Instructions:** The tablet may be crushed and taken without regard to meals. If a stimulating effect occurs: (1) necessary dose increases should be made in the morning; (2) the last daily dose should be taken in the afternoon (3 to 4 P.M.) to avoid insomnia and disturbed dreaming.

Author's note: The information in this profile has been shortened to make room for more widely used medicines.

PYRAZINAMIDE (peer a ZIN a mide)

Introduced: 1968 **Class:** Anti-infective, antituberculosis drug **Prescription:** USA: Yes **Controlled Drug:** USA: No; Canada: No **Available as Generic:** USA: Yes; Canada: No
Brand Names: ✸PMS Pyrazinamide, Rifater, ✸Tebrazid

BENEFITS versus RISKS	
Possible Benefits	*Possible Risks*
EFFECTIVE ADJUNCTIVE TREATMENT OF TUBERCULOSIS	DRUG-INDUCED HEPATITIS—rare
	Activation of gouty arthritis and porphyria
	Decreased platelets and hemoglobin

▷ **Principal Uses**
As a Single Drug Product: Uses currently included in FDA-approved labeling: Treatment of active tuberculosis, in combination with other antitubercular drugs.
Other (unlabeled) generally accepted uses: (1) Combination therapy of *My-*

cobacterium xenopi infections; (2) combination therapy of resistant tuberculosis; (3) combination therapy of tuberculosis in AIDS.

As a Combination Drug Product [CD]: This medicine is combined with two other
antituberculosis medicines(isoniazid and rifampin) in order to attack tuberculosis with combination treatment with a single dose form.

How This Drug Works: This drug is ideal for killing tuberculosis organisms
that are in acid environments, such as in some kinds of white blood (macrophages) cells.

Available Dose Forms and Strengths
Tablets — 500 mg

▷ **Recommended Dose Ranges** (Actual dose and schedule must be determined for
each patient individually.)

Infants and Children: 7.5 to 15 mg per kg of body mass, twice daily; or 15 to
30 mg per kg of body mass, once daily. Total daily dose should not exceed
1.5 g.

12 to 60 Years of Age: For tuberculosis—15 to 30 mg per kg of body mass (up to
a maximum of 2000 mg) daily. Some patients do better with twice-weekly
dosing: 50 to 70 mg per kg of body mass (up to 4000 mg).

**Author's Note: Because of the current resistant tuberculosis problem,
most clinicians start all patients on a four-drug regimen until laboratory culture results are available.**

Over 60 Years of Age: Same as 12 to 60 years of age.

Conditions Requiring Dosing Adjustments

Liver Function: This drug should be used with caution and in decreased doses
by patients with liver compromise. Contraindicated in patients with severe
liver dysfunction.

Kidney Function: For patients with endstage renal failure, the dose **must** be adjusted. One researcher recommends 60 mg per kg of body mass, twice
weekly. The dose of pyrazinamide should be given at least 24 hours before
any given dialysis session. Patients should be closely monitored.

▷ **Dosing Instructions:**   The tablet may be crushed and taken with or following
food to reduce stomach irritation. Take the full course prescribed. This drug
should be taken concurrently with other antitubercular drugs to prevent the
development of drug-resistant strains of tuberculosis bacteria.

Usual Duration of Use: Use on a regular schedule for 2 months usually determines effectiveness in controlling active tuberculosis. Long-term use of antitubercular drugs (6 months) requires periodic physician evaluation.

Possible Advantages of This Drug
May reduce the period of drug treatment from 9 to 6 months in responsive infections.

▷ **This Drug Should Not Be Taken If**
- you have had an allergic reaction to it previously.
- you have permanent liver damage with impaired function.
- you have active gout.
- you have active peptic ulcer disease.

▷ **Inform Your Physician Before Taking This Drug If**
- you have had an allergic reaction to ethionamide, isoniazid, or niacin (nicotinic acid).

- you have a history of liver disease.
- you have a history of peptic ulcer or porphyria.
- you tried to take medicines for tuberculosis before, but did not complete the prescribed therapy.
- you have gout or diabetes.
- you have impaired kidney function.

Possible Side Effects (natural, expected, and unavoidable drug actions)
Increased blood uric acid levels. Fever.

▷ **Possible Adverse Effects** (unusual, unexpected, and infrequent reactions)
If any of the following develop, consult your physician promptly for guidance.

Mild Adverse Effects
Allergic reactions: skin rash, itching, fever.
Loss of appetite, mild nausea, vomiting—frequent.
Joint pain—frequent.
Acne—rare.

Serious Adverse Effects
Idiosyncratic reactions: rare sideroblastic anemia.
Decreased blood platelets—rare.
Seizures—rare.
Drug-induced porphyria or pellagra—case reports.
Kidney problems (interstitial nephritis)—case reports.
Drug-induced hepatitis, with and without jaundice (see Glossary)—case reports.
Gouty arthritis, due to increased blood uric acid levels—possible.

▷ **Possible Effects on Sexual Function:** None reported.

▷ **Adverse Effects That May Mimic Natural Diseases or Disorders**
Drug-induced hepatitis may suggest viral hepatitis.

Natural Diseases or Disorders That May Be Activated by This Drug
Gout, peptic ulcer, porphyria.

Possible Effects on Laboratory Tests
Complete blood cell counts: decreased red cells, hemoglobin, and platelets.
INR (prothrombin time): increased.
Blood uric acid level: increased.
Liver function tests: increased enzymes (ALT/GPT, AST/GOT, alkaline phosphatase), or bilirubin.
Urine ketone tests: false-positive test result with Acetest and Ketostix.

CAUTION
1. When this drug is used alone, tuberculosis bacteria rapidly develop resistance to it. To be effective, this drug must be used in combination with other effective antitubercular drugs, such as isoniazid and rifampin.
2. This drug may interfere with control of diabetes.

Precautions for Use
By Infants and Children: Safety and effectiveness for those under 12 years of age are not established. The rare occurrence of drug-related seizure has been reported in a 2-year-old child.
By Those Over 60 Years of Age: No specific information available.

▷ **Advisability of Use During Pregnancy**

Pregnancy Category: C. See Pregnancy Risk Categories at the back of this book.

Animal studies: No information available.

Human studies: Adequate studies of pregnant women are not available.

Use this drug only if clearly needed. Ask your physician for guidance.

Advisability of Use If Breast-Feeding

Presence of this drug in breast milk: Yes.

Avoid drug or refrain from nursing.

Habit-Forming Potential: None.

Effects of Overdose: Nausea, vomiting, malaise.

Possible Effects of Long-Term Use: Liver damage.

Suggested Periodic Examinations While Taking This Drug (at physician's discretion)

Complete blood cell counts.

Liver function tests.

Uric acid blood levels.

▷ **While Taking This Drug, Observe the Following**

Foods: No restrictions.

Beverages: No restrictions. May be taken with milk.

▷ *Alcohol:* Use sparingly to minimize liver toxicity.

Tobacco Smoking: No interactions expected. I advise everyone to quit smoking.

▷ *Other Drugs:*

Pyrazinamide may *decrease* the effects of

- allopurinol (Zyloprim).
- BCG vaccine.
- cyclosporine (Sandimmune).
- probenecid (Benemid).
- sulfinpyrazone (Anturane).

Pyrazinamide *taken concurrently* with

- phenytoin (Dilantin) may lead to phenytoin toxicity.
- zidovudine (AZT) may lead to low pyrazinamide levels.

▷ *Driving, Hazardous Activities:* No restrictions.

Aviation Note: The use of this drug is probably *not a disqualification* for piloting. Consult a designated aviation medical examiner.

Exposure to Sun: Use caution—this drug may cause photosensitivity (see Glossary).

Discontinuation: If tolerated, this drug is usually taken for a minimum of 2 months. Do not stop it without your physician's knowledge and guidance.

PYRIDOSTIGMINE (peer id oh STIG meen)

Introduced: 1962   **Class:** Anti-myasthenic   **Prescription:** USA: Yes
Controlled Drug: USA: No; Canada: No   **Available as Generic:** USA: No;
Canada: No

Brand Names: ♣Anaplex SR, Mestinon, Mestinon-SR, Mestinon Timespan, Regonol

---

BENEFITS versus RISKS

Possible Benefits	*Possible Risks*
MODERATELY EFFECTIVE TREATMENT OF OCULAR AND MILD FORMS OF MYASTHENIA GRAVIS (symptomatic relief of muscle weakness)	Cholinergic crisis (overdose): excessive salivation, nausea, vomiting, stomach cramps, diarrhea, shortness of breath (asthma-like wheezing), excessive weakness

---

▷ **Principal Uses**

As a Single Drug Product: Uses currently included in FDA-approved labeling: (1) Used to treat the ocular and milder forms of myasthenia gravis by providing temporary relief of muscle weakness and fatigability (most useful in long-term treatment when there is little or no swallowing difficulty); (2) used to reverse muscle relaxants.

Other (unlabeled) generally accepted uses: (1) Combination therapy in chronic pain; (2) may help in combination therapy of Huntington's chorea and Lambert-Eaton syndrome; (3) adjunctive use with scopolamine to prevent side effects of scopolamine in treating motion sickness; (4) used in war zones to treat the effects of nerve gas; (5) may have a role in treating nonepidemic parotitis.

How This Drug Works: This drug inhibits cholinesterase, the enzyme that destroys acetylcholine. This results in higher levels of acetylcholine, the nerve transmitter that facilitates the stimulation of muscular activity. The net effects are increased muscle strength and endurance.

Available Dose Forms and Strengths

Syrup — 60 mg/5 ml (5% alcohol)
Tablets — 30 mg, 60 mg
Tablets, prolonged action — 180 mg

▷ **Usual Adult Dose Range:** Myasthenia gravis: Initially one to six normal-release tablets, spaced throughout the day when maximum strength is needed. Maintenance varies with the severity of the disease: one to three extended-release tablets taken every 6 hours. Some patients may need to supplement the extended-release tablets with the 30-mg, immediate-release tablets or the syrup in order to best control symptoms.

Nerve gas or agent protection: 30 mg every 8 hours when the threat of a nerve agent attack is present.

Note: Actual dose and schedule must be determined for each patient individually.

Conditions Requiring Dosing Adjustments

Liver Function: No dosing changes are defined in liver compromise.

Kidney Function: This drug is primarily eliminated in the urine; however, specific guidelines for dose adjustments in renal compromise are not available.

▷ **Dosing Instructions:** Take with food or milk to reduce the intensity of side effects. Larger portions of the daily maintenance dose should be timed according to the pattern of fatigue and weakness. The syrup will permit a finer adjustment of dose. The regular tablet may be crushed. Prolonged-action tablet should be taken whole (not altered).

Usual Duration of Use: Use on a regular schedule (with dose adjustment) for 10 to 14 days usually determines effectiveness in relieving myasthenia symptoms. Long-term use (months to years) requires periodic physician evaluation.

▷ **This Drug Should Not Be Taken If**
  • you are known to be allergic to bromide compounds.
  • you have a urinary obstruction or mechanical intestinal obstruction.

▷ **Inform Your Physician Before Taking This Drug If**
  • you have heart rhythm disorders or bronchial asthma.
  • you are sensitive to bromides.
  • you have recurrent urinary tract infections.
  • you have prostatism (see Glossary).
  • you will have surgery with general anesthesia.

Possible Side Effects (natural, expected, and unavoidable drug actions)
  Small pupils (miosis), watering of eyes, slow pulse, excessive salivation, nausea, vomiting, stomach cramps, diarrhea, urge to urinate, increased sweating, increased bronchial secretions.

▷ **Possible Adverse Effects** (unusual, unexpected, and infrequent reactions)
  If any of the following develop, consult your physician promptly for guidance.
  Mild Adverse Effects
  Allergic reactions: skin rash.
  Nervousness, anxiety, unsteadiness, muscle cramps or twitching—infrequent.
  Loss of scalp hair (alopecia)—case report.
  Serious Adverse Effects
  Confusion, slurred speech, seizures, difficult breathing (asthmatic wheezing).
  Increased muscle weakness or paralysis—case report.
  Psychosis—rare.
  Excessive vomiting or diarrhea may cause low potassium levels (hypokalemia). This accentuates muscle weakness.

▷ **Possible Effects on Sexual Function:**   None reported.

▷ **Adverse Effects That May Mimic Natural Diseases or Disorders**
  Seizures may suggest the possibility of epilepsy.

Natural Diseases or Disorders That May Be Activated by This Drug
  Latent bronchial asthma.

Possible Effects on Laboratory Tests
  None reported.

CAUTION
  1. Some drugs block this drug, reducing effectiveness in treating myasthenia gravis (see "Other Drugs" below). Ask your doctor before starting any other medicine.
  2. Variations in response may occur from time to time. Because generalized muscle weakness is a major symptom of both myasthenia crisis (underdose) and cholinergic crisis (overdose), it may be difficult to recognize the correct cause. As a rule, weakness that starts an hour after taking this drug probably represents overdose; weakness that begins 3 or more hours after taking this drug is probably due to underdose. Watch these relationships and tell your doctor.

3. During long-term use, watch for development of resistance to the therapeutic action (loss of effect). Ask your doctor if the drug should be stopped for a few days to see if response can be restored.

Precautions for Use

By Infants and Children: The syrup form of this drug permits greater precision of dose adjustment and ease of administration in this age group. Neonates have received 5 mg every 4 to 6 hours. Since this is often self-limiting in neonates, the medicine can frequently be tapered and stopped.

By Those Over 60 Years of Age: The natural decline of kidney function with aging may require smaller doses to prevent accumulation of this drug to toxic levels.

▷ **Advisability of Use During Pregnancy**

Pregnancy Category: C. See Pregnancy Risk Categories at the back of this book. Animal studies: No information available.

Human studies: Adequate studies of pregnant women are not available.

There are no reports of birth defects due to the use of this drug during pregnancy. However, there are reports of significant muscular weakness in newborn infants whose mothers had taken this drug during pregnancy. Ask your physician for guidance.

Advisability of Use If Breast-Feeding

Presence of this drug in breast milk: Yes, as roughly 0.01% of the mother's dose. Monitor nursing infant closely and discontinue drug or nursing if adverse effects develop.

Habit-Forming Potential: None.

Effects of Overdose: Generalized muscular weakness, blurred vision, very small pupils, slow heart rate, difficult breathing (wheezing), excessive salivation, nausea, vomiting, stomach cramps, diarrhea, muscle cramps or twitching. This syndrome constitutes the cholinergic crisis.

Possible Effects of Long-Term Use: Development of tolerance (see Glossary) with loss of therapeutic effectiveness.

Suggested Periodic Examinations While Taking This Drug (at physician's discretion)

Assessment of drug effectiveness and dose schedule for optimal therapeutic results.

▷ **While Taking This Drug, Observe the Following**

Foods: No restrictions.

Beverages: No restrictions. May be taken with milk.

▷ *Alcohol:* Use caution until the combined effects are determined. Weakness and unsteadiness may be accentuated.

Tobacco Smoking: No interactions expected. I advise everyone to quit smoking.

▷ *Other Drugs:*

Pyridostigmine *taken concurrently* with

• disopyramide (Norpace) may help the decreased sweating, difficulty urinating, and other anticholinergic effects.

The following drugs may *decrease* the effects of pyridostigmine:

• adrenocortical steroids (see Drug Classes).

• atropine (belladonna).

• clindamycin (Cleocin).

- guanadrel (Hylorel).
- guanethidine (Esimil, Ismelin).
- procainamide (Procan SR, Pronestyl).
- quinidine (Cardioquin, Duraquin, etc.).
- quinine (Quinamm).

▷ *Driving, Hazardous Activities:* This drug may cause blurred vision, confusion, or generalized weakness. Restrict activities as necessary.

Aviation Note: The use of this drug *is a disqualification* for piloting. Consult a designated aviation medical examiner.

Exposure to Sun: No restrictions.

Exposure to Heat: Use caution—this drug may cause excessive sweating and increased weakness.

Exposure to Environmental Chemicals: Avoid excessive exposure (inhalation, skin contamination) to the insecticides Baygon, Diazinon, and Sevin. These can worsen potential drug toxicity.

Discontinuation: Do not stop this drug abruptly without your doctor's knowledge and guidance.

QUAZEPAM (KWAH zee pam)

Introduced: 1982   **Class:** Hypnotic, benzodiazepines   **Prescription:** USA: Yes   **Controlled Drug:** USA: C-IV*
Available as Generic: USA: No
Brand Names: Doral, Dormalin
Author's Note: The National Institute of Mental Health has a new information page on anxiety. It can be found on the World Wide Web at www.nimh.nih.gov/anxiety. The information in this profile has been abbreviated to make room for more widely used medicines.

QUINAPRIL (KWIN a pril)

Introduced: 1984   **Class:** Antihypertensive, ACE inhibitor
Please see the new angiotensin-converting enzyme (ACE) inhibitor combination profile for more information.

QUINIDINE (KWIN i deen)

Introduced: 1918   **Class:** Antiarrhythmic   **Prescription:** USA: Yes
Controlled Drug: Canada: No; USA: No   **Available as Generic:** Yes
Brand Names: ✦Apo-Quinidine, ✦Biquin Durules, Cardioquin, Cin-Quin, Duraquin, ✦Natisedine, ✦Novoquinidine, Quinaglute Dura-Tabs, ✦Quinate, Quinatime, Quinidex Extentabs, ✦Quinobarb [CD]*, Quinora, Quin-Release, SK-Quinidine sulfate

---

*See Controlled Drug Schedules at the back of this book.
*Quinobarb contains phenylethylbarbiturate, a sedative of the barbiturate class.

```
BENEFITS versus RISKS
```

Possible Benefits	Possible Risks
EFFECTIVE TREATMENT OF SELECTED HEART RHYTHM DISORDERS	NARROW TREATMENT RANGE FREQUENT ADVERSE EFFECTS NUMEROUS ALLERGIC AND IDIOSYNCRATIC REACTIONS Dose-related toxicity Provocation of abnormal heart rhythms Abnormally low blood platelet count Hemolytic anemia Kidney or liver toxicity

▷ **Principal Uses**

As a Single Drug Product: Uses currently included in FDA-approved labeling: (1) Helps control the following types of abnormal heart rhythm: atrial fibrillation and flutter, paroxysmal atrial tachycardia, paroxysmal ventricular tachycardia, premature atrial and ventricular contractions; (2) intravenous treatment of malaria in people who cannot take medicine by mouth.

Other (unlabeled) generally accepted uses: None.

As a Combination Drug Product [CD]: This drug is available (in Canada) in combination with a barbiturate, a mild sedative that is added to allay the anxiety and nervous tension that often accompany heart rhythm disorders.

How This Drug Works: Slows activity of the heart pacemaker and delays electrical impulses through the heart conduction system, restoring normal heart rate and rhythm.

Available Dose Forms and Strengths

Capsules — 200 mg, 300 mg
Injections — 80 mg/ml, 200 mg/ml
Tablets — 100 mg, 200 mg, 275 mg, 300 mg
Tablets, prolonged action — 250 mg, 300 mg, 324 mg, 330 mg

▷ **Usual Adult Dose Range:** Premature atrial or ventricular contractions: 200 to 400 mg every 4 to 6 hours.

Paroxysmal atrial tachycardia: 400 to 600 mg every 2 to 3 hours until paroxysm is terminated.

Atrial flutter: Digitalize first; then individualize dose schedule as appropriate.

Atrial fibrillation: Digitalize first; then try 200 mg every 2 to 3 hours for five to eight doses; increase dose daily until normal rhythm is restored or toxic effects develop.

Maintenance schedule: 200 to 300 mg three or four times daily. Total daily dose should not exceed 4000 mg.

Note: Actual dose and schedule must be determined for each patient individually.

Conditions Requiring Dosing Adjustments

Liver Function: This drug is extensively metabolized in the liver. Blood levels should be obtained to guide dosing. A larger loading dose and a 50% decreased maintenance dose may be indicated.

Kidney Function: Blood levels should be obtained, and used to guide dosing. Quinidine should be used with caution in renal compromise.

▷ **Dosing Instructions:**   This drug is preferably taken on an empty stomach to achieve high blood levels rapidly. However, it may be taken with or following food to reduce stomach irritation. The regular tablets may be crushed and the capsules opened. Prolonged-action forms should be swallowed whole without alteration.

Usual Duration of Use: Use on a regular schedule for 2 to 4 days usually determines effectiveness in correcting or preventing responsive abnormal rhythms. Long-term use (months to years) requires physician supervision and periodic evaluation.

▷ **This Drug Should Not Be Taken If**
- you have had an allergic or idiosyncratic reaction to it previously.
- you currently have an acute infection of any kind.
- you have taken too much digoxin (digoxin toxicity).
- you have myasthenia gravis.
- you have abnormal heart rhythms caused by an escape mechanism (ask your specialist).

▷ **Inform Your Physician Before Taking This Drug If**
- you have coronary artery disease or myasthenia gravis.
- you have a history of excessive thyroid function (hyperthyroidism).
- you usually have very low blood pressure.
- you have had a deficiency of blood platelets in the past from any cause.
- you are now taking, or have taken recently, any digitalis preparation (digitoxin, digoxin, etc.).
- you will have surgery with general anesthesia.
- you have acute rheumatic fever or subacute bacterial endocarditis (SBE).

Possible Side Effects (natural, expected, and unavoidable drug actions)
Drop in blood pressure—may be marked in some patients and cause passing out (syncope).

▷ **Possible Adverse Effects** (unusual, unexpected, and infrequent reactions)
If any of the following develop, consult your physician promptly for guidance.

Mild Adverse Effects
Allergic reactions: skin rash, hives, itching, drug fever—rare.
Irritation of the esophagus (esophagitis)—possible.
Nausea, vomiting, diarrhea—infrequent.

Serious Adverse Effects
Allergic reactions: severe skin reactions, hemolytic anemia (see Glossary), joint and muscle pains, anaphylactic reaction (see Glossary), reduced blood platelet count, drug-induced hepatitis-like reaction (see Glossary).
Idiosyncratic reactions: skin rash, fast heart rate, delirium, difficult breathing.
Dose-related toxicity (cinchonism): blurred vision, ringing ears, hearing loss, heart arrest.
Drug-induced myasthenia gravis, systemic lupus erythematosus (SLE), or carpal tunnel syndrome—case reports.
Swelling of the lymph glands in the inguinal area (lymphadenopathy)—case report.
Kidney toxicity—case reports.
Heart conduction abnormalities—case reports.
Optic neuritis, impaired vision—case report.

Abnormally low white blood cell count: fever, sore throat, infections—case reports.

Abnormally low platelet count—case reports.

▷ **Possible Effects on Sexual Function:**   None reported.

▷ **Adverse Effects That May Mimic Natural Diseases or Disorders**
Drug-induced hepatitis may suggest viral hepatitis.

Natural Diseases or Disorders That May Be Activated by This Drug
Systemic lupus erythematosus, myasthenia gravis, psoriasis (in sensitive individuals).

Possible Effects on Laboratory Tests
Complete blood cell counts: decreased red cells, hemoglobin, white cells, and platelets; increased eosinophils (allergic reaction); marked increase of white blood cells in association with "quinidine fever"—very rare.

Antinuclear antibodies (ANA): positive.

INR (protime): increased (when taken concurrently with warfarin).

Liver function tests: increased enzymes (ALT/GPT, AST/GOT, alkaline phosphatase) or bilirubin.

CAUTION
1. Dose adjustments must be based upon individual reaction.
2. Prudent to carry a card noting that you take this drug.

Precautions for Use
By Infants and Children: A test for drug idiosyncrasy should be made before starting treatment with this drug. If there is no beneficial response after 3 days of adequate dose, this drug should be discontinued.

By Those Over 60 Years of Age: Small doses are mandatory until your individual response has been determined. Watch for the development of light-headedness, dizziness, weakness, or sense of impending faint. Use caution to prevent falls.

▷ **Advisability of Use During Pregnancy**
Pregnancy Category: C. See Pregnancy Risk Categories at the back of this book.

Animal studies: No information available.

Human studies: Adequate studies of pregnant women are not available. No birth defects have been reported following use of this drug during pregnancy.

Use this drug only if clearly needed.

Advisability of Use If Breast-Feeding
· Presence of this drug in breast milk: Yes.

Avoid drug or refrain from nursing.

Habit-Forming Potential: None.

Effects of Overdose: Nausea, vomiting, ringing in the ears, headache, jerky eye movements, double vision, altered color vision, confusion, delirium, hot skin, seizures, coma.

Possible Effects of Long-Term Use: None reported.

Suggested Periodic Examinations While Taking This Drug (at physician's discretion)
Complete blood cell counts, electrocardiograms, blood levels.

▷ **While Taking This Drug, Observe the Following**

Foods: No restrictions.

Beverages: No restrictions. May be taken with milk.

▷ *Alcohol:* Use caution—alcohol may enhance the blood-pressure-lowering effects of this drug.

Tobacco Smoking: Nicotine can increase irritability of the heart and aggravate rhythm disorders. Avoid all forms of tobacco.

▷ *Other Drugs:*

Quinapril **taken concurrently** with
- aspirin may prolong the bleeding time.
- beta-blockers may result in additive and undesirable beta-blockade. Lower starting doses may be needed for both medicines.
- codeine may blunt the effectiveness of codeine.
- grepafloxacin (Raxar) or sparfloxacin (Zagam) may lead to abnormal heart beats.
- tricyclic antidepressants (see Drug Classes) may result in antidepressant toxicity.
- venlafaxine (Effexor) may result in venlafaxine toxicity.

Quinidine may **increase** the effects of
- anticoagulants (Coumadin, etc.), and increase the risk of bleeding. More frequent INR (prothrombin time or protime) testing is needed.
- digitoxin and digoxin (Lanoxin), and cause digitalis toxicity.
- disopyramide (Norpace).
- metformin (Glucophage).
- tricyclic antidepressants (doxepin).

The following drugs may **increase** the effects of quinidine:
- amiodarone (Cordarone).
- cimetidine (Tagamet).
- itraconazole (Sporonox).
- ketoconazole (Nizoral).
- ritonavir (Norvir), and perhaps other protease inhibitors (see Drug Classes). Do not combine.
- sertraline (Zoloft).
- verapamil (Verelan).

The following drugs may **decrease** the effects of quinidine:
- barbiturates (phenobarbital, etc.).
- phenytoin (Dilantin).
- rifampin (Rifadin, Rimactane).
- rifabutin (Mycobutin).
- sucralfate (Carafate).

▷ *Driving, Hazardous Activities:* This drug may cause dizziness and alter vision. Restrict activities as necessary.

Aviation Note: The use of this drug **may be a disqualification** for piloting. Consult a designated aviation medical examiner.

Exposure to Sun: Use caution—this drug may cause photosensitivity (see Glossary).

RALOXIFENE (rah LOX i feen)

Introduced: 1997   **Class:** Antiestrogen, selective estrogen receptor inhibitor (SERM), anti-osteoporosis   **Prescription:** USA: Yes   **Controlled Drug:** USA: No; Canada: No   **Available as Generic:** No
Brand Name: Evista

BENEFITS versus RISKS	
Possible Benefits	*Possible Risks*
EFFECTIVE PREVENTION OF POSTMENOPAUSAL OSTEOPOROSIS	Changes in blood clotting Hot flashes (flushes)
REDUCED LDL CHOLESTEROL	
Possible benefits on heart health (being studied)	
Possible benefits in preventing breast cancer (being studied)	

▷ **Principal Uses**

As a Single Drug Product: Uses currently included in FDA-approved labeling: Helps prevent osteoporosis in women after menopause.

Other (unlabeled) generally accepted uses: (1) May have a role in preventing cancer of the breast (two studies found a 50% decreased risk); (2) because of LDL lowering, may have a role in maintaining heart (cardiovascular) health; (3) may be used to treat osteoporosis (more study needed).

How This Drug Works: Works similar to estrogen itself on the bone (increasing bone density) and on LDL cholesterol (lowering it). (This led to the news media deeming raloxifene a designer estrogen.) May block use (uptake) of estrogen (estradiol) and remove one stimulus for breast cancer.

Available Dose Forms and Strengths

Tablets — 60 mg

▷ **Usual Adult Dose Range:**   Prevention of postmenopausal osteoporosis: 60 mg once daily. **Note: Actual dose and schedule must be determined for each patient individually.**

Conditions Requiring Dosing Adjustments

Liver Function: Extensively changed (metabolized) in the liver. Dose decreases are not yet defined in liver disease although lower doses appear prudent.

Kidney Function: Not studied in people with kidney disease or compromise.

▷ **Dosing Instructions:**   The tablet may be crushed and taken without regard to food.

Usual Duration of Use: Use in clinical trials compared two years of raloxifene use to calcium use alone. These trials used measures of bone mineral density (BMD) to check the benefits of this drug. It appears prudent to check BMD before starting this medicine, and then to recheck markers of bone turnover and BMD once the medicine has been started to make sure that it is working.

Long-term use requires physician supervision.

▷ **This Drug Should Not Be Taken If**
- you had a serious allergic or adverse reaction to it before.
- you have a history of blood clots (clot in the retinal vein, DVT or pulmonary embolism [PE]).
- you are pregnant.
- you have a history of breast cancer.

▷ **Inform Your Physician Before Taking This Drug If**
- you are taking estrogen (not studied with this drug).
- you have a history of thrombophlebitis or pulmonary embolism.
- you have impaired liver function.
- you plan to have surgery or will be immobilized (prolonged rest in bed) in the near future.
- your diet is low in calcium or vitamin D.

Possible Side Effects (natural, expected, and unavoidable drug actions)

Hot flashes—may be frequent.

▷ **Possible Adverse Effects** (unusual, unexpected, and infrequent reactions)

If any of the following develop, consult your physician promptly for guidance.

Mild Adverse Effects

Allergic reactions: skin rash.

Insomnia, migraine or depression—infrequent.

Weight gain—infrequent

Indigestion (dyspepsia), nausea or vomiting—infrequent

Cough, sinusitis or pharyngitis—infrequent.

Joint or muscle pain—infrequent.

Swelling of the ankles or wrists (edema)—infrequent.

Serious Adverse Effects

Increased uterine cancer risk was found in mice and rats. How this applies to humans is not known.

Chest pain—infrequent.

Blood clots (thromboembolism)—twofold increased risk of lung (PE) and 3.4-fold increased risk of clots in veins.

▷ **Possible Effects on Sexual Function:**   None reported.

Possible Effects on Laboratory Tests

Markers of bone turnover (bone specific alkaline phosphatase): decreased.

Bone mineral density (BMD): increased.

LDL cholesterol: decreased (a very positive result).

Liver function tests: may be increased (questionable cause).

CAUTION

1. Calcium supplements should be added to your diet if your diet does not include enough calcium. Talk to your doctor about the need for vitamin D.
2. Research has not been done combining this medicine with estrogen.
3. Ask your doctor about how to decrease risk factors for osteoporosis. Also ask about an exercise program appropriate to your degree of bone loss.
4. One researcher questioned mouse and rat data that showed raloxifene causing cancer of the ovaries in those animals. The manufacturer said that cancer in rodents did not correspond to the risk of cancer in humans.

5. Has not been studied for use in men.
6. Has not been approved for use BEFORE menopause.
7. A head-to-head trial of tamoxifen and raloxifene will start in 1998 for benefits and risks.

▷ **Advisability of Use During Pregnancy**

Pregnancy Category: X. See Pregnancy Risk Categories at the back of this book.

Human studies: Studies of pregnant women will not be done.

This drug should NOT be used during pregnancy.

Advisability of Use If Breast-Feeding

Presence of this drug in breast milk: Unknown.

Avoid drug or refrain from nursing.

Habit-Forming Potential: None.

Effects of Overdose: A dose of 600 mg was tolerated in clinical trials.

Possible Effects of Long-Term Use: Increased bone mineral density.

Suggested Periodic Examinations While Taking This Drug (at physician's discretion)

Bone mineral density (BMD) testing. Laboratory tests of bone turnover. Periodic liver function tests. Check for blood clots. **Must** have regular gynecological examinations.

▷ **While Taking This Drug, Observe the Following**

Foods: No restrictions.

Beverages: No restrictions. May be taken with milk.

▷ *Alcohol:* No interactions expected.

Tobacco Smoking: No interactions expected. I advise everyone to quit smoking.

▷ *Other Drugs:*

The following drugs may *decrease* the effects of raloxifene:

- ampicillin (Polycillin, Principen).
- ampicillin/sulbactam (Unasyn).
- cholestyramine (Questran).

Raloxifene *taken concurrently* with

- other highly protein-bound medicines (such as diazepam [Valium], indomethacin [Indocin], naproxen [Naprosyn], or others) should be done only with great caution.
- warfarin (Coumadin) may lower benefits of warfarin. Increased frequency of INR (prothrombin time or protime) testing is needed.

▷ *Driving, Hazardous Activities:* No restrictions thought to be needed.

Aviation Note: The use of this drug *is probably not a disqualification* for piloting. Consult a designated aviation medical examiner.

Exposure to Sun: No restrictions.

RAMIPRIL (ra MI pril)

Introduced: 1985   **Class:**   Antihypertensive, ACE inhibitor
Author's note: Please see the new angiotensin-converting enzyme (ACE) inhibitor family profile for more information.

RANITIDINE (ra NI te deen)

Author's Note: ALL of the four available histamine (H₂) receptor blocking drugs are now available without prescription. See the new histamine (H₂) blocking drugs profile for further information.

REPAGLINIDE (ra PAG lyn ide)

Introduced: 1998   **Class:** Antidiabetic, meglitinide   **Prescription:** USA: Yes   **Controlled Drug:** USA: No; Canada: No   **Available as Generic:** No

Brand Name: Prandin

BENEFITS versus RISKS	
Possible Benefits	*Possible Risks*
HELPS REGULATE BLOOD SUGAR in type 2 DIABETES (adjunctive to appropriate diet and weight control)	Hypoglycemia (less common than sulfonylureas)
MAY BE COMBINED WITH METFORMIN IF BLOOD SUGAR CONTROL IS NOT ACCEPTABLE	Possible increased risk of heart (cardiovascular) problems (based on a 1970 UGDP study)
Absorbed well and cleared quickly from the blood	

▷ **Principal Uses**

As a Single Drug Product: Uses currently included in FDA-approved labeling: (1) Regulates type 2 diabetes mellitus (adult, maturity-onset) that does not require insulin, but can't be adequately controlled by diet alone; (2) used in combination treatment with metformin in people who do not have an adequate blood sugar response from repaglinide alone.

Other (unlabeled) generally accepted uses: None.

How This Drug Works: Stimulates secretion of insulin (closes ATP-sensitive potassium channels in beta cells).

Available Dose Forms and Strengths

Tablets — 0.5 mg, 1 mg, 2 mg

▷ **Usual Adult Dose Range:** People with a hemoglobin A1C (HGB A1C or glycosylated hemoglobin) less than 8% or who have not been treated: 0.5 mg before meals.

Previously treated patients or those with HGB A1C more than 8%: One to two mg is given before meals. Adjustments should be made based on ongoing blood sugar and HGB A1C.

Note: Actual dose and schedule must be determined for each patient individually.

Conditions Requiring Dosing Adjustments

Liver Function: Blood levels are higher and stay longer in moderate to severe liver failure. Decreased doses and more frequent fingerstick blood sugar testing is prudent.

Kidney Function: The same starting dose is used in kidney disease or compromise.

Any subsequent dose increases should be made cautiously.

▷ *Other Drugs:*

The following drugs may ***increase*** the effects of repaglinide:
- cimetidine (Tagamet).
- erythromycins (see *macrolide antiobiotics* in Drug Classes).
- itraconazole (Sporonox).
- ketoconazole (Nizoral).
- mibefradil (Posicor) (recently removed from the US market).
- nelfinavir (Viracept), and perhaps other protease inhibitors (see Drug Classes), may increase blood levels.
- Any medicine that interferes with cytochrome (CYP3A4) will potentially increase repaglinide blood levels. In some cases, I expect that repaglinide dosing will need to be adjusted.

The following drugs may ***decrease*** the effects of repaglinide:
- rifampin (Rifadin, Rimactane).
- rifabutin (Mycobutin).

Author's note: Information in this profile will be broadened in the next edition of this book.

RIFABUTIN (RIF a byu tin)

Introduced: 1993   **Class:** Anti-mycobacterial agent (antitubercular)
Prescription: USA: Yes   **Controlled Drug:** USA: No; Canada: No   **Available as Generic:** USA: No; Canada: No

Brand Name: Mycobutin

Warning: Rifabutin prophylaxis must not be taken by people with active tuberculosis.

BENEFITS versus RISKS	
Possible Benefits	*Possible Risks*
PREVENTION OF DISSEMINATED *MYCOBACTERIUM AVIUM-INTRACELLULARE COMPLEX* IN PEOPLE WITH ADVANCED HIV INFECTION	NEUTROPENIA Low platelet counts

▷ **Principal Uses**

As a Single Drug Product: Uses currently included in FDA-approved labeling: (1) Prevention of disseminated *Mycobacterium avium-intracellulare complex* in patients with advanced HIV infection; (2) combination treatment of *Mycobacterium avium-intracellulare complex* infection.

Other (unlabeled) generally accepted uses: None.

How This Drug Works: Rifabutin inhibits DNA-dependent RNA polymerase (an enzyme critical to cells that are dividing) in *E. coli*. The exact mechanism of action of rifabutin in *Mycobacterium avium* or *Mycobacterium avium-intracellulare complex* is not known.

Available Dose Forms and Strengths
Capsules — 150 mg

How to Store: Keep at room temperature and avoid exposure to excessive humidity.

▷ **Recommended Dose Ranges** (Actual dose and schedule must be determined for each patient individually.)

Infants and Children: Safety and effectiveness of rifabutin in *Mycobacterium avium-intracellulare complex* prophylaxis has not clearly been established. Safety data comes from a trial of 22 children who were HIV positive.

Infants 1 year of age—18.5 mg per kg of body mass per day.

Children 2–10 years—8.6 mg per kg of body mass per day.

Adolescents up to 14 years—4.0 mg per kg of body mass per day.

14 to 60 Years of Age: 300 mg once a day. Those prone to nausea and vomiting may take 150 mg two times a day with food.

Over 60 Years of Age: Same as 12 to 60 years of age.

Conditions Requiring Dosing Adjustments
Liver Function: At present, clear adjustments of dose in hepatic compromise are not defined, but the drug should be used with caution.

Kidney Function: Elimination of rifabutin may actually be increased in people with compromised kidneys, yet the clinical effect is as yet unknown.

Author's note: The information in this profile has been shortened to make room for more widely used medicines.

RIFAMPIN (ri FAM pin)

Other Name: Rifampicin

Introduced: 1967   **Class:** Antibiotic, rifamycins   **Prescription:** USA: Yes   **Controlled Drug:** USA: No; Canada: No   **Available as Generic:** Yes

Brand Names: Rifadin, Rifadin IV, Rifamate [CD], Rifater [CD], Rimactane, Rimactane/INH Dual Pack [CD], ✳Rofact

BENEFITS versus RISKS	
Possible Benefits	*Possible Risks*
EFFECTIVE TREATMENT OF TUBERCULOSIS in combination with other drugs	DRUG-INDUCED KIDNEY OR LIVER DAMAGE
EFFECTIVE PREVENTION OF MENINGITIS	Blood cell or coagulation disorders
COMBINATION TREATMENT OF SOME STAPH INFECTIONS	Colitis (pseudomembranous)

▷ **Principal Uses**

As a Single Drug Product: Uses currently included in FDA-approved labeling: (1) Treats active tuberculosis (usually given concurrently with other antitubercular drugs to enhance its effectiveness); (2) treats tuberculosis in coal workers with good outcomes when combined with other antitubercular drugs; (3) used to prevent tuberculosis in people exposed to patients with active disease; (4) also used to eliminate the meningitis germ (meningococcus) from the throats of healthy carriers so it cannot be spread to others.

Other (unlabeled) generally accepted uses: (1) Second-line agent in combination with doxycycline in treatment of brucellosis; (2) has a place in preventing *Haemophilus influenzae* infections in people exposed to patients with active disease; (3) combination therapy of lepromatous leprosy; (4) used with cotrimoxazole to eliminate methicillin-resistant *Staphylococcus aureus* (MRSA) from people who have the bacteria; (5) used with other drugs to treat staph endocarditis.

As a Combination Drug Product [CD]: This drug is available in combination with isoniazid, another antitubercular drug that delays the development of drug-resistant strains of the tuberculosis germ.

How This Drug Works: It prevents the growth and multiplication of susceptible tuberculosis organisms by blocking specific enzyme systems that are involved in the formation of essential proteins.

Available Dose Forms and Strengths

Capsules — 150 mg, 300 mg

▷ **Usual Adult Dose Range:**   For tuberculosis: 10 mg per kg of body mass per day, up to 600 mg once daily.

For meningococcus carriers: 600 mg once daily for 4 days. The total daily dose should not exceed 600 mg.

Note: Actual dose and schedule must be determined for each patient individually.

Conditions Requiring Dosing Adjustments

Liver Function: This drug can cause liver damage, and patients should be followed closely. In severe failure, the dose should be limited to 6 to 8 mg per kg of body mass twice a week.

Kidney Function: For patients with a creatinine clearance (see Glossary) of 10 to 50 ml/min, one researcher suggests that 50–100% of the usual dose should be given.

▷ **Dosing Instructions:**   This drug is preferably taken with 8 ounces of water on an empty stomach (1 hour before or 2 hours after eating). However, it may be taken with food if necessary to reduce stomach irritation. The capsule may be opened and the contents mixed with applesauce or jelly to take it.

Usual Duration of Use: Use on a regular schedule for several months usually determines effectiveness in promoting recovery from tuberculosis. Long-term use (possibly 1 to 2 years) requires ongoing physician supervision and periodic evaluation.

▷ **This Drug Should Not Be Taken If**

- you have had an allergic reaction to it previously.

▷ **Inform Your Physician Before Taking This Drug If**

- you are pregnant.
- you have a history of liver disease or impaired liver function.
- you have active liver disease.
- you consume alcohol daily.
- you are taking an oral contraceptive. (An alternate method of contraception is advised.)
- you are taking an anticoagulant.

Possible Side Effects (natural, expected, and unavoidable drug actions)

Red, orange, or brown discoloration of tears, sweat, saliva, sputum, urine, or stool. Yellow coloring of the skin (not jaundice). Note: In the absence of illness symptoms, any discoloration is a harmless drug effect and does not mean toxicity.

Possible fungal superinfections (see Glossary).

▷ **Possible Adverse Effects** (unusual, unexpected, and infrequent reactions)

If any of the following develop, consult your physician promptly for guidance.

Mild Adverse Effects

Allergic reactions: skin rash, hives, itching, drug fever (see Glossary).

Headache, dizziness, blurred vision, impaired hearing, vague numbness and tingling—infrequent.

Joint and muscle pain—infrequent and often subsides after a few weeks.

Loss of appetite, heartburn, nausea, vomiting, abdominal cramps, diarrhea—infrequent.

Serious Adverse Effects

Skin problems (Stevens-Johnson syndrome or toxic epidermal necrolysis)—case reports.

Flu-like syndrome: fever, headache, dizziness, musculoskeletal pain, difficult breathing—case reports.

Drug-induced liver damage, with or without jaundice—frequent.

Kidney damage—infrequent.

Drug-induced porphyria, pancreatitis, gallstones, or pseudomembranous colitis—case reports.

Excessively low blood platelet count: abnormal bleeding or bruising—rare.

Blood clotting problems (disseminated intravascular coagulopathy)—case report.

Hemolytic anemia—case reports.

Suppression of the adrenal gland—possible.

▷ **Possible Effects on Sexual Function:** Altered timing and pattern of menstruation—case reports.

Decreased effectiveness of oral contraceptives.

▷ **Adverse Effects That May Mimic Natural Diseases or Disorders**

Liver reactions may suggest viral hepatitis.

Kidney reactions may suggest an infectious nephritis.

Possible Effects on Laboratory Tests

Complete blood cell counts: decreased red cells, hemoglobin, white cells, and platelets; increased eosinophils (allergic reaction).

INR (protime): increased (when taken with warfarin).

Liver function tests: increased liver enzymes (ALT/GPT, AST/GOT, and alkaline phosphatase), increased bilirubin.

CAUTION

1. This drug may permanently discolor soft contact lenses.
2. May reduce the effects of oral contraceptives—pregnancy could occur. An alternate method of contraception is advised.
3. Resistance may develop rapidly if this drug is used alone to treat tuberculosis. Only used with other antitubercular drugs.
4. TAKE THE FULL course prescribed; this may be months or years.

Precautions for Use

By Infants and Children: Monitor closely for possible liver toxicity or deficiency of blood platelets.

By Those Over 60 Years of Age: Natural changes in body composition and function make you more susceptible to the adverse effects of this drug. Report promptly any indications of possible drug toxicity.

▷ **Advisability of Use During Pregnancy**

Pregnancy Category: C. See Pregnancy Risk Categories at the back of this book.
Animal studies: Cleft palate and spinal defects reported in rodent studies.
Human studies: Adequate studies of pregnant women are not available.
If possible, avoid use of drug during the first 3 months.

Advisability of Use If Breast-Feeding

Presence of this drug in breast milk: Yes.
Avoid drug or refrain from nursing.

Habit-Forming Potential: None.

Effects of Overdose: Nausea, vomiting, drowsiness, unconsciousness, severe liver damage, jaundice.

Possible Effects of Long-Term Use: Superinfections, fungal overgrowth of mouth or tongue.

Suggested Periodic Examinations While Taking This Drug (at physician's discretion)

Complete blood cell counts, liver and kidney function tests.
Hearing acuity tests if hearing loss is suspected.

▷ **While Taking This Drug, Observe the Following**

Foods: No restrictions.

Beverages: No restrictions.

▷ *Alcohol:* It is best to avoid alcohol completely to reduce the risk of liver toxicity.

Tobacco Smoking: No interactions expected. I advise everyone to quit smoking.

▷ *Other Drugs:*

Rifampin *taken concurrently* with
• halothane anesthesia may result in serious liver damage.

Rifampin may *decrease* the effects of
• antianxiety agents such as diazepam, and perhaps other benzodiazepines (see Drug Classes).
• anticoagulants such as warfarin (Coumadin).
• anticonvulsant drugs such as phenytoin (Dilantin).
• barbiturates (see Drug Classes).
• BCG live-attenuated vaccine.
• beta-blockers such as metoprolol or propranolol (see Drug Classes).
• birth control pills (oral contraceptives).
• some calcium channel blockers (see Drug Classes).
• carbamazepine (Tegretol), and may lead to carbamazepine toxicity.
• chloramphenicol (Chloromycetin).
• clofibrate (Atromid-S).
• cortisonelike drugs (see *adrenocortical steroids* in Drug Classes).
• cyclosporine (Sandimmune).

- dapsone.
- digitalis preparations (Lanoxin, others).
- disopyramide (Norpace).
- enalapril (Vasotec).
- fluconazole (Diflucan).
- some HMG-CoA reductase inhibitors (fluvastatin)
- indinavir (Crixivan).
- itraconazole (Sporanox).
- ketoconazole (Nizoral).
- methadone (Dolophine).
- montelukast (Singulair).
- mexiletine (Mexitil).
- narcotics such as methadone (see opioids in Drug Classes).
- nifedipine (Adalat).
- oral hypoglycemic agents (sulfonylureas such as tolbutamide—see Drug Classes).
- phenytoin (Dilantin).
- progestins.
- quinidine (Quinaglute, others).
- repaglinide (Prandin).
- ritonavir (Norvir)—this combination may also lead to rifampin toxicity.
- sildenafil (Viagra).
- theophylline (Theo-Dur, others).
- tricyclic antidepressants (see Drug Classes).
- verapamil (Verelan).
- warfarin (Coumadin). Increased INR testing is needed.
- zidovudine (AZT); the therapeutic effect will be lessened by a decreased drug level.

The following drug may *decrease* the effects of rifampin:

- *para*-aminosalicylic acid (PAS), and reduce its antitubercular effectiveness.

▷ *Driving, Hazardous Activities:* This drug may cause dizziness, drowsiness, impaired vision, and impaired hearing. Restrict activities as necessary.

Aviation Note: The use of this drug *may be a disqualification* for piloting. Consult a designated aviation medical examiner.

Exposure to Sun: No restrictions.

Discontinuation: It is advisable not to interrupt or stop this drug without consulting your physician. Intermittent use can increase risk of developing allergic reactions.

RISPERIDONE (RIS peer i dohn)

Introduced: 1993   **Class:** Antipsychotic agent   **Prescription:** USA: Yes
Controlled Drug: USA: No; Canada: No   **Available as Generic:** USA: No;
Canada: No
Brand Name: Risperdal

```
┌─────────────────────────────────────────────────────────────┐
│                    BENEFITS versus RISKS                      │
│      Possible Benefits                  Possible Risks        │
│  TREATMENT OF SCHIZOPHRENIA     Change in heart function      │
│     REFRACTORY TO OTHER         Involuntary movement disorder │
│     AGENTS                      Neuroleptic malignant syndrome│
│  DECREASED SIDE EFFECTS                                       │
│     COMPARED TO OTHER                                         │
│     AVAILABLE DRUGS                                           │
│  EFFECTIVE TREATMENT OF                                       │
│     CERTAIN PSYCHOTIC                                         │
│     DISORDERS                                                 │
└─────────────────────────────────────────────────────────────┘
```

▷ **Principal Uses**

As a Single Drug Product: Uses currently included in FDA-approved labeling: (1) Manages psychotic disorders such as chronic schizophrenia; (2) treats AIDS-related psychosis.

Other (unlabeled) generally accepted uses: (1) Treats acute schizophrenia; (2) treatment of aggression; (3) treatment of Tourette's syndrome; (4) can have a role in helping behavioral problems in people with mental retardation; (5) helps treatment-resistant obsessive-compulsive disorder.

How This Drug Works: Balances two nerve transmitters (dopamine and serotonin) helping restore more normal thinking and mood.

Available Dose Forms and Strengths

    Oral solution   1 mg/ml

      Tablets — 1 mg, 2 mg, 3 mg, 4 mg

▷ **Recommended Dose Ranges** (Actual dose and schedule must be determined for each patient individually.)

Infants and Children: Safety and effectiveness for those less than 18 years of age are not established.

18 to 60 Years of Age: Past starting dose was 1 mg taken twice daily. Newly approved dosing has shown doses up to 8 mg once daily to be effective.

Doses in the twice daily (BID) approach may be increased as needed and tolerated by 1 mg on the second and third day, for a total of 3 mg twice daily by the third day. If further dose changes are needed, they should be made at 1-week intervals. Doses greater than 8 mg per day are not recommended.

Over 60 Years of Age: Therapy is started with 0.5 mg twice daily. The dose is increased if needed and tolerated by 0.5 mg twice daily. Doses greater than 1.5 mg daily are achieved by small increases made at 1-week intervals. Careful attention must be paid to blood pressure and development of adverse effects.

Conditions Requiring Dosing Adjustments

Liver Function: The starting dose must be decreased and adjusted as for those over 60 years old. Additionally, there may be an increased amount of the active drug that results from each dose (increased free fraction), and as such a greater than expected effect may be seen.

Kidney Function: The starting dose must be decreased and adjusted as for those over 60 years old.

▷ **Dosing Instructions:**   The tablet may be crushed, and the medication's effect is not changed by food.

Usual Duration of Use: Use on a regular schedule for 1 to 2 weeks usually determines effectiveness in helping control chronic schizophrenia. If long-term use is attempted, the lowest effective dose should be used. Periodic physician evaluation of response and dose is required.

Possible Advantages of This Drug
Treatment of schizophrenia refractory to other therapy.

▷ **This Drug Should Not Be Taken If**
- you had an allergic reaction to it previously.
- you had neuroleptic malignant syndrome (ask your doctor).

▷ **Inform Your Physician Before Taking This Drug If**
- you have a history of breast cancer.
- you have liver or kidney compromise.
- you are pregnant or plan to become pregnant or are breast-feeding your infant.
- you have had tardive dyskinesia in the past.
- you have a history of Parkinson's disease or seizures.
- you have a history of heart rhythm disturbances.
- you are unsure how much to take or how often to take it.

Possible Side Effects (natural, expected, and unavoidable drug actions)
Increased prolactin levels may result in male and female breast tenderness and swelling. Sleepiness. Orthostatic hypotension (see Glossary)—rare. Weight gain—infrequent.

▷ **Possible Adverse Effects** (unusual, unexpected, and infrequent reactions)
If any of the following develop, consult your physician promptly for guidance.
Mild Adverse Effects
Allergic reactions: skin rash.
Difficulty in concentrating—rare.
Headache or increased dreaming—rare to infrequent.
Constipation, diarrhea, or nausea—infrequent.
Palpitations—rare.
Increased urination—rare.
Serious Adverse Effects
Allergic reactions: anaphylactic reactions.
Abnormal heart function (prolonged QT interval)—rare.
Tardive dyskinesia (see Glossary) or neuroleptic malignant syndrome (see Glossary)—case reports.
Low sodium—rare.
Seizures—rare.
Lowered white blood cells or platelets—case reports.
Abnormal liver function—rare.

▷ **Possible Effects on Sexual Function:** Diminished sexual desire; delayed or absent orgasm; erectile dysfunction including priapism; male or female breast tenderness or swelling; dry vagina or menstrual changes (hypermenorrhea)—rare. Ejaculation failure—case reports.

Possible Delayed Adverse Effects: Swelling and tenderness of male and female breast tissue.

Natural Diseases or Disorders That May Be Activated by This Drug

Some human cancers depend on prolactin for growth, and since risperidone increases prolactin, it should be used with caution by people with previously diagnosed breast cancer.

Possible Effects on Laboratory Tests

Liver function tests: increased SGPT, SGOT, and LDH.

Complete blood counts: decreased platelets, white blood cells, and hemoglobin.

Prolactin: increased.

CAUTION

1. This drug should be used with great caution, if at all, by patients with cancer.
2. Call your doctor promptly if you have an increased tendency to infection or abnormal bleeding or bruising while taking this drug.
3. This drug should be used with great caution, if at all, by patients with a history of seizures.

Precautions for Use

By Infants and Children: Safety and effectiveness for those under 18 years of age are not established.

By Those Over 60 Years of Age: The starting dose of 0.5 mg twice daily is used for patients who are elderly or debilitated, and slower increases in dose as needed and tolerated are indicated. Great care should be taken by those with heart disease. You may be more likely to experience orthostatic hypotension (see Glossary) and problems with motor skills. Those with prostate problems may have increased risk of urine retention.

▷ **Advisability of Use During Pregnancy**

Pregnancy Category: C. See Pregnancy Risk Categories at the back of this book.

Animal studies: Increased rat pup death during the first few days of lactation.

Human studies: Adequate studies of pregnant women are not available. One case report of lack of formation of the corpus callosum of the brain in a fetus exposed to this drug while in the uterus.

Ask your doctor for guidance.

Advisability of Use If Breast-Feeding

Presence of this drug in breast milk: Yes.

Avoid drug or refrain from nursing.

Habit-Forming Potential: None.

Effects of Overdose: Drowsiness, hypotension, tachycardia, low sodium and potassium, ECG changes (prolonged QT interval), and seizure.

Suggested Periodic Examinations While Taking This Drug (at physician's discretion)

Liver function tests. Electrolytes (sodium and potassium).

ECG. Prolactin levels.

▷ **While Taking This Drug, Observe the Following**

Foods: No restrictions.

Beverages: No restrictions.

▷ *Alcohol:* Patients should avoid alcohol while taking risperidone.

Tobacco Smoking: No interactions expected. I advise everyone to quit smoking.

Marijuana Smoking: Increased somnolence.

▷ *Other Drugs:*
Risperidone may *decrease* the effects of
• levodopa (Sinemet, others).
Risperidone *taken concurrently* with
• carbamazepine (Tegretol) will decrease the drug level and perhaps the therapeutic effects of risperidone.
• clozapine (Clozaril) may decrease the therapeutic effects of risperidone.
• other centrally acting medicines may result in increased central effects.
• lithium (Lithobid, others) may lead to increased adverse effects.
• ritonavir (Norvir), and perhaps other protease inhibitors (see Drug Classes), may lead to toxicity.
• tramadol (Ultram) may increase seizure risk.
• venlafaxine (Effexor) may increase risperidone toxicity risk.

▷ *Driving, Hazardous Activities:* This drug may cause drowsiness and difficulty in concentrating. Restrict activities as necessary.
Aviation Note: The use of this drug *is a disqualification* for piloting. Consult a designated aviation medical examiner.
Exposure to Sun: Use caution—this drug may cause photosensitivity.
Discontinuation: Consult your doctor before stopping this medication.

SALMETEROL (sal ME ter ohl)

Introduced: 1994   **Class:** Antiasthmatic (Bronchodilator)   **Prescription:**
USA: Yes   **Controlled Drug:** USA: No; Canada: Not available   **Available as**
Generic: USA: No
Brand Names: Aeromax, Serevent

BENEFITS versus RISKS	
Possible Benefits	*Possible Risks*
LONG-ACTING RELIEF OF BRONCHIAL ASTHMA PREVENTION OF NOCTURNAL ASTHMA SYMPTOMS	Rapid heart rate (tachycardia)

▷ **Principal Uses**
As a Single Drug Product: Uses currently included in FDA-approved labeling: (1) Treatment and prevention of bronchospasm in asthma; (2) prevention of nocturnal asthma; (3) prevention of exercise-induced bronchospasm.
Other (unlabeled) generally accepted uses: May have a role in treating chronic obstructive pulmonary disease (COPD).

How This Drug Works: Acts at specific sites (beta-2) in the lung and opens the airways (bronchodilation), decreases airway reactivity, and increases movement of mucus. It also blocks release of chemicals from cells (mast) that worsen asthma.

Available Dose Forms and Strengths
Inhaler — 13-g canister that (gives 21 mcg of salmeterol per use)
Serevent Diskus — 50 mcg of salmeterol per use.

▷ **Recommended Dose Ranges** (Actual dose and schedule must be determined for each patient individually.)

Infants and Children: Safety and effectiveness in those less than 12 years of age not established.

12 to 60 Years of Age: For prevention of asthma: Two inhalations (42 mcg) twice daily in the morning and evening. Doses are taken 12 hours apart.

For prevention of exercised-induced asthma: Two inhalations at least 30 to 60 minutes **before** exercise. Additional doses of salmeterol should **not** be taken for 12 hours.

Over 60 Years of Age: Same as 12 to 60 years of age.

Conditions Requiring Dosing Adjustments

Liver Function: Use with caution, as the drug may accumulate in liver failure.

Kidney Function: Salmeterol has not been studied in kidney failure patients.

▷ **Dosing Instructions:**   Follow written instructions closely. This drug has not been studied with a spacer. Shake well before using.

Usual Duration of Use: Use on a regular schedule for 4 to 6 weeks usually determines effectiveness in preventing asthma attacks. Long-term use (months to years) requires periodic physician evaluation of response and dose adjustment.

Possible Advantages of This Drug

Longer-acting beta-2 agent than previously available.

▷ **This Drug Should Not Be Taken If**
- you had an allergic reaction to it previously.
- you currently have an irregular heart rhythm.
- you are taking, or have taken within the past 2 weeks, any monoamine oxidase (MAO) type A inhibitor (see Drug Classes).
- you are having sudden (acute) symptoms or worsening (exacerbation) of your asthma.

▷ **Inform Your Physician Before Taking This Drug If**
- your breathing does not improve after taking this drug.
- you have an overactive thyroid (hyperthyroidism).
- you have diabetes.
- you have a history of heart problems.
- you have abnormally high blood pressure.
- you are unsure how much to take or how often to take it.

Possible Side Effects (natural, expected, and unavoidable drug actions)

Dryness or irritation of the mouth or throat, altered taste. Nervousness, tremor, or palpitations.

▷ **Possible Adverse Effects** (unusual, unexpected, and infrequent reactions)

If any of the following develop, consult your physician promptly for guidance.

Mild Adverse Effects

Allergic reactions: skin rash and urticaria.

Rhinitis and laryngitis—possible.

Rapid heart rate (tachycardia)—case reports.

Headache, tremor, dizziness, and nervousness—infrequent.

Serious Adverse Effects

Allergic reactions: not defined.

Paradoxical bronchospasm.

Respiratory arrest—case reports.

▷ **Possible Effects on Sexual Function:**   Not defined.

Possible Delayed Adverse Effects: None defined at present.

▷ **Adverse Effects That May Mimic Natural Diseases or Disorders**
Rapid heart rate may mimic heart disease. Bronchospasm may mimic asthma.

Natural Diseases or Disorders That May Be Activated by This Drug
Latent coronary artery disease. Diabetes or high blood pressure.

Possible Effects on Laboratory Tests
Blood cholesterol profile: may be increased.
Blood glucose level: increased.

CAUTION
1. Use of this drug by inhalation with beclomethasone aerosol (Beclovent, Vanceril) may increase the risk of fluorocarbon propellant toxicity. Use salmeterol aerosol 20 to 30 minutes before beclomethasone aerosol to reduce toxicity and enhance penetration of beclomethasone into the lungs.
2. Serious heart rhythm problems or cardiac arrest can result from excessive and prolonged use.
3. Call your doctor if asthma symptoms appear more often than usual, or if you begin to increase use of the immediate bronchodilator.
4. *Guidelines for the Diagnosis and Management of Asthma* from the National Institutes of Health state that salmeterol should NOT be used for acute symptoms or asthma exacerbations.

Precautions for Use
By Infants and Children: Safety and effectiveness for those under 12 not established.
By Those Over 60 Years of Age: Avoid increased use. If asthma is not controlled as it has been in the past, call your doctor.

▷ **Advisability of Use During Pregnancy**
Pregnancy Category: C. See Pregnancy Risk Categories at the back of this book.
Animal studies: Rabbit studies have revealed cleft palate, limb and paw flexures, and delayed bone formation.
Human studies: Adequate studies of pregnant women are not available.
Ask your doctor for guidance.

Advisability of Use If Breast-Feeding
Presence of this drug in breast milk: Yes, but extent not defined.
Avoid drug or refrain from nursing.

Habit-Forming Potential: None.

Effects of Overdose: Exaggeration of pharmacological effects: tachycardia and/or arrhythmia, muscle cramps, cardiac arrest, and death.

Suggested Periodic Examinations While Taking This Drug (at physician's discretion)
Blood pressure checks, evaluations of heart (cardiac) status.

▷ **While Taking This Drug, Observe the Following**
Foods: No restrictions.
Beverages: Avoid excessive caffeine as in coffee, tea, cola, and chocolate.
▷   *Alcohol:* No interactions expected.
Tobacco Smoking: No interactions expected. Asthma may be worsened by irritation from smoking. I advise everyone to quit smoking.

▷ *Other Drugs:*
Salmeterol *taken concurrently* with
- monoamine oxidase (MAO) type A inhibitor drugs (see Drug Classes) can cause extreme increases in blood pressure and heart stimulation.
The following drugs may *increase* the effects of salmeterol:
- methylxanthines such as caffeine or theophylline.
- tricyclic antidepressants.

▷ *Driving, Hazardous Activities:* This drug may cause nervousness or dizziness. Restrict activities as necessary.
Aviation Note: The use of this drug *is a disqualification* for piloting. Consult a designated aviation medical examiner.
Exposure to Sun: No restrictions.
Heavy Exercise or Exertion: Use caution—this may stress protective effects of this drug.

SELEGILINE (se LEDGE i leen)

Other Name: Deprenyl

Introduced: 1981   **Class:**   Anti-parkinsonism, monoamine oxidase (MAO) type B inhibitor   **Prescription:**   USA: Yes   **Controlled Drug:**   USA: No; Canada: No   **Available as Generic:**   USA: Yes

Brand Name: Eldepryl

BENEFITS versus RISKS

Possible Benefits	*Possible Risks*
EFFECTIVE INITIAL TREATMENT OF PARKINSON'S DISEASE when started at the onset of symptoms	ABNORMAL INVOLUNTARY MOVEMENTS
	HALLUCINATIONS
ADDITIVE RELIEF OF SYMPTOMS OF PARKINSON'S DISEASE when used concurrently with levodopa/carbidopa	INITIAL FALL IN BLOOD PRESSURE/ORTHOSTATIC HYPOTENSION
PERMITS REDUCTION IN SINEMET DOSE	
May have a role in Alzheimer's disease	

▷ **Principal Uses**
As a Single Drug Product: Uses currently included in FDA-approved labeling: (1) Used to start drug treatment of very early Parkinson's disease (soon after onset of symptoms), thus delaying the use of levodopa/carbidopa; (2) also used as an adjunct to levodopa/carbidopa treatment of Parkinson's disease if intolerable abnormal movements (dyskinesia) and/or increasing "on-off" episodes occur. Addition of selegiline (1) permits reduction of the daily dose of levodopa with consequent lessening of dyskinesia and erratic drug response, and (2) provides additional relief of parkinsonian symptoms.
Other (unlabeled) generally accepted uses: (1) Some improvement achieved in Alzheimer's disease (some trials also used high-dose vitamin E) in patients treated with this drug; (2) treatment of narcolepsy.

How This Drug Works: By (1) inhibiting monoamine oxidase type B, the enzyme that inactivates dopamine in the brain, and by (2) slowing the restorage of released dopamine at nerve terminals, this drug helps correct dopamine deficiency responsible for rigidity, tremor, and sluggish movement characteristic of Parkinson's disease.

Available Dose Forms and Strengths
　　Capsules — 5 mg
　　Tablets — 5 mg
Author's Note: The capsule form of this medicine will eventually replace the tablet form, and is an astute attempt by the company to help avoid confusion with other white tablets or counterfeit copies of Eldepryl.

▷ **Usual Adult Dose Range**
　　Parkinsonism: 5 mg once or twice daily. The usual maintenance dose is 5 mg after breakfast and 5 mg after lunch. Daily dose of 10 mg is adequate to achieve optimal benefit. Higher doses do not result in further improvement and are not advised. During gradual introduction of selegiline, dose of levodopa/carbidopa (Sinemet) may be cautiously decreased. Sinemet dose should be reduced by 10 to 20% when selegiline is started. **Note: Actual dose and schedule must be determined for each patient individually.**

Conditions Requiring Dosing Adjustments
　　Liver Function: This drug is extensively metabolized in the liver. Patients with liver compromise should be followed closely.
　　Kidney Function: No dosing changes thought to be needed. It can cause prostatic enlargement (hypertrophy). Used with urine outflow problems.

▷ **Dosing Instructions:** The tablet may be crushed and taken with food or milk to reduce stomach irritation.

Usual Duration of Use: Use on a regular schedule for 4 to 6 weeks usually determines effectiveness in controlling the symptoms of Parkinson's disease and permitting reduction of levodopa/carbidopa dose. Long-term use (months to years) requires periodic physician evaluation.

Possible Advantages of This Drug
　　It may provide a more effective and uniform control of parkinsonian symptoms and a significant reduction of some adverse effects associated with long-term levodopa therapy. It does not lose its effectiveness with long-term use, and does not require avoidance of foods containing tyramine, as is necessary with monoamine oxidase (MAO) type A inhibitors.

▷ **This Drug Should Not Be Taken If**
　　• you have had an allergic reaction to it previously.
　　• you have Huntington's disease, hereditary (essential) tremor, or tardive dyskinesia (see Glossary).
　　• you are pregnant or breast-feeding.
　　• you take meperidine (Demerol).

▷ **Inform Your Physician Before Taking This Drug If**
　　• you have constitutionally low blood pressure.
　　• you have peptic ulcer disease.
　　• you are taking levodopa.
　　• you have a history of heart rhythm disorder.

- you are taking any antihypertensive drugs or antipsychotic drugs (see Drug Classes).

Possible Side Effects (natural, expected, and unavoidable drug actions)
Weakness, orthostatic hypotension (see Glossary), dry mouth, insomnia—all rare.

▷ **Possible Adverse Effects** (unusual, unexpected, and infrequent reactions)
If any of the following develop, consult your physician promptly for guidance.

Mild Adverse Effects
Headache, dizziness, blurred vision, agitation—rare.
Palpitations, fainting—rare.
Altered taste—rare.
Nausea and vomiting, stomach pain, anorexia—common.

Serious Adverse Effects
Dyskinesias: abnormal involuntary movements—infrequent.
Confusion and hallucinations, depression, psychosis, vivid dreams—rare.
Aggravation of peptic ulcer, gastrointestinal bleeding—rare.
Growth of the prostate—rare.

▷ **Possible Effects on Sexual Function:**   Transient decreases in penile sensation and anorgasmia have rarely been reported if doses exceed 10 mg per day. Increased libido may occur.

▷ **Adverse Effects That May Mimic Natural Diseases or Disorders**
Effects on mental function and behavior may resemble psychotic disorders.

Natural Diseases or Disorders That May Be Activated by This Drug
Peptic ulcer disease.

Possible Effects on Laboratory Tests
None reported.

CAUTION
1. This drug can start dyskinesias and intensify existing dyskinesias. Watch carefully for tremors, twitching, or abnormal, involuntary movements of any kind. Report these promptly.
2. This drug potentiates the effects of levodopa. When added to current levodopa treatment, adverse effects of levodopa may develop or be intensified. Levodopa dose must be reduced by 10–20% when treatment with selegiline begins.
3. Tell your doctor promptly if you become pregnant or plan pregnancy. The manufacturer does not recommend the use of this drug during pregnancy.

Precautions for Use
By Infants and Children: This drug is not utilized by this age group.
By Those Over 60 Years of Age: This drug is well tolerated by the elderly. Observe closely for any tendency to light-headedness or faintness, especially on arising from a lying or sitting position.

▷ **Advisability of Use During Pregnancy**
Pregnancy Category: C. See Pregnancy Risk Categories at the back of this book.
Animal studies: No birth defects due to this drug were found in rat studies.
Human studies: Adequate studies of pregnant women are not available.
The manufacturer advises that this drug should not be taken during pregnancy.

Advisability of Use If Breast-Feeding

Presence of this drug in breast milk: Unknown.

Avoid drug or refrain from nursing.

Habit-Forming Potential: None.

Effects of Overdose: Nausea, vomiting, palpitations, low blood pressure, agitation, severe involuntary movements, hallucinations.

Possible Effects of Long-Term Use: None reported.

Suggested Periodic Examinations While Taking This Drug (at physician's discretion)

Regular evaluation of drug response, heart function, and blood pressure status.

▷ **While Taking This Drug, Observe the Following**

Foods: Caution should be used regarding foods containing tyramine (see Glossary for a list), although the reaction with this drug may not be as severe as that seen with other MAO inhibitors.

Beverages: No restrictions. May be taken with milk.

▷ *Alcohol:* Use caution until the combined effects have been determined. Alcohol may exaggerate the blood-pressure-lowering and sedative effects of this drug.

Tobacco Smoking: No interactions expected. I advise everyone to quit smoking.

Marijuana Smoking: Additive drowsiness may occur.

▷ *Other Drugs:*

Selegiline *taken concurrently* with

- albuterol (Ventolin, others) may result in increased adverse vascular effects.
- amphetamine (Dexedrine) can cause a severe increase in blood pressure.
- antidepressants (see Drug Classes) such as amitriptyline (Elavil) may cause neurotoxic reactions such as seizures.
- antihypertensive drugs (and other drugs that can lower blood pressure) require careful monitoring for excessive drops in pressure. Dose adjustments may be necessary.
- benzodiazepines (see Drug Classes) may result in increased central nervous system depression.
- bupropion (Wellbutrin) may cause seizures.
- buspirone (Buspar) may result in increases in blood pressure.
- carbamazepine (Tegretol) may result in high fevers and seizures. Still, some studies found benefits in resistant depression.
- dextromethorphan (various), a cough suppressant used in many nonprescription cough medicines, has been reported to cause toxicity with low blood pressure, spasms, high fevers, and some deaths. These medicines should not be combined.
- ephedrine (various) can result in severe increases in temperature.
- fluoxetine (Prozac) may cause serotonin toxicity syndrome.
- fluvoxamine (Luvox) may result in extreme agitation, rigidity, excessive temperatures, and coma. DO NOT combine these medicines.
- lithium (Lithobid) may increase risk of the serotonin toxicity syndrome.
- meperidine (Demerol) may cause a life-threatening reaction of unknown cause; avoid this combination.
- mirtazapine (Remeron) may lead to adverse seizures.
- oral hypoglycemic agents (see *oral antidiabetic drugs* in Drug Classes) may cause very low blood sugars.

- paroxetine (Paxil) may result in central nervous system toxicity.
- phenothiazines (see Drug Classes) may result in increased occurrence of movement disorders.
- phenylpropanolamine (various) can cause severe increases in temperature and blood pressure. DO NOT combine.
- pseudoephedrine (various) can cause severe increases in temperature and blood pressure. DO NOT combine.
- sertraline (Zoloft) may result in central nervous system toxicity.
- sibutramine (Meridia) may lead to toxicity.
- sumatriptan (Imitrex) may lead to toxicity.
- tramadol (Ultram) may lead to seizures.
- tryptophan may cause a fatal serotonin syndrome.
- venlafaxine (Effexor) can result in central and autonomic nervous system toxicity.

The following drugs may *decrease* the effects of selegiline and diminish its effectiveness:

- chlorprothixene (Taractan).
- haloperidol (Haldol).
- metoclopramide (Reglan).
- phenothiazines (see Drug Classes).
- reserpine (Ser-Ap-Es, etc.), in high doses.
- thiothixene (Navane).

▷ *Driving, Hazardous Activities:* This drug may cause dizziness, drowsiness, impaired coordination, or fainting. Restrict activities as necessary.

Aviation Note: The use of this drug *is a disqualification* for piloting. Consult a designated aviation medical examiner.

Exposure to Sun: Use caution—photosensitivity has been reported.

Exposure to Heat: Use caution until the combined effects have been determined. Hot environments can cause lowering of blood pressure.

Discontinuation: Do not stop this drug abruptly. Sudden withdrawal can cause prompt increase in parkinsonian symptoms and deterioration of control. Consult your physician regarding a schedule for gradual withdrawal and concurrent adjustment of Sinemet or other appropriate drugs.

SERTRALINE (SER tra leen)

Introduced: 1986   **Class:** Antidepressant   **Prescription:** USA: Yes
Controlled Drug: USA: No; Canada: No   **Available as Generic:** USA: No
Brand Name: Zoloft

BENEFITS versus RISKS	
Possible Benefits	*Possible Risks*
EFFECTIVE TREATMENT OF MAJOR DEPRESSIVE DISORDERS	Male sexual dysfunction Seizures
TREATS PANIC DISORDER	
TREATMENT OF OBSESSIVE COMPULSIVE DISORDER	

▷ **Principal Uses**

As a Single Drug Product: Uses currently included in FDA-approved labeling: Treats (1) major depression; (2) obsessive-compulsive disorder; (3) panic disorder.

Other (unlabeled) generally accepted uses: (1) May have a role in treating obesity (rat studies have shown a decrease in eating that depends on the dose that is taken; studies in humans are being conducted); (2) may help some kinds of sexual problems.

How This Drug Works: This drug relieves depression by slowly restoring to normal levels a specific constituent of brain tissue (serotonin) that transmits nerve impulses.

Available Dose Forms and Strengths

Tablets — 25 mg, 50 mg, 100 mg

▷ **Recommended Dose Ranges** (Actual dose and schedule must be determined for each patient individually.)

Infants and Children: In children 6 to 12 years old 25 mg once daily has been approved to treat obsessive-compulsive disorder.

12 to 60 Years of Age: Initially 50 mg once daily, taken in the morning or evening. The dose is then slowly increased, as needed and tolerated, in increments of 50 mg at intervals of 1 week. The total daily dose should not exceed 200 mg.

Over 60 Years of Age: Same as 12 to 60 years of age. Adjust dose as appropriate for impaired liver or kidney function.

Conditions Requiring Dosing Adjustments

Liver Function: Drug is a rare cause of liver damage. Patients with liver disease should be watched closely, and lower doses used.

Kidney Function: The role of the kidneys is unknown.

▷ **Dosing Instructions:**   The tablet may be crushed and is best taken with food to enhance absorption, but may be taken at any time with or without food.

Usual Duration of Use: Use on a regular schedule for 4 to 8 weeks usually determines (1) effectiveness in relieving depression; (2) pattern of both favorable and unfavorable drug effects. Long-term use requires periodic physician evaluation.

Possible Advantages of This Drug

Does not cause weight gain, a common side effect of tricyclic antidepressants.

Less likely to cause dry mouth, constipation, urinary retention, orthostatic hypotension (see Glossary), and heart rhythm disturbances than tricyclic antidepressants.

Does not cause Parkinson-like reactions.

▷ **This Drug Should Not Be Taken If**

• you have had an allergic reaction to it previously.
• you took a monoamine oxidase (MAO) type A inhibitor (see Drug Classes) in the last 14 days.

▷ **Inform Your Physician Before Taking This Drug If**

• you had any adverse effects from antidepressant drugs.
• you have impaired liver or kidney function.
• you have Parkinson's disease.
• you have had a recent heart attack.

- you have a seizure disorder.
- you are pregnant or plan pregnancy while taking this drug.

Possible Side Effects (natural, expected, and unavoidable drug actions)
Decreased appetite, weight loss (average 1 to 2 lb).

▷ **Possible Adverse Effects** (unusual, unexpected, and infrequent reactions)
If any of the following develop, consult your physician promptly for guidance.
Mild Adverse Effects
Allergic reactions: skin rash, itching—rare.
Headache, nervousness, insomnia, fatigue, tremor, dizziness, impaired concentration—rare; abnormal vision, numbness, and tingling—rare; confusion—rare; hallucinations—rare to infrequent.
Chest pain and increased blood pressure—rare.
Paresthesias—rare.
Dry mouth, altered taste, nausea, vomiting, diarrhea, tongue ulceration—rare to infrequent.
Serious Adverse Effects
Allergic reactions: dermatitis (various forms)—rare.
Drug-induced seizures—rare.
Hemorrhage into the anterior chamber of the eye or anemia—rare.
Increased blood cholesterol (hypercholesterolemia)—infrequent.
Low blood sugar—case reports.
Bronchospasm—infrequent.
Movement disorders (extrapyramidal reactions)—case reports.
Low blood sodium—rare; case reports of SIADH (may also occur with other selective serotonin reuptake inhibitors).

▷ **Possible Effects on Sexual Function:**   Male sexual dysfunction: delayed ejaculation—may be frequent; female sexual dysfunction: inhibited orgasm—rare.
Swelling and tenderness of male and female breast tissue—case reports. Infrequent dysmenorrhea, intermenstrual bleeding, or atrophic vaginitis.
May help some kinds of sexual disorders.

Natural Diseases or Disorders That May Be Activated by This Drug
Latent epilepsy.

Possible Effects on Laboratory Tests
Blood total cholesterol and triglyceride levels: increased—infrequent.
Blood uric acid levels: decreased.
Hemoglobin or hematocrit: decreased—rare.
Liver function tests: increased liver enzymes (ALT/GPT, AST/GOT, and alkaline phosphatase).
Blood sodium: decreased (with rare SIADH).

CAUTION
1. If any type of skin reaction develops (rash, hives, etc.), discontinue this drug and inform your physician promptly.
2. If dryness of the mouth develops and persists for more than 2 weeks, consult your dentist for guidance.
3. Ask your doctor or pharmacist before taking any other prescription or over-the-counter drug while taking sertraline.

4. If you are advised to take any monoamine oxidase (MAO) type A inhibitor drug (see Drug Classes), allow an interval of 5 weeks after discontinuing this drug before starting the MAO inhibitor.
5. It is advisable to withhold this drug if electroconvulsive therapy (ECT, "shock" treatment) is to be used to treat your depression.

Precautions for Use

By Infants and Children: Safety and effectiveness for those under 12 years of age are not established.

By Those Over 60 Years of Age: The lowest effective dose should be used for maintenance treatment and adjusted as needed for reduced kidney function.

▷ **Advisability of Use During Pregnancy**

Pregnancy Category: C. See Pregnancy Risk Categories at the back of this book.
   Animal studies: Delayed bone development due to this drug found in rat and rabbit studies.
   Human studies: Adequate studies of pregnant women are not available.
   Use this drug only if clearly needed. Ask your physician for guidance.

Advisability of Use If Breast-Feeding

Presence of this drug in breast milk: Yes, in variable amounts.
One small study found undetectable blood levels in infants who were breast-fed while their mothers were taking sertraline. Another found detectable levels.
Discuss breast feeding with your doctor.

Habit-Forming Potential: None.

Effects of Overdose: Agitation, restlessness, excitement, nausea, vomiting, seizures.

Possible Effects of Long-Term Use: None reported.

Suggested Periodic Examinations While Taking This Drug (at physician's discretion)
   None.

▷ **While Taking This Drug, Observe the Following**

Foods: May increase peak blood level.
Beverages: No restrictions. May be taken with milk.
▷   *Alcohol:* Avoid completely.
Tobacco Smoking: No interactions expected. I advise everyone to quit smoking.
▷   *Other Drugs:*
   Sertraline may *increase* the effects of
   • dextromethorphan (in many cough "DM" suppressants).
   • diazepam (Valium) and perhaps other benzodiazepines (see Drug Classes).
   • diltiazem (Cardizem).
   • sibutramine (Meridia) may lead to toxicity (serotonin syndrome).
   • tolbutamide (Orinase).
   • warfarin (Coumadin) and related oral anticoagulants. More frequent INR (prothrombin time or protime) testing is needed. Ongoing warfarin doses should be based on INR results.
   Sertraline *taken concurrently* with
   • antidiabetic drugs (insulin, oral hypoglycemics—see *oral antidiabetic drugs* in Drug Classes) may increase the risk of hypoglycemic reactions; monitor blood and urine sugar levels carefully.

- cimetidine (Tagamet, Tagamet HB 200) may lead to sertraline toxicity.
- flecainide (Tambocor) may lead to flecainide toxicity.
- metoclopramide (Reglan) may lead to sertraline toxicity.
- monoamine oxidase (MAO) type A inhibitor drugs (see Drug Classes) may cause confusion, agitation, high fever, seizures, and dangerous elevations of blood pressure. Avoid the concurrent use of these drugs.
- ritonavir (Norvir), and perhaps other protease inhibitors (see Drug Classes), may lead to toxicity.
- terfenadine (Seldane) may lead to toxicity.
- tramadol (Ultram) may lead to seizures.

▷ *Driving, Hazardous Activities:* This drug may cause drowsiness, dizziness, impaired judgment, and altered vision. Restrict activities as necessary.

Aviation Note: The use of this drug *is a disqualification* for piloting. Consult a designated aviation medical examiner.

Exposure to Sun: Use caution—this drug may (rarely) cause photosensitivity (see Glossary).

Discontinuation: The slow elimination of this drug from the body makes it unlikely that any withdrawal effects will result from abrupt discontinuation. However, call your doctor if you plan to stop this drug for any reason.

SIBUTRAMINE (si BUTE rah meen)

Introduced: 1998 **Class:** Serotonin reuptake inhibitor, anorexiant, weight-loss agent **Prescription:** USA: Yes **Controlled Drug:** USA: Yes, C-IV*; Canada: Yes **Available as Generic:** USA: No
Brand Name: Meridia

BENEFITS versus RISKS	
Possible Benefits	*Possible Risks*
EFFECTIVE WEIGHT LOSS FOR ONE YEAR	SIGNIFICANT INCREASES IN BLOOD PRESSURE
	Increased premature (asymptomatic) heart contractions

▷ **Principal Uses**

As a Single Drug Product: Uses currently included in FDA-approved labeling: Used to manage obesity, including weight loss and maintaining weight loss in people on a reduced calorie diet (used in those with an initial body mass index—BMI; see Glossary—greater than or equal to 30 kg per square meter or 27 kg per square meter if there are other risk factors, such as diabetes, hyperlipidemia, or hypertension).

Other (unlabeled) generally accepted uses: May have a role in depression.

How This Drug Works: This medicine helps treat obesity by decreasing the desire to eat by blocking reuptake of nerve transmitters (norepinephrine, serotonin, and dopamine) in brain synapses. People who took the drug in clinical studies were satisfied more quickly when they ate. Since metabolism is also increased, they used more of the food that they did eat than patients

*See Controlled Drug Schedules at the back of this book.

not receiving the medicine. Most of this effect comes from two active compounds (metabolites) that the body changes sibutramine into (M1 and M2).

Available Dosage Forms and Strengths

Capsules — 5 mg, 10 mg, 15 mg

▷ **Recommended Dose Range** (Actual dose and schedule must be determined for each patient individually.)

Dosing is started at 10 mg once a day in the morning. This dose may be decreased to 5 mg daily if not tolerated (using blood pressure and heart rate as guides). If weight loss does not reach goals after 4 weeks, the dose can be increased to 15 mg daily. The daily maximum is 15 mg.

Conditions Requiring Dosing Adjustments

Liver Function: This drug is changed in the liver; however, dose changes are not thought to be needed in mild to moderate liver failure. Drug should NOT be used in severe liver failure.

Kidney Function: No changes needed in mild to moderate kidney failure. Drug should NOT be used in severe kidney failure.

▷ **Dosing Instructions:**   Capsule may be taken before or following food. It was usually taken in the morning in clinical trials. If the starting dose of 10 mg isn't tolerated (using heart rate and blood pressure as guides) discuss this with your doctor. The dose is usually then lowered to 5 mg daily in those cases.

Usual Duration of Use: This medicine has only been used up to a year in clinical studies.

Longer-term use should be discussed with your doctor. Safety and effectiveness for longer than 1 year have NOT been determined. Ongoing use requires periodic physician follow-up.

▷ **This Drug Should Not Be Taken If**
- you had an allergic reaction to any form of it previously.
- you've had a stroke.
- you have a history of abnormal heart rhythms.
- you have pulmonary hypertension.
- you have poorly controlled or uncontrolled high blood pressure.
- you have congestive heart failure or disease of the coronary arteries.
- other causes of obesity such as untreated low thyroid function (hypothyroidism) were not ruled out.
- you are anorexic.
- you have glaucoma.
- you take or have taken a monoamine oxidase (MAO) inhibitor (see Drug Classes) within the last 14 days.
- you have severe kidney or liver disease.

▷ **Inform Your Physician Before Taking This Drug If**
- you have heart (cardiovascular) disease or have had an unfavorable reaction to any serotonin reuptake inhibitor.
- you have narrow-angle glaucoma.
- you have a history of abnormal heart rhythms.
- you have a history of kidney or liver compromise.
- you have a history of psychiatric disorders or drug abuse.
- you have taken other weight loss medicines (anorexiants) in the last year.

- you have a seizure disorder.
- you develop unexplained difficulty in breathing, fainting, chest pain, or swelling of the ankles. These may be early symptoms of pulmonary hypertension.

Possible Side Effects (natural, expected, and unavoidable drug actions)

> Since some weight-loss agents that cause increased levels of serotonin have been associated with development of a fatal lung problem (primary pulmonary hypertension—PPH), it is prudent to talk about this with your doctor. It is unknown if sibutramine can cause this problem.

▷ **Possible Adverse Effects** (unusual, unexpected, and infrequent reactions)

> **If any of the following develop, consult your physician promptly for guidance.**

Mild Adverse Effects

Allergic reaction: skin rash.

Headache and anorexia—frequent

Sleep disturbances—infrequent.

Dry mouth or constipation—frequent

Palpitations or tachycardia leading to stopping the drug—rare.

Fast heart rate (tachycardia)—infrequent.

Increased liver enzymes—frequent (questionable cause).

Serious Adverse Effects

High blood pressure (increased up to 30% of the level present before starting the medicine)—infrequent.

Low blood platelets—case reports.

Primary pulmonary hypertension (PPH)—not reported.

▷ **Possible Effects on Sexual Function:**   Painful menstruation—infrequent.

Natural Diseases or Disorders That May Be Activated by This Drug

> High blood pressure controlled by other medicines may be increased. Untreated high blood pressure may be worsened.

Possible Effects on Laboratory Tests

> Drug testing: may cause false **positive** tests for amphetamines.

CAUTION

1. It is best to carry a card noting that you are taking this drug. A medicine alert bracelet is also a good idea.
2. This medicine may cause false positive urine drug tests for amphetamines.
3. Other conditions (organic causes) leading to obesity (such as low activity of the thyroid gland—hypothyroidism) should be ruled out prior to starting this medicine.
4. Safety and efficacy of use of sibutramine with other weight loss agents have NOT been established. Combination therapy is NOT recommended.
5. This medicine has not been found to cause lung problems (primary pulmonary hypertension, or PPH); however, other drugs that increase serotonin were subsequently found to do this.

   If you develop unexplained difficulty in breathing, fainting, chest pain, or swelling of the ankles, call your doctor. These may be early symptoms of pulmonary hypertension.
6. Because of the increased risk of increased blood pressure, periodic checks of blood pressure are prudent.

7. Nonprescription medicines such as pseudoephedrine, ephedrine, or phenylpropanolamine can increase heart rate or blood pressure. Talk with your pharmacist or doctor BEFORE you combine any type of decongestant, cough, allergy, or cold medicine.

Precautions for Use

By Infants and Children: Safety and effectiveness have not been established in those less than 16 years old.

By Those Over 60 Years of Age: The drug levels this medicine achieves and the places in the body where this medicine goes are no different for those over 60 than those under 60. Caution should be used (as with all medicines active in the central nervous system) in treating elderly patients with sibutramine. Since there is also a higher occurrence of high blood pressure and heart disease, caution and lower doses appear prudent.

▷ **Advisability of Use During Pregnancy**

Pregnancy Category: C. See Pregnancy Risk Categories at the back of this book.
Human studies: Adequate studies of pregnant women are not available.
NOT recommended for pregnant women.

Advisability of Use If Breast-Feeding

Presence of this drug in breast milk: Unknown in humans.
Avoid drug or refrain from nursing.

Habit-Forming Potential: The possibility of physical dependence is low. Further study is needed to confirm an accurate probability of dependence risk. There was no evidence of addictive or drug-seeking behavior in premarketing studies.

Effects of Overdose: Few cases of overdose have been reported. Rapid heart rate was seen in one overdose.

Possible Effects of Long-Term Use: Weight loss (the desired effect). Increased blood pressure.

Suggested Periodic Examinations While Taking This Drug (at physician's discretion)

Periodic weigh-ins, liver function tests, and checks for early signs of primary pulmonary hypertension are prudent. Periodic blood pressure checks are prudent.

▷ **While Taking This Drug, Observe the Following**

Foods: Follow prescribed portion control and menu choices. Tryptophan (found in some health food stores) increases risk of serotonin syndrome.

Nutritional Support: Dietary counseling and physician- or dietitian-directed menus and portion control are suggested.

Beverages: No restrictions except as described in your dietary guidelines.

▷ *Alcohol:* The manufacturer does not recommend use of excessive alcohol and sibutramine.

Tobacco Smoking: No interactions are described in current literature. I advise everyone to quit smoking.

▷ *Other Drugs:*

Sibutramine *taken concurrently* with

- anti-migraine agents (such as sumatriptan or Imitrex) and dihydroergotamine may rarely result in a serotonin syndrome. DO NOT combine.
- central nervous system active medicines such as benzodiazepines, opioids

(fentanyl, etc.), phenothiazines, and others (see Drug Classes) may have additive effects. Caution is advised.

- dextromethorphan (various brands of cough medicine) may increase risk of serotonin syndrome. DO NOT COMBINE.
- lithium (Lithobid, others) increases risk of serotonin syndrome. DO NOT combine.
- meperidine (Demerol, others) increases risk of serotonin syndrome. DO NOT combine.
- monoamine oxidase (MAO) inhibitors (see Drug Classes) may result in serious, even fatal reactions. Fourteen days should pass after stopping a MAO inhibitor before starting sibutramine.
- pentazocine (Talwin, others) increases risk of serotonin syndrome. DO NOT combine.
- selective serotonin reuptake inhibitors (SSRIs) increases risk of serotonin syndrome. DO NOT COMBINE.
- tricyclic antidepressants such as desipramine (Norpramin) and amitriptyline (Elavil) increase serotonin syndrome risk.
- tryptophan (various) increases risk of serotonin syndrome. DO NOT combine.

Sibutramine *taken concurrently* with the following may result in increased sibutramine levels:

- erythromycins (see *macrolide antibiotics* in Drug Classes).
- itraconazole (Sporonox).
- ketoconazole (Nizoral).
- mibefradil (Posicor) (recently removed from the US market).
- nelfinavir (Viracept), and perhaps other protease inhibitors (see Drug Classes); may increase blood levels.
- sildenafil (Viagra) and any medicine that interferes with cytochrome (CYP3A4) is removed from the body by this enzyme and will potentially increase sibutramine blood levels. Sibutramine dosing will need to be adjusted.

The following drugs may *decrease* the effects of sibutramine:

- rifabutin (Mycobutin).
- rifampin (Rifadin, Rimactane).

▷ *Driving, Hazardous Activities:* Use caution.

Aviation Note: The use of this drug *may be a disqualification* for piloting. Consult a designated aviation medical examiner.

Exposure to Sun: No restrictions at present.

Occurrence of Unrelated Illness: Since weight loss may modify the need for medicines used to control blood pressure and lipids, the medicines used in these conditions may need to be adjusted.

Discontinuation: Ask your doctor for help if you are considering stopping this medicine.

SILDENAFIL CITRATE (sill DEN ah fill)

Introduced: 1998   **Class:** Anti-impotence   **Prescription:** USA: Yes   **Controlled Drug:** USA: No; Canada: No   **Available as Generic:** USA: No; Canada: No   **Brand Name:** Viagra

BENEFITS versus RISKS	
Possible Benefits	*Possible Risks*
SUCCESSFUL ACHIEVEMENT OF AN ERECTION	Drug-induced vision changes
	Headache
SUFFICIENT ERECTION TO ACHIEVE INTERCOURSE	

▷ **Principal Uses**

As a Single Drug Product: Uses currently included in FDA-approved labeling: (1) Treats difficulties getting or maintaining an erection (erectile dysfunction); (2) clinical trials that led to FDA approval for this medicine also showed better success rates for sexual intercourse for those using sildenafil versus placebo.

Other (unlabeled) generally accepted uses: Many anecdotal reports of improvement in sexuality (enhancement) and benefits in females have been made, but well-designed scientific studies have not been performed.

How This Drug Works: Causes smooth muscle in the penis to relax, increasing blood flow into the penis, resulting in erection. Sildenafil causes release of nitric oxide (NO) in part of the penis called the corpus cavernosum. This then increases an enzyme called guanylate cyclase. This enzyme increases cyclic guanosine monophosphate (CGMP). The CGMP causes the smooth muscle in the penis to relax. Once smooth muscle relaxes, blood flows into the penis, resulting in erection.

Available Dose Forms and Strengths

Tablets — 25 mg, 50 mg, 100 mg

▷ **Recommended Dose Ranges** (Actual dose and schedule must be determined for each patient individually.)

Infants and Children: Not used in this age group.

18 to 65 Years of Age: Fifty mg is used once daily about an hour before sexual activity.

The manufacturer says that the medicine can be taken from 30 minutes to four hours before sexual activity.

Over 65 Years of Age: Because plasma levels of sildenafil may be increased in this age group, doses should be reduced to 25 mg once daily. The drug can be taken 30 minutes to 4 hours before intercourse, as for those 18 to 65.

Conditions Requiring Dosing Adjustments

Liver Function: A starting dose of 25 mg is prudent in liver disease.

Kidney Function: Caution is advised as one measure of drug levels is doubled in those with compromised kidneys.

▷ **Dosing Instructions:**   The tablet may be crushed and taken without regard to eating (high fat meals decreased absorption, but not to a clinically significant degree). It can be taken an hour before sexual activity (the manufacturer mentions an acceptable range of half an hour to four hours before sexual activity).

Usual Duration of Use: Use is only recommended ONCE daily. If use is to be ongoing on a daily basis, this should be discussed with your doctor.

Possible Advantages of This Drug
> Avoids direct injections into the penis.
> Avoids surgical placement of an implant.

▷ **This Drug Should Not Be Taken If**
- you have had an allergic reaction to it previously.
- you are taking any nitrate (see Drug Classes). NEVER combine these medicines.

▷ **Inform Your Physician Before Taking This Drug If**
- you have liver or kidney disease.
- the drug was prescribed for you without a complete medical history or physical examination.
- you have a history of heart disease.
- you are over 65 and a 50 mg dose has been prescribed.
- you have vision changes while taking this medicine.
- you have cataracts or impaired vision.
- you have had structural damage to the penis (Peyronie's disease—see Glossary).
- you are taking a medicine that blocks or enhances the liver cytochrome system (CYP3A4 or 2C9) (TALK TO YOUR DOCTOR OR PHARMACIST ABOUT THIS).
- you have retinal disease (retinitis pigmentosa).
- you are prone to heartburn, or have other stomach conditions.
- you do not have any improvement in erections or sexual performance while taking this medicine.
- you are unsure of how much to take or how often to take it.

Possible Side Effects (natural, expected, and unavoidable drug actions)
> Changes in vision (blue tint) or dry eyes—up to 3% in clinical trials.

▷ **Possible Adverse Effects** (unusual, unexpected, and infrequent reactions)
> **If any of the following develop, consult your physician promptly for guidance.**
> *Mild Adverse Effects*
> Allergic reactions: rash.
> Headache—infrequent.
> Flushing—infrequent to frequent.
> Indigestion—infrequent.
> Sensitivity to light or blurred vision—possible to infrequent.
> Inability to distinguish between blue and green—possible and may be dose related.
> *Serious Adverse Effects*
> Not defined except for drug interactions.

▷ **Possible Effects on Sexual Function:**   No negative sexual function effects reported.

Possible Delayed Adverse Effects: None reported to date.

Natural Diseases or Disorders That May Be Activated by This Drug
> Patient perception of any preexisting retinal disease may be worsened if sildenafil haze or bluish vision tinting happens.

Possible Effects on Laboratory Tests
> None reported.

CAUTION

Author's Note: Case reports of 6 deaths were reviewed by the FDA in May 1998. A total of 30 deaths were reviewed as of June 1998. Based on the review, Viagra itself was NOT found to be the cause of the deaths and NO CHANGES were made to the package insert.

1. Because of the possibility of SERIOUS drug interactions, keep a card in your purse or wallet or get a medicine alert bracelet to wear that says you are taking sildenafil.
2. If this medicine does not help you to get or maintain an erection, it is important that you follow up with your doctor.
3. Safety and efficacy of sildenafil combined with other treatments for erectile problems (dysfunction) have not been established and are not recommended.
4. Some people use illegal poppers which are actually ampules of alkyl nitrites to enhance sexual activity. These should NEVER be combined with Viagra.
5. The American Academy of Ophthalmology recommended further studies of slidenafil's long-term effects on the eyes, and also warned that those with conditions of the retina should take the drug in the lowest effective dose and with caution. Promptly report altered or impaired vision so that appropriate evaluation can be made.
6. The manufacturer notes that it is important to have a physical exam and medical history taken to properly diagnose problems with erections (erectile dysfunction) and to identify (where possible) any underlying disease or condition that may actually be the cause of the problem (such as diabetes).

Precautions for Use

By Infants and Children: Safety and effectiveness for those under 18 not established.

By Those Over 60 Years of Age: Because this medicine is more slowly removed from the body in this age group, drug levels may be higher. Twenty-five mg is the recommended starting dose.

▷ **Advisability of Use During Pregnancy**

Pregnancy Category: B. See Pregnancy Risk Categories at the back of this book.

Human studies: Adequate studies of pregnant women are not available. NOT indicated for use in pregnant women.

Advisability of Use If Breast-Feeding

Presence of this drug in breast milk: Unknown.

Avoid drug or refrain from nursing.

Habit-Forming Potential: None.

Effects of Overdose: Not defined.

Possible Effects of Long-Term Use: Not defined.

Suggested Periodic Examinations While Taking This Drug (at physician's discretion)

Follow-up on success in achieving an erection and having intercourse.

Complete eye examination at beginning of treatment and at any time that significant change in vision occurs. Ask your doctor for help.

▷ **While Taking This Drug, Observe the Following**

Foods: Grapefruit juice can be an inhibitor of CYP3A4. Do NOT combine.

Beverages: Grapefruit juice can be an inhibitor of CYP3A4. Do NOT combine. May be taken with milk or water.

▷ *Alcohol:* Excess alcohol intake may blunt the benefits of this medicine.

Tobacco Smoking: No interactions expected. I advise everyone to quit smoking.

Marijuana Smoking: The active ingredient (cannabinoids) found in marijuana can act as inhibitors of the principle enzyme (CYP3A4) that removes sildenafil from the body. COMBININATION IS NOT recommended.

▷ *Other Drugs:*

Sildenafil may ***increase*** the effects of
- nitrates (see Drug Classes)—NEVER COMBINE.

The following drugs may ***increase*** the effects of sildenafil:
- cimetidine (Tagamet).
- erythromycins (see *macrolide antibiotics* in Drug Classes).
- itraconazole (Sporonox).
- ketoconazole (Nizoral).
- metronidazole (Flagyl).
- mibefradil (Posicor) (recently removed from the US market).
- nelfinavir (Viracept), and perhaps other protease inhibitors (see Drug Classes), may increase blood levels.
- Any medicine such as sibutramine (Meridia) that interferes with cytochrome (CYP3A4—major; or 2C9—minor). Such medicines will potentially increase sildenafil blood levels. In some cases, sildenafil dosing will need to be adjusted; in others, the combination should be avoided.
- sertraline (Zoloft).

Sildenafil ***taken concurrently*** with
- glipizide (Glucotrol) has resulted in serious interactions. DO NOT COMBINE.
- medicines that cause vision changes (see Section Six: Table Four) may result in additive vision problems.

The following drugs may ***decrease*** the effects of sildenafil:
- carbamazepine (Tegretol).
- phenytoin (Dilantin).
- rifampin (Rifadin, Rimactane).
- rifabutin (Mycobutin).
- troglitazone (Rezulin).

Author's Note: Some clinicians are beginning to question the combination of Viagra with any medicines for high blood pressure.

▷ *Driving, Hazardous Activities:* No restrictions.

Aviation Note: The use of this drug ***may be a disqualification*** for piloting. Consult a designated aviation medical examiner.

Exposure to Sun: May increase sensitivity of your eyes to sunlight. Talk to your doctor about sunglasses or other protective measures.

Discontinuation: Talk to your doctor about your results from taking this drug.

SIMVASTATIN (sim vah STA tin)

Introduced: 1986   **Class:** Anticholesterol (HMG-CoA reductase inhibitor)
Prescription: USA: Yes   **Controlled Drug:** USA: No; Canada: No   **Available as Generic:** USA: No; Canada: No
Brand Name: Zocor

<table>
<tr><td colspan="2" align="center">BENEFITS versus RISKS</td></tr>
<tr><td align="center">Possible Benefits</td><td align="center">Possible Risks</td></tr>
<tr><td>EFFECTIVE REDUCTION OF TOTAL
  BLOOD CHOLESTEROL AND LDL
  CHOLESTEROL
REDUCES RISK FROM CORONARY
  DISEASE
REDUCES DEATH FROM
  CORONARY
  REVASCULARIZATION
REDUCES NONFATAL
  MYOCARDIAL INFARCTIONS
REDUCES RISK OF STROKES</td><td>Drug-induced liver problems
  (hepatitis)
Drug-induced muscle damage
  (myositis)</td></tr>
</table>

▷ **Principal Uses**

As a Single Drug Product: Uses currently included in FDA-approved labeling: (1) Used by patients with elevated cholesterol to reduce death from heart disease and decrease the number of nonfatal heart attacks; (2) treats high total blood cholesterol levels in people with types IIa and IIb hypercholesterolemia (used in conjunction with a cholesterol-lowering diet; it should not be used until an adequate trial of nondrug methods for lowering cholesterol has proved to be ineffective); (3) stops progression and decreases number of deaths of patients with coronary artery disease; (4) decreases risk of strokes.

Other (unlabeled) generally accepted uses: (1) May help reduce lipid disorders that occur in kidney (nephrotic syndrome) problems; (2) has a role in combination therapy to prevent gallstones.

How This Drug Works: Blocks the liver enzyme starting production of cholesterol. Reduces low-density lipoproteins (LDL), the fraction of cholesterol thought to increase risk of coronary heart disease. May also increase high-density lipoproteins (HDL), the cholesterol fraction that reduces the risk of heart disease.

Available Dose Forms and Strengths

Tablets — 5 mg, 10 mg, 20 mg, 40 mg

Author's Note: The maker of this medicine is planning a double-strength version of simvastatin.

▷ **Recommended Dose Ranges** (Actual dose and schedule must be determined for each patient individually.)

Infants and Children: Under 2 years of age—do not use this drug.

2 to 20 years of age—dose not established.

20 to 60 Years of Age: Initially 5 to 10 mg daily, taken at bedtime. Dose is increased as needed to reach desired goals (such as decreased LDL-C percent).

More aggressive goals may require the 10-mg starting dose. The drug is then increased as needed and tolerated by increments of 5 to 10 mg at intervals of 4 weeks. The total daily dose should not exceed 40 mg.

Over 60 Years of Age: Initially 5 mg daily. Increase dose as needed and tolerated by increments of 5 mg at intervals of 4 weeks. The total daily dose should not exceed 20 mg.

Conditions Requiring Dosing Adjustments

Liver Function: This drug achieves a high concentration in the liver, and is subsequently eliminated in the bile. It can be a rare cause of liver damage, and patients should be followed closely.

Kidney Function: In severe kidney failure, the dose should be started at 5 mg, and the patient closely followed.

▷ **Dosing Instructions:** The tablet may be crushed and taken without regard to eating, preferably taken at bedtime (the highest rates of cholesterol production occur between midnight and 5 A.M.).

Usual Duration of Use: Use on a regular schedule for 4 to 6 weeks usually determines effectiveness in reducing blood levels of total and LDL cholesterol. Long-term use (months to years) requires periodic physician evaluation of response and dose adjustment. Consult your physician on a regular basis.

Possible Advantages of This Drug

Recent studies indicate that HMG-CoA reductase inhibitors are more effective and better tolerated than other drugs currently available for reducing total and LDL cholesterol.

▷ **This Drug Should Not Be Taken If**
- you have had an allergic reaction to it previously.
- you have active liver disease.
- you are pregnant or breast-feeding your infant.

▷ **Inform Your Physician Before Taking This Drug If**
- you have previously taken any other drugs in this class: lovastatin (Mevacor) or pravastatin (Pravachol).
- you have a history of liver disease or impaired liver function.
- you are not using any method of birth control, or you are planning pregnancy.
- you regularly consume substantial amounts of alcohol.
- you have cataracts or impaired vision.
- you have any type of chronic muscular disorder.
- you develop muscle pain, weakness, or soreness that is unexplained while taking this medicine.
- you plan to have major surgery in the near future.

Possible Side Effects (natural, expected, and unavoidable drug actions)
Development of abnormal liver function tests without associated symptoms.

▷ **Possible Adverse Effects** (unusual, unexpected, and infrequent reactions)
If any of the following develop, consult your physician promptly for guidance.

Mild Adverse Effects
Allergic reactions: rash.
Headache—infrequent.

Nausea, excessive gas, constipation, diarrhea—rare to infrequent.

Lowering of blood pressure—possible.

Serious Adverse Effects

Marked and persistent abnormal liver function tests with focal hepatitis—rare.

Acute myositis (muscle pain and tenderness)—infrequent.

Rhabdomyolysis—rare.

Potential for cataracts—based on animal data, not reported in humans.

Depression—rare.

Protein in the urine—rare.

Lichen planus skin rash—rare.

▷ **Possible Effects on Sexual Function:**   Impotence—case reports.

Possible Delayed Adverse Effects: None reported to date. Doses 15 to 33 times the human dose given to rats caused an increase in liver cancers.

Natural Diseases or Disorders That May Be Activated by This Drug

Latent liver disease.

Possible Effects on Laboratory Tests

Blood alanine aminotransferase (ALT) enzyme level: increased (with higher doses of drug).

Blood total cholesterol, LDL cholesterol, and triglyceride levels: decreased.

Blood HDL cholesterol level: increased.

CAUTION

1. If pregnancy occurs while taking simvastatin, stop taking this drug immediately and call your physician.
2. Report promptly any development of muscle pain or tenderness, especially if accompanied by fever or weakness (malaise).
3. Promptly report altered or impaired vision so that appropriate evaluation can be made.

Precautions for Use

By Infants and Children: Safety and effectiveness for those under 20 years of age are not established.

By Those Over 60 Years of Age: Inform your physician regarding any personal or family history of cataracts. Comply with all recommendations regarding periodic eye examinations. Report promptly any alterations in vision.

▷ **Advisability of Use During Pregnancy**

Pregnancy Category: X. See Pregnancy Risk Categories at the back of this book.

Animal studies: Mouse and rat studies reveal skeletal birth defects due to a closely related drug of this class.

Human studies: Adequate studies of pregnant women are not available.

This drug should be avoided during entire pregnancy.

Advisability of Use If Breast-Feeding

Presence of this drug in breast milk: Unknown.

Avoid drug or refrain from nursing.

Habit-Forming Potential: None.

Effects of Overdose: Increased indigestion, stomach distress, nausea, diarrhea.

Possible Effects of Long-Term Use: Abnormal liver function with focal hepatitis.

Suggested Periodic Examinations While Taking This Drug (at physician's discretion)

Blood cholesterol studies: total cholesterol, HDL, and LDL fractions.

Liver function tests before treatment, and at 6-month intervals for 1 year. In patients who have had an increase in liver enzymes, testing should continue at 6-month intervals until 1 year after the last liver function test elevation.

Complete eye examination at beginning of treatment and at any time that significant change in vision occurs. Ask your doctor for help.

▷ **While Taking This Drug, Observe the Following**

Foods: Follow a standard low-cholesterol diet.

Beverages: No restrictions. May be taken with milk.

▷ *Alcohol:* No interactions expected. Use sparingly.

Tobacco Smoking: No interactions expected. I advise everyone to quit smoking.

▷ *Other Drugs:*

Simvastatin may *increase* the effects of
- digoxin (Lanoxin).
- warfarin (Coumadin); more frequent testing of INR (prothrombin time or protime) will be needed.

Simvastatin *taken concurrently* with
- clofibrate (Atromid-S) or other fibrates may result in increased risk of serious muscle toxicity.
- cyclosporine (Sandimmune) can result in kidney failure and myopathy.
- gemfibrozil (Lopid) may alter absorption and excretion of simvastatin. DO NOT COMBINE.
- mibefradil (Posicor) may increase risk of toxicity.
- niacin may cause an increased frequency of muscle problems (myopathy) when combined with a related medicine (lovastatin). Caution is advised.
- ritonavir (Norvir) may lead to simvastatin toxicity.

The following drug may *decrease* the effects of simvastatin:
- cholestyramine (Questran) may reduce absorption of simvastatin; take simvastatin 1 hour before or 4 hours after cholestyramine.

▷ *Driving, Hazardous Activities:* No restrictions.

Aviation Note: The use of this drug *may be a disqualification* for piloting. Consult a designated aviation medical examiner.

Exposure to Sun: No restrictions.

Discontinuation: Do not stop this drug without your physician's knowledge and guidance. There may be significant increase in blood cholesterol levels following discontinuation of this drug.

SPIRONOLACTONE (speer on oh LAK tohn)

Introduced: 1959   **Class:** Diuretic   **Prescription:** USA: Yes   **Controlled Drug:** USA: No; Canada: No   **Available as Generic:** USA: Yes

Brand Names: Alatone, Aldactazide [CD], Aldactone, ✦Apo-Spirozide, ✦Novospiroton, ✦Novospirozine [CD], ✦Sincomen, Spironazide

---

BENEFITS versus RISKS

Possible Benefits	*Possible Risks*
EFFECTIVE PREVENTION OF POTASSIUM LOSS when used adjunctively with other diuretics	ABNORMALLY HIGH BLOOD POTASSIUM LEVEL with excessive use
EFFECTIVE DIURETIC IN REFRACTORY CASES OF FLUID RETENTION when used adjunctively with other diuretics	Enlargement of male breast tissue
	Masculinization effects in women: excessive hair growth, deepening of the voice
	Hepatitis

▷ **Principal Uses**

As a Single Drug Product: Uses currently included in FDA-approved labeling: (1) Manages congestive heart failure and disorders of the liver and kidney that are accompanied by excessive fluid retention (edema); (2) also used with other measures to treat high blood pressure where prevention of potassium loss is needed; (3) used to decrease fluid in patients who have failed glucocorticoid treatment and have nephrotic syndrome.

Other (unlabeled) generally accepted uses: (1) May have an adjunctive role in treating acne; (2) can help treat lung problems (bronchopulmonary dysplasia) and slow the disease process; (3) can help precocious puberty in females; (4) eases fluid buildup in premenstrual syndrome; (5) may help women with excessive facial hair growth (hirsutism).

As a Combination Drug Product [CD]: This drug is available in combination with hydrochlorothiazide, a different kind of diuretic that promotes the loss of potassium from the body. Spironolactone is used in this combination to counteract the potassium-wasting effect of the thiazide diuretic.

How This Drug Works: By inhibiting the action of aldosterone (an adrenal gland hormone), this drug prevents the reabsorption of sodium and the excretion of potassium by the kidney. Thus the drug promotes the excretion of sodium (and water with it) and the retention of potassium.

Available Dose Forms and Strengths

Tablets — 25 mg, 50 mg, 100 mg

▷ **Usual Adult Dose Range:**   For edema: Initially 100 mg per day in one dose or divided into several doses. The dose is then adjusted according to individual response. The usual maintenance dose is 50 to 200 mg daily, divided into two to four doses. If response is not adequate after 5 days, a second fluid medicine (diuretic) is added. **Note: Actual dose and schedule must be determined for each patient individually.**

Conditions Requiring Dosing Adjustments

Liver Function: This drug can be a rare cause of liver damage, and patients should be followed closely.

Kidney Function: For patients with mild kidney failure, the drug can be taken every 12 hours in the usual dose. In moderate kidney failure, spironolactone can be taken every 12 to 24 hours in the usual dose. In severe kidney failure, this drug should **not** be taken. Spironolactone is contraindicated in acute renal failure and severe chronic renal compromise.

▷ **Dosing Instructions:** The tablet may be crushed and taken with or following meals to promote absorption of the drug and reduce stomach irritation.
Author's note: The information in this profile has been shortened to make room for more widely used medicines.

STAVUDINE (STAV u dine)

Other Names: D4T

Introduced: 1994 **Class:** Anti-AIDS drug **Prescription:** USA: Yes
Controlled Drug: USA: No; Canada: No **Available as Generic:** USA: No; Canada: No

Brand Name: Zerit

BENEFITS versus RISKS	
Possible Benefits	*Possible Risks*
INCREASED CD4 COUNTS IN ADULTS WITH ADVANCED HIV	PERIPHERAL NEUROPATHY
THERAPEUTIC OPTION VERSUS AZT OR OTHER NUCLEOSIDE ANALOGS	Pancreatitis
LESS LIKELY THAN OTHER AGENTS TO DEVELOP RESISTANCE	
EFFECTIVE COMBINATION THERAPY OF HIV	
PART OF A COMBINATION REGIMEN REDUCING HIV TO UNDETECTABLE LEVELS	

▷ **Principal Uses**
As a Single Drug Product: Uses currently included in FDA-approved labeling: Treatment of HIV in adults and children.
Author's Note: *The Panel on Clinical Practices for Treatment of HIV Infection Report* says that the preferred regimen is two nucleoside analogs and one potent protease inhibitor. Single-agent therapy (with the exception of AZT use in preventing HIV transmission from mother to fetus) was rejected by the panel.
Other (unlabeled) generally accepted uses: Combination therapy may offer a durable increase in CD4 count and decrease in viral load.

How This Drug Works: This drug inhibits HIV reproduction (replication) by: (1) Inhibiting an HIV enzyme (reverse transcriptase), which blocks the ability of the virus to make nuclear material; (2) inhibiting an enzyme (DNA polymerase-gamma and -beta), which blocks the ability to make DNA in the mitochondria.

Available Dose Forms and Strengths
Capsules — 15 mg, 20 mg, 30 mg, 40 mg
Powder — 1 mg/ml

▷ **Recommended Dose Ranges** (Actual dose and schedule must be determined for each patient individually.)

Infants and Children: Children weighing less than 30 kg are given 2 mg per kg per day.

Those greater than 30 kg are given the adult dose.

18 to 60 Years of Age: Patients with a body mass of 60 kg (132 lb) or more should take 40 mg twice daily. Patients with a body mass of less than 60 kg should take 30 mg twice daily.

For those who have had to stop because of peripheral neuropathy (after complete resolution of symptoms): 20 mg twice daily for patients with a body mass of 60 kg or more; 15 mg twice daily for those with a body mass less than 60 kg.

Over 65 Years of Age: This drug has **not** been studied in those over 65.

Conditions Requiring Dosing Adjustments

Liver Function: If liver enzymes increase significantly, therapy may need to be stopped, then reintroduced with 20 mg daily for those patients greater than 60 kg and 15 mg daily for those less than 60 kg.

Kidney Function: Patients with mild kidney compromise (creatinine clearance greater than 50 ml/min) failure take the usual weight-adjusted dose for adults. Mild to moderate failure (creatinine clearance 26 to 50 ml/min) should take one-half of the usual weight-adjusted dose every 12 hours. In severe kidney compromise (creatinine clearance 10 to 25 ml/min) one-half the usual weight-adjusted dose should be taken every 24 hours.

▷ **Dosing Instructions:**   This drug may be taken without regard to food.

Usual Duration of Use: Use on a regular schedule for several months usually determines effectiveness in slowing AIDS progression and increasing CD4 counts. Long-term use (months to years) requires periodic physician evaluation of response (viral burden and CD4).

Possible Advantages of This Drug

More favorable side-effect profile than other nucleoside analogs. Favorable profile for combination therapy.

▷ **This Drug Should Not Be Taken If**
  • you had an allergic reaction to it previously.

▷ **Inform Your Physician Before Taking This Drug If**
  • you have had peripheral neuropathy caused by other drugs before.
  • you have kidney or liver compromise.
  • you have had pancreatitis.
  • your bone marrow is depressed.
  • you have vitamin B_{12} deficiency or folic acid deficiency.
  • you are unsure how much to take or how often to take it.

Possible Side Effects (natural, expected, and unavoidable drug actions)

Chills or fever—infrequent. Peripheral neuropathy—infrequent to frequent. Pancreatitis—infrequent.

▷ **Possible Adverse Effects** (unusual, unexpected, and infrequent reactions)

If any of the following develop, consult your physician promptly for guidance.

Mild Adverse Effects

Allergic reactions: skin rash.

Nausea and vomiting or abdominal pain—infrequent.

Increased liver enzymes—frequent.

Serious Adverse Effects

Allergic reactions: anaphylactic reactions—rare.

Anemia—case reports.

Low white blood cell or platelet counts—rare to infrequent in phase three data, not found in later data.

▷ **Possible Effects on Sexual Function:**   Impotence—rare in phase three data.

Possible Delayed Adverse Effects: Peripheral neuropathy.

▷ **Adverse Effects That May Mimic Natural Diseases or Disorders**

Increased liver function tests may mimic hepatitis.

Possible Effects on Laboratory Tests

Liver function tests: increased.

Amylase: increased.

Complete blood counts: decreased platelets and white blood cells—possible.

CAUTION

1. Stavudine has not been shown to decrease the risk of giving (transmission) HIV to others through sexual contact or blood contamination.
2. Promptly report the development of stomach pain and vomiting; this could indicate pancreatitis.
3. Report development of pain, numbness, or tingling or burning in the hands or feet, as this may be peripheral neuropathy.

Precautions for Use

By Infants and Children: Watch carefully for adverse effects.

By Those Over 65 Years of Age: Age-related decline in kidney function may require dosing changes.

▷ **Advisability of Use During Pregnancy**

Pregnancy Category: C. See Pregnancy Risk Categories at the back of this book.

Animal studies: Clinical doses in rats have not revealed teratogenicity; however, doses of 399 times those used in humans have resulted in skeletal problems. Increased early rat death has also occurred at 399 times the human dose.

Human studies: Adequate studies of pregnant women are not available.

Ask your doctor for guidance.

Advisability of Use If Breast-Feeding

Presence of this drug in breast milk: Yes.

Refrain from nursing if you are HIV positive or are taking this drug.

Habit-Forming Potential: None.

Effects of Overdose: Adults treated with 12 to 24 times the recommended daily dose revealed no acute toxicity.

Possible Effects of Long-Term Use: Peripheral neuropathy and hepatic toxicity.

Suggested Periodic Examinations While Taking This Drug (at physician's discretion)

Liver function tests, amylase and complete blood counts.

CD4 or viral load measurement.

▷ **While Taking This Drug, Observe the Following**
Foods: No restrictions.
Beverages: No restrictions.
▷ *Alcohol:* No interactions expected.
Tobacco Smoking: No interactions expected. I advise everyone to quit smoking.
▷ *Other Drugs:*
Stavudine *taken concurrently* with
• other drugs such as metronidazole (Flagyl) that can cause peripheral neuropathy should be avoided if possible.
Stavudine may *increase* the effects of
• didanosine (Videx) at specific drug concentration ratios.
• zidovudine (AZT) at specific drug concentration ratios.
Stavudine may *decrease* the effects of
• didanosine (Videx) at specific drug concentration ratios.
• zidovudine (AZT) at specific drug concentration ratios.
▷ *Driving, Hazardous Activities:* This drug may cause dizziness. Restrict activities as necessary.
Aviation Note: The use of this drug *may be a disqualification* for piloting. Consult a designated aviation medical examiner.
Exposure to Sun: No restrictions.
Discontinuation: Do not stop this drug without your doctor's knowledge and guidance.

STRONTIUM-89 (STRON tee um)

Introduced: 1993   **Class:** Systemic radionuclide, pain syndrome modifier
Prescription: USA: Yes   **Controlled Drug:** USA: No; Canada: No   **Available as Generic:** USA: No; Canada: No
Brand Name: Metastron

BENEFITS versus RISKS	
Possible Benefits	*Possible Risks*
EFFECTIVE RELIEF OF PRIMARY OR METASTATIC BONE CANCER PAIN	BONE MARROW TOXICITY (decreased white blood cells and platelets) Transient increase in bone pain

▷ **Principal Uses**
As a Single Drug Product: Uses currently included in FDA-approved labeling: Used to treat metastatic bone cancer pain.
Other (unlabeled) generally accepted uses: None at present.
How This Drug Works: This radiopharmaceutical is selectively taken up by areas of bone cancer. Once it accumulates in cancerous areas, it emits radiation directly at the site of the cancer.
Available Dose Forms and Strengths
Injection — 10.9 to 22.6 mg of strontium in a total of 1 ml of water
▷ **Recommended Dose Ranges** (Actual dose and schedule must be determined for each patient individually.)

Infants and Children: Safety and effectiveness for those less than 18 years old are not established.

18 to 60 Years of Age: A dose of 4 MCi (148 MBq) is given intravenously over 1 to 2 minutes. The dose may also be calculated using 40 to 60 mcCI/kg. The dose may be repeated at 90-day intervals, if needed.

Over 60 Years of Age: Same as 18 to 60 years of age.

Conditions Requiring Dosing Adjustments

Liver Function: Dosing changes in liver compromise do not appear to be needed.

Kidney Function: This agent is primarily removed by the kidneys; however, decreases in doses are not presently defined.

▷ **Dosing Instructions:** You may eat and drink as you normally would. During the first week after injection, strontium-89 will be present in the blood and the urine. A normal toilet should be used in preference to a urinal.

Usual Duration of Use: Use of previously prescribed pain medicine will be expected for 7 to 20 days after the injection. A maximum of 20 days after injection has been needed to determine peak effectiveness in controlling bone cancer pain. The dose may be repeated (if blood tests are acceptable) 90 days after the prior dose was given. See your physician on a regular basis.

Possible Advantages of This Drug

Effective control of bone cancer pain without the risks or compromise of narcotics.

▷ **This Drug Should Not Be Taken If**
- you had an allergic reaction to it previously.
- you have cancer that does not involve the bone.

▷ **Inform Your Physician Before Taking This Drug If**
- you have a history of low platelets or white blood cell counts.
- you take other drugs that may lower white cells or platelets.
- you do not understand how to appropriately dispose of your urine or vomit.

Possible Side Effects (natural, expected, and unavoidable drug actions)

May cause a calciumlike flushing when injected. May cause transient (up to 72 hours) increase in bone pain.

▷ **Possible Adverse Effects** (unusual, unexpected, and infrequent reactions)

If any of the following develop, consult your physician promptly for guidance.

Mild Adverse Effects

Allergic reactions: chills and fever.

Serious Adverse Effects

Allergic reactions: none defined.

Bone marrow toxicity: 20–30% decrease in white cell or platelet counts—may be dose related.

Bacterial infection of blood (septicemia) following drug-induced decreases in white blood cells—possible.

Animal data shows that this drug is a possible carcinogen.

▷ **Possible Effects on Sexual Function:** None reported.

Possible Delayed Adverse Effects: Lowering of white blood cells (recovery in up to 6 months) and blood platelets (lowest count 5 to 16 weeks after therapy).

Natural Diseases or Disorders That May Be Activated by This Drug

Aplastic anemia.

Possible Effects on Laboratory Tests

White blood cell counts: decreased.

Platelet counts: decreased.

CAUTION

1. Promptly report any signs of infection (lethargy, temperature, sore throat).
2. It may take up to 20 days for this agent to work. Narcotics will need to be continued.
3. Your blood and urine will contain radioactive strontium for 7 days after injection. Ask you doctor for help on appropriate disposal.
4. This drug is a potential carcinogen.
5. Promptly report any abnormal bleeding or bruising.

Precautions for Use

By Infants and Children: Safety and effectiveness for those under 18 years of age are not established.

By Those Over 60 Years of Age: Specific changes are not presently needed.

▷ **Advisability of Use During Pregnancy**

Pregnancy Category: D. See Pregnancy Risk Categories at the back of this book.
Animal studies: Adequate studies evaluating potential to cause birth defects have not been performed.
Human studies: Adequate studies of pregnant women are not available.
This drug may cause fetal harm. Ask your doctor for advice.

Advisability of Use If Breast-Feeding

Presence of this drug in breast milk: This drug acts like calcium and is expected to be present in breast milk.
Avoid drug or refrain from nursing.

Habit-Forming Potential: None.

Effects of Overdose: May result in acute radiation syndrome with initial nausea and vomiting followed by depressed white cells and platelets, and tendency to infections. Careful dose calculations are indicated, as this drug emits beta-radiation.

Possible Effects of Long-Term Use: Not indicated for long-term use.

Suggested Periodic Examinations While Taking This Drug (at physician's discretion)

Complete blood counts should be tested once every other week during therapy.

▷ **While Taking This Drug, Observe the Following**

Foods: No restrictions.

Beverages: No restrictions.

▷   *Alcohol:* No interactions expected.

Tobacco Smoking: No interactions expected. I advise everyone to quit smoking.

Marijuana Smoking: No interactions expected.

▷   *Other Drugs:*

Strontium-89 *taken concurrently* with

- medications that lower white blood cells or platelets may result in severe decreases.

▷   *Driving, Hazardous Activities:* This drug may cause a transient increase in bone pain. Restrict activities as necessary.

Aviation Note: The use of this drug *may be a disqualification* for piloting. Consult a designated aviation medical examiner.

Exposure to Sun: No restrictions.

Discontinuation: Dosing may be repeated if blood counts are acceptable.

SUCRALFATE (soo KRAL fayt)

Introduced: 1978   **Class:** Antiulcer, gastrointestinal drug   **Prescription:** USA: Yes   **Controlled Drug:** USA: No; Canada: No   **Available as Generic:** Yes

Brand Names: Carafate, ✢Sulcrate

BENEFITS versus RISKS	
Possible Benefits	*Possible Risks*
EFFECTIVE TREATMENT IN DUODENAL ULCER DISEASE No serious adverse effects	Constipation Skin rash, hives, itching Aluminum toxicity in kidney compromise

▷ **Principal Uses**

As a Single Drug Product: Uses currently included in FDA-approved labeling: Treats and prevents recurrence of duodenal ulcer disease in adults and children. Effective when used alone, but may be used with antacids for pain relief.

Other (unlabeled) generally accepted uses: (1) May be useful in treating stomach (gastric ulcers) if other therapy isn't tolerated; (2) can reduce the frequency of diarrhea caused by radiation therapy; (3) may have a role as a douche in promoting healing of vaginal ulcerations that are resistant to other measures; (4) can ease the pain and spasms associated with tonsillectomy.

How This Drug Works: Promotes ulcer healing by (1) forming a protective coating over the ulcer and ulcer margins, preventing further damage; (2) inhibiting the digestive action of pepsin; (3) stimulating active healing (tissue repair).

Available Dose Forms and Strengths
Tablets — 1 g
Suspension — 1 g/10 ml

▷ **Usual Adult Dose Range:** 1 g four times daily. Note: Actual dose and schedule must be determined for each patient individually.

Conditions Requiring Dosing Adjustments
Liver Function: Sucralfate is not absorbed.
Kidney Function: Sucralfate is not absorbed.

▷ **Dosing Instructions:** Take with water on an empty stomach at least 1 hour before or 2 hours after each meal and at bedtime. Swallow the tablets whole; do not alter or chew. Take the full course prescribed.

Usual Duration of Use: Use on a regular schedule for 6 to 8 weeks is usually needed for peak effect in promoting the healing of ulcers. Use beyond 8 weeks must be determined by your physician.

▷ **This Drug Should Not Be Taken If**
  • you have had an allergic reaction to it previously.
▷ **Inform Your Physician Before Taking This Drug If**
  • you have chronic constipation.
  • you have chronic kidney failure.
  • you are taking any other drugs at this time.
Possible Side Effects (natural, expected, and unavoidable drug actions)
  Constipation—infrequent.
▷ **Possible Adverse Effects** (unusual, unexpected, and infrequent reactions)
  If any of the following develop, consult your physician promptly for guidance.
  Mild Adverse Effects
  Allergic reactions: skin rash, hives, itching.
  Dizziness, light-headedness, drowsiness—infrequent.
  Dry mouth, indigestion, nausea, cramping, diarrhea—infrequent.
  Serious Adverse Effects
  Increased risk of aluminum toxicity (seizures, jerks, and encephalopathy) with patients in end-stage kidney failure.
  Bezoar (a clumping of food) formation in the esophagus or proximal stomach—possible.
▷ **Possible Effects on Sexual Function:**   None reported.
Possible Effects on Laboratory Tests
  None reported.
CAUTION
  1. If antacids are needed to relieve ulcer pain, do not take them within half an hour before or 2 hours after the dose of sucralfate.
  2. This drug may impair the absorption of other drugs if they are taken close together. Avoid taking any other drugs within 2 hours of taking sucralfate. This applies especially to cimetidine (Tagamet), phenytoin (Dilantin), and tetracyclines.
Precautions for Use
  By Infants and Children: This drug has been used to treat reflux esophagitis or long-standing (chronic) duodenal ulcers in those 3 months to 13 years. In esophagitis, 500 mg was used four times daily in those less than 6 years old. Adult dose and interval was used for those 6 or older. Duodenal ulcer treatment used adult doses.
  By Those Over 60 Years of Age: Specific changes not presently needed.
▷ **Advisability of Use During Pregnancy**
  Pregnancy Category: B. See Pregnancy Risk Categories at the back of this book.
  Animal studies: No birth defects reported in mouse, rat, and rabbit studies.
  Human studies: Adequate studies of pregnant women are not available.
  This drug should be used only if clearly needed. Ask your physician for guidance.
Advisability of Use If Breast-Feeding
  Presence of this drug in breast milk: Unknown.
  Watch nursing infant closely and stop drug or nursing if adverse effects develop.
Habit-Forming Potential: None.

Effects of Overdose: Nausea, stomach cramping, possible diarrhea.

Possible Effects of Long-Term Use: Deficiencies of vitamins A, D, E, and K due to impaired absorption from the intestine.

Suggested Periodic Examinations While Taking This Drug (at physician's discretion)

Follow-up on resolution of ulcer symptoms.

▷ **While Taking This Drug, Observe the Following**

Foods: No restrictions. Follow diet prescribed by your physician.

Beverages: No restrictions. This drug is preferably taken with water.

▷ *Alcohol:* No interactions with drug expected. However, alcohol is best avoided because of its irritant effect on the stomach.

Tobacco Smoking: Nicotine can delay ulcer healing and reduce the effectiveness of this drug. Avoid all forms of tobacco.

▷ *Other Drugs:*

Sucralfate may *decrease* the effects of

- cimetidine (Tagamet).
- ciprofloxacin (Cipro).
- digoxin (Lanoxin).
- enoxacin (Penetrex).
- fleroxacin (Megalone).
- grepafloxacin (Raxar).
- ketoconazole (Nizoral).
- lomefloxacin (Maxaquin).
- norfloxacin (Noroxin).
- ofloxacin (Floxin) or temafloxacin (Omniflox).
- phenytoin (Dilantin, etc.).
- quinidine (Quinaglute).
- sparfloxacin (Zagam).
- trovafloxacin (Trovan).
- tetracycline (Achromycin, Tetracyn, etc.).
- warfarin (Coumadin, etc.), and reduce its anticoagulant effect. Increased frequency of INR testing (prothrombin time or protime) is needed.

▷ *Driving, Hazardous Activities:* This drug may cause dizziness or drowsiness. Restrict activities as necessary.

Aviation Note: The use of this drug *may be a disqualification* for piloting. Consult a designated aviation medical examiner.

Exposure to Sun: No restrictions.

SULFAMETHOXAZOLE (sul fa meth OX a zohl)

See the new sulfonamide antibiotic family profile for more information.

SULFASALAZINE (sul fa SAL a zeen)

Introduced: 1949   **Class:** Bowel anti-inflammatory, sulfonamides   **Prescription:** USA: Yes   **Controlled Drug:** USA: No; Canada: No   **Available as Generic:** USA: Yes; Canada: No

Brand Names: Azaline, Azulfidine, Azulfidine EN-Tabs, ✦PMS Sulfasalazine, ✦PMS Sulfasalazine E.C., ✦Salazopyrin, ✦Salazopyrin EN, ✦SAS-Enema, ✦SAS Enteric-500, SAS-500

BENEFITS versus RISKS	
Possible Benefits	*Possible Risks*
EFFECTIVE SUPPRESSION OF INFLAMMATORY BOWEL DISEASE	Allergic reactions: mild to severe skin reactions
SYMPTOMATIC RELIEF OF REGIONAL ENTERITIS AND ULCERATIVE COLITIS	Blood cell disorders: aplastic anemia, hemolytic anemia, abnormally low white cell or platelet counts
HELPFUL IN REFRACTORY RHEUMATOID ARTHRITIS	Drug-induced liver damage
	Drug-induced kidney damage
	Seizures

▷ **Principal Uses**

As a Single Drug Product: Uses currently included in FDA-approved labeling: Treats inflammatory disease of the lower intestinal tract: regional enteritis (Crohn's disease) and ulcerative colitis. It is usually taken by mouth, but may also be used in retention enemas.

Other (unlabeled) generally accepted uses: (1) Short-term use in therapy of ankylosing spondylitis; (2) treatment of mild to moderate psoriasis; (3) helps rheumatoid arthritis.

How This Drug Works: Suppresses the formation of prostaglandins (and related compounds), tissue substances that induce inflammation, tissue destruction, and diarrhea.

Available Dose Forms and Strengths

Oral suspension — 250 mg/5-ml

Tablets — 500 mg

Tablets, enteric coated — 500 mg

▷ **Usual Adult Dose Range:** Ulcerative colitis: Initially 1 to 2 g every 6 to 8 hours until symptoms are adequately controlled. For maintenance, 500 mg every 6 hours. The total daily dose should not exceed 12 g. If diarrhea occurs, the dose is often decreased to the earlier dose that worked and did not cause diarrhea.

Rheumatoid arthritis (when salicylates or NSAIDs have not worked): 2 to 3 grams daily is taken in equally divided doses. If the delayed-release form (Azulfidine EN-Tabs) is used, 500 mg is taken for 1 week in the evening, then 500 mg twice daily for a week, then 500 mg in the morning and 1 g in the evening for a week, and continuing with 1 g twice a day.

Note: Actual dose and schedule must be individually determined.

Conditions Requiring Dosing Adjustments

Liver Function: This drug can be a cause of liver damage, and patients should be followed closely.

Kidney Function: Empiric decreases in doses should be considered. This drug should be used with caution in kidney compromise.

▷ **Dosing Instructions:** This drug is preferably taken with 8 ounces of water on an empty stomach, 1 hour before or 2 hours after eating. However, it may be taken with or following food to reduce stomach irritation. Intervals between doses (day and night) should be no longer than 8 hours. The regular tablet may be crushed; the enteric-coated tablet should be swallowed whole without alteration.

Usual Duration of Use: Use on a regular schedule for 1 to 3 weeks usually determines effectiveness in controlling the symptoms of regional enteritis or ulcerative colitis. Benefits in rheumatoid arthritis may be seen in 4 to 12 weeks. Long-term use (months to years) requires physician supervision.

▷ **This Drug Should Not Be Taken If**
- you are allergic to *any* sulfonamide drug (see Drug Classes), or aspirin (or other salicylates).
- you are in the final month of pregnancy.
- it has been prescribed for an infant less than 2 years old.
- you have a urinary or intestinal obstruction or porphyria.
- you are breast-feeding.

▷ **Inform Your Physician Before Taking This Drug If**
- you are allergic to any sulfonamide—acetazolamide, thiazide diuretics, or sulfonylurea antidiabetics (see Drug Classes).
- you are allergic by nature (history of hay fever, asthma, hives, eczema).
- you have asthma.
- you have impaired liver or kidney function.
- you have a glucose-6-phosphate dehydrogenase (G6PD) deficiency.
- you have a personal or family history of porphyria.
- you have had a drug-induced blood cell or bone marrow disorder.
- you currently take any oral anticoagulant, antidiabetic drug, or phenytoin.
- you plan to have surgery under pentothal anesthesia soon.

Possible Side Effects (natural, expected, and unavoidable drug actions)
Brownish coloration of the urine, of no significance. Skin pigmentation. Superinfections (see Glossary), bacterial or fungal.

▷ **Possible Adverse Effects** (unusual, unexpected, and infrequent reactions)
If any of the following develop, consult your physician promptly for guidance.
Mild Adverse Effects
Allergic reactions: skin rashes, hives, itching.
Headache—frequent; dizziness—infrequent.
Discoloration of contact lenses—possible.
Ringing in the ears—case reports.
Loss of appetite, irritation of mouth or tongue, nausea, vomiting, diarrhea—infrequent to frequent.
Taste disorders—rare.
Serious Adverse Effects
Allergic reactions: drug fever (see Glossary), swollen glands, painful joints, anaphylatic reaction (see Glossary). Allergic pneumonitis, allergic hepatitis. Severe skin reactions (Stevens-Johnson syndrome or toxic epidermal necrolysis).
Idiosyncratic reactions: hemolytic anemia (see Glossary).
Bone marrow depression (see Glossary): fever, sore throat, abnormal bleeding/bruising—rare to infrequent.
Pancreatitis, myopathy, or drug-induced lupus erythematosus—case reports.
Folic acid deficiency—possible.

Kidney damage—case reports.

Peripheral neuritis (see Glossary)—case reports.

Inflammation of tissue around the heart (pericarditis)—case reports.

▷ **Possible Effects on Sexual Function:**   Decreased production of sperm, reversible infertility—case reports.

▷ **Adverse Effects That May Mimic Natural Diseases or Disorders**

Liver reactions may suggest viral hepatitis. Lung reactions may suggest an infectious pneumonia.

Natural Diseases or Disorders That May Be Activated by This Drug

Goiter, acute intermittent porphyria.

Possible Effects on Laboratory Tests

Complete blood cell counts: decreased red cells, hemoglobin, white cells, and platelets; increased eosinophils (allergic reaction).

Liver function tests: increased enzymes (ALT/GPT, AST/GOT, alkaline phosphatase) or bilirubin.

Sperm count: decreased; abnormal sperm common; effects reversible on discontinuation of drug.

CAUTION

1. A large intake of water (up to 2 quarts daily) is necessary to ensure an adequate volume of urine.
2. Shake liquid dose forms well before measuring each dose.

Precautions for Use

By Infants and Children: Safety and effectiveness for those under 2 years of age are not established.

By Those Over 60 Years of Age: Watch for the development of reduced urine volume, fever, sore throat, abnormal bleeding or bruising, or skin irritation with itching, particularly in the anal or genital regions.

▷ **Advisability of Use During Pregnancy**

Pregnancy Category: B; however, this drug should **not** be used near the time of the birth of the baby. See Pregnancy Risk Categories at the back of this book.

Animal studies: Cleft palate and skeletal birth defects due to sulfonamides reported in mice and rats.

Human studies: No increase in birth defects reported in 4,584 exposures to various sulfonamides during pregnancy.

Avoid use of drug during the final month of pregnancy because of possible adverse effects on the newborn infant.

Advisability of Use If Breast-Feeding

Presence of this drug in breast milk: Yes.

Avoid drug or refrain from nursing.

Habit-Forming Potential: None.

Effects of Overdose: Headache, dizziness, nausea, vomiting, abdominal cramping, toxic fever, coma, jaundice, kidney failure.

Possible Effects of Long-Term Use: Development of goiter, with or without hypothyroidism. An orange-yellow discoloration of the skin has been reported. This is *not* jaundice.

Suggested Periodic Examinations While Taking This Drug (at physician's discretion)

Complete blood cell counts, weekly for the first 8 weeks.

Urine analysis weekly.

Liver and kidney function tests.

▷ **While Taking This Drug, Observe the Following**

Foods: No restrictions. Follow prescribed diet.

Beverages: No restrictions. May be taken with milk.

▷ *Alcohol:* Use caution. Sulfonamide drugs can increase the intoxicating effects of alcohol.

Tobacco Smoking: No interactions expected. I advise everyone to quit smoking.

▷ *Other Drugs:*

Sulfasalazine may *increase* the effects of

- anticoagulants (Coumadin, etc.), and increase bleeding risk. More frequent INR (prothrombin time) testing is needed.
- sulfonylureas or other oral hypoglycemic agents (see *sulfonylureas* and *oral antidiabetic drugs* in Drug Classes), and increase the risk of hypoglycemia.

Sulfasalazine may *decrease* the effects of

- digoxin (Lanoxin).

Sulfasalazine *taken concurrently* with

- ampicillin and perhaps other penicillins (see Drug Classes) may lower therapeutic benefits from sulfasalazine.
- calcium supplements (Calcium Gluconate) may result in decreased therapeutic benefits from sulfasalazine.
- iron salts or calcium may decrease sulfasalazine's benefits.
- some barbiturates (see Drug Classes) may result in decreased sulfasalazine therapeutic benefits.

▷ *Driving, Hazardous Activities:* This drug may cause dizziness. Restrict activities as necessary.

Aviation Note: The use of this drug *may be a disqualification* for piloting. Consult a designated aviation medical examiner.

Exposure to Sun: Use caution—some sulfonamide drugs can cause photosensitivity (see Glossary).

SULFONAMIDE ANTIBIOTIC FAMILY

Sulfamethoxazole (sul fa meth OX a zohl)   **Sulfisoxazole** (sul fi SOX a zohl)

Introduced: 1961, 1949, respectively   **Class:** Anti-infective, sulfonamides
Prescription: USA: Yes   **Controlled Drug:** USA: No; Canada: No   **Available as Generic:** Yes

Brand Names: Sulfamethoxazole: ✤Apo-Sulfamethoxazole, ✤Apo-Sulfatrim [CD], ✤Apo-Sulfatrim DS [CD], Azo Gantanol [CD], Bactrim [CD], Bactrim DS [CD], Bethaprim [CD], Comoxol [CD], Cotrim [CD], Gantanol, ✤Novo-Trimel [CD], ✤Novo-Trimel DS [CD], ✤Nu-Cotrimox, ✤Protrin [CD], ✤Protrin DF [CD], ✤Roubac [CD], Septra [CD], Septra DS [CD], Sulfatrim [CD], ✤Uro Gantanol [CD], Uroplus DS [CD], Uroplus SS [CD], Vagitrol; Sulfisoxazole: Azo Gantrisin [CD], Azo-Sulfisoxazole, Eryzole [CD], Gantrisin, Gulfasin, Lipo Gantrisin, ✤Novosoxazole, Pediazole [CD], SK-Soxazole, Sulfalar

---

BENEFITS versus RISKS

Possible Benefits	*Possible Risks*
EFFECTIVE ANTIMICROBIAL ACTION against susceptible bacteria and protozoa	Allergic reactions: mild to severe skin reactions, anaphylaxis, myocarditis
Effective adjunctive prevention and treatment of *Pneumocystis carinii* pneumonia (AIDS-related— sulfamethoxazole)	Blood cell disorders: aplastic anemia, hemolytic anemia, abnormally low white cell or platelet counts
	Drug-induced liver or kidney damage

▷ **Principal Uses**

As a Single Drug Product: Uses currently included in FDA-approved labeling: (1) Used to treat a variety of bacterial and protozoan infections (chancroid, cystitis, and other infections of the urinary tract); (2) sulfisoxazole is used in treating ear infections and toxoplasmosis.

Note: Sulfamethoxasole should not be used to treat group A streptococcal infections.

Other (unlabeled) generally accepted uses: (1) *Chlamydia* infections; (2) combination therapy of resistant *Mycobacterium kansasii* infections; (3) sulfisoxazole may work in long-term prevention of ear infections.

As a Combination Drug Product [CD]: These medicines are available in combination with phenazopyridine, an analgesic to ease discomfort associated with acute urethral infections. Sulfamethoxazole is also available in combination with another antibacterial drug, trimethoprim; in some countries this combination is given the generic name cotrimoxazole. This combination is quite effective in the treatment of certain types of middle ear infection, bronchitis, pneumonia, and certain infections of the intestinal tract and urinary tract. It is now used as primary prevention and treatment for *Pneumocystis carinii* pneumonia associated with AIDS.

How These Drugs Work:　Prevents the growth and multiplication of susceptible bacteria or protozoa by interfering with their formation of folic acid, an essential nutrient.

Available Dose Forms and Strengths

Sulfamethoxazole:

> Oral suspension — 500 mg/5 ml
> Tablets — 500 mg, 1 g

Sulfisoxazole:

Emulsion, prolonged action — 1 g/5 ml
Eyedrops — 4%
Eye ointment — 4%
Injection — 400 mg/ml
Pediatric suspension — 500 mg/5 ml
Syrup — 500 mg/5 ml
Tablets — 500 mg

▷ **Recommended Dose Ranges:**　Sulfamethoxazole: Children over 2 months—50 to 60 mg per kg of body mass to start, then 25 to 30 mg per kg of body mass every 12 hours, up to a maximum of 75 mg per kg of body mass daily. Adults—Initially 2 g, then 1 g every 8 to 12 hours, depending upon the severity of the infection. The total daily dose should not exceed 3 g.

Sulfisoxazole: Children over 2 months—50 mg per kg of body mass to start, then 100 mg per kg of body mass per day, divided into equal doses given two to four times daily. Adults—Initially 2 to 4 g, then 750 to 1500 mg (1.5 g) every 4 hours, or 1 to 2 g every 6 hours, depending upon the severity of the infection. The total daily dose should not exceed 8 g.

Note: Actual dose and schedule must be determined for each patient individually.

Conditions Requiring Dosing Adjustments

Liver Function: Patients with compromised livers should be followed closely; however, specific guidelines for decreasing doses are not defined. Sulfisoxazole may cause liver damage.

Kidney Function: Doses should be decreased for patients with compromised kidneys. For patients with mild to moderate kidney failure, sulfisoxazole can be taken every 6 hours in the usual dose. In moderate to severe kidney failure, it can be taken every 12 to 24 hours in the usual dose. In severe kidney failure, it can be taken once a day. Increased elimination of this drug may be seen in patients with alkaline urine. It should be used with caution in renal compromise.

▷ **Dosing Instructions:**   The tablet may be crushed and is preferably taken on an empty stomach, 1 hour before or 2 hours after eating. However, both drugs may be taken with or following food to reduce stomach irritation. Be certain to drink liberal amounts of water while taking these medicines if you are not restricted from doing so.

Usual Duration of Use: Use on a regular schedule for 4 to 7 days usually determines effectiveness in controlling responsive infections. Treatment should be continued until the patient is free of symptoms for 48 hours. Limit treatment to no more than 14 days if possible. Preventive use of trimethoprim/sulfamethoxazole will be ongoing.

Currently a "Drug of Choice"

Sulfamethoxazole (when combined with trimethoprim) for preventing pneumonia (due to *Pneumocystis carinii*) in patients with AIDS.

▷ **These Drugs Should Not Be Taken If**
- you are allergic to any sulfonamide drug (see Drug Classes).
- you are in the final month of pregnancy.
- you are breast-feeding your infant.
- it has been prescribed for an infant less than 2 months old (unless congenital toxoplasmosis is being treated—sulfisoxazole).

▷ **Inform Your Physician Before Taking These Drugs If**
- you are allergic to any sulfonamide derivative—acetazolamide, thiazide diuretics, sulfonylurea antidiabetics (see Drug Classes).
- you are allergic by nature (history of hay fever, asthma, hives, eczema).
- you have impaired liver or kidney function.
- you have a personal or family history of porphyria.
- you have had a drug-induced blood cell or bone marrow disorder.
- you have a glucose-6-phosphate dehydrogenase (G6PD) deficiency in your red blood cells (ask your doctor).
- you currently take any oral anticoagulant, antidiabetic drug, or phenytoin.
- you plan to have surgery under pentothal anesthesia while taking this drug.

Possible Side Effects (natural, expected, and unavoidable drug actions)
Brownish coloration of the urine, of no significance. Superinfections (see Glossary), bacterial or fungal.

▷ **Possible Adverse Effects** (unusual, unexpected, and infrequent reactions)
If any of the following develop, consult your physician promptly for guidance.

Mild Adverse Effects
Allergic reactions: skin rashes, hives, itching, localized swellings, reddened eyes.
Myopia—infrequent.
Headache, dizziness, unsteadiness, ringing in the ears—possible.
Loss of appetite, irritation of mouth or tongue, nausea, vomiting, abdominal pain, diarrhea—infrequent.

Serious Adverse Effects
Allergic reactions: drug fever (see Glossary), swollen glands, painful joints, anaphylactic reaction (see Glossary). Allergic reaction in the heart muscle (myocarditis), allergic pneumonitis, allergic hepatitis. Severe skin reactions—rare.
Idiosyncratic reactions: hemolytic anemia (see Glossary)—possible.
Bone marrow depression (see Glossary): fatigue, weakness, fever, sore throat, abnormal bleeding or bruising—case reports.
Liver damage—rare.
Pancreatitis—case reports.
Kidney damage: bloody or cloudy urine, reduced urine volume—possible.
Psychotic reactions, hallucinations, seizures, hearing changes (loss or vestibular symptoms), peripheral neuritis (see Glossary)—case reports.
Severe hypoglycemia—case report (sulfamethoxazole).
Methemoglobinemia—rare.
Drug-induced lupus erythematosus or blood clotting problems (hypoprothrombinemia)—rare.
Drug-induced disulfiram-like reaction (sulfisoxazole)—possible.

▷ **Possible Effects on Sexual Function:**   None reported.

▷ **Adverse Effects That May Mimic Natural Diseases or Disorders**
Liver reactions may suggest viral hepatitis. Lung reactions may suggest an infectious pneumonia.

Natural Diseases or Disorders That May Be Activated by These Drugs
Goiter, acute intermittent porphyria, polyarteritis nodosa, systemic lupus erythematosus (questionable).

Possible Effects on Laboratory Tests
Complete blood cell counts: decreased red cells, hemoglobin, white cells, and platelets; increased eosinophils (allergic reaction).
INR (prothrombin time): increased (when taken concurrently with warfarin).
Liver function tests: increased enzymes (ALT/GPT, AST/GOT, alkaline phosphatase), or bilirubin.

CAUTION
1. A large intake of water (up to 2 quarts daily) is necessary to ensure an adequate volume of urine.
2. Shake liquid dose forms well before measuring each dose.

Precautions for Use

By Infants and Children: These drugs should not be used in infants under 2 months of age.

By Those Over 60 Years of Age: Small doses taken at longer intervals often achieve adequate blood and tissue drug levels. Watch for the development of reduced urine volume, fever, sore throat, abnormal bleeding or bruising, or skin irritation with itching, particularly in the anal or genital regions.

▷ **Advisability of Use During Pregnancy**

Pregnancy Category: C; however, these drugs **SHOULD NOT BE TAKEN** (are contraindicated) near the time of the birth of the baby. See Pregnancy Risk Categories at the back of this book.

Animal studies: Cleft palate and skeletal birth defects reported in mice and rats.

Human studies: No increase in birth defects reported in 4,584 exposures to various sulfonamides during pregnancy.

Avoid use of drug during the final 3 months of pregnancy because of possible adverse effects on the newborn infant.

Advisability of Use If Breast-Feeding

Presence of this drug in breast milk: Yes.

Avoid drug or refrain from nursing.

Habit-Forming Potential: None.

Effects of Overdose: Headache, dizziness, nausea, vomiting, abdominal cramping, toxic fever, coma, jaundice, kidney failure.

Possible Effects of Long-Term Use: Superinfections, bacterial or fungal. Development of goiter, with or without hypothyroidism. Excessive loss of vitamin C via urine.

Suggested Periodic Examinations While Taking This Drug (at physician's discretion)

Complete blood cell counts, weekly for the first 8 weeks.

Urine analysis weekly.

Liver and kidney function tests.

▷ **While Taking This Drug, Observe the Following**

Foods: No restrictions.

Beverages: No restrictions. May be taken with milk. Note recommendations for increased fluid intake.

▷   *Alcohol:* Use caution. Sulfonamide drugs can increase the intoxicating effects of alcohol.

Tobacco Smoking: No interactions expected. I advise everyone to quit smoking.

▷   *Other Drugs:*

These medicines may *increase* the effects of

- amantadine (Symmetrel), and cause abnormal heart rhythms and CNS stimulation (confusion, disorientation).
- anticoagulants (Coumadin, etc.), and increase the risk of bleeding. More frequent INR testing (prothrombin time or protime) is needed. Ongoing warfarin doses should be decided based on laboratory results.
- methotrexate (Mexate), and cause severe blood toxicity.
- sulfonylureas (see Drug Classes) or other oral hypoglycemic agents, and increase the risk of excessively low blood sugar (hypoglycemia).
- zidovudine (AZT), and result in zidovudine toxicity.

These medicines may *decrease* the effects of
- birth control pills (oral contraceptives).
- cyclosporine (Sandimmune), and reduce its immunosuppressive effect.
- penicillins (see Drug Classes).

▷ *Driving, Hazardous Activities:* These drugs may cause dizziness. Restrict activities as necessary.

Aviation Note: The use of these drugs **may be a disqualification** for piloting. Consult a designated aviation medical examiner.

Exposure to Sun: Use caution. Some sulfonamide drugs can cause photosensitivity (see Glossary).

SULINDAC (sul IN dak)

See the acetic acids (nonsteroidal anti-inflammatory drugs) profile for further information.

SUMATRIPTAN (soo ma TRIP tan)

Introduced: 1993   **Class:** Anti-migraine drug, serotonin-1-receptor agonist
Prescription: USA: Yes   **Controlled Drug:** USA: No; Canada: No   **Available as Generic:** USA: No; Canada: No
Brand Name: Imitrex

BENEFITS versus RISKS	
Possible Benefits	*Possible Risks*
RAPID AND EFFECTIVE RELIEF OR PREVENTION OF MIGRAINE	Fainting
GENERALLY WELL TOLERATED	Myocardial infarction (probably secondary to coronary vasospasm)
NEWLY AVAILABLE IN A NASAL SPRAY FORM	Serious atrial and ventricular arrhythmias
Relieves photophobia (light sensitivity)	
Relieves phonophobia (sound sensitivity)	
Relieves nausea and vomiting	

▷ **Principal Uses**
As a Single Drug Product: Uses currently included in FDA-approved labeling: Acute treatment of migraine with or without aura in adults.
Other (unlabeled) generally accepted uses: (1) Treatment of cluster headache; (2) may have a role in treating post-traumatic headaches.

How This Drug Works: Sumatriptan acts on blood vessels to cause vasoconstriction (shrinking of the blood vessels). This relieves swelling, thought to be the cause of migraine. The drug binds to receptor arteries such as the basilar artery and in vasculature (blood vessels) associated with the dura mater (part of the lining of the brain).

Available Dose Forms and Strengths
Nasal spray — 5 mg/100 mcl, 20 mg/100 mcl

Sumatriptan succinate (Imitrex) injection: SELFdose system kit, which has two syringes with 6 mg in 0.5 ml of liquid in a 1-ml size syringe, a dosing device, and instructions.

Unit-of-use syringes with 6 mg in 0.5 ml of liquid in a 1-ml syringe in a carton of two syringes.

6 mg single-dose vials with 0.5 ml of liquid in a 2-ml vial.

All the liquid should be a colorless to pale yellow clear solution. Particles or precipitates should NEVER appear.

Tablets — 25 mg, 50 mg

How To Store

Keep out of reach of children. Store at room temperature in a room where the temperature will not exceed 86 degrees F (30 degrees C). Keep away from heat and light.

▷ **Recommended Dose Ranges** (Actual dose and schedule must be determined for each patient individually.)

Infants and Children: The safety and effectiveness in pediatrics have **not** been determined.

18 to 60 Years of Age: Subcutaneous: Maximum adult dose is 6 mg. The dose should be taken as soon as possible after the symptoms of acute migraine are recognized. Controlled clinical trials have failed to demonstrate a benefit of repeated injections if the initial injection is unsuccessful. If symptoms return, a second 6-mg injection may be taken 12 hours after the first injection. If side effects occur, use the lowest dose in the approved dose range that is effective for you. Daily maximum is 12 mg.

Oral: Newly labeled dosing notes that doses of 50 mg may be more effective than 25 mg. The dose chosen must balance possible benefit of the higher dose with increased risk of adverse effects of higher doses. Take the dose your doctor prescribes as soon as headache pain starts. If the headache returns or if there is a partial response, single tablets can be taken at least two hours after the first dose (up to 100 mg a day). Maximum daily oral dose is 100 mg. There is evidence that 100 mg doses do not provide more relief than 50 mg doses.

Nasal: 5 to 20 mg as a one-time dose. Newly labeled dosing notes that more patients taking the 20 mg dose had headache relief.

The dose chosen must balance possible benefit of the higher dose with increased risk of adverse effects of higher doses. Take the dose prescribed as soon as headache pain starts. For example, 10 mg may be taken by 5 mg in each nostril. A 20 mg dose can be taken as 10 mg in each nostril. Data exists that shows that single doses more than 20 mg do not give additional benefit.

If symptoms return, the dose can be taken once again, but the daily maximum of 40 mg must not be exceeded. Safety in treating more than 4 headaches in 30 days is unknown with any dosage form.

Over 65 Years of Age: Safety and effectiveness have **not** been evaluated in this age group. Since declines in renal and hepatic function and coronary artery disease are more common in those over 65, the possibility of an increase in side effects would be expected.

Conditions Requiring Dosing Adjustments

Liver Function: Oral tablets will give unpredictable variations in blood levels if used in liver disease. Maximum dose is 50 milligrams.

Kidney Function: No changes in dose thought to be needed in kidney disease.

▷ **Dosing Instructions:**   The injection form must be given subcutaneously, **not intravenously.** Intravenous injection must be avoided because of potential to cause coronary vasospasm (constriction of the blood vessels that supply the heart). This medicine should be colorless to pale yellow and clear. Particles should never be present. There is extensive information on self-injection available from your doctor or pharmacist. The first dose is usually given in the doctor's office. The tablet form may take more than an hour to work. The tablet form may be taken with food. Follow directions for the nasal form closely.

Usual Duration of Use: The maximum dose is two 6-mg doses (injections) in 24 hours. This medication relieves existing migraines, and will not change the frequency or number of attacks. Recurring use of this medicine will be needed. If your migraines increase in frequency or severity, consult your doctor. If this medicine is not effective in helping your migraine, call your doctor.

Possible Advantages of This Drug

Effective subcutaneous treatment of acute nonbasilar, nonhemiplegic migraine. Better side-effect profile and treatment of migraine-associated nausea and vomiting, phonophobia, and photophobia than other currently available agents.

Currently a "Drug of Choice"

For nonbasilar, nonhemiplegic migraine.

▷ **This Drug Should Not Be Taken If**
- you had an allergic reaction to it previously.
- you are unfamiliar with the subcutaneous route. Particular care must be taken to avoid intravenous use because this may lead to coronary vasospasm (constriction of the blood vessels that supply the heart).
- you have ischemic heart disease with symptoms such as angina pectoris or silent ischemia, or history of MI (myocardial infarction).
- you have Prinzmetal's angina (a specific kind of chest pain).
- you have uncontrolled hypertension (high blood pressure).
- you have basilar or hemiplegic migraine.
- you have taken a monoamine oxidase (MAO) inhibitor within the last 2 weeks.
- you have (within 24 hours) taken an ergotamine preparation.

▷ **Inform Your Physician Before Taking This Drug If**
- you are pregnant or plan to become pregnant.
- you are breast-feeding your infant.
- you have high blood pressure.
- you have chest pain, heart disease, or irregular heartbeats.
- you have had a heart attack.
- you have taken or have prescriptions for other migraine medications.
- you have allergies or trouble taking other medications, whether prescription or over the counter.
- you have liver or kidney disease.
- you are uncertain of how much to take or when to take this medicine.
- you do not understand the subcutaneous injection technique.
- you have Raynaud's phenomenon.

Possible Side Effects (natural, expected, and unavoidable drug actions)
Excessive thirst and frequent urination. Transient rises in blood pressure. Vision changes—rare. Taste changes—frequent.

▷ **Possible Adverse Effects** (unusual, unexpected, and infrequent reactions)
If any of the following develop, consult your physician promptly for guidance.
Mild Adverse Effects
Allergic reactions: red, itching skin; skin rash and tenderness.
Atypical sensations such as tingling (rare with injection, infrequent with tablet form).
Confusion and other mental changes or dizziness—rare.
Flushing—rare; tightness in the chest or jaw—infrequent.
Gastroesophageal reflux and diarrhea—case report.
Pain at the injection site; joint pain, weakness, and stiffness—rare.
Serious Adverse Effects
Allergic reactions: anaphylactic reactions.
Syncope (fainting), CVA, dysphasia, seizure—rare.
Serious changes in heart rate and rhythm—rare.
Raynaud's phenomenon, dyspnea (difficulty breathing)—rare.
Kidney stones (renal calculi)—rare.
Prinzmetal's angina—rare.
Heart attack (myocardial infarction)—rare.

▷ **Possible Effects on Sexual Function:** Dysmenorrhea, erection problems—case reports.

Possible Delayed Adverse Effects: None identified.

▷ **Adverse Effects That May Mimic Natural Diseases or Disorders**
Changes in heart rate and rhythm may mimic a number of cardiac conditions. Drug-induced acute renal failure (ARF) may mimic non-drug-induced ARF. Drug-induced hypertension may mimic hypertension from other causes. Urological symptoms may mimic benign prostatic hypertrophy. Sumatriptan can mimic Raynaud's phenomenon.

Natural Diseases or Disorders That May Be Activated by This Drug
Hypertension.

Possible Effects on Laboratory Tests
Liver function tests: rare increases in SGOT and SGPT.

CAUTION
1. Do not use sumatriptan if you are pregnant.
2. Call your doctor if you have any pain or tightness in the chest or throat when you use this medicine.
3. Do not use sumatriptan if you have used an ergotamine preparation within the last 24 hours.
4. This medication is not to be used intravenously.
5. If you are diagnosed as having ischemic heart disease after sumatriptan has been prescribed for you, do not use the medicine again.

Precautions for Use
By Infants and Children: Safety and effectiveness for those under 18 years of age are not established.
By Those Over 65 Years of Age: Not established.

▷ **Advisability of Use During Pregnancy**
   Pregnancy Category: C. See Pregnancy Risk Categories at the back of this book.
     Animal studies: Sumatriptan has been lethal to rabbit embryos when given in
     doses that were threefold higher than those produced by a 6-mg dose. Term
     fetuses from rabbits treated with sumatriptan exhibited an increase in cer-
     vicothoracic vascular defects and minor skeletal abnormalities.
   Human studies: Adequate studies of pregnant women are not available.
   Ask your physician for guidance.

Advisability of Use If Breast-Feeding
   Presence of this drug in breast milk: Yes.
   Use of this medication by nursing mothers is a benefit-to-risk decision to be
     made by a physician.

Habit-Forming Potential: Not clearly defined.

Effects of Overdose: Patients have received doses of 8 to 12 mg without adverse
   effects. Healthy volunteers have taken up to 16 mg subcutaneously without
   serious adverse events. Coronary vasospasm has resulted from intravenous
   doses. Animal data presents convulsions, tremor, flushing, decreased
   breathing and activity, cyanosis, ataxia, and paralysis.

Possible Effects of Long-Term Use: Not defined.

Suggested Periodic Examinations While Taking This Drug (at physician's discretion)
   Liver function tests, electrocardiogram.

▷ **While Taking This Drug, Observe the Following**
   Foods: No restrictions; however, some foods or additives such as monosodium
     glutamate or chocolate may be a risk factor for migraines. Skipping meals
     can also be a risk factor for migraines.
   Beverages: No restrictions.
▷ *Alcohol:* May cause additive sedation. Alcohol may also be a precipitating fac-
     tor for migraine.
   Tobacco Smoking: No interactions expected. I advise everyone to quit smoking.
   Marijuana Smoking: May cause additive dizziness, drowsiness, and lethargy;
     may cause additive increases in blood pressure.
▷ *Other Drugs:*
   Sumatriptan *taken concurrently* with
   • dexfenfluramine (Redux) may cause serotonin syndrome. DO NOT com-
     bine.
   • ergot derivatives (see Drug Classes) may result in additive vasospasm (pro-
     longed constriction of the blood vessels). These medicines should not be
     taken within 24 hours of any sumatriptan dose.
   • fluoxetine (Prozac) may result in coordination problems.
   • fluvoxamine (Luvox) may result in coordination problems.
   • monoamine oxidase (MAO) inhibitors (see Drug Classes) may result in toxic
     levels of sumatriptan. MAO inhibitors and sumatriptan should never be
     combined. It is important that 14 days go by after your last dose of an MAO
     inhibitor before you take any form of sumatriptan.
   • paroxetine (Paxil) may result in coordination problems.
   • sertraline (Zoloft) may result in coordination problems.
   • venlafaxine (Effexor) may result in coordination problems.

▷ *Driving, Hazardous Activities:* This drug may cause dizziness and drowsiness. Restrict activities as necessary.

Aviation Note: The use of this drug **may be a disqualification** for piloting. Consult a designated aviation medical examiner.

Exposure to Sun: No restrictions.

Exposure to Cold: Use caution until tolerance is determined. Cold may enhance sumatriptan vasoconstriction.

Heavy Exercise or Exertion: Strenuous exercise can be a risk factor for migraines in some patients.

Special Storage Instructions: Keep this medicine out of reach of children. Store at room temperature in a room where the temperature will not exceed 86 degrees F (30 degrees C). Keep away from heat and light.

Observe the Following Expiration Times: There is an expiration date printed on the treatment package. Throw the medication away if it has expired. The autoinjector may be used again.

TACRINE (TA kreen)

See the new anti-Alzheimer's drug family profile for more information.

TAMOXIFEN (ta MOX i fen)

Introduced: 1973   **Class:** Antiestrogen, anticancer   **Prescription:** USA: Yes   **Controlled Drug:** USA: No; Canada: No   **Available as Generic:** Yes

Brand Names: ✦Alpha-Tamoxifen, ✦Apo-Tamox, Nolvadex, ✦Nolvadex-D, ✦Novo-Tamoxifen, ✦Tamofen, ✦Tamone

BENEFITS versus RISKS	
Possible Benefits	*Possible Risks*
EFFECTIVE ADJUNCTIVE TREATMENT IN ADVANCED BREAST CANCER	UTERINE CANCER
	Severe increase in tumor or bone pain—transient
MAY INCREASE THE CHANCES OF BREAST CONSERVATION	Thrombophlebitis, pulmonary embolism
	Abnormally high blood calcium levels
	Eye changes: corneal opacities, retinal injury

▷ **Principal Uses**

As a Single Drug Product: Uses currently included in FDA-approved labeling: (1) An alternative to estrogens and androgens (male sex hormones) to treat advanced breast cancer in postmenopausal women; (2) treats advanced breast cancer in men that has spread (metastasized) from a prior site; (3) used to delay the recurrence of breast cancer in women.

Other (unlabeled) generally accepted uses: (1) May have a role in treating cancer of the liver or lung; (2) used to stimulate ovulation in premenopausal women with infertility; (3) used to treat rare desmoid tumors; (4) helps prevent osteoporosis in women in whom the drug is being used to prevent the recurrence of cancer; (5) can help retroperitoneal fibrosis; (6) could have a role in treating tenderness and swelling of male breast tissue (gynecomastia) of unknown cause (idiopathic); (7) helps lipid (cholesterol) levels; (8) helps PREVENT breast cancer in those at risk.

Author's Note: tamoxifen reduced breast cancer rates by almost half in a very large (13,388 patients) cancer prevention study performed by the National Cancer Institute over 6 years.

There is a new listing of cancer medicine trials on the WorldWide Web at www.cancertrials.nci.nih.gov

How This Drug Works: It is thought that by blocking the uptake of estradiol (estrogen), this drug removes or reduces a stimulus to breast cancer cells.

Available Dose Forms and Strengths
Tablets — 10 mg, 15.2 mg (in Canada), 20 mg (in Canada), 30.4 mg (in Canada)

▷ **Usual Adult Dose Range:**   Breast cancer: 10 to 20 mg two to three times a day for 2 to 5 years. Prevention of breast cancer: At this time, a consensus statement with recommended dosing guidelines is being prepared.

Note: Actual dose and schedule must be determined for each patient individually.

Conditions Requiring Dosing Adjustments
Liver Function: Dose decreases are not defined in liver disease.
Kidney Function: Dose decreases are not thought to be needed in mild to moderate kidney disease. No studies are available in severe disease.

▷ **Dosing Instructions:**   The tablet may be crushed and taken either on an empty stomach or with food.

Usual Duration of Use: Use on a regular schedule for 4 to 10 weeks usually determines effectiveness in controlling growth and spread of advanced breast cancer. In the presence of bone involvement, treatment for several months may be required to evaluate effectiveness. Long-term use (months to years) requires physician supervision and periodic evaluation.

▷ **This Drug Should Not Be Taken If**
   • you had a serious allergic or adverse reaction to it before.
   • you have active phlebitis.
   • you have a significant deficiency of white blood cells or blood platelets.
   • you are pregnant.

▷ **Inform Your Physician Before Taking This Drug If**
   • you have a history of thrombophlebitis or pulmonary embolism.
   • you have a history of abnormally high blood calcium levels.
   • you have a history of any type of blood cell or bone marrow disorder.
   • you have cataracts or other visual impairment.
   • you have impaired liver function.
   • you plan to have surgery in the near future.

Possible Side Effects (natural, expected, and unavoidable drug actions)
Hot flashes—frequent, fluid retention, weight gain.

▷ **Possible Adverse Effects** (unusual, unexpected, and infrequent reactions)
   If any of the following develop, consult your physician promptly for guidance.
Mild Adverse Effects
Allergic reactions: skin rash.

Visual impairment—infrequent.

Increased calcium—infrequent.

Headache, dizziness, drowsiness, depression, fatigue, confusion—infrequent.

Nausea, vomiting—frequent; itching in genital area, loss of hair—infrequent.

Serious Adverse Effects

Initial "flare" of severe pain in tumor or involved bone—possible.

Development of thrombophlebitis, risk of pulmonary embolism—increased risk.

Eye changes: corneal opacities, retinal injury—case reports.

Delusions—rare.

Increased uterine cancer risk (increased karyopyknotic index of vaginal epithelium)—possible, but many researchers now believe that the benefits far outweigh the risks.

Development of abnormally high blood calcium levels—possible.

Transient decreases in white blood cells and blood platelets—frequent.

Neutropenia or decrease in all blood cells (pancytopenia)—case reports.

Liver toxicity—rare.

▷ **Possible Effects on Sexual Function:** Premenopausal: Altered timing and pattern of menstruation. Postmenopausal: Vaginal bleeding. Decreased libido. Abnormal and painful erections (priapism)—case reports.

This drug may be effective in treating the following conditions:

• male infertility due to abnormally low sperm counts.

• male breast enlargement and tenderness.

• chronic female breast pain (mastodynia).

Possible Effects on Laboratory Tests

Complete blood cell counts: decreased red cells, hemoglobin, white cells, and platelets.

Blood calcium level: increased.

Blood thyroid hormone levels: T_3, T_4, and free T_4 increased.

Liver function tests: increased liver enzyme (AST/GOT), increased bilirubin (one case report).

Sperm count: increased or decreased.

CAUTION

1. If this drug is used prior to your menopause, it may induce ovulation and predispose to pregnancy. Since this drug should not be used during pregnancy, some method of contraception (other than oral contraceptives) is advised.

2. Do not take any form of estrogen while taking this drug; estrogens can inhibit tamoxifen's effectiveness.

3. Tamoxifen has been shown to cause an increased risk of uterine cancer. Women who have received or are receiving this drug should have regular gynecological examinations. Report menstrual irregularity, abnormal vaginal bleeding or vaginal discharge, pelvic pain or pressure promptly to your doctor.

▷ **Advisability of Use During Pregnancy**

Pregnancy Category: D. See Pregnancy Risk Categories at the back of this book.

Animal studies: No birth defects due to this drug reported.

Human studies: Adequate studies of pregnant women are not available.

This drug can have estrogenic effects. It should not be used during pregnancy.

Advisability of Use If Breast-Feeding
Presence of this drug in breast milk: Unknown.
Avoid drug or refrain from nursing.

Habit-Forming Potential: None.

Effects of Overdose: Severe extension of the pharmacological effects.

Possible Effects of Long-Term Use: Development of abnormally high blood calcium levels.

Suggested Periodic Examinations While Taking This Drug (at physician's discretion)
Complete blood cell counts, measurements of blood calcium levels.
Complete eye examinations if impaired vision occurs.
Women who have been given or are now receiving tamoxifen **must** have regular gynecological examinations.

▷ **While Taking This Drug, Observe the Following**
Foods: No restrictions.
Beverages: No restrictions. May be taken with milk.
▷ *Alcohol:* No interactions expected.
Tobacco Smoking: No interactions expected. I advise everyone to quit smoking.
Marijuana Smoking: Animal studies show an increased suppression of the immune system; significance in humans is not known.
▷ *Other Drugs*
The following drugs may *decrease* the effects of tamoxifen:
• estrogens.
• oral contraceptives (those that contain estrogens).
Tamoxifen *taken concurrently* with
• allopurinol (Zyloprim) may worsen allopurinol toxicity to the liver.
• cyclophosphamide (Cytoxan) may increase blood clot (thromboembolism) risk.
• cyclosporine (Sandimmune) may increase cyclosporine levels and cause toxicity.
• methotrexate (Mexate) may increase blood clot (thromboembolism) risk.
• mitomycin will cause increased risk of hemolytic uremic syndrome.
• pneumococcal, and perhaps other vaccines, will blunt the vaccine's immune response (benefit).
• ritonavir (Norvir), and perhaps other protease inhibitors (see Drug Classes), may lead to toxicity.
• warfarin (Coumadin) presents an increased risk of bleeding. Increased frequency of INR (prothrombin time or protime) testing is needed.
Driving, Hazardous Activities: This drug may cause dizziness or drowsiness. Restrict activities as necessary.
Aviation Note: The use of this drug *may be a disqualification* for piloting. Consult a designated aviation medical examiner.
Exposure to Sun: No restrictions.

TAMSULOSIN (TAM su low sin)

Introduced: 1997 **Class:** Antiprostatism, alpha 1 (A) blocker **Prescription:** USA: Yes **Controlled Drug:** USA: No **Available as Generic:** No
Brand Name: Flomax

BENEFITS versus RISKS	
Possible Benefits	*Possible Risks*
EFFECTIVE TREATMENT OF BENIGN PROSTATIC HYPERPLASIA	Headache
	Runny Nose
ONCE-DAILY DOSING	

▷ **Principal Uses**
As a Single Drug Product: Uses currently included in FDA-approved labeling: Treats symptomatic benign prostatic hyperplasia (BPH).
Other (unlabeled) generally accepted uses: None at present.

How This Drug Works: Relaxes smooth muscle around the bladder neck and prostate (by binding to a very specific 1A receptor), allowing opening of the urethra and increased urine flow.

Available Dose Forms and Strengths
Capsules — 0.4 mg

▷ **Usual Adult Dose Range:** Started with 0.4 mg once daily. If response is not acceptable after 2 to 4 weeks, the dose can be increased to 0.8 mg once a day.
Note: Actual dose and schedule must be determined for each patient individually.

Conditions Requiring Dosing Adjustments
Liver Function: Dose should be decreased in severe liver disease.
Kidney Function: Dose changes not needed in those with creatinine clearance (see Glossary) as low as 10 ml/min. Not studied in worse kidney failure.

Author's note: Information in this profile will be broadened in subsequent editions.

TERAZOSIN (ter AY zoh sin)

Introduced: 1987 **Class:** Antihypertensive **Prescription:** USA: Yes
Controlled Drug: USA: No **Available as Generic:** No
Brand Name: Hytrin

BENEFITS versus RISKS	
Possible Benefits	*Possible Risks*
EFFECTIVE TREATMENT OF MILD TO MODERATE HYPERTENSION	First-dose drop in blood pressure with fainting
LOWERED LOW-DENSITY LIPOPROTEINS AND TOTAL CHOLESTEROL	Fluid retention
LOWERED TRIGLYCERIDE LEVELS	
TREATS BENIGN PROSTATIC HYPERPLASIA	

▷ **Principal Uses**

As a Single Drug Product: Uses currently included in FDA-approved labeling: (1) Treats mild to moderate hypertension or used with other drugs to treat moderate to severe hypertension; (2) treats symptomatic benign prostatic hyperplasia (BPH).

Other (unlabeled) generally accepted uses: (1) Used to help correct symptoms in congestive heart failure; (2) may have a beneficial effect in lowering cholesterol levels.

How This Drug Works: Blocks some actions of the sympathetic nervous system, causing opening of blood vessel walls and lower blood pressure. In BPH it relaxes smooth muscle around the bladder neck and prostate, allowing opening of the urethra and increased urine flow.

Available Dose Forms and Strengths

Tablets — 1 mg, 2 mg, 5 mg, 10 mg

▷ **Usual Adult Dose Range:**   Started with a test dose of 1 mg. Patient response is observed for 2 hours (some doctors have the medicine taken at bedtime). If terazosin is tolerated, dose can be slowly (as needed and tolerated) increased to 5 mg daily. Daily maximum is 20 mg.

Benign prostatic hyperplasia: 1 mg is taken at bedtime. This dose is gradually increased as needed and tolerated to the desired response. Many patients need 10 mg for 4 to 6 weeks in order to get symptom relief.

Note: Actual dose and schedule must be determined for each patient individually.

Conditions Requiring Dosing Adjustments

Liver Function: Dose should be decreased in severe liver disease.

Kidney Function: Dose changes not needed in severe kidney failure.

▷ **Dosing Instructions:**   The tablet may be crushed and taken without regard to food. It is best taken at bedtime to avoid orthostatic hypotension (see Glossary).

Usual Duration of Use: Use on a regular schedule for 6 to 8 weeks usually determines effectiveness in hypertension; 4 to 6 weeks of scheduled use are needed in benign prostatic hyperplasia (BPH). See your doctor regularly.

Possible Advantages of This Drug

May be used to initiate treatment.

Usually effective with once-a-day dose.

Rarely causes depression or impotence.

Does not alter blood cholesterol, potassium, or sugar.

▷ **This Drug Should Not Be Taken If**

• you have had an allergic reaction to it previously.

• you are experiencing mental depression.

• you have angina (active coronary artery disease) and are not taking a beta-blocking drug (see your physician).

▷ **Inform Your Physician Before Taking This Drug If**

• you have experienced orthostatic hypotension (see Glossary).

• you have a history of mental depression.

• you have impaired circulation to the brain or a history of stroke.

• your job requires alertness or dexterity in operating heavy machinery (this medicine may cause somnolence or drowsiness).

- you have coronary artery disease.
- you have impaired liver or kidney function.
- you plan to have surgery under general anesthesia soon.

Possible Side Effects (natural, expected, and unavoidable drug actions)
Orthostatic hypotension—rare; drowsiness, salt and water retention, dry mouth, nasal congestion, constipation.

▷ **Possible Adverse Effects** (unusual, unexpected, and infrequent reactions)
If any of the following develop, consult your physician promptly for guidance.

Mild Adverse Effects
Allergic reactions: skin rash.
Headache, dizziness, fatigue, nervousness, sweating, numbness/tingling, blurred vision—rare to infrequent.
Weight gain—case reports.
Palpitation, rapid heart rate, shortness of breath—infrequent.
Nausea, vomiting, diarrhea—infrequent.

Serious Adverse Effects
Mental depression—rare.

▷ **Possible Effects on Sexual Function:**   Impotence—rare.

Natural Diseases or Disorders That May Be Activated by This Drug
Latent coronary artery insufficiency.

Possible Effects on Laboratory Tests
Blood total cholesterol, LDL and VLDL cholesterol levels: decreased.
Blood HDL cholesterol level or blood triglyceride levels: increased or no effect.

CAUTION
1. A first-dose precipitous drop in blood pressure, with or without fainting, can occur (usually within 30 to 90 minutes). Limit initial doses to 1 mg at bedtime (for first 3 days); lie down and do not get up after taking trial doses.
2. Nonprescription therapy for allergic rhinitis or head colds can cause serious drug interactions. Ask your doctor or before combining any medicine with terazosin.

Precautions for Use
By Infants and Children: Safety and effectiveness for those under 12 years of age are not established.
By Those Over 60 Years of Age: Therapy is started with no more than 1 mg/day for the first 3 days. Any dose increases must be very gradual and closely supervised by your physician. Orthostatic hypotension can cause falls and injury. Sit or lie down promptly if you feel light-headed or dizzy. Report dizziness or chest pain promptly.

▷ **Advisability of Use During Pregnancy**
Pregnancy Category: C. See Pregnancy Risk Categories at the back of this book.
Animal studies: No birth defects found in rat or rabbit studies.
Human studies: Adequate studies of pregnant women are not available.
Use this drug only if clearly needed. Ask your physician for guidance.

Advisability of Use If Breast-Feeding
Presence of this drug in breast milk: Unknown.
Watch infant closely and stop drug or nursing if adverse effects start.

Habit-Forming Potential: None.

Effects of Overdose: Orthostatic hypotension, headache, flushing, fast heart rate, extreme weakness, irregular heart rhythm, circulatory collapse.

Possible Effects of Long-Term Use: None reported.

Suggested Periodic Examinations While Taking This Drug (at physician's discretion)

Measurements of blood pressure in lying, sitting, and standing positions.

Measurements of body weight to detect fluid retention.

▷ **While Taking This Drug, Observe the Following**

Foods: No restrictions. Avoid excessive salt intake.

Beverages: No restrictions. May be taken with milk.

▷ *Alcohol:* Alcohol can exaggerate the blood-pressure-lowering actions of this drug and cause excessive reduction. Use with extreme caution.

Tobacco Smoking: Nicotine can intensify this drug's ability to worsen coronary insufficiency. Avoid all forms of tobacco.

▷ *Other Drugs*

The following drugs may ***increase*** the effects of terazosin:

• beta-adrenergic-blocking drugs (see Drug Classes); severity and duration of the first-dose response may be increased.

• ritonavir (Norvir)—may lead to toxicity.

• verapamil (Verelan, Calan, others), and cause excessive lowering of blood pressure.

The following drugs may *decrease* the effects of terazosin:

• estrogens (see Drug Classes).

• indomethacin (Indocin) and other NSAIDs (see *nonsteriodal anti-inflammatory drugs* in Drug Classes).

▷ *Driving, Hazardous Activities:* This drug may cause dizziness or drowsiness. Restrict activities as necessary.

Aviation Note: The use of this drug *is a disqualification* for piloting. Consult a designated aviation medical examiner.

Exposure to Sun: No restrictions.

Exposure to Cold: Cold environments may increase this drug's ability to cause coronary insufficiency (angina) and hypothermia (see Glossary). Use caution.

Heavy Exercise or Exertion: Excessive exertion can increase likelihood of chest pain.

Discontinuation: Do not stop this medicine abruptly if it is being used to treat congestive heart failure. Ask your physician for guidance.

TERBUTALINE (ter BYU ta leen)

Introduced: 1974   **Class:** Antiasthmatic, bronchodilator   **Prescription:** USA: Yes   **Controlled Drug:** USA: No; Canada: No   **Available as Generic:** No

Brand Names: Brethaire, Brethine, Bricanyl, ✚Bricanyl Spacer

```
┌─────────────────────────────────────────────────────────────────┐
│                    BENEFITS versus RISKS                          │
│        Possible Benefits              Possible Risks              │
│  VERY EFFECTIVE RELIEF OF      Increased blood pressure           │
│    BRONCHOSPASM               Fine hand tremor                    │
│                               Irregular heart rhythm (with excessive │
│                                 use)                              │
└─────────────────────────────────────────────────────────────────┘
```

▷ **Principal Uses**

As a Single Drug Product: Uses currently included in FDA-approved labeling: (1) Relieves acute bronchial asthma and reduces frequency and severity of chronic, recurrent asthmatic attacks; (2) relieves reversible bronchospasm associated with chronic bronchitis and emphysema.

Other (unlabeled) generally accepted uses: (1) May have a role in helping ease fetal distress in some patients; (2) used to help stop premature labor; (3) an alternative to intravenous isoproterenol in therapy of status asthmaticus.

How This Drug Works: Stimulates sympathetic nerve terminals, dilating constricted bronchial tubes and improving the ability to breathe.

Available Dose Forms and Strengths

Aerosol — 0.2 mg per actuation, 0.25 mg per actuation (Canada)
        Injection—1 mg/ml
Tablets — 2.5 mg, 5 mg

▷ **Usual Adult Dose Range:**   Aerosol: 0.4 mg taken in two separate inhalations 1 minute apart; repeat every 4 to 6 hours as needed.

Tablets: 2.5 to 5 mg taken every 6 hours. The total daily dose **should not** exceed 15 mg.

Note: Actual dose and schedule must be determined for each patient individually.

Conditions Requiring Dosing Adjustments

Liver Function: Extensively metabolized in the liver; however, dosing guidelines in liver disease are not available.

Kidney Function: For patients with moderate to severe kidney failure, 50% of the usual dose can be taken at the usual time. In severe failure, the drug should not be used.

▷ **Dosing Instructions:**   Tablets may be crushed and taken on an empty stomach or with food or milk. For aerosol, follow the written instructions carefully. Do not overuse.

Usual Duration of Use: Individualized. Do not use beyond the time necessary to terminate episodes of asthma.

Possible Advantages of This Drug

Rapid onset of action.
Long duration of action.
Highly effective relief of asthma.

▷ **This Drug Should Not Be Taken If**

• you had an allergic reaction to any form of it previously.
• you currently have an irregular heart rhythm.
• you took a monoamine oxidase (MAO) type A inhibitor (see Drug Classes) in the last 14 days.

▷ **Inform Your Physician Before Taking This Drug If**
- you are overly sensitive to other drugs that stimulate the sympathetic nervous system.
- you are currently using epinephrine (Adrenalin, Primatene Mist, etc.) to relieve asthmatic breathing.
- you have a seizure disorder.
- you have liver or kidney failure.
- you have any type of heart or circulatory disorder, especially high blood pressure or coronary heart disease.
- you have diabetes or an overactive thyroid gland (hyperthyroidism).
- you are taking any form of digitalis or any stimulant drug.

Possible Side Effects (natural, expected, and unavoidable drug actions)
Aerosol: dryness or irritation of mouth or throat, altered taste. Tablet: nervousness, tremor, palpitation.

▷ **Possible Adverse Effects** (unusual, unexpected, and infrequent reactions)
If any of the following develop, consult your physician promptly for guidance.

Mild Adverse Effects
Headache, dizziness, drowsiness, restlessness, insomnia—infrequent.
Rapid, pounding heartbeat; increased sweating; muscle cramps in arms and legs—infrequent to frequent.
Nausea, heartburn, vomiting—rare with oral form, frequent with IV.
Increased blood sugar—frequent (40% abnormal one-hour glucose).

Serious Adverse Effects
Rapid or irregular heart rhythm, intensification of angina, increased blood pressure—infrequent.
Lowered blood calcium or potassium (especially with intravenous use)—possible.
Liver toxicity—case reports.
Severe lowering of blood pressure (hypotension)—case reports.
Increased blood sugar—infrequent.

▷ **Possible Effects on Sexual Function:**   None reported.

Natural Diseases or Disorders That May Be Activated by This Drug
Latent coronary artery disease, diabetes, or high blood pressure.

Possible Effects on Laboratory Tests
Blood total cholesterol and LDL cholesterol levels: no effect.
Blood HDL cholesterol level: increased.
Blood triglyceride levels: no effect.
Blood thyroid hormone levels: T_3—increased; T_4—decreased; free T_4—no effect.
Glucose tolerance test: abnormal test.
Liver function tests: may be elevated.

CAUTION
1. Combination of this drug by aerosol with beclomethasone aerosol (Beclovent, Vanceril) may increase risk of fluorocarbon propellant toxicity. Best to use this aerosol 20 to 30 minutes before beclomethasone aerosol. This reduces toxicity risk and will help beclomethasone get into the lungs.
2. Avoid excessive use of aerosol inhalation. Excessive or prolonged inhala-

tion use can reduce effectiveness and cause serious heart rhythm disturbances, including cardiac arrest.

3. Do not use this drug with epinephrine. These two drugs may be used alternately provided that 4 hours is allowed between doses.

4. If you do not respond to your usually effective dose, ask your doctor for
help. Do not increase the size or frequency of the dose without your physician's approval.

Precautions for Use

By Infants and Children: Safety and effectiveness for those under 12 years of age
are not established.

By Those Over 60 Years of Age: Avoid excessive and continual use. If acute asthma
is not relieved promptly, other drugs will be needed. Watch for nervousness,
palpitations, irregular heart rhythm, and muscle tremors. Use with extreme
caution if you have hardening of the arteries, heart disease, or high blood
pressure.

▷ **Advisability of Use During Pregnancy**

Pregnancy Category: B. See Pregnancy Risk Categories at the back of this book.
Animal studies: No significant birth defects reported in mouse and rat studies.
Human studies: Adequate studies of pregnant women are not available.
Use only if clearly needed. Ask your physician for guidance.

Advisability of Use If Breast-Feeding

Presence of this drug in breast milk: Yes.
Monitor nursing infant closely and discontinue drug or nursing if adverse effects develop.

Habit-Forming Potential: None.

Effects of Overdose: Nervousness, palpitation, rapid heart rate, sweating,
headache, tremor, vomiting, chest pain.

Possible Effects of Long-Term Use: Loss of effectiveness. See "CAUTION"
above.

Suggested Periodic Examinations While Taking This Drug (at physician's discretion)
Blood pressure measurements, evaluation of heart status.

▷ **While Taking This Drug, Observe the Following**

Foods: No restrictions.

Beverages: Avoid excessive use of caffeine-containing beverages: coffee, tea, cola,
chocolate.

▷ *Alcohol:* No interactions expected.

Tobacco Smoking: No interactions expected. I advise everyone to quit smoking.

▷ *Other Drugs*

Terbutaline *taken concurrently* with

- monoamine oxidase (MAO) type A inhibitor drugs (see Drug Classes) may
cause excessive increase in blood pressure and undesirable heart stimulation.
- theophylline (Theo-Dur, others) may cause decreased theophylline effectiveness.

The following drugs may *decrease* the effects of terbutaline:

- beta-blocker drugs (see Drug Classes)—may impair terbutaline's effectiveness.

▷ *Driving, Hazardous Activities:* Usually no restrictions. Use caution if excessive nervousness or dizziness occurs.

Aviation Note: The use of this drug *is a disqualification* for piloting. Consult a designated aviation medical examiner.

Exposure to Sun: No restrictions.

Heavy Exercise or Exertion: Use caution—excessive exercise can induce asthma in some patients.

TERFENADINE (ter FEN a deen)

See the new minimally sedating antihistamines profile for further information.

TETRACYCLINE ANTIBIOTIC FAMILY (te trah SI kleen)

Introduced: 1953, 1967   **Class:** Antibiotic, tetracyclines   **Prescription:** USA: Yes   **Controlled Drug:** USA: No; Canada: No   **Available as Generic:** Yes

Brand Names: Doxycycline: Apo-Doxy, Apo-Doxy-Tabs, Atridox (gum line delivery form), ✦Doryx, Doryx, Doxy 100, 200, Doxy Caps, Doxy Tabs, Doxychel, ✦Doxycin, Doxy-Lemmon, Novopharm, Vibramycin, Vibra-Tabs, ✦Vibra-Tabs C-Pak; Tetracycline: Achromycin, Achromycin V, ✦Acrocidin, ✦Apo-Tetra, Actisite, Aureomycin, Contimycin, Cyclinex, Cyclopar, Lemtrex, ✦Medicycline, Mysteclin-F [CD], ✦Neo-Tetrine, ✦Nor-Tet, ✦Novo-Tetra, ✦Nu-Tetra, Panmycin, Retet, Robitet, SK-Tetracycline, Sumycin, Teline, Tetra-C, Tetracap, Tetra-Con, Tetracyn, Tetralan, Tetram, Tropicycline

BENEFITS versus RISKS	
Possible Benefits	*Possible Risks*
EFFECTIVE TREATMENT OF INFECTIONS due to susceptible bacteria and protozoa	ALLERGIC REACTIONS, mild to severe: ANAPHYLAXIS, DRUG-INDUCED HEPATITIS
	Drug-induced colitis
	Superinfections (bacterial or fungal)
	Blood cell disorders: hemolytic anemia, abnormally low white cell and platelet counts
	Kidney toxicity

▷ **Principal Uses**

As a Single Drug Product: Uses currently included in FDA-approved labeling: (1) Treats a broad range of infections caused by susceptible bacteria and protozoa (short-term use); (2) treats severe, resistant pustular acne (long-term use) (tetracycline); (3) used in a sustained-release form (Actisite) to treat gum disease (periodontitis) (tetracycline) in adults; (4) doxycycline treats syphilis in penicillin-allergic people; (5) helpful in acne; (6) helps prevent malaria in travelers.

Other (unlabeled) generally accepted uses: (1) Combination antibiotic treatment of duodenal ulcers caused by *Helicobacter pylori*; (2) used in vaginal and vulval cysts (Gartner's) and in vaginal hydrocele; (3) topical tetracycline is useful in chronic eye problems (blepharitis); (4) treats cancer (malignant) fluid (pericardial effusion) buildup around the heart; (5) used to treat stage one Lyme disease; (6) has a role in acne rosacea in decreasing the number of papules or nodules; (7) doxycline: (a) treats early Lyme disease; (b) treats sexual assault victims; (c) treats prostatitis; (d) can help in some cases of PMS; (e) may treat some cases of male infertility of unexplained origin.

As a *Combination Drug Product* [CD]: Tetracycline is available combined with amphotericin B, an antifungal antibiotic that is provided to reduce the risk of developing an overgrowth of yeast organisms (superinfection) of the gastrointestinal tract.

How These Drugs Work: Prevent growth and multiplication of susceptible organisms by interfering with formation of essential proteins.

Available Dose Forms and Strengths
Doxycycline:

Capsules — 50 mg, 100 mg
Capsules, coated pellets — 100 mg
Capsule, delayed release — 100 mg
Injection — 100 mg per vial, 200 mg per vial
Oral suspension — 25 mg/5 ml
Syrup — 50 mg/5 ml
Tablets — 50 mg, 100 mg

Tetracycline:

Capsules — 100 mg, 250 mg, 500 mg
Ointment — 3%
Ointment, ophthalmic — 10 mg/g
Periodontal fiber — 12.7 mg per fiber
Solution, topical — 2.2 mg/ml
Suspension, ophthalmic — 10 mg/ml
Suspension, oral — 125 mg/5 ml
Tablets — 250 mg, 500 mg

▷ **Usual Adult Dose Range:**   Doxycycline: 100 mg every 12 hours the first day, then 100 mg once daily. Some severe infections may require ongoing therapy of 100 mg every 12 hours. Total daily dose should not exceed 300 mg. Tetracycline: 250 to 500 mg every 6 hours, or 500 to 1000 mg every 12 hours. The total daily dose should not exceed 4000 mg (4 g).

Note: Actual dose and schedule must be determined for each patient individually.

Conditions Requiring Dosing Adjustments
Liver Function: Doxycycline: Patients with both liver and kidney compromise should have the dose decreased. Drug can cause liver problems, and a benefit-to-risk decision should be made for people with liver disease.
Tetracycline: Is a possible cause of hepatoxicity. A benefit-to-risk decision should be made for patients with compromised livers to use this drug. Daily maximum in liver disease is 1 g a day.
Kidney Function: Patients with mild to moderate kidney failure can take the usual dose every 8 to 12 hours. Patients with moderate to severe kidney fail-

ure take the usual dose every 12 to 24 hours. In severe kidney failure (creatinine clearance less than 10 ml/min), tetracycline should be avoided.

Malnutrition: Doxycycline: Lower than expected levels may occur in patients with malnutrition. If clinical progress is not as expected, the dose may need to be increased.

▷ **Dosing Instructions:**   The tablet may be crushed and the capsule opened and preferably taken on an empty stomach, 1 hour before or 2 hours after eating. However, to reduce stomach irritation these drugs may be taken with crackers that contain insignificant amounts of iron, calcium, magnesium, or zinc. Avoid all dairy products for 2 hours before and 2 hours after taking these drugs. (Unlike other tetracyclines, doxycycline absorption is not significantly changed by food or milk.) Take at the same time each day, with a full glass of water. Take the full course prescribed.

Usual Duration of Use: The time required to control the acute infection and be free of fever and symptoms for 48 hours. This varies with the nature of the infection. Long-term use (months to years, as for treatment of acne) requires supervision and periodic evaluation. Treatment of stage one Lyme disease requires 3 to 4 weeks in adults.

▷ **These Drugs Should Not Be Taken If**
- you are allergic to any tetracycline (see Drug Classes).
- you are pregnant or breast-feeding.
- you have severe liver disease.

▷ **Inform Your Physician Before Taking This Drug If**
- it is prescribed for a child under 8 years of age.
- you have a history of liver or kidney disease.
- you have systemic lupus erythematosus.
- you are taking any penicillin drug.
- you are taking any anticoagulant drug.
- you will have surgery with general anesthesia.

Possible Side Effects (natural, expected, and unavoidable drug actions)
Superinfections (see Glossary), often due to yeast organisms. These can occur in the mouth, intestinal tract, rectum, and/or vagina, resulting in rectal and vaginal itching.
Tooth discoloration (when used in children less than 8 years old). Metallic taste.

▷ **Possible Adverse Effects** (unusual, unexpected, and infrequent reactions)
If any of the following develop, consult your physician promptly for guidance.
Mild Adverse Effects
Allergic reactions: skin rash, hives, itching of hands and feet, swelling of face or extremities.
Loss of appetite, stomach irritation, taste disorders, nausea, vomiting, diarrhea—infrequent.
Warts—very rare and of questionable causality (tetracycline).
Irritation of mouth or tongue, "black tongue," sore throat, abdominal cramping or pain—infrequent.
Serious Adverse Effects
Allergic reactions: anaphylactic reaction (see Glossary), asthma, fever, swollen joints and lymph glands.

Serious skin problems (Stevens-Johnson syndrome, Jarisch-Herxheimer reaction)—case reports.

Drug-induced hepatitis with jaundice—case reports.

Permanent discoloration and/or malformation of teeth if taken by children under 8, including unborn child and infant.

Drug-induced colitis, myasthenia gravis, or pancreatitis—case reports.

Worsening of existing systemic lupus erythematosus—case reports.

Rare blood cell disorders: hemolytic anemia (see Glossary); abnormally low white blood cell count, causing fever and infections; abnormally low blood platelet count—case reports.

Impairment of blood clotting—case reports.

Increased intracranial pressure (pseudotumor cerebri) or kidney problems—rare (tetracycline).

Drug-induced porphyria, esophageal ulcers, or low blood potassium—case reports (tetracycline).

▷ **Possible Effects on Sexual Function:**   Decreased effectiveness of oral contraceptives taken concurrently (several case reports of pregnancy).

Decreased male fertility—case reports (tetracycline).

▷ **Adverse Effects That May Mimic Natural Diseases or Disorders**

Drug-induced hepatitis may suggest viral hepatitis.

Natural Diseases or Disorders That May Be Activated by This Drug

Systemic lupus erythematosus.

Possible Effects on Laboratory Tests

Complete blood cell counts: decreased red cells, hemoglobin, white cells, and platelets; increased eosinophils (allergic reaction).

Blood lupus erythematosus (LE) cells: positive.

Blood amylase level: increased (toxic effect in pregnant women).

Liver function tests: increased enzymes (ALT/GPT, AST/GOT, alkaline phosphatase) or bilirubin.

Kidney function tests: increased blood creatinine and urea nitrogen (BUN) levels (kidney damage).

Urine sugar tests: false-positive results with Benedict's solution and Clinitest.

CAUTION

1. Antacids, dairy products, and preparations containing aluminum, bismuth, calcium, iron, magnesium, or zinc can prevent adequate absorption and reduce effectiveness significantly.
2. Troublesome and persistent diarrhea can occur. If diarrhea persists for more than 24 hours, call your doctor.
3. If general anesthesia is required while taking these drugs, the choice of anesthetic agent must be selected carefully to prevent kidney damage.

Precautions for Use

By Infants and Children: If possible, tetracyclines should not be given to children under 8 years of age because of the risk of permanent discoloration and deformity of the teeth. Rarely, infants may develop increased intracranial pressure within the first 4 days of receiving this drug. Tetracyclines may inhibit normal bone growth and development.

By Those Over 60 Years of Age: Dose must be carefully individualized based on kidney function. Natural skin changes may predispose to severe and prolonged itching reactions in the genital and anal regions.

▷ **Advisability of Use During Pregnancy**

Pregnancy Category: D. See Pregnancy Risk Categories at the back of this book.

Animal studies: Tetracycline causes limb defects in rats, rabbits, and chickens.

Human studies: Information from studies of pregnant women indicates that this drug can cause impaired development and discoloration of teeth and other developmental defects.

It is advisable to avoid these drugs completely during entire pregnancy.

Advisability of Use If Breast-Feeding

Presence of this drug in breast milk: Yes.

Avoid drug or refrain from nursing.

Habit-Forming Potential: None.

Effects of Overdose: Stomach burning, nausea, vomiting, diarrhea.

Possible Effects of Long-Term Use: Superinfections; impairment of bone marrow, liver, or kidney function—rare.

Suggested Periodic Examinations While Taking This Drug (at physician's discretion)

Complete blood cell counts, liver and kidney function tests.

During extended use, sputum and stool examinations may detect early superinfection due to yeast organisms.

▷ **While Taking This Drug, Observe the Following**

Foods: Avoid cheeses, yogurt, ice cream, iron-fortified cereals and supplements, and meats for 2 hours before and 2 hours after taking this drug. Calcium and iron can combine with these drugs and reduce absorption significantly.

Beverages: Avoid all forms of milk for 2 hours before and 2 hours after taking.

▷ *Alcohol:* Reduces doxycycline blood levels. Alcohol should be avoided with doxycycline, and perhaps another tetracycline substituted, particularly for those who have drinking problems. Alcohol is also best avoided if you have active liver disease.

Tobacco Smoking: No interactions expected. I advise everyone to quit smoking.

▷ *Other Drugs*

Tetracyclines may ***increase*** the effects of

- cyclosporine (Sandimmune, Neoral).
- digoxin (Lanoxin), and cause digitalis toxicity.
- lithium (Eskalith, Lithane, etc.), and increase the risk of lithium toxicity.
- oral anticoagulants such as warfarin (Coumadin), and make it necessary to reduce their dose. Increased INR (prothrombin time or protime) testing is needed.

Tetracyclines may ***decrease*** the effects of

- birth control pills (oral contraceptives), and impair their effectiveness in preventing pregnancy.
- penicillins (see Drug Classes) and impair their effectiveness in treating infections.

Tetracyclines ***taken concurrently*** with

- furosemide (Lasix) increases blood urea nitrogen (BUN).
- isotretinoin (Accutane) may worsen tetracycline-caused increased intracranial pressure and cause additive toxicity.

- methoxyflurane anesthesia may impair kidney function.
- theophylline (Theo-Dur) may result in variable changes in drug levels. More frequent theophylline blood levels are needed if these medicines are to be combined.
- warfarin (Coumadin) poses an increased risk of bleeding. INR (prothrombin time or protime) testing should be checked more frequently, and doses adjusted if needed.

The following drugs may *decrease* the effects of tetracyclines:

- antacids (aluminum or magnesium preparations, sodium bicarbonate, etc.)—may reduce drug absorption.
- bismuth subsalicylate (Pepto-Bismol, others).
- calcium supplements (various brands).
- cholestyramine (Questran) and other cholesterol-lowering resins.
- colestipol (Colestid).
- iron, zinc, magnesium, and mineral preparations—may reduce drug absorption.
- phenobarbital.
- phenytoin (Dilantin).
- rifampin (Rifadin, others).
- sucralfate (Carafate).
- zinc salts.

▷ *Driving, Hazardous Activities:* Usually no restrictions. However, this drug may cause nausea or diarrhea. Restrict activities as necessary.

Aviation Note: The use of these drugs **may be a disqualification** for piloting. Consult a designated aviation medical examiner.

Exposure to Sun: Use caution—some tetracyclines can cause photosensitivity (see Glossary).

THEOPHYLLINE (thee OFF i lin)

Introduced: 1900   **Class:** Antiasthmatic, bronchodilator; xanthines   **Prescription:** USA: Yes   **Controlled Drug:** USA: No; Canada: No   **Available as Generic:** Yes

Brand Names: Accurbron, ✦Acet-Am, A.E.A., Aerolate, Aminodrox-Forte, ✦Apo-Oxtriphylline, ✦Aquaphyllim, ✦Asbron [CD], Asmalix, Azpan, Brocomar, Bronchial Gelatin Capsule, Broncomar, Bronkotabs, Bronkaid Tablets [CD], Bronkodyl, Bronkolixir [CD], Bronkotabs [CD], Constant-T, Duraphyl, Elixicon, Elixomin, Elixophyllin, For-Az-Ma [CD], Isuprel Compound [CD], Labid, Lanophyllin, Lixolin, Lodrane, Lodrane CR, Marax [CD], Marax DF [CD], Mudrane GG Elixir [CD], Phedral [CD], Phyllocontin, Physpan, ✦PMS Theophylline, Primatene, ✦Pulmophylline, Quadrinal [CD], Quibron [CD], Quibron-300 [CD], Quibron Plus [CD], Quibron-T Dividose, Quibron-T/SR, Respbid, Slo-bid, Slo-bid Gyrocaps, Slo-Phyllin, Slo-Phyllin GG [CD], Slo-Phyllin Gyrocaps, Somophyllin, Sompphyllin-12, Sustaire, Tedral [CD], Tedral SA [CD], T.E.H. [CD], T.E.P., Thalfed, Theobid Duracaps, ✦Theo-Bronc, Theochron, Theoclear, Theoclear L.A., Theocord, Theo-Dur, Theo-Dur Sprinkle, Theolair, Theolair-SR, Theolate [CD], Theolixir, Theomar [CD], Theomax DF, Theon, Theophyl-SR, Theo-24, Theospan-SR, Theo-SR,

Theo-Time, Theovent, Theox, Theozine, Therex [CD], Uni-Dur, ✦Uniphyl, Vitaphen [CD]

BENEFITS versus RISKS

Possible Benefits	*Possible Risks*
EFFECTIVE PREVENTION AND RELIEF OF ACUTE BRONCHIAL ASTHMA	NARROW TREATMENT RANGE
	FREQUENT STOMACH DISTRESS
MODERATELY EFFECTIVE CONTROL OF CHRONIC, RECURRENT BRONCHIAL ASTHMA	Gastrointestinal bleeding
	Central nervous system toxicity, seizures
Moderately effective symptomatic relief in chronic bronchitis and emphysema	Heart rhythm disturbances

---

▷ **Principal Uses**

As a Single Drug Product: Uses currently included in FDA-approved labeling: (1) Used to relieve shortness of breath and wheezing of acute bronchial asthma, and to prevent the recurrence of asthmatic episodes; (2) useful in relieving asthmatic-like symptoms associated with some types of chronic bronchitis, chronic obstructive pulmonary disease, and emphysema.

Other (unlabeled) generally accepted uses: (1) May have a role in combination therapy of cystic fibrosis; (2) can help decrease excessive production of red blood cells in kidney transplant patients; (3) may have a role in helping decrease the risk of sudden infant death syndrome (SIDS); (4) may have a supportive role with steroids and other agents in helping prevent rejection of transplanted kidneys; (5) can help ease essential tremor; (6) decreases risk of breathing cessation in neonatal apnea; (7) helps in treating SIDS children; (8) may have a role in treating sleep apnea; (9) one small study found it effective in stopping ACE inhibitor (see Drug Classes) cough.

As a Combination Drug Product [CD]: Available combined with several other drugs that manage bronchial asthma and related conditions. Ephedrine is added to enhance opening of the bronchi (bronchodilation); guaifenesin is added to thin mucus in the bronchial tubes (an expectorant effect); and mild sedatives such as phenobarbital are added to allay anxiety often seen in acute attacks of asthma.

How This Drug Works: By inhibiting the enzyme phosphodiesterase, this drug produces an increase in the tissue chemical cyclic AMP. This causes relaxation of the muscles in the bronchial tubes and blood vessels of the lung, resulting in relief of bronchospasm, expanded lung capacity, and improved lung circulation.

Available Dose Forms and Strengths

Capsules — 100 mg, 200 mg, 250 mg, 260 mg

Capsules, prolonged action — 50 mg, 60 mg, 65 mg, 75 mg, 100 mg, 125 mg, 130 mg, 200 mg, 250 mg, 260 mg, 300 mg

Elixir — 27 mg/5 ml, 50 mg/5 ml

Oral solution — 27 mg/5 ml, 53.3 mg/5 ml

Oral suspension — 100 mg/5 ml

Syrup — 27 mg/5 ml, 50 mg/5 ml

Tablets — 100 mg, 125 mg, 200 mg, 250 mg, 300 mg
Tablets, prolonged action — 50 mg, 60 mg, 65 mg, 75 mg, 100 mg,
125 mg, 130 mg, 200 mg, 225 mg, 250 mg,
260 mg, 300 mg, 350 mg, 400 mg, 450 mg,
500 mg, 600 mg

▷ **Recommended Dose Ranges** (Actual dose and schedule must be determined for
each patient individually.)

Infants and Children: Sudden asthma attack: (not currently taking theophylline)—loading dose of 5 mg per kg of body mass. For acute attack while
currently taking theophylline—a single dose of 2.5 mg per kg of body mass,
if no signs of theophylline toxicity. Check blood levels of theophylline.

For ongoing use during acute attack—dose is based on age. Up to 6 months
of age—0.07 for each week of age + 1.7 = the mg per kg of body mass,
given every 8 hours. 6 months to 1 year of age—0.05 for each week of age
+ 1.25 = the mg per kg of body mass, given every 6 hours. 1 to 9 years of
age—5 mg per kg of body mass, every 6 hours. 9 to 12 years of age—4 mg
per kg of body mass, every 6 hours. 12 to 16 years of age—3 mg per kg of
body mass, every 6 hours.

For ongoing use to prevent asthma—dose is based on age. Once slow dosing
increase is accomplished, daily doses are adjusted to reach blood levels of
10 to 15 mcg/ml.

16 to 60 Years of Age: For acute attack of asthma (not currently taking theophylline)—loading dose of 5 mg per kg of body mass.

For acute attack while currently taking theophylline—a single dose of 2.5 mg
per kg of body mass, if no indications of theophylline toxicity. Monitor
blood levels of theophylline.

For maintenance during acute attack—for nonsmokers: 3 mg per kg of body
mass, every 8 hours; for smokers: 4 mg per kg of body mass, every 6 hours.

For chronic treatment to prevent recurrence of asthma—initially 6 to 8 mg per
kg of body mass, in three or four divided doses at 6- to 8-hour intervals, up
to a maximum of 400 mg daily. Increase dose as needed and tolerated by increments of 25% every 2 to 3 days. The total daily dose should not exceed
13 mg per kg of body mass or 900 mg, whichever is less.

Prolonged-action formulations may allow twice-daily dosing with good results.

Over 60 Years of Age: Theophylline is removed some 30% more slowly than in
younger patients. Decreased doses and more frequent blood levels are prudent.

Conditions Requiring Dosing Adjustments

Liver Function: The dose **must** be lowered, and blood levels obtained frequently.
Doses may need to be decreased by 50% in some cases.

Kidney Function: Lower doses and more frequent blood levels are indicated.

▷ **Dosing Instructions:**   May be taken with or following food to reduce stomach irritation. The regular capsules may be opened and the regular tablets may be
crushed. The prolonged-action forms should be swallowed whole and not
altered. Shake the oral suspension well before measuring each dose. Do
not refrigerate liquid dose forms.

Usual Duration of Use: Use on a regular schedule for 48 to 72 hours usually determines effectiveness in controlling the breathing impairment associated

with bronchial asthma and chronic lung disease. Long-term use requires supervision and periodic physician evaluation.

▷ **This Drug Should Not Be Taken If**
- you have had an allergic reaction to it, or to aminophylline, dyphylline, or oxtriphylline.
- you have active peptic ulcer disease.
- you have an uncontrolled seizure disorder.
- you had a blood level drawn and is in the "toxic" range.

▷ **Inform Your Physician Before Taking This Drug If**
- you have had an unfavorable reaction to any xanthine (see Drug Classes).
- you have a seizure disorder of any kind.
- you have a history of peptic ulcer disease.
- you have a history of underactive thyroid (hypothyroidism).
- you have impaired liver or kidney function.
- you take any of the drugs listed in the "Other Drugs" section below.
- you have hypertension, heart disease, or any type of heart rhythm disorder.

Possible Side Effects (natural, expected, and unavoidable drug actions)
Nervousness, insomnia, rapid heart rate, increased urine volume.

▷ **Possible Adverse Effects** (unusual, unexpected, and infrequent reactions)
If any of the following develop, consult your physician promptly for guidance.

Mild Adverse Effects
Allergic reactions: skin rash, hives.
Headache, dizziness, irritability, tremor, fatigue, weakness—infrequent.
Loss of appetite, nausea, vomiting (may be an early warning of toxicity), abdominal pain, diarrhea, excessive thirst—infrequent.
Flushing of face—case reports.

Serious Adverse Effects
Allergic reactions: severe skin rash (Stevens-Johnson syndrome)—case reports.
Idiosyncratic reactions: marked anxiety, confusion, behavioral disturbances.
Central nervous system toxicity: muscle twitching, seizures—dose related.
Heart rhythm abnormalities, rapid breathing, low blood pressure—variable and dose related.
Gastrointestinal bleeding—rare.
Defects in clotting (coagulation)—case reports.
Drug-induced abnormal urine production (SIADH) or porphyria—case reports.
Worsening of ulcers—possible.
Liver toxicity—case reports.

▷ **Possible Effects on Sexual Function:**   None reported.

Natural Diseases or Disorders That May Be Activated by This Drug
Latent peptic ulcer disease.

Possible Effects on Laboratory Tests
Blood uric acid level: increased.
Fecal occult blood test: positive (large doses may cause stomach bleeding).

CAUTION
1. This drug should not be taken at the same time as other antiasthmatic drugs unless your doctor prescribes the combination. Serious overdose could result.

2. Influenza vaccine may delay the elimination of this drug and cause accumulation to toxic levels.

Precautions for Use

By Infants and Children: Do not exceed recommended doses. Watch for toxicity: irritability, agitation, tremors, lethargy, fever, vomiting, rapid heart rate and breathing, seizures. Blood levels are needed during long-term use.

By Those Over 60 Years of Age: Small starting doses are indicated. You may be at increased risk for stomach irritation, nausea, vomiting, or diarrhea. When used concurrently with coffee (caffeine) or nasal decongestants, this drug may cause excessive stimulation and a hyperactivity syndrome.

▷ **Advisability of Use During Pregnancy**

Pregnancy Category: C. See Pregnancy Risk Categories at the back of this book. Animal studies: Significant birth defects due to this drug reported in mice. Human studies: Adequate studies of pregnant women are not available. No increase in birth defects reported in 394 exposures to this drug.

Avoid this drug during the first 3 months. Use it otherwise only if clearly needed. Ask your physician for guidance.

Advisability of Use If Breast-Feeding

Presence of this drug in breast milk: Yes.

Avoid drug or refrain from nursing.

Habit-Forming Potential: None.

Effects of Overdose: Nausea, vomiting, restlessness, irritability, confusion, delirium, seizures, high fever, weak pulse, coma.

Possible Effects of Long-Term Use: Gastrointestinal irritation.

Suggested Periodic Examinations While Taking This Drug (at physician's discretion)

Periodic testing of blood theophylline levels (see "Therapeutic Drug Monitoring" in chapter 2). Time to sample blood for theophylline level: 2 hours after regular (standard) dose forms; 5 hours after sustained-release dose forms. Recommended therapeutic range: 10 to 20 mcg/ml.

▷ **While Taking This Drug, Observe the Following**

Foods: No restrictions.

Beverages: Avoid excessive use of caffeine-containing beverages: coffee, tea, cola, or chocolate. This combination could cause nervousness and insomnia.

▷ *Alcohol:* Large doses may decrease removal by up to 30%. May have additive effect on stomach irritation.

Tobacco Smoking: May hasten the elimination of this drug and reduce its effectiveness. I advise everyone to quit smoking.

Marijuana Smoking: May hasten the elimination of this drug and reduce its effectiveness. Higher doses may be necessary to maintain a therapeutic blood level.

▷ *Other Drugs*

Theophylline may *decrease* the effects of

• benzodiazepines (See Drug Classes).

• lithium (Lithane, Lithobid, etc.), and reduce its effectiveness.

Theophylline *taken concurrently* with

- halothane (anesthesia) may cause heart rhythm abnormalities.
- phenytoin (Dilantin) may cause decreased effects of both drugs. Monitor blood levels and adjust doses as appropriate.

The following drugs may *increase* the effects of theophylline:

- allopurinol (Lopurin, Zyloprim).
- amiodarone (Cordarone).
- birth control pills (oral contraceptives—estrogens).
- cimetidine (Tagamet).
- ciprofloxacin (Cipro).
- clarithromycin (Biaxin).
- disulfiram (Antabuse).
- doxycycline and other tetracyclines (see Drug Classes).
- enoxacin (Penetrex).
- ephedrine.
- erythromycin (E-Mycin, Erythrocin, etc.).
- famotidine (Pepcid).
- flu vaccine (influenza vaccine).
- fluvoxamine (Luvox).
- furosemide (Lasix).
- grepafloxacin (Raxar).
- imipenem/cilastatin (Primaxin).
- interferon alfa.
- isoniazid (INH).
- methotrexate (Mexate)
- mexiletine (Mexitil).
- nicotine (Nicorette, Pro-Step, others).
- norfloxacin (Noroxin).
- ofloxacin (Floxin).
- pentoxifylline (Trental).
- ranitidine (Zantac).
- tacrine (Cognex).
- thiabendazole.
- ticlopidine (Ticlid).
- troleandomycin (TAO).
- trovafloxacin (Trovan).
- verapamil (Calan, Verelan).
- viloxazine.
- zileuton (Zyflo); may require 50% dose decreases.

The following drugs may *decrease* the effects of theophylline:

- barbiturates (phenobarbital, etc.).
- beta-blocker drugs (see Drug Classes).
- carbamazepine (Tegretol).
- isoproterenol.
- primidone (Mysoline).
- rifampin (Rifadin, Rimactane, etc.).
- ritonavir (Norvir), and perhaps other protease inhibitors (see Drug Classes), may lead to toxicity.
- sulfinpyrazone (Anturane).

▷ *Driving, Hazardous Activities:* This drug may cause dizziness. Restrict activities as necessary.

Aviation Note: The use of this drug *may be a disqualification* for piloting. Consult a designated aviation medical examiner.

Exposure to Sun: No restrictions.

Occurrence of Unrelated Illness: Sudden viral respiratory infections or fever may slow drug removal. Watch for signs of toxicity, as dosing **must** be changed if this occurs. More frequent blood levels are needed. Seizure disorders may be worsened by this medicine. Used with extreme caution by seizure patients. Theophylline used with extreme caution in active peptic ulcer disease or heart arrhythmias (cardiac, not including slow or bradyarrhythmias).

Discontinuation: Avoid prolonged or unnecessary use of this drug. When your asthma resolves, withdraw this drug gradually over several days.

THIAZIDE DIURETIC FAMILY PROFILE

Bendroflumethiazide (ben droh meh THI a zide)   **Hydrochlorothiazide** (hi droh klor oh THI a zide)   **Hydroflumethiazide** (hi droh flu meh THI a zide)   **Chlorothiazide** (klor oh THI a zide)   **Methyclothiazide** (METH i klo THI a zide)   **Trichlormethiazide** (tri klor me THI a zide)   **Chlorthalidone** (KLOR thal i dohn)   **Metolazone** (me TOHL a zohn)

Introduced: 1960, 1959, 1961, 1957, 1959, 1962, 1960, 1974, respectively   **Class:** Antihypertensive, diuretic, thiazides   **Prescription:** USA: Yes   **Controlled Drug:** USA: No; Canada: No   **Available as Generic:** USA: Yes—hydrochlorothiazide (also in combination with Triamterine); Canada: Yes

Brand Names: Bendroflumethiazide: Naturetin; Hydrochlorothiazide: Aldactazide [CD], Aldoril-15/25 [CD], Aldoril D30/D50 [CD], ✦Apo-Amilzide, ✦Apo-Hydro, ✦Apo-Methazide [CD], ✦Apo-Triazide [CD], Apresazide [CD], Apresoline-Esidrix [CD], Capozide [CD], ✦Co-Betaloc [CD], Diaqua, ✦Diuchlor H, Dyazide [CD], Esidrix, Ezide, H-H-R, H.H.R., HydroDiuril, Hydromal, Hydro-Par, Hydropres [CD], Hydroserpine [CD], Hydroserpine Plus [CD], Hydro-T, Hydro-Z-50, Inderide [CD], Inderide LA [CD], ✦Ismelin-Esidrix [CD], Lopressor HCT [CD], Maxzide [CD], Maxzide-25 [CD], M Dopazide [CD], Microzide, Mictrin, ✦Moduret [CD], Moduretic [CD], ✦Natrimax, ✦Neo-Codema, Normozide [CD], ✦Novo-Doparil [CD], ✦Novo-Hydrazide, ✦Novo-Spirozine [CD], ✦Novo-Triamzide [CD], Oretic, Oreticyl [CD], ✦PMS Dopazide [CD], Prinzide [CD], Ser-Ap-Es [CD], Serpasil-Esidrix [CD], SK-Hydrochlorothiazide, Thiuretic, Timolide [CD], Trandate HCT [CD], Unipres [CD], ✦Urozide, Vaseretic [CD], ✦Viskazide [CD], Zestoretic [CD], Ziac, Zide; Chlorothiazide: Aldochlor [CD], Diachlor, Diupres [CD], Diurigen, Diuril, SK-Chlorothiazide, ✦Supres [CD]; Hydroflumethiazide: Diucardin, Saluron; Methyclothiazide: Aquatensen, ✦Duretic, Enduron; Trichlormethiazide: Diurese, Marazide II, Metahydrin, Naqua, Naquival [CD]; Chlorthalidone: ✦Apo-Chlorthalidone, Combipress [CD], Demi-Regroton [CD], Hygroton, ✦Hygroton-Resperpine [CD], Hylidone, ✦Novothalidone, Regroton [CD], Thalitone, Tenoretic; Metolazone: ✦Uridon, Diulo, Microx, Mykrox, Zaroxolyn

BENEFITS versus RISKS	
Possible Benefits	*Possible Risks*
EFFECTIVE, WELL-TOLERATED DIURETICS	Loss of body potassium and magnesium (especially with higher doses)
POSSIBLY EFFECTIVE IN MILD HYPERTENSION	
ENHANCE EFFECTIVENESS OF OTHER ANTIHYPERTENSIVES	Cardiac arrhythmias caused by decreased electrolytes (studied in chlorthalidone and hydrochlorothiazide)
Beneficial in treatment of diabetes insipidus	Increased blood sugar, uric acid, or calcium
	Rare blood cell disorders
	Rare liver toxicity (chlorothiazide or hydrochlorothiazide)

▷ **Principal Uses**

As a Single Drug Product: Uses currently included in FDA-approved labeling: (1) Increases the volume of urine (diuresis) to correct fluid retention (edema) seen in congestive heart failure, corticosteroid or estrogen use, and certain types of liver and kidney disease; (2) starting therapy for high blood pressure (hypertension).

Author's Note: One large study shows that hydrochlorothiazide achieves benefits (outcomes) in decreasing left ventricular size equal to more expensive agents such as ACE inhibitors. A recent review of ten studies found that diuretics, as opposed to beta-blockers, should be the first-line medicines for treating high blood pressure in the elderly.

Other (unlabeled) generally accepted uses: (1) Prevention of kidney stones that contain calcium; (2) may help decrease the frequency of hip fractures in the elderly; (3) methyclothiazide has been used to help maintain blood calcium levels in Paget's disease; (4) may have a role in helping prevent osteoporosis (by correcting abnormally high elimination of calcium in the urine or hypercalciuria); (5) used in diabetes insipidus (nephrogenic) in decreasing the urine volume.

As Combination Drug Products [CD]: Used to treat blood pressure that has not responded to single-drug therapy.

How These Drugs Work: By increasing removal of salt and water in the urine, these drugs reduce fluid volume and body sodium. They also relax walls of smaller arteries. The combined effect of these two actions (reduced blood volume in expanded space) lowers blood pressure.

Available Dose Forms and Strengths

Bendroflumethiazide:
        Tablets — 5 mg, 10 mg
Hydrochlorothiazide:
        Solution — 50 mg/5 ml
 Solution, intensol — 100 mg/ml
        Tablets — 12.5 mg, 25 mg, 50 mg, 100 mg
Chlorothiazide:
        Injection — 500 mg/20 ml
 Oral suspension — 250 mg/5 ml
        Tablets — 250 mg, 500 mg

Methyclothiazide:
> Tablets — 2.5 mg, 5 mg

Trichlormethiazide:
> Tablets — 2 mg, 4 mg

Chlorthalidone:
> Tablets — 25 mg, 50 mg, 100 mg

Metolazone:
> Tablets — 0.5 mg, 2.5 mg, 5 mg, 10 mg

▷ **Usual Adult Dose Range:**   Bendroflumethiazide: As antihypertensive—12.5 to 5 mg daily, in a single dose.

Hydrochlorothiazide: As antihypertensive—12.5 to 100 mg daily initially; 12.5 to 200 mg daily for maintenance. As diuretic—variable; 12.5 to 200 mg daily. Many patients require 100 to 200 mg; the smallest effective dose should be determined (see "CAUTION" below). The total daily dose should not exceed 200 mg. Microzide is a new once-daily formulation (12.5 mg) of this medicine.

Author's Note: Many patients with mild to moderate high blood pressure get acceptable blood-pressure-lowering results from 12.5 mg of hydrochlorothiazide. If results are obtained with this dose, it can minimize loss of potassium and magnesium as well!

Chlorothiazide: As antihypertensive—500 to 1000 mg per day to start and 500 to 2000 mg daily as a maintenance dose. As a diuretic—500 to 2000 mg per day, using the smallest effective dose. Daily maximum is 2000 mg.

Methyclothiazide: As antihypertensive or diuretic—2.5 to 5 mg daily. Maximum daily diuretic dose is 10 mg. Pediatric dose—0.05 to 0.2 mg per kg of body mass daily.

Trichlormethiazide: As antihypertensive or diuretic—therapy may be started with 1 to 4 mg twice daily. Usual maintenance dose is 1 to 4 mg once daily.

Chlorthalidone: As antihypertensive—25 to 50 mg daily to start therapy, then 50 to 100 mg for maintenance. As a diuretic—50 to 100 mg daily, then maintenance with the smallest effective dose (see "CAUTION" below). Daily maximum is 200 mg; however, this may change with recently published data.

Note: Actual dose and schedule must be determined for eachpatient individually.

Conditions Requiring Dosing Adjustments

Liver Function: Electrolyte balance is critical in liver failure. These drugs may precipitate encephalopathy. Hydrochlorothiazide and chlorothiazide are also a rare cause of cholestatic jaundice and should be used with caution in liver failure.

Kidney Function: These drugs can be used with caution by patients with mild kidney failure, and are not effective for patients with moderate failure. They should not be used in severe kidney failure; they can be a rare cause of kidney damage.

▷ **Dosing Instructions:**   The tablets may be crushed and taken with or following meals to reduce stomach irritation. They are best taken in the morning to avoid nighttime urination.

Usual Duration of Use: Regular use for 2 to 3 weeks determines benefits in lowering high blood pressure. Long-term use requires follow up with your doctor.

Possible Advantages of These Drugs

Hydrochlorothiazide was studied in more than 1,100 Veterans Administration patients with mild to moderate high blood pressure. It was found to have met blood pressure reduction goals while offering decreased left ventricular mass. These outcomes or results were accomplished using low-dose therapy, avoiding many of the undesirable changes in blood chemistry that can be seen with higher doses. This was also accomplished at a fraction of the cost of ACE inhibitors or calcium channel blockers.

▷ **These Drugs Should Not Be Taken If**
- you had an allergic reaction to any form previously.
- your kidneys are not making urine.

▷ **Inform Your Physician Before Taking These Drugs If**
- you are allergic to any form of "sulfa" drug.
- you are pregnant or planning to become pregnant.
- you have a history of kidney or liver disease.
- you have a history of pancreatitis.
- you have asthma or allergies to other medicines.
- you have had testing of electrolytes ordered by another physician, which your doctor has not seen.
- you develop muscle cramps, weakness, or abnormal heartbeats while taking one of these medicines.
- you have diabetes, gout, or lupus erythematosus.
- you are allergic to the dye tartrazine, as some of these medicines contain it.
- you take any form of cortisone, digitalis, oral antidiabetic drug, or insulin.
- you will have surgery with general anesthesia.

Possible Side Effects (natural, expected, and unavoidable drug actions)

Light-headedness on arising from sitting or lying position (see **Orthostatic Hypotension** in Glossary).

Increased blood sugar or uric acid level; decreased blood potassium or magnesium level. Decreased blood magnesium, combined with loss of potassium, may lead to increased risk of sudden cardiac death (high doses for extended periods).

▷ **Possible Adverse Effects** (unusual, unexpected, and infrequent reactions)

If any of the following develop, consult your physician promptly for guidance.

Mild Adverse Effects

Allergic reactions: skin rashes, hives, drug fever (see Glossary).

Headache, dizziness, blurred or yellow vision—infrequent.

Reduced appetite, indigestion, nausea, vomiting, diarrhea—infrequent.

Serious Adverse Effects

Allergic reactions: hepatitis with jaundice (see Glossary), anaphylactic reaction (see Glossary), severe skin reactions.

Inflammation of the pancreas—case reports.

Bone marrow depression (see Glossary): fever, sore throat, abnormal bleeding/bruising—case reports.

Data from studies of hydrochlorothiazide and chlorthalidone suggest that potassium and magnesium loss associated with higher-dose therapy increases the risk of sudden cardiac death.

Acute gout in some patients (because these medicines decrease uric acid removal).

Loss of blood glucose control—possible.

Short-term (less than 1 year) increase in serum lipids (returns to pretreatment
levels in about 1 year).

▷ **Possible Effects on Sexual Function:** Decreased libido (hydrochlorothiazide,
chlorthalidone); impotence (bendroflumethiazide, chlorothiazide, hydrochlorothiazide)—case reports.

▷ **Adverse Effects That May Mimic Natural Diseases or Disorders**
Liver reaction may suggest viral hepatitis.

Natural Diseases or Disorders That May Be Activated by These Drugs
Diabetes, gout, systemic lupus erythematosus. Those with asthma or drug allergies are more likely to have allergic reactions.

Possible Effects on Laboratory Tests
Complete blood counts: decreased red cells, hemoglobin, white cells, and
platelets.

Blood amylase level: increased (possible pancreatitis).

Blood calcium or uric acid level: increased.

Blood sodium and chloride levels: decreased.

Blood cholesterol and triglyceride levels: increased, short term.

Blood glucose level: increased.

Glucose tolerance test (GTT): decreased.

Blood lithium level: increased.

Blood potassium and magnesium level: decreased.

Blood urea nitrogen (BUN) level: increased with long-term use.

Liver function tests (hydrochlorothiazide and chlorothiazide): increased liver
enzymes (ALT/GPT, AST/GOT, and alkaline phosphatase), increased bilirubin.

CAUTION

1. One study found a strong association between higher doses of hydrochlorothiazide and chlorthalidone and combination drugs containing these diuretics and electrolyte loss and sudden cardiac death. This
appeared to be a result of magnesium and potassium loss, and may be cir-
cumvented by close following of those electrolytes.

2. Take these medicines exactly as prescribed. Excessive loss of sodium and
potassium can lead to loss of appetite, nausea, fatigue, weakness, confusion, and tingling in the extremities.

3. If you take digitalis (digitoxin, digoxin), adequate potassium is critical.
Periodic testing and high-potassium foods may be needed to prevent
potassium deficiency—a potential cause of digitalis toxicity (see Table
13, "High-Potassium Foods," in Section Six).

Precautions for Use
By Infants and Children: Overdose could cause serious dehydration. Significant
potassium loss can occur within the first 2 weeks of drug use.

By Those Over 60 Years of Age: Starting doses may be as low as 12.5 mg. Increased risk of impaired thinking, orthostatic hypotension, potassium loss,
and blood sugar increase. Overdose or extended use can cause excessive loss
of body water, thickening (increased viscosity) of blood, and increased ten-

dency for the blood to clot—predisposing to stroke, heart attack, or thrombophlebitis (vein inflammation with blood clot).

▷ **Advisability of Use During Pregnancy**

Pregnancy Category: Metolazone: B by manufacturer, D by other researchers. All other thiazides in this class are D. See Pregnancy Risk Categories at the back of this book.

Animal studies: No birth defects found in rat studies.

Human studies: Reports are conflicting and inconclusive. Use of thiazides can cause maternal complications that may cause adverse fetal effects, including death. They should not be used in pregnancy unless a very serious complication occurs for which these drugs works. Ask your doctor for guidance.

Advisability of Use If Breast-Feeding

Presence of these drugs in breast milk: Yes.

Avoid drugs or refrain from nursing.

Habit-Forming Potential: None.

Effects of Overdose: Dry mouth, thirst, lethargy, weakness, muscle cramping, nausea, vomiting, drowsiness progressing to stupor or coma.

Possible Effects of Long-Term Use: Impaired balance of water, salt, magnesium, and potassium in blood and body tissues. Impaired tolerance of glucose. Pathological changes in parathyroid glands with increased blood calcium levels and decreased blood phosphate levels.

Suggested Periodic Examinations While Taking These Drugs (at physician's discretion)

Complete blood cell counts; measurements of blood levels of sodium, potassium, chloride, magnesium, sugar, and uric acid.

Kidney and liver function tests.

▷ **While Taking These Drugs, Observe the Following**

Foods: Ask your doctor if you need to eat foods rich in potassium. See Table 13, "High-Potassium Foods," in Section Six, if needed. Follow your physician's advice regarding the use of salt. Magnesium should be routinely checked and supplemented if these medicines have lowered blood levels.

Beverages: No restrictions. This drug may be taken with milk.

▷ *Alcohol:* Use with caution—alcohol may exaggerate the blood-pressure-lowering effects of these drugs and cause orthostatic hypotension.

Tobacco Smoking: No interactions expected. I advise everyone to quit smoking.

▷ *Other Drugs*

These drugs may *increase* the effects of

- fluconazole (Diflucan).
- lithium (Lithobid, others), and cause lithium toxicity.
- other antihypertensive drugs; dose adjustments may be necessary to prevent excessive lowering of blood pressure.

These drugs may *decrease* the effects of

- oral anticoagulants such as warfarin (Coumadin). Increased frequency of INR (prothrombin time) testing is needed.
- oral antidiabetic drugs (sulfonylureas—see Drug Classes); dose adjustments may be needed for better blood sugar control.

These drugs *taken concurrently* with

- allopurinol (Zyloprim) may decrease kidney function.
- amphotericin B (Fungizone) may result in additive potassium loss. Increased frequency of laboratory testing is needed.
- calcium may result in the milk-alkali syndrome with increased calcium, alkalosis, and kidney failure.
- carbamazepine (Tegretol) may result in low sodium levels and symptomatic hyponatremia.
- cortisone or other corticosteroid medicines may result in excessive potassium loss with resultant heart rhythm changes and lethargy.
- cyclophosphamide (Cytoxan) may increase immunosuppression.
- digitalis preparations (digitoxin, digoxin) requires careful monitoring and dose changes to prevent low potassium levels and serious disturbances of heart rhythm.
- methotrexate (Mexate) may increase immunosuppression.
- nonsteroidal anti-inflammatory drugs (NSAIDS—see Drug Classes) such as sulindac (Clinoril) and naproxen (Naprosyn, Aleve, Anaprox, others) may result in decreased thiazide effectiveness.

The following drugs may *decrease* the effects of these thiazides:
- cholestyramine (Cuemid, Questran)—may interfere with its absorption.
- colestipol (Colestid)—may interfere with its absorption.

Take cholestyramine and colestipol 1 hour before any oral diuretic.

▷ *Driving, Hazardous Activities:* Use caution until the possible occurrence of orthostatic hypotension, dizziness, or impaired vision has been determined.

Aviation Note: The use of these drugs *may be a disqualification* for piloting. Consult a designated aviation medical examiner.

Exposure to Sun: Use caution until sensitivity has been determined. These drugs can cause photosensitivity (see Glossary).

Exposure to Heat: Caution—excessive perspiring could cause additional loss of salt and water from the body.

Heavy Exercise or Exertion: Avoid exertion that produces light-headedness, excessive fatigue, or muscle cramping. Isometric exercises can raise blood pressure significantly. Ask your doctor for help regarding participation in this form of exercise.

Occurrence of Unrelated Illness: Vomiting or diarrhea can produce a serious imbalance of important body chemistry. Ask your doctor for help.

Discontinuation: These drugs should not be stopped abruptly following long-term use; sudden discontinuation can cause serious thiazide-withdrawal fluid retention (edema). The dose should be reduced gradually. It may be advisable to discontinue this drug 5 to 7 days before major surgery. Ask your physician, surgeon, and/or anesthesiologist for guidance.

THIORIDAZINE (thi oh RID a zeen)

Introduced: 1959   **Class:** Antipsychotic; tranquilizer, major; phenothiazines
Prescription: USA: Yes   **Controlled Drug:** USA: No; Canada: No   **Available as Generic:** USA: Yes; Canada: Yes
Brand Names: ✦Apo-Thioridazine, Mellaril, Mellaril-S, Millazine, ✦Novoridazine, ✦PMS-Thioridazine SK-Thioridazine

```
┌─────────────────────────────────────────────────────────────────┐
│                      BENEFITS versus RISKS                        │
│      Possible Benefits                  Possible Risks            │
│  EFFECTIVE CONTROL OF ACUTE      TARDIVE DYSKINESIA (SERIOUS       │
│    MENTAL DISORDERS                TOXIC BRAIN EFFECT with long-   │
│  Relief of anxiety, agitation, and  term use)                     │
│    tension                        NEUROLEPTIC MALIGNANT           │
│  Treats behavior problems that are  SYNDROME                      │
│    resistant to other medicines   Liver damage with jaundice      │
│                                     (infrequent)                  │
│                                   Blood cell disorder: abnormally low │
│                                     white blood cell count        │
└─────────────────────────────────────────────────────────────────┘
```

▷ **Principal Uses**

As a Single Drug Product: Uses currently included in FDA-approved labeling: (1) Helps manage symptoms of psychotic disorders as well as moderate to marked depression with significant anxiety and nervous tension and agitation, anxiety, depression, and exaggerated fears in the elderly; (2) used in severe behavioral problems in children characterized by hyperexcitability, short attention span, and rapid swings in mood (temper tantrums).

Other (unlabeled) generally accepted uses: (1) May have a role in treating alcohol withdrawal in patients who cannot tolerate benzodiazepines; (2) can be used to treat unexplained infertility; (3) may help control premature ejaculation and nocturnal emissions in men; (4) can help borderline personality disorder; (5) of use in some chronic pain syndromes; (6) may be of use in hypersexuality.

How This Drug Works: Inhibits the action of dopamine in some brain centers, correcting an imbalance of nerve impulse transmissions thought to be responsible for certain mental disorders. May help control premature ejaculation by inhibiting the muscle (longitudinal) that controls the vas deferens.

Available Dose Forms and Strengths
>   Concentrate — 30 mg/ml, 100 mg/ml
>   Oral suspension — 25 mg/5 ml, 100 mg/5 ml
>   Tablets — 10 mg, 15 mg, 25 mg, 50 mg, 100 mg, 150 mg, 200 mg

▷ **Usual Adult Dose Range:**   Initially 25 to 100 mg three times daily. Dose may be increased by 25 to 50 mg at 3- to 4-day intervals as needed and tolerated. Usual dose range (psychosis) is 200 to 800 mg daily, divided into two to four doses. The total daily dose should not exceed 800 mg. **Note: Actual dose and schedule must be determined for each patient individually.**

Conditions Requiring Dosing Adjustments
Liver Function: Extensively changed (metabolized) in the liver. Used with caution in liver disease, and the patient closely watched.
Kidney Function: Patients with compromised kidneys should be closely followed.

▷ **Dosing Instructions:**   The tablets may be crushed and taken with or following meals to reduce stomach irritation.

Usual Duration of Use: Regular use for 3 to 4 weeks usually determines benefits in controlling psychotic disorders. If not beneficial in 6 weeks, it should be stopped. Long-term use requires periodic follow-up by your doctor.

▷ **This Drug Should Not Be Taken If**
- you are allergic to any of the brand name drugs listed above.
- you have active liver disease.
- you have cancer of the breast.
- you have a constitutionally low blood pressure.
- you have a current blood cell or bone marrow disorder.

▷ **Inform Your Physician Before Taking This Drug If**
- you are allergic or abnormally sensitive to any phenothiazine (see Drug Classes).
- you have impaired liver or kidney function.
- you have any type of seizure disorder.
- you have diabetes, glaucoma, or heart disease.
- you have a history of lupus erythematosus.
- you are taking any drug with sedative effects.
- you will have surgery with general or spinal anesthesia.

Possible Side Effects (natural, expected, and unavoidable drug actions)
Drowsiness (usually during the first 2 weeks), orthostatic hypotension (see Glossary), blurred vision, dry mouth, nasal congestion, constipation, impaired urination. Pink or purple coloration of urine, of no significance.

▷ **Possible Adverse Effects** (unusual, unexpected, and infrequent reactions)
If any of the following develop, consult your physician promptly for guidance.
Mild Adverse Effects
Allergic reactions: skin rash, hives, low-grade fever.
Lowering of body temperature, especially in the elderly (see *hypothermia* in Glossary)—possible.
Abnormal body hair growth (hirsutism)—case reports.
Urinary incontinence—possible.
Increased appetite and weight gain—case reports.
Inflammation of the parotid gland—case reports.
Weakness, agitation, insomnia, impaired day and night vision—infrequent.
Chronic constipation, fecal impaction—infrequent.
Serious Adverse Effects
Allergic reactions: hepatitis with jaundice (see Glossary), severe skin reactions (Stevens-Johnson syndrome or erythema multiforme).
Idiosyncratic reactions: neuroleptic malignant syndrome (see Glossary)—possible.
Depression, disorientation, seizures, loss of peripheral vision—case reports.
Rapid heart rate, heart rhythm disorders—case reports.
Blood cell disorders: reduced white blood cell count—more common in the elderly.
Excessive production of urine (SIADH) or pituitary tumors—case reports.
Nervous system reactions: Parkinson-like disorders (see Glossary), severe restlessness, muscle spasms involving the face and neck, tardive dyskinesia (see Glossary)—case reports.
Retinopathy—case reports.
Liver toxicity (cholestatic jaundice)—infrequent.
Abnormally low blood pressure—possible.

▷ **Possible Effects on Sexual Function:** Decreased male and female libido; inhibited ejaculation; impotence—frequent; impaired female orgasm; priapism (see Glossary)—infrequent.

Male breast enlargement and tenderness (gynecomastia), female breast enlargement with milk production—case reports.

Altered timing and pattern of menstruation. False positive pregnancy test results—case reports.

May help control premature ejaculation and nocturnal emissions.

▷ **Adverse Effects That May Mimic Natural Diseases or Disorders**

Nervous system reactions may suggest true Parkinson's disease.

Liver reactions may suggest viral hepatitis.

Reactions resembling systemic lupus erythematosus can occur.

Natural Diseases or Disorders That May Be Activated by This Drug

Latent epilepsy, glaucoma, diabetes mellitus, prostatism (see Glossary).

Possible Effects on Laboratory Tests

Complete blood cell counts: decreased red cells, hemoglobin, white cells, and platelets.

Liver function tests: increased enzymes (ALT/GPT, AST/GOT, alkaline phosphatase) or bilirubin.

Urine pregnancy tests: false-positive result with Prognosticon.

CAUTION

1. Many over-the-counter medications (see Glossary) for allergies, colds, and coughs contain drugs that can interact unfavorably with this drug. Ask your doctor or pharmacist for help before using any such medications.

2. Antacids that contain aluminum and/or magnesium can limit drug absorption and benefits.

3. Call your doctor if you develop any change in vision.

Precautions for Use

By Infants and Children: NOT recommended for children under 2 years of age. Do not use this drug in the presence of symptoms suggestive of Reye syndrome (see Glossary). Children with acute infectious diseases (flu-like infections, chicken pox, measles, etc.) are more prone to develop muscular spasms of the face, back, and extremities when this drug is given for any reason.

By Those Over 60 Years of Age: Small starting doses are advisable. You may be more susceptible to drowsiness, lethargy, constipation, lowering of body temperature (hypothermia), and orthostatic hypotension (see Glossary). This drug can worsen existing prostatism (see Glossary). You may also be more susceptible to Parkinson-like disorders and/or tardive dyskinesia (see discussion of these terms in Glossary). These reactions must be recognized early since they may become unresponsive to treatment and permanent.

▷ **Advisability of Use During Pregnancy**

Pregnancy Category: C. See Pregnancy Risk Categories at the back of this book.

Animal studies: The results of rodent studies are conflicting.

Human studies: No increase in birth defects reported in 23 exposures. Adequate studies of pregnant women are not available.

Avoid drug during the first 3 months. Use it otherwise only if clearly needed. Ask your physician for guidance.

Advisability of Use If Breast-Feeding
>Presence of this drug in breast milk: Yes, in minute amounts.
>Monitor nursing infant closely and discontinue drug or nursing if adverse effects develop.

Habit-Forming Potential: None.

Effects of Overdose: Marked drowsiness, weakness, tremor, agitation, unsteadiness, deep sleep, coma, convulsions.

Possible Effects of Long-Term Use: Opacities in the cornea or lens of the eye, pigmentation of the retina. Tardive dyskinesia (see Glossary).

Suggested Periodic Examinations While Taking This Drug (at physician's discretion)
>Complete blood cell counts, especially between the 4th and 10th weeks of treatment.
>Liver function tests, electrocardiograms.
>Complete eye examinations—eye structures and vision.
>Careful tongue inspection for early symptoms of fine, involuntary, wavelike movements (could be beginnings of tardive dyskinesia).

▷ **While Taking This Drug, Observe the Following**
>*Foods:* No restrictions.
>*Nutritional Support:* A riboflavin (vitamin B$_2$) supplement should be taken with long-term use.
>*Beverages:* No restrictions. May be taken with milk.

▷ *Alcohol:* Avoid completely. Alcohol can increase the sedative action of phenothiazines and accentuate their depressant effects on brain function and blood pressure. Phenothiazines can increase the intoxicating effects of alcohol.

>*Tobacco Smoking:* There may be a reduction of drowsiness from this drug if you smoke. I advise everyone to quit smoking.

>*Marijuana Smoking:* Moderate increase in drowsiness; accentuation of orthostatic hypotension; increased risk of precipitating latent psychoses, confusing the interpretation of mental status and drug responses.

▷ *Other Drugs*
>Thioridazine may *increase* the effects of
>• all atropinelike drugs, and cause nervous system toxicity.
>• all sedative drugs, especially meperidine (Demerol), and cause excessive sedation.

>Thioridazine may *decrease* the effects of
>• amphetamines.
>• bromocriptine (Parlodel).
>• guanethidine (Ismelin, Esimil), and reduce its effectiveness in lowering blood pressure.
>• oral hypoglycemic agents (see *oral antidiabetic drugs* in Drug Classes).

>Thioridazine *taken concurrently* with
>• ascorbic acid (vitamin C) may result in decreased thioridazine therapeutic benefits.
>• grepafloxacin (Raxar) or sparfloxacin (Zagam) may result in abnormal heart beats.
>• lithium (Lithobid, Lithotabs) may impair the effectiveness of lithium and cause nervous system toxicity.

- monoamine oxidase (MAO) inhibitors (see Drug Classes) may lead to prolonged thioridazine effects.
- phenytoin (Dilantin) may increase or decrease blood levels.
- ritonavir (Norvir), and perhaps other protease inhibitors (see Drug Classes), may lead to toxicity.
- tramadol (Ultram) may increase seizure risk.

The following drugs may *decrease* the effects of thioridazine:

- antacids containing aluminum and/or magnesium.
- barbiturates (see Drug Classes).
- benztropine (Cogentin).
- disulfiram (Antabuse).
- trihexyphenidyl (Artane).

▷ *Driving, Hazardous Activities:* This drug can impair mental alertness, judgment, and physical coordination. Avoid hazardous activities.

Aviation Note: The use of this drug *is a disqualification* for piloting. Consult a designated aviation medical examiner.

Exposure to Sun: Use caution—some phenothiazines can cause photosensitivity (see Glossary).

Exposure to Heat: Use caution and avoid excessive heat as much as possible. This drug may impair the regulation of body temperature and increase the risk of heatstroke.

Exposure to Cold: Use caution and dress warmly. This drug can increase the risk of hypothermia in the elderly.

Discontinuation: After long-term use, do not stop this drug suddenly. Gradual withdrawal over 2 to 3 weeks under physician supervision is recommended. Do not discontinue this drug without your physician's knowledge and approval.

THIOTHIXENE (thi oh THIX een)

Introduced: 1967   **Class:** Antipsychotic; Tranquilizer, major; thioxanthenes
Prescription: USA: Yes   **Controlled Drug:** USA: No; Canada: No   **Available as Generic:** USA: Yes; Canada: No
Brand Name: Navane

BENEFITS versus RISKS	
Possible Benefits	*Possible Risks*
EFFECTIVE CONTROL OF ACUTE MENTAL DISORDERS	SERIOUS TOXIC EFFECTS ON BRAIN with long-term use
	Liver damage with jaundice
	Blood cell disorder: abnormally low white blood cell count

▷ **Principal Uses**

As a Single Drug Product: Uses currently included in FDA-approved labeling: Relieves psychotic thinking and behavior associated with acute psychoses, episodes of mania and paranoia, and acute schizophrenia.

Other (unlabeled) generally accepted uses: Can be of use in significant borderline personality disorder.

How This Drug Works: By inhibiting dopamine, this drug corrects an imbalance of nerve impulse transmissions (at both D1 and D2 receptors) that is thought to be responsible for certain mental disorders.

Available Dose Forms and Strengths
> Capsules — 1 mg, 2 mg, 5 mg, 10 mg, 20 mg
> Concentrate — 5 mg/ml
> Injections — 2 mg/ml, 5 mg/ml

▷ **Usual Adult Dose Range:**   Initially 2 to 5 mg two or three times daily. Dose may be increased by 2 mg at 3- to 4-day intervals as needed and tolerated. Usual dose range is 20 to 30 mg daily. The total daily dose should not exceed 60 mg. **Note: Actual dose and schedule must be determined for each patient individually.**

Conditions Requiring Dosing Adjustments
Liver Function: This drug should be used with caution in liver compromise.
Kidney Function: Patients with compromised kidneys should be closely followed.

▷ **Dosing Instructions:**   The capsules may be opened and taken with or following meals to reduce stomach irritation. The liquid concentrate must be diluted just before dosing by adding it to 8 ounces of water, milk, fruit juice, or carbonated beverage.

Usual Duration of Use: Use on a regular schedule for several weeks usually determines control of psychotic disorders. If not beneficial within 6 weeks, it should be stopped. Long-term use (months to years) requires periodic physician evaluation of response, appropriate dose adjustment, and consideration of continued need.

▷ **This Drug Should Not Be Taken If**
- you have had an allergic reaction to it previously.
- you have active liver disease.
- you have cancer of the breast.
- you have a current blood cell or bone marrow disorder.

▷ **Inform Your Physician Before Taking This Drug If**
- you are allergic or abnormally sensitive to other thioxanthene drugs or any phenothiazine drug (see Drug Classes).
- you have impaired liver or kidney function.
- you have any type of seizure disorder.
- you have diabetes, glaucoma, or heart disease.
- you have a history of lupus erythematosus.
- you have Parkinson's disease.
- you have had neuroleptic malignant syndrome.
- you are taking any drug with sedative effects.
- you drink alcohol daily.
- you plan to have surgery under general or spinal anesthesia in the near future.

Possible Side Effects (natural, expected, and unavoidable drug actions)
> Mild drowsiness (usually during the first 2 weeks), orthostatic hypotension (see Glossary), blurred vision, dry mouth, nasal congestion, constipation, impaired urination.

▷ **Possible Adverse Effects** (unusual, unexpected, and infrequent reactions)
> **If any of the following develop, consult your physician promptly for guidance.**

Mild Adverse Effects

Allergic reactions: skin rash, hives, itching.

Lowering of body temperature, especially in the elderly (see **hypothermia** in Glossary).

Fluid retention, weight gain—possible.

Dizziness, weakness, agitation, insomnia, impaired vision—infrequent to frequent.

Nausea, vomiting—infrequent.

Serious Adverse Effects

Allergic reactions: rare hepatitis with jaundice (see Glossary), anaphylactic reaction (see Glossary).

Idiosyncratic reactions: paradoxical worsening of psychotic symptoms. Development of the neuroleptic malignant syndrome (see Glossary).

Abnormal production of urine and loss of blood sodium (SIADH)—case reports.

Depression, disorientation, seizures—case reports.

Deposits in cornea and lens of the eye—infrequent.

Abnormal fixed eye positioning (oculogyric crisis)—frequent extrapyramidal effect.

Rapid heart rate, heart rhythm disorders—possible.

Systemic lupus erythematosus or blood cell disorders: reduced white blood count—case reports.

Nervous system reactions: Parkinson-like disorders (see Glossary), severe restlessness, muscle spasms involving the face and neck, tardive dyskinesia (see Glossary)—infrequent.

Severe reduction in blood pressure—rare.

▷ **Possible Effects on Sexual Function:**   Altered timing and pattern of menstruation.

Impotence, priapism, and retrograde ejaculation—rare.

Male breast enlargement and tenderness (gynecomastia)—case reports.

Female breast enlargement with milk production—rare.

▷ **Adverse Effects That May Mimic Natural Diseases or Disorders**

Nervous system reactions may suggest true Parkinson's disease or Reye syndrome (see Glossary). Liver reactions may suggest viral hepatitis.

Natural Diseases or Disorders That May Be Activated by This Drug

Latent epilepsy, glaucoma, prostatism (see Glossary).

Possible Effects on Laboratory Tests

Complete blood cell counts: decreased red cells, hemoglobin, white cells, and platelets; increased eosinophils.

Blood glucose level: increased and decreased (fluctuations).

Liver function tests: increased enzymes (ALT/GPT, AST/GOT, alkaline phosphatase) or bilirubin.

Urine pregnancy tests: false-positive result with some tests.

CAUTION

1. Many over-the-counter medications (see Glossary) for allergies, colds, and coughs contain drugs that can interact unfavorably with this drug. Ask your doctor or pharmacist for help before using any such medications.

2. Antacids that contain aluminum and/or magnesium may limit drug absorption and effectiveness.
3. Call your doctor if vision changes while taking this drug.

Precautions for Use

By Infants and Children: Use of this drug is not recommended for children under 12 years of age. Do not use this drug in the presence of symptoms suggestive of Reye syndrome (see Glossary). Children with acute infectious diseases (flu-like infections, chicken pox, measles, etc.) are more prone to develop muscular spasms of the face, back, and extremities when this drug is given.

By Those Over 60 Years of Age: Small starting doses are advisable. Increased risk of drowsiness, lethargy, constipation, lowering of body temperature (hypothermia), and orthostatic hypotension (see Glossary). This drug can worsen existing prostatism (see Glossary). You may also be more susceptible to the development of Parkinson-like disorders and/or tardive dyskinesia (see discussion of these terms in Glossary). These reactions must be recognized early since they may become unresponsive to treatment and irreversible.

▷ **Advisability of Use During Pregnancy**

Pregnancy Category: C. See Pregnancy Risk Categories at the back of this book.
Animal studies: No birth defects reported in rats, rabbits, or monkeys.
Human studies: Adequate studies of pregnant women are not available.
Avoid drug during the first 3 months if possible. Avoid during the final month (possible effects on the newborn).

Advisability of Use If Breast-Feeding

Presence of this drug in breast milk: Expected in small amounts, but no data are available.
Avoid drug or refrain from nursing.

Habit-Forming Potential: None.

Effects of Overdose: Marked drowsiness, weakness, tremor, agitation, unsteadiness, deep sleep, coma, convulsions.

Possible Effects of Long-Term Use: Opacities in the cornea or lens of the eye, pigmentation of the retina. Tardive dyskinesia (see Glossary).

Suggested Periodic Examinations While Taking This Drug (at physician's discretion)

Complete blood cell counts, especially between the 4th and 10th weeks of treatment.
Liver function tests, electrocardiograms.
Complete eye examinations—eye structures and vision.
Careful inspection of the tongue for early evidence of fine, involuntary, wave-like movements that could indicate the beginning of tardive dyskinesia.

▷ **While Taking This Drug, Observe the Following**

Foods: No restrictions.
Beverages: No restrictions. May be taken with milk.
▷ *Alcohol:* Avoid completely. Alcohol can increase the sedative action of thiothixene and accentuate its depressant effects on brain function and blood pressure. Thiothixene can increase the intoxicating effects of alcohol.
Tobacco Smoking: No interactions expected, but I advise everyone to quit smoking.

Marijuana Smoking: Moderate increase in drowsiness; accentuation of orthostatic hypotension; increased risk of precipitating latent psychoses, confusing the interpretation of mental status and drug responses.

▷ *Other Drugs*

Thiothixene may *increase* the effects of
- all atropinelike drugs, and cause nervous system toxicity.
- all sedative drugs, especially barbiturates and narcotic analgesics, and cause excessive sedation.

Thiothixene may *decrease* the effects of
- guanethidine (Ismelin, Esimil), and reduce its effectiveness in lowering blood pressure.

Thiothixene *taken concurrently* with
- ketorolac (Toradol) may result in hallucinations.
- lithium (Lithobid, others) may result in exaggerated neurotoxicity (rigidity and tremor).
- monoamine oxidase (MAO) inhibitors (see Drug Classes) may result in worsening of the depressive effects of thiothixene on the central nervous system and breathing.
- tramadol (Ultram) may increase seizure risk.

The following drugs may *decrease* the effects of thiothixene:
- antacids containing aluminum and/or magnesium.
- barbiturates (see Drug Classes).
- benztropine (Cogentin).
- trihexyphenidyl (Artane).

▷ *Driving, Hazardous Activities:* This drug can impair mental alertness, judgment, and physical coordination. Avoid hazardous activities.

Aviation Note: The use of this drug *is a disqualification* for piloting. Consult a designated aviation medical examiner.

Exposure to Sun: Use caution until sensitivity has been determined. This drug can cause photosensitivity (see Glossary).

Exposure to Heat: Use caution and avoid excessive heat as much as possible. This drug may impair the regulation of body temperature and increase the risk of heatstroke.

Exposure to Cold: Use caution and dress warmly. This drug can increase the risk of hypothermia in the elderly.

Discontinuation: After a period of long-term use, do not stop this drug suddenly. Gradual withdrawal over 2 to 3 weeks under physician supervision is recommended. Do not discontinue this drug without your physician's knowledge and approval. The relapse rate of schizophrenia after discontinuation is 50 to 60%.

TICLOPIDINE (ti KLOH pi deen)

Introduced: 1985   **Class:** Antiplatelet   **Prescription:** USA: Yes
Controlled Drug: USA: No; Canada: No   **Available as Generic:** USA: No
Brand Name: Ticlid

BENEFITS versus RISKS	
Possible Benefits	*Possible Risks*
SIGNIFICANT REDUCTION IN THE RISK OF STROKE FOR THOSE WITH TRANSIENT ISCHEMIC ATTACK (TIA) OR PREVIOUS STROKE	SIGNIFICANT REDUCTION IN WHITE BLOOD CELL COUNTS— uncommon Increased total blood cholesterol level Drug-induced hepatitis with jaundice

▷ **Principal Uses**

As a Single Drug Product: Uses currently included in FDA-approved labeling: Used in selected individuals (who are intolerant to aspirin) to prevent recurrent stroke following initial thrombotic stroke.

Other (unlabeled) generally accepted uses: (1) Used in some patients with peripheral vascular disease and intermittent claudication to prevent blood clots (thrombosis); (2) used by people who have had bypass surgery to help prevent clot formation and keep the graft working; (3) may slow progression of eye problems (retinopathy) in diabetics; (4) combined with other agents to keep patients with angina from having heart attacks; (5) combination therapy to lessen the symptoms of rheumatoid arthritis; (6) may help prevent strokes in patients who have experienced transient ischemic attacks (TIAs); (7) helps patients with kidney failure stop building up phosphate, urea, and creatinine.

How this Drug Works: By inhibiting clumping of blood platelets, this drug prevents the beginning of processes that lead to blood clot formation within atherosclerotic vessels (arterial thrombosis).

Available Dose Forms and Strengths

Tablets — 250 mg

▷ **Recommended Dose Ranges** (Actual dose and schedule must be determined for each patient individually.)

Infants and Children: Dose not established.
18 to 60 Years of Age: 250 mg twice daily, 12 hours apart, taken with food.
Over 60 Years of Age: Same as 18 to 60 years of age.

Conditions Requiring Dosing Adjustments

Liver Function: NOT to be used in patients with severe liver disease. Doses may need to be decreased for people with compromised livers.
Kidney Function: Dosing changes do not appear to be needed.

▷ **Dosing Instructions:** The tablet may be crushed and is best taken with meals to enhance absorption and reduce stomach irritation.

Usual Duration of Use: Use on a regular schedule for 6 to 12 months usually determines benefits in preventing stroke. Long-term use (months to years) requires periodic physician evaluation.

Possible Advantages of This Drug

A reduction in risk of initial stroke during first year following TIA (in contrast to aspirin). Decreased risk of recurrent stroke the first year after initial stroke. Works in both men and women.

▷ **This Drug Should Not Be Taken If**
• you have had an allergic reaction to it previously.
• you have a bone marrow, blood cell, or bleeding disorder.

- you have active peptic ulcer disease, Crohn's disease, or ulcerative colitis.
- you have severely impaired liver function.
- you are taking aspirin, anticoagulants, or cortisonelike drugs.

▷ **Inform Your Physician Before Taking This Drug If**
- you have a history of a drug-induced bone marrow depression or blood cell disorder.
- you have gastric or duodenal ulcers.
- you have impaired liver or kidney function.
- you plan to have surgery in the near future; this drug should be discontinued 10 to 14 days prior to surgery.

Possible Side Effects (natural, expected, and unavoidable drug actions)
Spontaneous bruising (purpura)—rare.

▷ **Possible Adverse Effects** (unusual, unexpected, and infrequent reactions)
If any of the following develop, consult your physician promptly for guidance.
Mild Adverse Effects
Allergic reactions: rash, itching—rare.
Dizziness, ringing in the ears—rare.
Loss of appetite, indigestion, nausea, vomiting, stomach pain, diarrhea—rare to infrequent.
Serious Adverse Effects
Allergic reactions: drug-induced hepatitis with jaundice (see Glossary)—rare. This usually occurs during the first 4 months of treatment.
Idiosyncratic reactions: decreased production of white blood cells (neutrophils and granulocytes): fever, sore throat, susceptibility to infection.
Thrombotic thrombocytopenic purpura (TTP)—rate unknown.
Aplastic anemia (see Glossary) or lupus erythematosus—case reports.

▷ **Possible Effects on Sexual Function:**   None reported.

▷ **Adverse Effects That May Mimic Natural Diseases or Disorders**
Drug-induced hepatitis may suggest viral hepatitis.

Possible Effects on Laboratory Tests
Complete blood cell counts: decreased red cells, hemoglobin, white cells, and platelets.
Bleeding time: increased.
Total cholesterol and triglyceride levels: increased.
Liver function tests: increased liver enzymes (ALT/GPT, AST/GOT, and alkaline phosphatase), increased bilirubin.

CAUTION
1. Low white blood cell counts may begin between 3 weeks and 3 months after treatment starts. White blood cell counts must be obtained every 2 weeks from the second week to the end of the third month of drug administration.
2. Report promptly any indications of infection: fever, chills, sore throat, cough, etc.
3. Report promptly any abnormal or unusual bleeding or bruising.
4. While taking this drug, do not take any type of aspirin or anticoagulant drug without your physician's approval.

5. Inform all health care professionals who prescribe medicines for you that you are taking this drug.

Precautions for Use

By Infants and Children: Safety and effectiveness for those under 18 years of age are not established.

By Those Over 60 Years of Age: You may be more susceptible to bone marrow depression and blood cell decreases. Watch carefully for any tendency to infections or unusual bleeding or bruising. Report such developments promptly.

▷ **Advisability of Use During Pregnancy**

Pregnancy Category: B. See Pregnancy Risk Categories at the back of this book.
Animal studies: No drug-induced birth defects found in mouse, rat, or rabbit studies.
Human studies: Adequate studies of pregnant women are not available.
Use this drug only if clearly needed. Ask your physician for guidance.

Advisability of Use If Breast-Feeding

Presence of this drug in breast milk: Unknown.
Avoid drug or refrain from nursing.

Habit-Forming Potential: None.

Effects of Overdose: Abnormal bleeding or bruising, dizziness, nausea, diarrhea.

Possible Effects of Long-Term Use: None reported.

Suggested Periodic Examinations While Taking This Drug (at physician's discretion)

Complete blood cell counts. See "CAUTION" above.
Liver function tests.

▷ **While Taking This Drug, Observe the Following**

Foods: High-fat meals may increase absorption by 20%.
Beverages: No restrictions. May be taken with milk.
▷ *Alcohol:* No interactions expected. Avoid if you have active peptic ulcer disease.
Tobacco Smoking: No interactions expected. I advise everyone to quit smoking.
▷ *Other Drugs*

Ticlopidine may *increase* the effects of
• aspirin.
• phenytoin (Dilantin).
• theophylline (Theo-Dur, others).
• warfarin (Coumadin), and also increase the risk of hepatitis. This combination is not recommended.

Ticlopidine may *decrease* the effects of
• cyclosporine (Sandimmune), and decrease its effectiveness.
• digoxin (Lanoxin).

The following drug may *increase* the effects of ticlopidine:
• cimetidine (Tagamet).

The following drugs may *decrease* the effects of ticlopidine:
• antacids—decrease absorption of ticlopidine.

▷ *Driving, Hazardous Activities:* This drug may cause dizziness. Restrict activities as necessary.
Aviation Note: The use of this drug *may be a disqualification* for piloting. Consult a designated aviation medical examiner.

Exposure to Sun: No restrictions.
Discontinuation: To be determined and guided by your physician.

TIMOLOL (TI moh lohl)

Introduced: 1972   **Class:** Anti-anginal, anti-glaucoma, antihypertensive, beta-blocker   **Prescription:** USA: Yes   **Controlled Drug:** USA: No; Canada: No   **Available as Generic:** USA: Yes; Canada: No

Brand Names: ✦Apo-Timolol, ✦Apo-Timop, Betimol, Blocadren, ✦Timolide [CD], Timoptic, Timoptic Ocudose, Timoptic-XE

BENEFITS versus RISKS	
Possible Benefits	*Possible Risks*
EFFECTIVE, WELL-TOLERATED ANTI-ANGINAL DRUG	CONGESTIVE HEART FAILURE in advanced heart disease
ANTI-GLAUCOMA DRUG	Worsening of angina in coronary
ANTIHYPERTENSIVE DRUG in mild to moderate hypertension	heart disease (if drug is abruptly withdrawn)
EFFECTIVE PREVENTION OF MIGRAINE HEADACHES	Masking of low blood sugar (hypoglycemia) in drug-treated
Effective adjunct in the prevention of recurrent heart attack (myocardial infarction)	diabetes
	Provocation of asthma

▷ **Principal Uses**

As a Single Drug Product: Uses currently included in FDA-approved labeling: (1) Treats classical effort-induced angina, certain types of heart rhythm disturbance, and high blood pressure; (2) lowers increased internal eye pressure in chronic open-angle glaucoma; (3) beneficial when taken within 24 hours and for 28 days thereafter in decreasing the size of the heart damage, decreasing arrhythmias, and preventing repeat heart attacks (myocardial infarction); (4) reduces frequency and severity of migraines.

Other (unlabeled) generally accepted uses: (1) Has been used by people who are afraid to fly on airplanes (air travel phobia); (2) may help decrease incidence of abnormal heart rhythms in the atria of the heart (atrial fibrillation and flutter); (3) helps prevent abnormally increased intraocular pressure after cataract surgery; (4) used in patients with detached (not torn) retinas.

As a Combination Drug Product [CD]: Available combined with hydrochlorothiazide to treat high blood pressure. Combination product includes two drugs with different mechanisms of action. This provides better effectiveness and convenience for long-term use.

How This Drug Works: Blocks certain actions of the sympathetic nervous system:
- reducing heart rate and contraction force, lowering blood ejection pressure and reducing oxygen needs of the heart.
- reducing degree of blood vessel wall contraction, lowering blood pressure.
- prolongs conduction time of nerve impulses through the heart, of benefit in managing certain heart rhythm disorders.

- slows formation of fluid (aqueous humor) in the anterior eye chamber, improving its drainage from the eye and thus lowering the internal eye pressure.

Available Dose Forms and Strengths
Eye solutions — 0.25%, 0.5%
Timoptic-XE — 2.5 mg per ml and 5 mg per ml
  Tablets — 5 mg, 10 mg, 20 mg

▷ **Usual Adult Dose Range:** Varies with indication.
  Anti-anginal and antihypertensive: Initially 10 mg two times daily; increase dose gradually every 7 days as needed and tolerated. Usual maintenance dose is 10 to 20 mg once a day or divided into two equal doses and taken twice daily. The total daily dose should not exceed 60 mg.
  Migraine headache prevention: Initially 10 mg two times daily; increase dose as needed to 10 mg in the morning and 20 mg at night.
  Preventing repeat heart attack: 10 mg twice daily.
  Anti-glaucoma: One drop in affected eye twice daily. Note: Timoptic-XE form is a clear gel and is used once daily.
  Note: Actual dose and schedule must be determined for each patient individually.

Conditions Requiring Dosing Adjustments
Liver Function: Prudent to decrease systemic (non-ophthalmic) doses in people with liver diseases.
Kidney Function: Patients with kidney compromise should be followed closely, and the dose decreased if the medication appears to be accumulating.

▷ **Dosing Instructions:** Preferably taken 1 hour before eating to maximize absorption. The tablet may be crushed. Do not stop this drug abruptly. Eyedrops or gel must be used on an ongoing basis.

Usual Duration of Use: Use on a regular schedule for 10 to 14 days usually determines effectiveness in preventing angina, controlling heart rhythm disorders, and lowering blood pressure. Peak benefit may require continual use for 6 to 8 weeks. The long-term use of pill forms will be determined by the course of your symptoms and response to an overall treatment program (weight reduction, salt restriction, smoking cessation, etc.). Ophthalmic forms start to work in 15 to 20 minutes, but require ongoing doses to keep eye pressure low. Follow-up with your doctor is mandatory.

▷ **This Drug Should Not Be Taken If**
- you have bronchial asthma or severe obstructive lung disease.
- you have had an allergic reaction to it previously.
- you have Prinzmetal's variant angina (coronary artery spasm).
- you have congestive heart failure.
- you have an abnormally slow heart rate or a serious form of heart block.
- you took a monoamine oxidase (MAO) type A inhibitor (see Drug Classes) in the last 14 days.

▷ **Inform Your Physician Before Taking This Drug If**
- you had an adverse reaction to a beta-blocker (see Drug Classes).
- you have a history of serious heart disease.
- you have a history of hay fever (allergic rhinitis), asthma, chronic bronchitis, or emphysema.

- you have a history of overactive thyroid function (hyperthyroidism).
- you have a history of low blood sugar (hypoglycemia).
- you have impaired liver or kidney function.
- you have Raynaud's phenomenon.
- you have diabetes or myasthenia gravis.
- you currently take digitalis, quinidine, or reserpine, or any calcium-channel-blocker drug (see Drug Classes).
- you plan to have surgery under general anesthesia in the near future.

Possible Side Effects (natural, expected, and unavoidable drug actions)
Lethargy and fatigability, cold extremities, slow heart rate, light-headedness in upright position (see *orthostatic hypotension* in Glossary).

▷ **Possible Adverse Effects** (unusual, unexpected, and infrequent reactions)
If any of the following develop, consult your physician promptly for guidance.

Mild Adverse Effects
Allergic reactions: skin rash, itching.
Loss of hair involving the scalp, eyebrows, and/or eyelashes. This effect can occur with use of the oral tablets or the eyedrops (used to treat glaucoma). Regrowth occurs with discontinuation of this drug.
Headache, dizziness, visual disturbances, vivid dreams—infrequent.
Indigestion, nausea, vomiting, diarrhea—infrequent.
Numbness and tingling in extremities, joint pain—case reports.

Serious Adverse Effects
Allergic reactions: laryngospasm, severe dermatitis.
Idiosyncratic reactions: acute behavioral disturbances—depression, hallucinations.
Chest pain, shortness of breath, precipitation of congestive heart failure—case reports.
Induction of bronchial asthma (in asthmatic individuals)—possible.
May mask warning signs of impending low blood sugar (hypoglycemia) in drug-treated diabetes.
Drug-induced myasthenia gravis—case reports.
Periodic cramping of the leg (intermittent claudication)—possible.
Stopping of breathing (respiratory arrest)—case report.
Author's note: Some of the eyedrops or eye gel form can get into your body. While the listed possible reactions are mainly for the forms taken by mouth (oral), they may possibly happen (although much less likely) with the eye forms.

▷ **Possible Effects on Sexual Function:**   Decreased libido, impaired erection, impotence. **Note: All of these effects can occur with the use of timolol eyedrops at recommended dose, albeit less often.**

▷ **Adverse Effects That May Mimic Natural Diseases or Disorders**
Reduced blood flow to extremities may resemble Raynaud's phenomenon (see Glossary).

Natural Diseases or Disorders That May Be Activated by This Drug
Prinzmetal's variant angina, Raynaud's disease, intermittent claudication, myasthenia gravis (questionable).

Possible Effects on Laboratory Tests
None reported.

CAUTION
1. *Do not stop this drug suddenly* without the knowledge and guidance of your doctor. Carry a note or card which states that you take this drug.
2. Ask your doctor or pharmacist before using nasal decongestants usually present in over-the-counter cold preparations and nose drops. These can cause sudden increases in blood pressure when taken concurrently with beta-blocker drugs.
3. Report development of tendency to emotional depression.

Precautions for Use

By Infants and Children: Safety and effectiveness for those under 12 years of age are not established. However, if this drug is used, watch for low blood sugar (hypoglycemia) during periods of reduced food intake.

By Those Over 60 Years of Age: High blood pressure should be reduced without creating risks associated with excessively low blood pressure. Small starting doses and frequent blood pressure checks are needed. Sudden, rapid, and excessive lowering of blood pressure can predispose to stroke or heart attack. Watch for dizziness, unsteadiness, falling, confusion, hallucinations, depression, or urinary frequency.

▷ **Advisability of Use During Pregnancy**

Pregnancy Category: C. See Pregnancy Risk Categories at the back of this book.
Animal studies: No significant increase in birth defects due to this drug.
Human studies: Adequate studies of pregnant women are not available.
Avoid use during the first 3 months if possible. Use only if clearly needed. Ask your physician for guidance.

Advisability of Use If Breast-Feeding

Presence of this drug in breast milk: Yes.
Monitor nursing infant closely and discontinue drug or nursing if adverse effects develop.

Habit-Forming Potential: None.

Effects of Overdose: Weakness, slow pulse, low blood pressure, fainting, cold and sweaty skin, congestive heart failure, possible coma and convulsions.

Possible Effects of Long-Term Use: Reduced heart reserve and eventual heart failure in susceptible people with advanced heart disease.

Suggested Periodic Examinations While Taking This Drug (at physician's discretion)
Complete blood cell counts (because of adverse effects of other drugs of this class). Measurements of blood pressure, evaluation of heart function. Lowering of eye (intraocular) pressure with ophthalmic forms.

▷ **While Taking This Drug, Observe the Following**

Foods: No restrictions. Avoid excessive salt intake.
Beverages: No restrictions. May be taken with milk.
▷ *Alcohol:* Use with caution. Alcohol may exaggerate drug's ability to lower blood pressure and may increase mild sedative effect.
Tobacco Smoking: Nicotine may reduce this drug's effectiveness. I advise everyone to quit smoking.
▷ *Other Drugs*
Timolol may **increase** the effects of

- amiodarone (Cordarone), and cause cardiac arrest and bradycardia.
- lidocaine (Xylocaine, etc.).
- other antihypertensive drugs, and cause excessive lowering of blood pressure. Dose adjustments may be necessary.
- reserpine (Ser-Ap-Es, etc.), and cause sedation, depression, slowing of the heart rate, and lowering of blood pressure.
- verapamil (Calan, Isoptin), and cause excessive depression of heart function; monitor this combination closely.

Timolol may *decrease* the effects of
- theophyllines (Aminophyllin, Theo-Dur, etc.), and reduce their antiasthmatic effectiveness.

Timolol *taken concurrently* with
- clonidine (Catapres) requires close monitoring for rebound high blood pressure if clonidine is withdrawn while timolol is still being taken.
- epinephrine (Adrenalin, etc.) may cause marked rise in blood pressure and slowing of the heart rate.
- insulin may hide the symptoms of hypoglycemia (see Glossary).
- oral hypoglycemic agents (see *oral antidiabetic drugs* in Drug Classes) such as acetohexamide (Dymelor) and glipizide (Glucotrol) may result in prolonged low blood sugar.
- venlafaxine (Effexor) may result in increased risk of timolol toxicity.

The following drugs may *increase* the effects of timolol:
- chlorpromazine (Thorazine, etc.).
- cimetidine (Tagamet).
- fluoxetine (Prozac).
- fluvoxamine (Luvox).
- methimazole (Tapazole).
- propylthiouracil (Propacil).
- ritonavir (Norvir), and perhaps other protease inhibitors (see Drug Classes).
- zileuton (Zyflo).

The following drugs may *decrease* the effects of timolol:
- antacids (when taken at the same time).
- barbiturates (phenobarbital, etc.).
- indomethacin (Indocin) and possibly other "aspirin substitutes," or NSAIDs—may impair timolol's antihypertensive effect.
- rifampin (Rifadin, Rimactane).

▷ *Driving, Hazardous Activities:* Use caution until the full extent of dizziness, lethargy, and blood pressure change have been determined.

Aviation Note: The use of this drug *may be a disqualification* for piloting. Consult a designated aviation medical examiner.

Exposure to Sun: No restrictions.

Exposure to Heat: Caution is advised. Hot environments can exaggerate the effects of this drug.

Exposure to Cold: Caution is advised. Cold environments can worsen circulatory deficiency in the extremities that may occur with this drug. The elderly should be careful to prevent hypothermia (see Glossary).

Heavy Exercise or Exertion: It is advisable to avoid exertion that produces lightheadedness, excessive fatigue, or muscle cramping. The use of this drug may intensify the hypertensive response to isometric exercise.

Occurrence of Unrelated Illness: Fever can lower blood pressure and require adjustment of dose. Nausea or vomiting may interrupt the dosing schedule. Ask your doctor for help.

Discontinuation: It is advisable to avoid sudden discontinuation of this drug in all situations; this is especially true in the presence of coronary artery disease. If possible, gradual reduction of dose over a period of 2 to 3 weeks is recommended. Ask your physician for specific guidance.

TOLBUTAMIDE (tohl BYU ta mide)

Introduced: 1956   **Class:** Antidiabetic, sulfonylureas   **Prescription:** USA: Yes   **Controlled Drug:** USA: No; Canada: No   **Available as Generic:** Yes

Brand Names: ✦Apo-Tolbutamide, ✦Mobenol, ✦Novobutamide, Oramide, Orinase, SK-Tolbutamide

Warning: The brand names Orinase, Ornade, and Ornex are similar; this can lead to serious medication errors. Orinase is tolbutamide, and is used to treat diabetes. Ornade is chlorpheniramine and phenylpropanolamine, and is used to treat nasal and sinus congestion. Ornex is acetaminophen and phenylpropanolamine, and is used to treat head colds and sinus pain. Make sure you get the correct drug.

BENEFITS versus RISKS	
Possible Benefits	*Possible Risks*
Assistance in regulating blood sugar in non-insulin-dependent diabetes (along with diet and weight control)	HYPOGLYCEMIA, severe and prolonged Drug-induced liver damage Bone marrow depression Hemolytic anemia

▷ **Principal Uses**

As a Single Drug Product: Uses currently included in FDA-approved labeling: (1) Helps control mild to moderate type 2 diabetes mellitus (adult, maturity-onset) that does not require insulin, but that cannot be adequately controlled by diet alone; (2) used intravenously to help diagnose tumors that secrete insulin.

Other (unlabeled) generally accepted uses: Not defined.

How This Drug Works: This drug (1) stimulates release of insulin (by a pancreas that is capable of responding to stimulation), and (2) enhances the utilization of insulin by appropriate tissues.

Available Dose Forms and Strengths

Tablets — 250 mg, 500 mg

▷ **Usual Adult Dose Range:** Dosing starts at 500 mg twice a day. May be increased every 48 to 72 hours until the minimum required for acceptable control is determined. Usual range is 500 to 2000 mg a day. 3 g (3000 mg) is the maximum daily dose. **Note: Actual dose and schedule must be determined for each patient individually.**

Conditions Requiring Dosing Adjustments
> *Liver Function:* The dose should be decreased in liver disease. Tolbutamide can be a rare cause of liver damage.
> *Kidney Function:* Dosing decreases are not needed in kidney compromise.

▷ **Dosing Instructions:**   May be taken with food (morning and evening meals) to reduce stomach irritation. The tablet may be crushed.

Usual Duration of Use: Regular use for 5 to 7 days weeks usually determines benefits in controlling diabetes. Failure to respond to maximal doses in 1 month is a primary failure. Up to 15% of those responding initially may develop secondary failure in the first year. Ongoing blood sugar testing is required. See your doctor regularly.

▷ **This Drug Should Not Be Taken If**
- you have had an allergic reaction to it previously.
- you have severe impairment of liver or kidney function.
- you are undergoing major surgery.
- you have a severe infection.
- you have diabetes complicated by formation of excess acid (acidosis).
- you are pregnant.

▷ **Inform Your Physician Before Taking This Drug If**
- you are allergic to other sulfonylurea, or "sulfa" drugs (see Drug Classes).
- your diabetes has been unstable or "brittle" in the past.
- you do not know how to recognize or treat hypoglycemia (see Glossary).
- you have an infection and a fever.
- you have a deficiency of glucose-6-phosphate dehydrogenase (G6PD) in your red blood cells (ask your doctor).
- you have a history of congestive heart failure, peptic ulcer disease, cirrhosis of the liver, hypothyroidism, or porphyria.

Possible Side Effects (natural, expected, and unavoidable drug actions)
> If drug dose is excessive or food intake is delayed or inadequate, abnormally low blood sugar (hypoglycemia) will occur.

▷ **Possible Adverse Effects** (unusual, unexpected, and infrequent reactions)
> **If any of the following develop, consult your physician promptly for guidance.**
> *Mild Adverse Effects*
> Allergic reactions: skin rash, hives, itching, drug fever (see Glossary).
> Headache, ringing in the ears, weakness—infrequent.
> Indigestion, heartburn, nausea, vomiting—infrequent.
> *Serious Adverse Effects*
> Allergic reactions: hepatitis with jaundice (see Glossary).
> Idiosyncratic reactions: hemolytic anemia (see Glossary); disulfiram-like reaction (see Glossary) with concurrent use of alcohol—infrequent with this drug.
> Seizures—case reports.
> Low blood sodium (SIADH), porphyria, or urinary tract stones (urolithiasis)—case reports.
> Bone marrow depression (see Glossary): fatigue, fever, abnormal bleeding or bruising—case reports.
> Abnormally low thyroid gland function (hypothyroidism)—case reports.

Increased risk of cardiovascular death versus management by diet or insulin (based on a single study).

▷ **Possible Effects on Sexual Function:**   None reported.

▷ **Adverse Effects That May Mimic Natural Diseases or Disorders**
Liver reactions may suggest viral hepatitis.

Natural Diseases or Disorders That May Be Activated by This Drug
Acute intermittent porphyria (see Glossary).

Possible Effects on Laboratory Tests
Complete blood cell counts: decreased red cells, hemoglobin, white cells, and platelets.
Blood glucose level: decreased.
Liver function tests: increased enzymes (ALT/GPT, AST/GOT, alkaline phosphatase) or bilirubin.

CAUTION
1. This drug is only one part of the total program for the management of your diabetes. It is not a substitute for a properly prescribed diet and regular exercise.
2. Over a period of time (usually several months), this drug may lose its effectiveness in controlling blood sugar levels. Periodic follow-up examinations are needed to monitor response to drug treatment.

Precautions for Use
By Infants and Children: This drug is not effective in type I (juvenile, growth-onset) insulin-dependent diabetes.
By Those Over 60 Years of Age: This drug should be used with caution in this age group. Newer medicines with a shorter half-life are preferred. Dosing starts with 500 mg/day with slow if any increases. Repeated episodes of hypoglycemia in the elderly can cause brain damage.

▷ **Advisability of Use During Pregnancy**
Pregnancy Category: C. See Pregnancy Risk Categories at the back of this book.
Animal studies: Ocular and bone birth defects reported in rat studies.
Human studies: Adequate studies of pregnant women are not available.
Because uncontrolled blood sugar levels during pregnancy are associated with a higher incidence of birth defects, many experts recommend that insulin (instead of an oral agent) be used as necessary to control diabetes during the entire pregnancy.
Use of this drug during pregnancy is not recommended by the manufacturer.

Advisability of Use If Breast-Feeding
Presence of this drug in breast milk: Yes.
Avoid drug or refrain from nursing.

Habit-Forming Potential: None.

Effects of Overdose: Symptoms of mild to severe hypoglycemia: headache, lightheadedness, faintness, nervousness, confusion, tremor, sweating, heart palpitation, weakness, hunger, nausea, vomiting, stupor progressing to coma.

Possible Effects of Long-Term Use: Reduced function of the thyroid gland (hypothyroidism). Reports of increased frequency and severity of heart and blood vessel diseases associated with long-term use of this class of drugs are highly controversial and inconclusive. A direct cause-and-effect relationship (see Glossary) is tenuous. Ask your physician for guidance.

Suggested Periodic Examinations While Taking This Drug (at physician's discretion)

Complete blood cell counts, liver function tests, thyroid function tests, periodic evaluation of heart and circulatory system.

▷ **While Taking This Drug, Observe the Following**

Foods: Follow the diabetic diet prescribed by your physician.

Beverages: As directed in the diabetic diet. May be taken with milk.

▷ *Alcohol:* Use with extreme caution. Alcohol can exaggerate this drug's hypoglycemic effect. This drug infrequently causes a marked intolerance of alcohol resulting in a disulfiram-like reaction (see Glossary): facial flushing, sweating, palpitation.

Tobacco Smoking: Decreased tolbutamide blood levels are found in smokers. I advise everyone to quit smoking.

▷ *Other Drugs*

The following drugs may *increase* the effects of tolbutamide:
- acarbose (Precose).
- aspirin and other salicylates.
- chloramphenicol (Chloromycetin).
- cimetidine (Tagamet).
- cisapride (Propulsid).
- clofibrate (Atromid-S).
- cotrimoxazole (Bactrim, others).
- fenfluramine (Pondimin).
- fluconazole (Diflucan).
- itraconazole (Sporanox).
- ketoconazole (Nizoral).
- monoamine oxidase (MAO) type A inhibitors (see Drug Classes).
- phenylbutazone (Butazolidin).
- ranitidine (Zantac).
- sulfonamide drugs (see Drug Classes).
- valproic acid (Depakene).

The following drugs may *decrease* the effects of tolbutamide:
- beta-blocker drugs (see Drug Classes).
- bumetanide (Bumex).
- corticosteroids (see *adrenocortical steroids* in Drug Classes).
- diazoxide (Proglycem).
- ethacrynic acid (Edecrin).
- furosemide (Lasix).
- phenytoin (Dilantin).
- rifampin (Rifadin, Rimactane).
- thiazide diuretics (see Drug Classes).
- thyroid hormones (see Drug Classes).

Tolbutamide *taken concurrently* with
- colestipol (Colestid) can result in decreased colestipol response.
- digoxin may result in increased risk of digoxin toxicity.
- insulin will result in additive lowering of the blood sugar.
- sulfonamides (see Drug Classes) may result in a greater than expected effect of tolbutamide. Caution against hypoglycemia is advised, along with consideration for lower tolbutamide doses while the medicines are combined.

▷ *Driving, Hazardous Activities:* Regulate your dose schedule, eating schedule, and physical activities very carefully to prevent hypoglycemia. Be able to recognize the early symptoms of hypoglycemia so you can avoid hazardous activities and take corrective measures.

Aviation Note: Diabetes *is a disqualification* for piloting. Consult a designated aviation medical examiner.

Exposure to Sun: Use caution—some drugs of this class can cause photosensitivity (see Glossary).

Occurrence of Unrelated Illness: Acute infections, illnesses causing vomiting or diarrhea, serious injuries, and surgical procedures can interfere with diabetic control and may require insulin. If any of these conditions occur, call your doctor promptly.

Discontinuation: Because of the possibility of secondary failure, it is advisable to evaluate the continued benefit of this drug every 6 months.

TOLCAPONE (TOHL ka poan)

Introduced: 1998 **Class:** Anti-parkinsoninism drug (COMT inhibitor) **Prescription:** USA: Yes **Controlled Drug:** USA: No **Available as Generic:** No

Brand Name: Tasmar
    Author's note: The information in this profile will be broadened in subsequent editions.

TOLMETIN (TOHL met in)

See the new acetic acids (nonsteroidal anti-inflammatory drugs) profile for further information.

TOLTERODINE (tol TER oh dyne)

Introduced: 1998 **Class:** Muscarinic receptor antagonist **Prescription:** USA: Yes **Controlled Drug:** USA: No **Available as Generic:** No

Brand Name: Detrol

BENEFITS versus RISKS	
Possible Benefits	*Possible Risks*
EFFECTIVE TREATMENT OF OVERACTIVE BLADDER	CONSTIPATION
CONTROLS URGE TO URINATE	Dry mouth
LOWERS FREQUENCY OF URINATION	Blurred vision
DECREASES UNEXPECTED URGENT DESIRE TO URINATE (URGE INCONTINENCE)	

▷ **Principal Uses**

As a Single Drug Product: Uses currently included in FDA-approved labeling: (1) Treats symptoms of overactive bladders; (2) used to decrease excessive urination (urinary frequency); (3) eases unexpected urgent desire to urinate followed by inability to control the bladder (urge incontinence).

Other (unlabeled) generally accepted uses: None at present.

How This Drug Works: Acts as an anticholinergic agent (competitive muscarinic receptor antagonist), with some selective action on the bladder. This effect increases volume of residual urine and decreases maximum detrusor pressure. This makes it more difficult to urinate, easing overactive bladder symptoms and helping urge incontinence.

Available Dose Forms and Strengths

Tablets — 1 mg, 2 mg

▷ **Usual Adult Dose Range:**   Started with 2 mg twice a day. The dose may be lowered to 1 mg twice a day if the higher dose is not tolerated. **Note: Actual dose and schedule must be determined for each patient individually.**

Conditions Requiring Dosing Adjustments

Liver Function: Dose should be decreased to 1 mg in liver disease.

Kidney Function: Used with caution. The drug was not studied in kidney disease.

▷ **Dosing Instructions:**   The tablet may be crushed and taken without regard to food (food does increase bioavailability—53% on average, but this is not thought to be clinically significant).

Usual Duration of Use: Initial response to this medicine happens in about an hour. The clinical trials leading to FDA approval showed some benefits of use on a regular schedule in one trial at 4 weeks, and peak and consistent benefits at 12 weeks. It is important to follow up with your doctor regarding side effects (dose may need to be decreased) and therapeutic benefits.

Possible Advantages of This Drug

May be more selective for the bladder than other medicines.

▷ **This Drug Should Not Be Taken If**

• you are allergic to tolterodine.
• you have retention of urine.
• you have a problem with retaining food or fluid in the stomach (gastric retention).
• you have narrow-angle glaucoma that is not controlled.

▷ **Inform Your Physician Before Taking This Drug If**

• you have liver disease.
• you have kidney disease.
• you have a history of ulcerative colitis.
• you have narrow-angle glaucoma controlled by medicines.
• your job requires visual acuity.
• you have heart or blood vessel disease.
• you have had a bowel obstruction.
• you are prone to constipation.
• you will have surgery under general anesthesia soon.

Possible Side Effects (natural, expected, and unavoidable drug actions)

Dry mouth, nasal congestion, constipation.

▷ **Possible Adverse Effects** (unusual, unexpected, and infrequent reactions)
If any of the following develop, consult your physician promptly for guidance.
Mild Adverse Effects
Allergic reactions: skin rash.
Blurred vision and increase light sensitivity—rare to infrequent.
Decreased salivation—infrequent.
Dryness of hands or feet—infrequent.
Serious Adverse Effects
Passing out (syncope)—case reports in clinical trials.
Urinary retention—case reports.

▷ **Possible Effects on Sexual Function:** None defined.

Natural Diseases or Disorders That May Be Activated by This Drug
Tendency to constipation may be worsened.
Narrow-angle glaucoma may be worsened.

Possible Effects on Laboratory Tests
None defined.

CAUTION
1. Some people (about 7% of the population) are poor metabolizers of this drug. This means that the medicine may accumulate, and more of an effect will be seen in those people from the same dose. Once this pattern is identified, doses will need to be decreased to avoid getting too much of the medicine from a "normal" dose.
2. Talk to your doctor or dentist about sugarless candy or other measures to take if dry mouth becomes a problem.

Precautions for Use
By Infants and Children: Safety and effectiveness not established in pediatrics.
By Those Over 60 Years of Age: No dosage change is recommended by the manufacturer. Mean blood concentrations of the drug and its metabolite were increased by 20 to 50%, but no overall safety differences were seen between older and younger patients who were studied.

▷ **Advisability of Use During Pregnancy**
Pregnancy Category: C. See Pregnancy Risk Categories at the back of this book.
Animal studies: No birth defects found in mice studies.
Human studies: Adequate studies of pregnant women are not available.
Use this drug only if clearly needed. Ask your doctor for help.

Advisability of Use If Breast-Feeding
Presence of this drug in breast milk: Yes in mice, unknown in humans.
Stop the medicine or discontinue nursing.

Habit-Forming Potential: None.

Effects of Overdose: Severe central anticholinergic effects.

Possible Effects of Long-Term Use: None reported.

Suggested Periodic Examinations While Taking This Drug (at physician's discretion)
Follow-up on decreased urination versus adverse effects.

▷ **While Taking This Drug, Observe the Following**
Foods: No restrictions.

Beverages: No restrictions. May be taken with milk.

▷　*Alcohol:* Alcohol can increase loss of water from the body. This can work against the action of this medicine.

Tobacco Smoking: Nicotine may work counter to this medicine. Avoid all forms of tobacco.

▷　*Other Drugs*

Other medicines have not been reported to cause any clinically significant interactions.

▷　*Driving, Hazardous Activities:* This drug may cause blurred vision. Restrict activities as necessary.

Aviation Note: The use of this drug **may be a disqualification** for piloting. Consult a designated aviation medical examiner.

Exposure to Sun: May increase sensitivity of your eyes to the sun.

Heavy Exercise or Exertion: Excessive exertion is cooled by sweating. This medicine may lead to drying of skin and decreased perspiration.

Discontinuation: Ask your physician for guidance.

TRAMADOL (TRAM ah doll)

Introduced: 1996　**Class:** Analgesic　**Prescription:** USA: Yes　**Controlled Drug:** USA: Yes; Canada: No　**Available as Generic:** USA: No; Canada: No

Brand Name: Ultram

BENEFITS versus RISKS	
Possible Benefits	*Possible Risks*
EFFECTIVE TREATMENT OF PAIN	DROWSINESS
MINIMAL SIDE EFFECTS VERSUS MORPHINE	May decrease the seizure threshold Constipation

▷ **Principal Uses**

As a Single Drug Product: Uses currently included in FDA-approved labeling: Used to provide symptomatic relief in all types of pain.

Other (unlabeled) generally accepted uses: May have a role in pain where depression is also a therapeutic problem.

How This Drug Works: Increases the availability of serotonin and norepinephrine in certain brain centers and also works at opioid (see Glossary) centers, thereby relieving pain.

Available Dose Forms and Strengths

Tablets — 50 mg

▷ **Usual Adult Dose Range:** 50 to 100 mg every 4 to 6 hours. Most patients respond to 150 to 300 mg daily. The total daily dose should not exceed 400 mg. German data uses 5.6 mg per kg of body mass per day as a maximum for those over 18 years of age. **Note: Actual dose and schedule must be determined for each patient individually.**

Conditions Requiring Dosing Adjustments

Liver Function: In patients with cirrhosis should be closely watched for adverse effects and may take only 50 mg every 12 hours.

Kidney Function: Patients with creatinine clearances less than 30 ml/min, usual dose is taken every 12 hours and the daily maximum is 200 mg.

▷ **Dosing Instructions:** May be taken without regard to meals. The tablet may be crushed. If excessive drowsiness or dizziness occurs, call your doctor.

Usual Duration of Use: Peak effect usually happens in half an hour. Use on a regular schedule depends on the condition treated. Many chronic pain syndromes are treated with combinations of medicines. Long-term use requires supervision by your doctor.

▷ **This Drug Should Not Be Taken If**
- you have had an allergic reaction to it previously.
- you are allergic to codeine or similar compounds.
- you are intoxicated by morphinelike drugs or alcohol.
- you are taking, or have taken within the last 14 days, a monoamine oxidase (MAO) inhibitor.

▷ **Inform Your Physician Before Taking This Drug If**
- you have a history of seizures or take medicines that may make seizures more likely.
- you have a history of alcoholism, epilepsy, narcotic addiction, or thyroid gland problems.
- you are prone to constipation.
- you have impaired liver or kidney function.
- you are pregnant or breast-feeding your infant.
- you plan to have surgery under general anesthesia in the near future.

Possible Side Effects (natural, expected, and unavoidable drug actions)
Drowsiness, light-headedness, blurred vision, dry mouth, constipation—infrequent to frequent.

▷ **Possible Adverse Effects** (unusual, unexpected, and infrequent reactions)
If any of the following develop, consult your physician promptly for guidance.
Mild Adverse Effects
Allergic reactions: skin rash.
Rapid heart rate, palpitations—case reports.
Nausea, vomiting, diarrhea—infrequent to frequent.
Sweating—frequent.
Urinary retention—possible.
Serious Adverse Effects
Allergic reactions: anaphylaxis—case reports.
Behavioral effects: confusion, hallucinations—case reports.
Seizures—increased risk, especially in those with seizure disorders.
Lowered blood pressure—possible and dose related.

▷ **Possible Effects on Sexual Function:** Decreased male or female libido—possible.

Possible Effects on Laboratory Tests
Liver enzymes: increased.

CAUTION
1. If you experience a significant degree of mouth dryness while using this drug, consult your dentist regarding the risk of gum erosion or tooth decay. Ask for guidance in ways to keep the mouth comfortably moist.

2. If you have breathing problems (such as chronic obstructive pulmonary disease [COPD]), you may be at greater risk for respiratory depression.
3. DO NOT take this medicine if you are allergic to codeine (more likely to have a serious reaction).

Precautions for Use

By Infants and Children: Safety and effectiveness for use by those under 16 years of age have not been established.

By Those Over 60 Years of Age: During the first 2 weeks of treatment, watch for confusion or disorientation. Be aware of possible unsteadiness and incoordination that may predispose to falling. This drug may enhance prostatism (see Glossary).

▷ **Advisability of Use During Pregnancy**

Pregnancy Category: C. See Pregnancy Risk Categories at the back of this book.
  Animal studies: Fetal deaths and birth defects reported at doses 3 to 15 times the human dose.
  Human studies: Adequate studies of pregnant women are not available.
  Avoid this drug completely during the first 3 months. Ask your physician for guidance.

Advisability of Use If Breast-Feeding

Presence of this drug in breast milk: Yes.
Avoid drug or refrain from nursing.

Habit-Forming Potential: May cause psychological or physical dependence.

Effects of Overdose: Marked drowsiness, weakness, confusion, tremors, stupor, coma, possible seizures.

Possible Effects of Long-Term Use: May increase likelihood of dependence.

Suggested Periodic Examinations While Taking This Drug (at physician's discretion)

Heart rate and blood pressure, bowel and bladder status, evaluation for tremor or hallucination. Liver function tests.

▷ **While Taking This Drug, Observe the Following**

Foods: No restrictions.

Beverages: No restrictions. May be taken with milk.

▷ *Alcohol:* Avoid completely. This drug can increase markedly the intoxicating effects of alcohol and accentuate its depressant action on brain functions.

Tobacco Smoking: No interactions expected. I advise everyone to quit smoking.

▷ *Other Drugs*

Tramadol may *increase* the effects of
  • antihypertensive drugs, and cause excessive lowering of blood pressure; dose adjustments may be necessary.
  • drugs with sedative effects (see *Antihistamines, Opioids, Antianxiety drugs,* etc., in Drug Classes), and cause excessive sedation.
  • tricyclic antidepressants (see Drug Classes), leading to seizures.
  • warfarin (Coumadin), requiring dose adjustment. More frequent INR (Protime) tests are prudent.

Tramadol *taken concurrently* with
  • clonidine will lessen clonidine's therapeutic effect.
  • digoxin (Lanoxin) may lead to digoxin toxicity. DO NOT combine.
  • fluoxetine (Prozac) may result in an increased seizure risk.

- fluvoxamine (Luvox) may result in an increased seizure risk.
- monoamine oxidase (MAO) inhibitors (see Drug Classes) may result in undesirable side effects.
- other drugs that cause central nervous system depression (see *Benzodiazepines, Opioids, and Tranquilizers* in Drug Classes) may have additive effects.
- other drugs that increase seizure risks may have additive effects.
- some phenothiazines (see Drug Classes) may result in excessively lowered blood pressure.
- ritonavir (Norvir), and perhaps other protease inhibitors (see Drug Classes), may lead to toxicity.
- sertraline (Zoloft) increases seizure risk.

▷ *Driving, Hazardous Activities:* This drug may cause dizziness or drowsiness. Restrict activities as necessary.

Aviation Note: The use of this drug *is a disqualification* for piloting. Consult a designated aviation medical examiner.

Exposure to Sun: No restrictions.

Discontinuation: It is advisable to discontinue this drug gradually. Ask your physician for guidance in dose reduction over an appropriate period of time.

TRAZODONE (TRAZ oh dohn)

Introduced: 1967   **Class:** Antidepressants   **Prescription:** USA: Yes
Controlled Drug: USA: No; Canada: No   **Available as Generic:** USA: Yes;
Canada: No
Brand Names: Desyrel, ✦Desyrel Dividose, Trialodine

BENEFITS versus RISKS	
Possible Benefits	*Possible Risks*
EFFECTIVE TREATMENT IN ALL TYPES OF DEPRESSIVE ILLNESS	Adverse behavioral effects Potential for causing heart rhythm disorders in people with heart disease

▷ **Principal Uses**

As a Single Drug Product: Uses currently included in FDA-approved labeling: Used to provide symptomatic relief in all types of depression.

Other (unlabeled) generally accepted uses: (1) May have a role in reducing the symptoms of agoraphobia; (2) may help drug-induced (such as MAO inhibitors) insomnia; (3) can have a role in combination therapy of some pain syndromes; (4) may be of help in essential tremor; (5) can ease bouts of repetitive screaming.

How This Drug Works: Increases availability of serotonin in certain brain centers and thereby relieves the symptoms of emotional depression.

Available Dose Forms and Strengths
Tablets — 50 mg, 100 mg, 150 mg, 300 mg

▷ **Usual Adult Dose Range:** Initially 50 mg three times daily. The dose may be increased by 50 mg daily at intervals of 3 or 4 days, as needed and tolerated.

The total daily dose should not exceed 400 mg. **Note: Actual dose and schedule must be determined for each patient individually.**

Conditions Requiring Dosing Adjustments

Liver Function: Blood levels should be obtained to guide dosing. May be a rare cause of liver damage, and patients should be followed closely.

Kidney Function: Metabolites are removed by the kidneys; however, dose adjustment in renal compromise is not defined.

▷ **Dosing Instructions:**   This drug is best taken with food to improve absorption. The tablet may be crushed. If excessive drowsiness or dizziness occurs, it is advisable to take a larger portion of the daily dose at bedtime and divide the remaining amount into two or three smaller doses to be taken during the day.

Usual Duration of Use: Use on a regular schedule for 2 to 4 weeks usually determines effectiveness in relieving the symptoms of depression. Long-term use (weeks to months) requires supervision and periodic evaluation by your physician.

▷ **This Drug Should Not Be Taken If**
- you have had an allergic reaction to it previously.
- you are recovering from a recent heart attack (myocardial infarction).
- you have carcinoid syndrome.
- you are taking, or have taken within the past 14 days, any monoamine oxidase (MAO) type A inhibitor (see Drug Classes).

▷ **Inform Your Physician Before Taking This Drug If**
- you have a history of alcoholism, epilepsy, or heart disease (especially heart rhythm disorders).
- you have impaired liver or kidney function.
- you are pregnant or breast-feeding your infant.
- you are taking any antihypertensive drugs.
- you will have surgery with general anesthesia.

Possible Side Effects (natural, expected, and unavoidable drug actions)

Drowsiness, light-headedness, blurred vision, weight gain, dry mouth, constipation.

▷ **Possible Adverse Effects** (unusual, unexpected, and infrequent reactions)

If any of the following develop, consult your physician promptly for guidance.

Mild Adverse Effects

Allergic reactions: skin rash.

Headache, dizziness, fatigue, impaired concentration, nervousness, tremors—infrequent.

Rapid heart rate, palpitations—rare.

Peculiar taste, stomach discomfort, nausea, vomiting, diarrhea—infrequent.

Urinary retention—possible.

Cavities (dental caries)—case reports.

Muscular aches and pains—infrequent.

Serious Adverse Effects

Allergic reactions: serious skin rashes (erythema multiforme).

Behavioral effects: confusion, anger, hostility, delusions, hallucinations, nightmares—case reports.

Irregular heart rhythms, low blood pressure, fainting—case reports.

Erythema multiforme—case reports.

Seizures—rare.

Liver toxicity—possible.

▷ **Possible Effects on Sexual Function:**   Decreased male libido; increased female libido.

Inhibited ejaculation, impotence, priapism (see Glossary), or altered timing and pattern of menstruation—case reports.

Possible Effects on Laboratory Tests

Liver enzymes: increased.

CAUTION

1. If you have significant mouth dryness while using this drug, ask your dentist about risk of gum erosion or tooth decay. Ask for help in ways to keep the mouth comfortably moist.
2. It is advisable to withhold this drug if electroconvulsive therapy (ECT) is to be used to treat your depression.

Precautions for Use

By Infants and Children: Safety and effectiveness for use by those under 18 years of age have not been established.

By Those Over 60 Years of Age: During the first 2 weeks of treatment, watch for the development of restlessness, agitation, excitement, forgetfulness, confusion, or disorientation. Be aware of possible unsteadiness and incoordination that may predispose to falling. This drug may enhance prostatism (see Glossary).

▷ **Advisability of Use During Pregnancy**

Pregnancy Category: C. See Pregnancy Risk Categories at the back of this book.

Animal studies: Fetal deaths and birth defects reported.

Human studies: Adequate studies of pregnant women are not available.

Avoid this drug completely during the first 3 months. Ask your physician for guidance.

Advisability of Use If Breast-Feeding

Presence of this drug in breast milk: Yes.

Avoid drug or refrain from nursing.

Habit-Forming Potential: None.

Effects of Overdose: Marked drowsiness, confusion, tremors, low blood pressure, rapid heart rate, stupor, coma, or seizures.

Possible Effects of Long-Term Use: None reported.

Suggested Periodic Examinations While Taking This Drug (at physician's discretion)

Complete blood cell counts. (This drug may cause slight reductions in white blood cell counts. This should be monitored closely if infection, sore throat, or fever develops.)

Serial blood pressure readings and electrocardiograms.

▷ **While Taking This Drug, Observe the Following**

Foods: No restrictions.

Beverages: No restrictions. May be taken with milk.

▷   *Alcohol:* Avoid completely. This drug can increase markedly the intoxicating effects of alcohol and accentuate its depressant action on brain functions.

Tobacco Smoking: No interactions expected. I advise everyone to quit smoking.

▷ *Other Drugs*

Trazodone may *increase* the effects of
- antihypertensive drugs, and cause excessive lowering of blood pressure; dose adjustments may be necessary.
- drugs with sedative effects, and cause excessive sedation.
- phenytoin (Dilantin), by raising its blood level; watch for phenytoin toxicity.
- tramadol (Ultram).

Trazodone *taken concurrently* with
- clonidine (Catapres) will lessen the therapeutic effect of clonidine.
- fluoxetine (Prozac) may result in an increased trazodone level and toxicity.
- monoamine oxidase (MAO) inhibitors (see Drug Classes) may result in undesirable side effects in some patients, and beneficial therapeutic effects in others.
- other drugs that cause central nervous system depression (see *benzodiazepines, opioids,* and *tranquilizers* in Drug Classes) may have additive effects.
- paroxetine (Paxil) may result in toxicity (serotonin syndrome).
- ritonavir (Norvir), and perhaps other protease inhibitors (see Drug Classes), may lead to toxicity.
- some phenothiazines (see Drug Classes) may result in excessively lowered blood pressure.
- warfarin (Coumadin) may result in decreased therapeutic benefits of warfarin. INR (prothrombin time or protime) should be checked more often if warfarin and trazodone are combined.

▷ *Driving, Hazardous Activities:* This drug may cause dizziness or drowsiness. Restrict activities as necessary.

Aviation Note: The use of this drug *is a disqualification* for piloting. Consult a designated aviation medical examiner.

Exposure to Sun: No restrictions.

Discontinuation: It is advisable to discontinue this drug gradually. Ask your physician for guidance in dose reduction over an appropriate period of time.

TRIAMCINOLONE (tri am SIN oh lohn)

Introduced: 1985   **Class:** Antiasthmatic, adrenocortical steroids (cortisonelike drugs)   **Prescription:** USA: Yes   **Controlled Drug:** USA: No; Canada: No   **Available as Generic:** Yes

Brand Name: Amcort, Aristocort, Aristocort R, Aristoform D, ✦Aristospan, Articulose LA, ✦Aureocort, Azmacort, Cenocort, Cenocort Forte, Flutex, ✦Kenacomb, Kenacort, Kenaject, Kenalog, Kenalog H, Kenalog IN, Kenalone, Mycogen II, Mycomar, Mytrex [CD], Nasacort, Nasacort AQ, SK-Triamcinolone, TAC-40, TAC-D, Triacet, ✦Triaderm Mild, ✦Triaderm Regular, Triam-A, Triam-Forte, Triamolone 40, Triderm, Tri-Kort, Trilog, Tristoject, ✦Viaderm-K.C.

BENEFITS versus RISKS

Possible Benefits	*Possible Risks*
EFFECTIVE CONTROL OF SEVERE, CHRONIC BRONCHIAL ASTHMA	Yeast infections of mouth and throat
EFFECTIVE SUPPRESSION OF A VARIETY OF INFLAMMATORY DISORDERS	Suppression of normal cortisone production
POSSIBLE REDUCTION IN SYSTEMIC STEROID USE	Euphoria and psychotic episodes
	Cushing's syndrome ("moon face," obesity, and "buffalo hump")
EFFECTIVE TREATMENT OF SEASONAL OR PERENNIAL ALLERGIC RHINITIS IN ADULTS AND CHILDREN	Muscle wasting (with long-term use)
	Osteoporosis (with long-term use)

▷ **Principal Uses**

As a Single Drug Product: Uses currently included in FDA-approved labeling: (1) Inhaler form is used to treat chronic bronchial asthma in people who require cortisonelike drugs for asthma control. This is better than cortisone taken by mouth (swallowed) or injection because it works more locally on the respiratory tract, not requiring systemic distribution. This helps prevent some serious adverse effects that usually result from the long-term use of cortisone taken for systemic effects; (2) tablet form can be used in a variety of inflammatory disorders; (3) tablet form is used to ease drug reactions; (4) used as part of combination treatment of acute lymphocytic leukemia in children; (5) used in autoimmune hemolytic anemia; (6) nasal inhaler form helps adults and children with symptoms of seasonal or perennial allergic rhinitis.

Other (unlabeled) generally accepted uses: (1) May have a role in postherpetic nerve pain (neuralgia); (2) corticosteroids may be of use with *Pneumocystis carinii* pneumonia in extreme cases where conventional therapy has not worked; (3) may help Guillain-Barré syndrome; (4) can help myasthenia gravis; (5) short-term therapy of psoriasis.

How This Drug Works: By increasing the amount of cyclic AMP in appropriate tissues, this drug may thereby increase the concentration of epinephrine, which is an effective bronchodilator and antiasthmatic. Additional benefit is due to the drug's ability to reduce local allergic reaction and inflammation in the lining tissues of the respiratory tract.

Available Dose Forms and Strengths

Inhalation aerosol — 0.1 mg per metered spray

Tablets — 1 mg, 2 mg, 4 mg, 8 mg

Topical cream — 0.1%, 0.25%, 0.5%

Topical ointment — 0.25%, 0.5%

▷ **Recommended Dose Ranges** (Actual dose and schedule must be determined for each patient individually.)

Infants and Children: Up to 6 years of age: dose not established.

6 to 12 years of age: 0.1 to 0.2 mg (one or two metered sprays) three or four times a day. Adjust dose as needed and tolerated. Limit total daily dose to 1.2 mg (12 metered sprays).

12 to 60 Years of Age: Initially 0.2 mg (two metered sprays) three or four times a day.

For severe asthma: 1.2 to 1.6 mg (12 to 16 metered sprays) per day, in divided doses. Adjust dose as needed and tolerated. It is usually used as two inhalations three to four times a day. Results are better when used in this fashion versus an as-needed basis. Limit total daily dose to 1.6 mg (16 metered sprays).

Nasacort AQ and Nasacort may prove effective with a starting dose of 220 mcg per day.

Tablets: 4 to 48 mg daily for inflammatory conditions.

Cream: 0.025% is usually applied to the affected area two to four times a day.

Over 60 Years of Age: Same as 12 to 60 years of age.

Conditions Requiring Dosing Adjustments

Liver Function: This drug is metabolized in the liver. Dosing changes in liver compromise are not defined.

Kidney Function: Dosing adjustments do not appear warranted for patients with compromised kidneys.

▷ **Dosing Instructions:**   Inhalation form: May be used as needed without regard to eating. Shake the container well before using. Carefully follow the printed patient instructions provided with the unit. Rinse the mouth and throat (gargle) with water thoroughly after each inhalation; do not swallow the rinse water. The Nasacort AQ form is water-based for treatment of allergic rhinitis and does not contain chlorofluorocarbon propellants.

Oral tablets: May cause stomach upset, and can be taken with meals or snacks.

Usual Duration of Use: Use on a regular schedule for 1 to 2 weeks usually determines effectiveness in controlling severe, chronic asthma. Long-term use requires the supervision and guidance of the physician.

▷ **This Drug Should Not Be Taken If**
- you have had an allergic reaction to it previously.
- you are having severe acute asthma or status asthmaticus that requires immediate relief.
- you have a form of nonallergic bronchitis with asthmatic features.
- you have a systemic fungal infection.

▷ **Inform Your Physician Before Taking This Drug If**
- you are now taking, or have recently taken, any cortisone-related drug (including ACTH by injection) for any reason (see *adrenocortical steroids* in Drug Classes).
- you have a history of tuberculosis of the lungs.
- you have chronic bronchitis or bronchiectasis.
- you have diabetes, glaucoma, myasthenia gravis, or peptic ulcer disease.
- you have had unexpected surgery (may delay wound healing).
- you have an underactive thyroid (hypothyroidism).
- you think you may have an active infection of any kind, especially a respiratory infection.
- you are taking any of the following drugs: warfarin, oral antidiabetic drugs, insulin, or digoxin.

Possible Side Effects (natural, expected, and unavoidable drug actions)

Yeast infections (thrush) of the mouth and throat. Irritation of mouth, tongue, or throat. May cause euphoria, manic-depressive illness, or paranoid states with long-term oral use. Can cause a syndrome (Cushing's) characterized by "moon face," obesity, and poorly controlled high blood pressure.

▷ **Possible Adverse Effects** (unusual, unexpected, and infrequent reactions)
If any of the following develop, consult your physician promptly for guidance.

Mild Adverse Effects

Allergic reactions: skin rash.

Easy bruising (ecchymosis)—infrequent.

Swelling of face, hoarseness, voice change, cough—possible to infrequent.

Serious Adverse Effects

Allergic Reactions—rare.

Bronchospasm, asthmatic wheezing—rare.

Can be a cause of high blood pressure with long-term use.

Edema or swelling, especially with kidney or heart vessel disease—infrequent.

Decrease of circulating T lymphocytes—possible.

Drug-induced seizures, ulcer development, pancreatitis, or osteoporosis—possible to infrequent.

Electrolyte disturbances (decreased blood potassium)—infrequent.

Excessive thyroid activity (hyperthyroidism).

Cataract formation or muscle wasting has occurred with long-term use.

Elevated blood sugar—possible.

Toxic megacolon—rare.

Toxic psychosis has occurred with other steroids.

Author's Note: The inhalation form and topical forms do not have many of the systemic side effects of the oral form.

▷ **Possible Effects on Sexual Function:**   None reported.

Natural Diseases or Disorders That May Be Activated by This Drug

Latent amebiasis, congestive heart failure, diabetes, glaucoma, hypertension, myasthenia gravis, peptic ulcer.

Cortisone-related drugs (used by inhalation) that produce systemic effects can impair immunity and lead to reactivation of "healed" or quiescent tuberculosis of the lungs. Individuals with a history of tuberculosis should be observed closely during use of cortisonelike drugs by inhalation.

Possible Effects on Laboratory Tests

Blood calcium levels: decreased.

Blood total cholesterol levels: increased.

Blood glucose or sodium levels: increased.

Blood potassium levels: decreased.

CAUTION

1. NOT for the immediate relief of acute asthma.
2. If you were using any cortisone-related drugs for asthma *before* switching to this inhaler, you may need to restart the former cortisone-related drug if you are injured, get an infection, or require surgery. Tell your doctor about prior use of cortisone-related drugs.
3. If you experience a return of severe asthma while using this drug, call your doctor immediately. Additional treatment with cortisone-related drugs by mouth or injection may be required.
4. Carry a card noting (if applicable) that you have used cortisone-related

drugs within the past year. During periods of stress, resumption of cortisone treatment may be required.

5. Approximately 5 to 10 minutes should separate the inhalation of bronchodilators such as albuterol, epinephrine, pirbuterol, etc. (which should be used first), and the inhalation of this drug. This sequence will permit greater penetration of triamcinolone into the bronchial tubes. This will also reduce the possibility of adverse effects from the propellants used in the two inhalers.

Precautions for Use

By Infants and Children: Safety and effectiveness for use of the oral inhaler by those under 6 years of age have not been established. To ensure adequate penetration of the drug and obtain maximal benefit, the use of a spacer device is recommended for inhalation therapy in children.

By Those Over 60 Years of Age: Individuals with chronic bronchitis or bronchiectasis should be observed closely for the development of lung infections.

▷ **Advisability of Use During Pregnancy**

Pregnancy Category: C. See Pregnancy Risk Categories at the back of this book.

Animal studies: Rat and rabbit studies reveal significant toxic effects on the embryo and fetus and multiple birth defects due to this drug.

Human studies: Adequate studies of pregnant women are not available.

Limit use to very serious illness for which no satisfactory treatment alternatives are available.

Advisability of Use If Breast-Feeding

Presence of this drug in breast milk: Unknown.

Ask your doctor for guidance.

Habit-Forming Potential: With recommended dose, a state of functional dependence (see Glossary) is not likely to develop.

Effects of Overdose: Indications of cortisone excess (due to systemic absorption)—fluid retention, flushing of the face, stomach irritation, nervousness.

Possible Effects of Long-Term Use: Significant suppression of normal cortisone production.

Suggested Periodic Examinations While Taking This Drug (at physician's discretion)

Inspection of mouth and throat for evidence of yeast infection.

Assessment of the status of adrenal gland function (cortisone production).

X ray of the lungs of individuals with a prior history of tuberculosis.

Bone mineral density tests to assess osteoporosis.

▷ **While Taking This Drug, Observe the Following**

Foods: No specific restrictions beyond those advised by your physician.

Beverages: No specific restrictions.

▷ *Alcohol:* No interactions expected.

Tobacco Smoking: No interactions expected. I advise everyone to quit smoking.

▷ *Other Drugs*

The following drugs may *increase* the effects of triamcinolone:

- inhalant bronchodilators—albuterol, bitolterol, epinephrine, pirbuterol, etc.
- oral bronchodilators—aminophylline, ephedrine, terbutaline, theophylline, etc.

The following drugs may *decrease* the effects of triamcinolone:
- carbamazepine (Tegretol)—increases triamcinolone metabolism and may result in decreased effectiveness.
- phenytoin (Dilantin)—increases triamcinolone metabolism and may result in decreased effectiveness.
- primidone (Mysoline)—increases steroid metabolism and may result in decreased triamcinolone metabolism.
- rifampin (Rifadin).

Triamcinolone *taken concurrently* with
- amphotericin B (Abelcet) may lead to additive potassium loss.
- aspirin may result in blunting of the therapeutic benefits of aspirin.
- cyclosporine (Sandimmune) may result in changes in the blood levels of both medicines.
- insulin (various) may lead to loss of glucose control.
- oral hypoglycemic agents (see *oral antidiabetic drugs* in Drug Classes) may result in loss of glucose control.
- thiazide diuretics (see Drug Classes) can result in loss of glucose control.
- vaccines (flu, rabies, others) may result in less than optimal vaccine response.
- warfarin (Coumadin) can result in variation in the degree of anticoagulation. Increased INR (prothrombin time or protime) testing is indicated.

▷ *Driving, Hazardous Activities:* No restrictions.

Aviation Note: The use of this drug and the disorder for which this drug is prescribed *may be disqualifications* for piloting. Consult a designated aviation medical examiner.

Exposure to Sun: No restrictions.

Occurrence of Unrelated Illness: Acute infections, serious injuries, and surgical procedures can create an urgent need for the administration of additional supportive cortisone-related drugs given by mouth and/or injection. Notify your physician immediately in the event of new illness or injury of any kind.

Discontinuation: If the regular use of this drug has made it possible to reduce or stop doses of cortisonelike drugs by mouth, *do not* discontinue this drug abruptly. Call your doctor if you must stop this drug for any reason. Restarting cortisone preparations may be required.

Special Storage Instructions: Store at room temperature. Avoid exposure to temperatures above 120 degrees F (49 degrees C). Do not store or use this inhaler near heat or open flame.

TRIAMTERENE (tri AM ter een)

Introduced: 1964   **Class:** Diuretic   **Prescription:** USA: Yes   **Controlled Drug:** USA: No; Canada: No   **Available as Generic:** Yes

Brand Names: ✚Apo-Triazide [CD], Dyazide [CD], Dyrenium, Maxzide [CD], Maxzide-25 [CD], ✚Novo-Triamzide [CD], ✚Nu-Triazide

```
┌────────────────────────────────────────────────────────────────┐
│                      BENEFITS versus RISKS                      │
│      Possible Benefits              Possible Risks              │
│  EFFECTIVE PREVENTION OF       ABNORMALLY HIGH BLOOD            │
│    POTASSIUM LOSS when used       POTASSIUM LEVEL with excessive │
│    adjunctively with other diuretics  use                       │
│  EFFECTIVE DIURETIC IN         Possible blood cell disorders:   │
│    REFRACTORY CASES OF FLUID      megaloblastic anemia, abnormally│
│    RETENTION when used            low white blood cell and platelet│
│    adjunctively with other diuretics  counts                    │
│                                Possible kidney stone formation  │
└────────────────────────────────────────────────────────────────┘
```

▷ **Principal Uses**

As a Single Drug Product: Uses currently included in FDA-approved labeling: (1) Used in combination with other drugs to treat high blood pressure, primarily in situations where it is advisable to prevent loss of potassium from the body; (2) used in combination therapy of congestive heart failure or liver and kidney disorders accompanied by excessive fluid retention (edema).

Other (unlabeled) generally accepted uses: None.

As a Combination Drug Product [CD]: Available in combination with hydrochlorothiazide, a different kind of diuretic that promotes potassium loss from the body. Triamterene is used to counteract the potassium-wasting effect of the thiazide diuretic.

How This Drug Works: By inhibiting the enzyme system that starts the sodium–potassium exchange process, this drug prevents reabsorption of sodium and excretion of potassium by the kidney. This leads to excretion of sodium (and water with it) and potassium retention.

Available Dose Forms and Strengths

Capsules — 50 mg, 100 mg

Dyazide capsules — triamterine 37.5 mg and hydrochlorothiazide 25 mg.

▷ **Usual Adult Dose Range:**   Hypertension: Initially 50 to 100 mg twice daily. The dose is then adjusted according to individual response. The usual ongoing dose is 100 to 200 mg daily, divided into two doses. The total daily dose should not exceed 300 mg.

Dyazide combination: One or two capsules daily for high blood Pressure.

Note: Actual dose and schedule must be determined for each patient individually.

Conditions Requiring Dosing Adjustments

Liver Function: Dose should be reduced and used with extreme caution in liver disease.

Kidney Function: Patients with mild to moderate kidney failure may take the usual dose every 12 hours. In severe or progressive kidney failure, this medication should **not** be used.

▷ **Dosing Instructions:**   May be taken with or following meals to promote absorption of the drug and reduce stomach irritation. The capsule may be opened. Intermittent or alternate-day use is recommended to minimize the risk of sodium and potassium imbalance.

Usual Duration of Use: Use on a regular schedule for 3 to 5 days usually determines effectiveness in clearing edema, and for 2 to 3 weeks to determine its effect on hypertension. Long-term use (months to years) requires physician supervision and periodic evaluation.

▷ **This Drug Should Not Be Taken If**
  • you have had an allergic reaction to it previously.
  • you have severely impaired liver or kidney function.
  • your kidney disease is progressive or you have a creatinine clearance greater than 2.5 mg/dl (ask your doctor).
  • your blood potassium level is significantly elevated (ask your doctor).

▷ **Inform Your Physician Before Taking This Drug If**
  • you have a history of liver or kidney disease.
  • you have diabetes or gout.
  • you are taking any of the following: antihypertensives, a digitalis preparation, another diuretic, lithium, or a potassium preparation.
  • you have a history of glucose-6-phosphate dehydrogenase (G6PD) deficiency (ask your doctor).
  • you have a history of blood cell disorders.
  • you will have surgery with general anesthesia.

Possible Side Effects (natural, expected, and unavoidable drug actions)   With excessive use: abnormally high blood potassium levels, abnormally low blood sodium levels, dehydration.
Blue coloration of the urine (of no significance).

▷ **Possible Adverse Effects** (unusual, unexpected, and infrequent reactions)
  If any of the following develop, consult your physician promptly for guidance.
  Mild Adverse Effects
  Allergic reactions: skin rash, itching.
  Headache, dizziness, unsteadiness, weakness, drowsiness, lethargy—infrequent.
  Dry mouth, nausea, vomiting, diarrhea—infrequent.
  Serious Adverse Effects
  Allergic reaction: anaphylactic reaction (see Glossary).
  Symptomatic potassium excess: confusion, numbness and tingling in lips and extremities, fatigue, weakness, shortness of breath, slow heart rate, low blood pressure—possible.
  Blood cell disorders: megaloblastic anemia, abnormally low white blood cell count, or abnormally low blood platelet count—case reports.
  Hemolytic anemia—in those with deficiency of G6PD in red cells.
  Abnormal urine production (SIADH)—case reports.
  Formation of kidney stones and kidney toxicity—rare.
  Liver toxicity—rare.

▷ **Possible Effects on Sexual Function:**   None reported.

Possible Effects on Laboratory Tests
  Complete blood cell counts: decreased red cells, hemoglobin, white cells, and platelets; increased eosinophils (allergic reaction).
  Blood glucose level: increased in diabetics.
  Blood lithium, potassium, or uric acid level: increased.
  Kidney function tests: increased blood creatinine and urea nitrogen (BUN) levels (kidney damage).

CAUTION
1. Do not take potassium supplements or increase your intake of potassium-rich foods while taking this drug.
2. Patients who take quinidine (Quinaglute, others) may have falsely increased laboratory test results if fluorescent measurement techniques are used.
3. Do not stop this drug abruptly unless abnormally high blood levels of potassium develop.
4. Avoid liberal use of salt substitutes with potassium in them (potential causes of potassium excess).

Precautions for Use
By Infants and Children: This drug is not recommended for use in children.
By Those Over 60 Years of Age: Natural decline in kidney function may predispose to potassium retention. Watch for potassium excess: slow heart rate, irregular heart rhythms, low blood pressure, confusion, drowsiness. Excessive use of diuretics can cause harmful loss of body water (dehydration), increased viscosity of the blood, and an increased tendency of the blood to clot, predisposing to stroke, heart attack, or thrombophlebitis.

▷ **Advisability of Use During Pregnancy**
Pregnancy Category: B by the manufacturer, D by one researcher. See Pregnancy Risk Categories at the back of this book.
Animal studies: No birth defects due to this drug reported.
Human studies: Adequate studies of pregnant women are not available.
This drug should not be used during pregnancy unless a very serious complication of pregnancy occurs for which this drug is significantly beneficial.

Advisability of Use If Breast-Feeding
Presence of this drug in breast milk: Yes.
Avoid drug or refrain from nursing.

Habit-Forming Potential: None.

Effects of Overdose: Thirst, drowsiness, fatigue, nausea, vomiting, confusion, irregular heart rhythm, low blood pressure.

Possible Effects of Long-Term Use: Potassium accumulation to abnormally high blood levels.

Suggested Periodic Examinations While Taking This Drug (at physician's discretion)
Complete blood cell counts.
Measurements of blood sodium, potassium, and chloride levels.
Kidney function tests.

▷ **While Taking This Drug, Observe the Following**
Foods: Diets high in high-potassium foods (see Table 13, Section Six) may cause problems. Avoid excessive restriction of salt.
Beverages: No restrictions. May be taken with milk.
▷ *Alcohol:* Use with caution. Alcohol may enhance the drowsiness and the blood-pressure-lowering effect of this drug.
Tobacco Smoking: No interactions expected. I advise everyone to quit smoking.
▷ *Other Drugs*
Triamterene may ***increase*** the effects of
• amantadine (Symmetrel).

- digoxin (Lanoxin).
- metformin (Glucophage).
- methotrexate (Mexate), leading to bone marrow toxicity.
- valsartan (Diovan), leading to potassium toxicity.

Triamterene **taken concurrently** with

- captopril (Capoten) or other ACE inhibitors may cause excessively high blood potassium levels.
- cyclosporine (Sandimmune) SHOULD NOT BE COMBINED.
- histamine (H$_2$) blockers (see Drug Classes) may decrease triamterene absorption and its therapeutic effects.
- indomethacin (Indocin) may increase the risk of kidney damage.
- lithium may cause accumulation of lithium to toxic levels.
- nonsteroidal anti-inflammatory drugs, or NSAIDs (see Drug Classes), may blunt the blood-pressure-lowering effect of triamterene.
- potassium preparations may cause excessively high blood potassium levels.

▷ *Driving, Hazardous Activities:* This drug may cause dizziness and drowsiness. Restrict activities as necessary.

Aviation Note: The use of this drug **may be a disqualification** for piloting. Consult a designated aviation medical examiner.

Exposure to Sun: Use caution—this drug may cause photosensitivity (see Glossary).

Discontinuation: With high dose or prolonged use, it is best to slowly withdraw this drug. Stopping it suddenly may cause rebound potassium removal and potassium deficiency. Ask your doctor for help.

TRICHLORMETHIAZIDE (tri KLOR meth i a zide)

See the thiazide diuretics profile for further information.

TRIFLUOPERAZINE (tri flu oh PER a zeen)

Introduced: 1958   **Class:** Tranquilizer, major; phenothiazines   **Prescription:** USA: Yes   **Controlled Drug:** USA: No; Canada: No   **Available as Generic:** USA: Yes; Canada: No

Brand Names: ✦Apo-Trifluoperazine, ✦Novo-Flurazine, ✦Solazine, Stelabid [CD], Stelazine, Suprazine, ✦Terfluzine

BENEFITS versus RISKS	
Possible Benefits	*Possible Risks*
EFFECTIVE CONTROL OF ACUTE MENTAL DISORDERS: beneficial effects on thinking, mood, and behavior	SERIOUS TOXIC EFFECTS ON BRAIN with long-term use
	Liver damage with jaundice (infrequent)
	Rare blood cell disorders: abnormally low red and white blood cell and platelet counts

▷ **Principal Uses**

As a Single Drug Product: Uses currently included in FDA-approved labeling: (1) Treats psychotic thinking and behavior seen in acute psychoses of unknown nature, mania, paranoid states, and acute schizophrenia (very effective in withdrawn and apathetic people and those with agitation, delusions, and hallucinations); (2) approved for treatment of anxiety disorders.

Other (unlabeled) generally accepted uses: May have a role in combination therapy of some kinds of chronic pain.

How This Drug Works: By inhibiting the action of dopamine, this drug corrects an imbalance of nerve transmissions thought to be responsible for certain mental disorders.

Available Dose Forms and Strengths

Concentrate — 10 mg/ml
Injection — 2 mg/ml
Tablets — 1 mg, 2 mg, 5 mg, 10 mg

▷ **Usual Adult Dose Range:**   Nonpsychotic anxiety: Initially 1 or 2 mg twice daily. The dose may be increased by 1 or 2 mg at 3- to 4-day intervals to a maximum dose of 4 mg for patients who are not in the hospital.

For psychosis: 2 to 5 mg twice a day. The dose is then increased every 3 or 4 days as needed and tolerated. Usual dose range is 15 to 20 mg daily. The total daily dose should not exceed 40 mg. Some rare cases have required 100 mg per day.

Note: Actual dose and schedule must be determined for each patient individually.

Conditions Requiring Dosing Adjustments

Liver Function: This drug should be used with caution in liver compromise.
Kidney Function: Patients with compromised kidneys should be closely followed.

▷ **Dosing Instructions:**   The tablets may be crushed and taken with or following meals to reduce stomach irritation.

Usual Duration of Use: Use on a regular schedule for several weeks usually determines effectiveness in psychotic disorders. If not significantly beneficial within 6 weeks, it should be stopped. Long-term use requires periodic physician evaluation.

▷ **This Drug Should Not Be Taken If**
- you are allergic to any form of trifluoperazine.
- you have active liver disease.
- you have cancer of the breast.
- you have a current blood cell or bone marrow disorder.

▷ **Inform Your Physician Before Taking This Drug If**
- you are allergic or abnormally sensitive to any phenothiazine drug (see Drug Classes).
- you have impaired liver or kidney function.
- you have a history of anginal pain (this drug may worsen it).
- you have any type of seizure disorder.
- you have diabetes, glaucoma, or heart disease.
- you have a history of lupus erythematosus.
- you are taking any drug with sedative effects.

- you have had neuroleptic malignant syndrome (ask your doctor).
- you will have surgery with general or spinal anesthesia.

Possible Side Effects (natural, expected, and unavoidable drug actions)
Drowsiness (usually during the first 2 weeks), orthostatic hypotension (see Glossary), blurred vision, dry mouth, nasal congestion, constipation, impaired urination.
Pink or purple coloration of urine, of no significance.

▷ **Possible Adverse Effects** (unusual, unexpected, and infrequent reactions)
If any of the following develop, consult your physician promptly for guidance.
Mild Adverse Effects
Allergic reactions: skin rash, hives, low-grade fever.
Lowering of body temperature, especially in the elderly (see **hypothermia** in Glossary).
Increased appetite and weight gain—possible.
Dizziness, weakness, agitation, insomnia, impaired day and night vision—infrequent.
Serious Adverse Effects
Allergic reactions: hepatitis with jaundice (see Glossary), severe skin reactions, anaphylactic reaction (see Glossary).
Idiosyncratic reactions: neuroleptic malignant syndrome (see Glossary).
Depression, disorientation, loss of peripheral vision—case reports.
Serious skin disorders (Stevens-Johnson syndrome)—rare.
Drug-induced glaucoma or abnormal eye positioning (oculogyric crisis)—case reports.
Drug-induced porphyrias, pituitary tumors, or seizures—case reports.
Rapid heart rate, heart rhythm disorders—possible.
Blood cell disorders: reduction in all cellular elements of the blood (see **bone marrow depression** in Glossary)—case reports.
Phenothiazine-induced sudden death syndrome—case reports.
Nervous system reactions: Parkinson-like disorders (see Glossary), severe restlessness, muscle spasms involving the face and neck, tardive dyskinesia (see Glossary)—rare to infrequent.

▷ **Possible Effects on Sexual Function:** Altered timing and pattern of menstruation.
Male breast enlargement and tenderness (gynecomastia).
Female breast enlargement with milk production.
Spontaneous male orgasm, paradoxical—one case reported. Inhibited ejaculation, painful ejaculation, painful and extended erections (priapism; see Glossary).
Delayed female orgasm—case reports.

▷ **Adverse Effects That May Mimic Natural Diseases or Disorders**
Nervous system reactions may suggest true Parkinson's disease. Liver reactions may suggest viral hepatitis.
Reactions resembling systemic lupus erythematosus may occur.

Natural Diseases or Disorders That May Be Activated by This Drug
Latent epilepsy, glaucoma, diabetes mellitus, prostatism (see Glossary).

Possible Effects on Laboratory Tests

Complete blood cell counts: decreased red cells, hemoglobin, white cells, and platelets.

Liver function tests: increased enzymes (ALT/GPT, AST/GOT, alkaline phosphatase) or bilirubin.

Urine pregnancy tests: falsely positive result with some tests.

CAUTION

1. Many over-the-counter medications (see Glossary) for allergies, colds, and coughs contain drugs that can interact unfavorably with this drug. Ask your doctor or pharmacist for help before using any such medications.
2. Antacids that contain aluminum and/or magnesium may prevent the absorption of this drug and reduce its effectiveness.
3. Call your doctor if your vision changes.

Precautions for Use

By Infants and Children: Use of this drug is not recommended in children under 6 years of age. Do not use this drug in the presence of symptoms suggestive of Reye syndrome (see Glossary). Children with acute infectious diseases (flu-like infections, chicken pox, measles, etc.) are more prone to develop muscular spasms of the face, back, and extremities when this drug is given.

By Those Over 60 Years of Age: Small starting doses are prudent to try to decrease risk of drowsiness, lethargy, constipation, lowering of body temperature (hypothermia), and orthostatic hypotension (see Glossary). This drug may enhance existing prostatism (see Glossary). You may also be more susceptible to Parkinson-like reactions and/or tardive dyskinesia (see discussion of these terms in Glossary). These reactions must be recognized early since they may become unresponsive to treatment and irreversible.

▷ **Advisability of Use During Pregnancy**

Pregnancy Category: C. See Pregnancy Risk Categories at the back of this book.

Animal studies: Significant birth defects reported in mouse and rat studies.

Human studies: No increase in birth defects reported in 700 exposures. Adequate studies of pregnant women are not available.

Avoid drug during the first 3 months; avoid during the final month because of possible adverse effects on the newborn infant.

Advisability of Use If Breast-Feeding

Presence of this drug in breast milk: Yes, in minute amounts.

Monitor nursing infant closely and discontinue drug or nursing if adverse effects develop.

Habit-Forming Potential: None.

Effects of Overdose: Marked drowsiness, weakness, tremor, agitation, unsteadiness, deep sleep, coma, convulsions.

Possible Effects of Long-Term Use: Tardive dyskinesia (see Glossary).

Suggested Periodic Examinations While Taking This Drug (at physician's discretion)

Complete blood cell counts, especially between the 4th and 10th weeks of treatment.

Liver function tests, electrocardiograms.

Complete eye examinations of eye structures and vision.

Careful inspection of the tongue for early evidence of fine, involuntary, wave-like movements that could indicate the beginning of tardive dyskinesia.

▷ **While Taking This Drug, Observe the Following**

Foods: No restrictions.

Nutritional Support: A riboflavin (vitamin B$_2$) supplement should be taken with long-term use.

Beverages: Caffeine may slightly blunt the calming effect of this medicine. May be taken with milk.

▷ *Alcohol:* Avoid completely. Alcohol can increase the sedative action of phenothiazines and accentuate their depressant effects on brain function and blood pressure. Phenothiazines can increase the intoxicating effects of alcohol.

Tobacco Smoking: I advise everyone to quit smoking.

Marijuana Smoking: Moderate increase in drowsiness; accentuation of orthostatic hypotension; risk of precipitating latent psychoses, confusing mental status exams and drug responses.

▷ *Other Drugs*

Trifluoperazine may *increase* the effects of
• all atropinelike drugs, and cause nervous system toxicity.
• all sedative drugs, especially narcotic analgesics (also see Drug Classes for opioids and benzodiazepines), and cause excessive sedation.

Trifluoperazine may *decrease* the effects of
• guanethidine (Ismelin, Esimil), and reduce its effectiveness in lowering blood pressure.

Trifluoperazine *taken concurrently* with
• ascorbic acid (vitamin C) may result in decreased therapeutic benefits from trifluoperazine.
• lithium (Lithobid, Lithotabs) may impair the effectiveness of lithium and cause nervous system toxicity.
• grepafloxacin (Raxar) or sparfloxacin (Zagam) may lead to abnormal heart beats.
• monoamine oxidase (MAO) inhibitors (see Drug Classes) may result in an increased risk of Parkinson-like disorders (see Glossary) reactions.
• oral hypoglycemic agents (see *oral antidiabetic drugs* in Drug Classes) will blunt the beneficial effects of the oral hypoglycemic agents.
• tramadol (Ultram) may increase risk of seizures.

The following drugs may *decrease* the effects of trifluoperazine:
• antacids containing aluminum and/or magnesium.
• barbiturates (see Drug Classes).
• benztropine (Cogentin).
• disulfiram (Antabuse).
• trihexyphenidyl (Artane).

▷ *Driving, Hazardous Activities:* This drug can impair mental alertness, judgment, and physical coordination. Avoid hazardous activities.

Aviation Note: The use of this drug *is a disqualification* for piloting. Consult a designated aviation medical examiner.

Exposure to Sun: Use caution—some phenothiazines can cause photosensitivity (see Glossary).

Exposure to Heat: Use caution and avoid excessive heat as much as possible. This drug may impair the regulation of body temperature and increase the risk of heatstroke.

Exposure to Cold: Use caution and dress warmly. This drug can increase the risk of hypothermia in the elderly.

Discontinuation: After a period of long-term use, do not stop this drug suddenly. Gradual withdrawal over 2 to 3 weeks by your doctor is prudent. Schizophrenia may recur if the medicine is stopped.

TRIMETHOPRIM (tri METH oh prim)

Introduced: 1966   **Class:** Anti-infective   **Prescription:** USA: Yes
Controlled Drug: USA: No; Canada: No   **Available as Generic:** USA: Yes; Canada: No

Brand Names: ✦Apo-Sulfatrim [CD], ✦Apo-Sulfatrim DS [CD], Bactrim [CD], Bactrim DS [CD], Bethaprim [CD], Comoxol [CD], ✦Coptin [CD], Cotrim [CD], ✦Novo-Trimel [CD], ✦Novo-Trimel DS [CD], ✦Nu-Cotrimox, Polytrim, Proloprim, ✦Protrin [CD], ✦Protrin DF [CD], ✦Roubac [CD], Septra [CD], Septra DS [CD], SMZ-TMP [CD], Sulfatrim D/S, Trimpex, Uroplus DS [CD], Uroplus SS [CD]

BENEFITS versus RISKS	
Possible Benefits	*Possible Risks*
EFFECTIVE TREATMENT OF INFECTIONS due to susceptible microorganisms Effective adjunctive prevention and treatment of *Pneumocystis carinii* pneumonia (AIDS related)	Blood cell disorders: megaloblastic anemia, methemoglobinemia, abnormally low white cells or platelets

▷ **Principal Uses**

As a Single Drug Product: Uses currently included in FDA-approved labeling: (1) Treats or prevents certain infections of the urinary tract not complicated by the presence of kidney stones or obstructions to the normal flow of urine; (2) treats eye infections caused by sensitive organisms.

Other (unlabeled) generally accepted uses: (1) Used in combination with dapsone to treat *Pneumocystis carinii* pneumonia in AIDS patients; (2) may have a role in combination therapy of resistant acne; (3) prevention (prophylaxis) of urinary tract infections.

As a Combination Drug Product [CD]: Available combined with sulfamethoxazole (cotrimoxazole is the name used in some countries to identify this combination). Treats certain urinary tract infections, middle ear infections, chronic bronchitis, acute enteritis, and certain types of pneumonia. It is now used as primary prevention and treatment of *Pneumocystis carinii* pneumonia associated with AIDS.

How This Drug Works: Prevents growth and multiplication of susceptible organisms by inactivating enzyme systems needed for formation of essential nuclear elements and cell proteins.

Available Dose Forms and Strengths
> Tablets — 100 mg, 200 mg
> Tablets — 80 mg combined with 400 mg of sulfamethoxazole
> Tablets — 160 mg combined with 800 mg of sulfamethoxazole
> Ophthalmic — 1 mg/ml
> Oral suspension — 40 mg combined with 200 mg of sulfamethoxazole per 5 ml

▷ **Usual Adult Dose Range:**   Orally for infections: 100 mg every 12 hours for 10 days. For certain pneumonias, the same dose is taken every 6 hours. The total daily dose should not exceed 640 mg.

Ophthalmic: one drop in the affected eye every 3 hours (up to six doses a day) for 7 to 10 days.

Note: Actual dose and schedule must be determined for each patient individually.

Conditions Requiring Dosing Adjustments
Liver Function: Used with caution by patients with both liver and kidney disease.
Kidney Function: Patients with mild kidney compromise can take the usual dose every 12 hours. Patients with moderate to severe kidney failure (creatinine clearances of 15 to 50 ml/min) can take the usual dose every 18 hours. Should NOT be used in severe or worsening kidney failure.

▷ **Dosing Instructions:**   The tablet may be crushed and taken without regard to meals. However, it may also be taken with or following food if necessary to reduce stomach irritation.

Usual Duration of Use: Use on a regular schedule for 7 to 14 days usually determines effectiveness in controlling responsive infections. The actual duration of use will depend upon the nature of the infection.

Currently a "Drug of Choice"
(When combined with sulfamethoxazole) for preventing pneumonia (due to *Pneumocystis carinii*) in patients with AIDS.

▷ **This Drug Should Not Be Taken If**
• you have had an allergic reaction to it previously.
• you have an anemia due to folic acid deficiency (megaloblastic anemia).

▷ **Inform Your Physician Before Taking This Drug If**
• you have a history of folic acid deficiency.
• you have impaired liver or kidney function.
• you are pregnant or breast-feeding.

Possible Side Effects (natural, expected, and unavoidable drug actions)
None with short-term use.

▷ **Possible Adverse Effects** (unusual, unexpected, and infrequent reactions)
If any of the following develop, consult your physician promptly for guidance.
Mild Adverse Effects
Allergic reactions: skin rash, itching, drug fever (see Glossary).
Headache, abnormal taste, sore mouth or tongue, nausea, vomiting, cramping, diarrhea—infrequent.
Serious Adverse Effects
Allergic reactions: severe dermatitis with peeling of skin (toxic epidermal necrolysis).

Blood cell disorders: megaloblastic anemia, methemoglobinemia, abnormally low white blood cell and platelet counts—rare.

Worsening of hyperkalemia (increased blood potassium)—possible.

Kidney or liver toxicity—rare.

Aseptic meningitis (of questionable causal relationship)—case reports.

▷ **Possible Effects on Sexual Function:**   None reported.

Possible Effects on Laboratory Tests

Complete blood cell counts: decreased red cells, hemoglobin, white cells, and platelets.

INR (prothrombin time): increased (when taken concurrently with warfarin).

CAUTION

1. Resistance may develop. If you do not show significant improvement within 2 days, call your physician.
2. Comply with your physician's request for periodic blood counts during long-term therapy.

Precautions for Use

By Infants and Children: Safety and effectiveness for those under 2 months of age are not established.

By Those Over 60 Years of Age: The natural decline in liver and kidney function may require smaller doses. If you develop itching reactions in the genital or anal areas, report this promptly.

▷ **Advisability of Use During Pregnancy**

Pregnancy Category: C. See Pregnancy Risk Categories at the back of this book.

Animal studies: Birth defects due to this drug reported in rat and rabbit studies.

Human studies: Adequate studies of pregnant women are not available.

Avoid use of drug during the first 3 months and during the final 2 weeks of pregnancy. Use this drug otherwise only if clearly needed. Ask your physician for guidance.

Advisability of Use If Breast-Feeding

Presence of this drug in breast milk: Yes.

Avoid drug or refrain from nursing.

Habit-Forming Potential: None.

Effects of Overdose: Headache, dizziness, confusion, depression, nausea, vomiting, bone marrow depression, possible liver toxicity with jaundice.

Possible Effects of Long-Term Use: Impaired production of red and white blood cells and blood platelets.

Suggested Periodic Examinations While Taking This Drug (at physician's discretion)

Complete blood cell counts.

▷ **While Taking This Drug, Observe the Following**

Foods: No restrictions.

Beverages: No restrictions. May be taken with milk.

▷ *Alcohol:* No interactions expected.

Tobacco Smoking: No interactions expected. I advise everyone to quit smoking.

▷ *Other Drugs*

Trimethoprim may ***increase*** the effects of

- ACE inhibitors (see Drug Classes), resulting in dangerously increased potassium levels.

- amantadine (Symmetrel), and also result in increased levels of trimethoprim, resulting in toxicity.
- cyclosporine (Sandimmune), and result in increased kidney toxicity.
- dapsone, and result in dapsone or trimethoprim toxicity.
- digoxin (Lanoxin), leading to toxicity.
- metformin (Glucophage) and other cationic drugs.
- methotrexate (Mexate), leading to toxicity.
- phenytoin (Dilantin), and cause phenytoin toxicity.
- procainamide (Procan SR) and result in procainamide toxicity.
- zidovudine (AZT), leading to increased toxicity risk.

The following drugs may *decrease* the effects of trimethoprim:
- cholestyramine (Questran) and perhaps other cholesterol-reducing medicines (see Drug Classes) of the same class—these will bind trimethoprim and blunt its beneficial effects by inhibiting absorption.
- rifampin (Rifadin, Rimactane).

▷ *Driving, Hazardous Activities:* No restrictions.
Aviation Note: The use of this drug is *probably not a disqualification* for piloting. Consult a designated aviation medical examiner.
Exposure to Sun: No restrictions.

TROGLITAZONE (troh GLIT a zoan)

Introduced: 1997   **Class:** Antidiabetic, thiazolidinedione   **Prescription:**
USA: Yes   **Controlled Drug:**   USA: No; Canada: No   **Available as Generic:**
No

Brand Name: Rezulin

BENEFITS versus RISKS	
Possible Benefits	*Possible Risks*
DECREASED INSULIN RESISTANCE	HYPOGLYCEMIA
EFFECTIVE CONTROL OF BLOOD SUGAR (GLUCOSE)	SERIOUS LIVER DAMAGE
POSSIBLE AVOIDANCE OF LONG-TERM EFFECTS (BLOOD VESSEL, NERVE, KIDNEY, HIGH BLOOD PRESSURE, AND HEART ADVERSE EFFECTS) FROM DIABETES	
Assistance in regulating blood sugar in insulin-dependent diabetes (adjunctive to appropriate diet and weight control)	
"Normalizing" some cancers	

▷ **Principal Uses**

As a Single Drug Product: Uses currently included in FDA-approved labeling: (1) Helps control mild to moderately severe Type 2 diabetes mellitus (adult, maturity-onset) with a glycoslylated hemoglobin greater than 8.5%, despite daily insulin injections; (2) helps people who have not responded to diet alone or to sulfonylureas.

Other (unlabeled) generally accepted uses: (1) Can help treatment of women who form multiple cysts on their ovaries (polycystic ovary syndrome); (2) experimental use "normalizing" some kinds of cancer cells (liposarcomas).

How This Drug Works: It is thought that this drug (1) improves how cells (target cells) respond to insulin; (2) decreases liver (hepatic) sugar (glucose) output, and (3) enhances the utilization of insulin (insulin-dependent functions) by appropriate tissues (skeletal muscle glucose disposal).

Available Dose Forms and Strengths

Tablets — 200 mg, 300 mg, 400 mg

▷ **Usual Adult Dose Range:**   Initially 200 mg once daily. The dose may be increased, if needed and tolerated, to 400 mg once daily after 2 to 4 weeks. Insulin doses should be decreased by 10 to 25% when fasting plasma glucose decreases to less than 120 mg/dl. 600 mg is the maximum daily troglitazone dose; this dose may be taken only for a maximum of one month. **Note: Actual dose and schedule must be determined for each patient individually.**

Conditions Requiring Dosing Adjustments

Liver Function: Used with caution by patients with liver damage.

Kidney Function: Dosing decreases are not needed in kidney compromise.

▷ **Dosing Instructions:**   Should be taken with a meal. The tablet may be crushed for administration.

Usual Duration of Use: Use on a regular schedule for 2 to 4 weeks usually determines peak effectiveness in controlling diabetes. Failure to respond after this period requires a dose increase. Insulin doses should be decreased by 10 to 25% when the fasting glucose decreases to less than 120 mg/dl. Effective use can only be determined by periodic measurement of the blood sugar. See your physician on a regular basis.

▷ **This Drug Should Not Be Taken If**

- you have had an allergic reaction to it previously.
- you have diabetes complicated by formation of excess acid (acidosis).

▷ **Inform Your Physician Before Taking This Drug If**

- you are over 60 years old.
- your diabetes has been unstable or "brittle" in the past.
- you are pregnant.
- you do not know how to recognize or treat hypoglycemia (see Glossary).
- you have an infection and a fever.
- you have a deficiency of red blood cells (anemia)—ask your doctor.
- you have liver damage.
- you take an oral hypoglycemic agent (not studied).
- you have NYHA class lll or IV heart failure (not studied).

Possible Side Effects (natural, expected, and unavoidable drug actions)

If drug dose is excessive or food intake is delayed or inadequate, abnormally low blood sugar (hypoglycemia) may occur.

▷ **Possible Adverse Effects** (unusual, unexpected, and infrequent reactions)

If any of the following develop, consult your physician promptly for guidance.

Mild Adverse Effects

Allergic reactions: skin rash—rare.

Hypoglycemia (more likely with use of insulin at the same time)—infrequent.

Decreased hemoglobin (mild and limited)—infrequent.

Increased liver enzymes—rare.

Increased blood urea nitrogen (BUN)—rare and not present in all studies.

Nausea, vomiting, or diarrhea—infrequent.

Serious Adverse Effects

Allergic reactions: not reported.

Idiosyncratic reactions: To date, 35 cases of severe liver reactions have been reported. Liver enzymes must be tested (see "Caution" and "Periodic Examinations" below).

Hypoglycemia—more likely with insulin use at the same time.

▷ **Possible Effects on Sexual Function:**　None reported.

▷ **Adverse Effects That May Mimic Natural Diseases or Disorders**

Liver reactions may suggest viral hepatitis.

Natural Diseases or Disorders That May Be Activated by This Drug

None reported.

Possible Effects on Laboratory Tests

Complete blood cell counts: decreased red cells, hemoglobin, and hematocrit—mild and stabilizes after 4 to 8 weeks.

Blood glucose or glycosylated hemoglobin level: decreased.

Liver function tests: increased liver enzymes (ALT/GPT, AST/GOT, and alkaline phosphatase).

Blood urea nitrogen (BUN): rarely increased in some clinical studies.

CAUTION

1. This drug must be regarded as only one part of the total program for the management of your diabetes. It is not a substitute for a properly prescribed diet, insulin, and regular exercise.

2. This medicine may reduce the effectiveness of birth control pills. Talk about alternative contraception options with your doctor. Periodic follow-up examinations are necessary.

3. Because of possible idiosyncratic liver reactions, liver function tests (serum transaminases) must be tested before treatment is started. Patients with alanine aminotransferase (ALT) of more than 1.5 times the upper normal limit should NOT be given troglitazone. Repeat ALT tests should be made monthly for eight months, every two months during the rest of the first year, and periodically thereafter. If ALT levels increase to more that 1.5 to 2 times the upper normal when retested, the ALT should be tested again in a week, and then weekly until ALT returns to normal or rises to more than three times the upper normal range. If ALT increases to more than three times the upper limit of normal, troglitazone MUST be stopped. Patients should also be told to report nausea, vomiting, abdominal pain, fatigue, anorexia, or dark urine to their doctor.

Precautions for Use

By Infants and Children: This drug is approved for Type 2 insulin-dependent diabetes.

By Those Over 65 Years of Age: This drug should be used with caution in this age group and monitored closely to prevent hypoglycemic reactions. Repeated episodes of hypoglycemia in the elderly can cause brain damage. Clinical trials did not reveal differences in safety or effectiveness in those over 65.

▷ **Advisability of Use During Pregnancy**
   Pregnancy Category: B. See Pregnancy Risk Categories at the back of this book.
   Animal studies: No effects were seen in rats given doses 10 or 20 mg per kg of body mass.
   Human studies: Adequate studies of pregnant women are not available.
   Because uncontrolled blood sugar levels during pregnancy are associated with a higher incidence of birth defects, many experts recommend that insulin (instead of an oral agent) be used as necessary to control diabetes during the entire pregnancy.
   Use of this drug during pregnancy is not recommended by the manufacturer.

Advisability of Use If Breast-Feeding
   Presence of this drug in breast milk: Yes, in rats; unknown in women.
   Avoid drug or refrain from nursing.

Habit-Forming Potential: None.

Effects of Overdose: Symptoms of mild to severe hypoglycemia: headache, light-headedness, faintness, nervousness, confusion, tremor, sweating, heart palpitation, weakness, hunger, nausea, vomiting, stupor progressing to coma.

Possible Effects of Long-Term Use: Not defined at present.

Suggested Periodic Examinations While Taking This Drug (at physician's discretion)
   Complete blood cell counts. Liver function tests (serum transaminases) must be given at the beginning of treatment and then every month for the first eight months, then every two months for the rest of the first year, and periodically thereafter. Follow-up tests (such as fingerstick testing) of blood sugar. Glycosylated hemoglobin.

▷ **While Taking This Drug, Observe the Following**
   Foods: Follow the diabetic diet prescribed by your physician.
   Beverages: As directed in the diabetic diet. May be taken with milk.
▷   *Alcohol:* Use with caution. Single doses of moderate amounts of alcohol did not increase risk of hypoglycemia.
   Tobacco Smoking: No interaction expected. I advise everyone to quit smoking.
▷   *Other Drugs*
   The following drugs may ***decrease*** the effects of troglitazone:
   • cholestyramine (Questran).
   • thiazide diuretics (see Drug Classes).
   • thyroid hormones (see Drug Classes).
   Troglitazone ***taken concurrently*** with
   • birth control pills (oral contraceptives) may decrease their effectiveness resulting in unwanted pregnancy.
   • insulin will result in additive lowering of the blood sugar.
   • oral hypoglycemic agents such as sulfonylureas (see Drug Classes) may further decrease fasting blood sugar. Caution is advised, as this combination was not well studied.
   • terfenadine (Seldane) may decrease terfenadine concentrations and lessen its therapeutic effect.

▷ *Driving, Hazardous Activities:* Regulate your dose schedule, eating schedule, and physical activities very carefully to prevent hypoglycemia. Be able to recognize the early symptoms of hypoglycemia so you can avoid hazardous activities and take corrective measures.

Aviation Note: Diabetes *is a disqualification* for piloting. Consult a designated aviation medical examiner.

Exposure to Sun: Not defined.

Occurrence of Unrelated Illness: Acute infections, illnesses causing vomiting or diarrhea, serious injuries, and surgical procedures can interfere with diabetic control and may require insulin. If any of these conditions occur, call your doctor promptly.

Discontinuation: Talk with your doctor before changing the dosing schedule of this medicine or considering stopping troglitazone.

VALACYCLOVIR (VALA si klo veer)

Introduced: 1996   **Class:** Antiviral   **Prescription:** USA: Yes   **Controlled Drug:** USA: No; Canada: No   **Available as Generic:** USA: No; Canada: No

Brand Name: Valtrex

BENEFITS versus RISKS	
Possible Benefits	*Possible Risks*
EFFECTIVE TREATMENT OF HERPES ZOSTER (SHINGLES)	Rare reports of thrombotic thrombocytopenic purpura (TTP) in
EFFECTIVE EPISODIC TREATMENT OF GENITAL	HIV and bone marrow or kidney transplant patients
HERPES	Nausea

▷ **Principal Uses**

As a Single Drug Product: Uses currently included in FDA-approved labeling: (1) Treats herpes zoster (shingles); (2) used in recurrent genital herpes in patients with intact immune systems.

Other (unlabeled) generally accepted uses: None at present; since this medicine is rapidly converted to acyclovir, see the acyclovir profile for some possible unlabeled uses.

How This Drug Works: This medicine is rapidly converted to acyclovir, and moves into the body to a much greater extent (dose to dose) than acyclovir. By blocking formation of genetic material by the virus, this medicine stops the ability of the virus to multiply and spread.

Available Dose Forms and Strengths

Caplets — 500 mg, 1000 mg

▷ **Usual Adult Dose Range** (Actual dose and schedule must be determined for each patient individually.)   Herpes zoster (shingles): Best started within 48 hours of the zoster rash. Dose is 1 g (1000 mg) three times a day for 7 days.

Genital herpes simplex: This medicine is best started within 24 hours of the onset of symptoms, and is taken as 500 mg twice daily for 5 days.

Conditions Requiring Dosing Adjustments
  Liver Function: Not recommended for people with cirrhosis.
  Kidney Function: Dosing changes **MUST** be made for patients with compromised kidneys, including the typical age-related decline in kidney function (ask your doctor about this if you are over 60 years old).

▷ **Dosing Instructions:**   May be taken without regard to meals.

Usual Duration of Use: Best started within 48 hours of onset of the zoster rash. Use on a regular schedule for 7 days for herpes zoster has been effective. Start therapy within 24 hours of signs of genital herpes; regular use for 5 days has been effective for genital herpes. Take the full course as prescribed.

Possible Advantages of This Drug
  Generally well-tolerated antiviral that decreases the length of time patients are in pain from genital herpes and herpes zoster. Achieves blood levels similar to INTRAVENOUS acyclovir with a medicine taken by mouth (the oral route). Patients do not have to take it as many times a day as acyclovir.

▷ **This Drug Should Not Be Taken If**
  • you have had an allergic reaction to it previously.
  • you have advanced HIV disease or have had a bone marrow or kidney transplant (increased risk of thrombotic thrombocytopenic purpura).

▷ **Inform Your Physician Before Taking This Drug If**
  • you have impaired liver or kidney function.
  • you are taking any other drugs at this time.
  • you think you are dehydrated.
  • you are unsure how much to take or how often to take it.

Possible Side Effects (natural, expected, and unavoidable drug actions)
  With use of caplets—none.

▷ **Possible Adverse Effects** (unusual, unexpected, and infrequent reactions)
  If any of the following develop, consult your physician promptly for guidance.
  Mild Adverse Effects
  Allergic reactions: skin rash.
  Headache, dizziness, nervousness, insomnia, depression, fatigue—infrequent.
  Nausea, vomiting, diarrhea—infrequent.
  Serious Adverse Effects
  Thrombotic thrombocytopenic purpura—rare and in immunocompromised patients.
  Kidney problems—reported with high doses of acyclovir and rare.

▷ **Possible Effects on Sexual Function:**   Altered timing and pattern of menstruation reported with acyclovir, not with valacyclovir.

Possible Effects on Laboratory Tests
  Complete blood cell counts: decreased red cells and hemoglobin.
  Blood urea nitrogen (BUN) or creatinine: increased.

CAUTION
  1. This drug does not eliminate all herpes virus and is not a cure. Recurrence is possible (with genital herpes use). Resume treatment at the earliest sign of infection.
  2. Avoid sexual intercourse if herpes blisters and swelling are present.
  3. Do not exceed the prescribed dose.

4. Tell your doctor if frequency (genital herpes) or severity (herpes zoster) doesn't improve.

Precautions for Use

By Infants and Children: Safety and effectiveness for use in pediatrics have not been established.

By Those Over 60 Years of Age: Avoid dehydration. Drink 2 to 3 quarts of liquids daily. Lower doses are required if you are over 60 years old and your kidneys have undergone the usual age-related decline in how well they work.

▷ **Advisability of Use During Pregnancy**

Pregnancy Category: B. See Pregnancy Risk Categories at the back of this book.

Animal studies: NOT teratogenic in rabbits or rats (up to 10 times the human dose).

Human studies: Adequate studies of pregnant women are not available.

Physicians should call 1-800-722-9292, extension 58465, to register their patients.

Advisability of Use If Breast-Feeding

Presence of this drug in breast milk: Yes (documented in two women; 0.6 to 4.1 times the plasma levels). Given to breast-feeding mothers with caution or not at all. Discuss the benefits versus risks with your doctor.

Habit-Forming Potential: None.

Effects of Overdose: Possible kidney damage (based on formation of crystals in the kidney with excessive doses).

Possible Effects of Long-Term Use: Development of acyclovir-resistant strains of genital herpes virus. Treatment will fail if this occurs.

▷ **While Taking This Drug, Observe the Following**

Foods: No restrictions.

Beverages: No restrictions. May be taken with milk. **Drink 2 to 3 quarts of liquids** (if not contraindicated for you) **daily.**

▷   *Alcohol:* Use caution; dizziness or fatigue may be accentuated.

Tobacco Smoking: No interactions expected. I advise everyone to quit smoking.

▷   *Other Drugs*

The following drugs may ***increase*** the effects of valacyclovir:

- cimetidine (Tagamet).
- cyclosporine (Sandimmune); may result in increased risk of kidney toxicity.
- probenecid (Benemid); may delay acyclovir elimination.

Valacyclovir ***taken concurrently*** with

- cimetidine (Tagamet) may caused decreased elimination by the kidney.
- meperidine may result in neurological problems (based on acyclovir data).
- varicella vaccine (Varivax) may blunt the vaccine's effectiveness (acyclovir data).
- zidovudine (AZT) may result in severe fatigue and lethargy with acyclovir, and may result in similar results with valacyclovir. An increased risk of thrombotic thrombocytopenic purpura (TTP) is possible in immunocompromised patients.

▷   *Driving, Hazardous Activities:* Use caution if dizziness or fatigue occurs.

Aviation Note: The use of this drug ***may be a disqualification*** for piloting. Consult a designated aviation medical examiner.

Exposure to Sun: No restrictions.

Discontinuation: Talk with your doctor or pharmacist about how long and how best to take this medicine.

VALPROIC ACID (val PROH ik a sid)

Introduced: 1967   **Class:** Anticonvulsant   **Prescription:** USA: Yes
Controlled Drug: USA: No; Canada: No   **Available as Generic:** USA: Yes; Canada: No
Brand Names: Depa, Depakene, Depakote (divalproex sodium), Deproic, ✤Epival

---

BENEFITS versus RISKS

Possible Benefits	*Possible Risks*
EFFECTIVE CONTROL OF MULTIPLE SEIZURE TYPES: ABSENCE SEIZURES, TONIC-CLONIC SEIZURES, MYOCLONIC SEIZURES, PSYCHOMOTOR SEIZURES, when used adjunctively with other antiseizure drugs	LIVER TOXICITY, infrequent but may be severe
	Reduction of blood platelets and impaired platelet function with risk of bleeding
HELPS CONTROL REFRACTORY MIGRAINES	Possible pancreatitis or liver toxicity
DIVALPROEX SODIUM HELPS MANIA	

▷ **Principal Uses**

As a Single Drug Product: Uses currently included in FDA-approved labeling: (1) Used to manage the following types of epilepsy: simple and complex absence seizures (petit mal), tonic-clonic seizures (grand mal), myoclonic seizures, complex partial seizures (psychomotor, temporal lobe epilepsy)—sometimes used adjunctively with other anticonvulsants as needed; (2) used for people who do not respond to medicine once they have a migraine or have more than two migraines a month; (3) divalproex sodium (Depakote) is now approved for use in treating mania.

Other (unlabeled) generally accepted uses: (1) Can help relieve the symptoms of trigeminal neuralgia; (2) can have a role in intractable hiccups; (3) some use in patients with epilepsy and hepatic porphyria; (4) may be of help for writer's cramp.

How This Drug Works: It is thought that by increasing the availability of the nerve impulse transmitter gamma-aminobutyric acid (GABA), this drug suppresses the spread of abnormal electrical discharges that cause seizures.

Available Dose Forms and Strengths

Capsules — 250 mg
Capsules, sprinkle — 125 mg
Syrup — 250 mg/5 ml
Tablets, enteric coated — 125 mg, 250 mg, 500 mg

▷ **Usual Adult Dose Range:**   Starting dose is 15 mg per kg of body mass per day. The dose is increased cautiously by 5 to 10 mg per kg of body mass daily, every 7 days as needed and tolerated. *The usual daily dose is from 1000* *mg to 1600 mg in divided doses.* The total daily dose should not exceed 60 mg per kg of body mass. Blood levels are used to guide ongoing dosing.

For migraines: Starting dose is 250 mg, which is then slowly increased, as needed and tolerated, to 500 to 750 mg daily in divided doses.

Note: **Actual dose and schedule must be determined for each patient individually.**

Conditions Requiring Dosing Adjustments

Liver Function: This medicine SHOULD NOT be taken by patients with significant liver compromise or liver disease.

Kidney Function: No dosing changes thought to be needed in kidney disease.

▷ **Dosing Instructions:** Preferably taken 1 hour before meals. However, it may be taken with or following food if necessary to prevent stomach irritation. The regular capsule should not be opened and the tablet should not be crushed. The sprinkle capsule may be opened and the contents sprinkled on soft food. Do not give the syrup in carbonated beverages. Dilute in water or milk.

Usual Duration of Use: Use on a regular schedule for 2 weeks usually determines effectiveness in reducing the frequency and severity of seizures. Long-term use (months to years) requires physician supervision and periodic evaluation.

▷ **This Drug Should Not Be Taken If**
- you have had an allergic reaction to it previously.
- you have active liver disease.
- you are pregnant.
- you have an active bleeding disorder.

▷ **Inform Your Physician Before Taking This Drug If**
- you have a history of liver disease or impaired liver function.
- you have a history of any type of bleeding disorder.
- you are pregnant or planning to become pregnancy.
- you have myasthenia gravis.
- you are taking anticoagulants; other anticonvulsants; antidepressants— either the tricyclic type or monoamine oxidase (MAO) type A inhibitors (see Drug Classes).
- you will have surgery or dental extraction.

Possible Side Effects (natural, expected, and unavoidable drug actions)
Drowsiness and lethargy.

▷ **Possible Adverse Effects** (unusual, unexpected, and infrequent reactions)
If any of the following develop, consult your physician promptly for guidance.

Mild Adverse Effects
Allergic reactions: skin rash—rare.
Headache, dizziness, confusion, unsteadiness, tremor—dose related; slurred speech—infrequent.
Nausea, indigestion, stomach cramps, diarrhea—infrequent.
Weight gain—case reports.
Bed-wetting at night—case reports.
Temporary loss of scalp hair—case reports.

Serious Adverse Effects

Idiosyncratic reactions: bizarre behavior, psychosis, hallucinations.

Drug-induced hepatitis with jaundice (see Glossary).

Children less than 2 years old have considerably increased risk of fatal hepatotoxicity.

Blood ammonia level or blood glucose—increased.

Drug-induced pancreatitis, porphyria, lowered thyroid gland function (hypothyroidism)—case reports.

Selenium levels—decreased.

Reduced formation of blood platelets, impaired platelet function, and anemia—case reports.

Increased pressure in the head (pseudotumor cerebri)—case reports.

Can cause a Reye-like syndrome.

▷ **Possible Effects on Sexual Function:**   Altered timing and pattern of menstruation.

Female breast enlargement with milk production.

Decreased libido—case reports.

Decreased effectiveness of oral contraceptives taken concurrently (6%).

▷ **Adverse Effects That May Mimic Natural Diseases or Disorders**

Liver reactions may suggest viral hepatitis.

Possible Effects on Laboratory Tests

Complete blood cell counts: decreased white cells and platelets.

Bleeding time or INR (prothrombin time): increased.

Blood amylase level: increased (possible pancreatitis).

Liver function tests: increased enzymes (ALT/GPT, AST/GOT, alkaline phosphatase) or bilirubin.

CAUTION

1. The capsules and tablets should be swallowed whole to avoid irritation of the mouth and throat.
2. This drug can impair normal blood clotting mechanisms. In the event of injury, dental extraction, or need for surgery, inform your physician or dentist that you are taking this drug.
3. Because this drug can impair the normal function of blood platelets, it is best to avoid aspirin (which has the same effect).
4. Over-the-counter drug products that contain antihistamines (allergy and cold remedies, sleep aids) can enhance sedation.

Precautions for Use

By Infants and Children: The concurrent use of aspirin with this drug can cause abnormal bleeding or bruising. Children with mental retardation, organic brain disease, or severe seizure disorders may be at increased risk for severe liver toxicity while taking this drug. Observe closely for the development of fever that could indicate the onset of a drug-induced Reye syndrome (see Glossary). Avoid concurrent use of clonazepam (Klonopin); the combined use could result in continuous petit mal episodes.

By Those Over 60 Years of Age: Start treatment with small doses and increase dose cautiously. Observe closely for excessive sedation, confusion, or unsteadiness that could predispose to falling and injury.

▷ **Advisability of Use During Pregnancy**

Pregnancy Category: D. See Pregnancy Risk Categories at the back of this book.

Animal studies: Palate and skeletal birth defects reported in mouse, rat, and rabbit studies.

Human studies: Adequate studies of pregnant women are not available. There have been several reports of birth defects attributed to the use of this drug during early pregnancy.

Consult your physician regarding the advantages and disadvantages of using this drug. If it is used, it is advisable to keep the dose as low as possible.

Advisability of Use If Breast-Feeding

Presence of this drug in breast milk: Yes.

Monitor nursing infant closely and discontinue drug or nursing if adverse effects develop.

Habit-Forming Potential: None.

Effects of Overdose: Increased drowsiness, weakness, unsteadiness, confusion, stupor progressing to coma.

Possible Effects of Long-Term Use: None reported.

Suggested Periodic Examinations While Taking This Drug (at physician's discretion)

Complete blood cell counts and baseline liver function tests should be done before treatment is started. During treatment, blood counts should be repeated every month and liver function tests repeated every 2 months.

▷ **While Taking This Drug, Observe the Following**

Foods: No restrictions.

Beverages: Do not administer the syrup in carbonated beverages; this could liberate the valproic acid and irritate the mouth and throat. This drug may be taken with milk.

▷ *Alcohol:* Alcohol can increase the sedative effect of this drug. Also, this drug can increase the depressant effects of alcohol on brain function.

Tobacco Smoking: No interactions expected. I advise everyone to quit smoking.

▷ *Other Drugs*

Valproic acid may *increase* the effects of

- anticoagulants (Coumadin, etc.), and increase the risk of bleeding. Increased frequency of INR (prothrombin time or protime) testing is needed.
- antidepressants, both monoamine oxidase (MAO) type A inhibitors and tricyclics, and cause toxicity.
- nimodipine (Nimotop),and cause nimodipine toxicity.
- phenobarbital, and cause barbiturate intoxication.
- phenytoin (Dilantin), and cause phenytoin toxicity.

Valproic acid *taken concurrently* with

- antacids (Maalox) will decrease absorption and their therapeutic benefits.
- antiplatelet drugs—aspirin, dipyridamole (Persantine), sulfinpyrazone (Anturane)—may enhance the inhibition of platelet function and increase the risk of bleeding.
- aspirin can lead to valproic acid toxicity.
- carbamazepine (Tegretol) may have a variable effect on blood levels. More frequent blood level testing is advised.
- clonazepam (Klonopin) may result in repeated episodes of absence seizures (absence status).

- cyclosporine (Sandimmune) may increase risk of liver toxicity.
- erythromycin (Ery-Tab, others) may increase the level of valproic acid and result in toxicity. The newer macrolides (azithromycin or clarithromycin) may also cause problems.
- felbamate (Felbatol) can lead to increased valproic acid levels.
- isoniazid (INH) can cause valproic acid or isoniazid toxicity.

▷ *Driving, Hazardous Activities:* This drug may cause drowsiness, dizziness, or confusion. Restrict activities as necessary.

Aviation Note: The use of this drug *is a disqualification* for piloting. Consult a designated aviation medical examiner.

Exposure to Sun: Caution: this drug has caused photosensitivity.

Discontinuation: **Do not stop this drug suddenly.** Abrupt withdrawal can cause repetitive seizures that are difficult to control.

VANCOMYCIN (van koh MI sin)

Introduced: 1974   **Class:** Anti-infective   **Prescription:** USA: Yes
Controlled Drug: USA: No; Canada: No   **Available as Generic:**   USA: Yes;
Canada: No

Brand Names: Vancocin, Vancoled, Vancor

Note: Vancomycin is used to treat a variety of serious infections. It is given intravenously to treat some infections and orally to treat others. In the past, the information provided in this profile was limited to the use of vancomycin taken by mouth. Since resistant organisms have increased the use of this medicine by vein (intravenously), this profile has been expanded to help patients understand vancomycin's broadened role in infectious disease.

BENEFITS versus RISKS	
Possible Benefits	*Possible Risks*
TREATS SERIOUS INFECTIONS CAUSED BY RESISTANT GRAM-POSITIVE ORGANISMS SUCH AS STAPH AND STREP TREATS ANTIBIOTIC-ASSOCIATED PSEUDOMEMBRANOUS COLITIS	Ringing in ears (tinnitus) Loss of hearing

▷ **Principal Uses**

As a Single Drug Product: Uses currently included in FDA-approved labeling: (1) Oral form is used in antibiotic-associated pseudomembranous colitis caused by *Clostridium difficile*; (2) the oral form is also used in enterocolitis caused by staphylococcal organisms; (3) the intravenous form is used to treat a variety of serious infections such those in heart valves, bones (osteomyelitis), endocarditis, and meningitis, including those caused by methicillin-resistant *Staphylococcus aureus* (MRSA).

Other (unlabeled) generally accepted uses: None.

How This Drug Works: By inhibiting the formation of bacterial cell walls and the production of RNA, this drug destroys susceptible strains of infecting bacteria.

Available Dose Forms and Strengths
   Capsules — 125 mg, 250 mg
   Intravenous — 500 mg/15 ml, 1 g/15 ml
   Oral solution — 250 mg/5 ml teaspoonful and 500 mg/5 ml

▷ **Recommended Dose Ranges** (Actual dose and schedule must be determined for
   each patient individually.)
   Infants and Children: 10 mg per kg of body mass every 6 hours, for 5 to 10 days.
   The total daily dose should not exceed 2000 mg (2 g). Repeat course as necessary.
   12 to 60 Years of Age: Many clinicians use a 15-mg-per-kg-of-body-mass loading
   dose and then calculate ongoing doses based on individual patient height,
   weight, kidney function, and suspected bacteria (bacterial pathogen). Calculations are made in order to attain a peak blood level of 30–40 mcg/ml
   and a lowest blood level (trough) of 5–10 mcg/ml.
   Oral dosing for pseudomembranous colitis caused by *Clostridium difficile*:
   125 mg by mouth every 6 hours for 10 days.
   Over 60 Years of Age: Intravenous dosing: The loading dose is the same as for
   younger patients. Ongoing doses may be much smaller and may need to be
   taken much less often than in younger patients (such as once a day or once
   every 2 days).
   For oral dosing: Same as 12 to 60 years of age (vancomycin in pseudomembranous colitis is not absorbed).

Conditions Requiring Dosing Adjustments
   Liver Function: The liver is not involved in the elimination of vancomycin.
   Kidney Function: Oral vancomycin is minimally absorbed. Intravenous vancomycin MUST be taken in decreased dose or increased interval in kidney
   failure. This drug is also a potential cause of kidney failure, and should
   only be taken if other alternatives are not available. Daily measures of kidney function and more frequent blood levels are indicated if this medicine
   is used by patients with compromised kidneys.

▷ **Dosing Instructions:**   Oral form may be taken with or following food to reduce
   stomach irritation. Because of this drug's unpleasant taste, it is preferable
   to swallow the capsule whole without alteration. Use a measuring device to
   ensure accuracy of dose when taking the oral solution. Observe the expiration date.

Usual Duration of Use: Oral use: Use on a regular schedule for 48 to 72 hours
   usually determines effectiveness in controlling infection in the colon. If response is prompt, limit treatment to 10 days. If symptoms warrant, continue treatment for 14 to 21 days. Consult your physician on a regular
   basis.
   For intravenous use, the length of treatment depends on the severity and site
   of the infection (for example, bone infections may take 6 weeks to cure).

Currently a "Drug of Choice"
   For treating metronidazole-treatment failures in antibiotic-associated
   pseudomembranous colitis caused by *Clostridium difficile*. Used in methicillin-resistant *Staphylococcus aureus* (MRSA).

▷ **This Drug Should Not Be Taken If**
   • you have had an allergic reaction to it previously.

▷ **Inform Your Physician Before Taking This Drug If**
- you have a history of Crohn's disease or ulcerative colitis.
- you have impaired kidney function.
- you are pregnant.
- you have any degree of hearing loss.
- you are taking cholestyramine (Questran) or colestipol (Colestid).

Possible Side Effects (natural, expected, and unavoidable drug actions)
Bitter, unpleasant taste for the oral form. Kidney damage with long-term, high-dose use of the intravenous form. Red-man syndrome (lowering of blood pressure; sudden rash of neck, chest, face, and extremities).

▷ **Possible Adverse Effects** (unusual, unexpected, and infrequent reactions)
If any of the following develop, consult your physician promptly for guidance.
Mild Adverse Effects
Allergic reactions: skin rash (with large doses or prolonged use).
Nausea, vomiting—infrequent with oral form and rare with intravenous form.
Chills—infrequent.
Serious Adverse Effects
Allergic reactions: anaphylaxis. Serious skin rashes (exfoliative dermatitis or Stevens-Johnson syndrome).
Ringing or buzzing in ears, sensation of ear fullness, loss of hearing—toxicity sign.
Lowering of white blood cells—reversible, and seen with the intravenous form.
Cardiac arrest—rare.
Hearing loss—may be reversible and more likely with high dose or long-term use.
Kidney toxicity—may be dose dependent and more likely with higher doses and long-term use.
Thrombophlebitis—infrequent with the intravenous form.

▷ **Possible Effects on Sexual Function:**   None reported.

Natural Diseases or Disorders That May Be Activated by This Drug
Latent hearing loss, kidney failure.

Possible Effects on Laboratory Tests
Serum creatinine: increased (a sign of kidney toxicity).

CAUTION
1. Report promptly the development of fullness, ringing, or buzzing in either ear. This may indicate the onset of nerve damage that could lead to hearing loss.
2. Do not take any medication to stop your diarrhea without calling your doctor. The bacterial toxin that causes colitis is eliminated by diarrhea; stopping the elimination could intensify and prolong your illness.
3. Blood levels MUST be used to guide dosing. Keep all appointments for laboratory work.

Precautions for Use
By Infants and Children: Some cases may require doses up to 50 mg per kg of body mass daily.

By Those Over 60 Years of Age: You may be more susceptible to drug-induced hearing loss. Use the minimum course of treatment required to cure your colitis or other infection.

▷ **Advisability of Use During Pregnancy**
    Pregnancy Category: C. See Pregnancy Risk Categories at the back of this book. Animal studies: Rat and rabbit studies reveal no drug-induced birth defects. Human studies: Adequate studies of pregnant women are not available. Use this drug only if clearly needed. Ask your doctor for help.

Advisability of Use If Breast-Feeding
    Presence of this drug in breast milk: Yes.
    Avoid drug or refrain from nursing.

Habit-Forming Potential: None.

Effects of Overdose: Possible nausea, vomiting, ringing in ears.

Possible Effects of Long-Term Use: Hearing loss.

Suggested Periodic Examinations While Taking This Drug (at physician's discretion)
    Hearing tests. Measures of kidney function and blood vancomycin levels with intravenous use.

▷ **While Taking This Drug, Observe the Following**
    Foods: No restrictions.
    Beverages: No restrictions. May be taken with milk.
▷   *Alcohol:* No interactions expected. Use sparingly; alcohol may aggravate colitis.
    Tobacco Smoking: No interactions expected. I advise everyone to quit smoking.
▷   *Other Drugs*
    The following drugs may *decrease* the effects of vancomycin:
      • cholestyramine (Questran).
      • colestipol (Colestid).
    Vancomycin *taken concurrently* with
      • aminoglycoside antibiotics (see Drug Classes) such as gentamicin or tobramycin may cause additive toxicity risk to the ears and kidneys.
      • cyclosporine (Sandimmune) may result in increased toxicity risk.
      • other medicines that cause kidney toxicity may pose an additive toxicity risk.
      • warfarin (Coumadin) may cause increased bleeding risk. Increased INR (prothrombin time or protime) testing is needed.
▷   *Driving, Hazardous Activities:* Usually no restrictions.
    Aviation Note: The use of this drug is *probably not a disqualification* for piloting. Consult a designated aviation medical examiner.
    Exposure to Sun: No restrictions.
    Discontinuation: To be determined by your physician.
    Special Storage Instructions: Refrigerate the oral solution. A home IV service will explain storage of the intravenous form.
    Observe the Following Expiration Times: Provided on your prescription label by your pharmacist.

VARICELLA VIRUS VACCINE (VAIR a sell ah)

Introduced: 1995   **Class:** Vaccine   **Prescription:** USA: Yes   **Controlled Drug:** USA: No; Canada: No   **Available as Generic:** USA: No; Canada: No

Brand Name: Varivax

BENEFITS versus RISKS	
Possible Benefits	*Possible Risks*
PREVENTION OF VARICELLA (chicken pox)	Rash Soreness at the injection site Anaphylactic reaction

▷ **Principal Uses**

As a Single Drug Product: Uses currently included in FDA-approved labeling: Prevention of chicken pox.

Other (unlabeled) generally accepted uses: Used in some cases after exposure to chicken pox to prevent it.

How This Drug Works: By stimulating the immune system, the vaccine prepares the body to fight any exposure to the wild-type virus.

Available Dose Forms and Strengths

Vaccine, multidose vial — a single-dose vial of vaccine (1500 PFU per dose)

How to Store

This product **must** be kept frozen prior to use.

Author's Note: The Center for Disease Control's (CDC) Immunization Practices Committee has recommended that all children 12 to 18 months old should be given varicella vaccine if they have not previously contracted chicken pox. The vaccine is also recommended by the committee for children 19 months to 13 years old. Finally, adults or adolescents who have not had chicken pox and are at risk for exposure should also be given the vaccine.

▷ **Recommended Dose Ranges** (Actual dose and schedule must be determined for each patient individually.)

Infants and Children 1 to 12 Years Old: Not indicated in infants. Children 1 year old or older are given 0.5 ml injected under the skin.

12 to 55 Years of Age: Same as the children's dose, providing the patient has not had chicken pox.

Over 55 Years of Age: Not studied.

Conditions Requiring Dosing Adjustments

Liver Function: Not a consideration.

Kidney Function: Not a consideration.

▷ **Dosing Instructions:**   This vaccine is to be injected under the skin. It may be given with measles, mumps, and rubella vaccine.

Usual Duration of Benefit: Exposure to chicken pox 5 years after vaccination may result in 20% of patients developing mild disease. More experience is needed before the question of repeat vaccination is answered. Immunity may last 10 years.

Possible Advantages of This Drug
Prevention of chicken pox.

Currently a "Drug of Choice"
For prevention of chicken pox.

▷ **This Drug Should Not Be Taken If**
- you had an allergic reaction to it previously.
- you have a history of anaphylactic reaction to neomycin.
- you have a history of blood diseases or leukemia, or have AIDS.
- you are taking medicines that suppress the immune system.
- you have tuberculosis that has not been treated.
- you are allergic to eggs.
- you are pregnant (avoid pregnancy for 3 months after vaccine).
- you have an active infection.

▷ **Inform Your Physician Before Taking This Drug If**
- you are planning a pregnancy in the near future.
- you have a condition that may require steroids.
- you take salicylates (aspirin, others) on a regular basis. This should NOT be done for 6 weeks following vaccination, as it is a risk for Reye syndrome.
- you live with someone who has a depressed immune system (such as an AIDS patient). Because this vaccine is a live-virus vaccine, you may be infectious to them.

Possible Side Effects (natural, expected, and unavoidable drug actions)
Pain at the injection site, fever—infrequent to frequent.

▷ **Possible Adverse Effects** (unusual, unexpected, and infrequent reactions)
If any of the following develop, consult your physician promptly for guidance.
Mild Adverse Effects
Allergic reactions: skin rash.
Varicellalike rash—infrequent.
Headache, irritability, fatigue, and loss of appetite—rare to infrequent.
Chills, stiff neck, and joint pain—infrequent.
Nausea, vomiting—rare.
Serious Adverse Effects
Allergic reactions: anaphylactic reaction.
Idiosyncratic reactions: none reported.
Febrile seizures—case reports.
Herpes zoster—possible.
Pneumonitis—case report and of questionable causation.
May be possible for a recently vaccinated person to transmit Varicella to a susceptible contact—one case report.

▷ **Possible Effects on Sexual Function:**   None reported.

Possible Delayed Adverse Effects: None reported.

▷ **Adverse Effects That May Mimic Natural Diseases or Disorders**
Rash may resemble chicken pox.

Natural Diseases or Disorders That May Be Activated by This Drug
None reported.

Possible Effects on Laboratory Tests
None reported.

CAUTION
1. Do not give aspirin or other salicylates to patients who have recently received the vaccine. The risk of Reye syndrome is associated with such aspirin use.

Precautions for Use

By Infants and Children: Safety and effectiveness for use by those under 12 months of age have not been established.

By Those Over 60 Years of Age: Not studied.

▷ **Advisability of Use During Pregnancy**

Pregnancy Category: C. See Pregnancy Risk Categories at the back of this book.
  Animal studies: Have not been conducted with this vaccine.
  Human studies: Information from adequate studies of pregnant women is not available. The manufacturer says that the vaccine should not be given to pregnant women and pregnancy should be avoided for 3 months following vaccination.

Advisability of Use If Breast-Feeding

Presence of this drug in breast milk: Expected.
  Avoid drug or refrain from nursing.

Habit-Forming Potential: None.

Effects of Overdose: Not defined.

Possible Effects of Long-Term Use: Not intended for long-term use.

Suggested Periodic Examinations While Taking This Drug (at physician's discretion)
  None suggested.

▷ **While Taking This Drug, Observe the Following**

Foods: No restrictions.

Beverages: No restrictions.

▷ *Alcohol:* No interactions expected.

Tobacco Smoking: No interactions expected. I advise everyone to quit smoking.

▷ *Other Drugs*

  Varicella vaccine *taken concurrently* with

  • acyclovir (Zovirax) may result in a blunted immune benefit from the vaccine.
  • aspirin or any salicylates (various) may result in Reye syndrome. DO NOT take aspirin for 6 weeks after vaccination.
  • adrenocortical steroids (see Drug Classes) may result in extreme reactions.
  • immune globulins (such as rabies or hepatitis immune globulin) may blunt beneficial response to the vaccine.
  • immunosuppressant medicines (such as cyclosporine—Sandimmune) may result in extreme reactions.
  • mesalamine (Asacol) may result in risk of Reye syndrome. DO NOT take salicylates for 6 weeks after vaccination.
  • olsalazine (Dipentum) may result in risk of Reye syndrome. DO NOT take salicylates for 6 weeks after vaccination.

▷ *Driving, Hazardous Activities:* This drug may cause soreness at the injection site. Restrict activities as necessary.

Aviation Note: The use of this drug *is probably not a disqualification* for piloting. Consult a designated aviation medical examiner.

Exposure to Sun: No restrictions.

Occurrence of Unrelated Illness: This vaccination should not be given in the presence of any other active infection.

Special Storage Instructions: This vaccine must be stored frozen.

Author's Note: There is now a Vaccine Adverse Event Reporting System (VAERS). The toll-free number is 1-800-822-7967.

VENLAFAXINE (ven la FAX een)

Introduced: 1993   **Class:** Antidepressant   **Prescription:** USA: Yes
Controlled Drug: USA: No; Canada: No   **Available as Generic:** USA: No
Brand Names: Effexor, Effexor XR

BENEFITS versus RISKS	
Possible Benefits	*Possible Risks*
EFFECTIVE TREATMENT OF DEPRESSION	INCREASED BLOOD PRESSURE
	Seizures
BETTER SIDE-EFFECT PROFILE THAN TRICYCLIC ANTIDEPRESSANTS	Constipation
	Increased heart rate
	Increased serum lipids
RAPID ONSET OF EFFECT	

▷ **Principal Uses**

As a Single Drug Product: Uses currently included in FDA-approved labeling: Treatment of depression.

Other (unlabeled) generally accepted uses: (1) May be useful in obsessive-compulsive disorder; (2) chronic fatigue syndrome.

How This Drug Works: This bicyclic (second-generation) antidepressant inhibits the return (reuptake) of nerve transmitters (serotonin, norepinephrine, and dopamine) and helps return normal mood and thinking.

Available Dose Forms and Strengths
Tablets — 25 mg, 37.5 mg, 50 mg, 75 mg, 100 mg
Tablets, extended release — 37.5 mg, 75 mg, 150 mg

▷ **Recommended Dose Ranges** (Actual dose and schedule must be determined for each patient individually.)

Infants and Children: Safety and effectiveness for those under 18 years of age are not established.

18 to 60 Years of Age: For depression: start with 75 mg per day, as 25-mg doses three times daily. If needed and tolerated, the dose may be increased at 4-day intervals up to a maximum of 225 mg per day. Some hospitalized patients have been given a maximum of 375 mg per day.

The XR form is started at 37.5 milligrams per day. Dose increases of 75 mg/day can be made at intervals of at least 4 days. Daily maximum is 225 mg per day.

Over 60 Years of Age: Low starting doses and slow increases are indicated. Natural declines in kidney function may lead to drug accumulation at higher doses. May worsen constipation.

Conditions Requiring Dosing Adjustments

Liver Function: Total daily dose must be reduced by 50% for patients with moderate liver compromise. Further dose decreases and individualized dosing is needed in liver cirrhosis.

Kidney Function: Patients with compromised kidneys (creatinine clearance of 10 to 70 ml/min) should take 75% of the usual daily dose.

▷ **Dosing Instructions:**   Food has no clinically significant effect on venlafaxine.

Usual Duration of Use: Regular use for 2 weeks usually determines benefits in treating depression. Long-term use requires follow-up by your doctor.

Possible Advantages of This Drug

Effective treatment of depression with fewer side effects than other currently available agents.

Starts to have a therapeutic effect more rapidly than other available agents.

▷ **This Drug Should Not Be Taken If**
- you had an allergic reaction to any form of it previously.
- you are taking a monoamine oxidase (MAO) inhibitor (see Drug Classes).

▷ **Inform Your Physician Before Taking This Drug If**
- you have a history of high blood pressure.
- you have recently had a heart attack.
- you have a history of abnormally increased lipids (hyperlipidemia).
- you are planning a pregnancy.
- you have a history of seizures.
- you have trouble sleeping.
- you have a history of hypomania or mania.
- you are unsure how much to take or how often to take it.

Possible Side Effects (natural, expected, and unavoidable drug actions)

Constipation and headache. Weight loss, dry mouth. Small increases in cholesterol (2–3 mg/dl).

▷ **Possible Adverse Effects** (unusual, unexpected, and infrequent reactions)

If any of the following develop, consult your physician promptly for guidance.

Mild Adverse Effects

Allergic reactions: not characterized.

Palpitations—rare.

Nausea and vomiting—infrequent.

Dizziness (may disappear without treatment), fatigue, and headache—infrequent to frequent.

Anxiety, somnolence or insomnia (may stop on its own).

Blurred vision—possible.

Sweating—possible.

Serious Adverse Effects

Allergic reactions: none reported.

Idiosyncratic reactions: none reported.

SIADH and very low sodium—case reports.

Increased blood pressure—case reports.

Seizures—very rare during premarketing studies.

▷ **Possible Effects on Sexual Function:**   Delayed orgasm, abnormal ejaculation, impotence, and erectile failure—all rare.

Possible Delayed Adverse Effects: None reported.

▷ **Adverse Effects That May Mimic Natural Diseases or Disorders**
None reported.

Natural Diseases or Disorders That May Be Activated by This Drug
None reported.

Possible Effects on Laboratory Tests
Serum cholesterol: increased slightly.

CAUTION
1. This drug should not be taken with monoamine oxidase (MAO) inhibitor (see Glossary) drugs. If you have recently stopped an MAO inhibitor, 14 days should pass before venlafaxine is started.

▷ **Advisability of Use During Pregnancy**
Pregnancy Category: C. See Pregnancy Risk Categories at the back of this book.
Animal studies: There was an increase in stillborn rats at 10 times the usual human dose.
Human studies: Adequate studies of pregnant women are not available.
Ask your doctor for guidance.

Advisability of Use If Breast-Feeding
Presence of this drug in breast milk: Unknown.
Monitor nursing infant closely and discontinue drug or nursing if adverse effects develop.

Habit-Forming Potential: None.

Effects of Overdose: Nausea, vomiting, constipation, seizure potential.

Possible Effects of Long-Term Use: None noted.

Suggested Periodic Examinations While Taking This Drug (at physician's discretion)
Blood pressure checks.

▷ **While Taking This Drug, Observe the Following**
Foods: No restrictions.
Nutritional Support: No special support indicated.
Beverages: Since venlafaxine is metabolized in the liver, and grapefruit juice has been shown to inhibit the removal (metabolism) of some other medications, caution is advised. Water is the best liquid to take this medicine with.
▷ *Alcohol:* May increase somnolence if combined.
Tobacco Smoking: No interactions expected. I advise everyone to quit smoking.
Marijuana Smoking: Additive effect on somnolence.
▷ *Other Drugs*
Venlafaxine *taken concurrently* with
- beta-blockers (see Drug Classes) may result in larger than expected pharmacological effects from the beta-blockers. Because these agents are metabolized in the liver, and venlafaxine may block this metabolism, caution is advised.
- calcium channel blockers (see Drug Classes) may result in toxicity. Because these agents are metabolized in the liver, and venlafaxine may block this metabolism, caution is advised.
- cimetidine (Tagamet) may lead to venlafaxine toxicity.
- drugs with sedative properties will increase those effects.
- MAO inhibitors may lead to undesirable side effects. Do not combine.
- quinidine (Quinaglute, others) may result in venlafaxine toxicity.
- ritonavir (Norvir) may lead to venlafaxine toxicity.

- sibutramine (Meridia) increases toxicity risk (serotonin syndrome). DO NOT combine.
- sumatriptan (Imitrex) may lead to incoordination and weakness. DO NOT combine.
- tricyclic antidepressants (see Drug Classes) may result in toxicity. Because these agents are metabolized in the liver, and venlafaxine may block this metabolism, caution is advised.
- warfarin (Coumadin) may result in bleeding. More frequent INR (prothrombin time or protime) testing is needed. Ongoing warfarin doses should be adjusted to laboratory results.
- zolmitriptan (Zomig) may lead to incoordination and weakness. DO NOT combine.

▷ *Driving, Hazardous Activities:* This drug may cause somnolence. Restrict activities as necessary.

Aviation Note: The use of this drug *is a disqualification* for piloting. Consult a designated aviation medical examiner.

Exposure to Sun: No restrictions.

Exposure to Heat: No restrictions.

Discontinuation: If this medicine is to be stopped, the dose should be slowly lowered over 2 to 3 weeks on your doctor's advice.

VERAPAMIL (ver AP a mil)

Introduced: 1967   **Class:** Anti-anginal, antiarrhythmic, antihypertensive, calcium channel blocker   **Prescription:** USA: Yes   **Controlled Drug:** USA: No; Canada: No   **Available as Generic:** USA: Yes (verapamil SR); Canada: No

Brand Names: ✦Apo-Verap, Calan, Calan SR, Isoptin, Isoptin SR, ✦Novo-Veramil, ✦Nu-Verap, Verelan

Controversies in Medicine: Medicines in this class have had many conflicting reports. The FDA has held hearings on the calcium channel blocker (CCB) class. A study called ALLHAT is comparing amlodipine, an ACE inhibitor, a diuretic, and an alpha blocker (see Drug Classes) and should clarify adverse effects, mortality, and other issues relating to CCBs.

Amlodipine got the first FDA approval to treat high blood pressure or angina in people with congestive heart failure. CCBs are currently second, line agents for high blood pressure, according to the JNC VI (see Glossary).

BENEFITS versus RISKS	
Possible Benefits	*Possible Risks*
EFFECTIVE PREVENTION OF BOTH MAJOR TYPES OF ANGINA	Congestive heart failure
	Low blood pressure (infrequent)
EFFECTIVE CONTROL OF HEART RATE IN CHRONIC ATRIAL FIBRILLATION AND FLUTTER	Heart rhythm disturbance
	Fluid retention
	Liver damage without jaundice
EFFECTIVE PREVENTION OF PAROXYSMAL ATRIAL TACHYCARDIA (PAT)	Swelling of male breast tissue
EFFECTIVE TREATMENT OF HYPERTENSION	

▷ **Principal Uses**

As a Single Drug Product: Uses currently included in FDA-approved labeling: Used to treat (1) angina pectoris due to coronary artery spasm (Prinzmetal's variant angina) that occurs spontaneously and is not associated with exertion; (2) classical angina-of-effort (due to atherosclerotic disease of the coronary arteries) in individuals who have not responded to or cannot tolerate the nitrates and beta-blocker drugs customarily used to treat this disorder; (3) abnormally rapid heart rate due to chronic atrial fibrillation or flutter; (4) recurrent paroxysmal atrial tachycardia; and (5) primary hypertension.

Other (unlabeled) generally accepted uses: (1) May help decrease keloid formation; (2) prevents abnormal heart rhythms that occur after surgery; (3) relieves symptoms and may help reverse hypertrophic cardiomyopathy; (4) may help decrease the severity or occurrence of cluster headaches; (5) helps control symptoms of panic attacks; (6) can be of use in post-ischemic-acute-kidney failure; (7) may stop the progression of abnormal buildup on the inside of blood vessels (atherosclerosis); (8) may help decrease severity and occurrence of nocturnal leg cramps; (9) can help stuttering; (10) may have a role in treating Tourette's syndrome.

How This Drug Works: By blocking passage of calcium through certain cell walls (which is necessary for the function of nerve and muscle tissue), this drug slows the spread of electrical activity through the heart and inhibits the contraction of coronary arteries and peripheral arterioles. As a result of these combined effects, this drug

- prevents spontaneous coronary artery spasm (Prinzmetal's type of angina).
- reduces heart rate and contraction force during exertion, thus lowering the oxygen requirement of the heart muscle; this reduces the occurrence of effort-induced angina (classical angina pectoris).
- reduces degree of contraction of peripheral arterial walls, resulting in relaxation and lowering of blood pressure. This further reduces the workload of the heart during exertion and contributes to the prevention of angina.
- slows the rate of electrical impulses through the heart and thereby prevents excessively rapid heart action (tachycardia).

Available Dose Forms and Strengths

Caplets, sustained release — 120 mg, 180 mg, 240 mg
Capsules, sustained release — 360 mg
　　　　　　　　　　　Injection — 5 mg/2 ml
　　　　　　　　　　　Tablets — 40 mg, 80 mg, 120 mg
Tablets, sustained release — 120 mg, 180 mg, 240 mg

▷ **Usual Adult Dose Range:** Hypertension: Initially 80 mg three times daily. The dose may be increased gradually at 1- to 7-day intervals as needed and tolerated. The usual maintenance dose is from 240 to 360 mg daily in three or four divided doses. The prolonged-action (sustained-release) dose forms permit once-a-day dosing. The total daily dose should not exceed 360 mg.

Once-a-day treatment may be initiated with one prolonged-action capsule of 120 mg or one tablet of 180 mg.

Note: Actual dose and schedule must be determined for each patient individually.

Conditions Requiring Dosing Adjustments

Liver Function: Blood levels should be obtained to guide dosing. In liver disease, dose should be decreased to 20–50% of usual doses at the usual times. This drug is also a rare cause of liver damage. Electrocardiogram changes may provide an early indication of increasing blood levels.

Kidney Function: In severe kidney compromise, the dose should be decreased by 50–75%.

▷ **Dosing Instructions:**   Preferably taken with meals and with food at bedtime. The regular tablet may be crushed for administration. The prolonged-action dose forms (capsules and tablets) should be swallowed whole and not altered. Verelan capsules may be taken without regard to food intake.

Usual Duration of Use: Use on a regular schedule for 2 to 4 weeks usually determines effectiveness in reducing the frequency and severity of angina. Reduction of elevated blood pressure may be apparent within the first 1 to 2 weeks. For long-term use (months to years), the smallest effective dose should be used. Periodic physician evaluation is needed.

Possible Advantages of This Drug

No adverse effects on blood levels of glucose, potassium, or uric acid.

Does not increase blood cholesterol or triglyceride levels.

Does not impair capacity for exercise.

The new 360-mg strength of Verelan allows once-daily dosing for those patients who require more than 240 mg daily. The company has noted that there is no increase in side effects when comparing the 240-mg capsules to the new 360-mg ones.

Currently a "Drug of Choice"

For treating hypertension in African-Americans.

▷ **This Drug Should Not Be Taken If**

- you have had an allergic reaction to it previously.
- you have active liver disease.
- you have a "sick sinus" syndrome (and do not have an artificial pacemaker).
- you have a fast heart rate (ventricular tachycardia) arising in the ventricles.
- you have been told that you have a second- or third-degree heart block.
- you have low blood pressure (systolic pressure below 90).
- you have advanced aortic stenosis (ask your doctor).

▷ **Inform Your Physician Before Taking This Drug If**

- you have had an unfavorable response to any calcium channel blocker.
- you are currently taking any other drugs, especially digitalis or a beta-blocker drug (see Drug Classes).
- you have had a recent stroke or heart attack.
- you have a history of congestive heart failure or heart rhythm disorders.
- you have poor circulation to your extremities, or gangrene.
- you have impaired liver or kidney function.
- you have a history of drug-induced liver damage.

Possible Side Effects (natural, expected, and unavoidable drug actions)

Low blood pressure, fluid retention—rare.

▷ **Possible Adverse Effects** (unusual, unexpected, and infrequent reactions)

If any of the following develop, consult your physician promptly for guidance.

Mild Adverse Effects

Allergic reactions: skin rash, hives, itching, aching joints.

Headache—frequent; dizziness, fatigue—infrequent.

Nausea, indigestion, constipation—rare.

Abnormal growth of the gums—infrequent.

Sensation of numbness or coldness in the extremities—case reports.

Serious Adverse Effects

Serious disturbances of heart rate and/or rhythm, congestive heart failure—rare.

Drug-induced liver damage without jaundice—case reports.

Antiplatelet effect and extended time to form blood clots—possible.

Excessive lowering of blood pressure—case reports.

Unmasking of parkinsonism—rare.

Low blood sugar—possible.

▷ **Possible Effects on Sexual Function:** Altered timing and pattern of menstruation.

Male breast enlargement and tenderness (gynecomastia)—case reports.

Impotence—frequent.

Possible Effects on Laboratory Tests

Blood total cholesterol and HDL cholesterol levels: no effect in some; decreased in others.

Blood LDL cholesterol or triglyceride level: no effect.

Glucose tolerance test (GTT): decreased.

Liver function tests: increased enzymes (ALT/GPT, AST/GOT), increased bilirubin (one case report).

CAUTION

1. Be sure to inform all physicians and other health care professionals who provide medical care for you that you take this drug. Note the use of this drug on your personal identification card.
2. You may use nitroglycerin and other nitrate drugs as needed to relieve acute episodes of angina pain. If angina attacks become more frequent or intense, call your doctor promptly.
3. If this drug is used concurrently with a beta-blocker drug, you may develop excessively low blood pressure.
4. This drug may cause swelling of the feet and ankles. This may not be indicative of either heart or kidney dysfunction.

Precautions for Use

By Infants and Children: Safety and effectiveness for those under 12 years of age are not established.

By Those Over 60 Years of Age: You may be more susceptible to weakness, dizziness, fainting, and falling. Take necessary precautions to prevent injury. Report promptly any changes in your pattern of thirst and urination.

▷ **Advisability of Use During Pregnancy**

Pregnancy Category: C. See Pregnancy Risk Categories at the back of this book.

Animal studies: Toxic effects on the embryo and retarded growth of the fetus (but no birth defects) reported in rat studies.

Human studies: Adequate studies of pregnant women are not available.

Avoid this drug during the first 3 months. Use during the final 6 months only if clearly needed. Ask your doctor for help.

Advisability of Use If Breast-Feeding

Presence of this drug in breast milk: Yes.

Discuss the benefits and risks of nursing your infant. Most clinicians find drug breast milk levels to be insignificant. Monitor infant for adverse effects.

Habit-Forming Potential: None.

Effects of Overdose: Flushed and warm skin, sweating, light-headedness, irritability, rapid heart rate, low blood pressure, loss of consciousness.

Possible Effects of Long-Term Use: None reported.

Suggested Periodic Examinations While Taking This Drug (at physician's discretion)

Evaluations of heart function, including electrocardiograms; liver and kidney function tests, with long-term use.

▷ **While Taking This Drug, Observe the Following**

Foods: Do NOT take this medicine with grapefruit or grapefruit juice.

Avoid excessive salt intake.

Beverages: Caffeine levels will be increased if caffeine-containing beverages are consumed while you are on verapamil. Do NOT take this medicine with grapefruit or grapefruit juice.

May be taken with milk.

▷ *Alcohol:* Use with caution until combined effects have been determined. Alcohol may exaggerate the drop in blood pressure, and change the elimination of alcohol (experienced by some patients).

Tobacco Smoking: Nicotine can reduce the effectiveness of this drug. Avoid all forms of tobacco.

Marijuana Smoking: Possible reduced effectiveness of this drug; mild to moderate increase in angina; possible changes in electrocardiogram, confusing interpretation.

▷ *Other Drugs*

Verapamil may *increase* the effects of

- carbamazepine (Tegretol), and cause carbamazepine toxicity.
- digitoxin and digoxin, and cause digitalis toxicity.

Verapamil *taken concurrently* with

- aspirin may result in bleeding.
- amiodarone (Cordarone) may result in cardiac arrest.
- beta-blocker drugs (see Drug Classes) may affect heart rate and rhythm adversely. Careful monitoring by your physician is necessary if these drugs are taken concurrently.
- calcium supplements (various) may blunt the therapeutic benefits of verapamil. Separate calcium and verapamil dosing by 2 hours.
- cyclosporine (Sandimmune) may result in cyclosporine toxicity and renal compromise.
- dantrolene will cause elevated blood potassium and depression of the heart.
- disopyramide (Norpace) can cause congestive heart failure.
- lithium (Lithobid, others) may result in lithium toxicity and mania.
- NSAIDs (nonsteroidal anti-inflammatory drugs; see Drug Classes) may blunt the therapeutic effect of verapamil on blood pressure.
- oral hypoglycemic agents (see *oral antidiabetic drugs* in Drug Classes) may lead to excessively low blood sugar.
- phenytoin (Dilantin) may result in decreased effectiveness of verapamil.
- quinidine (Quinaglute, others) can result in quinidine toxicity.

- rifampin (Rifadin, others) will decrease the therapeutic benefits of verapamil.
- sulfinpyrazone increases the removal of verapamil and lessens its therapeutic effects.
- terazosin (Hytrin) can lead to excessive decreases in blood pressure.
- theophylline (Theo-Dur, others) can lead to theophylline toxicity.

The following drugs may *increase* the effects of verapamil:

- cimetidine (Tagamet) and other histamine (H_2) blocking drugs (see Drug Classes).
- ritonavir (Norvir), and perhaps other protease inhibitors (see Drug Classes).
- tricyclic antidepressants (see Drug Classes).

▷ *Driving, Hazardous Activities:* Usually no restrictions. This drug may cause dizziness. Restrict activities as necessary.

Aviation Note: Coronary artery disease *is a disqualification* for piloting. Consult a designated aviation medical examiner.

Exposure to Sun: Use caution until sensitivity has been determined. This drug may cause photosensitivity (see Glossary).

Exposure to Heat: Caution is advised. Hot environments can exaggerate the blood-pressure-lowering effects of this drug. Watch for light-headedness or weakness.

Heavy Exercise or Exertion: This drug may improve your ability to be more active without resulting angina pain. Use caution and avoid excessive exercise that could impair heart function in the absence of warning pain.

Discontinuation: Do not stop this drug abruptly. Consult your physician regarding gradual withdrawal to prevent the development of rebound angina.

WARFARIN (WAR far in)

Introduced: 1941　**Class:** Anticoagulant, coumarins　**Prescription:**
USA: Yes　**Controlled Drug:** USA: No; Canada: No　**Available as Generic:**
USA: Yes; Canada: No

Brand Names: Coumadin, Warfarin Sodium

BENEFITS versus RISKS	
Possible Benefits	*Possible Risks*
EFFECTIVE PREVENTION OF BOTH ARTERIAL AND VENOUS THROMBOSIS	NARROW TREATMENT RANGE Dose-related bleeding Skin and soft tissue hemorrhage with tissue death
EFFECTIVE PREVENTION OF EMBOLIZATION IN THROMBOEMBOLIC DISORDERS	
HELPS PREVENT RECURRENCE OF HEART ATTACK	
HELPS PREVENT STROKES IN PATIENTS WITH ATRIAL FIBRILLATION	

▷ **Principal Uses**

As a Single Drug Product: Uses currently included in FDA-approved labeling: Used in (1) acute thrombosis (clot) or thrombophlebitis of the deep veins; (2) acute pulmonary embolism, resulting from blood clots that originate anywhere in the body; (3) atrial fibrillation, to prevent clotting of blood inside the heart that could result in embolization of small clots to any part of the body; (4) acute myocardial infarction (heart attack), to prevent clotting and embolization and therefore a recurrence of heart attack; (5) mitral valve replacement; (6) helps prevent blood clots in the lungs (pulmonary embolism) that may start after hip replacement surgery.

Other (unlabeled) generally accepted uses: (1) Helps prevent embolization from the heart in individuals with artificial heart valves; (2) may help patients with low blood platelets caused by heparin.

How This Drug Works: The coumarin anticoagulants interfere with the production of four essential blood clotting factors by blocking the action of vitamin K. This leads to a deficiency of these clotting factors in circulating blood and inhibits blood clotting mechanisms.

Available Dose Forms and Strengths

Injection — 5 mg

Tablets — 1 mg, 2 mg, 2.5 mg, 5 mg, 7.5 mg, 10 mg

▷ **Usual Adult Dose Range:** Initially 2 to 5 mg daily for 2 to 3 days. A large loading dose is inappropriate and may be hazardous. For ongoing use, the dose is decided based on INR (prothrombin time or protime) results and the condition being treated. In many conditions an INR of 2 to 3 is considered therapeutic. **Note: Actual dose and schedule must be determined for each patient individually.**

Conditions Requiring Dosing Adjustments

Liver Function: Blood testing (prothrombin times) should be obtained to guide dosing. This drug is contraindicated in patients with liver disease.

Kidney Function: This drug should be used with caution in renal compromise, as warfarin may cause microscopic kidney stones.

▷ **Dosing Instructions:** The tablet may be crushed and is preferably taken when the stomach is empty, and at the same time each day to ensure uniform results.

Usual Duration of Use: Use on a regular schedule for 3 to 5 days usually determines effectiveness in providing significant anticoagulation. An additional 10 to 14 days is required to determine the optimal maintenance dose for each individual. Long-term use (months to years) requires physician supervision.

▷ **This Drug Should Not Be Taken If**

- you have had an allergic reaction to it previously.
- you have an active peptic ulcer or active ulcerative colitis.
- you are pregnant.
- you have had recent anesthesia (lumbar block) to the spine.
- you have arterial aneurysm.
- you have low blood platelets.
- you have infective pericarditis.
- you have liver disease.

- you have esophageal varices (ask your doctor).
- you have had a recent stroke.

▷ **Inform Your Physician Before Taking This Drug If**
- you are now taking *any other drugs*, either prescription drugs or over-the-counter drug products.
- you are planning pregnancy.
- you have a history of a bleeding disorder.
- you have high blood pressure.
- you have abnormally heavy or prolonged menstrual bleeding.
- you have diabetes.
- you are using an indwelling catheter.
- you have impaired liver or kidney function.
- you will have surgery or dental extraction.

Possible Side Effects (natural, expected, and unavoidable drug actions)
Minor episodes of bleeding may occur even though dose and prothrombin times are well within the recommended range.

▷ **Possible Adverse Effects** (unusual, unexpected, and infrequent reactions)
If any of the following develop, consult your physician promptly for guidance.
Mild Adverse Effects
Allergic reactions: skin rash, hives.
Loss of scalp hair—case reports.
Loss of appetite, nausea, vomiting, cramping, diarrhea—case reports.
Serious Adverse Effects
Allergic reactions: drug fever (see Glossary).
Idiosyncratic reactions: bleeding into skin and soft tissues, causing gangrene of breast, toes, and localized areas anywhere—rare.
Hereditary warfarin resistance—rare.
Abnormal bleeding from nose, gastrointestinal tract, lungs, urinary tract, or uterus—possible and dose related.
Pericardial tamponade—case reports.
Hemolytic anemia—rare.
Sudden nerve damage (femoral neuropathy)—case reports.
Kidney problems (tubulointerstitial nephritis)—case reports.
Liver toxicity (viral hepatitis-like syndrome)—case report.

▷ **Possible Effects on Sexual Function:**   None reported.

▷ **Adverse Effects That May Mimic Natural Diseases or Disorders**
Drug-induced fever may suggest infection.

Natural Diseases or Disorders That May Be Activated by This Drug
Bleeding from "silent" peptic ulcer, intestinal or bladder polyp or tumor.

Possible Effects on Laboratory Tests
Complete blood cell counts: decreased red cells, hemoglobin, and white cells.
Bleeding time: increased.
INR (prothrombin time): increased.
Blood uric acid level: increased (in men).
Liver function tests: increased liver enzymes (ALT/GPT, AST/GOT, and alkaline phosphatase).

CAUTION

1. Always carry a personal identification card that includes a statement that *you are taking an anticoagulant drug.* A medicine alert bracelet is also prudent.
2. While taking this drug, always consult your physician *before* starting any new drug, changing the dose schedule of any drug, or stopping any drug.
3. Data from the Agency for Health Care Policy and Research have shown that expanded use of warfarin could cut in half the 80,000 strokes that occur every year in patients who have atrial fibrillation.
4. If you start taking the brand name form, it is prudent to keep taking the brand name form. Conversely, if you have your anticoagulation adjusted using the generic form, it is prudent to continue the generic form. Changing from one form to the other may result in differences in degree of anticoagulation.
5. If you choose to use acetaminophen while taking this medicine, talk to your doctor about adjusting the warfarin dose or more frequent INR testing.

Precautions for Use

By Those Over 60 Years of Age: Small starting doses are mandatory. Watch regularly for excessive drug effects: prolonged bleeding from shaving cuts, bleeding gums, bloody urine, rectal bleeding, excessive bruising. Some study data reveal that the beneficial effects of this medicine are not as widely known as needed and it is underprescribed for those over 60.

▷ **Advisability of Use During Pregnancy**

Pregnancy Category: X. See Pregnancy Risk Categories at the back of this book.
Animal studies: Fetal hemorrhage and death due to this drug reported in mice.
Human studies: Information from studies of pregnant women indicates fetal defects and fetal hemorrhage due to this drug.
The manufacturers state that this drug is contraindicated during entire pregnancy.

Advisability of Use If Breast-Feeding

Presence of this drug in breast milk: Yes.
Avoid drug or refrain from nursing.

Habit-Forming Potential: None.

Effects of Overdose: Episodes of bleeding, ranging from minor surface bleeding (nose, gums, small lacerations) to major internal bleeding (vomiting blood, bloody urine or stool).

Possible Effects of Long-Term Use: None reported.

Suggested Periodic Examinations While Taking This Drug (at physician's discretion)

Regular determinations of INR (prothrombin time or protime) are essential to safe dose and proper control. Urine analyses for blood.

▷ **While Taking This Drug, Observe the Following**

Foods: A larger intake than usual of foods rich in vitamin K may reduce the effectiveness of this drug and make larger doses necessary. Foods rich in vitamin K include asparagus, bacon, beef liver, cabbage, fish, cauliflower, and green leafy vegetables. Vitamin E may increase risk of bleeding.

Beverages: No restrictions. May be taken with milk.
▷ *Alcohol:* Limit alcohol to one drink daily. Note: Heavy users of alcohol with liver damage may be very sensitive to anticoagulants and require smaller than usual doses.

Tobacco Smoking: Heavy smokers may require relatively larger doses of this drug. I advise everyone to quit smoking.
▷ *Other Drugs*

Warfarin may ***increase*** the effects of
- oral hypoglycemic agents (see *oral antidiabetic drugs* in Drug Classes).
- phenytoin (Dilantin).

The following drugs may ***increase*** the effects of warfarin:
- acetaminophen (Tylenol, others).
- allopurinol (Zyloprim).
- amiodarone (Cordarone).
- androgens (see Drug Classes).
- aspirin and some other NSAIDs (see *nonsteroidal anti-inflammatory drugs* in Drug Classes).
- azithromycin (Zithromax).
- bismuth subsalicylate (Pepto-Bismol).
- carbamazepine (Tegretol).
- cephalosporins (see Drug Classes).
- chloral hydrate (Noctec).
- chloramphenicol (Chloromycetin).
- cimetidine (Tagamet).
- ciprofloxacin and other quinolone antibiotics.
- cisapride (Propulsid).
- clarithromycin (Biaxin).
- clofibrate (Atromid-S).
- cotrimoxazole (Bactrim).
- dextrothyroxine.
- dirithromycin and other macrolide antibiotics (see Drug Classes).
- disopyramide (Norpace).
- disulfiram (Antabuse).
- enoxaparin (Lovenox)
- erythromycin (various).
- felbamate (Felbatol).
- fluconazole (Diflucan).
- fluoxetine (Prozac).
- fluvastatin (Lescol), and perhaps similar drugs.
- fluvoxamine (Luvox).
- gemfibrozil (Lopid).
- glucagon.
- grepafloxacin (Raxar).
- HMG CoA-reductase inhibitors (see Drug Classes).
- influenza vaccine (various).
- isoniazid (INH).
- itraconazole (Sporanox).
- ketoconazole (Nizoral).
- mesna (Mesnex).
- metronidazole (Flagyl).

- miconazole (Monistat).
- nonsteroidal anti-inflammatory drugs (NSAIDs; see Drug Classes).
- omeprazole (Prilosec).
- pravastatin (Pravachol).
- propranolol (Inderal).
- quinidine (Quinaglute).
- ranitidine (Zantac).
- ritonavir (Norvir), and perhaps other protease inhibitors (see Drug Classes).
- salicylates (aspirin, etc.).
- sertraline (Zoloft).
- simvastatin (Zocor).
- streptokinase.
- sulfinpyrazone (Anturane).
- sulfonamides (see Drug Classes).
- tamoxifen (Nolvadex).
- tetracyclines (see Drug Classes).
- thyroid hormones (various).
- tramadol (Ultram).
- tricyclic antidepressants (see Drug Classes).
- vancomycin (Vancoled).
- vitamin E.
- zafirlukast (Accolate).
- zileuton (Zyflo).

The following drugs may *decrease* the effects of warfarin:
- azathioprine (Imuran).
- barbiturates (see Drug Classes).
- birth control pills (oral contraceptives).
- carbamazepine (Tegretol).
- cholestyramine (Questran).
- estrogens (unclear, but possible).
- ethchlorvynol (Placidyl).
- glutethimide (Doriden).
- griseofulvin (Gris-PEG).
- phytonadione (vitamin K).
- primidone (Mysoline).
- some penicillins (see Drug Classes).
- spironolactone.
- sucralfate (Carafate).
- rifampin (Rifadin).
- thiazide diuretics (see Drug Classes).
- vitamin K.

▷ *Driving, Hazardous Activities:* No restrictions.

Aviation Note: The use of this drug *is a disqualification* for piloting. Consult a designated aviation medical examiner.

Exposure to Sun: No restrictions.

Discontinuation: Do not stop this drug abruptly unless abnormal bleeding occurs. Ask your physician for guidance regarding gradual reduction in dose over a period of 3 to 4 weeks.

ZALCITABINE (zal SIT a been)

Other Names: Dideoxycytidine, DDC

Introduced: 1987   **Class:** Antiviral, anti-AIDS drug   **Prescription:** USA: Yes   **Controlled Drug:** USA: No; Canada: No   **Available as Generic:** USA: No

Brand Name: Hivid

BENEFITS versus RISKS	
Possible Benefits	*Possible Risks*
DELAYED PROGRESSION OF DISEASE IN HIV-INFECTED PATIENTS	DRUG-INDUCED PERIPHERAL NEURITIS
PART OF EFFECTIVE COMBINATION REGIMENS	Drug-induced pancreatitis, esophageal ulcers, or arthritis
	Drug-induced cardiomyopathy/congestive heart failure

▷ **Principal Uses**

As a Single Drug Product: Uses currently included in FDA-approved labeling: (1) This drug is approved for advanced (CD4 cell count less than or equal to 300 cells per cubic mm) HIV infection in adults who do not tolerate alternative antiretroviral therapy or have progression of their disease while taking alternative antiretrovirals; (2) used in combination therapy with zidovudine in patients with limited prior treatment with zidovudine (< 3 months); (3) pediatric AIDS. Note: This drug is not a cure for AIDS.

Author's Note: *The Panel on Clinical Practices for Treatment of HIV Infection Report* says that the preferred regimen is two nucleoside analogs and one potent protease inhibitor. Single-agent therapy was rejected by the panel.

Other (unlabeled) generally accepted uses: Combination therapy with protease inhibitors.

How This Drug Works: By interfering with essential HIV enzyme systems, this drug is thought to prevent the growth and reproduction of HIV particles within infected cells, thus limiting the severity and extent of HIV infection.

Available Dose Forms and Strengths

Tablets — 0.375 mg, 0.75 mg

▷ **Recommended Dose Ranges** (Actual dose and schedule must be determined for each patient individually.)

Infants and Children: Under investigation.

12 to 60 Years of Age: The recommended combination regimen is one 0.75-mg tablet every 8 hours. In combination therapy: one 0.75-mg tablet orally, to be taken with 200 mg of zidovudine every 8 hours. The total daily dose for both drugs then becomes 2.25 mg of zalcitabine and 600 mg of zidovudine. The initial dose does not need to be reduced unless the patient has a body mass of less than 30 kg (66 lb).

Conditions Requiring Dosing Adjustments

Liver Function: Liver toxicity more likely in people with a prior history of alcohol abuse or liver damage. Patients should watched closely, and dose reduced or drug interrupted if toxicity occurs. Those with liver function enzymes more than five times the upper limit of the normal range should stop the drug.

Kidney Function: Patients with moderate kidney failure can take 0.75 mg of zalcitabine every 12 hours. In severe kidney failure, the patient can take 0.75 mg every 24 hours.

▷ **Dosing Instructions:**   When combination therapy is being given, dose adjustments must be based on the toxicity profiles for each drug. For example: if peripheral neuropathy or severe oral ulcers occur, the zalcitabine dose should be decreased or interrupted. Second, if the patient experiences anemia or granulocytopenia, the zidovudine dose should be decreased or interrupted. If the zalcitabine is interrupted or stopped, the zidovudine dose should be changed from 200 mg every 8 hours to 100 mg every 4 hours. If zalcitabine is stopped, the physician **must** consider alternative antiretroviral therapy.

The largest peak concentration, the time that it takes for the peak to be achieved, and the amount absorbed are all changed if this drug is taken with food. It is better to take this medication on an empty stomach.

Usual Duration of Use: Use on a regular schedule for several months usually determines effectiveness in slowing the progression of AIDS. Long-term use (months to years) requires periodic physician evaluation of response (viral load and CD4) and dose adjustment.

Possible Advantages of This Drug

Does not cause serious depression of bone marrow function (production of blood cells).

▷ **This Drug Should Not Be Taken If**
- you have had an allergic reaction to it previously.
- you have had pancreatitis recently.
- you have severe myelosuppression (ask your doctor).

▷ **Inform Your Physician Before Taking This Drug If**
- you have had allergic reactions to any drugs in the past.
- you are taking any other drugs currently.
- you have a history of pancreatitis or peripheral neuritis.
- you have a history of severe myelosuppression (ask your doctor).
- you have a history of esophageal ulcers.
- you have congestive heart failure or cardiac muscle damage (cardiac myopathy).
- you have a history of alcoholism.
- you have impaired liver or kidney function.

Possible Side Effects (natural, expected, and unavoidable drug actions)

Mild and infrequent decreases in red blood cell, white blood cell, and platelet counts.

▷ **Possible Adverse Effects** (unusual, unexpected, and infrequent reactions)
   If any of the following develop, consult your physician promptly for guidance.

Mild Adverse Effects

Allergic reactions: skin rash and itching.

Fever, joint pains—infrequent.

Ringing in the ears—case reports.

Mouth sores, nausea, vomiting, diarrhea, stomach pain—infrequent.

Serious Adverse Effects

Allergic reactions: anaphylaxis—rare.

Drug-induced peripheral neuritis (see Glossary), usually occurring after 7 to 18 weeks of treatment. This is more frequent and severe with high doses, and less frequent and mild with low doses.

Drug-induced cardiomyopathy/congestive heart failure—infrequent.

Drug-induced pancreatitis (may happen in the first 6 months of treatment)— rare.

Electrolyte changes (lowered phosphorous, sodium, magnesium, or calcium)—rare to infrequent.

Ototoxicity and hearing loss—rare.

Lowered white blood cell counts—infrequent.

Worsening of preexisting liver disease or hepatotoxicity—rare.

▷ **Possible Effects on Sexual Function:**   None reported.

▷ **Adverse Effects That May Mimic Natural Diseases or Disorders**

None reported to date.

Possible Effects on Laboratory Tests

Complete blood cell counts: decreased red cells, white cells, and platelets (infrequent and mild).

Blood amylase level: increased (infrequent).

Blood glucose level: increased.

Liver function tests: increased (SGOT, SGPT, and LDH).

CD4: increased.

Viral burden: decreased.

CAUTION

1. This drug does not cure HIV infection.
2. Call your doctor right away if stomach pain with nausea and vomiting occurs; this could indicate the onset of pancreatitis. It may be necessary to discontinue this drug.
3. MOST clinicians advocate combination therapy.
4. Pain, numbness, tingling, or burning in the hands or feet should prompt a call to your doctor; this could indicate the onset of peripheral neuritis. Drug may need to be stopped.
5. Best to avoid all other drugs known to cause pancreatitis or peripheral neuritis; ask your physician for guidance.

Precautions for Use

By Infants and Children: Safety and effectiveness for use by this age group have not been established. Children may also be at risk for developing drug-induced pancreatitis and peripheral neuritis; monitor closely for significant symptoms.

By Those Over 60 Years of Age: Reduced kidney function may require dose reduction.

▷ **Advisability of Use During Pregnancy**

Pregnancy Category: C. See Pregnancy Risk Categories at the back of this book.

Animal studies: This drug has been shown to be teratogenic in mice at doses of 1,365 and 2,730 times of the maximum recommended human dose

(MRHD). Increased embryolethality was observed in mice with doses of 2,730 times the MRHD.

Human studies: Information from adequate studies of pregnant women is not available. The manufacturer recommends that fertile women should not receive zalcitabine unless they are using effective contraception during therapy.

Consult your physician for specific guidance.

Advisability of Use If Breast-Feeding

Presence of this drug in breast milk: Unknown.

Avoid drug or refrain from nursing.

Note: HIV has been found in human breast milk. Breast-feeding may result in transmission of HIV infection to the nursing infant.

Habit-Forming Potential: None.

Effects of Overdose: Nausea, vomiting, stomach pain, diarrhea, hand and foot pain.

Possible Effects of Long-Term Use: Peripheral neuritis (see Glossary).

Suggested Periodic Examinations While Taking This Drug (at physician's discretion)

Complete blood cell counts before starting treatment and weekly thereafter until tolerance is established.

Blood amylase levels, fractionated for salivary gland and pancreatic origin.

Triglyceride levels should be tested at baseline (before therapy is started) and periodically during therapy.

Assessment of CD4 counts and viral load. These tell of pending failure and reason to change to other agents.

▷ **While Taking This Drug, Observe the Following**

Foods: No restrictions.

Beverages: No restrictions.

▷ *Alcohol:* No interactions expected.

Tobacco Smoking: No interactions expected. I advise everyone to quit smoking.

▷ *Other Drugs*

Zalcitabine may ***increase*** the effects of
- zidovudine (Retrovir), and enhance its antiviral effect against HIV. Serious patient reactions to either of these medicines should be reported to the FDA.

Zalcitabine ***taken concurrently*** with
- cimetidine (Tagamet) may result in toxic zalcitabine levels.
- didanosine (Videx) may result in additive neurotoxicity.
- metoclopramide (Reglan) may result in lowered blood levels of zalcitabine and reduced therapeutic benefits.
- other drugs that cause neurotoxicity or pancreatitis—this combination is best avoided.
- probenecid (Benemid) may lead to zalcitabine toxicity.
- saquinavir (Invirase) did not change drug levels of saquinavir, zalcitabine, and zidovudine (in combination therapy).

▷ *Driving, Hazardous Activities:* This drug may cause pain and weakness in the extremities. Restrict activities as necessary.

Aviation Note: The use of this drug ***is a disqualification*** for piloting. Consult a designated aviation medical examiner.

Exposure to Sun: No restrictions.

Discontinuation: Do not stop this drug without your physician's knowledge and guidance.

ZIDOVUDINE (zi DOH vyoo deen)

Other Names: AZT, azidothymidine, Compound S, ZDV

Introduced: 1987 **Class:** Antiviral, anti-AIDS drugs **Prescription:** USA: Yes **Controlled Drug:** USA: No; Canada: No **Available as Generic:** USA: No; Canada: No

Brand Name: Retrovir, Combivir

BENEFITS versus RISKS	
Possible Benefits	*Possible Risks*
DELAYED PROGRESSION OF DISEASE IN HIV-INFECTED PATIENTS WHEN COMBINATION TREATMENT IS USED REDUCED INCIDENCE OF INFECTIONS WITH COMBINATION THERAPY	SERIOUS BONE MARROW DEPRESSION Brain toxicity Lip, mouth, and tongue sores

▷ **Principal Uses**

As a Single Drug Product: Uses currently included in FDA-approved labeling: (1) Used to treat selected patients who have acquired immunodeficiency syndrome (AIDS); (2) approved to help prevent transmission of HIV from mother to infant; (3) approved for combination therapy with other agents; (4) approved for children 3 months or older who have laboratory values that indicate HIV infection or HIV immunosuppression; (5) approved for use in HIV-positive patients who are as yet asymptomatic. Note: This drug is not a cure for AIDS, and it does not reduce the risk of transmission of AIDS infection to others through sexual contact or contamination of blood.

Author's Note: *The Panel on Clinical Practices for Treatment of HIV Infection Report* says that the preferred regimen is two nucleoside analogs and one potent protease inhibitor. Single-agent therapy (with the exception of AZT use in preventing HIV transmission from mother to fetus) was rejected by the panel. One researcher has questioned the effects zidovudine may have in decreasing later benefits of other HIV medicines. Further research is needed.

Other (unlabeled) generally accepted uses: (1) Used to treat Kaposi's sarcoma; (2) helps remove hairy leukoplakia in the mouth; (3) used to treat heart dysfunction in people with HIV; (4) may prevent HIV in health care workers exposed to the AIDS virus (combined with other HIV medicines); (5) appears to increase AIDS-related low platelet counts; (6) may have a role in treating adult T-cell leukemia or lymphoma with interferon alpha.

Author's Note: Although this drug has historically been used as a single drug to treat AIDS, a medical consensus has developed that limits the use of this drug to combination therapy.

How This Drug Works: By interfering with essential enzyme systems, this drug is thought to prevent the growth and reproduction of HIV particles within tissue cells, thus limiting the severity and extent of HIV infection.

Available Dose Forms and Strengths

> Capsules — 100 mg
> Injection — 10 mg/ml
> Syrup — 50 mg/5 ml
> Tablet (Combivir) — lamivudine 150 mg
> — zidovudine 300 mg

▷ **Usual Adult Dose Range:**   HIV infection: The product information insert for zidovudine recommends 600 mg daily, divided into equal doses in combination with other antiretroviral agents. Further, 500 mg as 100 mg every 4 hours while awake or 600 mg daily divided into equal doses is suggested for monotherapy.

Research into twice daily dosing is ongoing.

Combivir form: One tablet twice daily.

For prevention of maternal fetal transmission in pregnancy: 100 mg by mouth five times per day until the start of labor. During labor, AZT is given intravenously (2 mg per kg of body mass), followed by 1 mg per kg of body mass per hour. This dose is continued until the umbilical cord is clamped. The infant then receives 1.5 mg per kg of body mass every 6 hours.

Note: Actual dose and administration schedule must be determined for each patient individually.

Author's Note: There is controversy as to the ideal time to start antiretroviral therapy. Many clinicians advocate "start early and hit hard."

Conditions Requiring Dosing Adjustments

Liver Function: Dose decreased by 50% or the dosing interval doubled in significant liver disease. Drug can be a rare cause of liver damage, and patients should be followed closely.

Kidney Function: Specific guidelines for dose adjustments in patients with compromised kidneys are not available. This drug should be used with caution in kidney compromise.

▷ **Dosing Instructions:**   Preferably taken on an empty stomach, but may be taken with or following food. Take exactly as prescribed. The capsule may be opened and the contents mixed with food just prior to taking it.

Best to take the capsule with at least 120 ml of water.

Usual Duration of Use: Use on a regular schedule for 10 to 12 weeks usually determines effectiveness in improving the course of symptomatic AIDS infection. Long-term use requires periodic physician evaluation of response (viral load and CD4) and dose adjustment.

▷ **This Drug Should Not Be Taken If**
  • you have had a serious allergic reaction to it previously.
  • you have a serious degree of uncorrected bone marrow depression.

▷ **Inform Your Physician Before Taking This Drug If**
  • you have a history of either folic acid or vitamin B$_{12}$ deficiency.
  • you have impaired liver or kidney function.
  • you take other drugs that can have a bad effect on the bone marrow (are myelosuppressive).

Possible Side Effects (natural, expected, and unavoidable drug actions)
None reported.

▷ **Possible Adverse Effects** (unusual, unexpected, and infrequent reactions)
If any of the following develop, consult your physician promptly for guidance.

Mild Adverse Effects

Allergic reactions: skin rash, hives, itching.

Headache, weakness, drowsiness, dizziness, nervousness, insomnia—infrequent.

Nausea, diarrhea, vomiting, altered taste, lip sores, swollen mouth or tongue—infrequent.

Paresthesias, muscle aches, fever, sweating—infrequent.

Serious Adverse Effects

Allergic reactions: one case report of toxic epidermolysis.

Confusion, loss of speech, twitching, tremors, seizures (representing brain toxicity)—infrequent.

Eye problems (macular edema)—case reports.

Muscle toxicity (myopathy)—infrequent.

Mania or seizures—rare.

Muscle toxicity of the heart (cardiomyopathy)—case reports.

Bone marrow depression (see Glossary): fatigue, weakness, fever, sore throat, abnormal bleeding or bruising. Anemia occurs most commonly after 4 to 6 weeks of treatment; abnormally low white blood cell counts occur after 6 to 8 weeks of treatment—infrequent.

Esophageal ulcers (patients should take this medicine with at least 120 ml of water and not lie down for an hour)—possible.

Liver toxicity—infrequent.

▷ **Possible Effects on Sexual Function: None reported.**

Possible Delayed Adverse Effects: Significant anemia and deficient white blood cell counts may develop after this drug has been discontinued. Myopathy.

▷ **Adverse Effects That May Mimic Natural Diseases or Disorders**
Seizures may suggest the possibility of epilepsy.

Possible Effects on Laboratory Tests
Complete blood cell counts: decreased red cells, hemoglobin, white cells, and platelets.

CAUTION

1. This drug is not a cure for AIDS, nor does it protect completely against other infections or complications. Follow your doctor's instructions. Take all medications exactly as prescribed.
2. This drug does not reduce the risk of transmitting AIDS to others through sexual contact or contamination of the blood. The use of an effective condom is mandatory. Needles for drug administration should not be shared.

Precautions for Use

By Infants and Children: Zidovudine syrup is used in HIV-infected pediatric patients who are greater than 3 months old. The usual dose is 180 mg per square meter.

By Those Over 60 Years of Age: Impaired kidney function will require dose reduction.

▷ **Advisability of Use During Pregnancy**

Pregnancy Category: C. See Pregnancy Risk Categories at the back of this book.

Animal studies: Rat studies reveal no birth defects.

Human studies: Adequate studies of pregnant women are not available.

Consult your physician for specific guidance. This medicine has been shown to dramatically reduce the transference of HIV from mother to infant. If the decision is made to use this medicine in pregnancy, cases should be reported to 1-800-722-9292, extention 8465.

Advisability of Use If Breast-Feeding

Presence of this drug in breast milk: Unknown.

Breast feeding may pass the HIV to the infant. Avoid nursing.

Habit-Forming Potential: None.

Effects of Overdose: Nausea, vomiting, diarrhea, bone marrow depression.

Possible Effects of Long-Term Use: Serious anemia and loss of white blood cells. Muscle toxicity (myopathy).

Suggested Periodic Examinations While Taking This Drug (at physician's discretion)

Complete blood cell counts before starting treatment and weekly thereafter until tolerance is established. Continual monitoring for bone marrow depression is necessary during entire course of treatment. Periodic CD4 counts or measurements of viral load are indicators that treatment is failing and demand change of antiretroviral therapy.

▷ **While Taking This Drug, Observe the Following**

Foods: No restrictions.

Beverages: No restrictions. May be taken with milk.

▷   *Alcohol:* No interactions expected.

Tobacco Smoking: No interactions expected. I advise everyone to quit smoking.

▷   *Other Drugs*

The following drugs may ***increase*** the effects of zidovudine and enhance its toxicity:

- acetaminophen (Tylenol, others).
- acyclovir (Zovirax).
- amphotericin B (Fungizone).
- aspirin.
- benzodiazepines (see Drug Classes).
- cimetidine (Tagamet).
- fluconazole (Diflucan).
- ganciclovir (Cytovene).
- indomethacin.
- interferon alpha, beta-1-A and natural.
- methadone (Dolophine).
- morphine (various).
- probenecid (Benemid).
- sulfonamides (see Drug Classes).

Zidovudine ***taken concurrently*** with

- didanosine may result in increased risk of myelosuppression.

- filgrastim (Neupogen) may help maintain the white blood cell count.
- nimodipine (Nimotop) can increase toxicity to nerves.
- other nucleoside analogs for HIV may lower the ability of other HIV treatment requiring phosphorylation to become active.
- rifampin (Rifadin) can lead to decreased zidovudine blood levels.
- ritonavir (Norvir) may lower zidovudine levels.
- stavudine (D4T) may lessen effectiveness, as both agents are cell cycle specific.
- trimexate may cause additive hematological toxicity.

▷ *Driving, Hazardous Activities:* This drug may cause dizziness or fainting. Restrict activities as necessary.

Aviation Note: The use of this drug *is a disqualification* for piloting. Consult a designated aviation medical examiner.

Exposure to Sun: No restrictions.

Discontinuation: Do not stop this drug without your physician's knowledge and guidance.

ZOLPIDEM (ZOL pi dem)

Introduced: 1993 **Class:** Hypnotic, imidazopyridine **Prescription:** USA: Yes **Controlled Drug:** USA: C-IV*; Canada: prescription **Available as Generic:** USA: No

Brand Name: Ambien

BENEFITS versus RISKS	
Possible Benefits	*Possible Risks*
GIVES SHORT-TERM RELIEF OF INSOMNIA WITH MINIMAL SLEEP DISRUPTION (REM)	Habit-forming potential with prolonged use

▷ **Principal Uses**

As a Single Drug Product: Uses currently included in FDA-approved labeling: Short-term treatment of insomnia in adults.

Other (unlabeled) generally accepted uses: Long-term (more than 1 year) treatment of insomnia has been accomplished successfully in limited trials.

How This Drug Works: This drug attaches (binds) to a specific receptor (omega-1) and reduces the time it takes to fall asleep, thus increasing total sleep time while producing a pattern and benefit of sleep that is similar to normal sleep patterns.

Available Dose Forms and Strengths

Tablets — 5 mg, 10 mg

▷ **Recommended Dose Ranges** (Actual dose and schedule must be determined for each patient individually.)

Infants and Children: Safety and effectiveness for those under 18 years of age are not established.

18 to 60 Years of Age: 10 mg is taken immediately before bedtime. Patients should be reevaluated after taking this drug for 7 to 10 days.

*See Controlled Drug Schedules at the back of this book.

Over 60 Years of Age: Therapy should be started with 5 mg taken at bedtime. The dose may be cautiously increased to 10 mg at bedtime.

Conditions Requiring Dosing Adjustments
Liver Function: The dose should be reduced by 50% in liver compromise.
Kidney Function: No changes thought to be needed.

▷ **Dosing Instructions:**   The tablet may be crushed. Best taken on an empty stomach. Do **not** stop this drug abruptly if taken more than 7 days.

Usual Duration of Use: Use on a regular schedule for 2 nights usually determines effectiveness in treating insomnia. Your physician should assess the benefit of this drug after 10 days.

Possible Advantages of This Drug
Low occurrence of adverse effects.
May produce less of an undesirable effect on normal sleep patterns.
Author's note: The National Institute of Mental Health has a new information page on anxiety. It can be found on the World Wide Web at www.nimh.nih.gov/anxiety

Currently a "Drug of Choice"
For short-term management of insomnia in adults.

▷ **This Drug Should Not Be Taken If**
 • you had an allergic reaction to it previously.

▷ **Inform Your Physician Before Taking This Drug If**
 • you have abnormal liver or kidney function.
 • you are pregnant or planning pregnancy.
 • you have a history of alcoholism or drug abuse.
 • you have a serious lung problem (respiratory impairment).
 • you have a history of serious depression or mental disorder.
 • you are unsure how much to take or how often to take it.

Possible Side Effects (natural, expected, and unavoidable drug actions)
Drowsiness and blurred vision, "hangover" effects following long-term use.

▷ **Possible Adverse Effects** (unusual, unexpected, and infrequent reactions)
If any of the following develop, consult your physician promptly for guidance.
Mild Adverse Effects
Allergic reactions: skin rash.
Drowsiness and dizziness—rare.
Nausea and diarrhea—infrequent.
Elevation of liver function tests—rare.
Muscle tremors—infrequent.
Blurred vision—infrequent.
Serious Adverse Effects
Allergic reactions: not defined.
Abnormal thoughts or hallucinations—case reports.
Paradoxical aggression, agitation, or suicidal thoughts—rare.

▷ **Possible Effects on Sexual Function:**   None reported.

Possible Effects on Laboratory Tests
Liver function tests: increased SGOT, SGPT, and CPK.

CAUTION

1. This drug works quickly. It is best to take it just before bedtime.
2. Do not drink alcohol while taking this drug.
3. Withdrawal may occur, even if this drug was only taken for a week or two. Ask your doctor for advice before stopping zolpidem.
4. You may experience trouble going to sleep for 1 or 2 nights after stopping this drug (rebound insomnia). This effect is usually short term.
5. Sleep disturbances may be a symptom of underlying psychological problems. Tell your doctor if unusual behaviors or odd thoughts occur.
6. Drugs that depress the central nervous system may produce additive effects with this drug. Ask your doctor or pharmacist before combining other prescription or nonprescription drugs with zolpidem.

Precautions for Use

By Infants and Children: Safety and effectiveness for those under 18 years of age are not established.

By Those Over 60 Years of Age: The starting dose should be decreased to 5 mg. Since this drug works quickly, it is best taken immediately before going to bed. You may be at increased risk for falls if the drug remains in your system in the morning. Watch for lethargy, unsteadiness, nightmares, and paradoxical agitation and anger.

▷ **Advisability of Use During Pregnancy**

Pregnancy Category: B. See Pregnancy Risk Categories at the back of this book.

Animal studies: In rats, abnormal skull bone formation was reported. In rabbits, abnormal bone formation was found.

Human studies: Adequate studies of pregnant women are not available.

Use during pregnancy is **not** advisable. Ask your doctor for guidance.

Advisability of Use If Breast-Feeding

Presence of this drug in breast milk: Yes.

Avoid drug or refrain from nursing.

Habit-Forming Potential: This drug may cause dependence (see Glossary).

Effects of Overdose: Marked change from lethargy to coma. Cardiovascular and respiratory compromise was also reported. The drug flumazenil may help reverse symptoms.

Possible Effects of Long-Term Use: Psychological and/or physical dependence.

Suggested Periodic Examinations While Taking This Drug (at physician's discretion)

Liver function tests.

▷ **While Taking This Drug, Observe the Following**

Foods: This drug should **not** be taken with food.

Beverages: Avoid caffeine-containing beverages: coffee, tea, cola, chocolate.

▷ *Alcohol:* This drug should **not** be combined with alcohol.

Tobacco Smoking: Nicotine is a stimulant and should be avoided. I advise everyone to quit smoking.

Marijuana Smoking: May cause additive drowsiness.

▷ *Other Drugs:*

Zolpidem *taken concurrently* with

• rifampin (Rifater, others) may decrease zolpidem benefits.

- ritonavir (Norvir), and perhaps other protease inhibitors (see Drug Classes), may lead to toxicity.

Zolpidem may *increase* the effects of

- chlorpromazine (Thorazine).
- narcotics or other CNS-depressant drugs (see Drug Classes for *opioids, phenothiazines, antihistamines,* and *benzodiazepines*).

▷ *Driving, Hazardous Activities:* This drug may cause drowsiness and impair coordination. Restrict activities as necessary.

Aviation Note: The use of this drug *is a disqualification* for piloting. Consult a designated aviation medical examiner.

Discontinuation: This drug should **not** be stopped abruptly, even after a week of use. Ask your doctor for help regarding an appropriate withdrawal schedule.

THE LEADING EDGE

This section is designed to help you become more fully aware of medicines that show promise for a variety of reasons. Some are novel applications or are now FDA approvable. "The Leading Edge" can also explain new information about concepts in how medicines are packaged for better delivery into the body. A few interesting medicines or therapeutic products still in early clinical trials are included as "stars on the horizon."

It is impossible to predict which medicines or delivery systems **will** achieve final FDA approval or will be used in specific medicines, but many successful ones will be covered in subsequent editions of this book. Finally, many medicines or delivery systems which could be covered in a given year may be omitted simply because of space limitations. The author will select those which in his opinion offer the most potential benefit to his readers.

AIDS VACCINE (AYDS)

Star on the Horizon

In the most promising AIDS vaccine development yet, a company called Vaxgen has been given the go-ahead by the FDA to begin testing its AIDS vaccine in humans. This is the first such vaccine to be allowed to be tested in large studies known as Phase III Clinical Trials. Actual widespread use and FDA approval are probably a long way off, but early results are promising.

ANGIOGENIC GENE THERAPY (ANJIE oh jen ik)

Star on the Horizon

I expected to tell you about use of gene therapy in cystic fibrosis as the first dramatic use of gene therapy. Instead, I'm pleased to tell you about use of gene therapy to actually cause new blood vessels to grow in a diseased heart.

The heart that was used was a pig heart (often used for research because it acts like a human heart) that had significant compromise in the blood vessels that supplied nourishment and oxygen to the heart itself. The company is called Collateral Therapeutics, and they've developed the genes and a system to deliver them to the heart. Unlike another blood vessel gene treatment, this method does NOT involve surgery. What this means is that the potential now exists for a way to tell the heart to resupply itself with life-giving blood circulation when the original circulation has become blocked or diseased. This is a potential fundamental change in the model (paradigm) now used to treat heart disease! Trials in humans are just underway.

ANGIOSTATIN AND ENDOSTATIN
(ANNE gee oh stat in) (EN doh stat in)

Stars on the Horizon

In the most promising news on cancer in years, angiostatin and Endostatin were found to stop blood from going to cancer that had spread (metastasized) from an original site to form a second tumor. Entremed is working with Bristol-Myers to develop the substances into working medicines.

CERVICAL CANCER VACCINE (SIR vi kal) (KAN sir)

Novel Approach

Is it possible to prevent cervical cancer with a vaccine? Researchers at Merck released information in New York about a study that will show if it is possible to PREVENT a widely occurring cancer in women. The vaccine will be directed against the human papilloma virus (HPV). While you may not have heard about this previously, this virus is the most common sexually transmitted disease in the United States. Some of those infected will get one of the strains of HPV that can cause cervical cancer. The vaccine will help those vaccinated avoid the virus, and avoid one cause of cervical cancer.

CHLAMYDIA PNEUMONIAE (KLA mid ee ah)

Novel Bacteria Effect

This bacteria, which has long been known to cause lung infections, has some research saying it may be involved in heart attacks. A study reported in *The Lancet* found that people who had heart attacks also were likely to be infected with this organism. Further research is needed to find out if the bacteria just happens to be there, or actually is the cause inflammation which somehow destabilizes fat and calcium buildup (atherosclerosis). The theory holds that once the buildup breaks off the inside of blood vessels, it goes on to block circulation of blood. Fortunately, the bacteria is relatively easy to kill, and if (like ulcers) some heart attacks are found to actually be infections, a simple blood test may be used to identify those at risk. Once the bacteria is found, a course of the right antibiotics may become a key to preventing heart attacks.

COX-II INHIBITOR (KOX too)

Stars on the Horizon
Osteoarthritis and rheumatoid arthritis are prevalent and often debilitating conditions. A new class of medicines interferes with th COX-II system and is very promising. I expect that the first medicine to be approved will be MK-966 which will be named Vioxx.

IC-351 (HYDROXYLASE) (HI DROX UL ACE)

Star on the Horizon
Sildenafil (Viagra) has been one of the most widely publicized medicines ever to be FDA approved. A new medicine for impotence is in clinical trials which activates the same blood flow system as the existing medicine. IC-351 may have an advantage in that is may cause fewer possible side effects.

INFLIXIMAB (AVAKINE) (Inn FLIX I mab) (AV a kyne)

Star on the Horizon
This medicine is FDA approvable for use in treating Crohn's disease.
Interestingly, it works to block the effects of a substance called tumor necrosis factor or TNF. This compound also causes some of the symptoms of some kinds of arthritis and wasting in AIDS. It appears that the original use may broaden considerably.

INSULIN INHALER (IN sue lyn)

Novel Application
What this amounts to is an insulin shot by inhalation. Pfizer has been testing the inhaler form in humans, and has found promising results. It looks like the insulin is absorbed into the blood, and may replace injections in those diabetics who only require a short-acting insulin.

INTEGRASE (IN ta grace)

Star on the Horizon
Research into integrases, and medicines that can interfere with it, has continued since my last edition. Four companies currently have drugs in clinical trials to interfere with its action. These potential drugs act at a different point in the life cycle of HIV than the presently available medicines. The hope here is that combining an integrase with currently available drugs (one investigational protease inhibitor—amprenavir [VX-1478]—appears to enter the central nervous system well, and may attack the virus in a place that has previously been hard to reach) might make HIV infection a long-term (chronic) illness—or even raise the possibility of a cure. Abacavir (Ziagen or 159U89) and efavirenz (Sustiva) are investigational

medicines that offer advantages in less frequent dosing which may also be extremely effective with an integrase.

INTRANASAL FLU VACCINE (INTRA na sal)

Novel Application

What this amounts to is a flu vaccine that will be able to be given as a nasal spray. This is something I referred to in my newsletter as a "flu shot in the nose." The company (Aviron) has worked closely with the National Institutes of Health (NIH) to test this approach. Speculation is that this approach will be available for the 1999 flu (influenza) season.

LEPTIN (LEP TIN)

Novel Application

Late in 1997, the news media started to cover a newly discovered hormone called leptin. The hormone appeared to work remarkably well in mice, but the effect in humans was yet to be discovered. Some recent human research shows that 6 months of leptin injections helped the people in the study lose up to 16 pounds when being given the highest dose that was studied. Further research is needed, but these first human results look very promising.

LIPOSOMES (LIP oh soams)

Medication Delivery

Once again liposomes, and the ability to place medications in them, appear to offer greatly improved results (outcomes) from medicines. This time, a company called the Liposome Company has moved forward with a liposomally encapsulated cancer medicine. The medicine is called doxorubicin and is currently the drug of choice for breast cancer. Unfortunately, adverse effects from the medicine make use of the currently available form very difficult. The liposomally enclosed form was recently found to offer the same clinical advantage of the original medicine, and was found to have far fewer side effects.

NESIRITIDE (NES ear ih tide)

Star on the Horizon

The first new medicine to treat congestive heart failure in a decade appears to be headed for FDA approval. The medicine is a genetically engineered form of a heart hormone called human b-type natriuretic peptide (BNP). This is part of the response of the body to heart failure, and will be able to help improve the way the heart works.

PAIN RELIEF IMPLANT

Novel Application

Dr. Stewart (Skip) Grossman is leading a team of researchers at Johns Hopkins University looking into actually implanting a pain medicine under the skin. Dr. Grossman originally envisioned use of the medicine in countries where clocks and time are less widely used concepts. It appears, however, that Dr. Grossman's team has identified a way to bring long-lasting relief (the insert may provide a reliable amount of medicine for up to a month) to chronic pain patients. The clear benefit here is that a reliable level of pain medicine could be regularly delivered while having a minimal impact on a patient's life. Even pain patients can have problems trying to remember to take a pill!

SNX 111 (S n x one eleven)

Star on the Horizon

A poisonous snail may have delivered a key to a new pain medicine. One of the active ingredients in the venom has been isolated, and a structurally similar compound is now being tested in clinical trials. Early information points to a benefit that is much more potent than morphine with few side effects.

TELOMERASE (TELL om er ace)

Star on the Horizon

A new enzyme has been discovered that appears to have a role in aging and may also be part of the cancer mystery. Much research needs to be done to see where this enzyme fits in.

VITAMIN E (VI da min)

Novel Application

While I mentioned this vitamin last year, I feel that the research and benefits continue to accumulate for this entry. The American Psychiatric Association developed clinical guidelines for treating Alzheimer's disease. These guidelines recommend vitamin E for delay in progression of symptoms in people with mild to moderate Alzheimer's disease. The vitamin is recommended both alone or in combination with donepezil (Aricept) as the first-line approach.

DRUG CLASSES

Throughout the drug profiles, I often refer you to various drug classes. Use this section to protect yourself and your family. Medicines in the same class often share important characteristics in their chemistry, how they work in the body, and even the problems or side effects that they may cause. *Any* drug (or *all* drugs) in a given class can be expected to behave in a similar way . This knowledge helps you prevent interactions or unanticipated or hazardous adverse effects.

Each Drug Class is named, followed by an alphabetic listing of the generic names of the drugs in the class. Following each generic name (and enclosed in parentheses) is the widely recognized brand name(s) of that particular drug. A complete listing is not possible. If your medicine is not present, call your doctor or pharmacist to get the generic name of the drug that concerns you. The generic name listings are sufficiently complete to serve the scope of this book.

Angiotensin-Converting Enzyme (ACE) Inhibitors

benazepril (Lotensin)
captopril (Capoten)
enalapril (Vasotec)
fosinopril (Monopril)
lisinopril (Prinivil, Zestril)

moexipril (Univasc)
quinapril (Accupril)
ramipril (Altace)
spirapril (Renormax)
trandolapril (Mavik)

Adrenocortical Steroids (Cortisonelike Drugs)

amcinonide (Cyclocort)
beclomethasone (Beclovent, Vanceril)
betamethasone (Celestone)
budesonide (Pulmicort)
cortisone (Cortone)
dexamethasone (Decadron)
fludrocortisone (Florinef)
flunisolide (AeroBid, Nasarel)
fluorometholone (FML)
fluticasone (Flonase)
halcinonide (Halog)

halobetasol (Ultravate)
hydrocortisone (Cortef)
medrysone (HMS Ophthalmic Suspension)
methylprednisolone (Medrol)
mometasone (Elocon)
paramethasone (Haldrone)
prednisolone (Delta-Cortef)
prednisone (Deltasone)
rimexalone (Vexol)
triamcinolone (Aristocort, Azmacort)

Alpha-Glucosidase Inhibitors

acarbose (Precose)

miglitol (Glyset)

Amebicides (Anti-Infectives)

chloroquine (Aralen)
emetine
iodoquinol (Yodoxin)

metronidazole (Flagyl)
paromomycin (Humatin)

Aminoglycosides (Anti-Infectives)

amikacin (Amikin)
gentamicin (Garamycin)
kanamycin (Kantrex)

neomycin (Mycifradin, Neobiotic)
paromomycin (Humatin)
tobramycin (Tobicin)

Amphetaminelike Drugs

amphetamine
benzphetamine (Didrex)
dextroamphetamine (Dexedrine)
diethylpropion (Tenuate, Tepanil)
methamphetamine (Desoxyn)
methylphenidate (Ritalin)

phendimetrazine (Adipost, Anorex, Plegine)
phenmetrazine (Preludin)
phentermine (Adipex-P, Fastin)
phentermine resin complex (Ionamin)
phenylpropanolamine (Dexatrim)

Analgesics

acetaminophen (Datril, Tylenol)
acetaminophen/propoxyphene (Darvocet-N
   100)
aspirin
lidocaine/prilocaine cream (Emla)

propoxyphene (Darvon)
tramadol (Ultram)
See also Nonsteroidal Anti-Inflammatory
   Drugs (NSAIDs) and Opioid Drugs

Androgens (Male Sex Hormones)

fluoxymesterone (Halotestin)
methyltestosterone (Android, Metandren,
   Oreton)

testosterone (Androderm, Depotest,
   Testone)

Angiotensin-2-Receptor Antagonists

candesartan (Atacand)
eprosartan (Teveten)
irbesartan (Avapro)

irbesartan and hydrochlorothiazide
losartan (Cozaar)
valsartan (Diovan)

Anorexiants (Appetite Suppressants)

mazindol (Mazanor, Sanorex)
sibutramine (Meridia)

See also Amphetaminelike Drugs

Anti-Acne Drugs

adapalene (Differin)
azelaic acid (Azelex)
benzoyl peroxide (Epi-Clear, others)
erythromycin (Eryderm)

isotretinoin (Accutane)
sodium sulfacetamide 10% lotion (Klaron)
tetracycline (Achromycin V)
tretinoin (Retin-A)

Anti-AIDS Drugs (Antiretrovirals)

abacavir (Ziagen) (investigational)
amprenavir (Agenerase or VX-1478)
   (investigational)
delavirdine (Rescriptor)
didanosine (DDI, Videx)
efavirenz (Sustiva) (investigational)
indinavir (Crixivan)
integrase (Zintevir) (investigational)

lamivudine (3TC, Epivir)
nelfinavir (Viracept)
nevirapine (Viramune)
ritonavir (Norvir)
saquinavir (Invirase)
stavudine (D4T, Zerit)
zalcitabine (dideoxycytidine, DDC, Hivid)
zidovudine (AZT, Retrovir)

Antialcoholism Drugs

disulfiram (Antabuse)

naltrexone (Trexan, ReVia)

Anti-Alzheimer's Drugs

donepezil (Aricept)
metrifonate (brand pending)

tacrine (Cognex)
vitamin E (various brands)

Anti-Anginal Drugs

bepridil (Vascor)
diltiazem (Cardizem)
nicardipine (Cardene)
nifedipine (Adalat, Procardia)

nitrates (see class below)
verapamil (Calan, Isoptin)
See also Beta-Blockers

Antianxiety Drugs (Mild Tranquilizers)

buspirone (Buspar)
chlormezanone (Trancopal)
hydroxyzine (Atarax, Vistaril)

lorazepam (Ativan)
meprobamate (Equanil, Miltown)
See also Benzodiazepines

Antiarrhythmic Drugs (Heart Rhythm Regulators)

acebutolol (Sectral)
adenosine (Adenocard)
amiodarone (Cordarone)
atenolol (Tenormin)
digitoxin (Crystodigin)
digoxin (Lanoxin)
disopyramide (Norpace)
flecainide (Tambocor)
ibutilide (Corvert)

lidocaine (Xylocaine)
mexiletine (Mexitil)
procainamide (Procan SR, Pronestyl)
propafenone (Rythmol)
propranolol (Inderal)
quinidine (Quinaglute, Quinidex, Quinora)
sotalol (Betapace)
tocainide (Tonocard)
verapamil (Calan, Isoptin)

Antiarthritics

aspirin
azathioprine (Imuran; rheumatoid only)
chloroquine (Aralen; rheumatoid only)
penicillamine (Cuprimine)

See also Nonsteroidal Anti-Inflammatory
   Drugs (NSAIDs) and Adrenocortical
   steroids

Antiasthmatic Drugs

Anti-Inflammatory Agents, Corticosteroids

beclomethasone (Beclovent, Vanceril)
flunisolide (AeroBid)

fluticasone (Flovent)
triamcinolone (Azmacort)

Anti-Leukotrienes

montelukast (Singulair)
zafirlukast (Accolate)

zileuton (Zyflo)

Bronchodilators

albuterol (Proventil, Ventolin)
aminophylline (Phyllocontin)
bitolterol (Tornalate)
dyphylline (Lufyllin)
ephedrine (Efed II)
epinephrine (Adrenalin, Bronkaid Mist,
    Primatene Mist)
ipratropium
isoetharine (Bronkosol, Dey-Lute)

isoproterenol (Isuprel)
metaproterenol (Alupent, Metaprel)
oxtriphylline (Choledyl)
pirbuterol (Maxair)
salmeterol (Serevent)
terbutaline (Brethaire, Brethine, Bricanyl)
theophylline (Bronkodyl, Elixophyllin, Slo-
    Phyllin, others)

Mast-Cell-Stabilizing Agents

cromolyn sodium (Gastrocrom, Intal)

nedocromil (Tilade)

Preventive Agents

cromolyn (Intal)

nedocromil (Tilade)

Xanthines

theophylline (Slo-bid, Theo-Dur)

Anti-Attention-Deficit-Hyperactivity-Disorder Drugs

clonidine (Catapres)
methylphenidate (Ritalin)

pemoline (Cylert)

Anti-Benign-Prostatic-Hyperplasia Drugs

doxazosin (Cardura)
finasteride (Proscar)
prazosin (Minipres)

tamsulosin (Flomax)
terazosin (Hytrin)

Antibiotics

See specific antibiotic class (Cephalosporins, Penicillins, Tetracyclines, etc.)

Topical, Anti-Infectives

mupirocin (Bactroban)

Anticancer Drugs (Antineoplastics or Chemotherapy)

chlorambucil (Leukeran)
cyclophosphamide (Cytoxan)
flutamide (Eulexin)
hydroxyurea (Hydrea)
liposomally encapsulated doxorubicin

(Evacet) (investigational)
mercaptopurine (Purinethol)
methotrexate (Rheumatrex)
tamoxifen (Nolvadex)

Anti-Canker-Sore Drugs

amlexanox (Apthasol)

Anticholesterol Drugs

See Cholesterol-Reducing Drugs

See HMG-CoA Reductase Inhibitors

Anticholinergic Drugs (Atropinelike Drugs)

atropine
belladonna
hyoscyamine
scopolamine
See also the specific drug class:

Antidepressant Drugs, Tricyclic
Antihistamines, some
Anti-Parkinsonism Drugs, some
Antispasmodics, Synthetic, some
Muscle Relaxants, some

Anticoagulant Drugs

anisindione (Miradon)
dicumarol

warfarin (Coumadin and generic)

Anticonvulsant Drugs (Antiepileptic Drugs)

acetazolamide (Diamox)
carbamazepine (Tegretol)
clonazepam (Klonopin)
clorazepate (Tranxene)
diazepam (Valium)
ethosuximide (Zarontin)
ethotoin (Peganone)
felbamate (Felbatol)
gabapentin (Neurontin)
lamotrigine (Lamictal)
mephenytoin (Mesantoin)

methsuximide (Celontin)
paramethadione (Paradione)
phenacemide (Phenurone)
phenobarbital (Luminal)
phensuximide (Milontin)
phenytoin (Dilantin)
primidone (Mysoline)
topiramate (Topamax)
trimethadione (Tridione)
valproic acid (Depakene)

Anti-Cystic-Fibrosis Agents (Recombinant DNase)

dornase alfa (Pulmozyme)

Antidepressant Drugs

Bicyclic Antidepressants

fluoxetine (Prozac)

venlafaxine (Effexor)

Tricyclic Antidepressants

amitriptyline (Elavil, Endep)
amoxapine (Asendin)
clomipramine (Anafranil)
desipramine (Norpramin, Pertofrane)
doxepin (Adapin, Sinequan)

imipramine (Tofranil)
nortriptyline (Aventyl, Pamelor)
protriptyline (Vivactil)
trimipramine (Surmontil)

Tetracyclic Antidepressants

maprotiline (Ludiomil)

mirtazapine (Remeron)

Other Antidepressants

bupropion (Wellbutrin, Wellbutrin SR)
fluvoxamine (Luvox)
Hypericum (St.-John's-wort)
nefazodone (Serzone)
paroxetine (Paxil)

sertraline (Zoloft)
trazodone (Desyrel)
See also Monoamine Oxidase (MAO)
  Inhibitors

Antidiabetic Drugs

Oral

See Alpha-Glucosidase Inhibitors, Biguanides, Meglitinides, Sulfonylureas, and
  Thiazolidinediones

Injectable

insulin

Antidiarrheal Drugs

loperamide

Antiemetic Drugs (Anti-Motion-Sickness, Antinausea Drugs)

chlorpromazine (Thorazine)
cyclizine (Marezine)
dimenhydrinate (Dramamine)
diphenhydramine (Benadryl)
granisetron (Kytril)
hydroxyzine (Atarax, Vistaril)

meclizine (Antivert, Bonine)
ondansetron (Zofran)
prochlorperazine (Compazine)
promethazine (Phenergan)
scopolamine (Transderm Scop)
trimethobenzamide (Tigan)

Antiepileptic Drugs

See Anticonvulsant Drugs

Antifungal Drugs (Anti-Infectives)

amphotericin B (Fungizone)
butenafine (Mentax)
fluconazole (Diflucan)
flucytosine (Ancobon)
griseofulvin (Fulvicin, Grifulvin, Grisactin)
itraconazole (Sporanox)

ketoconazole (Nizoral)
lipid-associated amphotericin B (Abelcet)
miconazole (Monistat)
nystatin (Mycostatin)
terbinafine (Lamisil)
tioconazole (Vagistat-1)

Anti-Glaucoma Drugs

acetazolamide (Diamox)
betaxolol (Betoptic)
brimonidine (Alphagan)
brinzolamide (Azopt)
dipivefrin (Propine)
dorzolamide (Trusopt)
dorzolamide and timolol (Cosopt)

epinephrine (Glaucon)
latanoprost (Xalatan)
levobunolol (Betagan)
metipranolol (Optipranolol)
pilocarpine (Pilocar)
timolol (Betimol, Timoptic, Timoptic-XE)

Anti-Gout Drugs

allopurinol (Zyloprim)
colchicine
diclofenac (Cataflam, Voltaren)
fenoprofen (Nalfon)
ibuprofen (Advil, Motrin, Nuprin, Rufin)
indomethacin (Indocin)
ketoprofen (Orudis)

mefenamic acid (Ponstel)
naproxen (Anaprox, Naprosyn)
oxaprozin (Daypro)
piroxicam (Feldene)
probenecid (Benemid)
sulfinpyrazone (Anturane)
sulindac (Clinoril)

Antihistamines

astemizole (Hismanal)
azatadine (Optimine)
azelastine (Astelin)
brompheniramine (Dimetane, others)
carbinoxamine (Clistin, Rondec)
cetirizine (Zyrtec)
chlorpheniramine (Chlor-Trimeton,
   Teldrin)
clemastine (Tavist)
cyclizine (Marezine)
cyproheptadine (Periactin)
dimenhydrinate (Dramamine)

diphenhydramine (Benadryl)
doxylamine (Unisom)
hydroxyzine (Atarax)
loratadine (Claritin, Claritin Extra)
meclizine (Antivert, Bonine)
orphenadrine (Norflex)
pheniramine (component of Triaminic)
promethazine (Phenergan, others)
pyrilamine (component of Triaminic)
tripelennamine (Pyribenzamine, PBZ)
triprolidine (component of Actifed and
   Sudahist)

Nonsedating or Minimally Sedating

astemizole (Hismanal)
cetirizine (Zyrtec)

fexofenadine (Allegra)
loratadine (Claritin)

Antihypertensive Drugs

amlodipine/benazepril (Lotrel)
bisoprolol/hydrochlorothiazide (Ziac)
carvediol (Coreg)
clonidine (Catapres)
doxazosin (Cardura)
enalapril/felodipine (Lexxel)
guanabenz (Wytensin)
guanadrel (Hylorel)
guanethidine (Ismelin)
guanfacine (Tenex)

hydralazine (Apresoline)
hydrochlorothiazide/benazepril (Lotensin)
methyldopa (Aldomet)
minoxidil (Loniten)
prazosin (Minipres)
reserpine (Serpasil)
terazosin (Hytrin)
See also ACE Inhibitors, Angiotensin-2-
   Receptor Antagonists, Beta-Blockers,
   Calcium Blockers, and Diuretics

Anti-Impotence Drugs

alprostadyl injection (Caverject)

sildenafil (Viagra)

Anti-Infective Drugs

See the specific anti-infective drug class:
Amebicides
Aminoglycosides
Antifungal Drugs
Antileprosy Drugs
Antimalarial Drugs
Antituberculosis Drugs

Antiviral Drugs
Cephalosporins
Fluoroquinolones
Macrolide Antibiotics
Penicillins
Sulfonamides
Tetracyclines

Miscellaneous Anti-Infective Drugs

atovaquone (Mepron)
chloramphenicol (Chloromycetin)
clindamycin (Cleocin)
colistin (Coly-Mycin S)
furazolidone (Furoxone)
lincomycin (Lincocin)

nalidixic acid (NegGram)
nitrofurantoin (Furadantin, Macrodantin)
novobiocin (Albamycin)
pentamidine (Pentam-300)
trimethoprim (Proloprim, Trimpex)
vancomycin (Vancocin)

Antileprosy Drugs (Anti-Infectives)

clofazimine (Lamprene)

dapsone

Antimalarial Drugs (Anti-Infectives)

chloroquine (Aralen)
doxycycline (Vibramycin)
hydroxychloroquine (Plaquenil)
mefloquine (Lariam)
primaquine

pyrimethamine (Daraprim)
quinacrine (Atabrine)
quinine
sulfadoxine/pyrimethamine (Fansidar)

Anti-Migraine Drugs

atenolol (Tenormin)
ergotamine (Ergostat)
methysergide (Sansert)
metoprolol (Lopressor)
nadolol (Corgard)
naratriptan (Amerge)
nifedipine (Procardia)

propranolol (Inderal)
rizatriptan (Maxalt, Maxalt MLT)
sumatriptan (Imitrex)
timolol (Blocadren)
verapamil (Calan, Isoptin)
zolmatriptan (Zomig)

Anti-Motion-Sickness/Antinausea Drugs

See Antiemetic Drugs

Anti-Myasthenics

neostigmine

Anti-Mycobacterial Agents

rifabutin (Mycobutin)

Anti-Osteoporotics

alendronate (Fosamax)
antiestrogens (SERM)
calcitonin (Miacalcin)
calcium (various brands)

estrogen (various brands)
raloxifene (Evista)
tiludronate (Skelid)

Anti-Parkinsonism Drugs

amantadine (Symmetrel)
benztropine (Cogentin)
bromocriptine (Parlodel)
diphenhydramine (Benadryl)

levodopa (Dopar, Larodopa)
levodopa/bensarazide (Prolopa)
levodopa/carbidopa (Sinemet, Sinemet CR)
pergolide (Permax)

pramipexole (Mirapex)
ropinirole (Requip)

selegiline (Eldepryl)
trihexyphenidyl (Artane)

Antiplatelet Drugs (Platelet Aggregation Inhibitors)

aspirin
clopidogrel (Plavix)
dipyridamole (Persantine)

sulfinpyrazone (Anturane)
ticlopidine (Ticlid)
tirofibran (Aggrastat)

Anti-Psoriatic Drugs

acitretin (Soriatane)
etretinate

methotrexate

Antipsychotic Drugs (Neuroleptics, Major Tranquilizers)

chlorprothixene (Taractan)
clozapine (Clozaril)
haloperidol (Haldol)
loxapine (Loxitane)
molindone (Moban)
olanzapine (Zyprexa)

pimozide (Orap)
quetiapine (Seroquel)
risperidone (Risperdal)
thiothixene (Navane)
See also Phenothiazines and
   Thienobenzodiazepines

Antipyretic Drugs (Fever-Reducing Drugs)

acetaminophen
aspirin

See also Nonsteroidal Anti-Inflammatory
   Drugs (NSAIDs)

Anti-Sickle-Cell-Anemia Drugs

hydroxyurea (Droxia, Hydrea)

Antispasmodics, Synthetic

anisotropine (Valpin)
clidinium (Quarzan)
glycopyrrolate (Robinul)
hexocyclium (Tral)
isopropamide (Darbid)

mepenzolate (Cantil)
methantheline (Banthine)
methscopolamine (Pamine)
propantheline (Pro-Banthine)
tridihexethyl (Pathilon)

Antituberculosis Drugs

aminosalicylate sodium (Sodium P.A.S.)
capreomycin (Capastat)
cycloserine (Seromycin)
ethambutol (Myambutol)
ethionamide (Trecator-SC)
isoniazid (Laniazid, Nydrazid)

pyrazinamide
rifampin (Rifadin, Rimactane)
rifabutin (Mycobutin)
rifapentine (Priftin)
streptomycin

Antitussive Drugs (Cough Suppressants)

benzonatate (Tessalon)
codeine (various brands)
dextromethorphan (Hold DM, Suppress)
diphenhydramine (Benylin)

hydrocodone (Hycodan)
hydromorphone (Dilaudid)
promethazine (Phenergan)

Antiulcer Drugs

Antacids

various brands

Antibiotics

amoxicillin
clarithromycin
metronidazole

tetracycline
See H₂ Blockers
See Proton Pump Inhibitors

Miscellaneous Antiulcer Drugs

amoxicillin/clarithromycin/lansoprazole
  (Prevpac)
bismuth subsalicylate (Pepto-Bismol,
  others)

misoprostol (Cytotec)
ranitidine bismuth citrate (Tritec)
sucralfate (Carafate)

Antiviral Drugs (Anti-Infectives)

acyclovir (Zovirax)
amantadine (Symmetrel)
amprenovir (VX-1478)
cidofovir (Vistide)
didanosine (Videx)
efavirenz (Sustiva)
famciclovir (Famvir)
foscarnet (Foscavir)
ganciclovir (Cytovene)
indinavir (Crixivan)
lamivudine (Epivir)
nelfinavir (Viracept)

nevirapine (Viramune)
penciclovir (Denavir)
ribavirin (Virazole)
rimantadine (Flumadine)
ritonavir (Norvir)
saquinavir (Invirase)
stavudine (Zerit)
valacyclovir (Valtrex)
vidarabine (Vira A)
zalcitabine (Hivid)
zidovudine (Retrovir)

Appetite Suppressants

See Anorexiants

Atropinelike Drugs

See Anticholinergic Drugs

Barbiturates

amobarbital (Amytal)
aprobarbital (Alurate)
butabarbital (Butisol)
mephobarbital (Mebaral)
metharbital (Gemonil)

pentobarbital (Nembutal)
phenobarbital (Luminal, Solfoton)
secobarbital (Seconal)
talbutal (Lotusate)

Benzodiazepines

alprazolam (Xanax)
bromazepam (Lectopam)
chlordiazepoxide (Libritabs, Librium)
clonazepam (Klonopin)
clorazepate (Tranxene)
diazepam (Valium, Vazepam)
flurazepam (Dalmane)

halazepam (Paxipam)
ketazolam (Loftran)
lorazepam (Ativan)
midazolam (Versed)
nitrazepam (Mogadon)
oxazepam (Serax)
prazepam (Centrax)

quazepam (Doral)
temazepam (Restoril)

triazolam (Halcion)

Beta-Blockers (Beta-Adrenergic-Blocking Drugs)

acebutolol (Sectral)
atenolol (Tenormin)
betaxolol (Kerlone)
bisoprolol (Zebeta)
bisoprolol/hydrochlorothiazide (Ziac)
carteolol (Cartrol)
carvedilol (Coreg)

labetalol (Normodyne, Trandate)
metoprolol (Lopressor)
nadolol (Corgard)
penbutolol (Levatol)
pindolol (Visken)
propranolol (Inderal)
timolol (Blocadren)

Biguanides (Oral Antidiabetic Drugs)

metformin (Glucophage)

Blood Flow Agents

pentoxifylline (Trental)

Bowel Anti-Inflammatory Drugs (Inflammatory Bowel Disease Suppressants)

azathioprine (Imuran)
infliximab (Avakine)
mesalamine (Rowasa, Asacol)

metronidazole (Flagyl)
olsalazine (Dipentum)
sulfasalazine (Azulfidine)

Bronchodilators

See Antiasthmatic Drugs

Calcium Blockers (Calcium-Channel-Blocking Drugs)

amlodipine (Norvasc)
bepridil (Vascor)
diltiazem (Cardizem, Tiazac)
felodipine (Plendil)
isradipine (DynaCirc)
mibefradil (Posicor) (removed by the

company)
nicardipine (Cardene, Cardene SR)
nifedipine (Adalat CC, Procardia XL)
nimodipine (Nimotop)
nisoldipine (Sular)
verapamil (Calan, Isoptin, Verelan)

Catechol O-Methyl Tranferase (COMT) Drugs

tolcapone (Tasmar)

Cephalosporins (Anti-Infectives)

cefaclor (Ceclor)
cefadroxil (Duricef, Ultracef)
cefamandole (Mandol)
cefazolin (Ancef, Kefzol, Zolicef)
cefepime (Maxipime)
cefixime (Suprax)
cefmetazole (Zefazone)
cefonicid (Monocid)

cefoperazone (Cefobid)
ceforanide (Precef)
cefotaxime (Claforan)
cefotetan (Cefotan)
cefoxitin (Mefoxin)
cefpodoxime (Vantin)
cefprozil (Cefzil)
ceftazidime (Fortaz, Tazidime, Tazicef)

ceftibuten (Cedax)
ceftizoxime (Cefizox)
ceftriaxone (Rocephin)
cefuroxime (Ceftin, Kefurox, Zinacef)
cephalexin (Keflex, Keftab)

cephalothin (Keflin)
cephapirin (Cefadyl)
cephradine (Anspor, Velosef)
loracarbef (Cefobid)
moxalactam (Moxam)

Cholesterol-Reducing Drugs

atorvastatin (Lipitor)
cerivastatin (Baycol)
cholestyramine (Questran, Prevalite)
clofibrate (Atromid-S)
colestipol (Colestid)
dextrothyroxine (Choloxin)
fenofibrate (Tricor)

fluvastatin (Lescol)
gemfibrozil (Lopid)
lovastatin (Mevacor)
niacin (Nicobid, Slo-Niacin, others)
pravastatin (Pravachol)
simvastatin (Zocor)

Cortisonelike Drugs

See Adrenocortical Steroids

Cough Suppressants

See Antitussive Drugs

Decongestants

ephedrine (Efedron, Ephedrol)
naphazoline (Naphcon, Vasocon)
oxymetazoline (Afrin, Duration, others)
phenylephrine (Neo-Synephrine, others)
phenylpropanolamine (Propadrine,

Propagest, others)
pseudoephedrine (Afrinol, Sudafed, others)
tetrahydrozoline (Tyzine, Visine, others)
xylometazoline (Otrivin)

Digitalis Preparations

deslanoside (Cedilanid-D)
digitoxin (Crystodigin)

digoxin (Lanoxicaps, Lanoxin)

Diuretics

acetazolamide (Diamox)
amiloride (Midamor)
bumetanide (Bumex)
chlorthalidone (Hygroton)
ethacrynic acid (Edecrin)
furosemide (Lasix)

indapamide (Lozol)
metolazone (Diulo, Zaroxolyn)
spironolactone (Aldactone)
triamterene (Dyrenium)
See also Thiazide Diuretics

Ergot Derivatives

bromocriptine (Parlodel)
ergotamine (Bellergal)

methysergide (Sansert)
pergolide (Permax)

Estrogens (Female Sex Hormones)

chlorotrianisene (Tace)
diethylstilbestrol (DES, Stilphostrol)

estradiol (Estrace, Estraderm, others)
estrogens, conjugated (Premarin)

estrogens, esterified (Estratab, Menest)
estrone (Theelin, others)
estropipate (Ogen)

ethinyl estradiol (Estinyl)
quinestrol (Estrovis)

Female Sex Hormones

See Estrogens and Progestins

Fever-Reducing Drugs

See Antipyretic Drugs

5-Alpha-Reductase Inhibitors

finasteride (Proscar)

Fluoroquinolones (Anti-Infectives)

ciprofloxacin (Cipro)
grepafloxacin (Raxar)
levofloxacin (Levaquin)
lomefloxacin (Maxaquin)

norfloxacin (Noroxin)
ofloxacin (Floxin)
sparfloxacin (Zagam)
trovafloxacin (Trovan)

Gastrointestinal Drugs

Miscellaneous

cisapride (Propulsid)
infliximab (Avakine)

metoclopramide (Reglan)

Ulcer Preventatives

misoprostol (Cytotec)

Histamine (H₂) Blocking Drugs (Histamine [H₂] Blocking Drugs)

cimetidine (Tagamet, Tagamet HB 200)
famotidine (Pepcid, Pepcid AC)

nizatidine (Axid, Axid AR)
ranitidine (Zantac, Zantac 75)

Hair Growth Stimulants

finasteride (Proscar, Propecia)

minoxidil (Rogaine)

Heart Rhythm Regulators

See Antiarrhythmic Drugs

Hematopoietic Agents

filgrastim (Neupogen)

HMG-CoA Reductase Inhibitors

atorvastatin (Lipitor)
cerivastatin (Baycol)
fluvastatin (Lescol)

lovastatin (Mevacor)
pravastatin (Pravachol)
simvastatin (Zocor)

Hormones

Miscellaneous

nafarelin (Synarel)

See also Androgens for male sex hormones,

Estrogens and Progestins for female sex hormones

Hypnotic Drugs (Sedatives/Sleep Inducers)

acetylcarbromal (Paxarel)
chloral hydrate (Aquachloral, Noctec)
estazolam (ProSom)
ethchlorvynol (Placidyl)
ethinamate (Valmid)
flurazepam (Dalmane)
glutethimide (Doriden)
methyprylon (Noludar)

paraldehyde (Paral)
propiomazine (Largon)
quazepam (Doral)
temazepam (Restoril)
triazolam (Halcion)
zolpidem (Ambien)
See also Barbiturates

Immunosuppressants

azathioprine (Imuran)
chlorambucil (Leukeran)
cyclophosphamide (Cytoxan)

cyclosporine (Sandimmune)
hydroxychloroquine (Plaquenil)

Macrolide Antibiotics (Anti-Infectives)

azithromycin (Zithromax)
clarithromycin (Biaxin)
dirithromycin (Dynabac)

erythromycin (E-Mycin, Ilosone, Erythrocin, E.E.S.)
troleandomycin (TAO)

Male Sex Hormones

See Androgens

Mast-Cell-Stabilizing Agents

See Antiasthmatic Drugs

Meglitinides

repaglinide (Prandin)

Monoamine Oxidase (MAO) Inhibitor Drugs (Type A: Antidepressants)

isocarboxazid (Marplan)
phenelzine (Nardil)

tranylcypromine (Parnate)

Muscarinic Receptor Antagonists (Anti-Incontinence)

tolteradine (Detrol)

Muscle Relaxants (Skeletal Muscle Relaxants)

baclofen (Lioresal)
carisoprodol (Rela, Soma, others)

chlorphenesin carbamate (Maolate)
chlorzoxazone (Paraflex, Parafon Forte)

cyclobenzaprine (Flexeril)
dantrolene (Dantrium)
diazepam (Valium)
meprobamate (Equanil, Miltown, others)

metaxalone (Skelaxin)
methocarbamol (Robaxin, others)
orphenadrine (Norflex, others)

Nitrates

amyl nitrate (Amyl Nitrate Vaporole,
  others)
erythrityl tetranitrate (Cardilate)
isosorbide dinitrate (Isordil, Sorbitrate,
  others)

isosorbide mononitrate (Ismo, Imdur)
nitroglycerin (Nitrostat, Nitrolingual,
  Nitrogard, Nitrong, others)
pentaerythritol tetranitrate (Duotrate,
  Peritrate)

Nonnucleoside Reverse Transcriptase Inhibitors

delavirdine (Rescriptor)

nevirapine (Viramune)

Nonsteroidal Anti-Inflammatory Drugs (NSAIDs) (Aspirin Substitutes)

Acetic Acids

bromfenac sodium (Duract)
diclofenac potassium (Cataflam)
diclofenac sodium (Voltaren)
etodolac (Lodine)
indomethacin (Indochron E-R, Indocin,

  Indocin SR)
ketorolac (Toradol)
nabumetone (Relafen)
sulindac (Clinoril)
tolmetin (Tolectin, Tolectin DS)

Fenamates

meclofenamate (Meclomen)

mefenamic acid (Ponstel)

Oxicams

piroxicam (Feldene)

Propionic Acids

diflunisal (Dolobid)
fenoprofen (Nalfon)
flurbiprofen (Ansaid)
ibuprofen
ketoprofen (Orudis, Oruvail)
naproxen (Naprosyn)

naproxen sodium (Aleve, Anaprox, Anaprox
  DS)
oxaprozin (Daypro)
oxyphenbutazone (Oxalid)
suprofen (Profenal)

Opioid Antagonists

naltrexone (ReVia)

Opioid Drugs (Narcotics)

alfentanil (Alfenta)
codeine
fentanyl (Sublimaze, Duragesic)
hydrocodone (Hycodan)
hydromorphone (Dilaudid)
levorphanol (Levo-Dromoran)
meperidine (Demerol)

methadone (Dolophine)
morphine (Astramorph, Duramorph, MS
  Contin, Roxanol)
oxycodone (OxyContin, Roxicodone)
oxymorphone (Numorphan)
propoxyphene (Darvon)
sufentanil (Sufenta)

Pain Syndrome Modifiers (also adjuvants)

carbamazepine (Tegretol)
gabapentin (Neurontin)
phenytoin (Dilantin)

strontium-89 (Metastron)
samarium-EDTMP (Quadramet)

Penicillinsm (Anti-Infectives)

amoxicillin (Amoxil, Larotid, Polymox, Trimox, others)
amoxicillin/clavulanate (Augmentin)
ampicillin (Omnipen, Polycillin, Principen, Totacillin)
ampicillin/sulbactam (Unasyn)
bacampicillin (Spectrobid)
carbenicillin (Geocillin, Geopen, Pyopen)
cloxacillin (Cloxapen, Tegopen)
dicloxacillin (Dynapen, Pathocil, Veracillin)

methicillin (Staphcillin)
mezlocillin (Mezlin)
nafcillin (Nafcil, Unipen)
oxacillin (Prostaphlin)
penicillin G (Pentids, others)
penicillin V (Pen Vee K, V-Cillin K, Veetids, others)
piperacillin (Pipracil)
ticarcillin (Ticar)
ticarcillin/clavulanate (Timentin)

Phenothiazines (Antipsychotic Drugs)

acetophenazine (Tindal)
chlorpromazine (Thorazine)
fluphenazine (Permitil, Prolixin)
mesoridazine (Serentil)
perphenazine (Trilafon)

prochlorperazine (Compazine)
promazine (Sparine)
thioridazine (Mellaril)
trifluoperazine (Stelazine)
triflupromazine (Vesprin)

Potassium Replacement Products

K-Dur

potassium chloride (various)

Progestins (Female Sex Hormones)

ethynodiol
hydroxyprogesterone (Duralutin, Gesterol L.A., others)
medroxyprogesterone (Amen, Curretab, Prempro, Premphase, Provera)

megestrol (Megace)
norethindrone (Micronor, Norlutate, Norlutin)
norgestrel (Ovrette)
progesterone (Gesterol 50, Progestaject)

Protease Inhibitors

aprenavir (VX-1478)
indinavir (Crixivan)
nelfinavir (Viracept)

ritonavir (Norvir)
saquinavir (Invirase)

Proton Pump Inhibitors (H/K ATPase Inhibitors)

lansoprazole (Prevacid)

omeprazole (Prilosec)

Radiopharmaceuticals

samarium-EDTMP (Quadramet)

strontium-89 (Metastron)

Salicylates

aspirin
choline salicylate (Arthropan)

magnesium salicylate (Doan's, Magan, Mobidin)

salsalate (Amigesic, Disalcid, Salsitab)
sodium salicylate

sodium thiosalicylate (Rexolate, Tusal)

Sedatives/Sleep Inducers

See Hypnotic Drugs

SERMs (Selective Estrogen Receptor Modulators)

raloxifene (Evista)

Smoking Cessation Adjuncts

bupropion (Zyban)
nicotine (Nicorette, various patch brands

such as Nicotrol)

Sulfonamides (Anti-Infectives)

multiple sulfonamides (Triple Sulfa No. 2)
sulfacytine (Renoquid)
sulfadiazine
sulfamethizole (Thiosulfil)

sulfamethoxazole (Gantanol)
sulfasalazine (Azulfidine)
sulfisoxazole (Gantrisin)

Sulfonylureas (Oral Antidiabetic Drugs)

acetohexamide (Dymelor)
chlorpropamide (Diabinese)
glimepiride (Amaryl)
glipizide (Glucotrol)

glyburide (DiaBeta, Micronase)
tolazamide (Ronase, Tolamide, Tolinase)
tolbutamide (Orinase)

Tetracyclines (Anti-Infectives)

demeclocycline (Declomycin)
doxycycline (Doryx, Doxychel, Vibramycin)
methacycline (Rondomycin)
minocycline (Minocin)

oxytetracycline (Terramycin)
tetracycline (Achromycin V, Panmycin,
  Sumycin)

Thiazide Diuretics

bendroflumethiazide (Naturetin)
benzthiazide (Aquatag, Exna, Marazide)
chlorothiazide (Diuril)
cyclothiazide (Anhydron)
hydrochlorothiazide (Esidrix, Hydrodiuril,

  Oretic)
hydroflumethiazide (Diucardin, Saluron)
methyclothiazide (Enduron, Aquatensen)
polythiazide (Renese)
trichlormethiazide (Metahydrin, Naqua)

Thiazolidinediones

troglitazone (Rezulin)

Thienobenzodiazepines

olanzapine (Zyprexa)

Thyroid Hormones

levothyroxine (Synthroid)

liothyronine (Cytomel)

1006 Drug Classes

Tranquilizers, Major

See Antipsychotic Drugs

Tranquilizers, Minor

See Antianxiety Drugs

Vaccines (Immune Modulators)

influenza vaccine (Fluogen, Flu-Shield, Fluzone)

Lyme disease vaccine
varicella virus vaccine (Varivax)

Vasodilators (Peripheral Vasodilators)

cyclandelate (Cyclospasmol)
ethaverine (Ethaquin, Isovex)
isoxsuprine (Vasodilan)

nylidrin (Arlidin)
papaverine (Cerespan, Pavabid)

Xanthines (Bronchodilators)

aminophylline (Phyllocontin, Truphylline)
dyphylline (Dilor, Lufyllin)
oxtriphylline (Choledyl)

theophylline (Bronkodyl, Slo-Phyllin, Theolair, others)

A GLOSSARY
OF
DRUG-RELATED TERMS

Glossary

addiction Addiction is generally recognized as intense drug dependence, with uncontrollable drug-seeking behavior, *tolerance* for pleasure-giving effects, and *withdrawal* if the drug is withheld. This is *physical dependence*—where the drug is incorporated into the fundamental biochemistry of the brain. (See the terms DEPENDENCE and TOLERANCE for accounts of physical and psychological dependence.)

adverse effect or reaction An abnormal, unexpected, infrequent, and often unpredictable injurious response to a drug. This does *not* include a pharmacological action, even though some may be undesirable and unintended. (See SIDE EFFECT.) Adverse reactions are: those due to drug *allergy*, individual *idiosyncrasy*, and *toxic* effects of drugs on tissues (see ALLERGY [DRUG], IDIOSYNCRASY, and TOXICITY).

allergy (drug) An abnormal drug response that happens after antibodies* are made to the drug itself. People with history of hay fever, asthma, hives, or eczema are more likely to develop drug allergies. Allergies can develop slowly, or they can appear suddenly and require life-saving medical attention.

alternative delivery system (ADS) A term describing a variety of health care forms other than the established fee-for-service model such as HMOs, PPOs and others.

analgesic A drug used to relieve pain. There are three types: (1) simple nonnarcotics, which block production of chemicals that cause or worsen pain (prostaglandins, etc.)—examples are acetaminophen, aspirin, and nonsteroidal anti-inflammatory drugs (Motrin or Advil, etc.); (2) narcotic analgesics or opioids, which relieve pain by blunting pain perception in the brain—examples are morphine, codeine, and hydrocodone (natural derivatives of opium), and meperidine or pentazocine (synthetic drug products); (3) local anesthetics, which relieve pain by making sensory nerve endings insensitive to pain—such as phenazopyridine (Pyridium).

anaphylactic (anaphylactoid) reaction Symptoms that are an extreme hypersensitivity to a drug. Anaphylactic reactions often involve several body systems. Mild symptoms include itching, hives, congestion, nausea, cramping, or diarrhea. Sometimes these precede severe problems such as choking, shortness of breath, and loss of consciousness (usually referred to as anaphylactic shock). Anaphylactic reactions can happen after a very small dose, may develop suddenly, and can be rapidly fatal. They are true medical emergencies. Any adverse effect appearing within 20 minutes after taking a drug should be considered an early sign of anaphylactic reaction. Get medical attention immediately! (See ALLERGY [DRUG], and HYPERSENSITIVITY.)

---

*Antibodies are proteins that combine with foreign substances. Protective antibodies destroy bacteria and neutralize toxins. Injurious antibodies react with foreign substances such as drugs to cause release of histamine, a chemical causing allergic reactions.

antihypertensive A drug used to lower high blood pressure. *Hypertension* describes blood pressure above a normal range. It is not nervous or emotional tension. Medicines to treat hypertension fall into three major groups:

1. drugs that increase urine production (the diuretics)
2. drugs that relax blood vessel walls
3. drugs that reduce sympathetic nervous system activity

Although high blood pressure often does not have any symptoms, You MUST treat it for life. Take your medicine EXACTLY as prescribed.

antipyretic A drug that lowers body temperature. They reduce fever by working on the hypothalamus of the brain. This leads to dilation of blood vessels (capillary beds) in the skin and brings heated blood to the skin surface for cooling. Sweat glands are also stimulated to cool the body through evaporation. An antipyretic may also be a pain reliever (analgesic) (acetaminophen), or analgesic and anti-inflammatory (aspirin).

aplastic anemia Also known as pancytopenia, where production of the three types of blood cells is seriously impaired. Aplastic anemia can occur from unknown causes, but about half of reported cases are caused by drugs or chemicals. A delay of 1 to 6 months may occur between the use of a drug and anemia. Symptoms include: lower red blood cells (anemia) resulting in fatigue and pallor; deficiency of white blood cells (leukopenia) predisposing to infections and low blood platelets (thrombocytopenia) can cause spontaneous bruising or bleeding. Treatment is difficult. Even with the best of care, half the cases may be fatal. Aplastic anemia is rare, but anyone taking a drug that can cause it should have periodic complete blood cell counts. For a listing of causative drugs, see Table 5, Section Six.

Bad Med Syndrome (BMS) The decreased quality of life, decrease in expected beneficial drug results, loss of time from work, unnecessary stays in the hospital or additional treatment resulting from medicines themselves or from the improper use of medicines.

Improper use includes: drug interactions resulting from inappropriate medicine combinations; too low a dose (subtherapeutic dosing); too high a dose (overdose); as well as taking the medicine "every once in a while" when it was prescribed for ongoing use.

No one intends to cause Bad Med Syndrome (BMS), yet patients, pharmacists, physicians, other health care providers, JCAHO, the FDA, and managed care organizations all contribute to it. I believe it will take a team effort to solve it.

bioavailability How fast and how much active drug is absorbed into the blood. Two types of measurements—blood levels after it was taken, and how long the drug stays in the blood—shows how much drug is available to work and how long it stays. The two major factors that govern bioavailability are the chemical and physical characteristics of the dose, and how well the digestive system of the person taking it works. A drug that falls apart quickly in a normal stomach or small intestine produces blood levels quite promptly. Such a drug product has good bioavailability. Drugs such as metoclopramide or cisapride that slow the gastrointestinal system may act to actually increase the amount of drug that gets into the body.

bioequivalence The ability of a drug product to cause its intended therapeutic effect is related to bioavailability. When a drug is made by several manufacturers, it is critical to pick the one that has the bioavailability needed to work. While the drug in medicines from different firms may the same chemical, don't assume that they are equally available.

Bioavailability depends mostly on physical characteristics of how a drug is made. These determine how well a drug falls apart and releases its active drug component(s). Drug products that have the same drug but are combined with different inert additives, coated with different substances, or enclosed in different capsules may or may not have the same bioavailability. Those that do are termed bioequivalent, and can be relied upon to give the same result.

If you consider having your prescription filled with a generic, ask your physician *and* pharmacist for help. This requires professional judgment in each case. In some cases, reasonable differences in bioavailability is acceptable. For serious illnesses, or because blood levels must be kept in a narrow range, it is essential to use the drug product that has been shown to have reliable bioavailability.

blood platelets The smallest of the blood cells made by bone marrow. Platelets are normally present in very large numbers. They are the basis of normal blood clotting and prevent excessive bruising or bleeding if you are injured. Platelets preserve smaller blood vessel walls. If there is damage, platelets seal small holes in vessel walls. Some drugs and chemicals may lower the platelet count. Many slow formation; other drugs hasten destruction. If the platelet count gets too low, blood begins to leak through the walls of smaller vessels. This shows as scattered bruises in skin of the thighs or legs and is called purpura. Bleeding happens anywhere, internally as well as into the tissues immediately beneath the skin. For a listing of causative drugs, see Table 5, Section Six.

body mass index (BMI) A calculation used to measure the relative degree of a patient's obesity. This measurement is used in deciding the appropriateness of using sibutramine (Meridia). BMI is calculated using weight in kilograms divided by the height in meters squared. If the BMI is greater than 30 kg per square meter or is 27 kg per square meter with other risk factors such as diabetes, sibutramine is approved for that use.

bone marrow depression A decrease in the ability of bone marrow to make blood cells. This can be an adverse reaction to drugs or chemicals. Bone marrow makes most of the body's blood cells: red blood cells (erythrocytes), white blood cells (leukocytes), and platelets or (thrombocytes). Each type of cell has one or more functions, critical to life and health.

Drugs that depress bone marrow may impair all types of blood cells right away or only one type selectively. Blood tests can show drug effects on bone marrow. If fewer red blood cells are made, anemia results, causing weakness, cold intolerance, and shortness of breath. Low white blood cells lowers resistance to infection (fever, sore throat, or pneumonia). If platelets fall to very low levels, the blood loses its ability to quickly clot. Bruising or prolonged bleeding may happen. Any of these symptoms require immediate studies of blood and bone marrow. For a listing of causative drugs, see Table 5, Section Six.

brand name The registered trade name given to a drug by its manufacturer. Each company creates a trade name to distinguish its brand of the generic drug from its competitors. A brand name designates a proprietary drug—one that is protected by patent or copyright. Generally, brand names are shorter, easier to pronounce, and more readily remembered than their generic counterparts.

capitation A system where a set amount of money is used to cover the cost of health care for a given person. For instance, a health plan or hospital is paid monthly on a negotiated per-person rate and the plan or hospital provides all health services for the people in the plan.

cause-and-effect relationship An association between a drug and a biological event— most commonly a side effect or an adverse effect. Important factors are: when the drug was given, use of multiple drugs and possible interactions, the effects of the disease being treated, physiological and psychological patient factors, and influences of unrecognized disorders or malfunctions.

The majority of adverse drug reactions occur sporadically, unpredictably, and infrequently in the general population. A *definite* cause-and-effect relationship between drug and reaction is shown when (1) the adverse effect immediately follows dosing of the drug; or (2) the adverse effect disappears after the drug is stopped (dechallenge) and reappears when the drug is used again (rechallenge); or (3) the adverse effects are clearly the expected and predictable toxic consequences of drug overdose.

There is also a large gray area of "probable," "possible," and "coincidental" associations. Clarification of cause-and-effect relationships requires observation over a long period of time, followed by sophisticated statistical analysis. Some news stories are based on suggestive but incomplete data. Though early warning is in the public interest, these stories should make clear whether the presumed relationship is based on definitive criteria or is inferred. It is critical to avoid losing valuable medicines because of poorly designed studies that find their way to the news.

The most competent techniques for evaluating cause-and-effect relationships of adverse drug reactions have been devised by the Division of Tissue Reactions to Drugs, a research unit of the Armed Forces Institute of Pathology:

No association	5.0%
Coincidental	14.5%
Possible	33.0%
Probable	30.0%
Causative	17.5%

It is significant that expert evaluation of 2,800 drug-related cases concluded that only 47.5% could be substantiated as causative or probably causative.

contraindication A condition or disease that precludes the use of a drug. Some contraindications are *absolute*, meaning that the drug should NEVER be used in a particular situation. Other contraindications are *relative*, meaning that using the drug requires expert consideration of all factors.

covered lives A term used by health maintenance organizations to indicate how many people have enrolled in their plan. From the HMO's point of view, a minimum number of covered lives is needed to support a certain number of family practice physicians, specialists, and so on. Understanding their logic helps explain why some HMOs have one specialist while others have several.

creatinine clearance A measure of how well the kidneys are eliminating waste, toxins, and impurities from the body. A low creatinine clearance (such as 20 ml per minute or ml/min) means poorer kidney function; a high creatinine clearance (such as 120 ml/min) means better kidney function. People who have low creatinine clearances often receive lower initial doses and smaller increases of medicines that the kidneys remove.

critical or clinical pathway An assortment of coordinated measures taken by a health care organization to effectively group care of specific diseases or conditions. All diagnostic tests, treatments, discharge plans, and other factors are carefully studied and practice is aimed at giving the best patient results in the most cost-effective manner.

dependence A term identifying *psychological dependence* (or *habituation*) and *physical dependence* (or *addiction*). In addition, *functional dependence*—the need to use a drug continuously in order to sustain a particular body function—is included.

Psychological dependence is a form of neurotic behavior—an "emotional" dependence. It is an obsession to satisfy a particular desire. Psychological dependence is also seen in many socially acceptable patterns such as entertainment, gambling, sports, and collecting. Unfortunately, we often see an increasing reliance on drugs to help cope with everyday problems: pills for frustration, nervous stomach, tension headache, and insomnia. This compulsive abuse shows little or no tendency to increase the dose (see TOLERANCE) and no or minor physical symptoms on withdrawal. Some clinicians include psychological dependence in the definition of addiction.

Physical dependence, which is true addiction, includes two elements: *tolerance* and *withdrawal*. Addicting drugs provide relief from anguish and pain, but can also cause a physiological tolerance requiring increased doses or repeated use to remain effective. These two features foster its becoming a functioning component in brain biochemistry. (Thus some authorities prefer *chemical dependence*.) Sudden removal of the drug causes a major upheaval in body chemistry provoking a withdrawal syndrome—the intense mental and physical pain that is the hallmark of addiction. True addiction is rare, and fear of addiction, even with potent narcotics, should never stand in the way of effective pain control.

Functional dependence differs from both psychological and physical dependence. It occurs when a drug relieves a distressing condition and provides a sense of well-being. Drugs that cause functional dependence are often used for symptom relief. The most familiar example of functional dependence is the "laxative habit." Some types of constipation are made worse by the wrong laxative, and natural bowel function fades as the colon becomes more and more dependent on the laxative drug.

disease management An approach to prevention and treatment of a specific condition that checks how often it happens in a population, organizes resources, and allocates money to reach the best balance of dollars spent and results achieved.

disulfiramlike (Antabuse-like) reaction Symptoms resulting from the interaction of alcohol and a drug causing the "Antabuse effect." Symptoms include intense facial flushing, severe throbbing headache, shortness of breath, chest pains, nausea, repeated vomiting, sweating, and weakness. If a large enough amount of alcohol is present, the reaction may progress to blurred vision, vertigo, marked drop in blood pressure, and loss of consciousness. Severe reactions may lead to convulsions and death. The reaction can last from 30 minutes to several hours, depending upon the amount of alcohol in the body. As the symptoms subside, the person is exhausted and often sleeps for several hours.

diuretic A drug that increases urine volume. Diuretics work in several ways to accomplish this. Diuretics are used to (1) remove excess water from the body (as in congestive heart failure and some types of liver and kidney disease), and (2) treat hypertension by promoting excretion of sodium from the body.

divided doses The total daily dose of a medicine is split into smaller individual doses over the course of a day.

dosage forms and strengths This information category in the individual Drug Profiles (Section Two) uses several abbreviations to designate measurements of weight and volume. These are:

mcg	=	microgram	= 1,000,000th of a gram (weight)
mg	=	milligram	= 1,000th of a gram (weight)
ml	=	milliliter	= 1,000th of a liter (volume)
gm	=	gram	= 1,000 milligrams (weight)

There are approximately 65 mg in 1 grain.
There are approximately 5 ml in 1 teaspoon.
There are approximately 15 ml in 1 tablespoon.
There are approximately 30 ml in 1 ounce.
1 milliliter of water weighs 1 g.
There are approximately 454 g in 1 pound.

drug, drug product Terms used interchangeably to describe a medicine (in any form) used in medical practice. The term *drug* refers to the single chemical that provokes a specific response when put in a biological system—the "active" ingredient. A *drug product* is the dosage form—tablet, capsule, elixir, etc.—that has the active drug mixed with inactive ingredients to provide convenient dosing. Drug products that have one active ingredient are called single-entity drugs. Drug products with two or more active ingredients are called combination drugs ([CD] in the brand names in the Drug Profiles, Section Two).

drug class A group of drugs that are similar in chemistry, method of action, and use. Because of their common characteristics, many drugs in a class will cause the same side effects and have similar potential for related adverse reactions and interactions. Variations among members within a drug class can occur. This permits choices to be made if certain benefits are desired or particular side effects are to be minimized. Examples: Antihistamines and phenothiazines (see Drug Classes, Section Four).

drug family A group of drugs that are similar in chemistry, method of action, and purpose. In *The Essential Guide*, drug families are identified by entries such as the Minimally Sedating Antihistamines Family. This allows you to easily compare the drugs meeting the criteria for listing in the book.

drug fever Increased body temperature caused by a medicine. Drugs can cause fever by allergic reactions, tissue damage, acceleration of tissue metabolism, constriction of skin blood vessels, and direct action on the brain. The most common form of drug fever is allergic. It may be the only allergic symptom, or may include skin rash, hives, joint swelling and pain, enlarged lymph glands, hemolytic anemia, or hepatitis. The fever usually appears about 7 to 10 days after starting the drug and varies from low-grade to alarmingly high levels. It may be sustained or intermittent, but usually lasts for as long as the drug is taken. Although many drugs can cause fever, the following are more commonly responsible:

allopurinol	novobiocin
antihistamines	*para*-aminosalicylic acid
atropinelike drugs	penicillin
barbiturates	pentazocine
coumarin anticoagulants	phenytoin
hydralazine	procainamide
iodides	propylthiouracil
isoniazid	quinidine
methyldopa	rifampin
nadolol	sulfonamides

extension effect An unwanted but predictable drug response that is a result of mild to moderate overdose. It is an exaggeration of the drug's pharmacological action; it can be thought of as a mild form of dose-related toxicity (see OVERDOSAGE and TOXICITY).

> *Example:* The continued "hangover" of mental sluggishness that persists in the morning is a common extension effect of a long-acting, sleep-inducing drug (hypnotic, such as Dalmane) taken the night before.

FDA approvable A stage in the Food and Drug Administration's review and approval process. A medicine is considered FDA approvable once the panel which reviewed the supporting data submitted to the FDA finds that data acceptable. In general, at this point only final details need to be resolved before the drug becomes FDA approved and is made available for general use.

generic name The official, common, or public name used to describe an active drug. Generic names are coined by committees of drug experts and are approved by governmental agencies for national and international use. Many drug products are marketed only under a generic name. The most commonly prescribed generics are listed below, ranked in descending order of new or refill prescriptions issued.

amoxicillin

hydrocodone/acetaminophen

furosemide

albuterol aerosol

trimethoprim/Sulfa

cephalexin

acetaminophen/codeine

propoxyphene-N/acetaminophen

triamterene/HCTZ

ibuprofen

genetic therapy Perhaps the most promising area of therapy in medicine today. Healthy genetic material is isolated and inserted into appropriate but diseased cells. For example, normal lung genes are given to a person with cystic fibrosis. Still very experimental, it may someday allow people suffering with genetically-based diseases or conditions to receive therapy that changes the affected genes and actually *cure* those conditions.

habituation A form of drug dependence based upon strong psychological gratification. Ongoing use of mood altering drugs or those relieving minor discomforts results from compulsive need to feel pleasure and satisfaction or to escape emotional distress. If these drugs are abruptly stopped, a withdrawal does not result. Thus habituation is a *psychological dependence*. (See DEPENDENCE for more on psychological and physical dependence.)

hemolytic anemia Lower red blood cells and hemoglobin caused by premature destruction (hemolysis) of red blood cells. One way that this happens is from a genetic lowering of glucose-6-phosphate dehydrogenase (G6PD), a needed enzyme. If patients with this condition are given antimalarial drugs, sulfa drugs, or others, red cells will be destroyed. One type of drug-induced hemolytic anemia is a form of allergy. Many drugs widely used drugs (such as quinidine and levodopa) can cause hemolytic destruction of red cells as an allergic reaction. Hemolytic anemia can occur abruptly or silently. The acute form lasts about 7 days and shows as fever, pallor, weakness, dark-colored urine, and varying degrees of jaundice. If drug-induced hemolytic anemia is mild, there may be no symptoms (see IDIOSYNCRASY and ALLERGY [DRUG]). For drugs that may cause this, see Table 5, Section Six.

hepatitislike reaction Some drugs may cause liver damage similar to viral hepatitis. Symptoms of drug-induced hepatitis and viral hepatitis are often so similar that only laboratory tests can tell the difference. Hepatitis from drugs may be an allergy, or it may be a toxic adverse effect. Serious liver reactions usually lead to jaundice (see JAUNDICE). For drugs that can cause this, see Table 8, Section Six.

HMO Abbreviation for Health Maintenance Organization: A health care system that provides a broad spectrum of medical therapies and services by a collective group of people in a common organization.

hypersensitivity Overresponsiveness to drugs. Used in this sense, it means that the response is appropriate but the degree of response is exaggerated. The term is more widely used today to identify an allergy. To have *hypersensitivity* to a drug is to be *allergic* to it (see ALLERGY [DRUG]). Some people develop cross-hypersensitivity. This means that allergy to one drug will also lead to a reaction to other closely related drugs.

> *Example:* A *hypersensitive* patient had seasonal hay fever and asthma since childhood. His *allergy* to penicillin developed after his third treatment. The *hypersensitivity* was a diffuse, measles-like rash. When he was later given acephalosporin antibiotic, he developed the same rash.

hypnotic A drug used to cause sleep. Classes include: antihistamines, barbiturates,

benzodiazepines, and several unrelated compounds. In the past 15 years, benzodiazepines have largely replaced barbiturates. In general, they are safer and have
lower dependence potential. Tolerance to the hypnotic effect can happen after several weeks of continual use, so hypnotics should be used for short periods of time.

hypoglycemia Sugar (glucose) in blood below the normal range. Since the brain only
runs on sugar, the brain can be seriously impaired by too low a sugar level. Early
warnings include: headache, mild drunkenness feeling, hunger, and an inability to
think clearly. If blood sugar falls further, nervousness and confusion develop.
Weakness, numbness, trembling, sweating, and rapid heartbeat follow. If blood
sugar drops further, impaired speech, and unconsciousness, with or without convulsions, will follow. Treatment for any low blood sugar (hypoglycemia) is important. If you take a drug that can cause hypoglycemia it is prudent to know the
symptoms and what to do if hypoglycemia occurs.

hypothermia A state that occurs when internal body temperature falls below 98.6 degrees F or 37 degrees C. By definition, hypothermia is a body temperature of less
than 95 degrees F or 35 degrees C. The elderly and debilitated are more prone to
hypothermia. Most cases are initiated by room temperatures below 65 degrees F
or 18.3 degrees C. This condition can develop suddenly, can mimic a stroke, and
has a mortality rate of 50%. Some drugs, such as phenothiazines, barbiturates, and
benzodiazepines may make hypothermia more likely.

idiosyncrasy An abnormal drug response that happens in people with a defect in body
chemistry (often hereditary) producing an effect totally unrelated to the drug's
normal action. This is not a form of allergy. Some defects responsible for idiosyncratic drug reactions are well understood; others are not.

Example: Some 100 million people in (including 10% of African-Americans)
have a low glucose-6-phosphate dehydrogenase (G6PD) in red blood cells. These
cells then disintegrate when exposed to sulfonamides (Gantrisin, Kynex), nitrofurantoin (Furadantin, Macrodantin), probenecid (Benemid), quinine, and quinidine. This can lead to a serious anemia.

immunosuppressive A drug that suppresses the immune system. Immunosuppression
maybe an intended drug effect such as cyclosporine preventing the rejection of a
transplanted kidney. In other cases, it is an unwanted side effect, such as the long-
term use of cortisonelike drugs (to control asthma) suppressing the immune system. Chronic disorders thought to be autoimmune—such as rheumatoid arthritis,
ulcerative colitis, and systemic lupus erythematosus—may be eased by immunosuppressive medicines.

interaction An change in a drug that results when a second drug (altering the action
of the first) is given to the same person. Some interactions can enhance the effect
of either drug, giving a response similar to overdose. Other interactions may reduce
drug effectiveness and cause inadequate response. A third interaction can produce an unrelated toxic response with no increase or decrease in the interacting
drugs. Many interactions can be anticipated, and appropriate adjustments in dose
can be made to prevent or minimize fluctuations in drug response.

jaundice A yellow color of skin (and the white portion of the eyes) that occurs when
bile accumulates in blood because of impaired liver function. Jaundice can happen
from a wide variety of diseases, or may be an adverse reaction to a drug. Jaundice
due to a drug is always a serious adverse effect. If you take a medicine that can
cause jaundice, watch closely for any change in urine or feces color. Dark discoloration of urine or pale (lack of color) stools may be early indication of developing jaundice. If this happen, call your doctor promptly. Lab tests can clarify the
nature of the jaundice. Table 8, Section Six lists causative drugs.

JNC VI A national committee of experts that meets to try to establish a framework of medicines used to treat high blood pressure. The committee reviews the currently available drugs and tries to organize possible treatments into a logical approach for lowering high blood pressure and prolonging lives.

lupus erythematosus (LE) A serious disease seen in two forms, one limited to skin (discoid LE) and the other involving several body systems (systemic LE). Both forms occur mostly in young women. About 5% of cases of discoid form convert to the systemic form. Systemic LE is an immune disorder that can be chronic, progressive inflammation destroying connective tissue of the skin, blood vessels, joints, brain, heart muscle, lungs, and kidneys. Altered proteins in the blood lead to antibody formation that attacks the person's own organs or tissues. Low white blood cells and platelets often occur. The course of systemic LE is usually quite protracted and unpredictable. There is no cure, but acceptable management may be achieved in some cases by judicious use of cortisonelike drugs.

Several drugs can start a form of systemic LE quite similar to that which occurs spontaneously. Symptoms may appear as early as 2 weeks or as late as several years after starting the drug. Initial symptoms are usually low-grade fever, skin rashes of various kinds, aching muscles, and multiple joint pains. Chest pains (pleurisy) are fairly common. Enlargement of the lymph glands occurs less frequently. Symptoms usually subside if the drug is stopped, but laboratory evidence of the reaction may persist for many months.

medication map (MM) A new concept in medicines pioneered by Dr. Rybacki. One of the flaws in current drug information is that it is provided for individual medicines when patients actually often take medicines during the same day and in combination as well. Patients are not given a schedule that organizes their medicines into a framework which works well with their usual day. The medication map seeks to organize any and all of the medicines a patient takes into a clear schedule using the best possible times, combinations, and results or outcomes data. A medication map helps avoid drug–drug, drug–food, and drug activity interactions, and gives the patient the best possible quality of life.

neuroleptic malignant syndrome (NMS) A rare, serious, sometimes fatal idiosyncratic reaction to neuroleptic (antipsychotic) drugs. The symptoms are hyperthermia (temperatures of 102 to 104 degrees F), marked muscle rigidity, and coma. Rapid heart rate and breathing, profuse sweating, tremors, and seizures can also occur. Two-thirds of cases happen in men, one-third in women. Mortality rate is 15 to 20%.

The following drugs may cause this reaction:

amitriptyline + perphenazine (Triavil)
amoxapine (Asendin)
chlorpromazine (Thorazine)
chlorprothixene (Taractan)
clomipramine (Anafranil)
fluphenazine (Permitil, Prolixin)
haloperidol (Haldol)
imipramine (Tofranil, etc.)
levodopa + carbidopa (Sinemet)
loxapine (Loxitane)

metoclopramide (Reglan, Octamide)
molindone (Moban)
perphenazine (Etrafon, Trilafon)
pimozide (Orap)
prochlorperazine (Compazine)
thioridazine (Mellaril)
thiothixene (Navane)
trifluoperazine (Stelazine)
trimeprazine (Temaril)

orthostatic hypotension A type of low blood pressure related to body position or posture (also called postural hypotension). People who get orthostatic hypotension may have normal blood pressure lying down, but on sitting upright or standing will feel light-headed, dizzy, and like they are going to faint. These symptoms come from inadequate blood flow (oxygen supply) to the brain.

Many drugs may cause orthostatic hypotension. Tell your doctor if you have this effect so that changes can be made. If this situation isn't corrected, severe falls or injury may result. It is prudent to avoiding sudden standing, prolonged standing, vigorous exercise, and exposure to hot environments. Alcoholic beverages should be used cautiously until combined effects with the drug in use have been determined.

outcomes research A concept in health care evaluation that considers the benefits (gauged by a variety of measures) of using a particular drug versus another. This may lead to the cheapest drug **not** being the drug of choice, because the outcomes from therapy don't stand up over time or may result in significant treatment failure.

overdose The meaning of this term is not limited to doses exceeding the normal range recommended by a manufacturer. The "best" dose of many drugs varies greatly from person to person. An average dose for most people can be an overdose for some and an underdose for others. Factors such as age, body size, nutritional status, and liver and kidney function have significant impacts on dosing.

Drugs with narrow safety margins often give signs of overdose if removal of the daily dose is delayed. Massive overdose—as in accidental ingestion of drugs by children or with suicides—is referred to as poisoning.

over-the-counter (OTC) drugs Medicines that can be bought without prescriptions. Many people do not look upon OTC medicines as drugs. It is important to remember that OTC medicines can have a variety of actions. OTC drugs may react with each other and can also react with prescription medicines. Serious problems can arise when (1) the patient fails to tell their doctor about OTC drug(s) he or she is taking ("because they really aren't drugs") and (2) the doctor fails to specify that his or her question about which drugs are being taken *includes all OTC drugs and herbal meds as well*. During any treatment, patients need to talk with their doctor or pharmacist about any OTC drug that he or she wishes to take. The major classes of OTC drugs for internal use include:

allergy medicines (antihistamines)	menstrual aids
antacids	motion sickness remedies
anti-worm medicines	pain relievers
aspirin and aspirin combinations	salt substitutes
aspirin substitutes	sedatives and tranquilizers
asthma aids	sleeping pills
cold medicines (decongestants)	smoking cessation products
cough medicines	stimulants (caffeine)
diarrhea remedies	sugar substitutes (saccharin)
digestion aids	tonics
diuretics	vaginal yeast infection medicines
heartburn medicines	vitamins
iron preparations	weight-reducing aids
laxatives	

paradoxical reaction A drug response that does not follow the known pharmacology of a drug. These effects are due to individual sensitivity and can occur at any age. They are seen more commonly in children and the elderly.

Example: An 80-year-old man was sent to a nursing home after his wife died. He had trouble adjusting to his new environment and was agitated and irritable. He was given diazepam (Valium) to relax him, starting with small doses. On the second day he became confused. The dose of diazepam was increased. On the third day he began to wander, talked incessantly, and was angry when attempts were made to help him. Suspecting a paradoxical reaction, his health care provider stopped the diazepam. All behavioral disturbances subsided in 3 days.

Parkinson-like disorders (parkinsonism) A group of symptoms resembling Parkinson's disease. The typical features of parkinsonism include a fixed, emotionless facial expression (mask like in appearance); trembling hands, arms, or legs; and stiffness of extremities that produces rigid posture and gait. Parkinsonism is a fairly common adverse effect that occurs in about 15% of patients who take large doses of phenothiazines or use them over an extended period. If found early, the Parkinson-like features will lessen or disappear with lower doses or different medicines. In some cases, Parkinson-like changes may become permanent.

peripheral neuritis (peripheral neuropathy) A group of symptoms that results from injury to nerve tissue in the extremities. A variety of drugs or chemicals can cause this. The sensation of numbness and tingling usually starts in the toes and fingers and toes and is accompanied by altered sensation to touch. Vague discomfort from aching sensations to burning pain is also seen. Severe forms of peripheral neuritis may include loss of muscular strength and coordination. Isoniazid can cause this condition.

If vitamin B_6 (pyridoxine) is not given with isoniazid, peripheral neuritis may occur. Vitamin B_6 can be both preventive and curative in this form of drug-induced peripheral neuritis.

Since peripheral neuritis can also be a late complication of many viral infections, care must be taken to avoid assigning a cause-and-effect relationship to a drug that is not responsible for the nerve injury (see CAUSE-AND-EFFECT RELATIONSHIP).

See Table 10, Section Six, for further discussion of drug-induced nerve damage.

Peyronie's disease A permanent deformity of the penis caused by dense fibrous (scarlike) tissue within in the penile vessels that become engorged with blood during an erection. During sexual arousal, inelastic fibrous tissue causes a painful downward bowing of the penis that hampers or precludes intercourse. This condition has been caused by phenytoin (Dilantin, etc.) and with most members of the beta-blocker drug family (see Drug Classes, Section Four). For a listing of causative drugs, see Table 11, Section Six.

pharmacoeconomics The discipline within pharmacology that studies the issues of costs versus benefits, utilizing a variety of measures: material and personnel costs, treatment outcomes, quality of patient life, etc. Study results are used in deciding where and how health care resources should be utilized.

pharmacology The medical science relating to development and use of drugs as well as their composition and action in animals and man. Used in its broadest sense, pharmacology embraces related sciences of medicinal chemistry, experimental therapeutics, and toxicology.

photosensitivity A drug-induced skin change resulting in a rash or exaggerated sunburn on exposure to the sun or ultraviolet lamps. The reaction is confined to uncovered areas of skin, giving a clue to the nature of its cause. For a list of causative drugs, see Table 2, Section Six.

porphyria Hereditary disorders characterized by the production of excessive amounts of respiratory pigments known as porphyrins. (One porphyrin is part of hemoglobin in red blood cells.) Two forms of porphyria—acute intermittent porphyria and cutaneous porphyria—can be activated by drugs. Acute intermittent porphyria involves nervous system damage. An attack can include fever, rapid heart rate, vomiting, pain in the abdomen and legs, hallucinations, seizures, paralysis, and coma. Some of the drugs that cause this condition include barbiturates, "sulfa" drugs, chlordiazepoxide (Librium), chlorpropamide (Diabinese), methyldopa (Aldomet), and phenytoin (Dilantin). Cutaneous porphyria involves skin and liver damage.

Symptoms include red and blistered skin, followed by crusting, scarring, and excessive hair growth. Repeated liver damage can lead to cirrhosis. This form of porphyria can be caused by chloroquine, estrogen, oral contraceptives, and excessive iron.

priapism Prolonged, painful erection of the penis usually on sexual arousal. It is caused by obstruction to drainage of blood through the veins at the root of the penis. Erection may last for 30 minutes to a few hours and then subside, or it may persist for up to 30 hours and require surgical drainage. More than half of the cases of priapism from drugs result in permanent impotence. Sickle cell anemia may predispose to priapism, and those with this disorder should avoid all drugs that may cause priapism.

Drugs reported to induce priapism include:

anabolic steroids (male hormonelike
    drugs: Anadrol, Anavar, Android,
    Halotestin, Metandren, Oreton,
    Testred, Winstrol)
chlorpromazine (Thorazine)
cocaine
guanethidine (Ismelin)
haloperidol (Haldol)
heparin
levodopa (Sinemet)
molindone (Moban)
prazosin (Minipres)
prochlorperazine (Compazine)
trazodone (Desyrel)
trifluoperazine (Stelazine)
warfarin (Coumadin)

prostatism The difficulties that happen with an enlarged prostate. As the prostate enlarges, it constricts the urethra (outflow passage) and impedes urination. This causes a lower size and force of the urinary stream, hesitancy, interruption, and incomplete bladder emptying. Atropine and drugs with atropinelike effects can impair the bladder's ability to compensate for the prostate gland, intensifying all of the above symptoms.

Raynaud's phenomenon Intermittent episodes of reduced blood flow to fingers or toes, with resulting paleness, discomfort, numbness, and tingling. Stress or exposure to cold can cause an attack. It can occur as part of a systemic disorder (lupus erythematosus, scleroderma) or it can occur without apparent cause (Raynaud's disease). Beta-adrenergic blockers and products that contain ergotamine can lead to Raynaud-like symptoms in predisposed people.

Reye (Reye's) syndrome A sudden, often fatal, childhood illness where the brain swells and the liver degenerates. It usually develops during a viral infection (flu), measles, or chicken pox. Cases have been seen with lupus (SLE). Symptoms include fever, headache, delirium, loss of consciousness, and seizures. It is one of the 10 major causes of death in children ages 1 to 10 years. Those younger than 18 may be affected. The syndrome may be due to combined effects of viral infection and chemical toxins in a genetically predisposed child. Drugs that have been used prior to symptoms include salicylates (aspirin) and drugs to control nausea and vomiting. This is why salicylates (aspirin and aspirinlike medicines) should be avoided in children with flu-like infections, chicken pox, or measles. Some clinicians question the use of any NSAID. Remember to look for salicylates in combination cold or flu products and inflammatory bowel drugs. Valproic acid (a seizure medicine) can cause a Reye-like syndrome. Acetaminophen appears to the medicine of choice in those less than 18 with fever from a sudden viral illness.

secondary effect A complication of drug use that does not occur as part of the drug's primary pharmacological activity. Secondary effects are unwanted consequences and are adverse effects.

    Example: Cramping of leg muscles can be a *secondary effect* of diuretic (urine-producing) drug treatment for high blood pressure. Excessive loss of potassium renders the muscle vulnerable to painful spasm during exercise.

side effect A normal, expected, and predictable response to a drug. Side effects are part of a drug's pharmacological activity and are unavoidable. Most side effects are undesirable. The majority cause minor annoyance and inconvenience; a few can be hazardous.

superinfection (suprainfection) A second infection superimposed on an initial infection. The superinfection is caused by organisms not killed by the drug(s) used to treat the original (primary) infection. This kind of infection usually happens during or following use of a broad-spectrum antibiotic. The disturbance of the normal balance of bacteria permits overgrowth of organisms usually found in numbers too small to cause disease. The superinfection may also require treatment, using those drugs that are effective against the offending organism.

Example: A woman is given an antibiotic for a sinus infection. This medicine changes the bacteria usually present in her vagina, allowing yeast to grow. The yeast infection must then be treated with a second medicine.

tardive dyskinesia A drug-induced nervous system disorder with involuntary and bizarre movements of eyelids, jaws, lips, tongue, neck, and fingers. It can happen after use of potent drugs for mental illness. It may occur in any age group, but is more common in the middle-aged and especially in chronically ill older women. Once it starts, it may be irreversible. To date, there is no way of identifying who may develop this reaction. The abnormal movement (dyskinesia) is not associated with decline in mental function.

tolerance A situation where the body adapts to a medicine, and reacts to it less vigorously over time. Tolerance can be beneficial or harmful in treatment.

Example: Beneficial tolerance happens when someone with hay fever finds that drowsiness from their antihistamine gradually disappears after 4 or 5 days of continuous use.

Harmful tolerance occurs when the patient with shingles (herpes zoster) finds that the usual dose of pain medicine no longer works to relieve pain.

toxicity Capacity of a drug to impair body functions or damage tissues. Most drug toxicity is related to total dose: the larger the dose, the greater the toxic effects. Some drugs are toxic in normal doses. Toxic effects due to overdose are often a harmful extension of normal pharmacological actions and may be predictable and preventable.

trough-to-peak ratio (T/P) A new concept that the FDA is currently using to check dosing of medicines for high blood pressure. The T:P ratio is calculated by dividing the blood pressure level immediately before the next drug dose (trough) by the largest blood pressure drop during the time between doses. A result greater than 50% means that the effect of the medicine over the entire time between doses is ideal.

tyramine A chemical present in many common foods and beverages which raises blood pressure. Normally, enzymes in the body (monoamine oxidase [MAO] type A) neutralize tyramine. If the action of MAO type A is blocked, substances like tyramine can cause alarming and dangerous increases in blood pressure.

Several drugs can block monoamine oxidase type A. They are called monoamine oxidase (MAO) type A inhibitors (see Drug Classes, Section Four). If you take one of these drugs and your diet includes foods or beverages high in tyramine, sudden increases in blood pressure may happen. Talk with your doctor or pharmacist about an appropriate diet and before combining any other medicine with an MAO inhibitor.

The following foods and beverages have been reported to contain varying amounts of tyramine. Unless their tyramine content is known to be insignificant, they should be avoided altogether while taking an MAO type A inhibitor drug.

FOODS	BEVERAGES
Aged cheeses of all kinds*	Beer (unpasteurized)
Avocado	Chianti wine
Banana skins	Sherry wine
Bean curd	Vermouth
Bologna	
"Bovril" extract	
Broad bean pods	
Chicken liver (unless fresh and used at once)	
Chocolate	
Figs, canned	
Fish, canned	
Fish, dried and salted	
Herring, pickled	
Liver, if not very fresh	
"Marmite" extract	
Meat extracts	
Meat tenderizers	
Pepperoni	
Raisins	
Raspberries	
Salami	
Shrimp paste	
Sour cream	
Soy sauce	
Yeast extracts	

Note: *Any* high-protein food that is aged or has undergone breakdown by putrefaction probably contains tyramine and could produce a hypertensive crisis in anyone taking MAO type A inhibitor drugs.

viral load or viral burden A term used in reference to AIDS patients to describe the amount of HIV virus present in the body at any given time. The amount of virus relates to how well drug therapy is working, and can be a reason to change drugs if the load increases.

WHO Pain Ladder A therapeutic scheme using increasing strengths and combinations of pain medicines (analgesics) that includes NSAIDs, opiates, and adjuvant drugs to control pain as specified by the World Health Organization. It is *not* an absolute treatment scheme, but should be used to organize the approach to effective pain prevention.

*Cottage cheese, cream cheese, and processed cheese are safe to eat.

TABLES OF DRUG INFORMATION

TABLE 1

Drugs That May Adversely Affect the Fetus and Newborn Infant

The thalidomide disaster of 1961 sparked concern about medicines causing problems if used during pregnancy (possible teratogens). Extremely effective medicines such as the HMG-CoA inhibitors for lowering cholesterol should NEVER be taken during pregnancy (Category X). Our understanding of how drugs can affect the fetus or newborn infant has grown, and the list of the drugs that can cause significant harm to the unborn and newborn child has gotten larger and larger. In many cases, it is not possible to clearly separate adverse effects due to the mother's disease or disorder from those that may be caused by medicines. Based on our current knowledge, it is strongly recommended that only those drugs that confer clear and essential benefits should be used during pregnancy.

Drugs that *probably* cause adverse effects when taken during the *first trimester*

aminopterin
anticonvulsants*
antithyroid drugs
cytarabine
danazol
diethylstilbestrol
ethanol (large amounts and for long periods)
etretinate

finasteride
fluorouracil
HMG-CoA reductase inhibitors*
iodides
isotretinoin
kanamycin
mercaptopurine
methotrexate

misoprostol
opioid analgesics*
progestins*
quinine
streptomycin
testosterone
warfarin

Drugs that *possibly* cause adverse effects when taken during the *first trimester*

angiotensin-converting enzyme inhibitors*
busulfan
chlorambucil
estrogens*

lithium
mebendazole
monoamine oxidase inhibitors*
oral contraceptives

piperazine
rifampin
tetracyclines*

Drugs that *probably* cause adverse effects when taken during the *second* and *third trimesters*

amiodarone
androgens*
angiotensin-converting enzyme inhibitors*
antithyroid drugs
aspirin
benzodiazepines*
chloramphenicol
estrogens*
ethanol (large amounts and for long periods)

finasteride
HMG-CoA reductase inhibitors*
iodides
kanamycin
lithium
nonsteroidal anti-inflammatory drugs (NSAIDs)*
opioid analgesics*
phenothiazines*

progestins*
rifampin
streptomycin
sulfonamides*
sulfonylureas*
tetracyclines*
thiazide diuretics*
tricyclic antidepressants*
warfarin

Drugs that *possibly* cause adverse effects when taken during the *second* and *third trimesters*

acetazolamide
clemastine
diphenhydramine

ethacrynic acid
fluoroquinolones*
haloperidol

hydroxyzine
promethazine

*See Drug Class, Section Four.

TABLE 2

Drugs That May Cause Photosensitivity on Exposure to the Sun

Some drugs can sensitize skin to ultraviolet light. This can cause the skin to react with a rash or exaggerated burn on exposure to sun or ultraviolet lamps. If you are taking any of the following drugs, ask your doctor for help about sun exposure and sunblocks.

acetazolamide
acetohexamide
alprazolam
amantadine
amiloride
aminobenzoic acid
amiodarone
amitriptyline
amoxapine
barbiturates
bendroflumethiazide
benzocaine
benzophenones
benzoyl peroxide
benzthiazide
captopril
carbamazepine
chlordiazepoxide
chloroquine
chlorothiazide
chlorpromazine
chlorpropamide
chlortetracycline
chlorthalidone
ciprofloxacin
clindamycin
clofazimine
clofibrate
clomipramine
cyproheptadine
dacarbazine
dapsone
demeclocycline
desipramine
desoximetasone
diethylstilbestrol
diflunisal
diltiazem
diphenhydramine
disopyramide

doxepin
doxycycline
enoxacin
estrogen
etretinate
flucytosine
fluorescein
fluorouracil
fluphenazine
flutamide
furosemide
glipizide
glyburide
gold preparations
griseofulvin
haloperidol
hexachlorophene
hydrochlorothiazide
hydroflumethiazide
ibuprofen
imipramine
indomethacin
isotretinoin
ketoprofen
lincomycin
lomefloxacin
maprotiline
mesoridazine
methacycline
methotrexate
methyclothiazide
methyldopa
metolazone
minocycline
minoxidil
nabumetone
nalidixic acid
naproxen
nifedipine
norfloxacin

nortriptyline
ofloxacin
oral contraceptives
oxyphenbutazone
oxytetracycline
para-aminobenzoic acid
perphenazine
phenelzine
phenobarbital
phenylbutazone
phenytoin
piroxicam
polythiazide
prochlorperazine
promazine
promethazine
protriptyline
pyrazinamide
quinidine
quinine
sulfonamides*
sulindac
tetracycline
thiabendazole
thioridazine
thiothixene
tolazamide
tolbutamide
tranylcypromine
trazodone
tretinoin
triamterene
trichlormethiazide
trifluoperazine
triflupromazine
trimeprazine
trimethoprim
trimipramine
triprolidine
vinblastine

TABLE 3

Drugs That May Adversely Affect Behavior

Medicines can alter mood and emotional stability. They can also cause unpredictable patterns of thinking or behavior. These responses are relatively infrequent, but the na-

*See Drug Class, Section Four.

ture and degree of mental disturbance can be alarming as well as dangerous for both patient and family.

Such paradoxical responses are often of an idiosyncratic nature, and someone with a history of a serious mental or emotional disorder is more likely to experience bizarre reactions. In some cases, it may be hard to separate the disorder being treated from an effect of one (or more) medicines the patient may be taking. If in doubt, it is best to talk with your doctor.

Drugs reported to impair *concentration* and/or *memory*

antihistamines*
anti-parkinsonism drugs*
barbiturates*
benzodiazepines*

isoniazid
monoamine oxidase
  (MAO) inhibitor drugs*
phenytoin

primidone
scopolamine

Drugs reported to cause *confusion, delirium,* or *disorientation*

acetazolamide
acyclovir
aminophylline
amphotericin B
anticholinergics
antidepressants*
antihistamines*
antipsychotics
atropinelike drugs*
barbiturates*
benzodiazepines*
beta-adrenergic blockers
  (some)*
bromides
carbamazepine
chloroquine
cimetidine

clonidine
cortisonelike drugs*
cycloserine
digitalis
digitoxin
digoxin
disulfiram
diuretics
ethchlorvynol
ethinamate
fenfluramine
fluoroquinolone
  antibiotics*
glutethimide
H_2-receptor antagonists
isoniazid
levodopa

meprobamate
methyldopa
metoclopramide
narcotic pain relievers
  (analgesics)
NSAIDs*
para-aminosalicylic acid
phenelzine
phenothiazines*
phenytoin
piperazine
primidone
propranolol
reserpine
scopolamine
theophylline
tricyclic antidepressants

Drugs reported to cause *paranoid thinking*

acyclovir
amphetaminelike
  medicines
anticholinergic drugs
benzodiazepines*

bromides
cortisonelike drugs*
diphenhydramine
disopyramide
disulfiram

isoniazid
levodopa
propafenone
tricyclic antidepressants*

Drugs reported to cause *schizophrenic-like behavior*

amphetamine-like drugs*
anabolic steroids
cimetidine (case reports
  and in elderly or

debilitated)
ciprofloxacin (case reports
  and idiosyncratic)
ephedrine

fenfluramine
phenmetrazine
phenylpropanolamine

Drugs reported to cause *manic-like behavior*

antidepressants*
clarithromycin (case
  reports)
cortisonelike drugs*
levodopa

metoclopramide (case
  reports)
monoamine oxidase
  (MAO) inhibitor drugs*
selective serotonin

reuptake inhibitors
(SSRIs) (when drug
stopped)

*See Drug Class, Section Four.

Some medicines have mood-altering *side effects*, although they are prescribed for altogether unrelated conditions. Emotional and behavioral secondary effects will be quite unpredictable and vary enormously from person to person. However, the following experiences have been seen with sufficient frequency to establish recognizable patterns.

Drugs reported to cause *nervousness* (anxiety and irritability)

amantadine
amphetaminelike drugs*
    (appetite suppressants)
anabolic steroids
antihistamines*
caffeine
chlorphenesin
cimetidine (case reports in
    elderly)
cocaine
cortisonelike drugs*

ephedrine
epinephrine
isoproterenol
levodopa
liothyronine (in excessive
    dosage)
methylphenidate
methysergide
monoamine oxidase
    (MAO) inhibitor drugs*
nylidrin

oral contraceptives
selective serotonin
    reuptake inhibitors
theophylline
thyroid (in excessive
    dosage)
thyroxine (in excessive
    dosage)

Drugs reported to cause *emotional depression*

amantadine
amphetamines* (on
    withdrawal)
baclofen
benzodiazepines*
beta-adrenergic-blocking
    drugs* (some)
calcium channel blockers*
    (case reports)
carbamazepine
chloramphenicol
cortisonelike drugs*
cycloserine
digitalis
digitoxin
digoxin
diphenoxylate

estrogens
ethionamide
fenfluramine (on
    withdrawal)
fluphenazine
guanethidine
haloperidol
HMG-CoA reductase
    inhibitors* (case reports)
indomethacin
isoniazid
isotretinoin
levodopa
methsuximide
methyldopa
methysergide
metoclopramide (case

reports)
metoprolol
oral contraceptives
phenylbutazone
procainamide
progesterones
propranolol
reserpine
sulfonamides*
thiazide diuretics* (may
    start after weeks to
    months)
vinblastine (possibly dose
    related)
vitamin D (in excessive
    dosage)

Drugs reported to cause *euphoria*

amantadine
aminophylline
amphetamines
antihistamines* (some)
antispasmodics, synthetic*
aspirin
barbiturates*
benzphetamine
cephalosporins (increased
    risk with kidney disease)
chloral hydrate

clorazepate
codeine
cortisonelike drugs*
diethylpropion
diphenoxylate
dronabinol
ethosuximide
flurazepam
haloperidol
levodopa
meprobamate

methysergide
monoamine oxidase
    (MAO) inhibitor drugs*
morphine
opioids*
pargyline
pentazocine
phenmetrazine
propoxyphene
scopolamine
tybamate

Drugs reported to cause *excitement*

acetazolamide
amantadine
amphetaminelike drugs*

antidepressants*
antihistamines*
atropinelike drugs*

*See Drug Class, Section Four.

Drugs reported to cause *excitement* (cont.)

barbiturates* (paradoxical response)
benzodiazepines* (paradoxical response)
cortisonelike drugs
cycloserine
diethylpropion
digitalis
ephedrine
epinephrine

ethinamate (paradoxical response)
ethionamide
glutethimide (paradoxical response)
isoniazid
isoproterenol
levodopa
meperidine and MAO inhibitor drugs*

methyldopa and MAO inhibitor drugs*
methyprylon (paradoxical response)
nalidixic acid
orphenadrine
quinine
scopolamine

TABLE 4

Drugs That May Adversely Affect Vision

A significant percentage of all adverse drug effects involve visual changes or eye damage. Some effects, such as blurring of vision or double vision, may occur shortly after starting a drug. More subtle and serious effects, such as cataract development or damage to the retina or optic nerve, may not happen until a drug has been in use for a long time. Some changes are irreversible. If you are taking a drug that can affect the eye, promptly report any eye discomfort or change in vision.

Drugs reported to cause *blurring of vision*

acetazolamide
antiarthritic/anti-inflammatory drugs
antidepressants*
antihistamines*
atropinelike drugs*

chlorthalidone
ciprofloxacin
cortisonelike drugs*
diethylstilbestrol
etretinate
fenfluramine

norfloxacin
oral contraceptives
phenytoin
sulfonamides*
tetracyclines*
thiazide diuretics*

Drugs reported to cause *double vision*

antidepressants*
antidiabetic drugs*
antihistamines*
aspirin
barbiturates*
benzodiazepines*
bromides
carbamazepine
carisoprodol
chloroquine
chlorprothixene
ciprofloxacin
clomiphene
colchicine
colistin
cortisonelike drugs*

digitalis
digitoxin
digoxin
ethionamide
ethosuximide
etretinate
guanethidine
hydroxychloroquine
indomethacin
isoniazid
levodopa
mephenesin
methocarbamol
methsuximide
morphine
nalidixic acid

nitrofurantoin
norfloxacin
oral contraceptives
orphenadrine
oxyphenbutazone
pentazocine
phenothiazines*
phensuximide
phenylbutazone
phenytoin
primidone
propranolol
quinidine
sedatives/sleep inducers*
thiothixene
tranquilizers*

Drugs reported to cause *farsightedness*

ergot
penicillamine

sulfonamides* (possibly)
tolbutamide (possibly)

*See Drug Class, Section Four.

Drugs reported to cause *nearsightedness*

acetazolamide
aspirin
carbachol
chlorthalidone
codeine
cortisonelike drugs*

ethosuximide
methsuximide
morphine
oral contraceptives
penicillamine
phenothiazines*

phensuximide
spironolactone
sulfonamides*
tetracyclines*
thiazide diuretics*

Drugs reported to *alter color vision*

acetaminophen
amodiaquine
amyl nitrite
aspirin
atropine
barbiturates*
belladonna
chloramphenicol
chloroquine
chlorpromazine
chlortetracycline
ciprofloxacin
cortisonelike drugs*
digitalis
digitoxin
digoxin
disulfiram
epinephrine
ergotamine
erythromycin

ethchlorvynol
ethionamide
fluphenazine
furosemide
hydroxychloroquine
indomethacin
isocarboxazid
isoniazid
mefenamic acid
mesoridazine
methysergide
nalidixic acid
norfloxacin
oral contraceptives
oxyphenbutazone
paramethadione
pargyline
penicillamine
pentylenetetrazol
perphenazine

phenacetin
phenylbutazone
primidone
prochlorperazine
promazine
promethazine
quinacrine
quinidine
quinine
reserpine
sodium salicylate
streptomycin
sulfonamides*
thioridazine
tranylcypromine
trifluoperazine
triflupromazine
trimeprazine
trimethadione

Drugs reported to cause *sensitivity to light* (photophobia)

antidiabetic drugs*
atropinelike drugs*
bromides
chloroquine
ciprofloxacin
clomiphene
digitoxin
doxepin
ethambutol

ethionamide
ethosuximide
etretinate
hydroxychloroquine
mephenytoin
methsuximide
monoamine oxidase
    (MAO) inhibitor drugs*
nalidixic acid

norfloxacin
oral contraceptives
paramethadione
phenothiazines*
quinidine
quinine
tetracyclines*
trimethadione

Drugs reported to cause *halos around lights*

amyl nitrite
chloroquine
cortisonelike drugs*
digitalis
digitoxin

digoxin
hydrochloroquine
nitroglycerin
norfloxacin
oral contraceptives

paramethadione
phenothiazines*
quinacrine
trimethadione

Drugs reported to cause *visual hallucinations*

amantadine
amphetaminelike drugs*
amyl nitrite
antihistamines*
aspirin

atropinelike drugs*
barbiturates*
benzodiazepines*
bromides
carbamazepine

cephalexin
cephaloglycin
chloroquine
cycloserine
digitalis

*See Drug Class, Section Four.

Drugs reported to cause *visual hallucinations* (cont.)

digoxin	isosorbide	primidone
disulfiram	levodopa	propranolol
ephedrine	nialamide	quinine
furosemide	oxyphenbutazone	sedatives/sleep inducers*
gabapentin	pargyline	sulfonamides*
griseofulvin	pentazocine	tetracyclines*
haloperidol	phenothiazines*	tricyclic antidepressants*
hydroxychloroquine	phenylbutazone	tripelennamine
indomethacin	phenytoin	

Drugs reported to impair the use of *contact lenses*

brompheniramine	dexbrompheniramine	oral contraceptives
carbinoxamine	dexchlorpheniramine	terfenadine
chlorpheniramine	dimethindene	tripelennamine
cyclizine	diphenhydramine	
cyproheptadine	furosemide	

Drugs reported to cause *cataracts* or *lens deposits*

allopurinol	methotrimeprazine	thioridazine
busulfan	perphenazine	thiothixene
chlorpromazine	phenmetrazine	trifluoperazine
chlorprothixene	pilocarpine	triflupromazine
cortisonelike drugs*	prochlorperazine	trimeprazine
fluphenazine	promazine	
mesoridazine	promethazine	

TABLE 5

Drugs That May Cause Blood Cell Dysfunction or Damage

All blood cells come from and mature in the bone marrow: red blood cells (erythrocytes), white blood cells (leukocytes), and blood platelets (thrombocytes). There are three kinds of white blood cells: granulocytes, monocytes (macrophages), and lymphocytes. Drugs that affect formation or development of blood cells can (1) act on any stage of cell production; (2) impair one cell type or line; (3) influence all cell lines. Some medicines can damage mature cells in the bloodstream.

Drugs that cause inevitable (dose-dependent) *aplastic anemia* (see Glossary)

actinomycin D	cytarabine	mercaptopurine
azathioprine	doxorubicin	methotrexate
busulfan	epirubicin	mitomycin
carboplatin	etoposide	mitoxantrone
carmustine	fluorouracil	plicamycin
chlorambucil	hydroxyurea	procarbazine
cisplatin	lomustine	thioguanine
cyclophosphamide	melphalan	thiotepa

Drugs that may cause idiosyncratic (dose-independent) *aplastic anemia*

amodiaquine	carbimazole	chlorpromazine
benoxaprofen	chloramphenicol	gold

*See Drug Class, Section Four.

Drugs that may cause idiosyncratic (dose-independent) *aplastic anemia* (cont.)

indomethacin
mepacrine
oxyphenbutazone
penicillamine
phenylbutazone

phenytoin
piroxicam
prothiaden
pyrimethamine
sulfonamides*

sulindac
thiouracils
trimethoprim/
   sulfamethoxazole

Drugs that may *impair red blood cell production* (only)

azathioprine
carbamazepine
chloramphenicol
chlorpropamide
dapsone
fenoprofen
gold
halothane

isoniazid
methyldopa
penicillin
pentachlorophenol
phenobarbital
phenylbutazone
phenytoin
pyrimethamine

sulfasalazine
sulfathiazol
sulfonamides*
sulfonylureas*
thiamphenicol
tolbutamide
trimethoprim/
   sulfamethoxazole

Drugs that may significantly *reduce granulocyte cell counts* (various mechanisms)

acetaminophen
acetazolamide
allopurinol
amitriptyline
amodiaquine
benzodiazepines*
captopril
carbamazepine
carbimazole
cephalosporins*
chloramphenicol
chloroquine
chlorothiazide
chlorpromazine
chlorpropamide
chlorthalidone
cimetidine
clindamycin
dapsone
desipramine
disopyramide

ethacrynic acid
gentamicin
gold
hydralazine
hydrochlorothiazide
imipramine
indomethacin
isoniazid
levamisole
meprobamate
methimazole
methyldopa
oxyphenbutazone
penicillamine
penicillins*
pentazocine
phenacetin
phenothiazines*
phenylbutazone
phenytoin
procainamide

propranolol
propylthiouracil
pyrimethamine
quinidine
quinine
ranitidine
rifampin
sodium aminosalicylate
streptomycin
sulfadoxine
sulfadoxine/
   pyrimethamine
sulfonamides*
tetracyclines*
tocainide
tolbutamide
trimethoprim/
   sulfamethoxazole
vancomycin

Drugs that may significantly *reduce blood platelet counts*

acetazolamide
actinomycin
allopurinol
alpha-interferon
amiodarone
ampicillin
aspirin
carbamazepine
carbenicillin
cephalosporins*
chenodeoxycholic acid

chloroquine
chlorothiazide
chlorpheniramine
chlorpropamide
chlorthalidone
cimetidine
cyclophosphamide
danazol
desferrioxamine
diazepam
diazoxide

diclofenac
digoxin
diltiazem
furosemide
gentamicin
gold
hydrochlorothiazide
imipramine
isoniazid
isotretinoin
levamisole

*See Drug Class, Section Four.

Drugs that may significantly *reduce blood platelet counts* (cont.)

meprobamate	penicillin	sodium aminosalicylate
methyldopa	phenylbutazone	sulfasalazine
mianserin	phenytoin	sulfonamides*
minoxidil	piroxicam	thioguanine
morphine	procainamide	trimethoprim/
nitrofurantoin	quinidine	sulfamethoxazole
oxprenolol	quinine	valproate
oxyphenbutazone	ranitidine	vancomycin
penicillamine	rifampin	

Drugs that cause *hemolytic anemia* due to glucose-6-phosphate dehydrogenase (G6PD) deficiency of red blood cells

acetanilid	pamaquine	sulfanilamide
methylene blue	phenazopyridine	sulfapyridine
nalidixic acid	phenylhydrazine	thiazolsulfone
naphthalene	primaquine	toluidine blue
niridazole	sulfacetamide	
nitrofurantoin	sulfamethoxazole	

Drugs that may cause *hemolytic anemia* by other mechanisms

antimony	methotrexate	quinidine
chlorpropamide	*para*-aminosalicylic acid	quinine
cisplatin	penicillamine	rifampin
mephenesin	phenazopyridine	sulfasalazine

Drugs that may cause *megaloblastic anemia*

acyclovir	metformin	primidone
alcohol	methotrexate	pyrimethamine
aminopterin	neomycin	sulfasalazine
azathioprine	nitrofurantoin	tetracycline
colchicine	nitrous oxide	thioguanine
cycloserine	oral contraceptives	triamterene
cytarabine	*para*-aminosalicylic acid	trimethoprim
floxuridine	pentamidine	vinblastine
fluorouracil	phenformin	vitamin A
hydroxyurea	phenobarbital	vitamin C (large doses)
mercaptopurine	phenytoin	zidovudine

Drugs that may cause *sideroblastic anemia*

alcohol	isoniazid	pyrazinamide
chloramphenicol	penicillamine	
cycloserine	phenacetin	

TABLE 6

Drugs That May Cause Heart Dysfunction or Damage

Drugs may damage both heart structure or function. Heart problems themselves often decide the nature of adverse drug effects. Some are direct pharmacological actions of a drug on heart tissues, and others are caused indirectly by altering chemical balances

*See Drug Class, Section Four.

that diminish how well the heart works (as with potassium or magnesium loss from diuretics).

Drugs that may cause or contribute to *abnormal heart rhythms* (arrhythmias)

aminophylline
amiodarone
amitriptyline
antiarrhythmic drugs*
bepridil
beta-adrenergic-blocking
  drugs*
beta-adrenergic
  bronchodilators
carbamazepine
chlorpromazine
cimetidine
digitoxin
digoxin

diltiazem
disopyramide
diuretics*
doxepin
encainide
fentolterol
flecainide
isoproterenol
ketanserin
lidocaine
maprotiline
methyldopa
mexiletine
milrinone

phenothiazines*
prenylamine
procainamide
quinidine
ranitidine
sotalol
terbutaline
theophylline
thiazide diuretics*
thioridazine
trazodone
tricyclic antidepressants*
verapamil

Drugs that may *depress heart function* (reduce pumping efficiency)

beta-adrenergic-blocking
  drugs*
cocaine
daunorubicin
diltiazem

disopyramide
doxorubicin
epinephrine
flecainide
fluorouracil

isoproterenol
nifedipine
verapamil

Drugs that may *reduce coronary artery blood flow* (reduce oxygen supply to heart muscle)

amphetamines*
beta-adrenergic-blocking
  drugs* (abrupt
  withdrawal)
cocaine

ergotamine
fluorouracil
nifedipine
oral contraceptives
ritodrine

vasopressin
vinblastine
vincristine

Drugs that may *impair healing of heart muscle* following heart attack (myocardial infarction)

adrenocortical steroids*
nonsteroidal anti-

inflammatory drugs
  (NSAIDs)*

Drugs that may cause *heart valve damage*

dexfenfluramine (Redux)
ergotamine
fen-phen (fenfluramine-

phenteramine) (recently
  outlawed in some states)
methysergide

minocycline (blue-black
  pigmentation)

Drugs that may cause *pericardial disease*

actinomycin D
anthracyclines
bleomycin
cisplatin
cyclophosphamide

cytarabine
fluorouracil
hydralazine
methysergide
minoxidil

phenylbutazone
practolol
procainamide
sulfasalazine

*See Drug Class, Section Four.

TABLE 7

Drugs That May Cause Lung Dysfunction or Damage

Lung damage from medicines may be difficult to distinguish from natural diseases or disorders that involve lung function or structure. Type A reactions are those due to known pharmacological drug actions. Type B reactions are unexpected and unpredictable allergic or idiosyncratic reactions.

Drugs that may adversely affect *blood vessels of the lung*

Drugs that may cause thrombo-embolism

estrogens*
oral contraceptives (high-
  estrogen type)

Drugs that may cause pulmonary hypertension

amphetamines*	fenfluramine	tryptophan
dexfenfluramine (Redux)	oral contraceptives	

Drugs that may cause vasculitis (blood vessel damage) with or without hemorrhage

aminoglutethimide	febarbamate	phenytoin
amphotericin	nitrofurantoin	
cocaine	penicillamine	

Drugs that may cause adult respiratory distress syndrome (ARDS)

bleomycin	heroin	naloxone
codeine	hydrochlorothiazide	ritodrine
cyclophosphamide	methadone	terbutaline
dextropropoxyphene	mitomycin	vinblastine

Drugs that may adversely affect the *bronchial tubes*

Drugs that may cause bronchoconstriction (asthma)

acetaminophen	griseofulvin	inflammatory drugs
aspirin	maprotiline	(NSAIDs)*
beta-adrenergic-blocking	methacholine	penicillins*
drugs*	methoxypsoralen	pilocarpine
carbachol	metoclopramide	propafenone
cephalosporins*	morphine	pyridostigmine
chloramphenicol	neomycin	streptomycin
deanol	neostigmine	tartrazine (coloring agent)
demeclocycline	nitrofurantoin	
erythromycin	nonsteroidal anti-	

Drugs that may cause bronchiolitis (with permanent obstruction of small bronchioles)

penicillamine	sulfasalazine

*See Drug Class, Section Four.

Drugs that may *damage lung tissues*

Drugs that may cause acute allergic-type pneumonitis

ampicillin
bleomycin
cephalexin
chlorpropamide
gold
imipramine
mephenesin
mercaptopurine
metformin

methotrexate
metronidazole
mitomycin
nalidixic acid
nitrofurantoin
nomifensine
nonsteroidal anti-
   inflammatory drugs
   (NSAIDs)*

para-aminosalicylic acid
penicillamine
penicillin
phenylbutazone
phenytoin
procarbazine
sulfonamides*
tetracycline
vinblastine

Drugs that may cause chronic pneumonitis and fibrosis (scarring)

amiodarone
bleomycin
bromocriptine
busulfan
carmustine
chlorambucil
cyclophosphamide

ergotamine
gold
hexamethonium
mecamylamine
melphalan
methysergide
nitrofurantoin

pentolinium
practolol
sulfasalazine
tocainide
tolfenamic acid

Drugs that may *damage the pleura*

bromocriptine

methysergide

practolol

TABLE 8

Drugs That May Cause Liver Dysfunction or Damage

The liver often changes drugs into forms easily removed from the body. Medicines can hurt liver structure or function. Reactions range from mild and transient changes in liver function tests to complete liver failure and death. Many drugs may affect the liver in more than one way. Careful liver monitoring is required.

Drugs that may cause *acute dose-dependent liver damage* (resembling acute viral hepatitis)

acetaminophen (overdose)
salicylates* (doses over 2 g
  daily)

Drugs that may cause *acute dose-independent liver damage* (resembling acute viral hepatitis)

acebutolol
allopurinol
atenolol
carbamazepine
cimetidine
dantrolene

diclofenac
diltiazem
disulfiram
enflurane
ethambutol
ethionamide

halothane
ibuprofen
indomethacin
isoniazid
ketoconazole
labetalol

*See Drug Class, Section Four.

maprotiline
metoprolol
mianserin
naproxen
nifedipine
para-aminosalicylic acid
penicillins*
phenelzine

phenindione
phenobarbital
phenylbutazone
phenytoin
piroxicam
probenecid
pyrazinamide
quinidine

quinine
ranitidine
rifampin
sulfonamides*
sulindac
tricyclic antidepressants*
valproic acid
verapamil

Drugs that may cause *acute fatty infiltration of the liver*

adrenocortical steroids*
antithyroid drugs
isoniazid
methotrexate

phenothiazines*
phenytoin
salicylates*
sulfonamides*

tetracyclines*
valproic acid

Drugs that may cause *cholestatic jaundice*

actinomycin D
amoxicillin/clavulanate
azathioprine
captopril
carbamazepine
carbimazole
cephalosporins*
chlordiazepoxide
chlorpromazine
chlorpropamide
cloxacillin
cyclophosphamide
cyclosporine
danazol
diazepam
disopyramide
enalapril
erythromycin (estolate)

estradiol
flecainide
flurazepam
flutamide
glyburide
gold
griseofulvin
haloperidol
ketoconazole
mercaptopurine
methyltestosterone
nafcillin
nifedipine
nitrofurantoin
nonsteroidal anti-
    inflammatory drugs
    (NSAIDs)*
norethandrolone

oral contraceptives
oxacillin
penicillamine
phenothiazines*
phenytoin
propoxyphene
propylthiouracil
rifampin
sulfonamides*
tamoxifen
thiabendazole
tolbutamide
tricyclic antidepressants*
trimethoprim/
    sulfamethoxazole
troleandomycin
verapamil

Drugs that may cause *liver granulomas* (chronic inflammatory nodules)

allopurinol
aspirin
carbamazepine
chlorpromazine
chlorpropamide
diltiazem
disopyramide

gold
hydralazine
isoniazid
methyldopa
nitrofurantoin
penicillin
phenylbutazone

phenytoin
procainamide
quinidine
ranitidine
sulfonamides*
tolbutamide

Drugs that may cause *chronic liver disease*

Drugs that may cause active chronic hepatitis

acetaminophen (chronic
    use, large doses)
dantrolene

isoniazid
methyldopa
nitrofurantoin

trazodone

*See Drug Class, Section Four.

Drugs that may cause liver cirrhosis or fibrosis (scarring)

methotrexate	nicotinic acid
methyldopa	vitamin A

Drugs that may cause chronic cholestasis (resembling primary biliary cirrhosis)

chlorpromazine/valproic acid (combination)	mycin (combination)	phenytoin
	imipramine	thiabendazole
chlorpropamide/erythro-	phenothiazines*	tolbutamide

Drugs that may cause *liver tumors* (benign and malignant)

anabolic steroids	oral contraceptives	thorotrast
danazol	testosterone	

Drugs that may cause *damage to liver blood vessels*

adriamycin	sporine (combination)	mitomycin
anabolic steroids	dacarbazine	oral contraceptives
azathioprine	herbal teas, some	thioguanine
carmustine	mercaptopurine	vincristine
cyclophosphamide/cyclo-	methotrexate	vitamin A (excessive doses)

TABLE 9

Drugs That May Cause Kidney Dysfunction or Damage

The kidneys perform two major drug functions: (1) alteration of the drug to help remove it; (2) elimination of the drug from the body in the urine. As with effects on the liver, many drugs can harm the kidneys in several ways. Careful monitoring is prudent when taking any of the drugs listed below.

Drugs that may primarily *impair kidney function* (without damage)

amphotericin	demeclocycline	nifedipine
angiotensin-converting enzyme (ACE) inhibitors* (with renal artery stenosis; with congestive heart failure)	diuretics/NSAIDs* (avoid this combination)	nitroprusside
	glyburide	nonsteroidal anti-inflammatory drugs (NSAIDs)*
	isofosfamide	
	lithium/tricyclic antidepressants* (avoid this combination)	rifampin
beta-adrenergic-blocking drugs*		vinblastine
colchicine	methoxyflurane	

Drugs that may cause *acute kidney failure* (due to kidney damage)

Drugs that may damage the kidney filtration unit (the nephron)

acetaminophen (excessive dosage)	cisplatin	penicillamine
	cyclosporine	phenytoin
allopurinol	enalapril	quinidine
aminoglycoside antibiotics*	ergometrine	rifampin
	hydralazine	streptokinase
amphotericin	metronidazole	sulfonamides*
bismuth thiosulfate	mitomycin	thiazide diuretics*
carbamazepine	oral contraceptives	

*See Drug Class, Section Four.

Drugs that may cause *acute interstitial nephritis*

allopurinol
amoxicillin
ampicillin
aspirin
azathioprine
aztreonam
captopril
carbamazepine
carbenicillin
cefaclor
cefoxitin
cephalexin
cephalothin
cephapirin
cephradine
cimetidine
ciprofloxacin
clofibrate
cloxacillin
diazepam

diclofenac
diflunisal
fenoprofen
foscarnet
furosemide
gentamicin
glafenine
ibuprofen
indomethacin
ketoprofen
mefenamate
methicillin
methyldopa
mezlocillin
minocycline
nafcillin
naproxen
oxacillin
penicillamine
penicillin

phenindione
phenobarbital
phenylbutazone
phenytoin
piroxicam
pirprofen
pyrazinamide
rifampin
sodium valproate
sulfamethoxazole
sulfinpyrazone
sulfonamides*
sulindac
thiazide diuretics*
tolmetin
trimethoprim
vancomycin
warfarin

Drugs that may cause muscle destruction and associated acute kidney failure

adrenocortical steroids*
alcohol
amphetamines*
amphotericin
carbenoxolone
chlorthalidone
clofibrate

cocaine
cytarabine
fenofibrate
haloperidol
halothane
heroin
lovastatin

opioid analgesics*
pentamidine
phenothiazines*
streptokinase
suxamethonium

Drugs that may cause *kidney damage resembling glomerulonephritis or nephrosis*

captopril
fenoprofen
gold
ketoprofen

lithium
mesalamine
penicillamine
phenytoin

practolol
probenecid
quinidine

Drugs that may cause *chronic interstitial nephritis and papillary necrosis* (analgesic kidney damage)

acetaminophen
aspirin

phenacetin
(All with long-term use)

Drugs that may cause or contribute to *urinary tract crystal or stone formation*

acetazolamide
acyclovir
cytotoxic drugs
dihydroxyadenine
magnesium trisilicate
mercaptopurine
methotrexate

methoxyflurane
phenylbutazone
probenecid
salicylates*
sulfonamides*
thiazide diuretics*
triamterene

uricosuric drugs
vitamin A
vitamin C
vitamin D
warfarin
zoxazolamine

*See Drug Class, Section Four.

TABLE 10

Drugs That May Cause Nerve Dysfunction or Damage

Medicines may affect any part of the nervous system from the brain to peripheral nerves. The extent of benefits or problems varies widely from person to person.

Drugs that may cause *significant headache*

amyl nitrate	indomethacin	sulindac
bromocriptine	labetalol	terbutaline
clonidine	naproxen	tetracyclines*
ergotamine (prolonged use)	nifedipine	theophylline
etretinate	nitrofurantoin	tolmetin
hydralazine	nitroglycerin	trimethoprim/
ibuprofen	perhexilene	sulfamethoxazole
	propranolol	

Drugs that may cause *seizures* (convulsions)

ampicillin	ether	penicillins* (synthetic)
atenolol	halothane	phenothiazines*
carbenicillin	indomethacin	pyrimethamine
cephalosporins*	isoniazid	terbutaline
chloroquine	lidocaine	theophylline
cimetidine	lithium	ticarcillin
ciprofloxacin	mefenamic acid	tricyclic antidepressants*
cycloserine	nalidixic acid	vincristine
disopyramide	oxacillin	

Drugs that may cause *stroke*

anabolic steroids	oral contraceptives
cocaine	phenylpropanolamine

Drugs that may cause features of *parkinsonism*

amitriptyline	diphenhydramine	methyldopa
amodiaquine	droperidol	metoclopramide
chloroquine	haloperidol	phenothiazines*
chlorprothixene	imipramine	reserpine
desipramine	levodopa	thiothixene
diazoxide	lithium	trifluperidol

Drugs that may cause *acute dystonias* (acute involuntary movement syndromes—AIMS)

carbamazepine	metoclopramide	propranolol
chlorzoxazone	phenothiazines*	tricyclic antidepressants*
haloperidol	phenytoin	

Drugs that may cause *tardive dyskinesia* (see Glossary)

haloperidol	phenothiazines*	thiothixene

Drugs that may cause *neuroleptic malignant syndrome* (NMS)

See this term in the Glossary for a list of causative drugs.

*See Drug Class, Section Four.

Drugs that may cause *peripheral neuropathy* (see Glossary)

amiodarone
amitriptyline
amphetamines*
amphotericin
anticoagulants*
carbutamide
chlorambucil
chloramphenicol
chloroquine
chlorpropamide
cimetidine
clioquinol
clofibrate
colchicine
colistin
cytarabine
dapsone
disopyramide

disulfiram
ergotamine
ethambutol
glutethimide
gold
hydralazine
imipramine
indomethacin
isoniazid
methaqualone
methimazole
methysergide
metronidazole
nalidixic acid
nitrofurantoin
nitrofurazone
penicillamine
penicillin

perhexiline
phenelzine
phenylbutazone
phenytoin
podophyllin
procarbazine
propranolol
propylthiouracil
stavudine
streptomycin
sulfonamides*
sulfoxone
thalidomide
tolbutamide
vinblastine
vincristine

Drugs that may cause a *myasthenia gravis* syndrome

aminoglycoside
  antibiotics*
beta-adrenergic-blocking

drugs*
penicillamine
phenytoin

polymixin B
trihexyphenidyl

TABLE 11

Drugs That May Adversely Affect Sexuality

Many commonly used drugs can cause obvious or subtle changes on one or more aspects of sexual expression. Patients may be unaware that sexual changes can be related to medicines, and are often reluctant to talk about it. Sexual dysfunction may also be a result of the disorder being treated or an undetected problem. Diabetes, kidney failure, hypertension, depression, and alcoholism may reduce libido and cause failure of erection. Many drugs used to treat these conditions may worsen subclinical sexual dysfunction. This requires the closest cooperation between therapist and patient in order to correctly assess possible cause-and-effect relationships and change therapy appropriately.

Possible Drug Effects on Male Sexuality

1. Increased libido
     androgens (replacement therapy in deficiency states)
     baclofen (Lioresal)
     chlordiazepoxide (Librium) (antianxiety effect)
     diazepam (Valium) (antianxiety effect)
     haloperidol (Haldol)
     levodopa (Larodopa, Sinemet) (may be an indirect effect due to improved
       sense of well-being)

2. Decreased libido
     antihistamines
     barbiturates
     chlordiazepoxide (Librium), sedative effect

*See Drug Class, Section Four.

chlorpromazine (Thorazine), 10 to 20% of users
cimetidine (Tagamet)
clofibrate (Atromid-S)
clonidine (Catapres), 10 to 20% of users
danazol (Danocrine)
diazepam (Valium), sedative effect
disulfiram (Antabuse)
estrogens (therapy for prostatic cancer)
fenfluramine (Pondimin)
finasteride (Propecia, Proscar)
heroin
licorice
medroxyprogesterone (Provera)
methyldopa (Aldomet), 10 to 15% of users
metoclopramide (Reglan), 80% of users
perhexilene (Pexid)
prazosin (Minipres), 15% of users
propranolol (Inderal), rarely
reserpine (Serpasil, Ser-Ap-Es)
spironolactone (Aldactone)
tricyclic antidepressants

3. Impaired erection (impotence)
anticholinergics*
antihistamines*
baclofen (Lioresal)
barbiturates* (when abused)
beta-blockers*
chlordiazepoxide (Librium) (in high dosage)
chlorpromazine (Thorazine)
cimetidine (Tagamet)
clofibrate (Atromid-S)
clonidine (Catapres), 10 to 20% of users
cocaine
diazepam (Valium) (in high dosage)
digitalis and its glycosides
disopyramide (Norpace)
disulfiram (Antabuse), uncertain
estrogens* (therapy for prostatic cancer)
ethacrynic acid (Edecrin), 5% of users
ethionamide (Trecator-SC)
fenfluramine (Pondimin)
finasteride (Propecia, Proscar)
furosemide (Lasix), 5% of users
guanethidine (Ismelin)
haloperidol (Haldol), 10 to 20% of users
heroin
hydroxyprogesterone (therapy for prostatic cancer)
licorice
lithium (Lithonate)
marijuana
mesoridazine (Serentil)
methantheline (Banthine)
methyldopa (Aldomet), 10% to 15% of users
metoclopramide (Reglan), 60% of users
monoamine oxidase (MAO) type A inhibitors,* 10 to 15% of users

*See Drug Class, Section Four.

perhexilene (Pexid)
prazosin (Minipres), infrequently
reserpine (Serpasil, Ser-Ap-Es)
spironolactone (Aldactone)
thiazide diuretics,* 5% of users
thioridazine (Mellaril)
tricyclic antidepressants*

4. Impaired ejaculation
anticholinergics*
barbiturates* (when abused)
chlorpromazine (Thorazine)
clonidine (Catapres)
estrogens* (therapy for prostatic cancer)
guanethidine (Ismelin)
heroin
mesoridazine (Serentil)
methyldopa (Aldomet)
monoamine oxidase (MAO) type A inhibitors*
phenoxybenzamine (Dibenzyline)
phentolamine (Regitine)
reserpine (Serpasil, Ser-Ap-Es)
thiazide diuretics*
thioridazine (Mellaril)
tricyclic antidepressants*

5. Decreased testosterone
adrenocorticotropic hormone (ACTH)
barbiturates*
digoxin (Lanoxin)
haloperidol (Haldol)
—increased testosterone with low dosage
—decreased testosterone with high dosage
lithium (Lithonate)
marijuana
medroxyprogesterone (Provera)
monoamine oxidase (MAO) type A inhibitors*
spironolactone (Aldactone)

6. Impaired spermatogenesis (reduced fertility)
adrenocorticosteroids (prednisone, etc.)
androgens (moderate to high dosage, extended use)
antimalarials*
aspirin (abusive, chronic use)
chlorambucil (Leukeran)
cimetidine (Tagamet)
colchicine
cotrimoxazole (Bactrim, Septra)
cyclophosphamide (Cytoxan)
estrogens* (therapy for prostatic cancer)
marijuana
medroxyprogesterone (Provera)
methotrexate
metoclopramide (Reglan)
monoamine oxidase (MAO) type A inhibitors*
niridazole (Ambilhar)
nitrofurantoin (Furadantin)

*See Drug Class, Section Four.

spironolactone (Aldactone)
sulfasalazine (Azulfidine)
testosterone (moderate to high dosage, extended use)
vitamin C (doses of 1 g or more)

7. Testicular disorders
Swelling
—tricyclic antidepressants*
Inflammation
—oxyphenbutazone (Tandearil)
Atrophy
—androgens* (moderate to high dosage, extended use)
—chlorpromazine (Thorazine)
—cyclophosphamide (Cytoxan) (in prepubescent boys)
—spironolactone (Aldactone)

8. Penile disorders
Priapism (see Glossary)
—anabolic steroids (male hormonelike drugs)
—chlorpromazine (Thorazine)
—clozapine (Clozaril)
—cocaine
—fluphenazine (Prolixin)
—guanethidine (Ismelin)
—haloperidol (Haldol)
—heparin
—hydralazine (Apresoline)
—levodopa (Sinemet)
—mesoridazine (Serentil)
—molindone (Moban)
—phenelzine (Nardil)
—phenytoin (Dilantin)
—prazosin (Minipres)
—prochlorperazine (Compazine)
—thioridazine (Mellaril)
—trazodone (Desyrel)
—trifluoperazine (Stelazine)
—warfarin (Coumadin)
Peyronie's disease (see Glossary)
—beta-blocker drugs*
—phenytoin (Dilantin, etc.)

9. Gynecomastia (excessive development of the male breast)
anabolic steroids
androgens* (partial conversion to estrogen)
busulfan (Myleran)
carmustine (BiCNU)
chlormadinone
chlorpromazine (Thorazine)
chlortetracycline (Aureomycin)
cimetidine (Tagamet)
clonidine (Catapres), infrequently
diethylstilbestrol (DES)
digitalis and its glycosides
estrogens* (therapy for prostatic cancer)
ethionamide (Trecator-SC)
finasteride (Propecia, Proscar)

*See Drug Class, Section Four.

fluphenazine
griseofulvin (Fulvicin, etc.)
haloperidol (Haldol)
heroin
human chorionic gonadotropin
isoniazid (INH, Nydrazid)
marijuana
mestranol
methyldopa (Aldomet)
metoclopramide (Reglan)
penicillamine
phenelzine (Nardil)
phenothiazines*
reserpine (Serpasil, Ser-Ap-Es)
spironolactone (Aldactone)
thioridazine (Mellaril)
tricyclic antidepressants*
vincristine (Oncovin)

10. Feminization (loss of libido, impotence, gynecomastia, testicular atrophy)
conjugated estrogens (Premarin, etc.)

11. Precocious puberty
anabolic steroids
androgens*
isoniazid (INH)

Possible Drug Effects on Female Sexuality

1. Increased libido
androgens*
chlordiazepoxide (Librium) (antianxiety effect)
diazepam (Valium) (antianxiety effect)
mazindol (Sanorex)
oral contraceptives (freedom from fear of pregnancy)

2. Decreased libido
See list of drug effects on male sexuality. Some of these *may* have potential for
reducing libido in the female. The literature is sparse on this subject.

3. Impaired arousal and orgasm
anticholinergics*
clonidine (Catapres)
methyldopa (Aldomet)
monoamine oxidase (MAO) inhibitors*
tricyclic antidepressants*

4. Breast enlargement
penicillamine
tricyclic antidepressants*

5. Galactorrhea (spontaneous flow of milk)
amphetamine
chlorpromazine (Thorazine)
cimetidine (Tagamet)
haloperidol (Haldol)
heroin
methyldopa (Aldomet)
metoclopramide (Reglan)

*See Drug Class, Section Four.

oral contraceptives
phenothiazines*
reserpine (Serpasil, Ser-Ap-Es)
sulpiride (Equilid)
tricyclic antidepressants*

6. Ovarian failure (reduced fertility)
anesthetic gases (operating room staff)
cyclophosphamide (Cytoxan)
cytostatic drugs
danazol (Danocrine)
medroxyprogesterone (Provera)

7. Altered menstruation (menstrual disorders)
adrenocortical steroids* (prednisone, etc.)
androgens*
barbiturates (when abused)
chlorambucil (Leukeran)
chlorpromazine (Thorazine)
cyclophosphamide (Cytoxan)
danazol (Danocrine)
estrogens*
ethionamide (Trecator-SC)
haloperidol (Haldol)
heroin
isoniazid (INH, Nydrazid)
marijuana
medroxyprogesterone (Provera)
metoclopramide (Reglan)
oral contraceptives
phenothiazines*
progestins*
radioisotopes
rifampin (Rifadin, Rifamate, Rimactane)
spironolactone (Aldactone)
testosterone
thioridazine (Mellaril)
vitamin A (in excessive dosage)

8. Virilization (acne, hirsutism, lowering of voice, enlargement of clitoris)
anabolic drugs
androgens*
haloperidol (Haldol)
oral contraceptives (lowering of voice)

9. Precocious puberty
estrogens* (in hair lotions)
isoniazid (INH, Nydrazid)

TABLE 12
Drugs That May Interact With Alcohol

Alcohol may interact with a wide variety of drugs. The most important problem happens when depressant action on the brain of sedatives, sleep-inducing drugs, tranquilizers, and narcotic drugs is intensified by alcohol. Alcohol may also reduce drug

*See Drug Class, Section Four.

benefits or lead to toxic effects. Some drugs may increase the intoxicating effects of alcohol, further impairing mental alertness, judgment, coordination, and reaction time.

The intensity and significance can vary greatly from one person to another and from one occasion to another. This is because many factors influence what happens when drugs and alcohol interact. Factors include variations in sensitivity to drugs, the chemistry and quantity of the drug, type and amount of alcohol consumed, and the sequence in which drug and alcohol are taken. If you need to use any of the drugs in the following table, ask your doctor for help about alcohol use.

Drugs with which it is advisable to avoid alcohol completely

Drug name or class	Possible interaction with alcohol
amphetamines	excessive rise in blood pressure with alcoholic beverages containing tyramine**
antidepressants*	excessive sedation, increased intoxication
barbiturates*	excessive sedation
bromides	confusion, delirium, increased intoxication
calcium carbimide	disulfiramlike reaction**
carbamazepine	excessive sedation
chlorprothixene	excessive sedation
chlorzoxazone	excessive sedation
disulfiram	disulfiramlike reaction**
ergotamine	reduced effectiveness of ergotamine
fenfluramine	excessive stimulation of nervous system with some beers and wines
furazolidone	disulfiramlike reaction**
haloperidol	excessive sedation
monoamine oxidase (MAO) inhibitor drugs*	excessive rise in blood pressure with alcoholic beverages containing tyramine**
meperidine	excessive sedation
meprobamate	excessive sedation
methotrexate	increased liver toxicity and excessive sedation
metronidazole	disulfiramlike reaction**
narcotic drugs	excessive sedation
oxyphenbutazone	increased stomach irritation and/or bleeding
pentazocine	excessive sedation
pethidine	excessive sedation
phenothiazines*	excessive sedation
phenylbutazone	increased stomach irritation and/or bleeding
procarbazine	disulfiramlike reaction**
propoxyphene	excessive sedation
reserpine	excessive sedation, orthostatic hypotension**
sleep-inducing drugs (hypnotics) —carbromal —chloral hydrate —ethchlorvynol	excessive sedation

*See Drug Class, Section Four.
**See Glossary

Drug name or class	Possible interaction with alcohol
sleep-inducing drugs (con't.)	
—ethinamate	
—glutethimide	
—flurazepam	
—methaqualone	
—methyprylon	
—temazepam	
—triazolam	
thiothixene	excessive sedation
tricyclic antidepressants*	excessive sedation, increased intoxication
trimethobenzamide	excessive sedation

Drugs with which alcohol should be used only in small amounts (use cautiously until combined effects have been determined)

Drug name or class	Possible interaction with alcohol
acetaminophen (Tylenol, etc.)	increased liver toxicity
amantadine	excessive lowering of blood pressure
antiarthritic/anti-inflammatory drugs*	increased stomach irritation and/or bleeding
anticoagulants (coumarins)*	increased anticoagulant effect
antidiabetic drugs (sulfonylureas)*	increased antidiabetic effect, excessive hypoglycemia**
antihistamines*	excessive sedation
antihypertensives*	excessive orthostatic hypotension**
aspirin (large doses or continuous use)	increased stomach irritation and/or bleeding
benzodiazepines*	excessive sedation
carisoprodol	increased alcoholic intoxication
diethylpropion	excessive nervous system stimulation with alcoholic beverages containing tyramine**
dihydroergotoxine	excessive lowering of blood pressure
diphenoxylate	excessive sedation
dipyridamole	excessive lowering of blood pressure
diuretics*	excessive orthostatic hypotension**
ethionamide	confusion, delirium, psychotic behavior
fenoprofen	increased stomach irritation and/or bleeding
griseofulvin	flushing and rapid heart action
ibuprofen	increased stomach irritation and/or bleeding
indomethacin	increased stomach irritation and/or bleeding
insulin	excessive hypoglycemia**
iron	excessive absorption of iron
isoniazid	decreased effectiveness of isoniazid, increased incidence of hepatitis
lithium	increased confusion and delirium (avoid all alcohol if any indication of lithium overdose)

*See Drug Class, Section Four.
**See Glossary

Drug name or class	Possible interaction with alcohol
methocarbamol	excessive sedation
methotrimeprazine	excessive sedation
methylphenidate	excessive nervous system stimulation with alcoholic beverages containing tyramine**
metoprolol	excessive orthostatic hypotension**
nalidixic acid	increased alcoholic intoxication
naproxen	increased stomach irritation and/or bleeding
nicotinic acid	possible orthostatic hypotension**
nitrates* (vasodilators)	possible orthostatic hypotension**
nylidrin	increased stomach irritation
orphenadrine	excessive sedation
phenelzine	increased alcoholic intoxication
phenoxybenzamine	possible orthostatic hypotension**
phentermine	excessive nervous system stimulation with alcoholic beverages containing tyramine**
phenytoin	decreased effect of phenytoin
pilocarpine	prolongation of alcohol effect
prazosin	excessive lowering of blood pressure
primidone	excessive sedation
propranolol	excessive orthostatic hypotension**
sulfonamides*	increased alcoholic intoxication
sulindac	increased stomach irritation and/or bleeding
tolmetin	increased stomach irritation and/or bleeding
tranquilizers (mild) —chlordiazepoxide —clorazepate —diazepam —hydroxyzine —meprobamate —oxazepam —phenaglycodol —tybamate	excessive sedation
tranylcypromine	increased alcoholic intoxication

Drugs capable of producing a disulfiramlike reaction** when used concurrently with alcohol

antidiabetic drugs (sulfonylureas)*	disulfiram	procarbazine
calcium carbimide	furazolidone	quinacrine
chloral hydrate	metronidazole	sulfonamides*
chloramphenicol	nifuroxime	tinidazole
	nitrofurantoin	tolazoline

TABLE 13

High-Potassium Foods

Drugs that cause loss of potassium are often used to treat conditions that also require a reduced intake of sodium. The high-potassium foods listed below have been selected

*See Drug Class, Section Four.
**See Glossary

for compatibility with a sodium-restricted diet (500 to 1000 mg of sodium daily). Water pills (diuretics) may also cause loss of magnesium. Make sure magnesium is tested if you take a diuretic, and the results discussed with your doctor.

Beverages

orange juice	skim milk	tomato juice
prune juice	tea	whole milk

Breads and Cereals

brown rice	muffins	waffles
cornbread	oatmeal	
griddle cakes	shredded wheat	

Fruits

apricot	fig	orange
avocado	honeydew melon	papaya
banana	mango	prune

Meats

beef	haddock	rockfish
chicken	halibut	salmon
codfish	liver	turkey
flounder	pork	veal

Vegetables

baked beans	parsnips	tomato
lima beans	radishes	white potato
mushrooms	squash	
navy beans	sweet potato	

TABLE 14
Your Personal Drug Profile

I have spoken to countless patients who were sure that they knew how much of their medicines to take, and when to take them, only to learn that they were not only taking the wrong dose, but had also been taking a second medicine too many or too few times a day. Knowing as much as possible about your body and your medicines can save your life. Please take the time to fill out this profile with the latest information. **Medicine never does you any good if you forget to take it.** Also make time to copy the Medication Map and have your doctor or pharmacist fill it in and discuss it with you. Make sure you work with your doctor to fit your medicines into your life.

Name:

Age:

Weight in kilograms: (pounds divided by 2.2)

Height in inches:

Prescription drug allergies:

Non-prescription drug allergies:

Food allergies:

My kidneys* are: normal_____

mildly_____   moderately_____   severely_____   compromised.

My liver* is: normal_____

mildly_____   moderately_____   severely_____   compromised.

Conditions or diseases that I have or have had:

Prescription and nonprescription medications I take regularly:

*Make certain your dose is decreased if the drug is eliminated by an organ (such as the liver or kidneys) with which you have a problem. To determine which organs are involved, refer to the drug profile and "Conditions Requiring Dosing Adjustments" section for each medication you are taking.

Prescription and nonprescription medications I take periodically:

I find it very difficult_____
                                          to remember to take medicines.
I find it very easy_____

I become constipated rarely_____   occasionally_____   never_____.

Urination is usually easy_____   rather difficult_____   difficult_____.

The phone number of the nearest Poison Control Center is _____. .

I sleep well_____   OK_____   poorly_____   little_____   on most nights.

I have_____   have never_____   had blood problems in the past.

I am considering becoming_____   might be_____   am_____   pregnant.

I want the medications which offer the best balance of **price** and **outcomes** for my specific medical history and present conditions.

TABLE 15

The Medication Map

Getting four new prescriptions often means that you will get four brief patient package inserts or papers stapled to the pharmacy bag when you pick up your prescriptions. Rarely does anyone take the time to understand YOUR INDIVIDUAL day, and select medicines based on how your day REALLY works or help you fit the medicines into the way that you actually live. I believe that this is a critical cause of drug interactions, irrational drug combinations, and taking the medicine incorrectly. It also dooms to failure what otherwise might be brilliant use of medicines.

This reality contributes to the 136 billion dollars spent EACH YEAR on treatment problems, and leads to the more than 100,000 deaths caused by medicines. I can't begin to count the number of times I've found that medicines prescribed to be taken three times a day were actually only taken twice a day or less. The cure can easily become the disease.

Use the map below to talk with your doctor or pharmacist to schedule your prescription, nonprescription, or herbal medicines as you really plan or are able to take them. Make sure the timing and combinations are okay! Important questions to ask include:

Have all of these medicines been checked for drug interactions?

Do I really need to take all of these medicines at this time?

Are there newer medicines that might have fewer possible side effects or that might treat the conditions or diseases being treated more effectively (get better results or outcomes)?

Are there medicines that only need to be taken twice or once daily that could be substituted for one or more of those I take now?

Can food react with any of the medicines I take?

Midnight	Medicine and dose planned:	
1 A.M.	Medicine and dose planned:	
2 A.M.	Medicine and dose planned:	
3 A.M.	Medicine and dose planned:	
4 A.M.	Medicine and dose planned:	
5 A.M.	Medicine and dose planned:	
6 A.M.	Medicine and dose planned:	
7 A.M.	Medicine and dose planned:	*Morning Meal Time is*:
8 A.M.	Medicine and dose planned:	
9 A.M.	Medicine and dose planned:	
10 A.M.	Medicine and dose planned:	
11 A.M.	Medicine and dose planned:	
12 noon	Medicine and dose planned:	*Lunch or Brunch Time*:
1 P.M.	Medicine and dose planned:	
2 P.M.	Medicine and dose planned:	
3 P.M.	Medicine and dose planned:	
4 P.M.	Medicine and dose planned:	
5 P.M.	Medicine and dose planned:	
6 P.M.	Medicine and dose planned:	*Evening Meal Time*:
7 P.M.	Medicine and dose planned:	
8 P.M.	Medicine and dose planned:	
9 P.M.	Medicine and dose planned:	*Snack (if any)*:
10 P.M.	Medicine and dose planned:	
11 P.M.	Medicine and dose planned:	

TABLE 16

Medicines Removed from the Market

Since the last edition of *The Essential Guide,* several medicines (some widely used) have been removed from the U.S. market. In fact, the addition of bromfenac to this list makes the fifth medicine that has been recalled in only nine months—the highest number of recalls ever. While this is somewhat disconcerting, it also shows that the Phase Four (reporting after a drug is FDA approved) system sometimes works. On the other hand, it means that more than ever, you need to be a partner in your health care! Talk to your doctor right away if you suspect you are having a reaction to one of your medicines.

The information in this table will be updated for each subsequent *Essential Guide* edition. The listings will give the general category to which the medicine belongs, the generic name and at least one brand name, and the reason for its removal.

Analgesics (Pain Relievers)

bromfenac (Duract)   Reason removed: Serious liver damage if taken for
                            more than 10 days.

Anti-Psoriatic Drugs (Psoriasis Treatments)

etretinate (Tegison)   Reason removed: Newer medicines available.

Cholesterol-Reducing Drugs

probucol (Lorelco)   Reason removed: More effective medicines available.

High Blood Pressure Medicines (Antihypertensives)

mibefradil (Posicor)   Reason removed: Serious drug interactions with
                            multiple drugs.

Minimally Sedating Antihistamines

terfenadine (Seldane)   Reason removed: Voluntarily withdrawn because of
                            serious drug interactions with multiple drugs.

Weight-Loss Agents (Anorexiants)

dexfenfluramine (Redux)   Reason removed: Heart valve damage.
fenfluramine (Pondimin)   Reason removed: Heart valve damage.

Sources

The following sources were consulted in the compilation and revision of this book:

Abramowicz, M., ed. 1997. *Drugs of Choice: The Medical Letter on Drugs and Therapeutics.* New Rochelle, NY: The Medical Letter.

Abramowicz, M., ed. 1998. *Some Drugs That Cause Psychiatric Symptoms: The Medical Letter on Drugs and Therapeutics.* New Rochelle, NY: The Medical Letter.

Abramowicz, M., ed. 1998. *The Choice of Antibacterial Drugs: The Medical Letter on Drugs and Therapeutics.* New Rochelle, NY: The Medical Letter.

Ackerman, B. H., and N. Kasbekar. 1997. Disturbances of taste and smell induced by drugs. *Pharmacotherapy* 17(3):482–496.

Advances in Osteoporosis. 1996, 1997.

AIDS Clinical Care. 1996, 1997, 1998. Boston: Massachusetts Medical Society.

American Board of Internal Medicine. 1996. *Caring for the Dying.* American Board of Internal Medicine.

American Family Physician. 1998. Kansas City, Mo: American Academy of Family Physicians.

American Pain Society. 1996. *Principles of Analgesic Use in the Treatment of Acute Pain and Cancer Pain.* 3rd ed. Glenview, IL: American Pain Society.

American Journal of Hospice and Palliative Care. 1998. Enk, R. ed. Weston, MA.

American Pharmaceutical Association. 1996. *Handbook of Nonprescription Drugs.* 11th ed. Washington, DC: American Pharmaceutical Association.

American Pharmaceutical Association. 1998. *APhA Special Report: A Review of the Sixth Report of the Joint National Committee on Prevention, Detection, Evaluation and Treatment of High Blood Pressure.* Washington, DC: American Pharmaceutical Association.

American Psychiatric Association. 1997. *Practice Guideline for the Treatment of Patients with Alzheimer's Disease and Other Dementias of Late Life.* Washington, DC: American Psychiatric Association.

American Society for Pharmacology and Experimental Therapeutics. 1990. *Rational Drug Therapy and Pharmacology for Physicians.* Bethesda, MD: American Society for Pharmacology and Experimental Therapeutics.

Annals of Pharmacotherapy. 1996–1998. Cincinnati, OH: Harvey Whitney Books.

Aparasu, R. R. and S. E. Flinginger. 1997. Inappropriate medication prescribing for the elderly by office-based physicians. *The Annals of Pharmacotherapy* 31(July/August 1997):823–836.

Archives of Internal Medicine. 1998. Chicago: The American Medical Association.

Avery's Drug Treatment. 4th ed. Auckland, NZ: Adis International.

Bartlett, J. 1996. *The Johns Hopkins Hospital 1996 Guide to Medical Care of Patients with HIV Infection.* Baltimore: Williams & Wilkins.

Bartlett, J. 1998. *Medical Management of HIV Infection: 1998 Edition.* Baltimore: Port City Press.

Berkow, R., ed. 1996. *The Merck Manual.* 15th ed. Rahway, NJ: Merck Sharp & Dohme Research Laboratories.

Bonnick, S. L. 1994. *The Osteoporosis Handbook.* Dallas: Taylor Publishing.

Briggs, G. G., T. W. Bodendorfer, R. K. Freeman, and S. J. Yaffee. 1983. *Drugs in Pregnancy and Lactation.* Baltimore: Williams & Wilkins.

Brooke, M. H. 1986. *A Clinician's View of Neuromuscular Diseases.* 2nd ed. Baltimore: Williams & Wilkins.

Canadian Pharmaceutical Association. 1991. *Compendium of Pharmaceuticals and Specialties.* 26th ed. Ottawa: Canadian Pharmaceutical Association.

Canadian Pharmaceutical Association, St. Paul's Hospital British Columbia Center of Excellence for HIV–AIDS. Vancouver, BC: Canadian Pharmaceutical Association, 1997, 1998.

Cape, R. 1978. *Aging: Its Complex Management.* Hagerstown, MD: Harper & Row.

Chest. 1998. Northbrook, IL: American College of Physicians.

Circulation. 1998. American Heart Association. Baltimore: Williams & Wilkins.

Classen, D. C., et al. 1997. Adverse drug events in hospitalized patients. *Journal of the American Medical Association* 277:301–306.

Clin-Alert. 1996–1997. Medford, NJ: Clin-Alert.

Clinisphere. 1997. Facts and Comparisons 1.0. Facts and Comparisons, St. Louis.

Cumming, R. G., et al. Use of inhaled corticosteroids and the risk of cataracts. *New England Journal of Medicine* 337(1):8–14, 1997.

Daniels, J. B., ed. 1997. *Infectious Disease in Clinical Practice.* Baltimore: Williams & Wilkins.

DiGregorio, J. G., et al. 1991. *Handbook of Pain Management.* Westchester, NY: Medical Surveillance.

Drug Information Journal. 1996–1997–1998.

Drug Interactions Newsletter. 1997. Spokane, WA: Applied Therapeutics.

DrugLink. 1998. St. Louis: J. B. Lippincott, Facts and Comparisons.

Drug Newsletter. 1998. St. Louis: J. B. Lippincott, Facts and Comparisons.

Drug Therapy: Physicians Prescribing Update. 1992. Lawrenceville, NJ: Excerpta Medica.

Drugs and Therapy Perspectives. 1996–1997.

Dukes, M. N. G., ed. 1988. *Meyler's Side Effects of Drugs.* 11th ed. Amsterdam: Excerpta Medica.

Eastell, R., et al. 1998. Treatment of Postmenopausal Osteoporosis. *New England Journal of Medicine* 338(11):736–746.

The Electronic Library of Medicine. 1996. Boston: Little, Brown.

Farrell, B., and B. Farrell, eds. 1996. *Pain in the Elderly.* International Association for the Study of Pain Press.

Favus, M., ed. 1996. *Primer on the Metabolic Bone Diseases and Disorders of Mineral Metabolism.* 3rd ed. Philadelphia, New York: Lippincott-Raven.

Fraunfelder, F. T. 1989. *Drug-Induced Ocular Side Effects and Drug Interactions.* 3rd ed. Philadelphia: Lea & Febiger.

Gleason, P. P., et al. 1997. Medical outcomes and antimicrobial costs with the use of the American Thoracic Society Guidelines for Outpatients with Community Acquired Pneumonia. *Journal of the American Medical Association* 278(1):32–39.

Goodman, L. S., and A. Gilman, eds. 1996. *The Pharmacological Basis of Therapeutics.* 9th ed. New York: Macmillan.

Graham, I. M., et al. 1997. Plasma homocysteine as a risk factor for vascular disease. *Journal of the American Medical Association* 277(22):1775–1781.

Griffiths, M. C., ed. 1988. *USAN 1989*. Rockville, MD: United States Pharmacopeial Convention.

Griffiths, M. C., ed. 1988. *The USP Dictionary of Drug Names*. Rockville, MD: United States Pharmacopeial Convention.

Handbook of Clinical Drug Data. 1993. Hamilton, IL: Drug Intelligence Publications.

Hansten, P. D. 1992. *Drug Interactions*. 6th Ed. Philadelphia: Lea & Febiger.

Hasketh, P. L., ed. 1998. *The Journal of Oncology*. Cedar Knolls, NJ: National Medical Information Network.

Heinonen, O. P., D. Slone, and S. Shapiro. 1977. *Birth Defects and Drugs in Pregnancy*. Littleton, MA: PSG Publishing.

Hollister, L. E. 1983. *Clinical Pharmacology of Psychotherapeutic Drugs*. 2nd ed. New York: Churchill Livingstone.

Hospice Journal. 1998. New York: The Haworth Press.

Hospital Pharmacy. 32(5). 1998.

Huff, B.B., ed. 1998. *The Physicians' Desk Reference*. 52nd ed. Montvale, NJ: Medical Economics.

International Drug Therapy Newsletter. 1997. Baltimore: Ayd Medical Communications.

Jefferson, J. W., and J. H. Greist. 1977. *Primer of Lithium Therapy*. Baltimore: Williams & Wilkins.

Journal of Acquired Immune Deficiency Syndromes. 1998. Hagerstown, MD: Lippincott-Raven.

Journal of Bone and Mineral Research. 1996–1997.

Journal of Bone and Mineral Research. 1998. Malden, MA: Blackwell Science, Inc.

Journal of the American Medical Association. 1997, 1998.

Journal of the National Cancer Institute. 1998. Cary, NC: Oxford University Press.

Journal Watch. 1996–1998. Waltham, MA: The Massachusetts Medical Society.

Journal Watch: Women's Health. 1996–1998, 1998. Waltham, MA: The Massachusetts Medical Society.

Kaplan, N. M. 1995. *Management of Hypertension*. 6th ed. Durant, OK: Essential Medical Information Systems.

Kazak, A. E., et al. 1998. Pharmacologic and Psychologic Interventions for Procedural Pain. *Pediatrics* 102(1):59–66.

Klippel, J. H., ed. 1997. Systemic Lupus Erythematosus demographics, prognosis and outcome. *J Rheumatol Suppl* 48:67–71.

Koda-Kimbal (Lloyd Yee Young). 1995. *Applied Therapeutics: The Clinical Use of Drugs*. 6th ed. Vancouver, WA: Applied Therapeutics.

Koller, W. C., ed. 1987. *Handbook of Parkinson's Disease*. New York: Marcel Dekker.

Kolodny, R. C., W. H. Masters, and V. E. Johnson. 1979. *Textbook of Sexual Medicine*. Boston: Little, Brown.

Lawrence, R. A. 1980. *Breast-Feeding*. St. Louis: Mosby.

Lieberman, M. L. 1988. *The Sexual Pharmacy*. New York: New American Library.

Long, J. W. 1984. *Clinical Management of Prescription Drugs*. Philadelphia: Harper & Row.

Long, J. W. 1997. *The Essential Guide to Chronic Illness*. New York: HarperCollins.

Maddin, S., ed. 1982. *Current Dermatologic Therapy*. Philadelphia: W. B. Saunders.

Mayo Clinic Proceedings. 1996–1998.

McEvoy, G. K., ed. 1997. *American Hospital Formulary Service: Drug Information 1997*. Bethesda, MD: American Society of Hospital Pharmacists.

The Medical Letter on Drugs and Therapeutics. 1997, 1998. New Rochelle, NY: The Medical Letter.

Melmon, K. L., and H. F. Morrelli. 1978. *Clinical Pharmacology*. 2nd ed. New York: Macmillan.

Michelson, M. D., et al. 1996. Bone mineral density in women with depression. *New England Journal of Medicine*, 335(16):1176–1181.

Micromedex: Drugdex. 1997. Englewood, CO: Computerized Clinical Information System.

Mohler, S. R. 1982. *Medication and Flying: A Pilot's Guide.* Boston: Boston Publishing.

Morbidity and Mortality Weekly Report: Report of the NIH Panel to Define Principles of Therapy of HIV Infection and Guidelines for the Use of Antiretroviral Agents in HIV-Infected Adults and Adolescents, April 24 1998. Washington, DC: U.S. Department of Health and Human Services. Atlanta: CDC.

Murphy, J. E. 1993. *Clinical Pharmacokinetics.* Bethesda, MD: American Society of Hospital Pharmacists.

National Institutes of Health (NIH, NHLBI). 1997. Guidelines for Diagnosis and Management of Asthma.

New England Journal of Medicine. 1997, 1998.

Olin, B. R., ed. 1992. *Patient Drug Facts.* St. Louis: J. B. Lippincott, Facts and Comparisons.

Olin, B. R., ed. 1997, 1998. *Facts and Comparisons.* St. Louis: J. B. Lippincott, Facts and Comparisons.

Pain Forum: Official Journal of the American Pain Society. 1997, 1998.

Pharmacotherapy: The Journal of Human Pharmacology and Drug Therapy. 1997, 1998.

Physician's GenRX. 1996. Version 96.1a. St. Louis: Mosby.

The Physician's Therapeutics and Drug Alert. 1996–1998.

Postgraduate Medicine: The Journal of Applied Medicine for the Primary Care Physician. 1998. '

Raj, P. P. 1986. *Practical Management of Pain.* Chicago: Year Book Medical Publishers.

Rakel, R. E., ed. 1992. *Conn's Current Therapy 1992.* Philadelphia: W. B. Saunders.

Reynolds, J. E. F., ed. 1997. *Martindale: The Extra Pharmacopoeia.* 29th ed. London: The Pharmaceutical Press.

Rogers, C. S., and J. D. McCue, eds. 1987. *Managing Chronic Disease.* Oradell, NJ: Medical Economics Books.

Rybacki, J. J. 1997. Letter to the editor. *Journal of the American Medical Association* 277(17):1351.

Sanford, J., et al. 1996. *The Sanford Guide to HIV/AIDS Therapy.* 5th ed. Antimicrobial Therapy, Inc. Vienna, VA: Lippincott-Raven.

Sauer, G. C. 1985. *Manual of Skin Diseases.* 5th ed. Philadelphia: J. B. Lippincott.

Scan Newsletter. 1996–1998. Norwich, NY: Society for Clinical Densitometry.

Schardein, J. L. 1976. *Drugs as Teratogens.* Cleveland: CRC Press.

Scientific American Medicine. 1998. CD-ROM. New York: Enigma Information Systems.

Semla, T. P., et al. 1993. *Geriatric Dosage Handbook.* Cleveland: Lexi-comp.

Shepard, T. H. 1989. *Catalog of Teratogenic Agents.* 6th ed. Baltimore: Johns Hopkins University Press.

Smith, L. H., and S. O. Thier. 1985. *Pathophysiology: The Biological Principles of Disease.* 2nd ed. Philadelphia: W. B. Saunders.

Sorensen, S. J., and S. R. Abel. 1997. Comparison of the ocular beta-blockers. *Annals of Pharmacotherapy* 30:43–54.

Spath, P. L., ed. 1994. *Clinical Paths, Tools for Outcomes Management.* Chicago: The American Hospital Association.

Speight, T. M., and N. H. G. Holford, eds. 1997.

Swash, M., and M. S. Schwartz. 1988. *Neuromuscular Diseases.* 2nd ed. Berlin: Springer-Verlag.

Tatro, D. S., ed. 1997. *Drug Interaction Facts.* St. Louis: J. B. Lippincott, Facts and Comparisons.

Thordsen, D. J., and Welty, T.E., eds. 1998. *Clinical Abstracts: Current Therapeutic Findings.* Cincinnati, OH: Harvey Whitney Books.

Tuchmann-Duplessis, H. 1975. *Drug Effects on the Fetus.* Sydney, Australia: ADIS Press.

United States Pharmacopeial Convention. 1997. *USP Dispensing Information 1997. Vol. 1: Drug Information for the Health Care Provider.* 12th ed. Rockville, MD: United States Pharmacopeial Convention.

U.S. Department of Health and Human Services. 1993. *Depression in Primary Care. Volume 1: Detection and Diagnosis.* Washington, DC: U.S. Department of Health and Human Services.

U.S. Department of Health and Human Services. 1993. *Sickle Cell Disease: Screening, Diagnosis, Management and Counseling in Newborns and Infants.* Washington, DC: U.S. Department of Health and Human Services.

U.S. Department of Health and Human Services. 1996. *Morbidity and Mortality Weekly Report: Immunization of Adolescents,* 22 November 1997. Washington, DC: U.S. Department of Health and Human Services.

U.S. Department of Health and Human Services, Food and Drug Administration. 1996–1997. *F.D.A. Drug Bulletin.* Rockville, MD: Department of Health and Human Services, Food and Drug Administration.

Utian, W. H. 1980. *Menopause in Modern Perspective.* New York: Appleton-Century-Crofts.

Wallach, J. B. 1996. *Interpretation of Diagnostic Tests.* 6th ed. Boston: Little, Brown.

Wilcox, S. M., et al. 1994. Inappropriate drug prescribing for the community-dwelling elderly. *Journal of the American Medical Association* 272(4):292–296.

Worley, R. J., ed. 1981. Menopause. *Clinical Obstetrics and Gynecology* 24(1):163–164.

Young, D. S. 1991. *Effects of Drugs on Clinical Laboratory Tests.* 1991 supplement. Washington, DC: AACC Press.

Young, L. L., ed. 1996. *Nonprescription Products: Formulations and Features, '96–97.* Washington, DC: American Pharmaceutical Association.

Index

    This index contains all the brand and generic drug names included in Section Two.

    Brand names of drugs appear in italic type and are capitalized.

    Each brand name is followed by its generic name. The generic name is the name under which you'll find the drug profile in Section Two.

    The symbol [CD] indicates that the brand name represents a combination drug that contains other generic drug components; see the Drug Profile for details on other components present. To be fully familiar with any combination drug [CD], it is necessary to read the Drug Profile of each component.

    The symbol ✿ before the brand name of a combination drug indicates that the brand name is used in both the United States and Canada, but that the ingredients in the combination product in each country differ. The Canadian drug is marked with the symbol ✿ to distinguish it from the American drug with the same name.

    A generic name with no page designation indicates an active component of a combination drug for which there is no Profile in Section Two. It is included to alert you to its presence, should you wish to consult your physician regarding its significance.

About the Authors

JAMES J. RYBACKI, Pharm. D., was born in Oneonta, New York. He received his prepharmacy education at Creighton University, and his Doctor of Pharmacy degree from the University of Nebraska Medical Center, College of Pharmacy, in Omaha. Over a quarter century of Dr. Rybacki's hospital and clinical experience includes early efforts in gas–liquid chromatography research characterizing human drug metabolites, and data collection for the College of American Pathologists to establish normal values for laboratory studies. He is a member of the clinical faculty at the University of Maryland School of Pharmacy and has provided clinical rounding and hospital experience for Pharm. D. and Bachelor students. He presently teaches a Drug Information rotation for Pharm. D. students at The Clearwater Group. He is board certified in pain management at the Diplomat level by the American Academy of Pain Management, and provides ongoing clinical pain management consulting nationwide. He is a member of the National Council of Hospice Professionals. Dr. Rybacki is actively involved in the postmarketing monitoring of medicines via the Drug Surveillance Network, a nationwide association of clinical pharmacists, and he is an approved External New Drug Application reviewer for the Canadian Drug Ministry. He lives on the eastern shore of Maryland.

Dr. Rybacki's efforts in drug information and clinical pharmacy include many years of active practice, eight of which were at Dorchester General Hospital in Cambridge, Maryland, including infectious disease, pharmacokinetic, nutrition support, pain management, and pharmacological consultations. Through the Occupational Health Unit, he has offered independent pain management and pharmacological consultations nationwide. He has also advised the World Health Organization's Expert Committee regarding revisions as well as selection of drugs to be listed in the next edition of *The Use of Essential Drugs* and is an assistant editor for the Drugdex drug information system. His past role as Vice President Clinical Services has bought him added expertise in overseeing Occupational Health, Physical Medicines, Laboratory Services, Imaging, Cardiology, Respiratory Therapy, Cancer Programs, and Continuing Medical Education. He served as conference coordinator for the first and second annual Dorchester General Hospital Pain Conferences, and seminar coordinator for the Eastern Shore of Maryland for the "Take Control" physician and public pain education programs with Johns Hopkins.

Dr. Rybacki is now president of The Clearwater Group, headquartered in Easton, Maryland, and provides drug information support and clinical pharmacy services to physician groups, consumers, and employers; holds seminars on medical cost containment, outcomes research, infectious disease, osteoporosis, pain management, and therapeutics; provides information support to insurance companies and HMOs; produces educational tapes on medicines; designs clinical programs; and conducts independent pharmacological evaluations. He was selected for full membership in the American College of Clinical Pharmacy, is a Certified Clinical Densitometrist (CCD) through the Society for Clinical Densitometry, and is also a board-certified Forensic Examiner. He was accepted as a Fellow to the American College of Forensic Examiners in 1997. He is a lifetime member of Who's Who in Global Business. Dr. Rybacki is also the director of clinical research, therapeutics, and outcomes at BoneSafe Osteoporosis Centers, an interdisciplinary osteoporosis testing, research, and consulting group.

Dr. Rybacki has been interviewed widely and is often a guest or guest host on numerous radio and television shows. He is presently working with the American Heart Association on a major campaign to encourage people to take medicines more effectively. He was featured on CNN's *Comcast Newsmakers* program, where he spoke of the importance of taking medicines correctly. Recent interviews include *Good Morning Arizona, The Bill Miller Show, The Madison Show, Retail Pharmacy News,* and *The Wall Street Journal.* He also participates in numerous medical speakers bureaus, including Merck, Miles, Dupont Pharma, and Glaxo. He has been a member of the Bristol-Myers Squibb Distinguished Speakers in HIV faculty since 1994 and lectures across the country. He has jointly authored several articles in professional journals on the use of medicines in infectious diseases, critical care, therapeutics, and cost containment. His letter on medication use in the United States appeared in the *Journal of the American Medical Association* (JAMA). *The Essential Guide to Prescription Drugs,* first published in 1977, was co-authored by Dr. Rybacki since 1994, before he assumed full authorship in 1996. "The Medicine Man," a nationwide live radio show, was developed, written, produced, and hosted by Dr. Rybacki in 1995. He is the original writer and host of the American Pharmaceutical Association's *The Pharmacist Minute* radio program, sponsored by a grant from Johnson and Johnson Merck (Pepcid AC$^{(R)}$). This program—which is broadcast from more than 2,000 locations—was the largest launch of a radio program, and is now heard in 141 countries worldwide. Dr. Rybacki believes that the new art of prescribing medicines lies in cost containment without sacrifice of clinical outcomes. He has created a site on the World Wide Web at www.medicineinfo.com.

JAMES W. LONG, M.D., was born in Allentown, Pennsylvania. He received his premedical education from the University of Maryland and his medical degree from the George Washington University School of Medicine in Washington, D.C. For 20 years he was in private practice of internal medicine in the Washington, D.C., metropolitan area, and for over 35 years he was a member of the faculty of the George Washington University School of Medicine. He has served with the Food and Drug Administration, the National Library of Medicine, and the Bureau of Health Manpower of the National Institutes of Health. Prior to his retirement, Dr. Long was director of Health Services for the National Science Foundation in Washington. He lives in Oxford, Maryland.

Dr. Long's involvement in drug information activities includes service on the HEW Task Force on Prescription Drugs, on the FDA Task Force on Adverse Drug Reactions, as a delegate-at-large to the U.S. Pharmacopeial Convention, as editorial consultant for *Hospital Formulary,* as a director of the

Drug Information Association, and as a member of the Toxicology Information Program Committee of the National Research Council/National Academy of Sciences. He was consultant to the Food and Drug Administration, serving as adviser to their staff on the development of patient package inserts. He is also the author of numerous articles in professional journals. *The Essential Guide to Prescription Drugs* is an outgrowth of his conviction that the general public needs and is entitled to practical drug information that is the equivalent of the professional "package insert." Dr. Long is the author of *The Essential Guide to Chronic Illness*, first published in 1997. He believes the patient can be reasonably certain of using medications with the least risk and greatest benefit only when the patient has all the relevant information about the drugs he or she is taking.

Controlled Drug Schedules

Schedule I: These medicines have a high abuse and dependence potential. Typically, the only use for these drugs is for research purposes. Examples include LSD and heroin. A prescription cannot be legally written for these drugs for medicinal use.

Schedule II: These medicines have therapeutic uses and the highest abuse and dependence potential for drugs with medicinal purposes. Examples include analgesics such as morphine (MS Contin) and meperidine (Demerol). A written prescription is required and refills are **not** allowed.

Schedule III: Medicines in this schedule have an abuse and dependence potential that is less than those in schedule II, but greater than those in schedule IV. These medicines have clear medicinal uses and include such medicines as codeine, or paregoric in combination. A common name is Tylenol Number 3 with codeine. A telephone prescription is permitted for medications in this class; however, it must be converted to a written form by a pharmacist. Prescriptions for these medicines may be refilled, but only five times in 6 months.

Schedule IV: This schedule contains medicines with less abuse and dependence potential than those in schedule III. Examples of medicines in this schedule include diazepam (Valium) and chlordiazepoxide (Librium). Prescriptions for these medicines may be refilled, but only five times in 6 months.

Schedule V: These medicines have the lowest abuse and dependence potential. Medicines in this class include diphenoxylate (Lomotil) and loperamide (Imodium). Drugs in this class which require a prescription are handled the same as any nonscheduled prescription medicine. Some drugs in this class do not require a prescription, and can be sold only with the approval of a pharmacist. The buyer may be required to sign a logbook when the drug is dispensed. Examples include codeine and hydrocodone in combination with other active nonnarcotic drugs, sold in preparations that have limited quantities of codeine or hydrocodone for control of diarrhea or cough.

Pregnancy Risk Categories

Definitions of FDA Pregnancy Categories

Category A: Adequate and well-controlled studies in pregnant women are **negative** for fetal abnormalities. Risk to the fetus is remote.

Category B: Animal reproduction studies are **negative** for fetal abnormalities, and data from adequate and well-controlled studies in pregnant women are not available.

OR:

Animal reproduction studies are **positive** for fetal abnormalities. Adequate and well-controlled studies in pregnant women are **negative** for fetal abnormalities, and fail to show a risk to the fetus.

Category C: Animal reproduction studies are **positive** for fetal abnormalities. Information from adequate and well-controlled studies in pregnant women is not available.

OR:

Information from animal reproduction studies **and** from adequate and well-controlled studies in pregnant women is not available.

Category D: Studies in pregnant women and/or premarketing (investigational) or postmarketing uses show **positive** evidence of human fetal risk. The drug is only used in serious disease or in life-threatening situations where safer medicines will not work or cannot be used. These situations may make the medicine acceptable despite its risks.

Category X: Animal reproduction studies and/or human pregnancy studies are **positive** for fetal abnormalities.

OR:

Studies in pregnant women and/or premarketing (investigational) or postmarketing (Phase Four) experience shows **positive** evidence of human fetal risk.

AND:

Potential fetal risks outweigh possible benefits of the drug. These medicines **should never** be used in pregnancy.

The FDA is currently evaluating these pregnancy categories, and may opt to modify them.